D1473813

THE
MERCK
MANUAL
OF
GERIATRICS

OTHER MERCK PROFESSIONAL HANDBOOKS

THE MERCK INDEX
First Edition, 1889

THE MERCK MANUAL OF DIAGNOSIS AND THERAPY
First Edition, 1899

THE MERCK VETERINARY MANUAL
First Edition, 1955

MERCK Professional Handbooks
are published on a nonprofit basis
as a service to the scientific community.

THE
MERCK
MANUAL
OF
GERIATRICS

William B. Abrams, M.D., and Robert Berkow, M.D., *Editors*

Andrew J. Fletcher, M.B., B. Chir., *Assistant Editor*

Editorial Board

Published by

MERCK SHARP & DOHME RESEARCH LABORATORIES

Division of

MERCK & CO., INC.

Rahway, N.J.

1990

MERCK & CO., INC.
Rahway, N. J.
U.S.A.

MERCK SHARP & DOHME
West Point, Pa.

MERCK SHARP & DOHME INTERNATIONAL
Rahway, N. J.

MERCK SHARP & DOHME RESEARCH LABORATORIES
Rahway, N. J.   *West Point, Pa.*

MSD AGVET DIVISION
Woodbridge, N. J.

HUBBARD FARMS, INC.
Walpole, N. H.

MERCK CHEMICAL MANUFACTURING DIVISION
Woodbridge, N. J.

MERCK PHARMACEUTICAL MANUFACTURING DIVISION
Rahway, N. J.

CALGON CORPORATION
Water Management Division
Pittsburgh, Pa.
Calgon Vestal Laboratories
St. Louis, Mo.

KELCO DIVISION
San Diego, Calif.

Library of Congress Catalog Card Number 89 – 63495
ISBN Number 9110910 – 32 – 8

First Printing – January 1990
Second Printing – April 1990

Printed in the U. S. A.

FOREWORD

THE MERCK MANUAL OF GERIATRICS is intended to provide information of clinical relevance to all physicians involved in the care of elderly patients. It follows the tradition set by THE MERCK MANUAL, which has been continuously published since 1899 and is the world's most widely used medical text.

The concept of a geriatric medical book was under consideration for several years. There was concern about whether there were sufficient important data to warrant a separate book on geriatric medicine. However, we became convinced that there is so much new information on both the structural and physiologic changes of normal aging and the clinical aspects of caring for elderly patients that it was not possible to include all that a practicing physician should know in a general textbook of medicine. Furthermore, even experienced clinicians are often not fully aware of much of this valuable information. Hence, this separate text seemed warranted.

The demographic imperative is clear: There are more Americans over 65 than under 25 for the first time in history and the average age is steadily increasing. People over 65 now represent about 12% of the US population and utilize about 30% of all health care resources; these figures are projected to reach over 20% and 50%, respectively, by 2030. It is also clear that gerontology, which includes the sciences describing the changes of normal aging as distinguished from disease effects, is becoming more sophisticated and prolific, while the practice of geriatrics is becoming increasingly specialized. Interest within the medical community is evidenced by the popularity of the examination, first offered in 1988, leading to a certificate of special competence in geriatrics.

In many individuals certain physiologic processes decline with age (eg, renal blood flow and glomerular filtration rate, maximal heart rate and cardiac output with exercise, glucose tolerance, cellular immunity), but other processes (eg, most liver functions and total lung capacity) remain unchanged. Secretion of ADH and response to osmolar stimuli actually increase with advancing age. The striking differences in how disease processes manifest themselves in the elderly, as compared to younger patients, are particularly important. For example, it has long been recognized that disorders such as hyperthyroidism may present in a masked or "apathetic" form, and that inflammatory intra-abdominal disorders such as appendicitis may not evoke typical symptoms and signs, requiring adjustments in the diagnostician's thinking. However, it is far less recognized that presenting symptoms in the elderly, while indicating that the patient is sick, may be totally misleading with regard to the nature and the primary location of the disease process. For example, when a patient presents with confusion, one thinks immediately of psychoactive drugs or a disease process primarily affecting the brain as a possible cause. In an elderly person, one must also consider such diverse factors as simple dehydration due to a wide variety of etiologies, infection, cardiac disorders producing subtle failure, intra-abdominal organ disease, etc. In short, diagnostic logic is different.

Similarly, the approach to therapeutics is far more complex in the elderly. Drug pharmacokinetics may be significantly different from those in younger adults, depending on the drug and the individual patient. Drug disposition may be altered by declines in kidney function and some liver metabolic activities, as well as by changes in body composition such as increased fat, decreased lean body mass, and reduced serum albumin levels. In addition, fluid stores such as plasma volume and total body water decline with age.

Nondrug therapy is more complex in this population and must take into account many factors; eg, rehabilitation strategies and the mobilization of a variety of community services. Furthermore, consideration of specific sites for optimal care and of the social, cultural, legal, financial, and ethical issues is important, complex, and evolving. Clearly, care of the elderly requires a substantially different approach to case management.

We have tried to provide a practical handbook covering all aspects of disease and the clinical management of elderly patients in a readily usable format. The book begins with a problem-oriented diagnostic approach to common presentations of illness in older patients. The second section deals with broad management approaches specific to the elderly. The third section addresses individual organ systems, with emphasis on age-related concerns. This is followed by a section dealing with epidemiologic, social, ethical, financial, and legal issues. Reference guides, with laboratory values and other data unique to the older population, are provided in the final section.

This book is designed to be comprehensive and authoritative, yet tightly edited to provide a large amount of information in a compact, handbook format. It is published by MERCK SHARP & DOHME RESEARCH LABORATORIES, a division of MERCK & CO., INC., on a not-for-profit basis in order to make the information available at a very modest cost, and thus accessible to students and nonmedical professionals involved in the care of older patients.

In developing this book, we have continued the tradition of THE MERCK MANUAL in seeking outstanding experts to serve as members of the Editorial Board, consultants, authors, and reviewers. We cannot adequately thank these contributors for the enormous effort and cooperation they provided to produce this book, but we know that they will feel sufficiently rewarded if their efforts serve your needs and those of the elderly for whom you care.

We hope THE MERCK MANUAL OF GERIATRICS will be compatible with your needs and worthy of frequent use. Suggestions for improvements will be warmly welcomed and carefully considered.

William B. Abrams, M.D., and Robert Berkow, M.D., *Editors*
MERCK SHARP & DOHME RESEARCH LABORATORIES
West Point, Pa. 19486

CONTENTS

GUIDE FOR READERS

- The **Contents** (p. vii) shows the pages where readers will find lists of Editorial Board Members, consultants, and contributors, as well as abbreviations and symbols, titles of sections (groupings of related chapters), and the index. **Thumb-tabs** with appropriate abbreviations mark each section, selected subsections, and the index.

- Each section, designated by the symbol §, and each subsection in Section 3 begins with its own table of contents, listing chapters and subchapters in that section.

- **Chapters** are numbered serially from the beginning to the end of the book.

- The **Index** contains many cross-entries; page numbers in bold type signify major discussions of the topics. In addition, the text gives numerous cross-references to other sections and chapters.

- Each **Page Head** carries the page number (page numbers and chapter numbers run serially from the beginning to the end of the book); left-hand pages contain the section or subsection title, and right-hand pages contain the chapter number and title.

- **Abbreviations and Symbols,** used throughout the book as essential space savers, are listed on pp. ix and x. Other abbreviations in the text are explained with their first use in the chapter or subchapter.

- The **Tables** and **Figures** found throughout the text are referenced appropriately in the index but are not listed in a table of contents.

- **Drugs** are designated in the text mainly by generic (nonproprietary) names.

- The authors, reviewers, editors, and publisher of this book have made extensive efforts to ensure that treatments, drugs, and dosage regimens are accurate and conform to the standards accepted at the time of publication. However, constant changes in information resulting from continuing research and clinical experience, reasonable differences in opinions among authorities, unique aspects of individual clinical situations, and the possibility of human error in preparing such an extensive text require that the reader exercise individual judgment when making a clinical decision and, if necessary, consult and compare information from other sources. In particular, the reader is advised to check the product information provided by the manufacturer of a drug product before prescribing or administering it, especially if the drug is unfamiliar or is used infrequently.

ABBREVIATIONS AND SYMBOLS

ADH	antidiuretic hormone	**GU**	genitourinary
ADL	activities of daily living	**h**	hour
ADP	adenosine diphosphate	**H$_2$**	histamine
AIDS	acquired immunodeficiency syndrome	**Hb**	hemoglobin
		HCO$_3$	bicarbonate
ALT	alanine aminotransferase (formerly SGPT)	**Hct**	hematocrit
		HF	heart failure
AST	aspartate aminotransferase (formerly SGOT)	**Hg**	mercury
		HI	hemagglutination-inhibition, inhibiting
bid	2 times a day		
BP	blood pressure	**HLA**	human leukocyte group A
BSA	body surface area	**Hz**	hertz (cycles/second)
C	Celsius; centigrade; complement	**IADL**	instrumental activities of daily living
Ca	calcium	**ICF**	intracellular fluid
CF	complement fixation, fixating	**IgA, etc**	immunoglobulin A, etc
		IM	intramuscular(ly)
CFU	colony-forming units	**in.**	inch; inches
Ch.	chapter	**IPPB**	inspiratory positive pressure breathing
Ci	curie		
CK	creatine kinase	**IU**	international unit
Cl	chloride; chlorine	**IV**	intravenous(ly)
cm	centimeter	**IVU**	intravenous urography
CO	carbon monoxide; cardiac output	**K**	potassium
		kcal	kilocalorie (food calorie)
CO$_2$	carbon dioxide	**kg**	kilogram
CPR	cardiopulmonary resuscitation	**L**	liter
		LDH	lactic dehydrogenase
CSF	cerebrospinal fluid	**LE**	lupus erythematosus
CT	computed tomography	**lt**	left
cu	cubic	**m, m^2**	meter, square meter
dL	deciliter (= 100 mL)	**M**	molar
D/W	dextrose in water	**MCH**	mean corpuscular hemoglobin
ECF	extracellular fluid		
ECG	electrocardiogram	**MCHC**	mean corpuscular hemoglobin concentration
ECT	electroconvulsive therapy		
EEG	electroencephalogram	**mCi**	millicurie
ESR	erythrocyte sedimentation rate	**MCV**	mean corpuscular volume
		mEq	milliequivalent
F	Fahrenheit	**mg**	milligram
fL	femtoliter	**Mg**	magnesium
ft	foot; feet (measure)	**MI**	myocardial infarction
FUO	fever of unknown origin	**MIC**	minimum inhibitory concentration
GFR	glomerular filtration rate		
GI	gastrointestinal	**min**	minute
gm	gram	**mIU**	milli-international unit

mL	milliliter	**rt**	right
mm	millimeter	**Sa$_{O_2}$**	arterial oxygen saturation
mM	millimole	**SBE**	subacute bacterial endocarditis
mo	month		
mol wt	molecular weight	**s.c.**	subcutaneous(ly)
mOsm	milliosmole	**sec**	second
MRC	Medical Research Council (units)	**SI**	International System of Units
MRI	magnetic resonance imaging	**SLE**	systemic lupus erythematosus
mV	millivolt		
N	nitrogen; normal (strength of solution)	**soln**	solution
		sp gr	specific gravity
Na	sodium	**sq**	square
NaCl	sodium chloride	**STS**	serologic test(s) for syphilis
ng	nanogram (= millimicrogram)		
		t$_{1/2}$	half-life
nm	nanometer (= millimicron)	**TB**	tuberculosis
OA	osteoarthritis	**tbsp**	tablespoon
OTC	over-the-counter (pharmaceuticals)	**tid**	3 times a day
		tsp	teaspoon
oz	ounce	**u.**	unit
P	phosphorus; pressure	**URI**	upper respiratory infection
P$_{CO_2}$	carbon dioxide pressure (or tension)	**US**	ultrasonography;ultrasound
		UTI	urinary tract infection
P$_{O_2}$	oxygen pressure (or tension)	**WBC**	white blood cell
		WHO	World Health Organization
Pa$_{CO_2}$	arterial carbon dioxide pressure	**wk**	week
		wt	weight
Pa$_{O_2}$	arterial oxygen pressure	**yr**	year
PA$_{O_2}$	alveolar oxygen pressure	**μ**	micro-
pg	picogram (= micromicrogram)	**μL**	microliter
		μm	micrometer; micron
po	orally	**mμ**	millimicron (= nanometer)
PPD	Purified Protein Derivative (tuberculin)	**μCi**	microcurie
		μg	microgram
ppm	parts per million	**μmol**	micromole
prn	as needed	**μOsm**	micro-osmole
q	every	**/**	per
q 4 h, etc	every 4 hours, etc	**<**	less than
		>	more than
qid	4 times a day	**$\leq$**	equal to or less than
R, r	roentgen	**$\geq$**	equal to or more than
RA	rheumatoid arthritis	**$\cong$**	approximately equal to
RBC	red blood cell	**$\pm$**	plus or minus
RF	rheumatic fever; rheumatoid factor	**§**	section

CONSULTANTS

Tom Arie, B.M., F.R.C.P., F.R.C. Psych., F.F.C.M.
Professor and Head, Department of Health Care of the Elderly, University of Nottingham, England

Psychiatric Disorders

Edward G. Lakatta, M.D.
Chief, Laboratory of Cardiovascular Science, Gerontology Research Center, National Institute on Aging; Professor of Medicine (Cardiology), The Johns Hopkins University

Cardiovascular Disorders

Marvin M. Schuster, M.D.
Professor of Medicine and of Psychiatry, The Johns Hopkins University; Director, Division of Digestive Diseases, Francis Scott Key Medical Center

Gastrointestinal Disorders

EDITORIAL STAFF

Shirley Claypool, Executive Editor
Barbara J. Masten, Medical Textbook Coordinator

ACKNOWLEDGMENTS

The publication of a book of this scope involves the efforts of a great many persons. Our gratitude is expressed to the Editorial Board, consultants, and contributors, whose names appear elsewhere in this manual.

We wish to acknowledge the editorial expertise of Medical Information Services, Inc., New York City, which played a significant role in the preparation of this manual. The MIS staff helped to effectively and efficiently transform manuscripts into finished pages. Among those who merit special thanks are Judith Ann Cohen, president; Phyllis Tish Harbus, executive editor; and Georgia Koumantzelis, editorial assistant.

We also wish to express our appreciation for the expert assistance provided by Laurie Dornbrand, M.D., Geriatric Research, Education, and Clinical Center, Palo Alto Veterans Administration Hospital, and Alan Laties, M.D., Scheie Eye Institute, in the chapters on Rehabilitation and Ophthalmologic Disorders, respectively.

Finally, we thank Gary Zelko and Pamela J. Barnes of Merck Professional Handbooks for their unfailing enthusiasm and guidance.

W.B.A. and R.B.

CONTRIBUTORS

Ronald D. Adelman, M.D.
Chief, Division of Geriatrics, Winthrop-University Hospital; Assistant Professor of Medicine, SUNY, Stony Brook

Mistreatment

Tom Arie, B.M., F.R.C.P., F.R.C. Psych., F.F.C.M.
Professor and Head, Department of Health Care of the Elderly, University of Nottingham, England

Acute Confusion

Shirley P. Bagley, M.S.
Assistant Director for Special Programs, National Institute on Aging

Preventive Strategies

John G. Bartlett, M.D.
Professor of Medicine and Chief, Division of Infectious Diseases, The Johns Hopkins University School of Medicine

Pneumonia and Tuberculosis

Bruce J. Baum, D.M.D., Ph.D.
Clinical Director and Chief, Clinical Investigations and Patient Care Branch, National Institute of Dental Research

Dental and Oral Disorders

Richard W. Besdine, M.D.
Travelers Professor of Geriatrics and Gerontology; Director, Travelers Center on Aging; Associate Professor of Internal Medicine and of Community Medicine, University of Connecticut

Introduction; Hyperthermia and Accidental Hypothermia; Establishing Therapeutic Objectives: Quality of Life Issues

Dan G. Blazer, II, M.D.
Professor of Psychiatry, Assistant Professor of Community and Family Medicine, and Head, Division of Geriatric Psychiatry, Duke University

Anxiety Disorders; Hypochondriasis; Depression; Alcohol Abuse and Dependence; Schizophrenia and Schizophreniform Disorders

Risa Breckman, M.S.W.
Co-director, Elder Abuse Training and Resource Center, New York City

Mistreatment

John C. Brocklehurst, M.D., F.R.C.P.
Professor of Geriatric Medicine and Director, Manchester University Unit for Biological Aging Research, University of Manchester, England

Disorders of the Lower Bowel

Jacob A. Brody, M.D.
Dean, School of Public Health; Research Professor of Medicine, College of Medicine, University of Illinois at Chicago

Epidemiology and Demographics

Reginald C. Bruskewitz, M.D.
Associate Professor of Surgery/Urology, University of Wisconsin Hospitals

Disorders of the Lower Genitourinary Tract: Bladder, Prostate, and Testicles

Larry M. Bush, M.D.
Clinical Assistant Professor of Medicine, The Medical College of Pennsylvania

Epidemiology and Pathogenesis of Infectious Diseases

Robert N. Butler, M.D.
Brookdale Professor of Geriatrics and Adult Development; Chairman, Ritter Department of Geriatrics and Adult Development, Mount Sinai School of Medicine

Sexuality; Senile Dementia of the Alzheimer Type; Living Alone

Ronald D. T. Cape, M.D., F.R.C.P.E., F.R.C.P.C.
Chairman, Committee of the National Research Institute of Gerontology and Geriatric Medicine, Victoria, Australia

Malnutrition, Weight Loss, and Anorexia; Obesity

Louis R. Caplan, M.D.
Professor and Chairman, Department of Neurology, Tufts University; Neurologist-in-Chief, New England Medical Center

Cerebrovascular Disease

Barbara J. Carroll, M.D.
Assistant Professor, Division of Geriatrics, George Washington University; Medical Director, Hospice of Washington

Care of the Dying Patient

Donald O. Castell, M.D.
Professor of Medicine and Chief, Section on Gastroenterology, The Bowman Gray School of Medicine

Upper Gastrointestinal Tract Disorders

Maxwell Chait, M.D.
Assistant Clinical Professor of Medicine, Albert Einstein College of Medicine; Adjunct Attending Physician, Memorial Sloan-Kettering Cancer Center

Gastrointestinal Neoplasms

Gene D. Cohen, M.D., Ph.D.
Deputy Director, National Institute on Aging; Clinical Professor, Department of Psychiatry, Georgetown University

Normal Changes and Patterns of Psychiatric Disease

Barry S. Collet, D.P.M., M.P.H.
Hebrew Rehabilitation Center for Aged, Boston

Foot Problems

Eugene Coodley, M.D., F.A.C.P.
Professor of Medicine, University of California, Irvine; Chief of Gerontology, VA Medical Center, Long Beach

Changes in Laboratory Values

Mayer B. Davidson, M.D.
Professor of Medicine, University of California, Los Angeles; Director, Diabetes Program, Cedars-Sinai Medical Center

Carbohydrate Metabolism and Diabetes Mellitus

John O. L. DeLancey, M.D.
Assistant Professor, Department of Gynecology and Obstetrics, The University of Michigan

Female Genitourinary Disorders

Ananias C. Diokno, M.D.
Clinical Professor, University of Michigan; Chief of Urology, William Beaumont Hospital

Urinary Incontinence

Nancy Neveloff Dubler, LL.B.
Associate Professor and Director, Department of Epidemiology and Social Medicine, Division of Legal and Ethical Issues in Health Care, Montefiore Medical Center/Albert Einstein College of Medicine

Legal Issues

Theodore C. Eickhoff, M.D.
Professor of Medicine, University of Colorado; Director, Internal Medicine, Presbyterian St. Luke's Medical Center

Vaccines and Immunization

Thomas A. Einhorn, M.D.
Associate Professor of Orthopedics and Director of Orthopedic Research, The Mount Sinai School of Medicine

Orthopedic Problems

Thomas Elkins, M.D.
Associate Professor, Department of Gynecology and Obstetrics, and Chief, Division of Gynecology, The University of Michigan

Female Genitourinary Disorders

W. Gary Erwin, Pharm.D.
Program Administrator, Geriatric Pharmacy Institute, and Associate Professor of Clinical Pharmacy, Philadelphia College of Pharmacy and Science

The Role of the Pharmacist

Walter H. Ettinger, M.D.
Associate Professor of Medicine and Head, Section on Internal Medicine and Gerontology, Wake Forest University

Joint and Soft Tissue Disorders

Jerome L. Fleg, M.D.
Staff Cardiologist, Laboratory of Cardiovascular Science, Gerontology Research Center, National Institute on Aging

Diagnostic Evaluation; Arrhythmias and Conduction Disorders

Marshal F. Folstein, M.D.
Eugene Meyer III Professor of Psychiatry and Medicine, The Johns Hopkins University

Mental Status Examination

Susan E. Folstein, M.D.
Associate Professor of Psychiatry and Director, Division of Psychiatric Genetics, The Johns Hopkins University

Mental Status Examination

Michael L. Freedman, M.D.
The Diane and Arthur Belfer Professor of Geriatric Medicine and Director, Division of Geriatrics, New York University

Normal Aging and Patterns of Hematologic Disease; Anemias; Malignancies and Myeloproliferative Diseases

Marsha D. Fretwell, M.D.
Assistant Professor of Medicine, Brown University

Comprehensive Functional Assessment

Sandor A. Friedman, M.D.
Director, Department of Medicine, Coney Island Hospital; Professor of Medicine, State University of New York, Health Science Center at Brooklyn

Peripheral Vascular Diseases

Edward D. Frohlich, M.D.
Alton Ochsner Distinguished Scientist and
Vice President for Academic Affairs,
Alton Ochsner Medical Foundation

Hypertension

Philip P. Gerbino, Pharm.D.
Professor, Clinical Pharmacy, Associate
Dean of Pharmacy, and Executive
Director, Geriatric Pharmacy Institute,
Philadelphia College of Pharmacy and
Science

The Role of the Pharmacist

Tobin N. Gerhart, M.D.
Clinical Instructor in Orthopedic Surgery,
Harvard Medical School

Fractures

Bernard J. Gersh, M.D., Ch.B., D.Phil.
Professor of Medicine, Mayo Medical
School; Consultant in Cardiovascular
Diseases and Internal Medicine, Mayo
Clinic

*Cardiovascular Surgery and Percuta-
neous Interventional Technics*

Gary Gerstenblith, M.D.
Associate Professor of Medicine, The
Johns Hopkins University

Coronary Artery Disease

Barbara A. Gilchrest, M.D.
Professor and Chairman, Department of
Dermatology, Boston University

Skin Changes and Disorders

Charles J. Glueck, M.D.
Director, Cholesterol Center, The Jewish
Hospital of Cincinnati, Inc.

Lipoprotein Metabolism

A. Julianna Gulya, M.D., F.A.C.S.
Associate Professor of Surgery, Division
of Otolaryngology-Head and Neck Surgery, The George Washington University

Ear Disorders

Paul A. L. Haber, M.D.
Regional Coordinator for Aging, VA
Medical Center, Washington, D.C.

Diagnostic and Therapeutic Technology

Charles O. Herrera, M.D.
Director, Sleep Disorders Program for
Middle Age and Older Adults, and
Assistant Professor, Department of Geri-
atrics and Adult Development, The
Mount Sinai School of Medicine

Sleep Disorders

Bruce E. Hirsch, M.D.
Instructor in Medicine, Cornell University

Normal Changes in Host Defense

Kathryn Hyer, M.P.P.
Associate Director, Office of Health
Policy and Aging Research, Mount Sinai
School of Medicine

Living Alone

Masayoshi Itoh, M.D.
Associate Professor of Clinical Rehabil-
itation Medicine, New York University;
Associate Director, Department of Re-
habilitation Medicine, Goldwater
Memorial Hospital

Rehabilitation

Robert J. Joynt, M.D., Ph.D.
Dean, School of Medicine and Dentistry, and Professor of Neurology, The University of Rochester

Normal Aging and Patterns of Neurologic Disease

Arthur D. Kay, M.D.
Director of Neurology, The Brookdale Hospital Medical Center; Assistant Professor of Neurology, State University Health Science Center at Brooklyn

Falls and Gait Disorders

Donald Kaye, M.D.
Professor and Chairman, Department of Medicine, The Medical College of Pennsylvania

Epidemiology and Pathogenesis of Infectious Diseases

Michael J. Klein, M.D.
Associate Professor of Pathology and Orthopedics, Mount Sinai School of Medicine

Orthopedic Problems

Mary Jane Koren, M.D.
Director, Bureau of Long-Term Care Services, New York State Department of Health; Adjunct Assistant Professor of Geriatrics, Mount Sinai School of Medicine

Site-Specific Care

Stanley G. Korenman, M.D.
Professor and Chair, Department of Medicine, UCLA San Fernando Valley Program; Chief, Medical Services, VA Medical Center, Sepulveda

Male Hypogonadism and Impotence

O. Dhodanand Kowlessar, M.D.
Professor of Medicine and Associate Chairman, Department of Medicine, Jefferson Medical College of Thomas Jefferson University

Diarrhea; Malabsorption Syndromes

Carl Kupfer, M.D.
Director, National Eye Institute, National Institutes of Health

Ophthalmologic Disorders

Edward G. Lakatta, M.D.
Chief, Laboratory of Cardiovascular Science, Gerontology Research Center, National Institute on Aging; Professor of Medicine (Cardiology), The Johns Hopkins University

Normal Changes of Aging

Mathew H. M. Lee, M.D.
Professor of Clinical Rehabilitation Medicine, New York University

Rehabilitation

Michael M. Lewis, M.D.
Professor and Chairman, Department of Orthopedics, The Mount Sinai School of Medicine

Orthopedic Problems

Myrna Lewis, A.C.S.W.
Instructor, Department of Community Medicine, The Mount Sinai School of Medicine

Sexuality

Leslie S. Libow, M.D.
Chief of Medical Services, The Jewish
Home & Hospital for Aged; Greenwall
Professor, The Mount Sinai School of
Medicine

History and Physical Examination

Lewis A. Lipsitz, M.D.
Assistant Professor of Medicine, Harvard
University; Director for Education and
Clinical Research, Hebrew Rehabilitation
Center for Aged, Boston

Syncope; Hypotension

David T. Lowenthal, M.D., Ph.D.
Professor of Medicine, Pharmacology, and
Exercise Science, University of Florida
College of Medicine; Director, Geriatric
Research, Education, and Clinical Center,
VA Medical Center, Gainesville

Clinical Pharmacology; Exercise

Marjorie Luckey, M.D.
Assistant Professor, Department of
Obstetrics, Gynecology, and Reproductive
Science, The Mount Sinai School of
Medicine

Metabolic Bone Disease

Joanne Lynn, M.D.
Associate Professor and Acting Director,
Center for Aging Studies and Services,
Department of Health Care Sciences and
Medicine, The George Washington Uni-
versity; Medical Director, The Washington
Home

Care of the Dying Patient; Ethical Issues

William J. MacLennan, M.D., F.R.C.P. (Glas.,
Ed., Lond.)
Professor, Department of Geriatric Med-
icine, University of Edinburgh, Scotland

*Giant Cell (Temporal) Arteritis and
Polymyalgia Rheumatica*

Gail Hills Maguire, Ph.D., O.T.R.
Professor, Department of Occupational
Therapy, Florida International University

Occupational Therapy

E. Gordon Margolin, M.D.
Professor of Medicine, University of
Cincinnati; Medical Director, Semmons
Center on Aging, The Jewish Hospital
of Cincinnati, Inc.

Lipoprotein Metabolism

Lila T. McConnell, M.D.
Assistant Professor, Department of
Health Care Sciences, Division of Geri-
atric Medicine, The George Washington
University

Ethical Issues

Edward J. McGuire, M.D.
Professor and Section Head, Section of
Urology, The University of Michigan

Female Genitourinary Disorders

Diane E. Meier, M.D.
Assistant Professor, Department of
Geriatrics and Adult Development, The
Mount Sinai School of Medicine

Metabolic Bone Disease

Geno J. Merli, M.D., F.A.C.P.
Clinical Associate Professor of Medicine
and Director, Division of Internal Medicine, Jefferson Medical College of
Thomas Jefferson University

Geriatric Emergencies

John R. Michael, M.D.
Associate Professor of Medicine and
Director, Medical Intensive Care Unit,
University of Utah

Pulmonary Embolism

Myron Miller, M.D.
Professor and Vice-Chairman, Department of Geriatrics and Adult Development, and Professor of Medicine, The Mount Sinai School of Medicine

Disorders of Water and Sodium Balance

Jonathan D. Moreno, Ph.D.
Professor of Pediatrics and of Medicine (Bioethics), SUNY Health Science Center at Brooklyn

Ethical Issues

Richard T. Moxley, M.D.
Professor of Neurology and of Pediatrics; Director, Neuromuscular Disease Center, University of Rochester

Muscular Disorders

Robert J. Nathan, M.D.
Professor, Department of Mental Health Sciences, Hahnemann University

Geriatric Psychiatric Consultation Services

S. Ragnar Norrby, M.D., Ph.D.
Professor and Chairman, Department of Infectious Diseases, University of Lund, Sweden

Urinary Tract Infection; Antimicrobial Agents

Marilyn Pajk, R.N., M.S.
Geriatric Nurse Specialist, Home Medical Service, University Hospital, Boston University Medical Center

Pressure Sores

Stuart W. H. Pang, M.D.
Department of Neurology, The Mount Sinai School of Medicine

Movement Disorders

Victoria W. Persky, M.D.
Associate Professor, Epidemiology and Biometry, School of Public Health, University of Illinois at Chicago

Epidemiology and Demographics

Tania J. Phillips, B.Sc., M.B.B.S., M.R.C.P.
Fellow in Geriatric Dermatology, Boston University

Skin Changes and Disorders

Russell K. Portenoy, M.D.
Director of Analgesic Studies, Pain Service, and Assistant Attending Neurologist, Memorial Sloan-Kettering Cancer Center; Assistant Professor of Neurology, Cornell University

Pain

Lawrence G. Raisz, M.D.
Professor of Medicine and Head, Division of Endocrinology and Metabolism, The University of Connecticut School of Medicine

Disorders of Mineral Metabolism

Joel E. Richter, M.D.
Associate Professor of Medicine, Section on Gastroenterology, Wake Forest School of Medicine

Functional Disorders of the Gastrointestinal Tract

John W. Rowe, M.D.
President, The Mount Sinai School of Medicine

Aging Processes; Renal System

Laurence Z. Rubenstein, M.D.
Associate Professor of Medicine, University of California, Los Angeles; Clinical Director, Geriatric Research, Education, and Clinical Center, VA Medical Center, Sepulveda

Assessment Instruments

Bruce M. Schechter, Pharm.D.
Assistant Program Administrator, Geriatric Pharmacy Institute, and Assistant Professor of Clinical Pharmacy, Philadelphia College of Pharmacy and Science

The Role of the Pharmacist

Mal Schechter, M.S.
Assistant Professor, Gerald and May Ellen Ritter Department of Geriatrics and Adult Development, Mount Sinai School of Medicine

Health Insurance

Steven Schenker, M.D.
Professor of Medicine and of Pharmacology, University of Texas Health Science Center; Staff Physician, VA Hospital, San Antonio

The Aging Liver

Isaac Schiff, M.D.
Joe Vincent Meigs Professor of Gynecology, Harvard University; Chief of Vincent Gynecology Service, Massachusetts General Hospital

Menopause and Ovarian Hormone Therapy

Edward L. Schneider, M.D.
Dean, Andrus Gerontology Center, University of Southern California

Aging Processes

Marvin M. Schuster, M.D.
Professor of Medicine and of Psychiatry, The Johns Hopkins University; Director, Division of Digestive Diseases, Francis Scott Key Medical Center

Influence of Aging on Gastrointestinal Disorders

David H. Solomon, M.D.
Professor of Medicine/Geriatrics, University of California, Los Angeles

Introduction (Metabolic and Endocrine Disorders); The Normal and Diseased Thyroid Gland

Perry J. Starer, M.D.
Assistant Professor, Department of Geriatrics and Adult Development, The Mount Sinai School of Medicine

History and Physical Examination

Trey Sunderland, M.D.
Chief, Unit on Geriatric Psychopharmacology, National Institute of Mental Health

Organic Brain Disorders

Peter B. Terry, M.D.
Associate Professor of Medicine, Environmental Health Sciences, Anesthesiology, and Critical Care Medicine, The Johns Hopkins Medical Institutions

Chronic Obstructive Pulmonary Disease

Rein Tideiksaar, Ph.D.
Assistant Professor of Geriatrics, The Mount Sinai School of Medicine and The Jewish Home and Hospital for Aged

Falls and Gait Disorders

Melvyn S. Tockman, M.D., Ph.D.
Associate Professor of Environmental
Health Sciences, The Johns Hopkins
University

The Effects of Age on the Lung

Ronald G. Tompkins, M.D., Sc.D.
Assistant Professor of Surgery, Harvard
University; Assistant Surgeon, Massa-
chusetts General Hospital

*Surgery: Preoperative Evaluation and
Intraoperative and Postoperative Care;
Surgery of the Digestive Tract*

Brian W. Walsh, M.D.
Instructor, Obstetrics and Gynecology,
Harvard University

*Menopause and Ovarian Hormone Ther-
apy*

John H. Wasson, M.D.
Professor of Clinical, Community, and
Family Medicine, Dartmouth College;
Associate Chief for Ambulatory Care, VA
Medical Center, White River Junction

*Disorders of the Lower Genitourinary
Tract: Bladder, Prostate, and Testicles*

Jerome D. Waye, M.D.
Chief, Gastrointestinal Unit, The Mount
Sinai Hospital and Lenox Hill Hospital,
New York City

Gastrointestinal Endoscopy

Jeanne Y. Wei, M.D., Ph.D.
Associate Professor of Medicine, Harvard
University; Acting Chief, Gerontology
Division, Beth Israel and Brigham and
Women's Hospitals

Heart Failure

Nancy T. Weintraub, M.D.
Clinical Assistant Professor in Internal
Medicine, State University of New York;
Attending Physician, Bellevue Medical
Center

*Normal Aging and Patterns of Hema-
tologic Disease; Anemias; Malignancies
and Myeloproliferative Diseases*

Howard H. Weitz, M.D.
Associate Director, Division of Internal
Medicine, and Clinical Assistant Professor of Medicine, Jefferson Medical College of Thomas Jefferson University

Geriatric Emergencies

Marc E. Weksler, M.D.
Wright Professor of Medicine and Director, Division of Geriatrics and Gerontology, Cornell University

Normal Changes in Host Defense

Claude E. Welch, M.D.
Senior Surgeon, Massachusetts General
Hospital; Clinical Professor of Surgery
(Emeritus), Harvard University

*Surgery: Preoperative Evaluation and
Intraoperative and Postoperative Care;
Surgery of the Digestive Tract*

Nanette K. Wenger, M.D.
Professor of Medicine (Cardiology),
Emory University; Director, Cardiac
Clinics, Grady Memorial Hospital

Valvular Heart Disease

Terrie Wetle, Ph.D.
Director of Research, Braceland Center
for Mental Health and Aging, Institute of
Living; Associate Professor of Community Medicine, University of Connecticut Health Center

Social Issues

Mary E. Wheat, M.D.
Assistant Service Leader, Montefiore Medical Center; Assistant Professor of Medicine and of Epidemiology and Social Medicine, Albert Einstein College of Medicine

Exercise

Thomas E. Whigham, M.D.
Assistant Professor, Gastroenterology and Nutrition, University of Texas Health Science Center, San Antonio

The Aging Liver

T. Franklin Williams, M.D.
Director, National Institute on Aging, National Institutes of Health

Preventive Strategies

William R. Wilson, M.D.
Chief, Division of Otolaryngology-Head and Neck Surgery, The George Washington University

Nose and Throat Disorders

Sidney J. Winawer, M.D.
Chief, Gastroenterology Service, and Member and Co-Head, Laboratory for Gastrointestinal Cancer Research, Memorial Sloan-Kettering Cancer Center

Gastrointestinal Neoplasms

Melvin D. Yahr, M.D.
Henry P. and Georgette Goldschmidt Professor of Neurology and Chairman, Department of Neurology, The Mount Sinai School of Medicine

Movement Disorders

Robert A. Zorowitz, M.D.
Department of Medicine, Long Island Jewish Medical Center, Albert Einstein College of Medicine

Metabolic Bone Disease

§1. A PROBLEM–ORIENTED APPROACH

1. INTRODUCTION

Richard W. Besdine

Among the many characteristics of geriatric medicine that differentiate it from the traditional medical specialties is the prominence of certain recurring clinical problems, which, though few in number, can originate in a wide array of organ system disorders. In older persons, predicting or identifying the locus of disease by these presenting symptoms or syndromes demands careful and comprehensive evaluation. These problems —anorexia, weight loss, fluid and electrolyte abnormalities, heat regulation disorders, syncope, gait disturbance, falls, immobility, confusion, incontinence, pain, sleep abnormalities, and pressure sores—are the bedeviling afflictions of the elderly. Their elucidation and treatment are critical to the well-being of older persons, and a thorough understanding of their associated organ systems is the blueprint to successful patient care for a geriatrician.

Restriction of independent functional ability is the final common outcome for many disorders in the elderly. Functional impairment means decreased ability to meet one's own needs (see also Ch. 15). In older individuals, unlike in younger ones, the first sign of a new illness or reactivated chronic disease is rarely a single, specific complaint that helps to localize the organ system or tissue in which the disease occurs. It is more likely to be one or more *nonspecific* problems, which themselves are only manifestations of impaired function.

These problems quickly impair independence in the previously self-sufficient elder, but do not necessarily produce the obvious, typical signs of illness, recognized by most lay and even general professional standards. The reason why disease in older persons manifests itself first as functional loss, usually in organ systems *unrelated* to the locus of illness, is not well understood. Apparently, disruption of homeostasis by any disease in previously independent, functional elderly persons is likely to be expressed in the most vulnerable, most delicately balanced systems. The result is functional problems in Activities of Daily Living **(ADL)** or Instrumental Activities of Daily Living **(IADL).**

Deterioration of functional independence in active, previously unimpaired elders *is an early, subtle sign of untreated illness characterized by the absence of typical symptoms and signs of disease.* Consequently, problems with mobility, cognition, continence, and nutrition require a problem-oriented approach to geriatric care, linking functional assessment with traditional clinical evaluation. If quality of life is to be maintained, a rapid, thorough clinical evaluation must be performed as soon as such functional impairments develop. These disease-generated impairments are usually treatable, if they are detected and evaluated promptly.

Although early functional assessment (Ch. 15) and prompt treatment of disease are often called "prevention" or "preventive geriatrics," they are tertiary prevention at best. Nevertheless, they are crucial to restoring independence. In addition, periodic formal reassessment and rapid response to detected declines in independence are essential for providing adequate geriatric care.

A problem-oriented approach to the impaired older person illuminates another phenomenon common in geriatric medicine, that of **poor correlation between type and severity of problem (functional disability) and the disease problem list.** Since the burden of illness and functional loss both increase with advancing age, the assumption is often made that the number of diseases or conditions on the problem list of an older person correlates with type and degree of functional disability. But accumulating a number of diseases does not necessarily result in serious loss of function. Rather, an independent, vigorous elderly person with a shockingly long list of serious diseases is more common.

The assumption that the diseased organ or tissue determines the specific functional impairment in older persons is also common but erroneous. For example, the assumption (causality principle) that mobility problems are caused by musculoskeletal or neurologic disorders, that confusion arises from brain disease, that incontinence results from bladder dysfunction, and so on, which is usually valid for disease in young and middle-aged persons, does not hold for aged patients. Certain vulnerable tissues and systems responsible for functional integrity in the elderly are especially likely to decompensate as a result of a systemic influence of disease anywhere in the body. For example, evaluation of an elderly man with urinary incontinence may show that his urinary tract is normal but that he is taking a diuretic, which is causing the problem.

The discovery of disease in an organ system does not necessarily indicate that the cause of functional loss can be attributed to that organ system. If prostatitis were found in an incontinent man, treatment of the infection may not alleviate the incontinence. Only the restoration of normal organ function by successful treatment of the disease in that system allows us to identify a causal relationship with certainty.

The severity of illness, as measured by objective data, does not necessarily determine the presence or severity of functional dependency. For example, cardiac arrhythmias may be discovered on routine ECG or Holter monitoring, or chronic elevation of alkaline phosphatase may be noted on multiphasic screening in an independent, fully functional older person. When a patient's laboratory study results are notably abnormal but functional disability is minimal, the functional evaluation can support withholding treatment, particularly if it involves considerable cost, discomfort, or health risk.

The lessons to be learned from these noncorrelations between function and diagnoses are crucial for good geriatric care. The following chapters in this section explore the functionally related problems to which the elderly are most vulnerable. Each chapter maintains a clinical focus on etiology of the presenting problem and considers the diagnostic and management approaches most useful in treating that problem. Many of the disease states provoking these problems are considered in detail in Section 3, in which diseases are discussed in relation to organ systems. The physician, however, should consider the problems discussed in this section, along with those described in Section 3, to ensure that older patients are receiving adequate care.

---

2. MALNUTRITION, WEIGHT LOSS, AND ANOREXIA

Ronald D. T. Cape

Malnutrition is *a negative imbalance between the nutrient supply to tissues and the requirement for that nutrient, whether from an inappropriate dietary intake or defective utilization by the body.* While the elderly are considered to be at risk for developing malnutrition, surveys suggest that the prevalence is low. According to one authority, about 3% of the elderly population in Great Britain suffers from malnutrition. While many more may consume a diet adequate in calories but unbalanced in mix of essential nutrients (protein, carbohydrate, fat, vitamins, minerals, certain electrolytes, and water), the number is unknown.

Malnutrition has, however, been documented frequently in hospitalized subjects, with prevalence rates ranging from 26% in 1 study of surgical patients at an English teaching hospital to 43% in a study of medical patients at the University of Alabama. Vitamin levels are also low in hospitalized patients. A possible explanation is that people are admitted to the hospital because they are ill and, usually, the malnutrition is a result of the illness. Clinical significance results from a lack of nutritional reserves and the risk of serious malnutrition in the presence of metabolic stress.

Effects of Aging

The lean body mass of an average man in his middle 20s is about 60 kg; by the time he reaches 75 or 80 yr of age, this falls to 48 kg. During the same period, the fat content of the body doubles from 13 to 26 kg. Loss of tissue occurs mainly from muscle, but some reduction occurs in the size of large organs, eg, the brain and liver. Similar changes occur in women but to a lesser degree. The net effect is that the total active cellular mass of the body is appreciably decreased, reducing the quantity of energy-producing food required by an older person.

The loss of active cell mass also accounts for a slow decline in **the basal metabolic rate** throughout life, with the change averaging 1.66 kcal/m^2/h/decade.

In an important study, rats placed on a diet (introduced at weaning) that contained all essential nutrients but was calorically less than the animals would have consumed ad lib lived longer and were healthier than control animals, although they remained smaller and weighed less. Other studies have demonstrated that restricting the diet of middle-aged animals may also yield gains in longevity, perhaps because the immune system of animals on a reduced diet remains more reactive. However, all these animals were fed a carefully controlled diet that contained adequate amounts of vitamins, minerals, and essential amino acids; thus, the significance of these data for human health is not clear. Undernourished patients tend to be malnourished. Furthermore, at least 1 study of elderly people in 7 countries found that those who were 10 to 20% "overweight" had the lowest mortality rates (see Ch. 43).

Further changes associated with aging are discussed under Risk Factors, below.

Essential Food Elements

The elderly consume fewer total calories per day. This is associated with a decline in fat and, less certainly, in protein intake. Like the general population, older persons have shifted their consumption of substances containing saturated fats to those containing poly- and mono-unsaturated fatty acids. Carbohydrate intake is well maintained in the elderly and may even increase slightly. Older individuals derive about 20% of their calories from protein and about 41 and 39% from carbohydrate and fat, respectively. Because these changes were noted in well-motivated adult men, they are thought to be age-related.

Carbohydrate is readily available in foods that are easily prepared, including many items that do not require cooking. Studies suggest it is a mainstay of the older person's diet. During the early 20th century, flour and rice became increasingly more refined as whiter bread and rice were introduced. This trend has slowed with the recognition of the advantages of fiber and whole-meal flour. As bread remains a staple ingredient of the older person's diet, whole-meal varieties should be recommended.

Protein: Accompanying the reduction in lean body mass with age is a progressive decrease in total body protein. While protein is constantly synthesized and broken down in the body, in older people with smaller stores, the total turnover is less. This process occurs more rapidly in organ protein than in muscle. Protein synthesis decreases and breakdown of protein occurs more rapidly in older people than in younger people, probably because of the reduced amount of muscle protein.

Although changes in protein metabolism follow the pattern of increasing loss of muscle during senescence, an accurate figure for protein demand is difficult to determine. For the healthy elderly person, 50 to 70 gm of protein in a diet containing between 1800 and 2400 kcal is considered adequate. No useful information is available about the protein constituents or whether some amino acids are more desirable than others.

Total intravascular and interstitial **albumin** decline in the elderly, with the former being reduced by 11% and the latter by 5%, and the total albumin pool, by about 20%. In a study of 48 subjects with low albumin levels (< 3.5 gm/dL), 19 had evidence of peripheral edema, but in only 3, the low albumin was considered to be related to hypoalbuminemia; factors such as heart failure were usually implicated. No consistent relationship has been shown between protein intake and serum albumin levels. Therefore, no satisfactory evidence exists that points to a clear advantage of a high-protein diet for individuals with low serum albumin levels, except in protein-energy malnutrition (see below).

Fat is useful because it produces more than twice the energy of either carbohydrate or protein. For most persons, 15 to 25 gm fat is adequate and allows for an adequate supply of fat-soluble vitamins. **Lipoproteins** are associated with the development of atherosclerosis (see Ch. 74), but their significance as a potential risk factor appears to diminish with increasing age.

Calcium absorption becomes less efficient in both men and women as they age; the reduction becomes significant during the 60s in women and the 70s in men. Dietary Ca is related to the inevitable loss of bone that accompanies aging from the 40s on (see Chs. 71 and 72).

Iron: Average Hb levels in large samples of community-dwelling elderly persons are lower than those found in younger persons, because this population has more cases of significant iron-deficiency anemia. In healthy individuals, normal Hb levels are maintained throughout life. Some studies suggest that reduced serum transferrin levels (eg, < 0.2 gm/dL) can be a diagnostic marker of malnutrition. However, from a practical point of view, the Hb level and the total iron-binding capacity are of more value. Nutrition alone does not govern the transferrin level.

Occult iron-deficiency anemia is unlikely if older persons consume a sensible, balanced diet, and routine iron prescribing is not justified. Anemia should be investigated in elderly as in younger patients. The possibility of occult loss of blood via the alimentary tract (eg, colonic neoplasm) is high.

Zinc: It has been suggested that zinc is particularly important in the elderly. The recommended daily allowance of zinc is 15 mg, although an average balanced diet in the USA is estimated to contain 10 to 15 mg. Many elderly persons living in institutions have low zinc intake. Intake of zinc is correlated with total caloric intake; thus, evidence of zinc deficiency may be an indicator of protein-calorie malnutrition. The tendency toward low zinc levels is increased in patients with cirrhosis or diabetes and those taking diuretics—all relatively common situations in old age. Checking zinc levels appears to offer little advantage, even in patients receiving diuretics, but normal serum levels are between 50 and 150 μg/dL.

Zinc plays a role in wound healing, appetite, and taste. Unfortunately, dysgeusia as a concomitant of zinc deficiency usually does not improve when zinc is given, and information on how and when to treat with zinc is lacking.

Although equivocal results are obtained when zinc is used for taste problems, a possible indication in the elderly is chronic skin ulcer. A trial of zinc supplementation, consisting of zinc sulfate 120 mg/day, might stimulate wound healing.

Magnesium: Muscular excitability, hyperreflexia, tetany, seizures, ataxia, tremors, weakness, and emotional lability are all relatively common in the geriatric population and may be manifestations of hypomagnesemia.

Magnesium is an essential element in the body; 70% of it is combined with phosphate and Ca in bone. The total amount in humans is between 20 and 25 gm. Normal nerve impulses and muscle contractions depend on an adequate level of magnesium. Whole blood contains 2 to 4 mg/dL, while serum levels have < 50% of that amount. Low serum magnesium levels are found in alcoholics and in patients with chronic malabsorption syndromes.

Foods rich in magnesium include whole grains, raw dried peas and beans, cocoa, various nuts, and some seafoods (100 to 400 mg/100 gm). Milk contains 12 mg/dL. The recommended daily intake is 350 mg. Magnesium aspartate tablets (500 mg) provide 40 mg elemental magnesium; 2 to 6 tablets may be given in cases of magnesium deficiency.

Vitamins: Vitamin requirements in the elderly remain largely undetermined. Much has been written on the subject, but variable conclusions have been drawn. Evidence exists that some elderly are deficient in $\geq$ 1 vitamin, chiefly B vitamins or vitamin C. Unequivocal cases of deficiency are, however, unusual. Methods for estimating B vitamins are technologically difficult and not in common laboratory use. Vague symptoms (eg, lack of well-being, loss of appetite, and general malaise) frequently are suggested as indications of nutritional deficiencies, but there is no proof that the problem is insufficient vitamin intake, and there can be many other causes of these common complaints. In general, a healthy skepticism about vague clinical symptoms is sensible, and megavitamin therapy should be avoided unless definitive clinical justification for it exists.

Since the 1950s, vitamin B_{12} deficiency has been reported to lead to dementia. Its frequency, however, is very low; 1 study found no association between below-normal levels of vitamin B_{12} and dementia. Furthermore, data on the reversibility of dementia with B_{12} treatment are unclear and controversial. Thus, keeping an open mind on the subject is prudent.

Nevertheless, institutional diets are often inadequate in the provision of vitamins, some of which may be destroyed by the cooking. For this reason, a higher index of clinical suspicion should be maintained in nursing home patients.

Fiber: The importance of dietary fiber has become increasingly evident over the past 10 to 20 yr. So-called convenience foods, used extensively by the elderly, are highly refined and notoriously lacking in fiber. Fiber is essential for a satisfactorily soft yet bulky stool. Constipation is common in the elderly and may be partly due to their intake of a more refined diet (see CONSTIPATION in Ch. 48).

Increased dietary fiber can alleviate the symptoms of diverticular disease and irritable bowel syndrome. Many people now consume bran as breakfast cereal or add it to soup or other foods to increase fiber intake. Although the results are difficult to assess, bran appears to have some beneficial effect. However, it may be more effective as a preventive measure and should begin to be used in younger persons.

There are many different types of fiber, some of which (eg, wheat bran) are useful for constipation, and others (eg, pectin) for reducing plasma cholesterol levels. However, indiscriminate use of fiber may cause deficiencies of trace minerals (eg, high-fiber cereals contain phytate, which binds these substances and makes them unavailable).

Risk Factors for Malnutrition

Disease factors: An association between ill health and malnutrition is important. While malnutrition may predispose one to some diseases, in most cases, ill health precedes the inadequate diet and consequent loss of good nutrition. **Almost any disease can cause poor food intake and weight loss.** Therefore, in the elderly, this presentation is not necessarily a clue to GI tract disorders but may signal subtle disease in *any* major organ system. Cancer, particularly if it is located in the upper alimentary tract, has a dramatic effect on nutrition and weight. Thyrotoxicosis occurs in about 1% of elderly persons and commonly presents atypically (eg, as a profound apathy, or apathetic thyrotoxicosis, akin to depression). Every elderly person who experiences chronic weight loss without an obvious cause should undergo thyroid function tests.

Aging factors: Activity level significantly reduces in the elderly, primarily because of less exercise, leading to a reduced intake of energy-producing foods containing primarily fats and carbohydrates. Evidence shows that the average caloric intake of older people is reduced from the 70s on, and most people $\geq$ 70 yr of age tend to lose weight.

Age-related physiologic changes that may lead to malnutrition can be divided into 2 groups: those that affect alimentary function and those that alter metabolism. Changes in alimentary function include problems of dentition, increased taste threshold (ie, reduced sense of taste and smell), decreased intestinal absorption, decreased GI secretion, and functional GI obstruction. Altered alimentary function associated with aging may be aggravated by specific disease states (eg, alterations in taste as a result of cancer, interference with absorption of certain nutrients as a result of motility and secretory disorders). Sensory input to the hypothalamus, which controls the hunger and satiety centers, also may become reduced. Alterations in metabolism include decreased protein synthesis, increased protein breakdown, impaired ability to enhance protein synthesis in response to increased amino acid intake, and decreased energy expenditure.

Neuropsychiatric factors: Bereavement may cause malnutrition by means of the reactive depression that frequently accompanies it. Individuals who lose a spouse or other close person should be closely monitored during the months following the loss. As a practical step, such individuals should be checked for anorexia and weight loss about 6 wk after the loss. **Depression** of any etiology may cause anorexia and undernutrition.

Two types of eating disorders may affect patients with **dementia:** loss of appetite with almost no food intake or voracious eating. It is not known whether these 2 extremes arise from loss of immediate memory or whether the organic brain syndrome interferes with the normal controlling influences of appetite.

Social factors: Because many older people live alone, they are commonly thought to be at risk for malnutrition, but evidence suggests that this is not the case unless additional factors (eg, poverty) enter the situation. Absence of socialization at mealtimes is likely to adversely affect nutrition, but the most significant causes of poor nutrition are poverty and associated chronic illness.

When active people living in a residential home or in their own home are compared with house-bound individuals, diet is poorest and evidence of malnutrition occurs in the latter group. The house-bound persons tend to have more disability and disease. Physicians should visit house-bound patients periodically and should be particularly aware of their nutritional state and try to prevent malnutrition.

Patients living in institutions are often fed unappetizing or cold food. At the least, food choices are limited and the cooking style is often different from what the patient is accustomed to.

The side effects of many drugs include nausea and dyspepsia, either of which could adversely affect nutrition. Therefore, inquiry into the drugs currently being taken should be one of the first investigative steps.

Diagnosis

The possibilities of weight loss and malnutrition should be considered in any elderly person who is not thriving. Relatives may ask whether an older person is sick, because they believe the person is not eating and is losing weight. Many older people are small and thin, but that does not mean they are undernourished. The reliability of a complaint should be checked before one embarks on other investigations; both subjective and objective criteria must be evaluated. Often, one can dispel the illusion that a person is losing weight by weighing the patient periodically over 2 to 3 wk. If the patient is hospitalized, a dietitian may check the amount of food actually consumed, as well as make daily observations of weight. The presence of peripheral edema, which can cause a misinterpretation of weight-loss or weight-gain patterns, must be noted.

Anthropometric measurements have been performed in the elderly to establish norms, but the ranges vary greatly for height, weight, triceps skinfold thickness, and upper-arm circumference. Such measurements can be taken only as a general guide and are not infallible in determining nutritional status.

The most important clue is progressive weight loss (eg, $\geq$ 10 lb in recent months). Clinical examination—in which the time of onset, number of pounds lost, rate of progression of weight loss, anorexia, decreased or altered food consumption, nausea, vomiting, diarrhea, and any indication of edema or chronic illness are noted—is the most effective means to estimate malnutrition. Risk factors (see above) also need to be assessed.

The physical examination should focus particularly on the presence of jaundice, cheilosis, glossitis, edema, obvious loss of subcutaneous fat, and muscle wasting. However, since weight loss and malnutrition are not diseases but result from a wide range of disorders, the physical examination must be complete.

Laboratory investigations should include determination of serum Hb, Ca, iron, transferrin, total iron-binding capacity, folate, B_{12}, and zinc levels, and evaluation of thyroid function. Skin tests to evaluate immune responses to common antigens should be performed, depending on the clinical circumstances, and the stool should be tested for occult blood.

If initial evaluation does not produce helpful information, the scope of investigation must be extended to search for evidence of a primary cancer, beginning with the lungs, breast, and alimentary system. This investigation should include consideration of the patient's physical and mental state and the level of capability that existed before the onset of the illness. Although these features are more important than age, a nonagenarian should not be submitted to extensive invasive testing simply to satisfy one's intellectual curiosity. Furthermore, patients with borderline nutritional status are at risk if food is withheld so that complex diagnostic evaluations can be performed.

This approach establishes a diagnosis and basis for rational therapy in up to 75% of patients, according to one study. In the remaining 25% there will not be a clear diagnosis, and one must speculate about the possibility of an occult tumor or a subtle imbalance of nutritional homeostasis, as described above. Explanation to the patient and family is necessary for reassurance, although the persistence of these symptoms carries a poor prognosis.

Any patient whose weight has fallen below the 15th percentile of an age-adjusted height and weight table should be considered to have **marasmus**. Such a patient has marked depletion of muscle mass and fat stores but normal visceral protein and organ function. Edema is absent; serum albumin and Hb levels, total iron-binding capacity, and tests of cell-mediated immune function are usually normal. The important point is that *the patient is depleted of nutritional reserves, and any additional metabolic stress (eg, surgery, infection, burn) may rapidly lead to* **hypoalbuminemic protein-energy malnutrition.** Characteristically, elderly patients deteriorate to this state more rapidly than do young patients; even relatively minor stress may be the cause. Usually, susceptible elderly patients are underweight at the outset, but even those who appear to have ample fat and muscle mass are susceptible if they have a history of recent rapid weight loss.

When protein-energy malnutrition is present, the serum albumin level is < 3.5 gm/dL and anemia, lymphocytopenia, and hypotransferrinemia (evidenced by a total iron-binding capacity < 250 μg/dL) are likely to be present. Anergy is often demonstrated, and edema is frequently present.

Treatment

In all cases of malnutrition, unexplained weight loss, and anorexia, the first concern must be to treat the underlying condition whenever possible. In a number of patients, however, even after extensive diagnostic evaluation, no specific cause is identified. What can one offer such patients?

First, one can use encouragement and gentle stimulation to persuade the individual to eat more. A dietitian should determine the patient's food preferences and create appropriate menus. Small, attractively served meals that tempt the appetite should be provided in a cheerful dining room with congenial company, if possible. If the person wishes, an aperitif, such as sherry, may be offered to stimulate the appetite. Flexibility in the timing of meals should be considered for anorectic patients.

Special nutritional supplements can be used to add specific components such as vitamins, minerals, and protein. For example, the Ensure® range of products, in vanilla, strawberry, or eggnog flavors, contain the required vitamins, Ca, iron, and some protein. These are most acceptable if not cold. Supplements may also be given by nasogastric tube.

Patients recovering from strokes may have difficulty swallowing as a result of partial paralysis of the muscles of deglutition or their uncoordinated action. Such cases pose difficult decisions to the physician. The following general principles apply. (See also Ch. 23.)

1. If possible, avoid long-term nasogastric tube feeding. Many patients dislike it, and it implies compulsion.

2. In most poststroke aphasic and dysphagic patients, an adequate swallowing reflex can be achieved by constant sucking stimulation with regular small servings of liquid feedings over 24 h. If a nasogastric tube must be used, withdrawal should be attempted early (ie, after 1 wk) to add the stimuli of hunger and thirst to the reacquisition of the swallowing reflex.

3. All feeding attempts must be made with the patient sitting as upright as possible, preferably in a chair. This helps prevent aspiration and encourages the swallowing reflex.

4. Discussion of this problem with the patient and the family at an early stage ensures a jointly agreed upon plan for the provision of adequate nutrition.

Patients with protein-energy malnutrition are always anorectic. Considering that they may need 2 to 4 times more calories and up to 4 times more proteins, dietary intervention alone is not sufficient, and more aggressive intervention may be required. The objective is to provide about 35 kcal/kg of ideal body weight (not actual weight). Enteral or parenteral hyperalimentation may be needed, but such decisions require clinical judgment; one plans differently for a patient who is obviously dying than for a patient who clearly requires long-term management or who needs only brief intervention. Furthermore, these interventions have risks as well as benefits.

Enteral hyperalimentation by nasogastric tube or by feeding gastrostomy or jejunostomy can have serious adverse effects. Fluid overload may cause edema or heart failure. Hyponatremia, hypocalcemia, hypophosphatemia, and hypomagnesemia may occur from electrolyte and fluid imbalances. Hyperglycemia and even diabetic coma may occur, and severe diarrhea is common. Patients requiring enteral hyperalimentation are often confused and may repeatedly pull out a nasogastric tube. This often leads to use of restraints, which adds to the distress of patient, family, and staff. In a long-term situation, such action may be an indication of the patient's refusal, and discontinuance of such feeding methods may be appropriate. Alternatively, changing to a feeding gastrostomy or jejunostomy or to parenteral nutrition may be necessary.

Parenteral feeding is most useful clinically in elderly patients undergoing acute metabolic stresses; eg, pre-and postoperative interventions (see Ch. 22). In other situations, however, parenteral nutrition can be useful and even lifesaving. It can be provided via a peripheral vein, although protein is difficult to infuse adequately by this route. A central line may be preferable, but either route risks thrombosis and sepsis.

Care should be taken to give all nutrients (protein, carbohydrate, fat, vitamins, electrolytes, and water) in adequate amounts and proper proportions. Restoring nutrition in this way may improve the patient's general condition to a point at which he accepts nasogastric or oral feedings. Thus, parenteral feeding is a potential adjuvant treatment in special situations in geriatric medicine.

3. GERIATRIC EMERGENCIES

Geno J. Merli and *Howard H. Weitz*

Rapid diagnosis and treatment of medical emergencies in older persons is often impaired because of altered responses to the stress of illness and coexisting medical and environmental problems. This chapter addresses the following common emergencies: chest pain, syncope, GI bleeding, infections, and impaired thermoregulation.

Other emergency situations that are important in the care of geriatric patients—eg, cardiac arrhythmias, changes in mental status, hyperosmotic-hyperosmolar nonketotic coma, perforation of peptic ulcer, and socially determined crises—are discussed elsewhere in the book.

Chest Pain

Acute chest pain has a variety of causes and the etiology often is quite difficult to identify. Chronic medical illnesses, dementia, delirium, and atypical presentation of illness may contribute to the difficulty. Because treatment is similar to that in younger patients, this discussion focuses on diagnosis.

Coronary artery disease is the most common cause of death in the elderly, but associated angina pectoris is often absent. Less than 50% of older patients have chest pain accompanying an acute **MI,** compared with 80% of younger patients. Dyspnea, confusion, paresthesias, or syncope may be the initial manifestations of MI, and physical findings are nonspecific. ECG findings are similar to those in the younger population. (See also Ch. 32.)

Thoracic aortic dissection is generally characterized by sudden, severe, tearing chest pain and should be suspected in the patient with a history of hypertension. Supporting this diagnosis are a murmur of aortic regurgitation (proximal aortic dissection), pulse deficits of the upper extremities (brachiocephalic vessel involvement), chest x-ray evidence of mediastinal widening, and an ECG without evidence of acute MI. The definitive diagnostic study is an aortic angiogram. (See also AORTIC DISSECTION in Ch. 36.)

Pulmonary embolism is signaled by chest pain that is typically pleuritic and usually associated with acute dyspnea. This diagnosis should be suspected in the patient who has been immobilized, has recently undergone surgery, or who has a malignancy. Tachycardia is common but may be absent if the patient is taking a β-blocking drug or has cardiac conduction system disease (eg, sick sinus syndrome). A pleural friction rub is characteristic but often difficult to detect. Suggestive laboratory findings are hypoxemia with hypocapnia and an ECG indicating right ventricular strain. The chest x-ray is nonspecific and may demonstrate diaphragmatic elevation; basal, platelike atelectasis; pleural effusion; pulmonary infiltrate; or, in massive embolism, decreased vascularity of the affected lung. The diagnosis is supported by a high-probability radionuclide lung scan, but the definitive diagnostic study is a characteristic pulmonary angiogram. (See also Ch. 41.)

Pneumothorax, *spontaneous rupture of the pleura with entry of air from the lung to the pleural space,* may cause acute chest pain with dyspnea. Emphysema is the most common pulmonary cause, but pulmonary fibrosis, chronic bronchitis, and asthma can also lead to pneumothorax. The diagnosis is supported by decreased breath sounds over the affected lung and is confirmed by evidence of lung collapse on an expiration chest x-ray.

Pneumonia may be associated with sharp, pleuritic chest pain and may present in an atypical fashion. (See Ch. 39 and under Infection, below.)

Pericarditis is a less common cause of chest pain. Idiopathic and viral pericarditis, usually following a URI, are the most common causes, but TB, collagen vascular disease, metastatic tumor, and acute MI must also be sought. Pain is stabbing in nature, increases with inspiration, and decreases while the patient is sitting up and leaning forward. The most supportive diagnostic study is the ECG, which typically reveals diffuse, concave upward ST-segment elevations in all leads (except aVR and V_1); these changes persist for several days.

Acute cholecystitis, peptic ulcer disease, and esophagitis are common, and the initial presentation may be nonspecific, including referred chest pain. Often, the medical history suggests the diagnosis, and a relation between meals and pain provocation can be identified. The physical examination may be nonspecific or may reveal evidence of right upper quadrant tenderness (cholecystitis) or epigastric tenderness (peptic ulcer disease, esophagitis). Laboratory and x-ray studies include testing stool for occult blood (peptic ulcer disease), upper GI series (peptic ulcer disease, esophagitis), oral cholecystogram (cholecystitis), abdominal ultrasonography (cholecystitis), and occasionally endoscopy.

Herpes zoster is common and is readily diagnosed by the characteristic vesicular eruption on an erythematous base along a cutaneous dermatome. Occasionally, pain along the dermatomal distribution *precedes* the skin rash by 3 to 4 days. This may cause chest pain, sometimes accompanied by chills, fever, and malaise.

Musculoskeletal disease also causes chest pain. While usually chronic, it may be acute and difficult to differentiate from more serious visceral causes. Diagnostic clues include reproducibility of pain by localized chest wall palpation, generalized chest wall tenderness, and relief of pain following injection of local anesthetics.

Syncope (see also Chs. 6 and 31)

A *transient loss of consciousness, characterized by unresponsiveness, loss of postural tone, and spontaneous recovery not requiring specific resuscitative procedures.* The most common cause is acutely decreased cerebral blood flow, which may be precipitated by cardiac arrhythmias, orthostatic hypotension, hypovolemia, vasodilation, cerebrovascular disease, cardiac outflow obstruction, or decreased cardiac output from left ventricular dysfunction.

The history of the episode, including precipitating events, symptoms, concomitant medical problems, and drugs (see TABLES 3-1 and 3-2), is crucial to presumptive diagnosis. Information from family members or witnesses can also be helpful.

Syncope preceded by sudden weakness, nausea, sweating, and warmth (especially in circumstances involving pain, fear, or prolonged standing, or associated with micturition, defecation, coughing, or swallowing) is usually due to enhanced vasovagal tone, resulting in bradycardia and/or peripheral vasodilation. This form of syncope does not occur in the supine position, and recovery is rapid. However, weakness, nausea, and sweating could represent myocardial ischemia, which can cause syncope in any position and is often associated with chest pain. Loss of con-

TABLE 3-1. CLINICAL MANIFESTATIONS IN SYNCOPE

Symptoms	Most Common Etiology
Nausea, sweating, anxiety, fever, warmth	Vasovagal or cardiac
Loss of consciousness without warning	Cardiac arrhythmia
Prolonged confusion, fatigue, postsyncope syndrome	Seizure

Signs	Most Common Etiology
Neck turning	Hypersensitive carotid sinus
Exertional	Aortic stenosis, hypertrophic cardiomyopathy, pulmonary hypertension
Change to standing position	Orthostatic hypotension

TABLE 3-2. DRUGS CAUSING SYNCOPE

Diuretics	Antiarrhythmics
Antihypertensives	Psychotropics
Nitrates	β-blockers
Ca channel blockers	Digitalis

sciousness without warning suggests a cardiac arrhythmia or a seizure disorder frequently associated with a prolonged recovery time or a post ictal state.

Information about the circumstances surrounding the syncopal episode should be elicited. Careful questioning about the position of the neck before the episode, ie, hyperextension, may provide a clue to carotid sinus hypersensitivity. Exertional syncope suggests a specific group of causes: aortic stenosis, hypertrophic cardiomyopathy, pulmonary hypertension, and exercise-induced arrhythmias. Syncope that develops within a few seconds after standing indicates orthostatic hypotension, which may be associated with autonomic dysfunction or certain drugs (eg, vasodilators, diuretics).

The additive effect of coexisting diseases (eg, heart failure, chronic renal failure, angina pectoris, anemia, chronic obstructive lung disease, venous and arterial insufficiency in the legs, and diabetes mellitus) and multiple drug regimens, may result in a critical threshold for CNS dysfunction. Antihypertensive, antianginal, or arrhythmogenic drugs frequently cause hypotension with syncope due to volume depletion, inadequate cardiac output, or peripheral vasodilation.

The physical examination begins with measurement of BP and pulse in the supine and standing positions, since orthostatic hypotension is more common in the elderly, although preexisting hypertension may be the primary cause. Symptoms appearing in association with the postural BP drop are required to implicate orthostatic hypotension as a cause of syncope. The carotid arteries should be examined for evidence of obstruction (ie, bruits or delayed upstroke) and to assess the presence of aortic stenosis (transmitted murmur and delayed upstroke). The latter is particularly difficult to detect because decreased vascular elasticity may mask typical physical findings (ie, delayed carotid upstroke and pulsus parvus et tardus). An ECG should be performed to rule out acute MI and continuous cardiac monitoring should be initiated if heart disease with arrhythmia is found or suspected. IV access should be maintained and supplemental O_2 at 2 to 4 L/min begun by nasal cannula. The following additional laboratory tests should be performed in all patients: measurement of glucose, electrolytes, BUN, and creatinine levels, and a CBC. Of assignable diagnoses, 60 to 85% are made on the basis of history, physical examination, and 12-lead ECG.

The need for hospital admission can best be determined by reviewing the mortality rates of specific risk groups (see TABLE 3–3). At lowest risk are patients < 60 yr of age with syncope of noncardiac or undetermined cause; these patients have a 2-yr mortality of 2 to 5%. Intermediate-risk patients are > 60 yr of age with a noncardiac or an unknown cause of syncope; they have a 2-yr mortality of 20%. Patients in the highest risk group are those of all ages whose syncope has a cardiac origin; their 2-yr mortality is 32 to 38%. However, *the underlying diseases causing syncope determine mortality, not the syncope* per se. High-risk patients should be admitted for evaluation and treatment. Lower-risk patients may or may not require hospitalization, depending on the presumed cause of syncope.

TABLE 3–3. TWO-YR MORTALITY RISK IN PATIENTS WITH SYNCOPE

Group	Age (yr)	Cause			Mortality (%)
		Cardiac	Noncardiac	Unknown	
High risk	All ages	+			32–38
Moderate risk	> 60		+	+	20
Low risk	< 60		+	+	2–5

GI Bleeding (see also GASTROINTESTINAL BLEEDING in Chs. 47, 48, and 53)

In the USA, GI bleeding in the elderly is associated with a mortality rate that approaches 10%. Clinical manifestations are diverse, ranging from change in mental status to syncope with hemodynamic collapse. Rapid assessment of blood loss, cardiac status, and cause of hemorrhage is essential.

GI hemorrhage may be categorized into 3 classes (see TABLE 3–4): **severe** (active hematemesis or hematochezia with shock); **moderate** (active hematemesis or hematochezia with orthostatic BP change); and **occult** (stool positive for occult blood, decreased Hb and Hct, fatigue, weakness, and BP stable). Patients with severe or moderate hemorrhage require emergency evaluation and stabilization. Those with occult GI blood loss may be evaluated as outpatients if they are hemodynamically stable.

TABLE 3–4. CATEGORIZATION OF GASTROINTESTINAL BLEEDING

Severe	Active hematemesis, hematochezia, shock
Moderate	Active hematemesis, hematochezia, orthostatic BP change
Occult	Stool positive for occult blood, decreased Hb and Hct, fatigue, weakness

Treatment is directed at intravascular volume repletion, hemodynamic stabilization, and localization of the bleeding site (see TABLE 3–5). A large-bore (16- to 18-gauge) IV catheter is inserted and fluids or blood administered. Blood loss can be estimated by serial determination of pulse and degree of shock. However, pulse rate may not be a sensitive indicator of hypovolemia because of the baroreflex blunting commonly seen. Hb and Hct levels may not reflect the degree of blood loss because of insufficient intravascular equilibration. The percentage of blood volume loss can be estimated as follows (see TABLE 3–6): 10 to 20% (BP > 90 mm Hg; pulse, 110/min, mild shock); 20 to 30% (BP > 70 to 80 mm Hg; pulse, 110 to 130/min, moderate shock); > 30% (BP < 70 mm Hg; pulse, > 130/min, severe shock).

TABLE 3–5. MANAGEMENT OF GASTROINTESTINAL BLEEDING

Categorize patient

Insert large-bore IV (16 to 18 gauge) catheter, administer NSS or Ringer's injection, lactated

Type and crossmatch 4 units packed red cells

Obtain determinations: CBC, PT, PTT, PLT, electrolytes, glucose, creatinine

Insert nasogastric tube (No. 16 F. or Ewald)

Obtain surgical consultation

NSS = normal saline solution; CBC = complete blood count; PT = prothrombin time; PTT = partial thromboplastin time; PLT = platelets.

TABLE 3–6. ESTIMATION OF BLOOD VOLUME LOSS

Blood Vol Loss (%)	BP (mm Hg)	Pulse	Shock Status
10–20	> 90	110/min	Mild
20–30	> 70–80	110–130/min	Moderate
> 30	< 70	> 130/min	Severe

If bleeding is severe or there is evidence of cardiac dysfunction, a pulmonary artery catheter may need to be inserted to monitor fluid management. The following laboratory studies should be performed: CBC (including platelet count); partial thromboplastin time; blood type and cross-match; and measurement of electrolyte, glucose, and creatinine levels. A nasogastric tube (No. 16 F. or Ewald) is placed to assess for upper GI bleeding; major causes are listed in TABLE 3–7.

TABLE 3–7. MAJOR CAUSES OF UPPER GASTROINTESTINAL TRACT
BLEEDING

Cause	%
Gastric ulcer	29
Duodenal ulcer	21
Gastritis	17
Esophagitis	14
Esophageal varices	12

If the nasogastric aspirate is bloody or has a coffee-ground appearance, the stomach is lavaged with 1 to 2 L iced saline until the aspirate clears. If the aspirate is negative, the nasogastric tube is removed.

If bright red blood from the rectum is noted, bleeding from the lower GI tract is likely and surgical consultation is obtained for possible immediate intervention. Diverticulitis and angiodysplasia are the most frequent causes of lower GI bleeding in the elderly. Causes of lower GI bleeding are listed in TABLE 3–8. (See also Ch. 48.)

TABLE 3–8. MAJOR CAUSES OF LOWER GASTROINTESTINAL TRACT
BLEEDING

Cause	%
Diverticulitis	43
Vascular ectasia of right colon	20
Undetermined	11
Radiation proctitis	6
Colorectal carcinoma	5
Colonic polyps	4
Other	11

After hemodynamic stabilization is achieved, immediate evaluation is begun to determine the cause of bleeding. Additional history of drug use or abdominal vascular surgery, previous bleeding problems, or concomitant illness is obtained.

Infection

Infection is a common problem necessitating emergency evaluation. Most infections occur in the urinary tract or the lungs, but diagnosis is often difficult because of atypical presentations.

UTIs are very common, with an incidence of substantial bacteriuria as high as 15% in the elderly, and bacteremia may occur in up to $\frac{1}{3}$ of these cases. (See also Ch. 56.) Several factors contribute to this high infection rate: (1) bladder outlet obstruction from prostatic hypertrophy, (2) upper urinary tract stones, (3) atrophic vaginitis, (4) immobilization,

(5) neuropathy resulting in poor bladder emptying, (6) instrumentation of the urinary tract and use of indwelling bladder catheters, (7) diabetes mellitus, (8) stroke, and (9) dementia with poor perianal hygiene. In younger patients, the usual manifestations of UTI are frequency, dysuria, suprapubic discomfort, fever, and flank pain, while in the elderly, incontinence, confusion, vague abdominal pain, anorexia, nausea, vomiting, azotemia, and uncontrolled diabetes may also occur. On occasion, the initial manifestations of urosepsis may be septic shock which, in the elderly, is associated with a mortality rate of 50 to 70%.

When the patient arrives in the emergency department, a history is obtained and a physical examination is performed. The presence of fever, chills, abdominal discomfort, or signs of cardiopulmonary compromise strongly suggests sepsis. A large-bore IV catheter is placed for administration of 5% dextrose and normal saline. If the urinary bladder is distended, an indwelling catheter is inserted and drained slowly to prevent bladder wall hemorrhage. A CBC, measurement of serum creatinine, and blood cultures are obtained. Urinalysis, urine culture and sensitivity, and Gram stain of sediment should be performed. Five organisms per high-power microscopic field corresponds with 95% confidence to bacteriuria at 10^5 organisms. Pyuria *without* bacteriuria should prompt consideration of renal calculi, papillary necrosis due to obstruction, diabetes mellitus, analgesic nephropathy, chronic prostatitis, or tuberculosis.

Therapy may be initiated in the emergency department on the basis of the Gram stain findings. If gram-negative organisms are noted, an aminoglycoside (gentamicin or tobramycin) or one of the third-generation cephalosporins (cefotaxime, cefoperazone, moxalactam) may be administered. Gram-positive cocci in chains may represent enterococcus, and the use of a penicillin (ampicillin) or vancomycin (for the penicillin-allergic patient) is necessary. A patient with gram-positive cocci in clumps suggesting *Staphylococcus* should be treated with a first-generation cephalosporin (cefazolin). The patient is admitted for a 10-day course of therapy and further evaluation of underlying problems.

Community-acquired pneumonia is a frequent cause of infection in the elderly, with an annual incidence of 20 to 44/1000. It is the principal cause of infectious-disease death in the elderly and overall the fourth leading cause of death in patients > 65 yr of age in the USA. (See also Ch. 39.)

Multiple factors predispose older persons to pneumonia. Aging leads to impairment of the respiratory system's bacterial defenses (ie, decreased vital capacity, chest wall compliance, and rib cage mobility; diminished cough effectiveness; and impaired mucociliary clearance). Gram-negative bacterial colonization of the oropharynx, underlying chronic medical conditions, and malnutrition also contribute. Patients requiring more skilled care have a higher percentage of oropharyngeal colonization with gram-negative organisms, resulting in an increased frequency of pneumonia caused by these bacteria. Chronic medical conditions (eg, chronic obstructive pulmonary disease, heart failure, stroke, and alcoholism) also result in decreased mobility, impaired host defenses, and poor nutrition.

Commonly used drugs may also contribute to the development of pneumonia. They include nonsteroidal anti-inflammatory drugs (NSAIDs), which may reduce pulmonary parenchymal recruitment of granulocytes and macrophages, and H_2-receptor antagonists, which decrease gastric acidity, resulting in gastric proliferation of gram-negative organisms; if aspirated, these bacteria cause gram-negative pneumonia.

Streptococcus pneumoniae is the most common cause of community-acquired pneumonia, occurring in 50% of cases. *Hemophilus influenzae* is seen more frequently in patients with chronic lung disease or lung cancer. Other causative organisms include *Legionella pneumophila, Staphylococcus aureus,* gram-negative bacilli, and anaerobic bacteria. Patients in long-term care facilities frequently have gram-negative pneumonia caused by *Klebsiella pneumoniae, Pseudomonas, E. coli, Proteus, Serratia, S. aureus,* and *L. pneumophila.*

Symptoms, Signs, and Diagnosis: The older patient with pneumonia may present with lethargy, mental confusion, anorexia, and deterioration of a preexisting medical condition. Usual features (eg, fever, chills, and productive cough) also may occur. After the history and physical examination are completed, the following laboratory and diagnostic findings should be obtained: CBC, serum electrolyte and creatinine levels, blood cultures, arterial blood gas levels, chest x-ray, and ECG. If an adequate sputum specimen (< 10 epithelial cells and > 25 polymorphonuclear leukocytes/low-power field) can be obtained, a Gram stain is useful to guide initial antibiotic therapy.

Treatment: If the patient appears to have cardiopulmonary compromise, IV fluids and nasal cannula O_2 should be administered. Antibiotic therapy may be initiated in the emergency department, depending on the clinical situation. If a sputum sample Gram stain exhibits gram-positive cocci in pairs or chains, *S. pneumoniae* is the most likely cause, and penicillin or erythromycin may be used. Gram-negative infections can be treated with an aminoglycoside or second-generation cephalosporin. If no sputum is available, broad antibiotic coverage should be provided (eg, ampicillin, a second- or third-generation cephalosporin, or erythromycin). If the patient is in a long-term care facility, an aminoglycoside plus a cephalosporin is required.

Because of the associated mortality, the elderly patient with pneumonia and concomitant illness must be hospitalized for monitoring of vital signs, hydration, and IV antibiotic therapy. (More details on pneumonia and its treatment are given in Chs. 39, 75, 76, and 77.)

Heat Stroke

Nonexertional **heat stroke** is *a disorder of thermoregulation usually occurring during summer heat waves and typically affecting elderly persons who are debilitated or taking drugs that alter fluid balance or tempera-*

ture regulation (see TABLE 3–9). Mortality reaches 80% in persons > 65 yr of age. The classic triad is *hyperpyrexia, severe CNS dysfunction,* and *anhidrosis.*

TABLE 3–9. AGENTS THAT IMPAIR RESPONSE TO HEAT

Types of Drugs
Hypohidrosis
Anticholinergics
Phenothiazines
Tricyclics
Antihistamines
Monoamine oxidase (MAO) inhibitors
Antiparkinsonian drugs
Butyrophenones
Thioxanthenes
Hypovolemia
Diuretics

The patient may have a decreased perception of temperature or may be limited in ability to remove clothing or to move to a cooler environment, thus impairing radiation and conduction of heat, which accounts for 78% of heat loss. Evaporation of sweat accounts for 22% of heat loss, but in the elderly, the sweat threshold increases and volume decreases. Concomitant cardiac, pulmonary, or metabolic diseases are adversely affected by the above changes.

The diagnosis is established when the clinical features of hyperpyrexia (temperature of 37.8 to 41.1 C [100 to 106 F]), impaired sensorium (altered mental status, seizures, focal neurologic deficits), and anhidrosis are present. Also common are hyperventilation, vomiting, diarrhea, fatigue, weakness, and headaches.

Treatment is initially directed at immediate reduction of elevated core temperature and support of vital organ systems. Vital signs are serially obtained to assess the degree of cardiovascular impairment secondary to thermal stress. A large-bore IV catheter (16 to 18 gauge) is placed for the delivery of normal saline or Ringer's injection, lactated, to maintain hemodynamic stability. A pulmonary artery catheter may be of value in the patient who requires careful monitoring of cardiac parameters during fluid administration. O_2 at 4 to 6 L/min is provided via nasal cannula or mask.

The following changes may occur in laboratory values and diagnostic tests that should be obtained to assess the degree of thermal injury: CBC (increased WBC, decreased Hb and Hct); partial thromboplastin time **(PTT)** and prothrombin time **(PT)** (increased in disseminated intravascular coagulation **[DIC]**); platelets (decreased in DIC); electrolyte levels (elevated K); creatinine clearance (increased); urinalysis (myoglobinuria); arterial blood gas **(ABG)** levels (decreased P_{O_2}, P_{CO_2}, and pH); ECG (tachycardia); and chest x-ray (adult respiratory distress syndrome [**ARDS**], aspiration).

While the above assessments and interventions are being completed, an ice-water tub is prepared and the patient immersed, to reduce core body temperature. If such a tub is not available, the patient can be wrapped in a sheet that is continuously wet with ice water. The temperature should be reduced to 38.8 C (102 F) to avoid overcooling and hypothermia. During cooling, seizures and aspiration may occur, so the airway must be closely monitored. Seizures should be treated with diazepam or phenytoin and the patient admitted to the intensive care unit for cardiovascular monitoring. (See also HYPERTHERMIA in Ch. 5.)

Hypothermia (see also Ch. 5)

Hypothermia is an often fatal environmental emergency. Exposure to cold, together with elderly persons' decreased ability to cope with the effects of changes in ambient temperature because of decreased metabolism and body fat, less efficient peripheral vasoconstriction, often poor nutrition, and concomitant medical disorders, presents a problem of significant dimension. The number of deaths from hypothermia is uncertain; one estimate indicates 17 per million. It is also estimated that persons > 75 yr of age are 5 times more likely to die from hypothermia than are those < 75 yr. Other factors contributing to the development of hypothermia are drugs, alcohol, metabolic disorders, stroke, and sepsis.

The physician should be aware of the following: (1) The ability to perceive cold diminishes with age. Thus, the ability to detect environmental temperature differences varies between 2.5 and 10 C (4.5 and 18 F) in the elderly as compared with a discrimination threshold of 0.8 C (1.4 F) in the young. (2) Body water acts as a thermal buffer and heat reservoir, but in the elderly, total body water is decreased (< 60%), reducing this protective mechanism. (3) Shivering occurs in only 10% of the elderly and, coupled with decreased resting metabolic rate, results in an inability to maintain normal core temperature. These 3 changes, together with concomitant problems (eg, heart failure, diabetes mellitus, hypothyroidism, parkinsonism, stroke, and various drugs) result in a mortality rate of approximately 50% in the elderly with hypothermia.

The diagnosis of hypothermia requires a high index of suspicion in conjunction with compatible history and physical and laboratory examinations. The history obtained from family and friends regarding home environment, drugs taken, and concomitant medical problems provides facts that may help explain a decreased core temperature. Because standard clinical thermometers do not record temperatures < 34.4 C (94 F), a special thermocouple should be used. Skin color is usually pale but may be pink. As the temperature decreases to < 34 C (93.2 F), ataxia, confusion, and disorientation increase significantly. Temperature < 31 C (88 F) results in stupor and coma.

Further decrements in temperature precipitate cardiovascular changes, such as hypotension; J (Osborn) waves on the ECG; bradycardia; atrial fibrillation; atrial flutter; ventricular ectopy; ventricular tachycardia; and ventricular fibrillation (the most frequent cause of death). Cardiac arrest occurs at 22 to 25 C (72 to 78 F). The pulmonary manifestations are slow, shallow breathing and a decreased cough reflex, frequently resulting in atelectasis and pneumonia.

Changes in laboratory and diagnostic tests include electrolytes (decreased CO_2), creatinine and glucose (increased), CBC (increased Hb, Hct, and WBC), platelets (decreased in DIC), PT and PTT (increased in DIC), ECG (J waves), and ABG (increased P_{O_2} and P_{CO_2} and decreased pH). A toxicology screen should also be obtained. A large-bore IV catheter is placed for the administration of 5% dextrose and normal saline solution. If the patient is comatose, naloxone 0.4 mg IV, thiamine 100 mg IV, and 1 ampule of 50% dextrose are administered.

Therapy for hypothermia is discussed in detail in Ch. 5.

4.   DISORDERS OF WATER AND SODIUM BALANCE

Myron Miller

Many diseases that appear with increasing frequency in advancing age present with disorders of fluid and electrolyte balance. Both fluid overload and plasma volume depletion, which are common in the hospitalized elderly, are often accompanied by alterations in serum Na concentration, especially hyponatremia. This chapter will deal with (1) the physiologic and pathophysiologic changes that predispose the elderly to disturbances of fluid balance and serum Na concentration, (2) the clinical consequences of such alterations, and (3) approaches to management.

PHYSIOLOGIC REGULATION OF WATER AND SODIUM

The ability to regulate the volume and tonicity of extracellular body water within narrow limits is important in the health maintenance of older persons. Aging is associated with impaired conservation of water and maintenance of Na balance, the 2 primary factors determining ECF volume and tonicity. Among the homeostatic mechanisms responsible are (1) **thirst perception;** (2) secretion of **ADH (vasopressin),** the major hormonal regulator of water balance; (3) secretion of **aldosterone and atrial natriuretic hormone,** hormonal regulators of Na excretion; (4) **renal hemodynamics** (BP, renal blood flow, and GFR); (5) **renal sympathetic nerve activity;** and (6) **renal response system** (proximal and distal tubules). Normally, these intake, hormonal, and effector systems operate so that wide variations in fluid or Na intake are modulated to maintain constancy of extracellular volume and tonicity. When the function of any component is impaired, water or Na balance can be seriously deranged, with clinical consequences.

In young, healthy adults, total body water **(TBW)** is approximately 60% of body weight, and the ECF and plasma volumes are approximately 20 and 5%, respectively. With aging, however, TBW decreases to approximately 45% of body weight, because of a proportionate increase in fat and a reduction in lean body mass.

The secretion of ADH by the neurohypophyseal system is the principal hormonal regulator of body water. Variations in secretion occur in response to several stimuli: changes in blood tonicity, blood volume, BP, and such factors as nausea, pain, emotional stress, and a variety of drugs. Osmoreceptors in the hypothalamus respond to minor changes in blood tonicity, resulting primarily from changes in serum Na. Increasing tonicity stimulates ADH release, while decreasing tonicity inhibits release, with accompanying antidiuresis or diuresis, respectively. This helps maintain plasma osmolality in the narrow range between 292 mOsm/kg (when maximal urine concentration occurs) and 282 mOsm/kg (when full diuresis is achieved).

Through volume receptors in the left atrium, a decrease in blood volume stimulates hormone release; an expansion of blood volume inhibits it. Similarly, ADH secretion responds to changes in BP through baroreceptors in the aorta and carotid arteries. A fall in BP provokes release of ADH; a rise inhibits its release.

Na and its accompanying anions are the major solutes of ECF, accounting for > 90% of osmolality. Serum osmolality can be estimated with the following formula:

$$\text{Osmolality} = 2[\text{Na}] + \frac{\text{BUN}}{2.8} + \frac{\text{glucose}}{18}$$

Body Na content is determined by the balance between dietary intake and renal excretion, since extrarenal losses in sweat and stool are, normally, minimal. Within 2 to 4 days of complete cessation of Na intake, urinary excretion normally decreases to < 5 mEq/L, while an increase in Na intake is promptly followed by a matching increase in excretion.

Under extreme circumstances, an alteration in Na intake can be reflected in a change in serum Na concentration as either hypo- or hypernatremia. *However, the serum Na concentration is primarily determined by the state of body water balance, so that hyponatremia usually results from excessive water retention, while hypernatremia results from water loss.* The magnitude of Na intake can influence the ECF volume; excessive Na leads to an expansion of ECF volume, and decreased Na results in contraction of ECF volume. Serum Na concentration alone, therefore, rarely provides information on the clinical state of Na balance.

ALTERATIONS OF WATER AND SODIUM REGULATION DURING AGING

Normal aging is accompanied by the following changes that can affect water and Na regulation: (1) impaired renal concentrating capacity; (2) increased ADH secretion; (3) impaired renal Na-conserving capacity; and (4) impaired thirst perception.

Studies in healthy men ranging from 40 to 101 yr of age demonstrate **impaired renal concentrating capacity** with increasing age. There is a decline in the maximal urine specific gravity attainable after 24 h of water deprivation. This decrease is slight in individuals 60 to 65 yr of age, greater in those > 65 yr, and even greater in those > 75 yr. Subsequent studies in healthy men 26 to 86 yr of age demonstrated a progressive age-related decline in the renal concentration response to vasopressin administered IV. More recent studies confirmed the progressive decline in maximal urine osmolality response to water deprivation with increasing age in healthy men. Thus, even in the absence of clinically identifiable renal disease, age predisposes an individual to fluid loss when fluid intake is limited, increasing the risk of dehydration. The basis for this effect appears to be resistance to the renal action of ADH, ie, a form of **acquired nephrogenic diabetes insipidus.**

The capacity of the neurohypophyseal system to secrete ADH increases with age. In response to the osmotic stimulus of IV hypertonic saline infusion, older persons (54 to 92 yr of age) show a greater increase in plasma ADH at any level of serum osmolality than do younger persons (21 to 49 yr of age). Similarly, IV ethanol is less effective in inhibiting the release of ADH in older than in younger individuals. These observations suggest that increased osmoreceptor sensitivity is a result of normal aging. There is some evidence that this heightened sensitivity may be due to impaired baroreceptor function, with a decline in the inhibitory activity on ADH release that is normally mediated by this neural pathway. Several studies have shown that the basal concentration of ADH in blood increases as a result of aging, becoming most evident in individuals > 60 yr of age. The increased concentrations of ADH, as well as an enhanced release in response to osmotic and perhaps other stimuli, increases the risk of developing hyponatremia when fluid intake is increased, leading to the **syndrome of inappropriate ADH secretion (SIADH).**

The ability of the kidney to conserve Na appears compromised in healthy aging men. In a study of 89 healthy subjects 18 to 76 yr old, restriction of dietary Na intake demonstrated that the capacity to decrease renal Na excretion is impaired with age. Subjects < 30 yr of age were able to decrease urinary Na excretion by 50% in a mean of 17.6 h, while those > 60 yr required a mean of 30.9 h. Although the basis for this decline in Na-conserving capacity is not fully understood, it may partly result from an age-related reduction in circulating renin and aldosterone, as well as decreased responsiveness to acute stimuli. An additional fac-

or is nephron loss with resultant increase in osmotic load per nephron and osmotic diuresis.

Preliminary studies indicate that atrial natriuretic factor **(ANF)** levels in blood are increased in the elderly, and these elevated levels may also play a role in the impaired Na-conserving ability of the aged kidney. These changes may result in continued renal loss of Na when intake is reduced because of illness or dietary modification, leading to Na depletion, decreased plasma volume, and hyponatremia.

A decline in thirst perception is less well recognized. Healthy older individuals deprived of fluid intake for 24 h have been found to have less subjective awareness of thirst than younger persons. Subsequently, when water was presented, the older persons ingested a strikingly lower amount, despite the demonstration that water deprivation increased plasma osmolality to a significantly higher level in this group. This loss of thirst perception again places the older individual at increased risk for volume depletion and dehydration.

VOLUME DEPLETION/DEHYDRATION

A loss of body water and sodium resulting in a decrease in ECF volume. **Dehydration** is *a relatively pure depletion of water alone.*

Symptoms and Signs

Volume depletion and dehydration may present in a variety of ways, but altered mental status, lethargy, light-headedness, and syncope are particularly common in elderly patients. On physical examination, evidence of decreased skin turgor, dry mucous membranes, tachycardia, and orthostatic hypotension provide further support for the clinical diagnosis, but these findings may be present in elderly individuals whose volume status is normal. Laboratory evidence of increased Hct, BUN, and serum creatinine also points to significant volume depletion. The serum Na concentration may be increased, normal, or low, depending on the mechanism underlying the volume depletion. Urinary Na excretion is usually < 20 mEq/L when Na intake has been chronically reduced or losses have occurred through vomiting or diarrhea.

Diagnosis

A history of decreased food or fluid intake, febrile illness, diabetes mellitus, vomiting, diarrhea, chronic renal disease, use of diuretic agents, or nasogastric suction should alert the physician to the possibility of volume depletion or dehydration. Adrenal insufficiency must always be considered, especially if there is evidence of a malignancy with predilection for metastasis to the adrenal gland. A urinary Na concentration > 20 mEq/L is consistent with this disorder, as well as with chronic renal disease with associated impaired Na-conserving capacity. Hypercalcemia, hypokalemia, and hyperglycemia, with consequent glycosuria leading to an osmotic diuresis, must be excluded as causes of impaired renal water-conserving ability.

Treatment

When volume depletion results almost entirely from water loss alone the fluid deficit can be estimated by the following calculation:

$$\text{Total body fluid volume (L)} = \frac{140\ \text{mEq/L} \times \text{basal body wt (kg)} \times 0.45}{\text{current serum Na (mEq/L)}}$$

where 0.45 represents the approximate proportion of body weight a water. This figure is then subtracted from the patient's estimated norma TBW (0.45 × basal body weight) to give the value for approximate wa ter deficit. This calculation is *not* valid if there has been a large loss of Na as well as water, with resultant hyponatremia.

When the volume deficit is modest (1 to 2 L), it can be corrected b oral intake of fluid, provided there is no accompanying GI disorder o impairment of mental status. If oral fluid cannot be given, or if the vol ume deficit is more significant, IV fluid therapy is required, preferabl with isotonic (0.9%) saline, provided the patient is not hypernatremi from dehydration. In the presence of hypernatremia, hypotonic flui (0.45% saline) should be used. The rate of administration should b such that once orthostatic hypotension and tachycardia have resolve the remaining deficit will be corrected over 2 to 3 days to avoid precip tating heart failure (HF). Useful clinical guidelines for determining effec tiveness of therapy are increases in skin turgor and decreases in hea rate, orthostatic BP, urine output, BUN, and creatinine. The presence o other deficits, including hypokalemia, hypomagnesemia, hypophos phatemia, and metabolic acidosis, should be considered.

HYPONATREMIA

The decrease in serum Na concentration to < 136 mEq/L that occur when there is an excess of water relative to total Na. Total ECF volum may be increased, normal, or decreased.

Older individuals are at increased risk for developing hyponatremi An analysis of 139 sets of plasma electrolyte values for healthy indivic uals demonstrated an age-related decrease of 1 mEq/L/decade from mean value of 141 ± 4 mEq/L in younger subjects. In ambulatory ind viduals 65 yr of age who were living at home and lacked evidence o acute illness, a 7% incidence of serum Na concentrations ≤ 137 mEq/ was observed. An increased prevalence of hyponatremia has also bee found in hospitalized patients. An analysis of 5000 consecutive sets o plasma electrolytes from hospitalized patients with a mean age of 54 y revealed a mean serum Na concentration of 134 mEq/L, with the value skewed toward the hyponatremic end of the frequency distributio curve. In elderly residents of long-term care institutions, an 18 to 22' prevalence of serum Na concentrations ≤ 135 mEq/L was observed. I the same population, patients followed on a longitudinal basis over 1 no displayed an incidence of hyponatremia of approximately 50%. While hyponatremia is common in the elderly, it is often without clinically apparent symptoms, especially when it is of mild degree.

Etiology and Pathophysiology

Hyponatremia may occur in association with combined Na and ECF volume depletion, eg, vomiting, diarrhea, GI suction, renal disorders, diuretic therapy, etc. In this circumstance, volume depletion stimulates ADH release so that water is retained in excess of Na. Hyponatremia resulting from these events is usually mild—rarely being < 125 mEq/L.

Disorders producing edematous states, eg, heart failure (HF), cirrhosis, nephrotic syndrome, or acute glomerulonephritis, are associated with an *elevated* total body Na content and normal or increased ECF volume. However, "effective" plasma volume is reduced, decreasing delivery of Na and water to the diluting segments of the nephron. Consequently, sodium-retaining mechanisms are activated as release of ADH is increased. The net effect over time is the retention of water in excess of Na, leading to dilutional hyponatremia.

In a form of hyponatremia common in the elderly, total body Na content is *normal* but water is retained because of increased ADH secretion, ie, the syndrome of inappropriate ADH secretion (SIADH). This syndrome, which has numerous causes (see TABLE 4–1), is defined by (1) inappropriate hypertonicity of the urine, with osmolality often hypertonic to plasma in the presence of plasma hypotonicity; (2) increased excretion of Na in the urine; (3) plasma volume dilution, as suggested by normal or low BUN and creatinine concentrations; and (4) absence of edema. Elderly patients with underlying disorders that may lead to SIADH often have normal serum Na concentrations, since fluid intake may not be sufficient to produce a dilutional hyponatremia. However, when fluid intake is increased (eg, when IV fluids are administered or when oral intake is encouraged during management of febrile illness), the increase in body water may lead to rapid development of hyponatremia. This is most likely to occur in institutionalized patients, whose fluid intake is not primarily determined by thirst or custom.

Another common cause of hyponatremia in elderly patients is the use of nutritional support with defined formula diets such as Isocal®, Ensure®, or Osmolite®. Such diets are almost universally low in Na content, containing approximately 20 to 30 mEq Na/1000 calories. These dietary sources should be supplemented with Na to provide a total intake of approximately 100 mEq daily.

Symptoms, Signs, and Diagnosis

The severity of symptoms and signs of hyponatremia is related to the magnitude of the hyponatremia and the rapidity with which the serum Na has declined. Mild chronic hyponatremia may be asymptomatic. When serum Na concentration falls to < 125 mEq/L, lethargy, fatigue,

TABLE 4-1. CAUSES OF SYNDROME OF INAPPROPRIATE
ANTIDIURETIC HORMONE SECRETION (SIADH)

Malignancy with ectopic hormone production
Small cell carcinoma of lung
Pancreatic carcinoma
Thymoma
Lymphosarcoma, reticulum cell sarcoma,
  Hodgkin's disease

Pulmonary disease
Pneumonia
Lung abscess
Tuberculosis

CNS disorders
Trauma
Tumor
Infectious diseases
Vascular diseases
Acute intermittent porphyria
Lupus erythematosus

Drugs (See also Ch. 18)
Chlorpropamide
Vincristine
Vinblastine
Cyclophosphamide
Carbamazepine
Thiazide diuretics
Narcotics
General anesthetics
Tricyclic antidepressants
Oxytocin
Phenoxybenzamine

Other
Hypothyroidism
Positive-pressure breathing

and muscle cramps may occur. GI symptoms (eg, anorexia and nausea) may be early features. *Of major importance are the CNS manifestations of hyponatremia,* ranging from disorientation to confusion, coma, and seizures, often related to the severity of the hyponatremia. *Serum Na values < 115 mEq/L may result in sudden death.* The overall mortality rate in patients with symptomatic hyponatremia and serum Na concentration < 120 mEq/L is approximately 40% and reaches approximately 70% when there is coexisting alcoholism or cachexia.

Physical examination may reveal signs related to hypovolemia in patients with volume depletion as the basis for hyponatremia or edema in patients with Na retention and decreased effective plasma volume.

Edema is rarely seen in patients with SIADH. Physical signs associated with CNS effects of hyponatremia are depressed sensorium, depressed deep tendon reflexes, hypothermia, Cheyne-Stokes respiration, pathologic reflexes, and seizures.

Measurements of serum BUN and creatinine are useful in determining the type of hyponatremia. These values are usually elevated in patients with combined Na and ECF volume depletion, as well as in those with decreased effective plasma volume. In patients with dilutional hyponatremia or SIADH, serum BUN and creatinine values are usually normal or low. Urinary Na concentration is usually low (ie, < 20 mEq/L) in patients with volume depletion or edema; it is usually > 20 mEq/L in patients with expanded ECF volume, such as occurs in SIADH.

An **oral water-loading test** may be of value in determining the diagnosis of SIADH. The test is performed by giving an oral water load of 20 mL/kg body weight over 15 to 30 min. The patient is kept recumbent for the next 5 h, except when voiding. Urine is collected at hourly intervals for 5 h, and volume and osmolality are measured in each sample. A normal response is excretion of > 80% of the water load in 5 h and a decrease in urine osmolality to < 100 mOsm/kg in at least 1 specimen, usually that collected during the 2nd h after administration of the water load. Patients with SIADH will have impaired ability to excrete the water load and dilute the urine. A normal response in a hyponatremic person whose clinical and laboratory findings indicate normal or expanded ECF volume suggests that the hyponatremia may be due to primary polydipsia or a low-set osmoreceptor mechanism. *The test should not be performed in patients who have serum Na concentrations < 125 mEq/L or who have clinical evidence of symptomatic hyponatremia, regardless of serum Na level.*

In evaluating the elderly patient with hyponatremia, other causative factors must be excluded. One such cause is hyperglycemia in association with diabetes mellitus. In this situation, the glucose-induced hyperosmolar state produces a shift of body water into the intravascular space, diluting serum Na by approximately 1.6 mEq/L for each 100 mg/dL elevation in the blood glucose value over normal. Correction of the hyperglycemia returns the serum Na value to normal.

Pseudohyponatremia may occur when there is marked hyperlipidemia or hyperproteinemia. In these conditions, the increased lipid or protein replaces a portion of Na-containing plasma so that measured Na concentration per liter of plasma is reduced. However, determination of plasma osmolality will reveal a normal value for solute concentration, since this measurement reflects solute concentration of plasma water.

A summary of the differentiating features of various types of hyponatremia is shown in TABLE 4–2.

Treatment

In hyponatremia due to Na and ECF volume depletion, treatment is based on correction of the volume deficit with isotonic saline solution.

TABLE 4–2. FEATURES OF VARIOUS TYPES OF HYPONATREMIA

Type of Hyponatremia	Edema	Serum BUN/Creatinine	Urine Na (mEq/L)	Response to Water Load
Na and ECF volume depletion	−	↑	< 20	Impaired
Decreased effective plasma volume	+	↑	< 20	Impaired
Dilutional SIADH	−	NL or ↓	> 20	Impaired
Primary polydipsia	−	NL or ↓	> 20	Normal
Low-set osmorecepter	−	NL	> 20	Normal

ECF = extracellular fluid; SIADH = syndrome of inappropriate antidiuretic hormone secretion; NL = normal limits.

If the serum Na concentration is < 125 mEq/L, a portion of the IV fluid should be given in the form of hypertonic saline. In patients with hyponatremia and decreased effective plasma volume who are edematous, treatment should be directed to the underlying cause—ie, congestive HF, cirrhosis, or nephrotic syndrome. Although diuretics (eg, furosemide) are often effective in reducing edema, they may cause a natriuresis of sufficient magnitude to produce a further decrease in the serum Na concentration. In this situation, moderate fluid restriction (eg, 1000 to 1500 mL/24 h) may be sufficient to correct the hyponatremia.

Symptomatic hyponatremia, particularly that resulting from a dilutional state, warrants prompt intervention. In the mildly symptomatic patient with serum Na > 125 mEq/L, restricting fluid to 800 to 1000 mL/day is usually sufficient. In patients with more severe symptoms, serum Na should be increased more rapidly by infusing hypertonic saline until symptoms begin to clear and the serum Na concentration has increased to approximately 120 to 125 mEq/L. A desired goal is elevation of the serum Na concentration at the rate of 2 mEq/L/h. This can usually be accomplished by administering 200 to 300 mL of 3% saline solution over 4 to 6 h. Patients with very low serum Na concentrations (< 105 mEq/L) and symptoms of seizure or coma may benefit from simultaneous administration of IV furosemide to promote diuresis. These patients may require larger amounts of hypertonic saline to compensate for the enhanced natriuresis and monitoring of serum electrolytes to avoid diuretic-induced hypokalemia and hypomagnesemia.

Overcorrection of hyponatremia must be avoided. Generally, restoration of the serum Na concentration to approximately 120 to 125 mEq/L is sufficient to correct major symptomatic consequences of hyponatremia. **Central pontine myelinolysis** may result from rapid treatment of severe hyponatremia in patients with alcoholism and severe malnutrition whose serum Na concentration has been rapidly increased to levels > 140 mEq/L.

The chronic management of hyponatremia is based on identification and correction of the underlying cause. Additional measures include fluid restriction to a level that will maintain a serum Na concentration > 130 mEq/L; this intake will usually range from 1000 to 1500 mL/day. In patients who do not respond or are unable to comply with fluid restriction, the tetracycline antibiotic demeclocycline 600 to 1200 mg/day is capable of inducing mild nephrogenic diabetes insipidus with polyuria of 2 to 4 L/24 h. Patients treated with this drug require careful monitoring of fluid balance to avoid excessive fluid loss. In addition, some individuals have markedly elevated serum BUN levels as a result of drug treatment.

HYPERNATREMIA

An increase in serum Na concentration to > 146 mEq/L as a result of a deficit of body water relative to total body Na content.

Hypernatremia is common in the elderly, with a reported incidence of approximately 1% in hospitalized patients ≥ 60 yr of age. A similar incidence was observed among the elderly residents of a long-term care institution, with the prevalence increasing to 18% when the population was evaluated over 12 mo.

The development of hypernatremia in an elderly patient portends a high risk of morbidity and mortality, often as a reflection of the severity of the predisposing disorder. CNS manifestations are common, often leading to depression of sensorium and chronic decline in functional status in those who survive the acute episode. A mortality rate of approximately 40% was reported in elderly hospitalized patients who developed hypernatremia with serum Na concentration > 148 mEq/L. The mortality rate was greatest in those with rapid onset of hypernatremia and those with a serum Na concentration > 160 mEq/L.

Etiology

The most common mechanism underlying hypernatremia is loss of body water in excess of Na losses in association with inadequate fluid intake (see TABLE 4–3). The TBW deficit can reach 11 L or 30% of TBW volume. Disorders leading to this degree of water depletion include febrile illness with increased insensible losses, tachypnea with increased water loss from the lungs, fever-related obtundation with decreased drinking, diarrhea from hyperosmolar tube feedings, polyuria from uncontrolled diabetes mellitus with glycosuria, and debilitating illness with inadequate oral fluid intake. Rarely, dehydration and hypernatremia are seen in elderly patients with central diabetes insipidus or with acquired vasopressin resistance as a result of chronic renal disease, hypercalcemia, or hypokalemia. An important common occurrence is

TABLE 4–3. CAUSES OF HYPERNATREMIA

Decreased fluid intake
  Physical impairment
  Mental impairment
  Obtundation
  Hypodipsia/adipsia

Increased water loss
  Increased insensible loss
    Fever
    Tachypnea
  Sweating
  Diarrhea
  Dialysis
  Renal water loss
    Loop diuretics
    Osmotic diuresis—
      glucose, mannitol, Na, urea
    Diabetes insipidus
    Nephrogenic diabetes insipidus
    Chronic renal disease
    Hypercalcemia
    Hypokalemia

Increased sodium intake
  Sodium bicarbonate therapy for metabolic acidosis
  Isotonic or hypertonic IV saline

excessive water depletion, which can result from the administration of potent loop diuretics.

Occasionally, hypernatremia occurs without accompanying dehydration as a result of high Na intake. This has been observed following sodium bicarbonate administration for cardiac arrest or metabolic acidosis, as well as following normal saline infusion for treatment of fluid loss or shock.

Symptoms and Signs

The symptoms of moderate hypernatremia may be nonspecific; weakness and lethargy are common. More severe hypernatremia, with serum Na concentration > 152 mEq/L, may be accompanied by obtundation, stupor, coma, and seizures. The clinical signs are those of volume depletion and dehydration, with weight loss, decreased skin turgor, dry mucous membranes, and orthostatic hypotension. The laboratory findings, in addition to the increase in serum Na concentration, are those of hemoconcentration, as reflected by increases in Hct, serum osmolality, BUN, and creatinine values. Urine osmolality may not be greatly increased because of age-associated impairment in renal concentrating capacity.

Treatment

Early recognition and treatment of mild hypernatremia and proper attention to fluid needs are of special importance in hospitalized elderly patients, since many cases of severe hypernatremia develop after admission and may rapidly evolve as a consequence of therapeutic interventions or progression of the underlying disease process.

The correction of hypernatremia requires the replacement of body water deficits with hypotonic fluid. The magnitude of the fluid deficit can be estimated as described under VOLUME DEPLETION/DEHYDRATION, above. Fluid in the form of hypotonic NaCl or 5% D/W should be administered at a rate that will correct the hypernatremia over approximately 48 h. *Overly rapid correction may lead to cerebral edema with either permanent brain damage or death;* the serum Na concentration should be lowered no more rapidly than 2 mEq/L/h. In the elderly patient with coexisting cardiac disease, attention must be paid to avoiding heart failure. When the cause of hypernatremia has been identified (eg, diabetes insipidus, diuretic administration, increased Na intake), specific treatment measures should be implemented.

---

5. HYPERTHERMIA AND ACCIDENTAL HYPOTHERMIA

Richard W. Besdine

HYPERTHERMIA

Abnormally high body temperature due to inadequate or inappropriate responses of heat-regulating mechanisms.

Pathophysiologic changes due to high environmental temperature represent an important health risk for older people, from both chronic diseases exacerbated by heat and heat stroke itself. Deaths due to most diseases increase during hot, humid weather, and the increase is borne disproportionately by those > 65 yr of age. Eighty percent of the mortality associated with heat stroke is reported in those > 50 yr of age.

Influence of Normal Aging on Temperature Regulation

Under usual environmental conditions, convection and radiation account for 65% of heat loss; evaporation from skin and lungs contributes another 30%. The hypothalamus regulates heat loss via neuroendocrine and autonomic mechanisms. Heat causes blood vessels in the skin to dilate, and increased sweating due to cholinergic discharge occurs. Vasodilation, in turn, increases heart rate and CO.

When environmental temperature exceeds body surface temperature, heat loss by convection and radiation stops and heat absorption begins. Evaporation of sweat becomes the last major means of heat loss, but increased humidity prevents cooling by this mechanism.

Aging appears to reduce the effectiveness of sweating in cooling the body. Many eccrine glands becomes fibrotic, and surrounding connective tissue becomes less vascular. In addition, the remaining anatomically normal eccrine glands may not function normally. Older individuals require a higher core temperature to initiate sweating and produce lower maximal sweat output per gland.

Because physiologic responses to heat include vasodilation and associated increases in cardiac work and output, the high prevalence of heart disease in older persons increases their risk of heat stress. Heart failure worsens with experimentally increased ambient heat and humidity. The greater the degree of cardiac impairment, the less the ability of the patient to withstand the environmental stress. Thus changes seen both with normal aging and as the consequence of diseases more common in the elderly combine to impair optimal heat regulation.

Risk Factors

During the summer of 1980, heat stroke rates in persons $\geq$ 65 yr of age were 12 to 13 times those in the younger population. Risk factors for heat stroke in older people include low socioeconomic status, impaired ability to perform self-care, alcoholism, mental illness, and unavailability of air-conditioning. Concomitant medical disorders (eg, cardiovascular or cerebrovascular disease, diabetes, or COPD) common in the elderly also increase risk. Deaths due to diabetes, lung disease, and hypertension increase by > 50% during heat waves; thus, mortality due to hyperthermia may depend more on severity of associated diseases than severity of heat stress.

Some drugs present special heat-related health risks. Many illnesses common in old age, particularly psychiatric problems, are treated with drugs that predispose the patient to heat stroke. Anticholinergic agents, phenothiazines, tricyclic antidepressants, antihistamines, and synthetic and belladonna alkaloids impair both hypothalamic function centrally and sweat output peripherally. By altering awareness of heat, these drugs, as well as narcotics, sedative-hypnotics, and alcohol, diminish the ability to respond to heat stress. Amphetamines can increase body temperature by direct action on the hypothalamus. Diuretics (by causing additional fluid loss) and β-adrenergic blockers (by impairing cardiovascular responsiveness) can increase the risk of heat stroke. Therefore, a careful drug history can be helpful in elucidating the cause of and preventing heat stroke.

Disorders Caused by Heat

Heat cramps (muscle cramps), preceded by profuse sweating and polydipsia without an elevation in body temperature, often occur during intense physical activity in hot, humid weather. Heat cramps probably result from sweat-induced fluid and electrolyte loss and replacement mainly with water.

Heat exhaustion consists of anorexia, nausea, vomiting, disorientation, and postural hypotension. Cramping may occur, and body temperature may be normal or elevated. Patients may be thirsty and weak and generally have some CNS signs—usually light-headedness, dizziness, or loss of consciousness. Two major forms of heat exhaustion are recognized: **water depletion,** which produces hypertonic dehydration, and **salt depletion,** which results from replacement of sodium chloride lost by sweating with free water (similar to patients suffering with heat cramps). Major complications or death are rare.

Heat stroke is a syndrome characterized by fever (generally > 41 C [> 106 F], although if other criteria are met, a lesser degree of fever is accepted), absence of sweating, and severe CNS disturbance. Prodromal light-headedness, dizziness, headache, weakness, dyspnea, and/or nausea, may appear transiently, but loss of consciousness may be the first manifestation. Heat stroke has a bimodal population distribution, occurring in younger people who overexert at high ambient temperatures and in older people, developing insidiously as the ability to dissipate heat declines.

Two patterns of cardiovascular response may occur with heat stroke. In the **hyperdynamic state,** generally seen in younger individuals, CO is normal or increased and elevated central venous pressure **(CVP)** is common. In the **hypodynamic response,** more typical in the elderly, hypovolemia is often present and capillary wedge pressure is normal. It has been hypothesized that the hypodynamic response in older people is due to an inability to respond to heat stress by sufficient increase in heart rate or appropriate change in peripheral vascular resistance. In addition, the slower development of heat stroke in older patients may result in greater fluid loss. Other **cardiovascular manifestations** include electrocardiographic ST-segment and T-wave changes, premature ventricular contractions, supraventricular tachycardias, and conduction abnormalities.

CNS signs may include lethargy, stupor, or coma. The EEG is usually normal initially, in the absence of seizures, and cerebrospinal fluid is unremarkable. Cerebellar symptoms may be permanent in a small number of those who recover. At autopsy, edema, patchy congestion, and diffuse petechial hemorrhages are found in the brain.

Renal manifestations range from mild proteinuria to acute tubular necrosis in 10 to 30% of cases. Rhabdomyolysis, which causes acute renal failure, has been described in both standard and exercise-induced heat stroke. Generally, heat stroke is accompanied by metabolic acidosis and an elevated lactate level with compensatory respiratory alkalosis.

Although **transient elevations of transaminases** are common and **jaundice** may be seen, there is usually no residual hepatic damage. **Coagulation defects** include elevated prothrombin and partial thromboplastin times and a decreased fibrinogen level; the full-blown syndrome of disseminated intravascular coagulation is rare. **Severe hypokalemia** is common and is thought to be secondary to increased aldosterone secretion.

Specific prognostic signs remain undefined, but elderly patients with the highest fever, the most severe hypotension, or the deepest neurologic impairment have the highest mortality.

Prevention

Heat stroke in the elderly, like many conditions, is caused by interaction of environmental factors and the normal physiologic changes of aging, often complicated by concomitant diseases and the effects of certain drugs. Prevention is preferable to treatment, since morbidity and mortality are high. Those who care for high-risk older individuals should be alerted to the symptoms of heat stroke and advised to move such individuals to an air-conditioned environment in very hot weather, if only for brief periods. Adequate fluid intake and avoidance of exercise are important.

Sensible environmental manipulation includes having the patient wear light clothing and opening and shading windows during night and day, respectively. Decreasing the doses of drugs that predispose one to heat stroke is advised during heat waves. At times of greatest risk, it may be necessary to move people to temporary shelters. Primary care physicians should be aware of the nonspecific presentation of heat stroke, and in times of heat stress, routine temperature monitoring is advisable. Heat stroke is both a public and an individual health problem, and only by increased awareness and action can morbidity and mortality be decreased.

Treatment

Heat stroke is a medical emergency. Normal body temperature must be restored as quickly as possible, since many metabolic and cardiovascular problems are temperature dependent. Core temperature should be continuously monitored with the use of a thermocouple while the patient is immersed in cool water. To avoid overcooling and hypothermia, the patient should be removed from the bath when body temperature reaches 38.8 C (102 F). The cooling process can then continue with wet sponging.

Heat stroke may be either hyperdynamic, often associated with pulmonary edema, or hypodynamic, with major fluid loss. Thus, CVP or pulmonary capillary wedge pressure monitoring is advisable, with fluid replacement as necessary. Close monitoring of hematologic and renal parameters during the acute event is mandatory, as is a search for predisposing factors, including infection.

ACCIDENTAL HYPOTHERMIA

The unintentional decrease in body temperature to < 35 C (95 F). Older persons may become hypothermic while at home in mildly cold environments, but most episodes are initiated by ambient temperatures near 15.5 C (60 F).

Current prevalence, incidence, and mortality data regarding accidental hypothermia are scanty, particularly in the USA. In a large community survey conducted in Great Britain during the winter of 1972, 10% of the elderly population experienced early morning core temperatures of ≤ 35.5 C (95.5 F). There was no correlation between low body temperature and living alone, being housebound, or lacking central heating or indoor plumbing. Thus increased urbanization does not appear to reduce the risk of hypothermia.

The only US data available are from a study done in Maine in which 97 elderly subjects (average age, 74 yr) from an internal medicine clinic were surveyed; many were poor or living in subsidized housing. No subject had a basal body temperature < 35.5 C (95.5 F). Estimates of mortality due to hypothermia are difficult to calculate, since there are no definitive clinical or pathologic findings. Also, since most dead bodies are cold when found, it is difficult to attribute death to hypothermia after the event. Accordingly, death certificate figures indicating that only a few hundred deaths each year in the USA are caused by hypothermia may underestimate the problem.

A high figure of 75,000 is attributed to "excess winter deaths" among the elderly. In addition to hypothermic deaths, this figure includes deaths associated with many other winter risks, eg, influenza and pneumonia. Among identified cases of hypothermia, the mortality rate is disturbingly high at 50%. Mortality correlates best with the presence and severity of associated illness, rather than with the degree of hypothermia.

US data support a substantially increased risk of hypothermic death in patients > 75 yr of age. Hypothermia may also result in significant morbidity. One British study showed that in malnourished patients, there was a midwinter peak in hip fracture incidence and a higher mortality after hip fracture. Malnourished patients were frequently hypothermic on admission to the hospital, whereas well-nourished patients had normal body temperatures. It is presumed that malnutrition leads to impaired heat generation and retention, hypothermia, lack of coordination, and subsequent injury.

Additionally, elderly diabetics have a sixfold greater risk of hypothermia, probably due to vascular disease that alters thermoregulatory mechanisms. Temperatures of elderly patients admitted to 2 London hospitals during 3 winter months of 1975 were accurately measured and revealed a 3.6% incidence of hypothermia in those ≥ 65 yr of age.

Etiology and Pathophysiology

The usual factors implicated in the genesis of accidental hypothermia are environmental cold, age-related physiologic changes in thermoregulation, drugs, and the diseases that either decrease heat production, increase heat loss, or impair thermoregulation (see TABLE 5–1). Ambient temperature only a few degrees colder than body temperature can cause hypothermia in elderly, severely debilitated individuals. A number of

TABLE 5-1. ETIOLOGY OF ACCIDENTAL HYPOTHERMIA

Environmental cold
Physiologic changes
    Diminished perception of cold
    Autonomic nervous system deterioration
        Decreased shivering
        Low resting peripheral blood flow
        Nonconstrictor response to cold
        Orthostatic hypotension
Drugs
    Tranquilizers
    Sedative/hypnotics
    Alcohol
Diseases
    Decreased heat production
        Myxedema
        Hypopituitarism
        Hypoglycemia
        Malnutrition/starvation
        Diabetic ketoacidosis
        Diminished activity
            Arthritis
            Parkinsonism
            Paralysis/stroke
            Dementia
            A fall
    Increased heat loss
        Inflammatory dermatitis
            Ichthyosis
            Psoriasis
            Exfoliation
        Paget's disease
        A-V shunt
    Impaired thermoregulation
        Primary CNS pathology
            Stroke
            Subarachnoid hemorrhage
            Subdural hematoma
            Tumor
            Head trauma
            Wernicke's encephalopathy
            Polio
            Sarcoidosis
        Systemic disease influencing hpothalamus
            Uremia
            CO poisoning
        Neuropathy
            Diabetes
            Alcoholism

(From R.W. Besdine: "Accidental hypothermia in the elderly," in *Medical Grand Rounds*, Vol. 1, p. 36, 1982. Used with permission of Plenum Publishing Corporation and the author.)

physiologic changes predispose elderly persons to hypothermia, including their diminished perception of cold. Changes in response to endogenous catecholamines in the elderly reduce the vasoconstrictor and shivering responses to cold.

Other factors that predispose older people to hypothermia include a reduction in physical activity and a decreased caloric intake, both of which reduce their ability to generate heat. A decrease in lean body mass reduces the efficiency of shivering in heat production. Finally, the frequent occurrence of multiple pathologic conditions in older patients adds to the physiologic risks.

A number of diseases and drugs may alter thermoregulatory mechanisms. Decreased heat production occurs with hypopituitarism, hypoglycemia, starvation, and malnutrition. Forced or involuntary inactivity (eg, as in Parkinson's disease, arthritis, paralysis, and dementia) decreases heat production and increases the risk of hypothermia. Increased heat loss can occur secondary to inflammatory skin disease, alcohol-induced vasodilation, cold exposure, Paget's disease, and reduction in insulating subcutaneous fat.

Central hypothalamic temperature regulation can be disturbed by a variety of pathologic processes, including stroke, subarachnoid hemorrhage, subdural hematoma, and brain tumor. Uremia and carbon monoxide poisoning may also affect thermoregulation. Many drugs, including phenothiazines, tricyclic antidepressants, benzodiazepines, barbiturates, reserpine, and narcotics, depress central thermoregulation and predispose patients to accidental hypothermia. Chlorpromazine, which inhibits shivering, is the best-known offender.

Symptoms and Signs

The symptoms of hypothermia are insidious and may be transient. While elderly people with body temperatures between 35 C (95 F) and 36.1 C (97 F) usually complain of being cold, patients with established hypothermia do not. Clinical findings are numerous but nonspecific; they can suggest stroke or metabolic disorder. The patient feels cool to the touch and has a history of confusion and sleepiness, which may have progressed to coma over the previous 2 to 3 days.

Neurologic findings include thick, slow speech; ataxic gait; and depressed reflexes. Pathologic reflexes and plantar responses may be present, and pupils may be dilated and sluggishly reactive. Focal signs, seizures, paralysis, and sensory loss have also been reported.

Although shivering may occur at temperatures > 35 C (> 95 F), most reports indicate that it is absent in hypothermic elderly patients. Instead, marked rigidity, accompanied by a generalized increase in muscle tone and, occasionally, a fine tremor, may be found.

Although cold extremities are common in winter, hypothermic patients have cold abdomens and backs as well. The skin has a cadaveric pallor and chill, and pressure points show erythematous, bullous, or purpuric patches. Subcutaneous tissues are firm, probably from edema, which also produces a puffy appearance, especially of the face.

The **cardiovascular system** is initially stimulated by cold, resulting in peripheral vasoconstriction, tachycardia, and BP elevation; however, as hypothermia progresses, the myocardium is depressed, producing hypotension and progressively slow sinus bradycardia. Severe hypothermia can reduce BP and heart beat to barely detectable levels, sometimes leading to an erroneous pronouncement of death. Various other cardiac arrhythmias also have been reported in cold temperatures, including atrial fibrillation and flutter, premature ventricular beats, and idioventricular rhythm.

The **GI response** to hypothermia consists of decreased peristalsis and ileus, producing abdominal distention and decreased or absent bowel sounds, and, less often, acute gastric dilation with vomiting. Pancreatitis may also occur but is usually not apparent until rewarming has been achieved. Because hepatic metabolism is depressed, the metabolism of many drugs may be sharply reduced.

Pulmonary findings include depression of respiration and cough reflex. Atelectasis is almost universal, and pneumonia is common. Pulmonary edema during recovery may be related to increased vascular permeability as well as to heart failure.

Early in hypothermia, increased heart rate and CO produce increased renal blood flow and diuresis. In addition, cold suppresses secretion of ADH and diminishes tubular responsiveness to its action, further increasing diuresis. Later, as volume depletion diminishes glomerular filtration and renal blood flow, oliguria and tubular necrosis follow.

Most **clinical laboratory data** are not specific for hypothermia. Hemoconcentration, leukocytosis, lactic acidosis, and thrombocytopenia are all common. The ECG can provide a major diagnostic clue. A junctional, or J, wave is a small deflection early in the ST segment, positive in the left and negative in the right ventricular leads. Although present in only about $\frac{1}{3}$ of hypothermic patients, this finding always indicates hypothermia. Another, more common ECG finding frequently seen in the nonshivering hypothermic patient is a regular oscillation of the baseline produced by the imperceptible tremor and increased muscle tone.

Blood glucose findings in hypothermia have been a point of confusion. Hypothermia produces hyperglycemia by increasing gluconeogenesis via increased corticosteroid and catecholamine release. Additionally, although the secretion of insulin is stimulated, cold interferes with its action, further raising glucose concentration. When hypothermic patients are hypoglycemic, the causality is reversed (ie, hypoglycemia, usually drug-induced, produces hypothermia).

Diagnosis

The diagnosis of accidental hypothermia depends on the ability to measure body temperature < 34.4 C (94 F). The usual clinical practice is to search for and exclude fever; thus, body temperature is usually recorded as high or normal. However, standard clinical thermometers are calibrated from 34.4 to 42.2 C (94 to 108 F), and 34.4 C (94 F) is the highest temperature for a patient considered hypothermic. Since these thermometers are usually shaken down to only between 35 C and 35.6 C (95 and 96 F) before measuring temperature, it is unlikely that they will detect hypothermia. A rectal thermometer calibrated from 28.9 to 42.2 C (84 to 108 F) is available from most hospital suppliers, although it is not commonly used. In the absence of a low-reading thermometer, more expensive thermistors or thermocouples have been used. Thus, hypothermia should be suspected if the history or physical examination is suggestive, and core temperature should be recorded using a low-reading instrument.

Prevention

Prevention of accidental hypothermia is preferable to treatment. Older persons with identifiable predisposing problems should have their household thermostats set at $\geq$ 18.3 C ($\geq$ 65 F) and should keep a reliable thermometer (separate from the thermostat) for determining room temperature where they can check it daily, especially during very cold weather. Additional indoor clothing, particularly covering for exposed areas (eg, hands, feet, and head) should be worn. Frequent periods of exercise can increase heat production, and adequate caloric intake is of prime importance. Drugs that may alter thermoregulatory mechanisms should be discontinued whenever possible.

Treatment

The elderly patient with accidental hypothermia usually is treated at the outset for some other disorder; either a cause or complication of hypothermia is the exclusive focus of treatment, or the symptoms and signs of hypothermia are erroneously attributed to some common geriatric disease. Therapeutic delay results in either case.

Once the temperature falls into the hypothermic range, thermoregulation becomes progressively impaired; hence, early during the temperature fall, regulatory mechanisms fail altogether and the patient behaves like a poikilotherm. Accordingly, *even mild accidental hypothermia should be regarded as a medical emergency, and patients should be monitored under hospital conditions* (usually in an intensive care setting) until recovery is complete.

Therapy for accidental hypothermia can be divided into primary treatment by rewarming and secondary treatment of the direct effects and complications of hypothermia. Primary measures aim to restore normal body temperature and to abort the pathophysiologic consequences of hypothermia. **In young, physiologically vigorous individuals,** especially those with hypothermia due to exposure, rapid active rewarming **(RAR)** is carried out by active heating.

Elderly individuals with accidental hypothermia, *when rewarmed actively and rapidly, often develop a syndrome of profound hypotension, new cardiac arrhythmias, and deteriorating metabolic abnormalities, culminating* *in death.* For this reason, recommendations favor slow spontaneous rewarming **(SSR)** for older hypothermia victims. By preventing further heat loss and conserving the heat still being produced by the patient, SSR allows the temperature to rise slowly to normal. The environmental temperature is kept > 21.1 C (> 70 F), and blankets or more sophisticated insulating materials are used to retain body heat. With the use of SSR, body temperature is carefully monitored and should rise approximately 0.6 C (1 F)/h. A more rapid rise in core temperature, even when SSR is used, has been associated with rewarming hypotension. If SSR does not produce a rise in temperature, RAR of the core is necessary in the elderly, usually by immersion in a warm-water bath heated to 37.7 to 43.3 C (100 to 110 F). Other easy and practical technics for core rewarming include the use of heated, moist inspired air and heated peritoneal dialysis.

When core rewarming is used in elderly patients, scrupulous, comprehensive intensive care must be taken. When ventricular fibrillation or cardiac standstill occurs at temperatures < 29.4 C (85 F), warming must be accomplished as quickly as possible, since the heart is unresponsive to electrical defibrillation at temperatures below this level. Bradycardia resulting from myocardial depression is not influenced by atropine. The need for ventilatory assistance, intracardiac monitoring and pacing, and full circulatory support should be anticipated, since collapse and profound hypotension associated with warming commonly occur under such conditions.

General medical care demands comprehensive evaluation, careful monitoring, and anticipation of likely complications. For the most part, treatment is guided by the problems present at the time of initial evaluation and by the complications that appear during rewarming. Laboratory evaluation should include CBC; platelet count; clotting studies; measurements of BUN, creatinine, electrolytes, blood glucose, and serum and urine amylase levels; thyroid and liver function tests; arterial blood gas studies; ECG with constant monitoring; chest and abdominal x-rays; and constant monitoring and recording of core temperature.

Although reports from various uncontrolled clinical studies have recommended the routine use of several drugs, including corticosteroids, thyroid hormone, anticoagulants, antibiotics, and digitalis, none of these agents has proved effective in the absence of specific indications for its use. Myxedema is, of course, a well-known cause of hypothermia, and when hypothermia and hypothyroidism occur together, they result in a very high mortality.

Ventricular arrhythmias, if not rapidly responsive to rewarming, should be suppressed with lidocaine. Both countershock and pacing are less effective than usual at low temperatures, but if critical arrhythmias appear, appropriate therapy should be administered while the patient is rewarmed. If cardiac arrest or ventricular fibrillation is unresponsive to usual measures, CPR should be continued until rewarming has been accomplished; treatment then should be repeated. All IV fluids should be warmed to normal or slightly above normal body temperature.

Although hyperglycemia is commonly present, insulin is rarely given to the hypothermic patient unless glucose levels are very high (> 400 mg/dL), since insulin is ineffective at low temperatures. Any previously administered insulin, combined with endogenous insulin, can produce severe hypoglycemia during rewarming. In general, most drugs are less active than usual during hypothermia, but produce exaggerated pharmacologic effects as body temperature rises.

Death usually results from cardiac arrest or ventricular fibrillation. The temperature at which each cardiac event appears is variable, but at temperatures < 29.4 C (85 F), lethal events are a major risk, particularly in patients with underlying heart disease. Movement or excessive stimulation of hypothermic patients may provoke arrhythmias and should be performed cautiously. *Resuscitation during rewarming should be aggressive and prolonged in patients who are profoundly hypothermic;* remarkable recoveries have been reported in such cases. Most authorities agree that these patients should not be pronounced dead until CPR is shown to be ineffective after body temperature has been raised to at least 35.8 C (96.5 F).

---

6. SYNCOPE
(Fainting)

Lewis A. Lipsitz

A sudden, transient loss of consciousness characterized by unresponsiveness and loss of postural control. Recovery usually is spontaneous and does not require resuscitation procedures. Syncope is not a disease but rather a symptom of numerous diseases.

Epidemiology

The prevalence and incidence of syncope in the elderly population have not been thoroughly investigated, but studies of older patients in institutions have indicated that about 25% have experienced syncope within the preceding 10 yr and that 6 to 7% do so each yr. In about 33% of cases, syncope is recurrent.

Syncope alone does not increase risk of mortality, but it is associated with physical disability and subsequent functional decline. Syncope and falls may be signs of a serious underlying disorder associated with high rates of morbidity and mortality.

Etiology and Pathophysiology

Syncope is the result of inadequate delivery of O_2 or metabolic substrate to the brain or of disorganized electrical activity in the brain. The elderly are subject to multiple age- and disease-related conditions that threaten cerebral blood flow or reduced O_2 content in the blood. An accumulation of these conditions may diminish cerebral O_2 delivery so that it is dangerously close to the threshold needed to maintain consciousness. Any additional stress that further reduces cerebral blood flow or blood O_2 content may precipitate the symptom.

For example, while numerous cardiovascular and neuroendocrine homeostatic mechanisms normally maintain BP at a level adequate for cerebral perfusion, the progressive decline in homeostatic capacity and cerebral blood flow associated with aging results in a blunted ability to adapt to hypotensive stress. Heart failure with dyspnea and hyperventilation can further decrease cerebral blood flow by as much as 40%. Other common conditions, such as chronic obstructive lung disease or anemia, can reduce cerebral O_2 delivery still further. At this point, development of pneumonia or cardiac arrhythmia, ingestion of a hypotensive drug, or even situational stress that reduces BP may produce syncope. Seemingly minor stresses (eg, taking medication, eating a meal, defecating, or changing posture) can precipitate syncope by interacting with coexisting clinical abnormalities to reduce cerebral blood flow below the critical threshold for the maintenance of consciousness (see Ch. 31).

Baroreflex sensitivity to both hyper- and hypotensive stimuli also decreases progressively with age, as demonstrated by the blunted heart rate response to postural change found in many elderly patients. Similarly, the elderly are less able to cardioaccelerate to compensate for the hypotensive effect of many drugs.

Progressive reductions in basal and stimulated renin levels and aldosterone production, which impair renal sodium conservation and maintenance of intravascular volume, also predispose to syncope. Elderly persons are more likely to become dehydrated and to experience hypotension in response to diuretics, acute febrile illness, or limited salt and water intake. Further, healthy elderly persons are less likely to experience thirst in response to hypertonic dehydration, which can lead to rapid volume depletion, orthostatic hypotension, and syncope.

Diseases causing syncope: The causes of syncope are listed in TABLE 6–1. Cardiovascular causes are more prevalent in elderly than in younger patients. Any **cardiac illness** that abruptly and momentarily diminishes CO can produce syncope. CO may be transiently compromised by the anatomic, myocardial, or electrical abnormalities listed in TABLE 6–1.

Orthostatic and postprandial hypotension are especially common among elderly persons. **Orthostatic hypotension,** which occurs in 20 to 30% of noninstitutionalized elderly persons, is *a drop in systolic BP of 20 mm Hg or greater upon standing.* Although it is usually asymptomatic, orthostatic hypotension is an important risk factor for syncope and falls, accounting for about 4% of falls that occur among the noninstitutionalized elderly. Causes include the age-related physiologic changes mentioned above, drugs, and autonomic insufficiency syndromes, eg, **idiopathic orthostatic hypotension, Shy-Drager syndrome** (distinguished by characteristic degeneration in the brain and spinal cord leading to parkinsonian symptoms and by failure of the CNS to activate the

TABLE 6-1. CAUSES OF SYNCOPE

Hypotension
  Vasomotor instability
    Orthostatic hypotension
    Carotid sinus syndrome
    Micturition, defecation, coughing, swallowing
    Vasovagal reflex
  Volume depletion
  Drugs

Metabolic Blood Abnormalities
  Hypoxemia
  Hypoglycemia

Cardiac Disease
  Anatomic
    Aortic stenosis
    Mitral prolapse and regurgitation
    Hypertrophic cardiomyopathy
    Myxoma
  Myocardial
    Ischemia and infarct
    Cardiomyopathy
  Electrical
    Tachyarrhythmia
    Bradyarrhythmia
    Heart block
    Sick sinus syndrome

Cerebral Disorders
  Vascular insufficiency
  Seizures

Pulmonary Embolism

autonomic nervous system), and **multiple cerebral infarctions.** Elderly persons are usually able to maintain postural BP homeostasis, but when exposed to mild volume depletion (eg, during diuretic therapy), they may experience a profound decline in postural BP.

Postprandial hypotension is a recently identified BP abnormality. In some elderly persons, BP declines an average of 11 mm Hg by 1 h after a meal. Although most of these individuals experience no symptoms, those who have a more profound decline may have syncopal episodes. Postprandial hypotension may be related to an inability to compensate for splanchnic blood pooling after a meal.

Vasodepressor reflexes are also common causes of syncope in the elderly, although typical **vasovagal syncope** is more common in younger persons. **Carotid sinus syncope, micturition and defecation syncope,** and the unusual syndromes of **cough** and **swallow syncope** are more prevalent with advancing age and increasing severity of illness.

Anemia may threaten cerebral O_2 delivery. When transient hypotension occurs, the anemic patient may not have sufficient O_2 in the blood to maintain cerebral function.

Other important causes of syncope are primary cerebral disorders, eg, vascular insufficiency and seizures. Syncope can be attributed to **cerebrovascular disease,** however, only if transient focal neurologic deficits are associated with the episode. Syncope may also be due to a **seizure disorder;** however, syncope due to nonepileptic causes may sometimes be associated with seizure activity. Clinical features (eg, occurrence of syncope while the patient is in the supine position, an olfactory or gustatory aura, tongue biting, fecal incontinence, and postictal confusion) all support a diagnosis of epilepsy.

Studies of the institutionalized elderly have shown that syncope is more likely to occur in patients who have 2 or more coexisting contributing factors, eg, CAD, postural BP reduction, aortic stenosis, a need for insulin therapy, or overall functional impairment.

Diagnosis

Because syncope in elderly persons is usually caused by multiple interacting abnormalities rather than by a single disease entity, the clinician must search for age- and disease-related abnormalities that impede cerebral O_2 delivery. The evaluation should begin with a thorough history and a complete physical examination, which are sufficient to identify underlying causes in most cases. Witnesses to the syncopal event should be asked to describe what the patient was doing immediately before its occurrence. Family members or caretakers should be asked about recent changes in the patient's clinical condition that may point to the underlying pathophysiology.

The **history** also should focus on evaluation of drugs ingested or used in any way, both prescription and OTC, including eye medications. Many OTC drugs have anticholinergic properties that cause tachyarrhythmias and may precipitate syncope. Similarly, certain eye medications have autonomic effects, and topical ophthalmic β-blockers have systemic effects (eg, bronchospasm and heart failure) that may be associated with syncope. The onset and nature of recovery from a syncopal event can also provide important clues to its etiology. Major precipitants of syncope include eating, medication, and straining while defecating. Vasovagal syncope is usually preceded by hunger, fatigue, emotional stress, and a typical autonomic prodrome. The recovery is usually rapid. In contrast, a seizure may have a sudden onset and slow recovery.

The **physical examination** should include *evaluation of postural vital signs to rule out orthostatic hypotension* by checking the BP and heart rate, with the patient supine after a 10-min rest period, then after 1 and 3 min of standing, if the patient is able to do so. Although a standing position is most effective for detecting immediate and delayed reduction in postural BP, sitting vital signs can be used if the patient is unable to stand. A diminished heart rate upon assuming an upright position may be a clue to baroreflex impairment. An excessive increase in heart rate on standing is uncommon in the elderly, but if present, it may indicate volume depletion.

The carotid arteries should be examined for evidence of flow abnormalities or bruits to rule out conditions contraindicating carotid sinus massage (see below), as well as to determine the quality of the carotid upstroke. Although the upstroke typically is slow and has a low amplitude in younger persons with **aortic stenosis,** it may be deceptively rapid in older patients with signficant stenosis. The brisk upstroke is caused by increased vascular rigidity that accompanies aging; when aortic stenosis intervenes, the intensity of the upstroke may diminish to a level that is normal for a younger person.

The heart should be examined for murmurs of **aortic stenosis, mitral regurgitation,** or **hypertrophic cardiomyopathy,** all of which are common in elderly patients. An apical heave; a loud, late-peaking aortic systolic murmur; and a diminished second aortic sound suggest significant aortic stenosis. Mitral regurgitation is marked by a holosystolic murmur at the cardiac apex, but such a murmur may also be present in elderly patients who have aortic stenosis or hypertrophic cardiomyopathy. If the patient can perform Valsalva's maneuver, accentuation of the systolic murmur may distinguish hypertrophic cardiomyopathy from aortic stenosis or mitral regurgitation.

The stool should be examined for blood to rule out the possibility of GI bleeding and associated anemia. Neurologic examination is essential to search for focal neurologic abnormalities that may indicate the presence of cerebrovascular disease or space-occupying lesions.

More specialized studies generally are undertaken only if indicated by findings in the history and physical examination. **Screening tests** are often useful, since disease presentations can be atypical in elderly patients. These tests include a WBC count to look for evidence of occult sepsis and a Hct to diagnose anemia. Electrolyte, BUN, and creatinine studies are helpful in assessing hydration status and ruling out electrolyte disorders. Serum glucose measurements are useful to exclude hypo- and hyperglycemia. The first sign of hyperosmolar dehydration with hyperglycemia may be syncope.

If the patient is taking antiarrhythmic, anticonvulsant, or bronchodilator drugs or lithium, measurements of **drug levels** are useful to determine whether the level is within therapeutic or toxic range. If the drug level is below the therapeutic range and syncope occurs, it may be the result of inadequate treatment of a known, predisposing condition, such as a seizure disorder.

An **ECG** should also be included in the evaluation of syncope. If the ECG reveals ischemic changes or the patient has a history of chest pain associated with a syncopal episode, cardiac enzyme and isoenzyme readings should be obtained to rule out myocardial infarction. Arrhythmias are a common cause of syncope in elderly patients. Although **24-h ambulatory cardiac monitoring** (Holter monitoring) is often used to evaluate syncope, the results are difficult to interpret, because they usually show a high prevalence of asymptomatic arrhythmias, which are rarely coincident with syncope. Also, empiric treatment of these arrhythmias with antiarrhythmic agents is often complicated by severe toxic effects. Thus, an ambulatory ECG recording should be obtained only in patients whose arrhythmias would be treated despite the risk of toxic reactions, eg, patients with underlying cardiovascular disease or who have recently experienced a myocardial infarction and are at highest risk for sudden death.

Carotid sinus massage should be performed only on patients who have *no* evidence of cerebrovascular disease (a carotid bruit, previous stroke, or transient ischemic attacks) or cardiac conduction abnormalities. Serious complications resulting from carotid massage have been reported in a few severely ill persons. In contrast, however, hundreds of elderly patients have been reported as having undergone carotid sinus massage without complication. Because this procedure can identify a treatable cause of syncope in elderly patients, it is indicated when no other apparent cause or contraindication is present.

The **carotid sinus syndrome**—defined as a sinus pause longer than 3 sec (cardioinhibitory response) or a drop in systolic BP of more than 50 mm Hg (vasodepressor response) during carotid sinus stimulation—occurs more frequently with advancing age and cardiovascular disease. This syndrome is detected by gentle circular massage of one carotid sinus at a time for 5 sec while the ECG is monitored. BP is measured before and immediately after each carotid sinus is massaged. Patients with carotid sinus syndrome usually can be helped by the elimination of cardioinhibitory or hypotensive drugs. If this is not effective, or drugs are not implicated, patients with the cardioinhibitory response can be treated with cardiac pacing; those with associated hypotension may benefit from pressor agents such as ephedrine.

Although an **EEG** and a **brain CT scan** are often ordered for the evaluation of syncope, recent studies suggest that they are of little value unless underlying focal abnormalities are found on neurologic examination.

The **phonocardiogram, cardiac ultrasound,** and **Doppler echocardiography** are often used to detect hemodynamically significant valvular heart disease as well as hypertrophic cardiomyopathy in patients with a cardiac murmur.

Invasive tests, eg, cerebral angiography, cardiac catheterization, and cardiac electrophysiologic studies, should not be used in the initial evaluation of syncope but may be useful in the confirmation of a clinical diagnosis. Use of electrophysiologic recording in the evaluation of unexplained syncope has detected occult sinus node disease, conduction disease, or inducible ventricular arrhythmias in more than half the patients in whom syncope was unexplained. Treatment of these abnormalities significantly reduces (but does not eliminate) recurrences of syncope.

The actual value of electrophysiologic studies is difficult to determine, however, because even those elderly patients who do not have syncope are likely to have electrophysiologic abnormalities and because patients who have syncope often stop fainting spontaneously. Elderly patients who have ECG or other clinical evidence of heart disease and recurrent episodes of unexplained syncope are most likely to benefit from such studies. Nevertheless, when the risks of the procedure are weighed against the relatively low mortality associated with unexplained syncope, use of electrophysiologic studies is hard to justify.

Treatment

The first step in the treatment of elderly patients with syncope is to identify and treat all primary causes as well as all predisposing pathologic conditions that might be contributory. Age alone is rarely a contraindication to therapy. Major interventions, such as aortic valve repair, are relatively well tolerated in otherwise healthy elderly persons and can significantly improve the quality of their lives. Similarly, pacemaker therapy, coronary artery bypass grafting, and carotid endarterectomy should be considered when appropriate; the patient's coexisting conditions rather than age should be the decisive factor in determining treatment.

In the absence of a clear primary cause of syncope, potential predisposing conditions should be treated. For example, anemic patients might benefit from vitamin or iron supplementation or transfusions, depending on the cause of anemia. The patient with orthostatic hypotension might benefit from increase of salt intake, use of support hose, and elevation of the head of the bed. Adjusting the time of hypotensive drug administration to avoid a peak effect after a meal may help ameliorate postprandial hypotension. The patient with ischemic heart disease and angina should be given antianginal therapy, providing a severe reduction in BP does not result. The drug regimens of patients with carotid sinus hypersensitivity or cardiac conduction disease should be carefully evaluated to ensure that cardioinhibitory drugs, eg, digoxin, β-blockers, methyldopa, or Ca channel blockers, are not contributing to these conditions.

In addition, patients should be taught to avoid common precipitants of syncope. For example, they should not arise from bed quickly (particularly in the middle of the night). Patients with orthostatic hypotension should sit at the side of the bed and flex their feet before standing. Those with postprandial hypotension should eat small, frequent meals and lie down after each meal. In general, elderly patients should learn how to avoid Valsalva's maneuver (straining) during defecation by using bowel softeners and altering their diet.

7.   FALLS AND GAIT DISORDERS

Arthur D. Kay and *Rein Tideiksaar*

As many as ⅓ of older persons residing in the community report a fall or tendency to fall. Up to 20% of hospitalized patients and 45% of residents in long-term–care facilities fall at some time during their stay. These figures represent conservative estimates at best, since most falls are either unreported by the elderly or undetected by health care professionals. Only falls resulting in physical injury that requires medical attention or leads to significant changes in functional status are likely to be reported or remembered. Elderly persons may forget or deny a falling episode, since it reminds them of increasing frailty, or they may attribute falls to the normal aging process. In addition, the elderly may hesitate to report a fall for fear of restriction of activities or placement in a nursing home.

Falls are the most common cause of accidents in people > 65 yr of age, and they are the leading cause of mortality due to injury in that age group. Complications frequently associated with falling include painful soft tissue injuries, hip fractures, Colles' fractures, subdural hematomas, and hot-water burns secondary to falling in the bathtub. Immobility secondary to a fall may contribute to hypothermia, deep venous thrombosis, dehydration, UTI, bronchopneumonia, joint contractures, and pressure sores. While most falls do not end in death or significant physical injury, they are not benign events. The psychologic damage due to loss of self-esteem and fear of falling can be severely debilitating and can create risks of future falls and self-protective immobility.

MORBIDITY AND MORTALITY

Although there has been a reduction in deaths attributable to falling (particularly in elderly females) due either to improvements in medical care and prevention of postfall complications or to changes in the methods of classification, older people continue to have an excess mortality associated with falling episodes. Accidental injury is the sixth leading cause of death in people ≥ 75 yr of age, and falls represent the single most common cause of accidental mortality, accounting for 70%. In persons ≥ 65 yr of age, falls cause more deaths than pneumonia or diabetes and all other types of accidents combined. Mortality due to falling increases with age and more than doubles with each decade of life; a death rate of < 50/100,000 at age 65 increases progressively to 150/100,000 at age 75 and to 525/100,000 in those > 85 yr of age.

Though the majority of falls do not result in death, falling is still associated with significant morbidity. Older people have the highest rate of acute-care hospitalization for injuries; the average stay for those who have fallen is 43 days vs. 25 days for those who have not. Approximately 47% of patients admitted to a hospital for falling become long-term care patients. Older persons also have a high incidence of head injuries attributable to falls. This may be explained by a diminished protective reflex of extending an outstretched hand to break a fall, as evidenced by a plateau in the incidence of wrist fractures in those > 65 yr of age. Eight to 40% of falls occurring in the community result in fracture, which is the most common fall-related injury. Approximately 40% of falls in women > 75 yr of age result in fracture, compared with 27% in men.

Hip fracture is the most common fall-related injury that leads to hospitalization, and the length of stay for hip fracture is almost double that for all other causes of hospital admission in the elderly. In the USA, approximately 200,000 hip fractures occur each year, with 84% in persons ≥ 65 yr of age. Between $1 and 2 billion is spent annually for acute medical care of the elderly with hip fractures. Approximately 25% of these patients die within 6 mo of injury. Approximately 60% have decreased mobility and 25% become more functionally dependent after a hip fracture.

Morbidity and mortality due to falls may be affected by the availability of emergency services and the length of time lying on the ground after a fall. In one study, as many as ⅔ of persons who fell received no first aid before reaching the hospital and the majority arrived by a means other than ambulance. Minor injuries that are not properly managed in the community may become major, requiring hospital treatment and resulting in greater morbidity and mortality. Patients who lie on the ground > 1 h after a fall experience greater difficulty ambulating independently and are more likely to die.

ETIOLOGIC CLASSIFICATION

The factors responsible for a fall can be either intrinsic (ie, related to the host) or extrinsic (ie, related to the environment). **Intrinsic factors** include age-related physiologic changes, diseases, and medications that place the aged at risk for falling. **Extrinsic factors** include environmental hazards such as slippery floors and poorly lit areas. It is important to analyze each fall with these 2 factors in mind. For example, a patient who falls only once may have 2 or 3 reasons for the fall, whereas those who repeatedly fall may have a different reason for each instance. Only by analyzing each fall separately can a management plan be developed.

Intrinsic Causes

Age-related changes: TABLE 7–1 lists the normal changes associated with aging that limit functional reserve, rendering the elderly more likely to fall when confronted with a pathologic process or environmental obstacle. **A decline in visual acuity** is one of the most significant. With age, pupillary size and response diminish. Entering a darkened room or going outside at night increases the elderly person's risk of falling, since the time needed for the aging eye to reach a level of light sen-

TABLE 7-1. AGE-RELATED PHYSIOLOGIC CHANGES THAT PREDISPOSE TO FALLS

Eye
  Decreases in accommodative capacity, near vision (presbyopia), visual acuity, night
    vision, peripheral vision, glare tolerance, and color vision (blue/green)
  Changes in contrast sensitivity

Ear
  Impaired speech discrimination
  Increase in pure-tone threshold (high-frequency sounds predominantly affected)
  Excessive wax accumulation

Nervous System
  Slower reaction time
  Diminished sensory awareness for light touch, vibration, temperature
  Increased body sway
  Impairment of righting reflexes

sitivity equal to a young person's is prolonged. As a result, older people require adequate illumination to ambulate safely.

With increasing age, the lens becomes more opaque, leading to glare intolerance and to a decline in depth perception. A fall can result from excessive glare caused by direct light radiating off highly waxed floors or from walking into a brightly lit room from a room more dimly lit. Altered depth perception can lead to falls associated with climbing or descending stairs. The yellowing of the lens with age results in the filtering out of the blue-green spectrum. This may cause the patient to have difficulty discriminating between the colors of various medications. Thus, a fall can be a sign of inappropriate medication administration. Age-related diseases of the eye, eg, macular degeneration, glaucoma, and cataracts, further compromise visual function.

Presbycusis, a decline in auditory acuity with age, can precipitate a fall when an individual is unable to hear the warning sounds of an approaching car, for example, and therefore does not have enough time to avoid an accident.

Postural instability increases with age and is manifested by a loss of righting reflexes and an increase in body sway. The maintenance of postural stability is a complex function that requires appropriate central integration of visual, vestibular, and proprioceptive senses, all of which suffer functional decline with age. Reaction time also increases with age, lengthening the interval between perceiving danger and acting to avoid it.

Pathologic states: TABLE 7-2 lists the pathologic states that can contribute to falls.

Cerebrovascular and neurologic disease: A frank stroke or a transient ischemic attack can cause a fall due to loss of motor or sensory function

TABLE 7–2. PATHOLOGIC STATES THAT PREDISPOSE TO FALLS

Neurologic
  Stroke
  Transient ischemic attack
  Parkinsonism
  Confusion
  Myelopathy
  Seizures
  Vertebrobasilar insufficiency
  Carotid sinus supersensitivity
  Cerebellar disorders
  Neuropathy
  Dementia

Cardiovascular
  Myocardial infarction
  Orthostatic hypotension
  Arrhythmia

Gastrointestinal
  Bleeding
  Diarrhea
  Defecation syncope
  Postprandial syncope

Metabolic
  Hypothyroidism
  Hypoglycemia
  Anemia
  Hypokalemia
  Dehydration
  Hyponatremia

Genitourinary
  Micturition syncope
  Incontinence

Musculoskeletal
  Arthritis
  Myositis
  Spinal deformity
  Muscle weakness
  Deconditioning

Psychologic
  Depression
  Anxiety

Drug Induced
  Pathologic states attributable to
    diuretics, antihypertensives,
    cardiotonics, hypnotics, sedatives,
    and psychotropics

in a lower extremity, sudden change in visual perception, alteration in level of consciousness, or seizure. Cerebrovascular disease involving the posterior (cerebellar) circulation gives rise to dizziness and ataxia. Similarly, carotid sinus supersensitivity may cause a fall due to syncope. Finally, the residuals of a prior stroke, eg, hemiparesis, ataxia, etc, may predispose to falls.

Dementia: In patients with acute or chronic dementia, frequency of falling increases because of misperception of environmental dangers and of the individual's own capabilities.

Parkinson's disease or secondary parkinsonism is common and associated with gait disturbance and postural imbalance, its major clinical manifestations. In addition, parkinsonian patients are slower to react to dangers in the environment and are frequently receiving medication that can cause confusion or orthostatic hypotension, leading to falls. Some of the parkinsonian states are themselves associated with primary orthostatic hypotension.

Orthostatic hypotension is defined as a drop of 20 mm Hg in systolic BP or 10 mm Hg in diastolic BP between the supine and standing positions. A smaller drop can also be significant if the patient has associated dizziness. Diabetic patients are frequently prone to orthostatic hypotension secondary to autonomic nervous system dysfunction. Large varicosities may cause postural drops in BP resulting from blood pooling in the legs. Postural hypotension may occur in patients who try to get up after being immobilized for a time and in those with intercurrent illness, such as infection and heart failure.

Dehydration, hemorrhage, and Na loss all cause changes in blood volume that predispose to postural hypotension. In addition, **drug treatment** may lead to orthostatic hypotension. Antihypertensive drugs, diuretics, tricyclic antidepressants, phenothiazines, and alcohol have been implicated.

Disorders of vagal response: Cough or micturition syncope may be responsible for falls. Cough syncope results from paroxysms of coughing in patients with chronic lung disease or bronchitis. Micturition syncope occurs most frequently in men with benign prostatic hypertrophy when they get up during the night to urinate. Hyperventilation can also cause a vasovagal response and result in falls. In patients who are hyperventilating, the possibility of diabetic acidosis, pulmonary embolism, heart failure, or respiratory failure must be considered.

Arrhythmia: A fall that occurs abruptly, with or without loss of consciousness, or that is preceded by dizziness or palpitations suggests a **cardiac arrhythmia.** Such falls are sometimes associated with exercise or with standing, if the patient has aortic stenosis causing diminished cerebral perfusion. Other cardiovascular problems responsible for falls include **heart block, sick sinus syndrome,** and **bradycardia,** which may be induced by drugs (eg, digoxin and β-blockers).

A fall may be the first sign of MI. Silent heart attacks are common in the aged, especially in those with diabetes.

Premonitory falls: *Any fall must be considered a possible sign of impending major illness.* Falls may be caused by any acute or chronic disease that results in weakness or dizziness. For example, MI, cerebrovascular accident **(CVA),** or GI bleeding may initially present as a fall. Of particular importance is the problem of atypical presentation of an infection. The elderly have a diminished febrile response, so a fall may be the first sign of an underlying infection, particularly of the urinary or respiratory tract or gallbladder.

Seizure: Patients with a history of epilepsy or recent stroke and those taking certain drugs (eg, neuroleptics, antidepressants, and theophylline) are at risk for developing seizures with syncopal episodes. The possibility of seizure should always be considered if there is reason to suspect that the patient has had repeated unwitnessed falls with involuntary voiding, or has a history of previous CVA.

Impaired gait: A variety of arthritic and pathologic neuromuscular changes can impair gait and increase the risk of falling. A description of some abnormal gait patterns can be found under EVALUATION, below. For example, Parkinson's disease greatly affects postural stability. Patients with this disease assume a forward-leaning, flexed posture and a shuffling gait, with the feet lifted slightly off the ground. Any irregularity in the floors, such as a door threshold, a curb, or a thick carpet, can cause these patients to trip. Parkinsonian patients are also prone to fall when getting in and out of chairs and when turning, since postural stability is compromised.

Proximal muscle weakness secondary to hypokalemia, osteomalacia, hyper- and hypothyroidism, polymyalgia rheumatica, and osteoarthritis of the knee joints contribute to a slow, cautious, steady gait, accompanied by waddling, difficulty in climbing stairs, and a propensity to fall. Pernicious anemia can lead to a loss of vibratory and proprioceptive sensation, which can in turn lead to falling. Patients with a history of partial gastrectomy or poor nutritional intake are at risk for developing this condition. Physicians should routinely inspect patients' feet for deformities, such as corns, calluses, and bunions, which can lead to impaired gait and predispose to falling.

Drugs: Studies indicate that elderly people who are receiving drug therapy fall more often than those who are not. Polypharmacy associated with multiple diseases and age-associated susceptibility to drug toxicity can lead to poor coordination, confusion, and cardiac arrhythmias. As mentioned previously, certain drugs pose a high risk of postural hypotension. Steroids, when taken for long periods, can lead to proximal muscle weakness. In addition, chronic steroid use can cause osteoporosis, a major reason for hip fracture following a fall.

Psychologic factors: Falls can be associated with **denial of physical limitations** imposed by aging. Older people who have not accepted their declining sensory and motor capabilities tend to fall as a result of overestimating their ability to perform youthful activities. To maintain an image of capability and independence, a person may refuse to use assistive devices or to accept assistance in performing activities (eg, getting out of bed or going to the bathroom). Many falls occur during periods of transient emotional stress. Preoccupation with illness or family relationships, declining vision or hearing, and admission to a hospital or nursing home are common reasons for emotional upheaval. As a result, patients become angry, anxious, disoriented, or depressed, and less alert to environmental hazards. Additionally, their capacity to halt a fall-in-progress declines.

Older people with **depression** often become confused and disoriented and lack awareness of the environment, which can lead to falls. Drugs used to treat psychiatric disorders may cause falls, either by producing confusion, sedation, or postural hypotension, or by lowering the seizure threshold.

Extrinsic Causes

TABLE 7–3 lists environmental obstacles that can predispose the patient to falls. In the community setting, a majority of falls occur at home. Important locations include stairwells, bedrooms, and living rooms. Common activities relating to falls include getting into and out of beds and chairs; tripping over household objects or floor coverings, such as carpets, rugs, and door thresholds; and slipping on wet surfaces or while wearing improper shoes or descending stairs.

In the hospital and nursing home, the most common site for falls is the patient's room. Most of these falls occur at the bedside, while the patient is getting into or out of bed. In a number of studies, bed rails were in the up position during falls out of bed. The falls resulted from climbing over the rail or over the footboard. The bathroom is another high-risk location in institutions, presumably the result of patients'

TABLE 7–3. EXTRINSIC CAUSES OF FALLS

Ground Surfaces
  Slippery floors
  Glare from highly polished/waxed floors
  Loose rugs
  Thick pile carpet

Lighting
  Excessive glare
  Inadequate illumination

Stairs
  Lack of handrails
  Poor lighting
  High steps
  Worn stair treads

Bathroom
  Slippery floor
  Slippery bathtub or shower
  Lack of grab bars
  Low toilet seats

Bedroom
  High bed
  Bed too far from bathroom
  Inadequate lighting
  Loose rugs
  Nonlocking bed wheels

Other Rooms
  Slippery floors
  Chairs at incorrect height
  No armrests on chairs
  Shelving too high

transferring themselves on or off toilets while hurrying to use the facility or slipping on the wet floor.

Chairs and wheelchairs have been implicated in falling episodes because of inappropriately designed equipment or poor transfer technics while the patient is sitting or rising. Falling over chairs that are difficult to see, tripping over chair legs or wheelchair footrests, and failing to lock wheelchair brakes on rising are other causes of falls. A causal relationship between falls and assistive ambulatory devices, such as walkers and canes, has been suggested by some researchers, while others have found either a reduction in serious falls in patients using such devices or no relationship between the devices and falls.

The number of staff members present has been discussed as a factor relating to falls in institutions. However, the data are contradictory, with reports indicating increases, decreases, and no relationship between falls in institutions and the number of staff present.

The peak incidence of falls in the nursing home and hospital varies with the length of stay, but most falls occur during the first week of admission. This is presumably related to such factors as anxiety over the new environment and unfamiliarity with the spatial organization of the environment.

EVALUATION

TABLE 7–4 outlines the medical approach to the patient who falls. First and foremost, assess and treat any acute injury such as a fracture. Then determine the probable causes of the fall. The evaluation should start with a detailed history. Inquire about previous falls, when and where the fall occurred, whether any assistive devices (eg, canes, walkers, or wheelchairs) were in use at the time of the fall, whether any associated symptoms (eg, shortness of breath, palpitations, or loss of consciousness) were present, and what activity the patient was engaged in when he fell.

Recurrent falls sometimes follow an established pattern that helps reveal the causative factors. For example, if an individual consistently falls immediately after getting up and this is associated with the complaint of light-headedness or other type of dizziness, orthostatic hypotension is a significant possibility. If a patient persistently loses consciousness at about the time of the fall and has other symptoms, eg, loss of urine or tongue biting, a seizure should be considered.

In obtaining the history, it is important to *avoid* open-ended questions such as, "What happened?" Elderly patients may be unreliable about the history of the fall, and direct questions about specific symptoms usually elicit more precise information. In addition, the history should include present and past medical problems and drug use. In cases involving patients who have difficulty communicating, physicians should contact witnesses and family members concerning the specifics of the fall.

TABLE 7–4. EVALUATION OF THE FALL

Assessment and treatment of acute injury
History
  Activity at time of fall
  Premonitory symptoms—ie, dizziness, palpitations, dyspnea, chest pain, weakness,
    confusion, incontinence, loss of consciousness, tongue biting
  Location of fall
  Witnesses to fall
  History of previous falls (of same or different character)
  Past medical history
  Drug use

Physical examination (full physical with special emphasis on the following)
  BP and pulse, supine and standing
  Visual acuity, visual fields, low-vision evaluation
  Cardiovascular
    Arrhythmia, murmur, bruits
  Extremities
    Degenerative joint disease, varicose veins, edema, podiatric problems, poorly fitting
      shoes
  Neurologic
    Includes gait and balance assessment—ie, getting in/out of chair, walking, bending,
      turning, reaching, ascending and descending stairs, standing with eyes closed
      (Romberg test), sternal push

The physical examination should be comprehensive enough to rule out intrinsic causes of falling. Emphasis should be placed on examining the cardiovascular, musculoskeletal, and neurologic systems (see Table 7–4). It is essential to measure BP in both the supine and standing position to rule out orthostatic hypotension. The presence of an arrhythmia should be considered during cardiovascular examination. If a standard ECG fails to demonstrate an arrhythmia in the presence of suggestive symptoms, a 24-h ambulatory ECG is appropriate. Carotid bruits that may implicate transient ischemic attacks and any heart murmur that may indicate such conditions as aortic stenosis also should be considered.

Symptoms of **dizziness or unsteadiness** may sometimes be elicited by backward flexion of the neck, as when the individual is looking up to reach something on a high shelf. To prevent such symptoms, the patient should be advised to minimize backward head flexion. Frequently, cervical collars are recommended to reduce neck bending. In the home, placing commonly used items (eg, kitchen utensils and clothing) at eye level can be helpful.

The diagnosis of carotid sinus supersensitivity is supported by reproducing the symptoms with gentle carotid massage under ECG monitoring. Emergency services must, of course, be immediately available.

The extremities should be evaluated for degenerative joint disease that could impair gait and posture and for any specific podiatric problem that may cause falling. Neurologic examination should be comprehensive. Impaired judgment secondary to dementia, delirium, or depression may be at the root of the falls. Examination of visual and auditory systems helps determine if a neurosensory deficit has contributed to falling. In addition, visual field defects suggest a focal brain lesion. Nystagmus might point to either a predisposing peripheral vestibular or brainstem problem.

One-sided weakness or sensory loss might indicate a focal brain lesion. Paraparesis or quadriparesis, especially when a sensory level is found, indicates a spinal cord lesion. Mild bilateral weakness in association with loss of proprioceptive and vibratory sense in the legs is a common finding in cervical spondylosis with myelopathy. Other symptoms and signs include occipital headache, vertigo, and loss of deep tendon reflexes in the arms, with increased reflexes in the lower extremities.

Distal weakness with stocking and glove anesthesia and loss of deep tendon reflexes suggests a peripheral neuropathy, and one must suspect a diabetic, alcoholic, or nutritional etiology. Proximal muscle weakness, in the absence of sensory findings, suggests such disorders as myositis, polymyalgia rheumatica, hypothyroidism, and hypokalemia. Symmetric appendicular muscle weakness without sensory findings with or without bulbar musculature involvement suggests either myasthenia gravis or amyotrophic lateral sclerosis. In the latter condition, muscle wasting, muscle fasciculations, and weight loss are additional findings.

In Parkinson's disease, an alteration in muscle tone, giving rise to the cogwheel phenomenon, is accompanied by a slowing of body movements (bradykinesia) and an involuntary resting tremor of 1 or more limbs. Sensation is intact. The extrapyramidal disorder in dementias such as Alzheimer's disease simulates Parkinson's disease, although tremor is not common in the former. Response to dopaminergic agents usually aids in differentiation. Evaluation of coordinated movements may reveal an appendicular or truncal ataxia, indicating a cerebellar disorder. The hereditary spinocerebellar disorders with onset in the senium present as cerebellar ataxia associated with parkinsonian and myelopathic features. Evidence of neuropathy also may be present.

GAIT

Evaluation of the **gait pattern** often proves instrumental in diagnosing a neurologic disorder. In the **circumduction gait,** the lower extremity assumes triple extension at the hip, knee, and ankle, and the individual has to swing the leg in an outward arc to ensure ground clearance. This type of gait is seen in patients with hemiplegia from a stroke or other focal brain lesion. With bilateral upper motor neuron lesions, the individual may manifest a **scissoring gait,** which is essentially a bilateral circumduction gait. The **festinating gait** is a symmetric shuffling of the feet with poor ground clearance, typically seen in Parkinson's disease. Frequently, the festination is seen only at the initiation of gait and upon reaching an obstacle or attempting a turn.

In addition, the parkinsonian patient tends to assume a forward-flexed posture, with reduced or absent associated arm movements during walking. Severe postural instability in the parkinsonian patient will lead to an inability to maintain stance when pushed from the back or front by the examiner, known as propulsion and retropulsion, respectively.

The **cerebellar gait** is broad-based with irregularity of steps. The patient veers to either side, forward, or backward. In severe cases, he will not be able to stand unsupported, even with the eyes open. This form of ataxia is common in chronic alcoholics and in patients with degenerative brain processes, such as the spinocerebellar atrophies or progressive supranuclear palsy. Multiple sclerosis and cerebellar tumors should be considered as well. The acute onset of such an ataxia in an older individual is almost always of vascular cause.

Frontal lobe apraxia causes a mild, broad-based gait that in other respects resembles the parkinsonian gait. The individual assumes a forward-flexed posture, and the steps are short, slow, and shuffling. The feet at times appear to be glued to the floor. At the same time, however, examination at the bedside will reveal normal power in the extremities, and the patient may be able to perform complex movements with the legs, such as drawing a figure 8 on the ground. Normal-pressure hydrocephalus **(NPH)** is a prime example of a neurologic disorder causing this type of gait. The gait disorder frequently precedes the dementia and incontinence that complete the NPH triad. Since the condition is potentially treatable with a shunt procedure, clinical suspicion should remain high in a patient with an apraxic gait.

Senile gait is a milder form of frontal lobe apraxia, manifested by a flexed posture, with short, shuffling steps that are especially prominent on making turns. These patients are particularly prone to retropulsion while making a turn. This gait is also known as a marche petit pas. Patients with this gait do not respond to antiparkinsonian drugs.

Sensory ataxia is a broad-based, foot-stamping gait. The individual constantly looks at his feet as he walks to compensate for lack of proprioceptive input with visual input. When asked to stand with his feet together, the patient is able to maintain stance with his eyes open. As his eyes are closed, however, he loses his balance. This is the positive Romberg test. In the elderly, the condition is caused by disorders affecting the posterior columns, such as vitamin B_{12} deficiency (posterolateral sclerosis), cervical spondylosis, and spinocerebellar degeneration. A **waddling gait** is usually seen in cases of severe degenerative disease of the hips or severe proximal muscle weakness, as in myositis or polymyalgia rheumatica.

In addition to observation for specific gait disorders, a performance-oriented mobility evaluation should be conducted. The patient should be observed performing activities of daily living (eg, getting into and out of a chair, turning around, bending down and picking up objects from the floor, reaching up to get something from a shelf, and descending or ascending stairs). Aside from documenting abnormalities that might not have been apparent on routine inspection of gait (eg, a proximal muscle weakness that may be apparent only when the subject is asked to bend), one may also gain an impression of the degree of daily living disability engendered by the disease process. This allows a better rehabilitation plan.

Laboratory examination need not be extensive but should be based on information obtained from the history and physical examination. For instance, an individual with physical evidence of orthostatic hypotension requires a CBC to rule out anemia and biochemical determinations for possible electrolyte or volume disturbance. An individual with cardiac symptoms at the time of the fall requires an ECG and possibly 24-h monitoring. Patients with focal neurologic signs or symptoms, or those suspected of having had a seizure, require an EEG and possibly a CT scan of the head. TABLE 7–5 lists these laboratory procedures and the diagnoses they attempt to elucidate.

Treatment

Since most falls involve many etiologic factors, the management plan should include an approach to both intrinsic and extrinsic causes. For example, a patient with Parkinson's disease may improve with dopaminergic drugs but continue to fall while at home if there are loose rugs and/or high door thresholds. Management of an intrinsic disorder will depend on the diagnosis. Recurrent transient ischemic attacks may respond to aspirin. Minimizing neck movement with a cervical collar may prevent vestibular symptoms.

Patients with orthostatic hypotension should sleep with the head of the bed slightly elevated and should dangle their legs over the edge for a few minutes before standing up to minimize sudden postural changes. Support stockings also may help. In severe cases, mineralocorticoids may be advised for orthostatic hypotension. Muscle weakness related to electrolyte or thyroid disturbance should respond to specific medical management. Transient arrhythmias may respond to medication or pacemaker implantation.

Patients with a neurologic dysfunction and associated gait disorder may benefit from management by rehabilitation experts such as physical and occupational therapists. Attempts should be made to correct or at least ameliorate any neurosensory deficits (eg, by provision of visual aids, cataract surgery, and hearing aids, as appropriate).

Attention to potential environmental obstacles is essential. This is especially important for persons with multiple chronic ailments, for whom the only workable approach is reduction of exposure to high-risk situations. Management includes environmental assessment, correction of potential hazards, and use of devices and furniture that minimize risk. Evaluation of the home environment will identify many potential hazards, with some presenting greater risk for a specific individual than others. A patient home-assessment checklist is presented in TABLE 7–6.

TABLE 7–5. LABORATORY PROCEDURES

Common Tests	Diagnosis
CBC	Anemia Infection
Biochemical determinations	Hyponatremia Hypoglycemia Hypokalemia Dehydration
Cardiac enzymes	Silent MI
Thyroid functions	Hypo- or hyperthyroidism
B_{12} level	Pernicious anemia
ESR	Myositis Polymyalgia rheumatica
ECG or Holter monitor	Arrhythmia
EEG	Seizure Metabolic encephalopathy
CT scan of head	Stroke Focal brain lesion Hydrocephalus Cerebellar degeneration
Less Common Procedures	Diagnosis
Myelogram or MRI of spine	Myelopathy
Electromyogram (EMG)	Peripheral neuropathy Neuromuscular disease
Echocardiogram	Valvular disease Mural thrombus
Noninvasive carotid studies	Extracranial cerebrovascular disease
Transcranial Doppler studies	Intracranial cerebrovascular disease

The patient should be observed walking from room to room and over different floor surfaces; climbing and descending stairs; transferring to and from beds, chairs, and toilets; getting into and out of bathtubs and showers; and reaching up and bending down to obtain objects in closets and from kitchen shelves. Environmental obstacles should be noted and corrective actions recommended. Principles of safety and function should prevail over esthetic appeal when selecting furniture, lighting, ground surfaces, and assistive devices.

TABLE 7–6. HOME-ASSESSMENT CHECKLIST FOR FALL HAZARDS

Area	Correction	Rationale
General Household		
Lighting		
Too dim	Provide ample lighting in all areas	Increased illumination improves visual acuity
Too direct, creating glare	Reduce glare with evenly distributed light, indirect lighting, translucent shades	
Light switches inaccessible	Install so they are immediately accessible on entering room	Reduces risk of falling when walking across darkened room
Carpets, rugs		
Torn	Repair or replace torn carpet	Prevent tripping and slipping by persons with decreased stepping-ability
Slippery	Provide rugs with nonskid backs; tack down to prevent curling	
Furniture		
Obstructs path	Arrange furnishings so that pathways are not obstructed; avoid cluttered hallways	Aids mobility in persons with impaired peripheral vision
Chairs, tables		
Unstable	Must be stable enough to support weight of person leaning on table edges or chair arms and backs	Balance-impaired persons use furniture for support
Lack of armrests	Provide chairs with armrests that extend forward enough for leverage in getting up or sitting down	Assists persons with proximal muscle weakness
Low-back chairs	High back provides support for neck and while transferring weight	Parkinsonian patients often begin rocking movement to assist in getting up; high chair back prevents falling backward
Heating		
Too cool	Maintain temperature at 72 F in winter	Prevents falls secondary to hypothermia

(Continued)

(Adapted from R. Tideiksaar: "Preventing falls: Home hazard checklist to help older patients protect themselves," in *Geriatrics,* Vol. 41, pp. 26–28, 1986. Reproduced with the permission of *Geriatrics.*)

TABLE 7–6. HOME-ASSESSMENT CHECKLIST FOR FALL HAZARDS
(Cont'd)

Area	Correction	Rationale
Kitchen		
Cabinets, shelves		
Too high	Keep frequently used items at waist level; install shelves, cupboards at accessible height	Reduces risk of falling because of frequent reaching or standing on unstable ladders or chairs
Floor		
Wet or waxed	Place rubber mat on floor in sink area; wear rubber-soled shoes in kitchen; use nonslip wax or buff paste wax thoroughly	Prevents slipping, especially if gait-impaired
Gas range		
Dial difficult to see	Clearly mark "on" and "off" positions on dials	Prevents a fall from being first sign of gas asphyxiation, especially if sense of smell is impaired
Chair		
Armrests lacking	Provide chairs with armrests and sturdy legs	Armrests assist in transfer
Legs unsound	Avoid chairs with wheels; repair legs that are loose	Sturdy, stable chairs do not slide away when transferring
Table		
Wobbly, unstable	Install table with sturdy legs of even length; avoid tripod or pedestal tables	Gait-impaired persons often use table for support
Bathroom		
Bathtub		
Slippery tub floor	Install skid-resistant strips or rubber mat; use shower shoes or bath seat	Prevents sliding on wet tub floor; if balance is impaired, sitting while showering prevents falls
Side of bathtub used for support or transfer	Use portable grab bar on side of tub	Aids transfers; portable grab bar can be taken along on travels
Towel racks, sink tops		
Unstable for use as support while transferring from toilet	Fix grab rails into wall studs next to toilet	Aids transfer to and from toilet

(Continued)

TABLE 7–6. HOME-ASSESSMENT CHECKLIST FOR FALL HAZARDS
(Cont'd)

Area	Correction	Rationale
Bathroom (cont'd)		
Toilet seat		
Too low	Use elevated toilet seat	Aids transfer to and from toilet
Medicine cabinet		
Inadequate lighting	Install brighter lighting	Helps avoid incorrect administration of medication, especially in visually impaired
Drugs improperly labeled	Label all drugs according to need for internal or external use; keep magnifying glass in or near cabinet	
Door		
Locks	Avoid locks on bathroom doors, or use only locks that can be opened from both sides of door	Permits access by others if fall occurs
Stairways		
Height		
Rise between steps is too high	Should be maximum of 6 in.	Reduces risk of tripping for persons with decreased stepping-ability height
Handrails		
Missing	Install and anchor well on both sides of stairway; use cylindric rails placed 1 to 2 in. away from wall	Ease of grasping with either hand
Improper length	Extend beyond top and bottom step, and turn ends inward	Signals that top or bottom step has been reached
Configuration		
Too steep, or too long	Provide stairways with intermediate landings	Rest stop especially convenient for cardiac or pulmonary patients
Condition		
Slippery	Place nonskid treads securely on all steps	Prevents slipping
Lighting		
Inadequate	Install adequate lighting at both top and bottom stairway; night lights or bright-colored adhesive strips can be used to clearly mark steps	Outlines location of steps, especially for persons with vision or perception impairment

Seven major environmental areas that contribute to falls are ground surfaces, lighting, stairs, bathrooms, beds, chairs, and shelves. Obstacles to safety in these areas should be identified and eliminated through environmental modification. **Ground surfaces** should not be wet or highly waxed. Thick pile carpet or area rugs without nonstick backings should be avoided. All **lighting** should be controlled by easily accessible wall switches. The color of the light-switch plates should contrast with the color of the wall to allow for easy visibility. Glare from sunlight through a window or from highly polished floors should be eliminated.

Stairways should be adequately illuminated; light switches should be positioned at both the top and bottom of the staircase. The placement of night lights by the first and last steps provides additional visual cues in darkness. Placing nonslip adhesive strips parallel to the step edges helps define the steps. Installation of handrails on both sides of the stairs helps older persons negotiate the stairs safely. The handrails should be round, located on the wall, approximately 30 in. higher than the stairs and set out far enough from the wall to allow for a good grasp. The ends of the handrails should be specially shaped to signal that the top or bottom of the stairs has been reached. Worn step runners and carpet should be repaired or replaced.

In **the bathroom,** towel bars should be replaced with nonslip grab bars. The grab bars must be securely fixed to the studs of the walls so they will not easily give way. The use of adjustable, raised toilet seats and toilet grab bars or grab bars located on the wall next to the toilet helps to minimize falls. Slip-resistant grab bars should be installed on the bathtub rim and in the shower. Nonslip adhesive rubber strips or a rubber mat with suction cups should be attached to the shower and bathtub floors. Tub or shower chairs or benches should be used if the patient lacks the power or the endurance to stand for long periods of time or to get up from a supine position.

The patient may fall while getting on and off **beds** that are too high or too low. A bed height of approximately 18 in. from the top of the mattress to the floor allows for safe transfer. **Chair** heights should be adjusted to ensure that when the patient is seated, his feet are firmly planted on the floor with knees flexed at 90°. Armrests should be horizontally placed approximately 7 in. above the seat and should extend beyond the seat edge by 1 to 2 in. to allow for maximal leverage.

Shelves that are too high or too low may contribute to the patient's loss of balance when he reaches up or bends down to retrieve objects. Frequently used items should be placed at levels that allow the person to avoid excessive bending, reaching, or climbing. Shelf storage in kitchens and closets should be between hip and eye level. The use of handheld "reachers" or grabbing devices allows the patient to reach objects from high or low places without compromising safety.

8. FRACTURES

Tobin N. Gerhart

Fractures are a major cause of morbidity and mortality in the elderly, differing in frequency, anatomic location within the bone, and fracture pattern from those found in a younger population. Most result from low-energy injuries and involve bone weakened by osteoporosis or other pathologic processes. The prognosis for uncomplicated healing also differs in elderly patients, who have a greater tendency to develop joint stiffness with immobilization and are at higher risk for medical complications with enforced bed rest. In order to avoid these complications and in view of their shorter anticipated life span, treatment goals in the elderly emphasize a rapid return to activities necessary for independent living rather than a more nearly perfect long-term result following prolonged casting or traction.

Most elderly persons need not perform strenuous work, and high-strength functional capabilities are not a priority. Because they place less stress on the musculoskeletal system, elderly people often do well with a fracture alignment or a prosthetic replacement that would be unsuitable in younger patients.

Descriptive and Anatomic Terms

A typical long bone is divided into 3 anatomic regions: (1) The **diaphysis,** or shaft, consists of a tube of cortical bone surrounding a medullary cavity of hematopoietic or fatty marrow; (2) the **epiphysis** lies at the end of the bone between the growth plate, or physis, and the articular surface; (3) the **metaphysis** is the intermediate, flared region joining the other 2. The skeleton consists of 2 forms of bone: **trabecular** and **cortical.** Trabecular, or porous, bone comprises most of the metaphysis and epiphysis. It varies widely in density and strength, depending on its skeletal location, the patient's age, and associated pathologic conditions (eg, osteoporosis). Cortical, or lamellar, bone comprises the diaphysis. Its dense histologic architecture of parallel haversian systems gives it great strength.

Standard terminology facilitates description of fracture patterns. Proximal, midshaft, or distal describes the location of a fracture. The orientation of a fracture line may be transverse, oblique, or spiral. Comminution refers to fragmentation. Open or closed indicates whether or not the fracture communicates to the outside through a soft tissue wound. (The archaic terms "simple" and "compound" should be avoided.) Alignment refers to the relative position of the main fracture fragments. Their apex may point anteriorly, posteriorly, laterally (varus angulation), or medially (valgus angulation). The bone ends may be overriding, distracted, or impacted.

Incidence and Epidemiology (see also Ch. 96)

About 225,000 hip fractures occur each year, with a large majority in persons > 70 yr old. As the population ages, the problem grows. One third of women and ¹/₆ of men who live to age 90 will sustain a hip fracture. There is an excess mortality rate of 12 to 20% during the first year following hip fracture. Of functionally independent patients who live at home prefracture, 15 to 25% will require institutional care for > 1 yr and another 25 to 30% will become dependent on mechanical aids or assistive personnel. The incidence of osteoporotic fractures occurring in the distal radius and in the spine during 1985 was estimated to be 172,000 and 538,000, respectively.

Only certain kinds of fractures increase in incidence with advancing age. Long-bone shaft fractures involve predominantly cortical bone and bear no positive correlation with age. In contrast, vertebral body and hip fractures have a low incidence until the 5th and 6th decades, when they increase dramatically. Fractures of the proximal humerus, wrist, tibia, and pubic rami follow a similar pattern. The sites of all of these fractures involve predominantly trabecular bone.

Etiology and Pathophysiology

Falls are the most common cause of fractures, accounting for an estimated 90% of geriatric hip, forearm, and pelvic fractures. The frequency of falling among the elderly is due in part to a high incidence of underlying medical conditions: failing vision, neurologic diseases and their sequelae, arthritis that impairs lower limb function, and the use of sedatives and other medications. In addition, slowed reflexes, decreased muscle strength, and impaired coordination may reduce the older patient's ability to dissipate the impact of a fall, thereby increasing the likelihood of fracture. Thus, most fractures in the elderly result from the relatively low-energy trauma incurred by a fall on level ground.

Biomechanics

The force required to break a bone depends on both its material properties and its geometry. Material properties determine the force per unit area required to cause failure of the material. These properties are referred to as ultimate tensile or ultimate compressive strength (expressed in metric units in megapascals [MPa], with 1 MPa equal to 145 lb/sq in.). The ultimate tensile strength of cortical bone decreases only slightly with aging from about 140 MPa in the 2nd decade to about 120 MPa in the 8th decade. Remodeling of the diaphysis occurs with aging, causing it to enlarge in cross section. Bone is resorbed from the inner, or endosteal, surface and is added to the outer, or periosteal, surface. This redistribution increases the resistance of the diaphysis to bending forces and compensates for the decrease in strength of the cortical bone. Thus fractures of the diaphysis do not occur more frequently with advancing age.

The ultimate compressive strength of trabecular bone is proportional to the density² and ranges between 1 and 10 MPa. Since normal cancellous bone has a density > 1.4 gm/cm^3, a density of 1 gm/cm^3 represents a halving of strength. Reduction in density cannot be detected on ordinary x-rays until at least 25% of bone mineral is lost. Fractures of the vertebrae and ends of the femur do not occur until bone density falls below a threshold of 1 gm/cm^3. Most fractures in the elderly occur in the metaphyseal region, which does not remodel with age and thus does not compensate for the decreased density of the trabecular bone.

Pathologic fracture refers to *any fracture involving abnormal (ie, weakened) bone,* eg, from underlying malignancy, benign bone tumor, metabolic disorder, infection, or osteoporosis. Thus any patient who presents with a fracture after minimal trauma must be suspected of having a pathologic fracture. There is usually a history of progressively increasing pain in the affected region, especially noticeable at night and on weight bearing. Diagnosis is important, since choice of treatment and prognosis for healing can be greatly altered, depending on the underlying pathologic condition.

Frequently, patients present with an impending pathologic fracture in which the bone has not yet broken entirely. Such patients have pain in the affected area associated with use of the limb. Rising out of a chair, for instance, can cause thigh pain in a patient with a lesion of the femur. Prophylactic internal fixation of such fractures with metal plates, rods, or prostheses is often indicated to prevent displacement, to provide pain relief, and to permit the patient to remain functional. If the impending fracture breaks through completely and becomes displaced, treatment is considerably more difficult, with increased morbidity and a poorer functional result.

Malignancy: Metastatic lesions account for most skeletal malignancies, with breast, lung, prostate, GI tract, kidney, and thyroid being the most common primary sites. The typical x-ray shows multiple lytic lesions. All can produce lucencies on x-ray; prostatic and breast metastases may also produce sclerosis. **Primary bone malignancies** occur with much less frequency. Multiple myeloma and lymphoma are the most common; osteosarcoma, fibrosarcoma, and chondrosarcoma are rare.

Osteopenia refers to abnormally decreased bone density. It is caused by 4 conditions that are indistinguishable on x-ray but involve different pathologic processes: **osteoporosis,** due to too little bone; **osteomalacia,** due to decreased mineralization; **hyperparathyroidism,** due to increased resorption; and **myeloma,** due to bone destruction by tumor. Consequently, patients with osteopenia require laboratory evaluation to exclude underlying endocrine or renal diseases. A thorough screening includes a CBC, ESR, serum Ca, P, alkaline phosphatase, BUN, blood glucose, SGOT, T$_4$, and serum immunoelectrophoretic studies. A bone scan may also be indicated. Osteoporosis causes no abnormal test results. It is most accurately detected and measured by specialized scanning technics, including photon absorptiometry and quantitative CT scanning. Because osteoporosis is so prevalent in the elderly, it is not considered a pathologic process in the usual sense. It has been estimated that about 90% of women > 75 yr of age have osteoporosis affecting the lumbar spine.

Normal Fracture Healing

Clinical management of fractures is based on an understanding of the physiology of bone repair. Fracture healing can be divided temporally into 3 overlapping phases: inflammation, repair, and remodeling. The inflammatory phase includes the initial response to injury and lasts for several days. The trauma that fractures the bone also injures the surrounding blood vessels, muscles, and other soft tissues. Hemorrhage at the fracture site forms a hematoma. Traumatic devascularization of the fractured ends and bony fragments results in nonviable or necrotic bone. All of this necrotic material elicits an immediate and intense acute inflammatory reaction. Clinically, the fracture site is swollen and tender. The reparative phase begins within 24 h postinjury and reaches peak activity after 1 to 2 wk.

Diaphyseal fractures that are not rigidly stabilized heal by formation around the fracture site of rapidly created new bone called the **external callus.** External callus is not visible radiographically until about 3 to 6 wk postinjury. Until sufficient external callus forms and provides stability—a process that can take several months in long-bone fractures—collapse and displacement of the fracture can occur. Metaphyseal fractures heal by direct union of the trabecular bone, a faster process that begins to occur within 2 to 3 wk. During the remodeling phase, the rapidly laid-down initial callus is slowly resorbed and replaced by mechanically stronger bone distributed to best resist load-bearing stresses. The events proceed slowly in the elderly and may account for many months of discomfort after a fracture.

DIAGNOSIS: GENERAL PRINCIPLES

Physical Examination

Most fractures are evident, due to swelling, deformity, or pain on attempted movement. Minimally displaced, stress, or impending fractures cause tenderness on palpation and pain on weight bearing or loading of the involved bone. In noncommunicative patients, refusal to move an extremity may be the only sign of a fracture or dislocation. Careful assessment of the sensory, motor, and circulatory status of the injured extremity is important prior to initiation of therapy. After application of a cast, splint, or traction or after manipulation of a fractured extremity, the neurovascular status of the limb should always be reevaluated.

When injury or lack of patient cooperation makes physical examination unreliable, x-rays are required to detect a fracture. For instance, the presence of a hip fracture can prevent an adequate examination of the contralateral leg because of pain caused by motion. Because coexisting injuries are not uncommon, the physician should obtain x-rays of both hips and the pelvis in all patients with a femoral or pelvic fracture to avoid missing additional injury.

Joint aspiration is a useful diagnostic and therapeutic maneuver in patients with suspected hemarthrosis. Acute effusion secondary to gout, pseudogout, or infection can be suggested by appearance of the fluid and confirmed by laboratory tests. Aspiration of blood confirms that an intra-articular injury (eg, fracture or torn ligament or meniscus) has occurred. The presence of fat globules admixed with blood, which can be seen easily when the aspirate is viewed in an open container, implies the existence of a fracture that allows fat from the marrow cavity to enter the joint.

X-rays

Routine x-ray evaluation of suspected fractures should always include both AP and lateral views. On a single view, the characteristic displacement, discontinuity in contour, or altered alignment of a fracture may be hidden because of overlap or projection. When standard views are equivocal, as sometimes occurs with minimally displaced spiral fractures, oblique views can be helpful. The trap of restricting the initial x-rays to too small an area should be avoided, since musculoskeletal pain is often referred or poorly localized. A patient complaining of thigh and knee pain, for instance, may actually have a hip fracture that would be missed unless x-rays of the entire femur were taken.

CT is a useful adjunct to plain x-rays in several circumstances. It allows visualization of occult fractures, particularly in areas in which difficulties arise because of overlying bony structures (eg, the cervical spine). CT is helpful in determining the extent to which articular surfaces have been disrupted in joint fractures and is also valuable in assessing suspected pathologic fractures for the presence of bone destruction and soft tissue masses.

Bone Scan

Total-body scanning, using ^{99m}Tc-labeled pyrophosphate or similar radioactive analogs, is performed to detect focal injury to bone from any cause. Uptake occurs wherever there is new bone formation (eg, in response to infection, arthritis, tumor, or fracture). A bone scan can reveal occult fractures not yet detectable on plain x-rays and is useful to differentiate conditions that mimic fractures by presenting with acute pain and swelling (eg, osteomyelitis and osteonecrosis). Patients with suspected pathologic fractures require bone scans for evaluation of metastatic and metabolic bone disease, both of which are evidenced by involvement of areas other than the fracture site.

Blood Tests

Measurement of the Hct is the most widely used clinical test for evaluating blood loss due to fractures. A 3 mL/dL drop in Hct corresponds to the loss of roughly 500 mL (1 u.) of blood in a normally hydrated patient. Patients with *acute* bleeding or dehydration may have a falsely normal or elevated Hct that falls when intravascular volume is replenished with IV fluids. Since elderly patients are generally at high risk for development of myocardial ischemia, their RBC volume should not be allowed to drop below a level suitable to maintain sufficient O_2 carrying capacity. As a clinical guideline, an Hct < 30 mL/dL indicates the need for blood transfusion, especially preoperatively. In hip fracture patients, the Hct should be monitored for at least 4 days following injury or surgery, since a 4- to 8-mL/dL drop can occur because of equilibration or continued bleeding.

A low Hct can also be a warning sign of a serious underlying medical condition with important implications in the fracture patient. For instance, GI bleeding can be exacerbated by anticoagulants routinely given to immobilized patients for prophylaxis of deep venous thrombosis **(DVT)**. Anemia may be the first sign of multiple myeloma or other malignancy that has weakened a bone enough to permit the occurrence of pathologic fracture.

Serum alkaline phosphatase is elevated when there is increased bone turnover. This occurs with normal fracture healing but may also indicate a malignancy or metabolic abnormality (eg, Paget's disease). The serum Ca is elevated with endocrine disturbances (eg, hyperparathyroidism) and with metastatic disease, especially breast carcinoma. When patients with Paget's disease are placed on bed rest, excessively rapid bone resorption can also elevate the serum Ca.

TREATMENT PRINCIPLES

Initial Immobilization of Fractures

Initial immobilization of injured extremities is important to prevent further damage before definitive stabilization can be achieved. Movement of sharp fracture ends can cause serious soft tissue trauma and even puncture the skin, converting a closed injury to an open one. Immobilization also aids patient transport and relieves pain, thus decreasing the need for narcotic analgesics.

Injuries located about or distal to the knee or elbow can usually be immobilized initially with splints. A wide variety of splints are available, including those made of preformed aluminum or plastic, inflatable clear plastic, and those that are easily adjustable with Velcro® closures. Plaster of Paris splints molded individually for each patient are perhaps the most comfortable for long-term use. All splints are best applied by an assistant while the injured extremity is held with gentle longitudinal traction.

Most injuries of the shoulder, upper arm, and elbow can be immobilized effectively by use of a sling. If further restraint is required, the arm can be kept close to the body by adding an elastic wrap or swath. Hip fractures can be immobilized by careful positioning with pillows or by light skin traction. Use of pillows beyond several days should be avoided to minimize risk of contracture.

Casts are used to control the alignment of a fracture while healing occurs. Traditionally, casts are made of rolls of stiff muslin impregnated with plaster of Paris (Ca sulfate hemihydrate). Inexpensive and easy to mold, plaster is often used for initial casts and for those that need frequent changing. Plaster casts are relatively heavy, deteriorate with excessive or prolonged use, and weaken if they become wet. Casting materials made of polymeric resins and fiberglass have recently been introduced. They are stronger, stiffer, and $1/2$ as heavy as plaster casts. Water will not weaken the cast itself, but if the underlying padding becomes wet, the cast must be changed to prevent skin maceration.

To provide effective immobilization, the cast must extend across 1 joint above and 1 joint below the fracture site. Thus for a distal radial fracture, the cast should theoretically extend from above the elbow to just proximal to the metatarsal joint. Because joint stiffness is a major problem in the elderly, this rule is often compromised by ending the cast below the elbow to allow joint motion.

Patients with casts must be given careful instructions. For the first 24 to 48 h postinjury, the casted limb should be elevated to prevent swelling. Rhythmic flexion and extension of the fingers or wiggling of the toes is encouraged to facilitate venous return. Progressive or unrelenting pain, pressure, or numbness in the casted extremity should be reported immediately. Swelling of an extremity within an unyielding circular cast can cause pressures high enough to stop tissue perfusion, thus creating a compartment syndrome (see below).

Traction is used in the elderly only when no satisfactory alternative exists. This may occur if the fracture is too fragmented for a cast or surgical stabilization or if the patient's medical condition will not permit an operation. Complications associated with traction include pressure sores, DVT, depression, disorientation, loss of appetite, atelectasis, and pulmonary infection. Meticulous, aggressive nursing care is required.

Skin traction is particularly hazardous in the elderly. Its only indication is to provide temporary, gentle restraint of the limb for comfort; > 5 lb should never be used. This is applied through foam boots or carefully wrapped moleskin strips. Vigilant monitoring is required. The strong and prolonged traction required to maintain the position of a fracture must be applied through skeletal pins. The proximal tibia is the preferred traction pin site for femoral and acetabular fractures.

Operative stabilization of fractures can offer compelling benefits in elderly patients. The risks of surgery are usually outweighed by the likelihood of complications resulting from enforced bed rest, especially with lower-extremity fractures, in which nonoperative treatment would entail a prolonged period of immobility. Patients with hip fractures, for instance, can usually begin ambulating within days after surgical stabilization.

Despite these advantages, surgical treatment of most fractures should be postponed until acute medical problems can be corrected. Only fractures associated with such limb-threatening conditions as an impending compartment syndrome, neurovascular compromise, or open wounds require urgent treatment. Furthermore, some conditions are relative contraindications to surgery. The presence of sepsis that could infect the operative site prohibits the use of metallic implants. Severely osteoporotic bone with poor mechanical properties is also a relative contraindication to internal fixation, since the hardware will become displaced if it cannot obtain a secure hold in the bone.

A deep postoperative wound infection is a serious complication that frequently necessitates removal of all implanted hardware, prolonged daily dressing changes, and weeks of IV antibiotics. Studies have shown that the use of prophylactic antibiotics can reduce the incidence of postoperative infections in hip fracture patients to about 1%. A cephalosporin is currently the agent of choice. An appropriate regimen is 1 gm cefazolin given IV during the hour prior to surgery, followed by 1 gm q 8 h for the next 24 h.

Ambulatory Aids (see Ch. 23)

COMPLICATIONS OF FRACTURES

Compartment Syndromes

A closed-space, or compartment, syndrome is the most frequent limb-threatening complication associated with extremity trauma. Swelling of injured muscle within a confined compartment surrounded by an unyielding envelope, such as fascia or a cast, can lead to elevated tissue pressures that block normal perfusion of the limb. The resulting tissue ischemia leads to further muscle injury and swelling and higher tissue pressures. The only solution to this ever-intensifying cycle is to completely remove all confining envelopes around the swollen muscular compartment. This means that casts, splints, and dressings should be thoroughly loosened immediately in all patients complaining of increasing pain or distal numbness in an immobilized, injured extremity. If the muscle swelling has increased to the point that the surrounding fascia has become a constricting envelope, an emergency fasciotomy must be performed. Even a few hours of muscle ischemia can lead to irreversible injury and necrosis.

The most reliable clinical signs of impending compartment syndrome are progressively increasing pain in an immobilized extremity, pain with passive flexion or extension of the toes or fingers, and numbness in a specific peripheral nerve distribution. The presence of pulses distally in a limb provides no assurance that a compartment syndrome has not developed. Muscle necrosis and irreversible nerve damage occur at tissue pressures much lower than those required to obliterate arterial inflow.

Thromboembolism

Pulmonary emboli are the most frequent fatal complications following lower-extremity trauma. By clinical diagnosis, about 50% of untreated hip fracture patients develop DVT; about 10%, pulmonary emboli; and in about 2%, the pulmonary emboli are fatal. The major predisposing factors for DVT are advanced age, trauma or surgery involving the lower extremities, history of DVT, immobilization, malignancy, and obesity. Sole reliance on clinical findings (eg, complaints of pain, swelling, tenderness, Homans' sign [pain on forced dorsiflexion of the foot], fever, and leukocytosis) leads to marked underdiagnosis of DVT. Only 5 to 30% of DVT cases can be detected by physical examination alone. By autopsy diagnosis, in 38% of patients who died after hip fracture, the cause of death was pulmonary emboli. Without autopsy, only 2% of patients dying after hip fracture were thought to have had fatal pulmonary embolism.

Ideally, thromboembolic disease should be treated prophylactically with anticoagulation begun at the **time of admission.** Studies in elective surgical patients show that 50% of thromboses develop by the end of an operation. For orthopedic patients at high risk for DVT (eg, those with hip fractures), warfarin and dextran are considered the most effective prophylactic agents. Neither aspirin, low-dose heparin, nor external pneumatic boot compression has been shown to provide as much protection. Anticoagulation should be started immediately upon hospitalization and continued until the patient is fully ambulatory. The initial dose of warfarin should be between 2.5 and 10 mg, depending on the patient's age and weight. Subsequently, daily doses are given with a goal of maintaining the prothrombin time in a range 1.5 times normal. Because GI, wound, CNS, and other bleeding complications can occur, a history of any of these is a relative contraindication to anticoagulation.

Fat Embolism Syndrome

Although microscopic fat emboli accompany most femoral fractures, overt symptoms and signs develop in only about 2%. Usually occurring 2 to 3 days after fracture, **fat embolism syndrome** presents with at least 1 of the following major signs: respiratory insufficiency, cerebral signs of drowsiness and confusion, or petechial rash. Minor signs include pyrexia, tachycardia, retinal changes, jaundice, renal changes, thrombocytopenia, and elevated ESR. Typically, chest x-ray shows variable streaks and infiltrates associated with overt pulmonary edema in $1/3$ of patients. Mild elevations in prothrombin time and activated partial thromboplastin time are also present. In some, the **adult respiratory distress syndrome (ARDS)** with noncardiac pulmonary edema and clinically significant **disseminated intravascular coagulation** may occur, or a **hyperacute syndrome** may result in death secondary to emboli to the coronary arteries and brain.

Treatment of fat embolism syndrome is aimed at respiratory support. Corticosteroids have been used in many cases, although their efficacy is unproved. The mortality rate is approximately 8%, compared to a 50% mortality associated with most other causes of ARDS.

Specific Fractures

Fractures of the proximal humerus, distal radius, pelvic rami, proximal femur, proximal tibia, and thoracic and lumbar vertebral bodies occur with disproportionate frequency in the elderly. These sites involve predominantly trabecular bone, often seriously weakened by osteoporosis. With the exception of hip fractures, most are treated nonoperatively. Nonetheless, rehabilitation is often prolonged and incomplete (see also Ch. 23). Usually, several months to a year pass before patients regain their preinjury capabilities.

PROXIMAL HUMERUS FRACTURES

Symptoms, Signs, and Diagnosis

The most common mechanism of injury is a fall on the outstretched hand. Patients present with shoulder pain and inability to move one arm. On x-ray, the proximal humerus may show as many as 4 separate fragments: eg, an articular fragment containing the humeral head, greater and lesser tuberosity fragments, and a distal fragment including the humeral shaft. These fragments are prone to displacement due to the pull of the supraspinatus, subscapularis, and pectoralis muscles. Fortunately, about 80% of proximal humeral fractures are minimally displaced, with < 45° angulation and < 1 cm displacement of any fragment. When displaced, the articular fragment may not lie in a satisfactory position above the humeral shaft on AP and lateral x-rays. Displaced fractures are classified according to increasing order of severity into 2-, 3-, and 4-part patterns. Those associated with a glenohumeral dislocation are usually the result of major trauma and constitute the most severe injuries.

Treatment and Prognosis

Treatment and prognosis depend upon the number of fracture fragments and the extent of displacement. Patients should be told to expect considerable swelling and discoloration in the lower arm. If the alignment and position of the fragments are satisfactory, the arm may be immobilized in a sling. Otherwise, closed reduction should be attempted. If satisfactory alignment cannot be achieved by manipulation, open reduction with internal fixation or insertion of a prosthetic replacement may be indicated.

The importance of beginning range-of-motion exercises as soon as possible cannot be overemphasized (see Ch. 23). The most common complication following a shoulder fracture is adhesive capsulitis resulting from approximation of the inflamed surfaces of the joint capsule. This can cause chronic pain as well as functional disability because of restricted motion.

For a stable 2-part fracture, active motion and use of the hand and wrist should be encouraged immediately. A physical therapist is indicated for instruction and monitoring of exercises. At 1 wk, pendulum exercises in the sling are started. The patient leans forward and, using the noninjured arm to assist, swings the injured arm like a pendulum, making circles with the elbow. The sling may be removed daily to allow bathing and elbow motion. By 2 wk, the patient should begin active and passive elevation of the arm. It may take several months to regain the ability to perform overhead activities such as combing the hair.

DISTAL RADIUS FRACTURES

In 1814, Abraham Colles first described the classic silver fork deformity of the wrist that bears his name. The dorsal trabecular bone of the distal radius impacts into itself, resulting in angulation and shortening. Patients present with pain, tenderness, and swelling of the wrist. The mechanism of injury is usually a fall on the outstretched hand.

Treatment and Prognosis

The severity and need for reduction are assessed radiographically. Shortening of the radial styloid should ideally be < 0.5 cm compared with the ulna on the AP view. On the lateral view, dorsal tilting of the distal radius articular surface should not go beyond neutral. Patients with minimally displaced fractures or low functional demands are treated with a short arm cast or splint. For fractures requiring closed reduction, some form of anesthesia is necessary. Aspiration of the hematoma and local injection of lidocaine may be sufficient, but regional or IV general anesthesia is superior for relaxation and pain relief. Fractures with severe shortening or intra-articular comminution may require application of an external fixator. In the operating room, pins are inserted through the skin into the metacarpals and proximal radius or ulna. Next, a metal external frame or plaster cast is applied to the pins, which then maintain the fracture reduction.

The most frequent complication of distal radius fractures is stiffness of the fingers and shoulder. For this reason, active motion of the fingers, elbow, and shoulder should be strongly encouraged. Elevation of the hand above the level of the heart is also important to minimize swelling. Cast immobilization is usually maintained for 3 to 8 wk, depending on the fracture's stability. Patients can expect gradually diminishing pain and weakness in the wrist for up to 6 to 12 mo postinjury. Physical therapy helps speed recovery. Most patients eventually regain satisfactory pain-free function.

PELVIC RAMUS FRACTURES

Symptoms, Signs, and Diagnosis

The usual mechanism of injury is a fall on level ground. Patients present with pain and inability to walk. Physical examination reveals localized tenderness in the groin and pain on movement of the legs. The clinical appearance mimics a proximal femoral fracture, and the diagnosis is made by x-ray. Usually only a single ramus is fractured, with the pubic ramus breaking twice as often as the ischiatic ramus. Less commonly, ≥ 2 rami are fractured, either on the same or on opposite sides of the symphysis pubis.

The weight-supporting function of the pelvis is borne mainly by strong bony arches in the ilium, with the pubic and ischiatic rami acting as secondary tie arches. When the pelvis is traumatized, the rami tend to fracture first. The secondary tie arches are weakened, but the main iliac weight-bearing arches remain intact.

Treatment and Prognosis

Hospitalization is required, since the patient is usually initially unable to stand or even sit without considerable pain. Analgesics and nonsteroidal anti-inflammatory drugs help symptomatically. In order to avoid the complications associated with bed confinement, patients should be encouraged to begin full weight-bearing ambulation as soon as possible. Most are able to use a walker by 1 wk. Pubic rami fractures typically heal without causing permanent functional disabilities.

HIP FRACTURES
(See also Ch. 23)

FEMORAL NECK FRACTURES

Symptoms, Signs, and Classification

These fractures can be classified as either occult, impacted, displaced, or nondisplaced. Occult fractures may occur in the elderly after minimal or even no apparent trauma. The patient complains of persistent groin pain on weight bearing, but initial x-rays of the hip reveal no fracture. A crack exists that is undetectable on x-ray and that can continue to propagate across the femoral neck with the cyclic stresses of walking. Weight bearing must be avoided, or eventually complete displacement can occur. Bone scans are positive before x-rays eventually reveal a fracture line.

Patients with impacted and nondisplaced femoral neck fractures also present with groin pain and no deformity on physical examination. X-rays of impacted (Garden I) fractures show the femoral head slightly tilted into valgus with an incomplete fracture line, leaving the medial cortex intact. Nondisplaced (Garden II) fractures extend completely across both cortices of the femoral neck and are more unstable. Patients with displaced femoral neck fractures (Garden III and IV) present with groin pain and a shortened, externally rotated leg that is too painful to move.

Classification of these fractures reflects varying degrees of disruption of the blood supply to the femoral head and has crucial implications for treatment and prognosis. Because the femoral head is intra-articular, its sole blood supply comes from vessels traversing 3 structures: the bone of the femoral neck, the surrounding hip capsule, and the ligamentum teres. A displaced fracture completely disrupts the blood vessels of the femoral neck and can also tear those of the hip capsule. The vessels in the ligamentum teres are nonfunctioning in $2/3$ of adults. Thus a displaced fracture often completely devascularizes the femoral head. Although a devascularized femoral head can heal if securely stabilized, the incidence of complications due to poor healing is considerable. Nonunion occurs in 15 to 20% of patients, and osteonecrosis of the femoral head, in another 15 to 30%.

Treatment and Prognosis

Occult, impacted, and nondisplaced femoral neck fractures are usually treated by internal fixation with multiple pins. This stabilization permits immediate full weight-bearing ambulation and prevents later displacement. Since the blood supply to the femoral head is not significantly disrupted, these fractures usually heal well.

Displaced fractures have 2 main treatment options—operative stabilization and prosthetic replacement—and each has advantages and disadvantages. Open reduction and internal fixation are usually reserved for vigorous patients < 70 yr of age who are able to comply with a postoperative regimen of limited weight bearing using crutches. The femoral head is preserved, and successful healing results in a nearly normal hip. However, if osteonecrosis or nonunion develops, the result is a painful, nonfunctional joint requiring a second procedure, total hip replacement, for correction. For this reason, elderly and less active patients with displaced fractures are often treated by primary prosthetic replacement of the femoral head, permitting immediate, full weight bearing and faster return to independent functioning.

The simplest prosthetic design (the Moore prosthesis) consists of a smooth metal sphere attached to a stem that is wedged into the medullary canal of the femur. Drawbacks include a tendency to cause wear of the acetabular articular surface and pain from a loose fit of the stem in the femoral medullary canal. More recent developments include use of acrylic cement and porous ingrowth to stabilize the stem of the prosthesis and an internal metal-polyethylene bearing to reduce acetabular wear. For patients who develop acetabular arthritis, total hip replacement may be performed as a secondary procedure. Primary total hip replacement in acute femoral neck fractures is reserved for patients with severe preexisting arthritis, since this more extensive operation has a higher associated morbidity than either hemiarthroplasty or internal fixation with pins.

INTERTROCHANTERIC HIP FRACTURES

Symptoms, Signs, and Classification

These fractures are usually caused by a fall, often on level ground. On physical examination of displaced fractures, the leg is found to be shortened and externally rotated from the pull of the leg muscles and gravity. Hemorrhage from multiple bone fragments and associated soft tissue injuries can be extensive and may cause hypovolemic shock.

Intertrochanteric hip fractures are classified according to the number of bony fragments present and whether the pattern is inherently stable or unstable with respect to weight-bearing forces. Typically, 2-part fractures have a single break, sloping obliquely between the greater and lesser trochanter on the AP x-ray view. Three-part fractures have, in addition, a lesser trochanteric fragment, and 4-part fractures include a greater trochanteric fragment. The stability of the fracture pattern depends on achievement of a reduction that maintains continuity of the weight-bearing medial femoral cortex. As a rule, 3- and 4-part fractures are inherently unstable because of comminution of the medial femoral cortex. Fractures involving the intertrochanteric region of the proximal femur usually allow satisfactory blood supply to be retained by all of the fragments, and therefore avascular necrosis and nonunion rarely occur.

Treatment and Prognosis

Intertrochanteric hip fractures are treated by surgical stabilization unless an absolute medical contraindication exists. Healing does occur with traction, but it usually requires 4 to 8 wk and involves all of the hazards of immobilization in bed. Furthermore, traction may not adequately control the deforming muscle forces around the hip, resulting in healing in a shortened and externally rotated position and a poor functional result.

Currently, the most commonly used fixation device is the sliding compression hip screw, which provides rigid stabilization together with impaction of the fracture fragments, thus ensuring healing. Postoperatively, most patients can begin immediate, full weight bearing with a walker. Usually 6 to 12 wk are required before they are able to use a cane.

TIBIAL PLATEAU FRACTURES

Symptoms, Signs, and Classification

Fractures of the proximal tibia usually result from a lateral bending force (eg, as when a pedestrian is struck from the side by an automobile). As the leg angulates, the femoral condyle drives the tibial articular surface down into the underlying metaphyseal bone, which gives way easily in the elderly because it is weakened by osteoporosis. Patients present with knee pain and effusion, proximal tibial tenderness, and inability to bear weight. Displaced fractures are readily apparent on standard AP and lateral x-rays. However, occult fractures can occur that are not well visualized on standard views. In such cases, oblique views are often helpful. The presence of fat globules in blood aspirated from the knee joint is also diagnostic of an occult fracture.

Prognosis and Treatment

Patients generally require hospitalization for elevation and observation of the leg to avoid neurovascular complications due to swelling of the surrounding soft tissues. Traction or continuous passive motion can be used initially to help mold the fragments, followed by restricted weight bearing in a long leg brace or cast for 8 to 12 wk. Patients need physical therapy to learn to walk using ambulatory aids (eg, crutches or walkers). Displacement of the articular surface $\leq$ 1 cm is usually acceptable in elderly patients. Severely displaced fractures require operative reduction of the articular surface, with inclusion of a bone graft to fill the void left by the impacted trabecular bone. Unfortunately, the leg must remain non–weight-bearing for 2 to 3 mo postoperatively, until healing has occurred.

The elderly are at less risk than young, active patients for developing osteoarthritis due to disruption of the joint surface, but total joint replacement is a good option if it does occur.

THORACIC AND LUMBAR VERTEBRAL-BODY COMPRESSION FRACTURES

Symptoms and Signs

Injury is usually caused by an activity that increases the compressive load on the spine (eg, lifting, forward bending, or a misstep while walking). Patients often present with acute pain that is exacerbated by sitting or standing. Physical examination reveals well-localized tenderness to percussion over a specific region of the spine. Associated neurologic deficits are rare.

Many vertebral-body fractures occur silently, however. Elderly patients often have x-ray evidence of fractures with no history of symptoms or antecedent injury. Osteoporosis weakens the trabecular bone of the vertebral bodies and leaves the posterior elements relatively unaffected. Excessive loads then compress the vertebral bodies into a wedge-shaped configuration as the trabecular bone impacts into itself.

Treatment and Prognosis

Vertebral-body compression fractures always heal. The trabecular bone is only impacted into itself, and the blood supply is not impaired. Neurologic deficits due to bony impingement rarely occur. These fractures are relatively stable, as the intact posterior elements prevent translational displacement. The primary clinical manifestation is progressive kyphotic deformity due to wedging and loss of height of the vertebral bodies.

Initially, hospitalization for bed rest may be necessary for pain relief. Analgesics, nonsteroidal anti-inflammatory drugs, and laboratory screening tests for other causes of osteopenia are indicated. Patients should be encouraged to begin sitting up and walking for short periods as soon as possible. They may require a week before returning to independent ambulation, and considerable back pain may persist for 6 to 12 wk. Sometimes, a month or more later, the pain shifts from the site of the original fracture to a higher or lower location, probably because of altered mechanical stresses caused by the deformity.

Bracing probably does little to prevent deformity, but it can help relieve pain and permit more rapid return to activities. Bracing is useful only for fractures of the lumbar and lower thoracic spine, since adequate support cannot be achieved above this level. While hyperextension braces (eg, the Jewett) are the most effective biomechanically, they are not the most comfortable. They apply 3-point stabilization of the spine through an anterior abdominal pad, a chest pad, and a posterior pad located at the level of the fracture. Corsets or abdominal binders are effective and better tolerated alternatives in patients with midlumbar fractures.

---

9. ACUTE CONFUSION

(Delirium; Acute Brain Syndrome; Acute Psychoorganic Syndrome; Acute Organic Reaction)

(See also Ch. 82)

Tom Arie

Confusion, or unclear thinking, is commonly the presenting or most prominent symptom in syndromes characterized by impaired cerebral function (see Symptoms and Signs, below). When *acute,* it is presumed to be potentially reversible.

Etiology

Confusional states are assumed to reflect disturbances in cerebral metabolism, probably mediated through disturbed arousal systems. The brain of an aging (particularly very elderly) person, like the immature brain, is prone to respond in this way at a lower threshold. Slowing of electrical activity on EEG is characteristic.

Confusional states can be provoked in the brain of the very elderly person by almost any physical derangement and by some psychologic disturbances, most notably depressive states. Even a sudden environmental change may precipitate an acute confusional state. The most common causes are listed in TABLE 9–1.

Symptoms and Signs

The acute confusional reaction is characterized by **clouding of consciousness,** *a level of awareness that fluctuates between the extremes of full alertness and coma.* Alertness and awareness are generally diminished, and drowsiness is most common. Key features are a relatively short history; a clouded sensorium; disorientation; agitation, with impaired attention span; impaired memory; and often anxiety and suspicion. Frank hallucinations and disrupted or delusional thinking may occur, and abnormalities of speech are common. Confusion is sometimes worse toward evening (**sundowner syndrome**) and quite variable. Other symptoms (eg, dyspnea, chest pain) may provide clues to the etiology of the acute confusion.

A complete physical examination is always required; signs such as impaired cardiopulmonary performance or neurologic findings may also provide clues to the etiology. The mental status examination follows

TABLE 9-1. COMMON CAUSES OF CONFUSION

Intracranial
    Tumors, subdural hematomas
    Cerebrovascular accidents
    Seizures, postictal states
    Infections (eg, meningitis, encephalitis)
Extracranial
    Infections (eg, respiratory, urinary tract)
    Metabolic (especially liver or kidney failure)
    Hypoxia
    Intoxication/withdrawal (eg, drugs, alcohol)*
    Hypoglycemia
    Hyperglycemia
    Myocardial infarction
    Giant cell arteritis
    Hypothermia
    Psychologic/environmental

* Drugs, particularly psychotropics, are a common cause.

standard lines; there is no specific test for clouding of consciousness. Observation of the total clinical picture—in which some, but rarely all, of the features listed in TABLE 9–2 occur—is required (see also Chs. 80 and 82).

Diagnosis

Since the causes include virtually any medical or psychologic condition, meticulous history taking and examination are essential. Confu-

TABLE 9-2. COMMON SYMPTOMS AND SIGNS OF ACUTE
CONFUSION

Short history
Clouding of consciousness
Reduced wakefulness
Disorientation of time and space
Increased motor activity: Restlessness,
    plucking, and picking
Impaired attention and concentration
Impaired memory (especially new learning and recall)
Anxiety, suspicion, agitation
Variability of symptoms
Symptoms worse at night
Misinterpretation, illusions, hallucinations
Disrupted thinking
Delusions (usually transient and primitive)
Speech abnormalities
Usually diffuse EEG slowing

sional states are often accompanied by other major, nonspecific presentations of disease in the elderly (eg, incontinence or instability and falls), and the patient may be smelly and unprepossessing, inspiring little therapeutic optimism. *Such patients must be viewed with an open mind, since the results of careful appraisal may mean the difference between life and death.*

Differentiation between acute confusion and dementia (chronic confusion, chronic brain syndrome) is important. Dementia implies chronic, progressive, and irreversible cerebral failure and must never be presumed to be present merely on the basis of an acute confusional state; a short history, in the absence of obvious causes of dementia (eg, previous cerebrovascular accident or trauma), virtually precludes the diagnosis of dementia. However, acute confusional reactions are more common in demented patients and are more often due to nonspecific or mild disorders, although specific causes (eg, infections) frequently precipitate confusion. In either case, the *acute* confusion can often be remedied effectively.

History: A confused patient rarely gives a useful history; therefore, a collateral information source is essential. Potential informants may be difficult to find once the patient has been admitted to the hospital. (If needed, admission should be to a general hospital where all investigatory facilities are readily available.) Whenever possible, therefore, the initial examination and history taking should be performed in the patient's normal setting (eg, during a home visit) when informants are most likely to be available. If the patient has been brought to the hospital, accompanying persons (relatives, friends, police, or neighbors) should be interviewed before they leave; their names, addresses, and telephone numbers should be noted.

The principles of history taking are routine, but the following factors must be considered: **Duration:** Has the duration of confusion been very short, indicating that it is almost certainly due to a specific cause? **Mode of onset:** Is the onset sudden or insidious? Is it associated with any possibly related events (eg, trauma; illness; development of specific symptoms, such as cough; UTI; changes in medication)? **Course:** Has the patient's condition been constant or variable, and is there a diurnal pattern? Are relatively lucid periods apparently associated with any specific factors? What appears to make the patient worse? **Recurrence:** Has the patient been in a state of confusion before? What caused it previously? To what treatment did it respond? Has there been previous depression? **Life-style:** Does the patient use standard drugs or abuse drugs or alcohol? What are the patient's patterns of nutrition and exposure to infection? What are the living circumstances, including heating?

Drugs, *prescribed by physicians or purchased over the counter, are among the most common causes of confusional states.* Anticholinergic agents are involved particularly often, and since many psychotropic drugs are anticholinergic, these should always be viewed with extreme suspicion. Many patients on standard drug regimens have problems with compliance, and it must never be assumed that an individual is actually taking what the physician intended; self-medication must not be overlooked.

Sometimes drugs used for treating the early stages of a confusional state actually exacerbate or perpetuate it. Antiparkinsonian drugs may be potent precipitants of confusion. Drug handling by the elderly body is often altered, even in the absence of specific disease, and high blood levels may occur even in patients taking normal or low doses. Polypharmacy is common in the elderly, and drug interactions may occur. Confusional states often are dramatically cured or alleviated by changes in or elimination of drug therapy.

Life events: Bereavements, actual or symbolic, are among the life events most commonly associated with the precipitation of depression. Depressive states may present as subacute confusion (possibly through disorders of arousal). Some cases of depressive **pseudodementia,** in which it is believed depression *mimics* dementia, would be better labeled **"depressive confusion,"** because the depression actually worsens the underlying (often unrecognized) dementia, precipitating an acute confusional state.

Laboratory Findings

The EEG is the only test that is regularly abnormal in an acute confusional state; however, this test is usually not necessary, since it provides no more information than can be determined clinically. The value of other laboratory tests depends on the clinical findings. The tests most often ordered are CBC, blood chemistry profile, urinalysis, and chest x-ray. Specific tests may be required in relation to certain conditions (see TABLE 9–1) or to diagnose other suspected disorders (eg, thyroid function tests, vitamin B_{12} levels, or brain CT). One must always remember to check whether the patient is febrile.

Treatment

A constant environment with, as far as possible, the same care givers minimizes exacerbations of confusion that derive from frequent changes. The room should either be well lighted or, when appropriate, dark; ambiguous lighting provokes illusions and even hallucinations. Confused patients need frequent repetition of information; patience on the part of the care giver is very important. Many elderly patients have impaired hearing, which makes communication more difficult, but shouting is inappropriate (hearing impairment responds to clear enunciation rather than to raised voices). Care givers should speak slowly, be prepared to repeat their remarks several times, and use the patient's name, which can be an important point of reference in the midst of confusion.

Dehydration and electrolyte imbalance are ever-present threats to ill older persons and may occur rapidly. Patients may die from these disorders, rather than from actual causes of confusion. Fluid intake must be meticulously charted (especially if the patient is febrile), and output must be sensibly estimated, even in the presence of urinary incontinence.

Blood chemistry reports must be obtained *promptly* from the laboratory *In the short term, hydration is much more important than nutrition.*

Observations: Detailed observations should be sought from nurses who are present around the clock. Depressive confusion may be mani fested by occasional facial expressions or utterances in an otherwise ex pressionless or virtually mute patient; these behaviors are likely to occur when the physician is not present. For example, a withdrawn disori ented patient may make revealing, self-deprecating utterances such as "I don't deserve this food" or "I'm a trouble to everyone."

Specific treatment depends on the cause of the confusion (eg, infection require specific therapy). Symptomatic treatment is often needed. Tran quilizers may break the vicious circle of confusion leading to anxiety and more confusion. Occasionally, a patient is so restless that sedation is needed to allow hydration and feeding; however, this is always a diffi cult course, for heavy sedation may increase risks. It is best to stick to a small, familiar range of drugs. Use of a regular regimen with close ob servation of results is best; drugs should almost never be prescribed or a prn basis. Proper titration of dosage is the responsibility of the physi cian, not the nurses.

All drugs have dangers, but in most cases phenothiazines (eg, thiorida zine 10 to 25 mg tid) or butyrophenones (eg, haloperidol 1.5 mg tid ini tially) are useful. The latter agents are less sedating but more likely to cause dystonic reactions. Promazine 25 mg tid is a useful mild tranquil izer that is usually free of dystonic effects. All these drugs should normally be given orally, and liquid forms are sometimes more accept able. Occasionally, an IM injection (eg, haloperidol 2.5 mg) may be re quired. Benzodiazepines are not usually useful as tranquilizers.

For sleep, chloral hydrate (eg, as syrup, 500 mg in 10 mL) may be given alone or combined with a phenothiazine in low dosage. Occasion ally, a shorter-acting benzodiazepine hypnotic (eg, triazolam 0.125 to 0.25 mg or lormetazepam 0.5 to 1 mg orally) may be needed, but even short-acting benzodiazepines have much longer half-lives in older peo ple.

Effective treatment of a patient's confusional state may still leave other unresolved disabilities or care needs. Proper management is not com plete until attention has been paid to *all* the patient's needs and appro priate arrangements have been made for continuing care.

---

10. URINARY INCONTINENCE

Ananias C. Diokno

Involuntary loss of urine was self-reported by 30% of community-dwell ing people $\geq$ 60 yr of age randomly surveyed in Washtenaw County Michigan. European surveys have reported that prevalence rates vary from 1.6 to 49%, the wide range attributable to differences in technics used in the surveys and in the definitions of urinary incontinence. The problem is more prevalent in the institutionalized elderly; about 50% of chronically institutionalized and 30% of unselected hospitalized elderly are incontinent. The prevalence is much higher in women than in men, with a ratio of about 2:1.

Urinary incontinence can be a cause of institutionalization and is a contributory factor in pressure sores, UTIs, and depression. The problem is closely associated with poor general health and with chronic medical conditions (eg, neurologic, GI, respiratory, and GU problems). In elderly women, parity alone does not correlate with urinary incontinence, unless the latter also occurred during a pregnancy.

The economic impact of urinary incontinence is considerable; costs of additional care required to manage incontinent institutionalized older persons have been estimated to be > $8 billion annually in the USA.

This condition in the elderly is poorly understood and neglected. Many persons incorrectly believe that aging per se causes urinary incontinence. A majority do not tell their doctor about involuntary urine loss. Even more distressing are reports that $1/2$ to $2/3$ of physicians do not institute even the most rudimentary evaluation when told of the problem. Educational programs for the public and for physicians are needed to provide accurate information and change misperceptions. With numerous treatment modalities available, every elderly person suffering from urinary incontinence should have an opportunity to control, if not correct, this problem.

Anatomy and Physiology of the Lower Urinary Tract

The 3 major lower urinary tract structures essential for maintenance of urinary continence, storage of urine in the bladder, and evacuation of urine from the bladder are the detrusor, the internal sphincter, and the external sphincter. The detrusor, or smooth muscle of the bladder, extends into the urethra and contributes to the bulk of its proximal wall (the internal sphincter).

The 3 structures are considered 1 anatomic and functional unit and have certain intrinsic contractile properties that are completely independent of CNS control. The smooth muscle and elastic tissue that make up these structures allow the bladder to accommodate a large volume of urine under low intravesical pressure.

The proximal urethra includes the prostatic and membranous urethra in men and the proximal $3/4$ of the urethra in women. Contraction of the internal sphincter prevents leakage of urine from the bladder. This resistance to leakage is the sum total of the forces originating from the mucosa, smooth muscle, blood vessels, and elastic tissue.

When high intravesical pressures occur as a result of increased intra-abdominal pressure (eg, coughing, straining, or laughing), the internal sphincter action is enhanced by the periurethral striated muscle (the external sphincter). This muscle, originating in the urogenital diaphragm and the levator ani, encircles the internal sphincter. Its greatest concentration of fibers is at the midurethra in women and the membranous urethra in men.

The detrusor and the sphincters are controlled by the cerebrospinal axis. Voluntary bladder control is thought to be achieved when the cerebral micturition center matures by the age of 2 to 4 yr. Prior to cortical maturation, or toilet training, micturition is uncontrolled.

The micturition center in the brain, located in the frontal lobe, is connected by axons to the pontine mesencephalic reticular formation. This pathway receives messages from the basal ganglia and the cerebellum. The fibers from the pontine mesencephalic reticular formation descend to and synapse at the spinal cord center located at sacral spinal cord segments 2, 3, and 4, where 2 important groups of neurons are located. Ventral (anterior) horn cells provide the pudendal nerves, and lateral horn cells produce the pelvic nerves.

The cerebral micturition center provides volitional control of urination by modulating the pontine mesencephalic center. Lesions in the cerebral area usually result in partial or complete release of the voluntary micturition reflex, leading to development of detrusor hyperreflexia. However, in certain cases, total or partial loss of the ability to initiate voiding is also seen, as in the early phase of cerebrovascular accident.

The pontine mesencephalic center is believed to control the development of a coordinated detrusor reflex of adequate temporal duration to ensure complete emptying of the bladder. The spinal cord micturition center at the sacral segments is believed to control the coordination between detrusor contraction and external sphincter relaxation, producing complete bladder emptying without any external sphincteric resistance.

The **pudendal nerve** is a somatic nerve that provides motor innervation of the external sphincter and sensory innervation of the perineum and genitalia. The **pelvic nerve** is a parasympathetic mixed nerve; its afferent fibers carry pain and stretch perception from the bladder.

Spinal segments T-10 through S-2 provide the neurons of the presacral, or hypogastric, nerves. The **presacral nerve,** a sympathetic nerve, innervates the bladder and the urethra. There are 2 distinct sympathetic receptors in the lower urinary tract: α-adrenergic receptors are highly concentrated in the trigone and the proximal urethra; β-adrenergic receptors are located in the bladder above the trigone. The α-adrenergic receptors mediate contraction of the internal sphincter, whereas β-adrenergic receptors cause relaxation of the smooth muscle of the bladder wall. These actions promote the storage of urine inside the bladder.

As the bladder fills with urine and stretches, proprioceptive endings are stimulated and send impulses to the pontine mesencephalic center, which in turn relays impulses to the spinal cord center. Motor neurons are then activated, transmitting impulses to the detrusor, causing it to contract. Just before measurable detrusor contractions or a rise in intravesical pressure, the periurethral striated muscle relaxes completely.

The detrusor contracts, and the proximal urethra opens. A strong continuous urinary stream is produced by the sustained detrusor contraction, relaxed external sphincter, and an open, funneled internal sphincter.

Pathophysiology

There is no evidence that normal aging causes urinary incontinence. However, aging does affect the lower urinary tract in ways that may make the elderly directly or indirectly more vulnerable. For example, studies have shown that maximal urethral closing pressure is reduced with age, but this reduction is not sufficient to produce incontinence, since it is seen in continent elderly people. However, superimposed insults to the lower urinary tract may have additive effects, leading to loss of control.

Involuntary urine loss occurs whenever the intravesical pressure equals or exceeds the maximal intraurethral pressure. This can be the result of an increase in intravesical pressure, a fall in intraurethral pressure, or a combination of these. In analyzing urinary incontinence, one should search for either detrusor dysfunction or sphincter dysfunction or both. Detrusor dysfunction can be categorized as overactivity, which may be caused by hyperreflexia or hypertonia, or as underactivity, which may be caused by areflexia/hyporeflexia or hypotonia.

Detrusor hyperreflexia, which is characterized by uncontrolled detrusor contractions caused by loss of cortical inhibition, is seen frequently in patients with cerebrovascular accidents, spinal cord injuries above sacral segments 2 to 4, parkinsonism, brain tumors, and multiple sclerosis. **Unstable bladder** describes uncontrolled detrusor contractions without any demonstrable neurologic lesion. It is suspected to be of intrinsic origin, presumably from detrusor instability as a consequence of prostatic enlargement or other local conditions.

Detrusor hypertonia is a condition of myogenic origin that produces a noncompliant detrusor. It is most often (1) a consequence of long-term indwelling catheter drainage with associated chronic cystitis, (2) secondary interstitial, radiation-induced, or cyclophosphamide-induced cystitis, or (3) rarely, secondary to carcinoma of the bladder. In these conditions, the small, contracted bladder cannot expand and accommodate urine under low intravesical pressure. As a result, high pressure develops at small volumes, overcoming the resistance at the urethral sphincter and causing involuntary urine loss. **Detrusor areflexia and hypotonia** are discussed under OVERFLOW INCONTINENCE, below.

Sphincter dysfunction can involve the internal or external sphincter or both and is the most common cause of stress incontinence (see below).

DIAGNOSTIC EVALUATION

A thorough **history** is needed. Urinary incontinence presents in many ways, and a preliminary classification of the problem may be formulated from **the patient's description of urine loss** (eg, urinary incontinence may be described as urge, precipitate, stress, or dribbling incontinence). These descriptive terms are based on subjective manifestations and should be considered the starting point rather than the end point of the evaluation process.

Data should be obtained regarding the history of urine loss; urologic, gynecologic, neurologic, and related medical and psychologic illnesses; and the use of medication. For example, incontinence may be a manifestation of polyuria due to diabetes mellitus.

The volume and frequency of urine loss should be assessed. Volume may be estimated by the number of pads used to contain the urine loss, but the type of pad used and the degree of wetness should be described before the pad is replaced. In stress incontinence, severity may be gauged by the degree of physical exertion needed to provoke urine loss. In urge incontinence, severity may be gauged by the frequency of the urge or the interval between wettings.

The patient should be asked about use of specific groups of drugs. **Diuretics,** especially the more powerful loop diuretics, may induce brisk diuresis and provoke incontinence, especially in patients with small functional bladder capacity. Drugs producing **anticholinergic** side effects (eg, major tranquilizers and antiparkinsonian agents) may induce urinary retention and overflow incontinence. **α-Adrenergic blockers** (eg, the antihypertensive prazosin) may reduce urethral resistance and induce stress incontinence. **Sedative/hypnotics** may affect the sensorium and depress the cerebral corticoregulatory tract, allowing detrusor contractions to "escape" control.

OTC drugs may also influence bladder and urethral function. **Adrenergic agonists,** eg, OTC decongestants, may induce worsening of obstructive symptoms or even urinary retention and overflow incontinence in men with chronic prostatism.

A helpful noninvasive technic to assess bladder function is **a patient-kept diary** that includes frequency of voluntary voiding, voided volumes, episodes and quantity of involuntary urine loss, and volume of fluid intake. This may help the physician assess functional bladder capacity, estimate the severity of incontinence, and evaluate the effects of behavior-modification therapy.

Physical examination should include pelvic, rectal, and neurologic examinations. In many patients, a distended urinary bladder is palpable. Percussion to detect the distended bladder may be helpful in the asthenic patient but is of little or no value in the obese patient. A normal finding should not be considered reliable, especially in a dribbling type of urinary incontinence.

Pelvic examination should include a search for signs of **atrophic vaginitis** (ie, thin, shiny, friable vaginal mucosa). The introitus is usually tight and narrow. A vaginal smear for a maturation index establishes the diagnosis. A distended bladder may be discovered during this examination. An **enlarged uterus** or an **abnormally flexed uterus** in either direction that is causing obstruction of the bladder neck or pressure on the body of the bladder should also be sought.

A **cystocele** or a **cystourethrocele** should be identified and the degree of movement assessed. The degree of cystocele, urethrocele, or rectocele should be determined by observing the specific structure as the patient strains or coughs. Incontinence may occur during this maneuver. However, although a cystocele or urethrocele is a sign of pelvic relaxation, it has no direct relationship to the occurrence of stress incontinence. In fact, a cystocele may have a protective effect because of its ability to absorb the transmitted increases in intravesical pressure.

Because cystocele repair itself may *cause* stress incontinence not previously present, urethral function should be evaluated prior to such surgery. The severity of a cystourethrocele in someone with stress incontinence is an important factor in deciding the appropriate surgical approach to the incontinence. (See also DISORDERS OF THE PELVIC-FLOOR SUPPORTING SYSTEM AND GENITOURINARY PROLAPSE in Ch. 57.)

Sensory testing of the perineum as well as testing the tone of the anal sphincter should be performed to identify possible pudendal nerve involvement. The finding of unilateral or bilateral saddle anesthesia or hypoesthesia may be the only sign of a neurogenic cause of incontinence. Weak or flaccid **anal tone** suggests a neurologic defect, although it may be a consequence of previous anal surgery.

On rectal examination, the possible presence of **fecal impaction** should be ascertained; this is a likely finding in the evaluation of acute-onset urinary incontinence, especially in nursing home patients. The impacted stool compresses the bladder outlet, leading to urine retention and subsequent overflow.

Digital examination of the prostate gland is an excellent method of screening for prostate carcinoma. An enlarged gland without tenderness or abnormal change in consistency is of no clinical significance unless it is associated with symptoms of urinary obstruction or bladder irritation. Conversely, the presence of symptoms in the absence of an enlarged prostate on rectal examination does not rule out an obstructing gland as the cause. The prostate can be enlarged externally without producing outlet obstruction, but it can also obstruct the outlet without external enlargement.

An evaluation of incontinence is incomplete without a urinalysis. If pyuria or bacteriuria is noted, contamination of the sample should be ruled out. A clean-catch urine sample is acceptable if the urine is normal. In men, the prepuce should be retracted and the glans penis rinsed adequately before collecting the midstream urine sample. Elderly women may have difficulty carrying out strict aseptic midstream collection of the urine sample. In this situation, sterile catheterization is the best and easiest way to obtain a sample that confirms the presence of urinary infection. It may also prevent unnecessary treatment for "multiple recurrent UTIs" diagnosed by urinary frequency and contaminated clean-catch specimens. Catheter-induced infection following a single sterile catheterization is extremely rare.

Whenever there is a question of urinary retention, a single sterile catheterization should be performed immediately after urination to measure the postvoiding residual volume. This is the only direct test for distinguishing urinary frequency and overflow incontinence from nonoverflow incontinence. Postvoiding residual volume also may be measured during cystometric examination or ultrasound study.

Urodynamic testing can be divided into basic and complex tests. **The basic tests include** uroflowmetry, cystometry, and sphincter electromyography.

Cystometry can confirm the presence of uncontrolled or uninhibited detrusor contraction or a noncompliant bladder. In patients with detrusor hyperreflexia or unstable bladder, uninhibited detrusor contractions are observed, while in detrusor hypertonia, a small-capacity, poorly compliant bladder is documented. Hyperreflexia can be distinguished from hypertonia by observing the effect of an anticholinergic agent on intravesical pressure. In hypertonia, the pressure remains unchanged, while in a hyperreflexic or unstable condition, the uninhibited contractions are suppressed or reduced.

More complex and dynamic tests include simultaneous pressure measurements of the bladder, urethra, and rectum at rest, with exertion, and during voiding. In conjunction with these measurements, urinary flow rates should be assessed, sphincter electromyography should be performed, and the bladder and urethra should be radiographically and fluoroscopically monitored at rest and during bladder filling, straining, and voiding. *Not all of these tests are needed to make an accurate diagnosis in most patients,* and should be reserved for complicated cases, when surgical procedures are contemplated, or when a trial of low-risk treatment has failed. Complicated cases include those with unexplained symptoms, previous anti-incontinence surgery, or postsurgical incontinence, or in which pharmacologic treatment has failed.

In patients with pure stress incontinence, a **cystometrogram** demonstrates a flattened curve without any sign of the uninhibited or uncontrolled contractions observed in patients with unstable bladder. In contrast to patients with overflow incontinence, those with pure stress incontinence void efficiently, with no residual urine.

To identify neurogenic bladder and sphincter as the cause of incontinence, a **Urecholine® supersensitivity test** and **needle sphincter electromyography** are performed. These are highly specific tests performed as part of the complex urodynamic assessment. The Urecholine® supersensitivity test of Lapides is based on the denervated bladder's hypersensitivity to cholinergic agents. It is used to confirm the presence of significant bladder denervation in patients with suspected paralytic bladder. The test is done in conjunction with standard cystometrography, usually using water or CO_2 as the infusing agent. The intravesical pressure is measured at 100 mL of volume, the patient is given bethanechol chloride 2.5 mg s.c., and the cystometrogram is repeated 15 to 20 min later.

A positive test is characterized by an increase in bladder pressure of 20 cm over the control intravesical pressure at 100 mL of volume. A response < 20 cm of water over baseline is considered normal. False-positive responses are observed in patients with azotemia; false-negative tests are seen in patients with very early or limited denervation of the bladder.

Urethrocystoscopy is mandatory in patients with possible obstructive incontinence as well as in all patients in whom urethral trauma or disease is suspected. The urethra should be carefully studied for strictures by bougienage, calibrating the entire urethra in women and the anterior (distal) urethra in men. The presence of scar tissue in the region of the membranous urethra usually suggests trauma or devascularization, and a rigid noncompliant tube is highly suggestive of an ineffective posterior (proximal) urethra. In patients with urinary stress incontinence, the incompetent proximal urethra can be visualized endoscopically, as can orifices of urethral diverticula.

TRANSIENT INCONTINENCE

All acute-onset urinary incontinence should be considered transient and reversible until proved otherwise. A specific cause should be sought and, whenever possible, treated aggressively. The most common cause is a patient's inability to get out of bed or to reach the urinal.

UTI should be treated while its underlying cause (eg, obstruction, stones, tumors, decompensated bladder, unstable bladder) is being sought and controlled or eliminated.

Drugs that may be inducing incontinence (eg, an α-adrenergic agonist decongestant in a man with borderline prostatism) should be discontinued or changed.

Atrophic vaginitis should be treated cyclically with conjugated estrogens 0.3 to 1.25 mg/day orally for 25 days followed by 5 days off drug. To counteract possible endometrial hyperplasia from unopposed estrogen (with the potential to cause endometrial carcinoma), medroxyprogesterone acetate 5 to 10 mg orally on days 13 to 25 of estrogen intake is recommended. An alternative is conjugated estrogens vaginal cream 2 gm intravaginally daily or every other day for 25 days. Treatment should be continued for 2 to 3 mo, followed by an assessment of the effects. In many cases, treatment is lifelong. (See also GENITAL ATROPHY in Ch. 72.)

Stool impaction should be relieved if present; the patient may have to be catheterized once to evacuate and decompress the bladder.

Specific metabolic derangements (eg, diabetes) should be managed aggressively; this usually leads to control of bladder function. If incontinence persists, further attention should be directed to identifying its cause.

URGE INCONTINENCE

The involuntary urine loss associated with a sudden strong desire to void.

Urge incontinence is caused by an overactive detrusor, due to hyperreflexia, instability, or hypertonia, resulting in increased intravesical pressure. Detrusor hyperreflexia and instability have identical mechanisms of urine loss: uncontrolled or uninhibited detrusor contraction. Detrusor hypertonia leads to urine loss from a noncompliant bladder. The preferred terms are **detrusor hyperreflexia** if there is a neurologic lesion and **detrusor instability** or **unstable bladder** if there is no neurologic etiology (see Pathophysiology, above).

Symptoms and Signs

The sudden desire to void is called urgency, often described as "There is not enough warning." The volume of urine lost ranges from a few drops to several hundred milliliters with complete bladder emptying. The timing of incontinence is usually unpredictable; it can occur in any position and at any time, day or night. Although there usually is preceding urgency, in some cases no warning occurs at all; this is usually termed **reflex incontinence. Precipitate incontinence** is *the sudden loss of a large amount of urine with or without preceding urgency or warning.*

Urge incontinence is usually associated with other voiding complaints, most often urinary frequency q 2 h or less, nocturia, and suprapubic discomfort. Dysuria indicates the presence of UTI or inflammation of the bladder or urethra.

Diagnosis

Diagnosis is suggested by the symptoms and signs; a patient-kept diary is helpful. A urinalysis and knowledge of postvoiding residual urine volume are essential for excluding other types of incontinence. Cystometry showing uninhibited detrusor contraction confirms the diagnosis.

Treatment

Primary treatment options include behavior modification, pharmacotherapy, and the use of absorbent pads and toilet supplements. When the primary options fail in the healthy elderly, electrical stimulation, vesical hydrodilation, augmentation cystoplasty and, as a last resort, bladder denervation may be considered. The most common initial treatment is pharmacotherapy plus behavior modification. Once urinary incontinence is controlled, drug therapy is gradually withdrawn to determine whether continence can be maintained by behavior modification alone.

Pharmacologic therapy is designed to inhibit uncontrolled detrusor contractions and to enlarge functional bladder capacity. Drugs are especially appropriate for long-term maintenance use, although they are not curative. They are effective in 80 to 85% of patients with uninhibited bladder contractions and symptoms of urinary frequency, urgency, and incontinence.

One of the most widely used drugs, approved specifically for control of uninhibited detrusor contractions, is **oxybutynin chloride,** an anticholinergic and antispasmodic agent. The dosage is 2.5 to 5.0 mg orally up to 4 times/day. In the elderly, starting with 2.5 mg bid to avoid anticholinergic side effects is prudent. **Propantheline,** a pure anticholinergic agent, is given in a dosage of 7.5 to 15 mg orally tid or qid. **Dicyclomine,** an anticholinergic and antispasmodic agent, has a recommended dosage of 20 mg orally tid. **Imipramine,** a very weak anticholinergic with indirect α-adrenergic agonist activity, prevents uptake of norepinephrine. The usual dosage is 25 mg orally tid, although starting at 10 mg tid and gradually increasing to tolerance is recommended.

Before initiation of therapy, patients should be warned about the usual anticholinergic side effects—dry mouth, blurred vision, and constipation. These side effects usually subside after a few days or with reduced dosage. *Anticholinergic agents should be used with caution,* since they can induce agitation or acute confusion in nondemented patients or aggravate these problems in demented patients.

Behavior-modification therapy includes maneuvers to adjust the intake of fluid, a planned schedule of voiding, provision of a bedside commode, biofeedback technics, and prompted voiding. The major objective of simple behavioral change is to reduce the chance of triggering an uninhibited detrusor contraction by regulating the frequency of voiding and preventing the bladder from being overstretched.

The use of a **daily diary** (see DIAGNOSTIC EVALUATION, above) helps modify the patient's behavior in terms of fluid intake, frequency of voiding, and prevention of incontinence. The diary also provides feedback for the patient and care givers in assessing the progress of management.

A frequent, regular toileting schedule may help physically restricted or confused incontinent patients, but prompting is always required. The prompting is offered by care givers, who remind the patient to void and provide any help needed. Once prompting is terminated, however, incontinence returns to its pretreatment level.

Adjunctive therapy: Throughout the trial of pharmacotherapy and behavior-modification therapy, the patient should be informed about, and (if necessary) taught to use, **superabsorbent pads** to catch urine loss from the urethra. These pads are available in a variety of disposable and reusable forms. The most commonly used is a pant insert, of which a menstrual "maxipad" is the most widely used. However, many disposable pant inserts are specifically designed to absorb urine. Some disposable pads are made with straps and have a waterproof backing that extends to the waist; they usually are held in place by washable elastic side straps.

In certain patients, eg, those with impaired mobility or sensorium, the use of toilet supplements is essential. These supplements include **bedside commodes, bedpans,** and **urinals.**

Electrostimulation of the perineal musculature reduces detrusor hyperactivity by inhibiting the voiding reflex arc. It also can help in other types of urinary incontinence by strengthening the pelvic musculature. However, there is no consensus regarding its effectiveness, and more research is needed.

Vesical hydrodilation is a technic of actively stretching the bladder wall to increase capacity and improve compliance. The technic used specifically for the hypertonic bladder is gravity hydrodilation under general or regional anesthesia. However, efficacy is limited, and when the technic is successful, improvement usually lasts no more than 6 to 12 mo. In these cases, the bladder may be redilated.

Bladder denervation, either at the level of the bladder or the spinal nerves, is used only in selected cases. Selective sacral rhizolysis, a percutaneous procedure, deactivates 1 or 2 of the nerve roots to the bladder. Another denervation technic is transection of the pelvic nerve at the posterior wall of the bladder at the level of the trigone. The long-term outcome of denervation is questionable because of nerve fiber regeneration. In the fit elderly, this technic should be considered before opting for the more involved diversionary procedure.

Bladder augmentation, a surgical technic for enlarging bladder capacity and improving compliance, is indicated for small-capacity, noncompliant bladders. Its use in the elderly is limited, since it is applicable mainly in noncompliant bladders of neuropathic origin and in highly selected cases of nonneurogenic noncompliant bladders.

In a few men who have had multiple strokes or other neurologic conditions, urinary incontinence is unresponsive to drugs and an external sheath catheter fails because of a retractile penis. In these patients, an **implantable semirigid penile prosthesis** in the corpora generally improves the fit of the external catheter and provides acceptable management of otherwise uncontrollable massive urinary incontinence. This device also eliminates the need for an indwelling Foley catheter.

OVERFLOW INCONTINENCE

Involuntary urine loss associated with an overdistended urinary bladder. This implies that the bladder is retaining urine that then overflows. The condition is characterized by a constant loss of small amounts of urine, either periodically or continuously **(dribbling incontinence)** in the presence of a distended bladder. Overflow incontinence (also called **paradoxic incontinence**) may mimic urge incontinence by presenting with urinary frequency and frequent small amounts of urine loss, usually occurring both during the day and at night. The chronic retention of urine may be observed in patients with an obstructing prostate gland, an areflexic type of neuropathic bladder, or a hypotonic bladder.

Etiology

Detrusor hypotonia and areflexia lead to chronic urinary retention from lack of voluntary sustained detrusor contraction to evacuate the bladder. The resultant chronic retention ultimately produces intravesical pressure equal to or exceeding that of intraurethral pressure. Areflexia is neurogenic in origin and is seen in spinal cord injury or lesions at or below sacral segments 2 to 4. Hypotonia may result from neurogenic retention or may be nonneurogenic, as in persons who void infrequently or who have recurrent, prolonged urinary retention. Hypotonia is usually the result of prolonged distention and overstretching of the detrusor and the elastic tissue of the bladder wall, which, in time, leads to loss of contractility.

Outlet obstruction, as in prostatism, can lead to urinary retention and produce overflow incontinence by a mechanism similar to that occurring with detrusor hypotonia or areflexia. Patients who chronically use **tranquilizers** of the phenothiazine family may present with large, hypotonic bladders.

Diagnosis

Diagnosis is suggested by the clinical picture. A patient-kept diary is helpful, and a urinalysis and knowledge of postvoiding residual urine volume are essential.

Urethrocystoscopy is mandatory to rule out anatomic obstruction (eg, an obstructing prostate gland or urethral strictures). In patients with suspected paralytic bladder, the Urecholine® supersensitivity test of Lapides can be performed in conjunction with urethrocystoscopy for confirmation. These procedures are described under DIAGNOSTIC EVALUATION, above. In complicated cases, more extensive urodynamic tests, such as a voiding pressure-flow study, may be necessary to determine the cause of chronic retention.

Treatment

Treatment should be directed at the cause of inadequate bladder emptying or urinary retention (eg, by prostatectomy or release of strictures) if at all possible. The transurethral approach is the most popular and least invasive in the elderly. Age alone is not a contraindication to surgery for relief of obstruction.

Most recently, the use of a balloon to dilate the obstructing prostatic urethra has been reported to be highly successful. Although experience with this new technic is still limited, it holds great promise, especially for the elderly. This new technic, when compared to the conventional transurethral resection procedure, requires less anesthesia (sedation only), can be performed as an outpatient procedure, and requires less postoperative recovery time.

For patients in whom surgical therapy is not feasible, and for those with a nonobstructive hypotonic bladder, the use of **clean intermittent catheterization** is the next treatment of choice. This safe, effective long-term treatment is preferable to long-term use of an indwelling Foley catheter and should be seriously considered for the alert, competent, ambulatory older person. Patients can be taught self-catheterization by a nurse, enterostomal therapist, or physician's assistant. **Indwelling urethral or suprapubic catheter drainage** is the last recourse.

Although the incidence of bacteriuria is high in patients undergoing intermittent catheterization or those with long-standing indwelling catheters, no attempt should be made to eradicate these bacteria, since resistant strains will emerge. Catheter-associated bacteriuria should be treated only prior to major instrumentation (eg, cystoscopy) or if the patient is symptomatic.

Occasionally, bladder emptying rehabilitation can be accomplished with the use of **a cholinergic agent** and **an α-adrenergic blocker,** along with intermittent catheterization. The aim is to stimulate the bladder with bethanechol chloride and relax the internal urethral sphincter with prazosin, an α-adrenergic blocker. The usual dosage of bethanechol in the elderly is 10 to 25 mg orally q 6 to 8 h, and the dosage of prazosin is 1 mg orally q 8 or 12 h. *Prazosin must be used with caution,* since it can cause postural hypotension, especially in the elderly. The lowest dose given at the longest interval should be used initially; the dose can gradually be increased and/or the time interval decreased, if necessary. These drugs should not be used in patients with cardiovascular or peptic ulcer disease or postural hypotension.

The use of an indwelling Foley catheter should be considered only as a last resort, when all of the above suggested treatments have failed, in patients with urinary retention and overflow incontinence. An indwelling Foley catheter may be used temporarily in patients with a pressure sore to prevent urine from bathing the wound.

STRESS INCONTINENCE

The involuntary loss of urine during physical exertion. The volume of urine lost varies from a few drops to massive amounts. Patients usually have no other urologic complaints.

Etiology

The most common cause of primary stress incontinence in women is sphincter dysfunction, believed to be due to pelvic musculofascial relaxation and reduction of urethral resistance. **In women,** a history of pregnancy, especially if associated with urinary incontinence, is generally essential for the development of pelvic relaxation and stress incontinence. Other causes include trauma to the proximal urethra following resections or incisions, a devascularized urethra, atrophic urethritis, and a paralytic external sphincter.

In men, sphincter incontinence is uncommon and is usually due to a defective or noncompliant membranous urethra resulting from pelvic trauma or radical prostatectomy, although it can occur after the transurethral procedure. External sphincter paralysis or injury may also lead to incontinence because of reduction of total urethral resistance.

Symptoms and Signs

Incontinence is usually reduced or absent at night while the patient is in bed, in contrast to the frequent wetting that occurs during the day while the patient is active. A thorough history helps distinguish stress incontinence from pure urge incontinence. Stress incontinence occurs simultaneously with exertion, such as coughing and lifting. In urge incontinence, leakage usually occurs several seconds after exertion has taken place, because it results from micturitional reflex activity stimulated by the sudden increase in intravesical pressure.

Diagnosis

The history and findings on physical examination suggest the diagnosis.

The simple, basic **provocative stress test** for stress incontinence can be performed while the patient is in the lithotomy position or standing (see also Ch. 57). The bladder should be full of urine or filled in retrograde fashion by catheter with room-temperature sterile water. The catheter is withdrawn once the bladder is filled to capacity (with the amount of fluid that the patient can hold comfortably). The patient is then asked to cough several times or "bear down."

The test is positive if urine or instilled fluid escapes from the urethra during exertion. If fluid leaks out a few seconds after the cough or exertion, the incontinence is probably due to a detrusor contraction rather than to true stress incontinence. In mild cases, a tissue paper or napkin pad may be placed between the patient's thighs to document the urine loss, which otherwise would not be visible to the examiner, especially when testing in the upright position. Additional stress test maneuvers are described under URINARY INCONTINENCE in Ch. 57.

Other aspects of a complete diagnostic evaluation, needed when the cause is uncertain or when planning surgical corrective procedures, are described under DIAGNOSTIC EVALUATION, above.

Treatment

Since stress incontinence is a manifestation of several pathologic processes, these processes must be identified before an irreversible or invasive form of therapy, such as a surgical procedure, can be considered. A history, physical examination, elimination of the diagnosis of overflow incontinence, and documentation of stress incontinence are sufficient for initiation of a reversible or noninvasive therapy. The patient and the family should be informed that this condition is not due to psychologic stress but rather to an exertional or physical type of stress.

Nonsurgical procedures consist of behavior modification, physical therapy, and pharmacologic intervention. **Behavior modification** includes altering fluid intake and voiding habits (see under URGE INCONTINENCE, above). **Physical therapy** consists of urethral sphincter exercises **(Kegel's exercises).** Although these exercises have been advocated for a long time, their benefits and long-term effects in elderly people are still not known. Designed specifically to exercise pelvic musculature, these exercises consist of contracting and relaxing the urogenital diaphragm 100 to 200 times/day to increase its tone and urethral resistance. Patients must be taught the location of these muscles to ensure that the exercises will be effective and should be cautioned about the possibility of developing pelvic pain and being sexually stimulated while performing the exercises.

Pharmacologic therapy is directed to the stimulation of the α-adrenergic receptors located at the trigone and internal sphincter. The α-adrenergic agonists are indicated for stress incontinence of mild to moderate degree; a 75% success rate can be expected. Recommended agents are phenylpropanolamine 50 to 75 mg orally bid or ephedrine 10 to 25 mg orally tid to qid. Starting at the lower dose and gradually increasing the dosage to tolerance is the preferred practice. These drugs are contraindicated in patients with uncontrolled hypertension or thyroid disease.

Surgical therapy can be divided into bladder-suspension procedures and urethral resistance-augmentation procedures. The standard treatment for stress incontinence due to pelvic relaxation is a bladder-suspension procedure. This operation can be accomplished through either a suprapubic, vaginal, or combined suprapubic and vaginal approach. A severe, symptomatic cystocele in the presence of stress incontinence is an indication for a vaginal surgical approach. However, if the cystocele is asymptomatic and nonprolapsing, the bladder-suspension procedure can be approached in a number of ways.

Regardless of approach, this procedure has a reported success rate of 85 to 90%. With the numerous simplified technics available to suspend the bladder, this procedure should not be denied elderly patients with simple stress incontinence who are good surgical and anesthesia risks.

In deciding whether to perform surgery, the anterior vaginal wall should be palpated. First, urethral diverticula should be sought; these appear as cystic, sometimes tender masses or indurated areas located in the anterior vaginal wall along the course of the urethra. When these masses are milked toward the introitus, a purulent discharge may be observed at the external urethral orifice. These findings are diagnostic of urethral diverticula, and urethral diverticulectomy may be indicated.

Second, the mobility of the anterior vaginal wall should be tested by lifting it superiorly, using the forefinger and middle finger at each side of the bladder neck. This maneuver not only allows determination of whether the bladder can be lifted and, therefore, suspended but also determines the elasticity of the anterior vaginal wall. In certain cases, the wall is very rigid and inelastic and, when lifted, provokes significant pelvic and vaginal pain. In such cases, the bladder-suspension procedure is probably **contraindicated.**

The artificial urinary sphincter is a device that can be implanted in men and women who have severe urinary incontinence due to a paralytic sphincter or a fibrous or traumatized urethra, and in men with postprostatectomy incontinence. This silicone rubber device is composed of

3 parts: a pressurized balloon, a deflating bulb, and a cuff. The parts are interconnected by an assembly unit that controls the flow of fluid within the system. The entire device is surgically implanted: the cuff, around the bulbous urethra or bladder neck; the deflating bulb, in the labia or hemiscrotum; and the pressurized balloon, in the prevesical space.

This semiautomatic device automatically pressurizes the cuff, occludes the urethra, and augments urethral resistance. The cuff is opened by squeezing the deflating bulb, causing a transfer of fluid from the cuff to the balloon. The overall success rate of this device is about 75 to 90%. Its mechanical failure rate is about 15%, but 95% of these failures are correctable. Implantation of an artificial urinary sphincter is **contraindicated** in patients who are unable to empty their bladder completely and in those who have a memory deficit.

An alternative procedure in women with defective or noncompliant sphincters is a **vaginal sling operation.** A strip of rectus fascia or a synthetic material is used to sling and lift the bladder neck, augmenting urethral resistance. Like the artificial sphincter, this procedure should be used only in cases in which the urethral wall is defective.

FUNCTIONAL INCONTINENCE

Urinary incontinence observed in patients with normal bladder and urethral function. This problem appears to be due to inability to comprehend the need to void or to communicate the sense of urgency or imminence of voiding. Consequently, large volumes are voided, with total emptying of the bladder, in inappropriate situations and environments. The patient may or may not be aware of the event.

Functional incontinence is typically seen in patients with severe dementia, closed head injuries, and in some cases, stroke. The diagnosis is usually obvious but occasionally is made only after the usual evaluation has been performed and other pathologic processes have been ruled out. Too often, the diagnosis of functional incontinence is made inappropriately, when the problem is really due to a patient's restricted mobility and failure of care givers to provide a urinal or bedpan or to get the patient to a commode.

Treatment

Treatment for functional incontinence (and for other forms of incontinence that fail to respond to standard treatment modalities) is directed at containing the urinary leakage with the use of external devices and superabsorbent lightweight pads. Men are better suited to external devices than women, and many such devices are available. In most instances, a double adhesive strip is wrapped around the penis. The condom portion is rolled over the strip and connected to the urinary drainage bag with a catheter. The device should be fit and applied initially by personnel who are familiar with its use.

For women and for men who cannot use the condom catheter, light-weight superabsorbent pads can be used. Gerontology nurses and enterostomal therapists can help in fitting such patients with the appropriate device or the best material to contain the involuntary urine loss.

A regular toileting technic (see Treatment under URGE INCONTI-NENCE, above) may help confused, incontinent patients or those with physical immobility.

COMPLEX INCONTINENCE

Incontinence secondary to combined urge and stress incontinence. This problem is prevalent in the elderly, especially women. The presenting complaint may be pure stress or urge incontinence, but generally symptoms of both can be obtained in the history. Usually, these patients have long-standing mild or moderate stress incontinence, with urge incontinence of more recent onset.

In general, the diagnosis can be suspected from the history and physical examination. Definitive diagnosis can be made by using the technics described above under DIAGNOSTIC EVALUATION. Complex urodynamic tests may be needed to establish this diagnosis.

Treatment

Treatment should focus on the most predominant symptom. Urge incontinence is usually the predominant component and should be managed as described above. If incontinence persists and is primarily stress related, it should be treated with a combination of anticholinergic and α-adrenergic agonist (see above). If stress incontinence persists, bladder suspension may be performed; urge incontinence should be controlled pharmacologically or by other means postoperatively.

When behavior-modification, pharmacologic, and surgical therapy fail in patients with complex incontinence, **superabsorbent pads** are the next choice. The skin should be protected from irritation, and the pads should be changed regularly. In most cases, this approach is satisfactory.

When all other methods have failed, the use of an indwelling Foley catheter is the only alternative. Attempts should be made periodically to wean patients from the catheter. **In women,** such catheterization is acceptable, although periodic urine loss around the catheter and expulsion of the catheter with the balloon still inflated are common problems.

The most common mistake made by care givers when these problems arise is to either increase the balloon volume to 10, 15, or even 30 mL or to increase the size of the catheter. However, the most common cause of urine leaking around the catheter or the balloon being extruded is bladder contractions pushing the urine and the catheter out of the urethra. The treatment, therefore, is to prevent the uninhibited bladder contractions with an anticholinergic/antispasmodic agent (see Treatment under URGE INCONTINENCE, above).

In men, the high incidence of epididymitis and urethritis warrant consideration of suprapubic cystostomy whenever prolonged permanent drainage is anticipated. If incontinence persists despite the cystostomy, bladder relaxants should be used.

11. PAIN

Russell K. Portenoy

Until recently, little attention has been given to the influence of aging on the incidence, clinical manifestations, and treatment of pain. However, new information provides a framework for rational nosology and therapeutic strategy.

Epidemiology

Although a recent survey found that persistent pain increased threefold between 18 and 80 yr of age, the largest survey of pain yet conducted revealed an age-related *reduction* in pain at all anatomic sites other than joints. Other studies have shown that analgesic use declines with age, the elderly constitute a relatively small proportion of pain-clinic admissions, and fewer pain complaints are recorded in older than in younger patients with MI.

A shift occurs in the relative frequency of disorders commonly associated with pain. Osteoarthritis is by far the most common painful disorder in the elderly. Neuropathic pain, notably trigeminal and postherpetic neuralgia, occurs often, while common, chronic nonmalignant pain syndromes (eg, atypical facial, failed low-back, and myofascial pain) appear to be infrequent.

The age-related reduction in pain incidence is unexplained but may be related to alterations in neural pathways involved in **nociception** (ie, *the sensation of a noxious stimulus*) or to differences in the psychologic disposition to report pain. The latter may reflect cautiousness in responding to any stimuli or stoicism toward pain. If neural changes are the cause, the lower incidence of pain accurately represents the experience of these patients. However, if the lower incidence derives from less reporting, pain may be underrecognized and inadequately assessed and treated.

Studies suggest that the neural apparatus involved in nociception does *not* decline with age. Therefore, comprehensive pain assessment is necessary to ensure that underlying conditions are not missed.

Chronic pain has an exaggerated impact in this population, and associated affective and behavioral disturbances may become particular problems. Depression often complicates pain in the older patient, who may deny overt mood disturbance but manifest profound vegetative signs (eg, sleep abnormalities and lassitude). The term **"abnormal illness be-**

havior" characterizes a syndrome of behavioral change commonly accompanying chronic pain (including social isolation, loss of interest in avocations, and inability to perform usual activities of daily living). Such consequences of chronic pain are especially urgent in older persons, who can rapidly become hopeless and disabled.

Assessment

The **history** is central. Stoicism or slowness to respond, at times compounded by mild cognitive deficits, compromises the reliability of the history. The clinician must be alert to this, spend adequate time with the patient, and obtain additional history from others.

The assessment of pain includes its location, severity, quality, duration and course, palliative and provocative factors, and associated somatic and psychosocial symptoms. A medical and drug history should include an attempt to evaluate compliance. A family history of chronic pain may clarify the patient's complaints. The patient's level of cognitive, psychologic, and social functioning must also be assessed.

One should distinguish **nociception** from **pain**, a perception only loosely related to nociception. The nociceptive focus (eg, an arthritic joint) must be identified so primary therapy can be instituted. However, pain can exist in the absence of a nociceptive focus, and conversely, profound tissue damage can be present without the *perception* of pain. In addition, the **concept of suffering** must be distinguished from both pain and nociception.

Suffering is *the aversive emotional state derived from the aggregate of negative perceptions, only one of which is pain.* Treatment directed only at pain or its nociceptive components will be ineffective in a patient whose complaints express more pervasive suffering (eg, loss of friends, withdrawal of family, financial concerns, and physical impairments).

Physical examination aims to identify underlying nociceptive factors; it includes observation and palpation of the painful region and functional testing, if indicated. Laboratory and special studies are determined by findings in the history and physical examination.

Classification

One classification distinguishes acute from chronic pain. **Acute pain** usually has a readily identifiable cause (eg, hip fracture) and signals tissue damage, enforcing immobility that may be essential for healing. The associated affect is anxiety, and the concomitant physiologic findings are those of sympathetic stimulation (eg, tachycardia, tachypnea, diaphoresis).

An important subgroup of acute pain syndromes is characterized by **recurrence;** eg, recurrent acute pain from arthritis, intermittent claudication, or decubitus ulcers.

Chronic pain is that lasting > 6 mo or persisting > 1 mo beyond the expected healing period. In contrast to acute pain, chronic pain loses its adaptive biologic function. Depression is common, and abnormal illness behavior often compounds the patient's impairment.

Chronic pain can be broadly divided into that which is **somatogenic** and that which is **predominantly psychogenic,** a distinction based on pathophysiologic considerations. A similar, more sophisticated classification designates chronic pain as **nociceptive,** or that which is commensurate with ongoing activation of pain-sensitive nerve fibers; neuropathic, or that which is **due to identifiable organic processes affecting afferent neural pathways;** and that which is **psychologic** (see TABLE 11–1). Although these distinctions may blur in the individual patient, this classification provides a practical clinical framework that aids diagnosis and management.

TABLE 11–1. PROPOSED PATHOPHYSIOLOGIC CLASSIFICATION OF PAIN

Type	Subtype	Example	Comment
Nociceptive	Somatic	Bone metastases	Due to chronic activation of nociceptive afferent neurons
	Visceral	Bowel obstruction	
Neuropathic			
Deafferentation	Peripheral	Phantom limb	Due to central reorganization of sensory processing after injury to an afferent pathway
	Central	Thalamic pain	
Sympathetic maintained		Causalgia	
Peripheral neuropathic	Compressive	Carpal tunnel	
	Neuroma	Stump pain	
	Neuralgic	Trigeminal neuralgia	
Psychogenic	Somatoform disorder	Psychogenic pain	Does not include factitious disorders, eg, malingering
	Chronic nonmalignant pain syndrome	Failed low-back	

Nociceptive pain can be somatic or visceral. Most chronic pain in the elderly is nociceptive and somatic; arthritis, cancer pain, and myofascial pain are most common. Relief requires removal of the peripheral cause (eg, reducing periarticular inflammation) and analgesic drugs are often effective. Therapeutic interruption of afferent nerve pathways may ameliorate the pain but is usually impractical and risky.

A subtype of neuropathic pain is related to reorganization of CNS processing of nociceptive information and persists in the absence of ongoing activation of pain-sensitive fibers. This pain, known collectively as the **deafferentation syndromes,** includes postherpetic neuralgia, central pain (which can result from a lesion at any level of the CNS), phantom-limb pain, and others. Another subtype, often called **sympathetic-main-**

tained pain, can be ameliorated by interruption of sympathetic nerves to the painful area; the prototypic disorder is reflex sympathetic dystrophy. The precise mechanisms involved in any of these disorders are conjectural, but all can produce an unfamiliar pain, often described as burning and stabbing. They usually respond poorly to analgesics.

Some patients have persistent pain in the absence of both nociceptive foci and evidence of central reorganization of afferent pathways. Many others have nociceptive lesions insufficient for the degree of their pain and disability. Psychopathologic processes may explain these complaints.

Many patients who have pain that is predominantly psychological in origin are best described by the generic diagnosis, **chronic nonmalignant pain syndrome,** a term denoting pain and disability disproportionate to an identifiable somatic cause and usually related to a more pervasive set of abnormal illness behaviors. Some of these patients have no organic illness; their problems can also be designated as one of the so-called **somatoform disorders.** Others have complaints that constitute a specific pain diagnosis, most commonly the failed low-back syndrome or atypical facial pain. Others have significant organic lesions (eg, lumbar arachnoiditis) but also a clear psychologic process that predominates. Diagnosis may be difficult, but the relative contributions of the organic and psychologic components of the pain must be defined.

The chronic nonmalignant pain syndrome is relatively rare in the elderly, whose persistent pain is usually associated with an organic lesion, either nociceptive (eg, osteoarthritis) or central (eg, postherpetic neuralgia). Nonetheless, profound psychosocial impairment is common and can have a devastating impact on function, regardless of whether it causes or is a reaction to the pain.

Another clinically useful classification of chronic pain is broadly syndromic. Chronic pain may be part of a medical illness (eg, cancer or arthritis). A mixture of pathophysiologic mechanisms may be involved (eg, tumor invasion of nerve and bone may cause deafferentation and somatic nociceptive pains, respectively), and psychologic factors may be prominent. The relationship between the pain and the underlying disease must be clarified to permit optimal management. Alternatively, a variety of specific organic syndromes exist that are characterized only by pain, eg, postherpetic neuralgia. Each diagnosis suggests specific therapeutic options.

Principles of Treatment

1. Treat the underlying problem, if possible. Particularly in cancer pain, recognition of the pain syndrome can lead to diagnosis of the primary disease and, possibly, to curative therapy. Although elimination of the underlying cause in nonmalignant pain syndromes is seldom feasible, primary treatment is often available for nociceptive pain (eg, prosthetic joint replacement for intractable hip or knee pain from osteoarthritis).

2. Address psychologic factors and functional impairment concurrently. This requires an accurate diagnosis.

3. Consider a multimodal approach. While some patients respond to only 1 form of therapy (eg, > 80% of patients with trigeminal neuralgia respond to carbamazepine), most require several concommitant analgesic approaches. Therapeutic modalities can be categorized as (1) pharmacologic, (2) neuroaugmentative, (3) anesthetic, (4) surgical, (5) physiatric, and (6) psychologic.

Pharmacologic Therapy

Pharmacotherapy, the mainstay of analgesia, involves the use of 3 categories of drugs: nonsteroidal anti-inflammatory drugs **(NSAIDs),** opioid analgesics, and the so-called adjuvant analgesics (see TABLE 11–2).

TABLE 11–2. ANALGESIC DRUGS

Opioid analgesics
NSAIDs
Adjuvant analgesics
Antidepressants
Anticonvulsants
Neuroleptics
Sympatholytic drugs
Calcium channel blockers
Corticosteroids
Antihistamines
Miscellaneous drugs
Baclofen
L-tryptophan

The aging process may dramatically alter the clinical pharmacology of all classes of analgesic drugs (see Ch. 18). Studies of several opioids have demonstrated some combination of diminished volume of distribution, prolonged half-life ($t_{1/2}$), and reduced clearance for each, *in every case leading to higher plasma levels than the same dose given to a younger patient.* Although the data on NSAIDs are less conclusive and those on adjuvant analgesics almost nonexistent, similar observations have been made about several compounds in each class.

Increased sensitivity to the adverse effects of all classes of analgesic drugs has been noted among the elderly. The relative contribution of pharmacokinetic factors (leading to higher plasma drug levels) and pharmacodynamic factors (increased sensitivity to drug effects independent of plasma level, presumably involving changes at a receptor level) remain undetermined.

General principles of pharmacologic management are as follows:

Choose an appropriate drug, depending on the severity and type of pain. In cancer pain, for example, mild pain is treated with an NSAID, moderate pain usually requires the addition of a "weak" opioid (eg, codeine), and severe pain mandates the use of a potent opioid (eg, morphine). Patients with deafferentation pain are less likely to respond to NSAIDs or opioids and should be treated early with adjuvant drugs, beginning with a tricyclic antidepressant. Patients with pain due to inflammation should be treated with an NSAID.

Choose a short-acting drug. Four to 5 $t_{1/2}$s are required to achieve steady-state plasma drug levels. This applies for initiation, discontinuance, or any change in dosage. A long $t_{1/2}$ drug thus presents a prolonged period before drug effects stabilize. For example, steady-state plasma levels are approached after 12 to 24 h with morphine, but more than a week may be required with methadone, which therefore has a far greater risk of delayed toxicity.

Prescribe 1 drug at a time. When combinations of drugs are needed, they should be started 1 at a time to avoid cumulative toxicity and to allow identification of the offending agent if an adverse effect occurs.

Begin with low doses. *For all analgesic drugs, starting doses administered to older patients should be lower than those administered to younger patients.* For example, an initial opioid dose equivalent to morphine 5 mg IM or 10 to 15 mg orally q 4 h is reasonable. Ibuprofen should be started at 400 mg tid or qid. The initial dose of analgesic antidepressants (amitriptyline, doxepin, or imipramine) should be 10 mg orally at bedtime.

Increase the dose incrementally until therapeutic effects or side effects occur. This guideline is absolute with opioid drugs and several of the adjuvant analgesics, specifically the tricyclic antidepressants and anticonvulsants. Given the **ceiling effect** (ie, a dose beyond which incremental increases fail to provide additive analgesia) characteristic of the NSAIDs and evidence of dose-related toxicity, upward dose titration of these drugs is finite. A useful empiric guideline for the NSAIDs is that the maximum reasonable dose is 1 ½ to 2 times the starting dose; if analgesia is not achieved after an adequate trial at this level, an alternative drug should be considered.

Be aware of additive effects from combinations of drugs. Sedation and confusion are the greatest problems, usually related to shared central depressant, antihistaminic, and anticholinergic effects of many drugs. Similarly, the hypotensive effects of antihypertensives and the vasodilator actions of many agents used in ischemic heart disease may be exaggerated by the α-blockade caused by tricyclic antidepressants or the venodilation caused by opioids.

Continue drug trials for an adequate duration. For virtually all nonopioid analgesic drugs, a minimum of 2 wk at an adequate dose is needed to judge efficacy.

NSAIDs—including aspirin and acetaminophen—are peripherally acting with varying and possibly disproportionate anti-inflammatory and analgesic effects. They can be classified into a weak acidic group and a nonacidic group (see TABLE 11–3). All share a ceiling effect, as noted above. Except for acetaminophen, all are anti-inflammatory, with variable potency. Although all are used empirically for pain, only aspirin, diflunisal, ibuprofen, naproxen, naproxen Na, fenoprofen, and mefenamic acid are currently approved as analgesics in the USA. There are few data relative to NSAID use in the elderly. Therefore, proper use depends on understanding their pharmacology and clinical experience, as follows:

Ensure that the indication is appropriate; eg, mild to moderate pain, particularly that caused by an inflammatory lesion. An NSAID also provides additive analgesia to chronic opioid therapy. NSAIDs should be prescribed cautiously in patients with preexistent renal disease, heart failure, hypertension, and bleeding diatheses, because of the risk of interstitial nephritis, Na retention, and platelet dysfunction shared to some degree by most of these drugs.

TABLE 11-3. NONSTEROIDAL ANTI-INFLAMMATORY DRUGS

Anti-inflammatory, Antipyretic, Acidic Analgesics		
Class	*Drug*	*Comment*

Salicylates	Aspirin
	Diflunisal
	Choline
	   magnesium
	   trisalicylate
	Salsalate
		Choline magnesium trisalicylate and
		  salsalate have no effect on GI tract or
		  platelet aggregation

Propionic acids	Ibuprofen Fenoprofen Naproxen Naproxen Na Ketoprofen	Ibuprofen available over the counter
Pyroles	Indomethacin Tolmetin Sulindac Suprofen	Potent anti-inflammatory effects; higher incidence of side effects
Fenamates	Mefenamic acid Meclofenamate	Use not recommended beyond 1 wk
Oxicams	Piroxicam	Very long $t_{1/2}$
Pyrazoles	Phenylbutazone Oxyphenbutazone	Considered to be most toxic; use supplanted by newer agents

Nonacidic, Antipyretic Analgesics		
Class	*Drug*	*Comment*

p-Aminophenyl
  derivatives
	Acetaminophen	Minimally anti-inflammatory; no effect on GI
		  tract or platelet aggregation

Nonacidic pyrazoles	Phenacetin Dipyrone	No longer used in USA

Choose an appropriate drug. Patient response to an individual agent is highly variable, and the initial choice of NSAID is largely empiric. However, several factors influence this decision. For the elderly, a drug with a short $t_{1/2}$ is generally preferred, although this guideline is less compelling for these analgesics than others. A better guide is a favorable prior experience with a specific drug. A history of ulcer disease or risk of ulcer or bleeding from any cause is an indication for selecting NSAIDs that least affect gastric mucosa and platelet function (ie, choline magnesium trisalicylate or salsalate).

Begin with a low initial dose and titrate to ceiling, as described above.

Switch to another class of analgesic if NSAIDs are ineffective. Drugs within a subclass may have similar efficacy and side effects. Thus, patients who fail to respond to a 2- to 3-wk trial of a salicylate at adequate doses should be switched to a drug in a different class (eg, a propionic acid).

Opioid analgesics are indicated primarily to relieve moderate to severe acute and chronic pain due to cancer. Response to these drugs is enhanced in the elderly, partly because of elevated plasma levels and prolonged clearance and partly because of increased tissue sensitivity. Dosage guidelines in this population are summarized as follows:

Ensure that the indication is appropriate. Severe acute pain, eg, that accompanying fractures, is the clearest indication. For chronic cancer pain, a so-called **analgesic ladder** has been advocated; mild pain is managed with an NSAID, moderate pain with the addition of a weak opioid (eg, codeine), and severe pain with a potent opioid. For nonmalignant pain, opioid maintenance is controversial and should be considered only after all other reasonable attempts at analgesia have failed.

Choose an appropriate drug. Opioid selection is based on empiric factors such as favorable prior experience, cost, availability of a certain formulation, and specific pharmacologic properties. Pharmacologic issues include the class of opioid, side effect liability of specific drugs, and pharmacokinetic differences among drugs.

Class of opioid. The opioids can be divided into pure agonists and agonist-antagonists (see TABLE 11-4). The latter are characterized by a balance of agonism and competitive antagonism at $\geq$ 1 type of opioid receptor site. Clinical characteristics of the agonist-antagonist opioids include a ceiling effect for respiratory depression, a lesser tendency to cause physical dependence, a relatively high incidence of psychotomimetic effects in the mixed agonist-antagonist subclass, and the ability to reverse opioid agonist effects and precipitate withdrawal in physically dependent patients. Because they reverse agonist effects, use of agonist-antagonists is limited to patients not already receiving opioid drugs (ie, as first-line agents only). The only drug in this class available in the USA in an oral formulation is pentazocine, which is likely to cause psychotomimetic effects.

TABLE 11–4. EQUIANALGESIC DOSES AND HALF-LIVES OF THE OPIOID ANALGESICS

Drug	*Route*	*Equianalgesic**	*t ½ (h)*
Opioid Agonists			
Morphine	IM	10	2–4
	po	20–60**	
Methadone	IM	10	15–>100
	po	20	
Levorphanol	IM	2	12–16
	po	4	
Hydromorphone	IM	1.5	2–3
	po	7.5	
Meperidine	IM	75	3–4
	po	300	
Oxymorphone	IM	1	2–3
	PR	10	
Oxycodone	IM	15	—
	po	30	
Codeine	IM	130	3–4
	po	200	
Opioid Agonist-Antagonists			
Mixed agonist-antagonists			
Pentazocine	IM	60	2–3
	po	180	
Nalbuphine	IM	10	5
Butorphanol	IM	2	2–4
Partial agonists			
Buprenorphine	IM	0.4	
	SL	0.3	

* Equianalgesic doses based on single-dose relative-potency assays.
** An IM:po relative potency of 1:6 is reported in single-dose studies of morphine, but uncontrolled data and clinical experience suggest that this changes to 1:2–3 with chronic dosing.

Agonist-antagonist drugs are *not* currently recommended for the treatment of chronic cancer pain and should be used for severe acute pain only when parenteral administration is necessary. None has compelling advantages over the agonists. A sublingual preparation of buprenorphine (not yet available in the USA) has a longer duration of action and may have a broader range of use. Older patients with pain requiring opioid analgesics usually can be adequately managed with pure agonists.

Specific drugs. Of the agonist drugs, meperidine causes a relatively high incidence of CNS hyperexcitability, including tremulousness, myoclonus, seizures, and dysphoria. This effect is caused by the accumulation in plasma of normeperidine, a toxic metabolite with a long $t_{1/2}$. Renal insufficiency is the major predisposing factor for this effect, suggesting that the elderly may be at particular risk. Thus, meperidine should generally be *avoided*.

Pharmacokinetic differences. The most important consideration is $t_{1/2}$. The preferred opioids are those that rapidly approach steady state and, therefore, are more easily monitored (eg, morphine, hydromorphone, and oxycodone).

Begin with the lowest dose that produces analgesia. In the nontolerant older patient, initial doses should be lower than those prescribed in younger patients. For example, opioid-naive patients with postoperative pain can be given morphine 5 mg or hydromorphone 0.75 mg IM q 3 to 4 h. Patients who have built up a tolerance require an initial dose based on their prior opioid exposure, converted to an equianalgesic dose as described below.

Titrate the dose to desired analgesic effect or to intolerance of side effects. If analgesia is *entirely* inadequate after the initial dose in the naive patient, the next dose should be doubled. If *partial* analgesia follows the initial dose of a short $t_{1/2}$ opioid, succeeding doses should be escalated by a smaller amount q 12 to 24 h, as steady-state plasma levels are approached. A useful approach to dose titration involves the concurrent prescription of a fixed dose (q 4 h) and a prn **"rescue dose"** (q 2 or 3 h). The latter should be a short-$t_{1/2}$ drug, the same as the drug used for fixed dosing if possible. This technic provides the patient some control over pain, allows transitory exacerbations of pain to be managed expeditiously, and can be the basis for upward titration of the fixed dose. The increment can equal the total of the rescue dose administered during the previous period or can be empirically chosen to be 25 to 50% of the current fixed dose. Analgesia provided by agonist opioids has no ceiling effect; upward dose titration should continue until analgesia occurs or limiting side effects develop.

Be aware of analgesic duration. Although buprenorphine and methadone are often effective with q 6 to 8 h dosing in some patients, other opioids usually require q 4 h dosing. Analgesic duration is largely independent of the pharmacologic $t_{1/2}$ of the drug.

Administer analgesics regularly. Generally, opioid drugs should be administered around the clock to provide consistent analgesia and reduce anticipatory anxiety and clock watching. Exceptions to this are: (1) In patients requiring long-term opioid use, several days of prn dosing can be used to determine the analgesic requirement. (2) With drugs possessing a long $t_{1/2}$, particularly methadone, dosing should always be initiated on a prn basis to reduce the risk of accumulation and toxicity as steady state is approached. (3) When the degree of nociception is likely to change rapidly, (eg, following certain operations or radiotherapy), prn dosing allows the patient to adjust the amount of analgesic needed. (4) A prn rescue dose is combined with a fixed dose during chronic opioid administration.

Choose an appropriate route of administration. The oral route is preferred for safety, ease of administration, and longer duration of action. If this route is unavailable or if pain is very severe and rapid dose titration is desired, a parenteral route should be used. Parenteral administration is *not* more effective than oral administration; if *equianalgesic* doses are used and all orally administered drug is absorbed, efficacy is the same, although onset of action is faster via the parenteral route. Opioids have a wide range of potential routes of administration (see TABLE 11–5).

Be aware of equianalgesic doses. TABLE 11–4 lists the equianalgesic doses for most opioid analgesics, relative to morphine 10 mg IM. This information must be used when switching drugs or routes of administration. For example, in switching a postoperative patient receiving 50 mg of meperidine IM to 50 mg orally, analgesic potency is abruptly reduced to $1/4$, resulting in undermedication. Conversely, if a patient with cancer pain receiving oral hydromorphone 8 mg q 3 h develops a bowel obstruction and is prescribed 8 mg IM, potency is increased 5 times, with

TABLE 11–5. ROUTES OF ADMINISTRATION FOR OPIOID DRUGS

Route	Comment
Oral	Preferred
Buccal	Not generally available
Sublingual	Buprenorphine effective but not yet available in USA; efficacy of morphine by this route suggested in 1 study, although absorption is variable; other drugs not tested
Rectal	Morphine, oxymorphone, and hydromorphone suppositories available; although very few studies, believed to be approximately equianalgesic with oral route
Subcutaneous Repetitive bolus Continuous infusion	Recent advent of ambulatory pumps allows outpatient continuous s.c. infusion
Intramuscular	—
Intravenous Repetitive bolus Continuous infusion Patient-controlled analgesia	Patient-controlled analgesia shown to provide analgesia with less drug in postoperative setting; however, cost and need for manual dexterity and intact cognitions limit its utility, particularly in the elderly and the severely ill
Epidural Repetitive bolus Continuous infusion	Spinal administration now well accepted and used for both cancer pain and postoperative pain, many controversies remain, especially in cancer pain, including indications, best drug, timing of therapy, and best site of administration
Intraventricular	Experimental technic for cancer pain

a serious risk of toxicity. Similar considerations apply when switching from 1 drug to another; since cross-tolerance between drugs is incomplete, the equianalgesic dose should be reduced by $\frac{1}{3}$ to $\frac{1}{2}$.

Anticipate and treat side effects. Constipation and sedation or confusion are the most common opioid side effects in older persons. **Constipation** should be addressed at the start of therapy and can be managed by (1) an osmotic laxative q 3 days (eg, magnesium citrate, magnesium sulfate, sodium citrate); (2) a daily contact laxative (senna, bisacodyl, or phenolphthalein) plus a stool softener (docusate); or (3) daily administration of lactulose 15 to 30 mL bid. **Sedation and confusion** are often transient and may improve if other contributing factors (eg, the use of nonopioid drugs with sedative effects) are reduced; if they persist, a switch to an alternative opioid may be salutary. The use of a psychostimulant (eg, methylphenidate or dextroamphetamine) to manage opioid-induced sedation should be only a last resort in the elderly.

Although **respiratory depression** is a serious potential adverse effect, tolerance to it develops rapidly, and it is rarely a problem if doses are increased cautiously. If it does develop, an alternative cause (eg, pulmonary embolism or pneumonia) should be sought. **Nausea** may be treated with antiemetic drugs (metoclopramide 20 mg orally qid, hydroxyzine 25 mg orally qid, or prochlorperazine 10 mg orally or 25 mg rectally qid). **Anticholinergic side effects** (eg, dry mouth, urinary retention, and accommodation difficulties) occur occasionally, particularly in patients receiving other drugs with similar effects. Nonessential drugs should be discontinued and a switch to an alternative opioid considered. **Pruritus,** an uncommon side effect, usually responds to antihistamines (eg, hydroxyzine 25 mg orally qid).

Use analgesic combinations cautiously. Drug combinations can enhance pain relief. Absent contraindications, an NSAID may be added to the opioid. One or more of the adjuvant analgesics may also be appropriate, depending on the nature of the pain. However, because *the older patient is at increased risk for side effects, particularly sedation or confusion,* these drugs should be added cautiously, at low initial doses and 1 drug at a time. Guidelines for their use are listed below.

Watch for the development of tolerance, *the need for increasing doses to maintain the same analgesic effect,* a poorly understood phenomenon. Although it can be reproducibly demonstrated in animals, it has a far more variable course in humans. The need to escalate doses could signal progressive disease or increased suffering, as well as the development of pharmacologic tolerance. The earliest indication of tolerance is the complaint of decreasing duration of analgesia after a dose. Clinically, tolerance is seldom a problem, since pain relief recurs with an increase in dose or reduction in the dosing interval. If rapid dose escalation becomes problematic, a switch to an alternative drug or route of administration may be useful.

Observe for signs of physical and psychologic dependence. Physical dependence is a *pharmacologic phenomenon in which a specific abstinence* *(withdrawal) syndrome occurs after abrupt discontinuance of an opioid drug or administration of an opioid antagonist.* Clinically, it poses no problem unless withdrawal is produced by noncompliance or inadvertent administration of a drug with antagonistic effects. In contrast, **psychologic dependence or addiction** *is a behavioral syndrome in which the drug craving is characterized by acquisition of the drug from multiple sources, unsanctioned dose escalation, and drug hoarding.* Although this is a risk with opioid drugs, the overwhelming majority of patients with acute pain and pain due to cancer do not develop such aberrant behaviors.

Opioid maintenance therapy in patients with chronic nonmalignant pain syndromes is controversial, especially in the elderly, but some patients benefit substantially from long-term use of opioids, without developing clinically significant tolerance, toxicity, or psychologic dependence. Guidelines for the management of opioid maintenance therapy are shown in TABLE 11–6.

TABLE 11–6. GUIDELINES FOR THE MANAGEMENT OF OPIOID MAINTENANCE THERAPY IN PATIENTS WITH NONMALIGNANT PAIN

Use only after all reasonable nonopioid therapies are exhausted

Formal consent required, specifically noting possibilities of side effects, minimal risk of addictive behaviors, and implications of physical dependence

Agreed-upon period of titration, aiming for at least partial relief of pain

After titration, agreed-upon monthly quantity of drug, with some leeway in daily dose but return to maintenance dose by month's end

Monthly visits

Return of function should continue to be the major emphasis

Drug hoarding and acquisition elsewhere should not be tolerated; if they occur, opioid drugs should be tapered and maintenance therapy discontinued

Rapid dose escalation or escalation without subsequent decrement suggests need for hospitalization

Adjuvant analgesics have other primary indications but are analgesic in certain settings. They are used as initial therapy in many nonmalignant pain syndromes and in combination with opioid drugs in patients receiving chronic opioid therapy.

Tricyclic antidepressants are used in patients with continuous neuropathic pain (eg, diabetic neuropathy and postherpetic neuralgia), chronic back pain, chronic headache, psychogenic pain, and others; 1 trial of imipramine has been effective in the pain of arthritis. Of those available in the USA, 3 have shown efficacy in controlled clinical trials: **amitriptyline, doxepin,** and **imipramine.** These are tertiary amine tricyclics with substantial anticholinergic and sedative effects. Clinical experience suggests that patients may respond to any of the 3, and those who fail to respond to 1 will usually respond to another. Doxepin is least anticholinergic and appears to be best tolerated by the elderly.

The regimens of amitriptyline, doxepin, and imipramine are similar: initially, 10 mg at bedtime, increasing over several weeks to 50 to 150 mg at bedtime. Higher doses may be needed for analgesia, as with depression.

These drugs should *not* be prescribed in patients with symptomatic urinary retention, narrow-angle glaucoma, or greater than first-degree heart block. They should be *used cautiously* in patients with mild dementia and in those receiving other drugs with similar side effects. A baseline ECG should be obtained and a repeat ECG when the daily dose reaches approximately 150 mg; conduction or rhythm disturbances mandate dose reduction or discontinuance of drug.

Secondary tricyclics (eg, desipramine and nortriptyline), or newer, structurally unrelated compounds (eg, trazodone) are sometimes administered as analgesics in patients unable to tolerate the first-line drugs or in those with relative contraindications to them. The literature provides meager support for the use of the former group and no support for the latter.

Anticonvulsants are advocated in neuropathic disorders characterized by lancinating pain, a use supported largely by controlled studies of **carbamazepine** in trigeminal neuralgia. There are anecdotal reports of carbamazepine, **phenytoin, valproate,** and **clonazepam** use in a wide variety of similar pain disorders, prescribed in the same dosage used to treat seizures.

Carbamazepine dosing in the elderly should be started at 100 mg orally bid, then increased gradually to the effective range of between 400 and 1000 mg/day in divided doses. A CBC should be performed prior to initial dosing and again at 2 wk, 4 wk, and periodically thereafter. **Phenytoin,** with an oral loading dose of 500 mg once, 300 mg that night and subsequent nights, may also be used. The initial dose of **clonazepam** is 0.5 mg/day, which is gradually increased; the usual effective dose is 0.5 to 5 mg bid. **Valproate** may be given at 250 mg once or twice daily and increased slowly to the usual range of 750 to 1500 mg/day in divided doses.

For all these drugs, doses should be increased until clinical efficacy or intolerance of side effects is achieved. Plasma drug levels should be monitored, if possible, to judge compliance, to identify patients who rapidly metabolize the drug, to evaluate changes when other drugs are taken, and to document an effective plasma level, which should not be considered maximal without side effects. Although not an anticonvulsant, **baclofen** is classified with these agents because of its documented efficacy in trigeminal neuralgia. When it is used in lancinating pain in the elderly, treatment should begin at 5 mg orally bid and dosage increased slowly, usually to the range of 15 to 40 mg/day in divided doses.

Neuroleptic drugs have been used in a variety of neuropathic pain states, despite a lack of evidence of efficacy in controlled clinical trials. *The risk of adverse effects, including tardive dyskinesia, is relatively high* *in the elderly. Neuroleptics should be viewed only as second-line agents,* to be considered in refractory neuropathic pain, such as postherpetic neuralgia or painful neuropathy. Clinical experience is greatest with **fluphenazine** 1 to 2 mg orally tid; **haloperidol** 0.5 to 5 mg orally tid is sometimes used.

Sympatholytic drugs have been used effectively in patients with sympathetic-maintained pain—specifically, reflex sympathetic dystrophy—according to anecdotal evidence. The oral drugs **phenoxybenzamine, prazosin, propranolol,** and **guanethedine** *should be considered only in unequivocal cases of reflex sympathetic dystrophy that have failed to respond to other measures.*

Calcium channel blockers may be used analgesically. **Nifedipine** has been used in refractory reflex sympathetic dystrophy, and both nifedipine (usually 10 mg orally tid) and **verapamil** 80 mg orally tid or qid may have efficacy in migraine prophylaxis. Recurrent migraine is rare in the elderly, and experience with these agents in this population is limited.

Corticosteroids have been used in reflex sympathetic dystrophy (prednisone 60 mg daily in divided doses, tapered over 2 wk); acute herpetic neuralgia in the immunocompetent host (see below); and malignant pain due to tumor invasion of bone or nerve trunks (empirically chosen as **methylprednisolone, prednisone,** or **dexamethasone** at a dose equivalent to 80 mg prednisone daily). The risks of a short course of therapy with these agents are generally low. Concurrent diseases, eg, diabetes or heart failure, may change these considerations.

Antihistamines (eg, **hydroxyzine, diphenhydramine,** and **orphenadrine**) may possess analgesic activity, although supporting data are limited. One of these agents may be selected for patients with pain and an associated indication for antihistamine therapy; eg, those with pain (particularly from a malignancy) plus anxiety or nausea may be given a trial of hydroxyzine 25 to 50 mg orally qid. The anticholinergic and sedative effects of these drugs in the elderly patient should always be considered.

L-tryptophan 3 to 5 gm daily in divided doses has demonstrated an analgesic effect in several controlled trials. Side effects, when they occur, are sedation and nausea. A trial in patients with chronic nonmalignant pain is reasonable, considering the relatively low risk.

Other Analgesic Approaches

Integration of pharmacologic approaches with other analgesic technics is the foundation of the multidisciplinary team approach successfully utilized by pain clinics in the treatment of refractory pain. Some elements of each of these approaches fall within the purview of nonspecialists (see TABLE 11–7).

Neuroaugmentative technics enhance afferent stimulation to provide segmental analgesia. They are useful for localized pain, particularly that of neuropathic origin. **Counterirritation,** or *brisk rubbing of the painful*

TABLE 11-7. NONPHARMACOLOGIC TECHNICS OF PAIN CONTROL
APPLICABLE BY THE NONSPECIALIST

Approach	Treatment	Indication
Neuroaugmentative	Counterirritation TENS*	Localized pain; neuropathic pain
Anesthetic	Trigger point injections	Myofascial pain with trigger points
Physiatric	Some physical therapy technics, eg, range-of-motion exercise program	Myofascial or joint pain; inactivity
Psychologic	Some cognitive technics, eg, relaxation, distraction; behavioral program	Predictable pain; muscle spasm; inactivity and abnormal illness behavior

* TENS = transcutaneous electrical nerve stimulation.

part, often preceded by application of a vapocoolant spray (fluorimethane or ethyl chloride), and **transcutaneous electrical nerve stimulation (TENS),** now widely available, can be applied by the nonspecialist. Although the analgesia provided is probably short-lived, and cognitive deficits and lack of manual dexterity may preclude their use in many older patients, the inherent safety of these technics recommends their use. Other neuroaugmentative technics, including **acupuncture, percutaneous electric nerve stimulation, dorsal column stimulation,** and **deep brain stimulation,** require special expertise.

Anesthetic approaches include trigger point injection, nitrous oxide inhalation in patients with advanced cancer, and a variety of somatic and sympathetic nerve blocks. **Trigger point injection** with saline or a local anesthetic is useful for myofascial pain. If palpation of a painful region reveals focally tender sites, injection may provide transitory relief, leading to improved physical activity, and occasionally, long-term analgesia. **Nerve blocks** (temporary or permanent, depending upon the solution injected) are most useful in the management of sympathetic-maintained and cancer pain and should be performed only by experienced personnel.

Surgical approaches. Joint replacement may cure intractable arthritic pain. Surgical lesions to manage cancer pain have been placed at every level of the nervous system, from peripheral nerve to cortex. Both chemical and surgical transsphenoidal pituitary ablation have been used to relieve cancer pain. The most common approach is cordotomy. These procedures should be considered only after failure of analgesic drugs and should be performed only by surgeons with expertise in cancer pain management.

Surgery for the purpose of analgesia is rarely appropriate in patients with nonmalignant pain syndromes. Occasionally, patients with reflex sympathetic dystrophy who obtain short-term relief from repeated temporary nerve blocks may be candidates for surgical sympathectomy. A new procedure, the dorsal root entry zone lesion, has been developed for the treatment of selected deafferentation pain syndromes. Early data suggest this procedure can be considered in patients with severe refractory postherpetic neuralgia and pain from root avulsion that is unresponsive to all other modalities.

Physiatric approaches: Many rehabilitative modalities may directly ameliorate pain as well as decrease the level of inactivity and reduce secondary myofascial complications that often accompany chronic pain. Orthoses may be useful in splinting the painful region, reducing so-called **incident pain** that occurs with movement or the assumption of certain positions. Participation of the elderly in physical therapy and exercise programs often improves psychologic outlook and social interaction, if not always the pain.

Psychologic approaches: These modalities include formal psychotherapy, cognitive technics (eg, relaxation training, distraction, biofeedback, and hypnosis), and behavioral therapy to reverse dysfunctional behaviors, eg, physical inactivity and social withdrawal. Many of these technics can be applied by nonspecialists. However, the elderly do not easily engage in these activities and are often not given the opportunity to do so, possibly because of clinician bias against such technics and the existence of subtle cognitive deficits and disinclination to trust psychologic procedures on the part of many elderly patients. For older patients who are willing to participate and appear capable of benefiting, a psychologic approach should be offered.

COMMON PAIN SYNDROMES

Certain pain syndromes are particularly common in the elderly. Their recognition and management should be viewed as a central focus of geriatric care.

NOCICEPTIVE SYNDROMES

Many pain syndromes are best understood as a consequence of ongoing nociceptive stimulation; eg, chronic lumbar pain due to degenerative arthritis and pain due to the failed low-back syndrome. They must be distinguished from others that result from similar organic lesions but are associated with such a degree of psychologic impairment that they are classified with the psychologic syndromes described below. Psychosocial factors are important in the nociceptive syndromes but are less compelling than in other syndromes.

Cancer Pain

This pain is usually nociceptive. A peripheral lesion activates pain-sensitive fibers, even in patients with mixed syndromes also characterized by a deafferentation component (usually caused by tumor infiltration of nerve trunks) or a prominent psychologic component.

Many cancer pain syndromes have been described (see TABLE 11–8). Primary therapy should be directed at the underlying cause, if possible. Most cancer pain can be managed pharmacologically (see Opioid Analgesics, above). Patients who fail to respond to pharmacologic management may be candidates for the invasive anesthetic, neurosurgical, or neuroaugmentative approaches available (see TABLE 11–9). In addition, newer technics of opioid administration (see TABLE 11–5) may be effective (eg, intraspinal administration is commonly used to relieve pain

TABLE 11–8. CANCER PAIN SYNDROMES

Associated with disease
    Bone
        Local pain at site of metastasis
        Generalized pain from multiple metastases
        Base-of-skull syndromes
        Vertebral body syndromes

    Nerve
        Epidural spinal cord compression
        Leptomeningeal metastasis
        Radiculopathy
        Lumbosacral or brachial plexopathy
        Painful polyneuropathy (eg, in
            paraproteinemias)
        Painful mononeuropathies

    Soft tissue infiltration

    Blood vessel infiltration

    Hollow viscus obstruction

Associated with therapy
    Postsurgical syndromes
        Post-thoracotomy
        Postmastectomy
        Phantom limb pain
        Postradical neck dissection

    Postchemotherapy syndromes
        Painful polyneuropathy
        Aseptic necrosis of femoral head
        Steroid pseudorheumatism

    Postradiation syndromes
        Radiation fibrosis of nerve plexus
        Radiation myelopathy
        Radiation necrosis of bone

below mid-thorax). All these technics require the guidance of persons with special expertise.

Osteoarthritis (See also Chs. 62 and 66)

Degenerative arthritis is the most common cause of nociceptive pain in the elderly. Several specific syndromes may occur. (1) Diffuse and focal joint pain is frequent, but some patients develop pain at only a single joint or bilaterally at only one level (usually, hips), while others develop only diffuse large and small joint pain. (2) Refractory low-back pain may be related to degenerative processes affecting facet joints and the intervertebral space. (3) An often unrecognized syndrome of occipital headache may occur, related to cervical osteoarthritis.

TABLE 11–9. INVASIVE PROCEDURES USED IN CANCER PAIN MANAGEMENT

Site	Procedure		Purpose
	Anesthetic	Neurosurgical*	Neuroaugmentative
For localized pain			
Pelvis/perineum[†]	Chemical rhizotomy	Bilateral cordotomy; midline myelotomy	Dorsal column stimulation
Epigastric	Celiac plexus block[‡]	—	—
Abdomen/chest[†]	Chemical neurectomy; chemical rhizotomy	Neurectomy; rhizotomy; cordotomy	Percutaneous electrical stimulation
Arms/legs[†]	Chemical rhizotomy	Neurectomy; rhizotomy; cordotomy	Percutaneous electrical stimulation
Head/neck	Chemical rhizotomy; chemical gangliolysis	Rhizotomy	—
For generalized pain			
	Chemical hypophysectomy	Bilateral cordotomy	Deep brain stimulation

* Other surgical procedures directed at the brainstem, specifically tractotomy and thalamotomy, can be done and may be useful for unilateral pain, especially that involving the face; other procedures, eg, lobotomy and cingulumotomy, are now seldom done and were designed to reduce suffering.
  [†] Spinal opioids commonly used in this setting.
  [‡] The risk:benefit ratio of celiac plexus block is such that it is often utilized early in the management of epigastric visceral pain without prior extensive trials of opioid drugs.

Since both anti-inflammatory and analgesic effects are desirable, NSAIDs are the primary treatment (see above). Occasionally, patients with virtually continuous pain or pain compounded by sleeplessness or depression will benefit from the addition of a tricyclic antidepressant. Patients with refractory pain can be considered for opioid maintenance therapy (see TABLE 11–6).

Physical therapy may forestall the development of secondary progressive ankylosis and contractures and helps prevent inactivity. Occasionally, orthoses (eg, a corset for lumbar pain, a soft collar for occipital or cervical pain, or a knee brace) may be useful.

Injections of local anesthetics and corticosteroids into joints, or epidurally for lumbar pain, are widely performed, despite a lack of well-controlled clinical trials establishing their efficacy. Dramatic benefits are often reported anecdotally, and the procedures should be considered if experienced personnel are available to perform them.

Joint replacement surgery is an option for intractable pain in some joints (see Ch. 66).

Other Nociceptive Syndromes

Myofascial pains, common in the elderly, may be acute or recurrent and conform to clear-cut etiologies; eg, bursitis, tendonitis, or sprains. Management usually relies on NSAIDs and local injection. Less well characterized is the **myofascial pain syndrome** (also known as **myofascitis, fibromyalgia,** and **fibromyositis**), which typically involves painful trigger points in muscle. Pathogenesis is obscure, but the syndrome may be related to overuse of a muscle. Pain may be referred and is usually reproduced by palpation of the causative trigger points. Inactivation of trigger points is accomplished by injection (dry needling, saline, or local anesthetic) or by a spray-and-stretch technic, in which a vapocoolant (fluorimethane or ethyl chloride) is applied until the skin is numb and the muscle then stretched through a full range of motion. Physical therapy and TENS may also reduce acute discomfort in these syndromes; continued activity without muscle overuse prevents recurrence.

DEAFFERENTATION SYNDROMES

These syndromes are less common than nociceptive pain syndromes in the elderly. The most prevalent is postherpetic neuralgia; rare causes are central pain, phantom limb pain, and pain from root avulsion. Also neuropathic in origin but representing different pathophysiologies, are sympathetic-maintained pains (eg, reflex sympathetic dystrophy), compressive neuropathies (eg, carpal tunnel syndrome), some painful polyneuropathies (most often diabetic), and trigeminal neuralgia. Adjuvant analgesics are the primary pharmacologic modalities for all of these disorders.

Postherpetic Neuralgia

Persistent pain following resolution of acute herpes zoster. The pathogenesis of this pain is unclear but presumed to involve central reorganization of afferent neural pathways. Persistent pain is present 1 yr after onset in 50% of patients 70 yr of age. Precisely when the pain of acute zoster neuralgia becomes postherpetic neuralgia is controversial, ranging from the time of lesion clearing to 6 mo. About 2 mo after the onset of the acute disease, treatment should be directed specifically to postherpetic neuralgia.

Primary prevention of postherpetic neuralgia may become possible with widespread use of a varicella vaccine. Prevention in patients with acute herpes zoster has been tried with corticosteroids and sympathetic blockade, but their efficacy is controversial. However, the data suggest a management scheme:

Immunocompetent patients > 50 yr of age with acute herpes zoster should be treated with corticosteroids (eg, prednisone 60 mg daily tapered over 2 wk or longer if pain flares on dose reduction). Immunocompromised patients should be treated with antiviral agents (usually, acyclovir); these agents prevent viral dissemination and reduce acute pain but have not been demonstrated to reduce the incidence of postherpetic neuralgia. If the pain is severe or persistent, sympathetic block with a local anesthetic may help. Other drugs that clear the rash or reduce the acute pain include amantadine 100 mg orally bid, levodopa, and adenine monophosphate. The risk:benefit ratio of the latter 2 in the older patient is unknown, and they are not recommended. The data for amantadine are limited to a single study, and its role remains undetermined.

The mainstay of pharmacologic therapy is a tricyclic antidepressant. A controlled trial with amitriptyline has been conducted, but as noted anecdotally, doxepin appears to be better tolerated in the elderly. Patients with a prominent lancinating component to their pain may benefit from the addition of an anticonvulsant. Dosing guidelines for these drugs are described above. L-tryptophan may boost the analgesia provided by antidepressants, and studies have demonstrated its primary analgesic effects; it is a reasonable addition in patients with persistent dysesthesias. Two to 4 gm/day are given orally in 3 to 4 divided doses; dosing should begin low (eg, 500 mg q 6 h) and be titrated upward. NSAIDs appear to have little effect on this and other neuropathic pains, but they help occasionally and are reasonable to try. Opioid maintenance therapy is controversial, but may ameliorate the pain in some patients.

A neuroaugmentative technic, usually TENS, and physical therapy to prevent secondary myofascial complications, should be considered, particularly if the pain affects an extremity. Psychologic interventions are often useful for secondary affective disturbances and abnormal illness behavior. Therapeutic goals should be individualized to restore normal day-to-day function, even when pain relief is incomplete.

Patients with refractory pain should be considered for a trial of temporary sympathetic blocks or subcutaneous injection of local anesthetic and steroid, technics supported only by uncontrolled survey data. All anesthetic and surgical neurolytic procedures carry too much risk to consider except in the most unusual circumstances of profound functional impairment caused by intractable pain alone. The dorsal root entry zone lesion is currently the procedure most accepted.

Central Pain

Persistent painful dysesthesias can complicate a lesion at any level of the nervous system. In the elderly, such central pain usually follows strokes affecting the posterior circulation of the brain; the thalamic syndrome is the best example (unilateral dysesthesias, often accompanied by sensory loss and sometimes by weakness and abnormal involuntary movements, occurring following a vascular insult to the contralateral thalamus). Lesions can be too small to be detected with current imaging technics, and the diagnosis often depends solely on clinical criteria.

Pharmacologic treatment of central pain is similar to that of postherpetic neuralgia. Maintenance of activity, physical therapy to retain the function of affected extremities, and treatment for concomitant psychologic disturbances are essential. Peripheral neuroaugmentative technics are seldom useful since the pain is diffuse (often hemibody), although deep brain stimulation has been used in specialized centers. Neurolytic technics are not useful.

Compressive Neuropathies

In addition to the pharmacologic approaches described above, splinting (eg, a nocturnal wrist splint for carpal tunnel syndrome) and occasionally, injection of a local anesthetic and a steroid into the site of compression may benefit these neuropathies. Oral steroids (prednisone 60 mg daily tapered over 1 to 2 wk) are used for acute carpal tunnel syndrome, although no controlled studies support this course.

Painful Polyneuropathy

Diabetes is the most common cause of neuropathic pains. **Diabetic polyradiculopathy,** a subtype of which is **diabetic amyotrophy,** can cause excruciating pain along multiple nerve roots, usually lumbar, at times accompanied by weight loss and lassitude almost suggestive of underlying malignancy. The pain is usually self-limited. In contrast, painful **diabetic polyneuropathy** is characterized by dysesthesias of the feet and calves that may be persistent and intractable.

The *acute* pain of diabetic polyradiculopathy can usually be managed with opioid drugs. Adjuvant analgesics are considered if the pain persists for more than several weeks. The diagnosis usually is reassuring to the patient and the severe pain is self-limited.

Chronic painful polyneuropathy is a far greater management problem. Psychologic interventions should be considered early to maintain activity and prevent abnormal illness behavior. Pharmacologic management is similar to that of other continuous neuropathic pains (see above). Occasionally, patients may benefit from the application of TENS to the calves of both legs.

Trigeminal Neuralgia

This disorder is believed to be caused by cross-compression of the proximal part of the trigeminal nerve (usually by an aberrant blood vessel), because an offending lesion is usually identified during surgery, and its removal or mechanical protection of the nerve is followed by pain relief. Other etiologies, including multiple sclerosis, are relatively rare, especially in the elderly.

Medical treatment of trigeminal neuralgia is usually successful. **Carbamazepine** and **baclofen** have been effective in controlled studies; the other anticonvulsants described above are used in patients who fail to respond to these or cannot tolerate them. Patients who fail with drug treatment are candidates for an invasive procedure. **Trigeminal gangliolysis** by a radio-frequency lesion or injection of glycerol or other neurolytic solution provides relief to about 80% of these patients for at least a year. Glycerol injection is now considered the safest of these procedures. **Suboccipital craniectomy** with microvascular decompression of the trigeminal nerve has a similar success rate but is a major operation requiring general anesthesia.

PSYCHOLOGIC PAIN

Chronic pain existing in the absence of any organic explanation or with an explanation insufficient to explain the degree of pain and disability. The presenting complaint may be headache, low back, atypical facial, pelvic, or other pain. Some organic component (eg, degenerative arthritis of the spine in chronic lumbar pain) also is usually present. *These pains are unequivocally experienced,* but psychologic factors predominate in their genesis. The term **chronic nonmalignant pain syndrome** is a general appellation for these conditions (see above).

From the start, therapy must emphasize the interrelatedness of physical impairment and psychologic state. While psychologic consultation is often needed, the nonspecialist can utilize principles of behavioral psychology to reduce the abnormal illness behavior and enhance function. The patient should keep a diary, recording the activities performed and the pain experienced (on a scale of 0 to 10) every hour during selected periods. Specific recommendations should be made for increasing activity; they should be time-contingent rather than pain-contingent. If pain is limiting, the amount of activity can be reduced and again made time-contingent. *The goal is to reduce the intense focus on symptoms and provide the patient with functional goals that can be accomplished.*

Simultaneously, maladaptive behaviors can be addressed with specific suggestions for gradual change; eg, for social withdrawal, a telephone call to a friend may be prescribed first, followed by a once-a-week outing, then by a visit to a senior center, and so on. The cooperation of the elderly patient may be difficult to obtain, but repeated interventions may yield small changes, with self-reinforcing cumulative improvement. Interventions aimed at similar maladaptive behaviors on the part of others in the patient's environment may be useful; eg, advising family members or care givers to encourage the patient to perform self-care activities and not to constantly ask the patient about pain, which only adds to the patient's ruminations.

Attempts to provide pain relief should not be neglected; nonpharmacologic methods should be stressed. Cognitive approaches (eg, relaxation training and distraction), TENS and counterirritation, trigger point injection, spray-and-stretch technics, and physical therapy may all be useful. Therapy with an NSAID and perhaps a tricyclic antidepressant may help. Opioid maintenance therapy can be considered in responsible patients willing to conform to strict management guidelines (see TABLE 11–6). Patients with profound abnormal illness behavior often benefit from referral to a pain clinic, which applies the same principles with greater resources.

---

12. SLEEP DISORDERS

Charles O. Herrera

SLEEP AND AGING

One misconception regarding the aging process is that the elderly require less sleep. While time spent sleeping does diminish as a function of age, the decline occurring from maturity to senescence is minimal.

Authorities disagree as to which changes are a natural part of aging and which are pathologic. Normal differences among individuals complicate this distinction. This chapter compares physiologic changes in sleep habits and common, specific pathologic problems. However, it should be understood that most sleep problems have not been rigorously investigated. Therefore, treatment recommendations are based on the best clinical knowledge available.

In objective studies, subjects exhibit a decreased amount of deep (Stages 3 and 4) sleep beginning during their late 40s and early 50s and experience a higher percentage of Stage 1 sleep, reflecting the numerous micro- and macroarousals that occur nocturnally. Rapid eye movement **(REM)** sleep is well preserved through senescence, although the absolute amount decreases as a function of decreased total sleep time. Sleep efficiency (the ratio of time spent asleep compared to total time in bed) decreases from 95% in adolescence to < 75% in old age.

Numerous surveys indicate that sleep problems are common and important in the elderly, who report spending increased time in bed not sleeping; frequent nocturnal arousals, with difficulty reinitiating sleep; shortened nocturnal sleep time; prolonged time falling asleep (sleep latency); and brief, recurring, involuntary, and often embarrassing day-time naps. Many complain that they awaken feeling unrefreshed and suffer fatigue during the day. Impaired cognition, compromised motor performance, and a generalized feeling of malaise and lassitude are also noted. These somatic symptoms are often *misinterpreted* as anxiety or depression and their origin believed to be psychogenic. However, sleep problems are not simply the result of normal aging. The elderly experience specific, diagnosable sleep disorders as well as medical/psychiatric problems that can cause difficulty sleeping (see below).

Hypnotics, OTC preparations, and alcohol are often consumed in excessive amounts to induce sleep. One survey indicates that the elderly, who account for about 12% of the population, receive 25% of the prescriptions for hypnotics. Surveys of long-term care institutions verify that an inordinate number of sedatives and tranquilizers are prescribed for these patients. Chronic administration of hypnotics is rarely recommended since efficacy decreases with prolonged use. In addition, dosage requirements are often lower than in younger individuals, and drug administration may be complicated and potentially dangerous.

There are other objections to a drug-oriented approach to sleep disturbances: First, the changes in sleep physiology associated with aging are not improved by hypnotics, nor are discrete entities that disturb sleep eliminated. Second, CNS depressants may adversely affect the already compromised physiologic function causing the sleep disturbance (eg, sleep apnea). Third, since the elderly use more drugs than do younger patients, they are at increased risk for potentially harmful drug interactions. Fourth, since the elderly may metabolize and excrete drugs less effectively, they often suffer prolonged pharmacologic effects (eg, daytime sedation and cognitive deficits). Last, since efficacy studies of hypnotics usually are performed in younger subjects for no more than 30 days, data on long-term use in older subjects are lacking.

SPECIFIC SLEEP DISORDERS

DISORDERS OF INITIATING AND MAINTAINING SLEEP

(The Insomnias)

Insomnia, *the inability to sleep,* is a common complaint, increasing linearly with age, and affecting postmenopausal women more than men. Insomnia is a symptom complex, not a diagnostic entity, and should signal the need for a more comprehensive evaluation. Patients may complain of difficulty falling asleep and maintaining sleep, frequent nocturnal awakening, early morning awakening with inability to reinitiate sleep, daytime fatigue, irritability, or problems concentrating or performing under stress. Insomnia is often accompanied by unwanted daytime naps. Many patients spend 10 to 12 h in bed at night trying to sleep. (NOTE: Sleep, as a function of circadian rhythms, and disturbances of the sleep-wake schedule are discussed separately below.)

TRANSIENT AND SITUATIONAL PSYCHOPHYSIOLOGIC INSOMNIA

The most common type of insomnia usually results from an acutely stressful situation (eg, hospitalization, surgery, retirement, bereavement, or other life events). Additionally, change in time zones can produce temporary insomnia, as in jet lag. The benign nature of this disturbance lies in its transient duration of 3-4 days.

Transient situational insomnia can lure the clinician into prescribing a soporific for longer than necessary. A hypnotic should be prescribed for no more than 2 or 3 nights, followed by intermittent use and eventual discontinuance of the drug.

The importance of ancillary measures to control this disorder cannot be overemphasized. Patients should avoid alcohol, OTC hypnotics, caffeine, and exercise before bed. They should urinate before going to bed. Clinicians should pay close attention to side effects of drugs and concurrent illnesses, with the goal of helping patients initiate and maintain a stable, consistent sleep schedule.

These therapeutic measures can help prevent transient insomnia from becoming chronic, a common phenomenon in geriatrics. Short- or intermediate-action benzodiazepines (eg, triazolam 0.125 mg or temazepam 15 mg at bedtime) are preferred to barbiturates, chloral hydrate, and antihistamines. A short-acting agent with no active metabolites is preferred for problems with sleep induction, while an intermediate-acting drug is recommended for problems with sleep maintenance. Patients should be observed for potentially harmful drug-drug interactions.

PERSISTENT PSYCHOPHYSIOLOGIC INSOMNIA

Persistent psychophysiologic insomnia resulting from temporary stress frequently occurs concurrently with incipient medical illness. The insomnia is often ignored while diagnosis and treatment of the primary complaint are initiated. As a result, the insomnia may become autonomous from the primary complaint. The patient comes to regard the bedroom as a place where comfortable sleep will not take place. Rather than sleeping when tired, the patient maintains a state of arousal and vigilance. The concept of retiring for bed produces anxiety and an inability to sleep. In addition, many patients have symptoms of depression, yet do not meet the criteria for a major affective disorder. A clue to the diagnosis lies in the improved sleep these patients enjoy while on vacation or when visiting others. Most have become psychologically dependent on hypnotics, to which they have developed tolerance.

The physician may feel frustrated treating these often unresponsive patients. If possible, patients should be gradually weaned from hypnotics, alcohol, and OTC preparations, with special attention given to withdrawal symptoms and so-called **rebound insomnia. Stimulus control,** a technic that advocates use of the bed for sleep and sexual activity only, involves having the patient get out of bed after 10 min if he has not fallen asleep. TABLE 12–1 lists recommendations for promoting sleep in insomniacs. Through stimulus control and other sleep hygiene measures (eg, gradual restriction of time in bed [sleep restriction therapy], consistent scheduling of sleep and wake periods), the patient can "unlearn" his negative associations concerning bed and sleep.

If the patient does not respond to these measures, referral to a sleep disorders center is appropriate. The Association of Professional Sleep Societies (604 Second St SW, Rochester, MN 55902; telephone 507/287-6006) can recommend a nearby facility. A polysomnographic recording may be needed to rule out sleep-related respiratory disturbances and periodic movements in sleep or other medical disorders exacerbated by or during sleep. Also, close supervision is needed if benzodiazepines are used to reestablish a stable sleep-wake cycle.

TABLE 12–1. TIPS FOR BETTER SLEEP

1. Go to bed and rise at about the same time every day. Establishing a schedule helps regulate the body's inner clock. Also, try to establish a sleep routine by following the same bedtime preparations each night, thereby telling yourself it is bedtime before you get into bed.

2. Make sure your sleep conditions, including your bed, are as comfortable as possible. If you share your bed with a snoring, cover-stealing, or restless partner, make separate, temporary sleeping arrangements until you reestablish a satisfactory sleeping pattern.

3. Wear loose-fitting night clothes. The more comfortable you are, the better.

4. Keep the bedroom dark. If street lights shine in your room or if you must sleep during the day, use room-darkening shades or blinds.

5. Occasional loud noises (eg, aircraft or traffic sounds) disturb sleep, even in people who do not awaken and who cannot remember the noise in the morning. Keep your bedroom as quiet as possible. If you cannot block outside noises, "cover" them with a familiar inside noise, such as the steady hum of a fan or other appliance. Heavy curtains or ear plugs might also be helpful for people who sleep near excessive noise.

6. Hunger may disturb sleep. A light snack (especially warm milk) seems to help individuals fall asleep. However, avoid late, heavy meals.

7. Although small amounts of alcohol (1 drink) may help induce sleep, the chronic use of large quantities leads to disturbed sleep and depression. Avoid taking an alcoholic drink directly before bedtime. When alcohol wears off during the night, you may experience periods of wakefulness.

8. Avoid too much mental stimulation during the hour or so before bedtime. Read a light novel or watch a relaxing television program. Do not finish office work or discuss family finances with your spouse.

9. Avoid using your bedroom for working or watching television. Learn to associate that room with sleep.

10. If you cannot sleep, get up and pursue some relaxing activity, such as reading or knitting, until you feel sleepy; do not lie in bed worrying about getting to sleep.

(Continued)

TABLE 12-1. TIPS FOR BETTER SLEEP *(Cont'd)*

11. Avoid daytime napping, which tends to fragment sleep at night.

12. Many beverages stimulate the body and disturb sleep. Avoid all caffeine-containing beverages after 12 noon. Remember that many soft drinks, as well as coffee and tea, contain caffeine.

13. Try to get some exercise each day. Regular walks, bicycle rides, or whatever exercise you enjoy may help you sleep better. However, avoid vigorous exercise immediately before bedtime.

14. Sleeping problems may indicate anxiety, depression, and many other medical and psychological disorders. Proper diagnosis and treatment of the underlying cause is of primary importance.

15. Sleep medications depress the CNS. Excessive use of alcoholic beverages and other depressant drugs taken with sleeping pills could prove extremely hazardous or even fatal.

16. Sleeping medications should be used with caution in special populations and situations: advanced age, pregnancy, respiratory or kidney disease, and liver impairment.

17. You should receive clear directions for the use of and warnings about any sleeping medication prescribed. Some have a prolonged effect and impair driving skill and coordination the next day.

18. Sleeping medications should be used ONLY for the short-term management of the sleep complaint. Chronic (nightly) use of sleeping pills is usually ineffective after a few weeks, and long-term nightly use may actually hinder good sleep. Do not self-medicate or independently increase your prescription doses. If you feel your medication is losing its effect, report this to your doctor.

(Adapted from *A to Zzzzz Guide to Better Sleep.* Copyright 1988 by The Better Sleep Council. Used with permission of The Better Sleep Council.)

INSOMNIA ASSOCIATED WITH DEPRESSION

Complaints of insomnia are often associated with psychiatric disturbances; the most common is depression, and its most prevalent symptom is insomnia. Although early morning arousal, with inability to return to sleep, is part of typical depression, in atypical depression patients complain of problems initiating sleep as well. The symptom of insomnia alone should prompt the clinician to ask about other complaints, especially when the insomnia becomes chronic and no other cause can be found. Successful therapy depends on treatment of the primary depression (see Ch. 89).

INSOMNIA ASSOCIATED WITH USE OF DRUGS

Chronic use of sedative-hypnotics reduces Stages 3, 4, and REM sleep, and efficacy generally wanes after 30 days. On return of the insomnia, dosage must be increased to produce the desired effect. Discontinuing sedatives often leads to rebound insomnia, which is generally transient but is often managed by reinstitution of sedatives, thus creating a vicious circle. Treatment strategy emphasizes assessment of the insomnia pattern and gradual tapering of drugs, reassuring the patient that rebound insomnia is transient. If after a drug-free period of 2 to 3 wk the patient is still unable to sleep, referral to a sleep disorders specialist may be appropriate.

INSOMNIA ASSOCIATED WITH SLEEP-RELATED RESPIRATORY DISTURBANCE (SRRD)

The coexistence of insomnia with SRRDs may be a cause-and-effect relationship or an epiphenomenon of aging. SRRDs increase with aging. Studies show that 35% of asymptomatic people > 65 yr of age have > 5 periods of apnea/h, mostly central (cessation of diaphragmatic and upper airway respiratory effort). **Central sleep apnea** occurs when there are at least 10 sec without air flow or respiratory effort. Apneic periods of 30 to 60 sec are not unusual. Upper airway occlusion is absent in the pure form of central apnea, although elderly patients often have mixed and obstructive apnea on overnight recording. Patients with central sleep apnea rarely complain of hypersomnolence, and their body habitus is closer to ideal than those with obstructive apnea. The diagnosis can be made only with certainty only by nocturnal polysomnography. On polysomnography, O_2 desaturation, cardiac arrhythmias, and swings in BP are uncommon. Central apnea is more common than obstructive apnea.

Most central sleep apnea is idiopathic, although certain entities (eg, heart failure, nasal obstruction, Shy-Drager syndrome, familial dysautonomia, diabetes mellitus, encephalitis, brainstem tumor, and cervical cordotomy) can precipitate it.

Treatment is largely unsatisfactory for the idiopathic type and is reserved for those with severe insomnia. Acetazolamide, a carbonic anhydrase inhibitor, produces metabolic acidosis and volume depletion and shifts hypercapnic ventilatory response to the left (more sensitive). Its therapeutic use remains experimental, and problems related to sulfonamide side effects arise with its use in an older population. Theophylline, naloxone, and progesterone are ineffective. Clomipramine, an antidepressant, was efficacious in a small study group but requires further investigation. Low-flow O_2 is currently being examined and should be tried in the sleep laboratory before use at home.

INSOMNIA ASSOCIATED WITH "RESTLESS LEGS" SYNDROME (RLS) AND PERIODIC MOVEMENTS IN SLEEP (PMS)

RLS is different from nocturnal leg cramps, in which the patient awakens from sleep with calf pain that is unrelieved by rubbing or analgesics. RLS occurs at bedtime and is described as "running in bed." Relief occurs with movement and symptoms occur when stationary. Symptoms are vague, with twitching and muscular discomfort.

PMS is often incorrectly referred to as nocturnal myoclonus. PMS occurs only during sleep and involves unilateral or bilateral flexion of the big toe, rapid ankle flexion, and partial flexion of the knee and hip. Movement lasts 2 to 4 sec and occurs consistently, sometimes as often as every 20 to 40 sec throughout the night. Incidence increases with age and peaks among 50- to 59-yr-olds. Patients are unaware that these movements are occurring; the information must be offered by a bed partner. Patients who have frequent periodic movements most often complain of insomnia. As in central sleep apnea, approximately 40% of noncomplaining elderly have PMS, while many patients who complain of insomnia may· have more or fewer movements. Drugs that have shown equivocal efficacy include clonazepam, γ-aminobutyric acid **(GABA),** 5-hydroxytryptophan, L-tryptophan, methysergide, levodopa, baclofen, diazepam, and valproic acid. Of these, benzodiazepines and L-tryptophan are most used. The others are considered experimental for this indication.

DISORDERS OF EXCESSIVE SOMNOLENCE

OBSTRUCTIVE SLEEP APNEA (OSA)

OSA is a complete cessation of breathing for $\geq$ 10 sec during sleep, secondary to obstruction of the upper airway. Diaphragmatic efforts persist in attempting to overcome the obstruction; nevertheless, periods of profound O_2 desaturation may occur, with systemic and pulmonary hypertension, cardiac arrhythmias (tachycardia-bradycardia, atrial arrhythmias, ventricular arrhythmias, etc.). OSA has been associated with sudden death at night and can lead to or exacerbate angina, renal dysfunction, stroke, or MI.

Prevalence has been estimated to be 5%. The male:female ratio is 30:1, although this relationship is modified with advancing age to reflect an increasing percentage of women with OSA. Generally, these patients have a high percentage of body fat. Hypertension is present in up to 80%. Thus, the typical OSA patient is an overweight man between the ages of 45 and 60 yr who has hypertension. His wife generally sleeps in another room because of his cacophonous snoring.

Although most cases are idiopathic, certain conditions can produce upper airway obstruction. These include hypothyroidism and acromegaly, which produce palatal enlargement, and micrognathia and retrognathia, which are often associated with trauma or rheumatoid arthritis. A cardinal sign of upper airway resistance is snoring. The site and mechanism of obstruction are variable, but they are usually in the oropharynx or hypopharynx.

The major symptoms of OSA include excessive daytime sleepiness, fatigue, loud snoring during sleep, cognitive impairment upon awakening, recurrent morning headaches, depression, automatic behavior, impotence, and reduced functional capacity. The bed partner observes periods during sleep when the patient is not breathing, followed by grunting or snorting sounds as breathing resumes. Odd sleeping postures are common and the patient can fall out of bed or sleepwalk. The snoring is cacophonous, yet the patient has no awareness of the apneic periods.

OSA is more dangerous than central apnea. Patients suspected of having OSA should be referred to a sleep disorders center for evaluation. **Diagnosis** is made by overnight polysomnography, with assessment of sleep, respiratory, muscular, and cardiac parameters. **Treatment** options are listed in TABLE 12–2. Procedures such as uvulopalatopharyngoplasty **(UPPP)** do not have proven long-term efficacy. Common sense measures, eg, termination of hypnotic, drug, or alcohol use and weight loss, are highly recommended.

TABLE 12–2. TREATMENTS FOR SLEEP-RELATED RESPIRATORY DISTURBANCES*

Drugs	*Other Options*
Acetazolamide	Continuous positive airway pressure (CPAP)
L-tryptophan	Avoidance of supine position
Medroxyprogesterone	Implanted phrenic pacemaker
Naloxone	Low-flow O_2
Protriptyline	Mandibular advancement
	Nasal surgery/adenotonsillectomy
	Patient-managed nasopharyngeal intubation
	Tongue-retaining device
	Tracheostomy
	Uvulopalatopharyngoplasty (UPPP)
	Weight loss

* The only measure that achieves total success is tracheostomy, a procedure reserved for the most severe cases. All others are only partially successful. For example, UPPP, which removes excess oropharyngeal tissue, resolves only about 50% of cases. CPAP abolishes the apneas, but they may return immediately if the patient discontinues use of the device. Some treatments are preferentially employed, depending on the type of apneas observed, eg, acetazolamide for central apnea and protriptyline for OSA. A 5- to 10-lb weight loss may be beneficial in elderly patients suffering from this syndrome.

(Bliwise D: Sleep-related respiratory disturbance in elderly persons. *Comprehensive Therapy* 1984; 10:8–14. Courtesy of The Laux Co., Inc. Maynard, MA.)

Narcolepsy, another cause of excessive daytime sleepiness, peaks in the late teens and 20s. It is differentiated from OSA by the presence of cataplexy, and by the absence of snoring, obesity, hypertension, and periods of apnea. Both OSA and narcolepsy can occur in the same patient.

Other causes: Kleine-Levin syndrome is a rare cause of excessive daytime sleepiness in young males, with sleep periods lasting up to 18 h/day. Other symptoms include hypersexuality and hyperphagia. Insufficient sleep, depression, sedating drugs, and alcohol can also cause excessive daytime sleepiness. Menstruation-associated daytime sleepiness occurs during the menstrual period; sleep time is otherwise normal.

The **depressive phase of bipolar depression** can produce hypersomnolence. Prolonged use of soporifics, anxiolytics, alcohol, and other drugs can cause daytime sleepiness. **Medical conditions,** such as brain tumors, cerebral hemorrhage, encephalitis, hypothyroidism, hypercapnia, or metabolic encephalopathies, can also cause excessive somnolence and are more commonly seen by the primary care clinician.

DISORDERS OF THE SLEEP-WAKE SCHEDULE

Like other animals, human beings exhibit species-specific rest-activity and sleep-wake cycles, controlled by the CNS. Social and environmental factors (eg, light, temperature) contribute to the varied expression of these cycles. The rest-activity cycle is rhythmic and manifests features such as length, frequency, and amplitude.

The term **"circadian rhythm"** (circa—about; diem—1 day) pertains to cyclic biologic activities of about 24 h (eg, the sleep-wake cycle). **Ultradian rhythm** describes rhythmic repetitions of a biologic phenomenon more frequent than once a day (eg, the 80- to 100-min alteration between rapid eye movement **[REM]** and non-rapid eye movement **[NREM]** sleep that occurs with each episode). An activity with an **infradian rhythm** occurs in cycles less frequently than once a day (eg, the menstrual cycle).

Normally, there is a predictable relationship between cycle control and body temperature. Two anatomically discrete pacemakers, labeled X (body temperature, REM sleep, and cortisol secretion) and Y (rest-activity, slow-wave sleep, and growth hormone), control these functions. These pacemakers are located in or around the suprachiasmatic nucleus of the hypothalamus and send afferent signals to anatomic areas that control various rhythms. The duration, internal organization, and timing of the sleep period within the 24-h day correlates with physiologic, biochemical, and hormonal rhythms. In an environment devoid of external time cues, human beings exhibit a sleep-wake cycle of 25.3 h; however, most people arrange for their consolidated period of sleep to occur at the same time within each 24-h cycle.

The increased incidence of sleep-wake schedule disturbances in the > 50 age group suggests loss in circadian control of the sleeping process. People tend to fall asleep and wake up progressively earlier as they age. In addition, notable changes occur in the frequency and amplitude of their temperature cycles in comparison with those of younger individuals. Internal desynchronization of the rest-activity and temperature rhythms is associated with extended sleep episodes and is more easily achieved in temporal isolation studies of the aged. Normal older individuals without a complaint of disturbed sleep are better able to adapt to changes in the internal organization of their sleep-wake cycle. Relative to transient sleep disorders, people in their 60s and 70s who fly take longer to recover, are more affected by jet lag, and tend to use sedatives inappropriately.

IRREGULAR SLEEP-WAKE PATTERN

Insomnia is often produced by constantly changing bedtime and waking time; daytime napping; spending inordinate amounts of time in bed, much of it awake; and going to bed earlier. Illness or hospitalization often leads to an irregular sleep cycle. This problem is difficult to treat because of a "change" in the ability of the biologic clock or its afferent systems to maintain a previously stable and predictable sleep-wake cycle. Conventional therapy, which attempts to restore cycle integrity by resetting the biologic clock with hypnotics, is often unsuccessful. To achieve 7 or 8 h of total sleep time, the patient must take short naps or spend more time in bed trying to sleep. Through the use of hypnotics, the clinician attempts to consolidate sleep into 1 nocturnal episode, and the adjustment period is often too rapid to solve the problem.

DELAYED SLEEP PHASE SYNDROME

Patients with this syndrome are unable to fall asleep for 4 to 5 h and then unable to awaken at the desired time, although their actual sleep duration is normal. When patients awaken at 11 AM or 12 noon on weekends, they are refreshed and able to function. During the week, however, they resort to hypnotics or alcohol to induce sleep at an earlier hour. Such patients often sleep normally while on vacation, since they are not forced to adhere to any particular schedule.

Diagnosis is based on the clinical picture. Sleep is polysomnographically normal. The use of a 2-wk sleep diary documents efficient but inappropriately timed sleep-wake periods. **Treatment** with soporifics, alcohol, or phase advancement (going to bed earlier) is ineffective and may make the problem worse. Chronotherapy (shifting bedtimes 3 h later each night) is safe and effective. Bedtime is moved around the clock until an appropriate time is reached.

ADVANCED SLEEP PHASE SYNDROME

Habitual sleep onset and wake times that occur earlier than desired. The individual cannot adhere to a standard sleep schedule. No pure case of this syndrome has been described in the literature, yet it has great relevance to the elderly patient. The aged have a tendency to go to bed earlier and wake up earlier. Although this syndrome does not meet the strict criteria of a disabling sleep disorder, sufferers complain of fatigue during the day and use excessive amounts of hypnotics or alcohol. **Treatment** includes sleep hygiene (TABLE 12–1), gradually restricting time in bed, and avoiding chronic use of hypnotics. Some patients may need referral to a sleep disorders center. The clinician should look for contributory factors (eg, depression, concomitant medical illness, drugs) that alter sleep physiology.

DYSFUNCTIONS ASSOCIATED WITH SLEEP (PARASOMNIAS)

These disorders occur during sleep or during partial arousal from sleep or are exacerbated by sleep.

Urinary Incontinence

Nocturnal urinary incontinence is found in 5 to 15% of elderly individuals in acute-care facilities and in 60% of those in nursing homes. No studies have addressed the issue of nocturnal bladder dysfunction in the older population. Diuretics given in the evening produce nocturia, thus fragmenting the sleep pattern; many patients have difficulty reinitiating sleep. Other drugs may contribute to incontinence (eg, sedative-hypnotics, tricyclic antidepressants, neuroleptics, anticholinergics, certain cardiotonic preparations that depress bladder contraction).

Management includes an appropriate urologic evaluation. Unnecessary drugs should be avoided; others may be given on different schedules. Fluids (particularly those that contain caffeine) taken close to bedtime should be eliminated, and the patient should go to the bathroom before retiring.

"Sundowning" in Dementing Illnesses

A peculiar phenomenon associated with dementing illness, "sundowning" encompasses *a spectrum of unusual but transiently disruptive behaviors, the etiology of which is poorly understood.* Treatment is based on the use of chemical or physical restraints. However, overreliance on drugs can lead to daytime sedation, nocturnal aspiration, accidents, and drug-drug interactions. Chronic use of physical restraints can lead to pressure sores, muscular contractions and atrophy, and venous stasis with the potential for pulmonary embolism. Sundowning is also referred to as nocturnal senile confusion, thus emphasizing confusion beyond the baseline as an important observation. Other descriptive terms for the syndrome include **nocturnal wandering, nocturnal hallucinosis,** and **nocturnal delirium.** All these terms describe various facets of the syndrome, which may occur in isolation or in combination. Despite its name, sundowning can occur at any time throughout the 24-h day. Patients with dementing illness are in a form of temporal isolation, having lost all sense of time and place.

Demented patients exhibit sundowning through purposeless motor activity and physical and verbal aggressiveness. They are generally uncooperative. Clouding of consciousness or speech impairment does not occur. The total pattern resembles a state of inappropriate hyperactivity with no obvious precipitating factor.

MEDICAL DISORDERS AND SLEEP

Medical illness and the resulting use of drugs can have an adverse impact on sleep. Drugs can blunt nocturnal breathing, exacerbate or cause apneic periods, produce unwanted arousals, and otherwise alter sleep physiology. In addition, many symptoms of diseases are worse during sleep.

Musculoskeletal pain/arthritis: Poor sleep frequently accompanies **fibrositis.** Polysomnography has revealed non-rapid eye movement **(NREM)** sleep disturbance with α-wave intrusions into Stages 2, 3, and 4. Symptomatic relief with analgesics, reassurance, behavioral modification, mild exercise, and avoidance of chronic hypnotic use may ameliorate the situation.

Patients with **osteoarthritis** may awaken with stiffness and pain, then have difficulty falling asleep again. The clinician should formulate a treatment plan based on behavioral change and the judicious use of analgesics, exercise, and other forms of physical activity.

Cardiovascular disorders: Many drugs for **hypertension** can have adverse effects on sleep. Diuretics can produce unwanted awakenings to urinate, with subsequent difficulty reinitiating sleep. β-Blockers, clonidine, reserpine, and α-methyldopa have CNS activity that can alter sleep physiology. Patients with insomnia related to use of antihypertensives may need to have their drug regimens altered.

Angina pectoris can prolong sleep latency and reduce the deep sleep of Stages 3 and 4. The pain of nocturnal angina disrupts sleep integrity, and the concomitant anxiety can lead to chronic insomnia and hypnotic dependency.

Chronic obstructive pulmonary disease (COPD) can decrease total sleep time, cause frequent awakenings, increase levels of lighter (Stage 1) sleep, and markedly reduce Stages 3, 4, and rapid eye movement **(REM)** sleep. Sympathomimetic bronchodilators, the mainstay of treatment for reversible bronchospasm, are CNS stimulants that can exacerbate insomnia.

Gastrointestinal disorders: In **ulcer disease,** acid secretion increases nocturnally, producing gastric discomfort that awakens patients and causes difficulty in initiating sleep. Recent studies support nocturnal use of H_2-receptor blockers. Newer agents are preferable to cimetidine, which can produce insomnia.

Renal disease: Patients undergoing renal dialysis experience chronically disturbed sleep. In uremic patients, long awakenings from all stages of sleep are common, total sleep time is decreased, and there is proportionally less deep sleep. Increased BUN levels correlate with the severity of the disturbance, which improves with dialysis, as Stages 3 and 4 increase.

Metabolic disorders: Sleepiness during the day and decreased functional capacity are prominent symptoms of **hypothyroidism.** Stages 3 and 4 sleep are reduced significantly but return to normal with thyroid replacement. In the elderly, it is unknown how long a sleep disturbance will persist after a euthyroid state is reached.

Hyperthyroid states increase Stages 3 and 4 sleep to almost 70% of total sleep time (25% is normal). When a euthyroid state returns, sleep stages become normal. As in hypothyroidism, little information exists regarding duration of sleep complaints in patients after treatment for hyperthyroidism.

Neurologic conditions: Both sleep initiation and maintenance are compromised by **Parkinson's disease.** Dopaminergic replacement with levodopa has produced variable effects on rapid eye movement **(REM)** and deep sleep, depending on dosage. Amantidine improves quantitative sleep, but its therapeutic effects are more modest.

Most nocturnal episodes of **migraine** begin during REM sleep. Patients may have problems establishing a stable sleep-wake cycle during exacerbations. Serotonin antagonists can produce insomnia severe enough for the patient to become noncompliant.

Institutionally Induced Insomnia

In hospitals, patients are awakened for checks throughout the night, and many find it difficult to reinitiate sleep without sedation. Such insomnia is often perpetuated after discharge through ongoing use of hypnotics that lose effectiveness after a short time.

---

13. PRESSURE SORES
(Decubitus Ulcers; Bedsores)

Marilyn Pajk

Ischemic damage and subsequent necrosis affecting the skin, the subcutaneous tissue, and often the muscle covering bony prominences when intense pressure is exerted over a short period or when low pressure is exerted for a longer time.

The terms **decubitus ulcer** and **bedsore** have been used to describe this problem. Translated literally from Latin, decubitus means "a lying down," which implies a specific positional predisposition to pressure sores. Although pressure sores usually occur from the waist down on bedridden patients, they can develop anywhere on the body (eg, in the nares or in the corners of the mouth from nasogastric or endotracheal tubes) and with the patient in any position. They may also occur interdigitally in patients whose hands are gnarled from rheumatoid arthritis and are common over the ischial tuberosities of patients who sit for prolonged periods. Therefore, **pressure sore** is the preferred term to describe this condition.

The incidence of pressure sores in hospitalized patients in the USA is not known precisely, but as many as 10 to 20% of patients are admitted with a pressure sore or develop one during hospitalization. Some 70 to 90% of all pressure sores are seen in patients > 65 yr of age. The incidence of pressure sores in nursing home residents has been reported to be as high as 24%.

The cost of medical and nursing care for these patients is difficult to estimate but has been assessed as ranging from $6,000 to $8,000/patient/mo for the healing of 1 sore.

The cost notwithstanding, pressure sores increase mortality in geriatric patients. Complications such as sepsis and osteomyelitis add to the length of the patient's hospital stay and the time needed for active rehabilitation. Furthermore, dollar value cannot be assigned to the effect on the individual's mental health and the stress placed on the family.

Etiology

Four physical factors contribute to skin breakdown: pressure, friction, shearing, and maceration.

Pressure is the most important external factor causing ischemic damage and tissue necrosis. Normal capillary BP at the arteriolar end of the vascular bed averages 32 mm Hg. When tissues are externally compressed, that pressure may be exceeded; blood supply to and lymphatic drainage of the affected area are reduced. In the seated or supine position, considerable pressure is exerted by the seat or bed surface on bony prominences. These **pressure points** are especially susceptible to the development of pressure sores (see TABLE 13–1). For example, in the sitting position, pressures > 300 mm Hg can be exerted against the ischial tuberosities, a common area of breakdown in those who sit for prolonged periods or are wheelchair bound.

TABLE 13–1. COMMON PRESSURE POINTS

Most Common Sites	Other Sites
Sacrum	Elbows
Greater trochanters	Scapulae
Ischium	Vertebrae
Medial and lateral condyles	Ribs
Malleolus	Ears
Heels	Back of head

Friction from the rubbing of skin against another surface results in the loss of epidermal cells (eg, when a patient slides down in bed or is pulled up in bed without the use of a pull sheet).

Shearing forces occur when 2 layers of skin slide upon each other, moving in opposite directions and causing damage to the underlying tissue. This may happen clinically when a patient is transferred from bed to stretcher, or when a patient slides down in a chair.

Maceration, caused by excessive moisture, softens the skin and reduces its resistance. This can occur with excessive perspiration, urinary or fecal incontinence, or grossly exudative wounds.

Risk factors in addition to the 4 physical factors described above, immobility, inactivity, incontinence (both fecal and urinary), poor or borderline nutritional status, and an altered mental status (decreased level of consciousness), are associated with the development of pressure sores. Medical conditions that may be associated with these risk factors or may occur alone and predispose to pressure sore formation include anemia, infections, peripheral vascular disease, edema, diabetes mellitus, cerebral vascular accidents, dementia, and malignancies. Other relevant factors include low body weight, smoking, and steroid use.

Classification

Severity of skin breakdown is commonly described by staging or classification systems. A useful staging system is similar to that for burn assessment (1st-, 2nd-, or 3rd-degree). This system provides a clear, objective way to describe the magnitude of tissue breakdown, a common language for all members of the health care team, and a basis for developing treatment protocols for each stage of breakdown.

Stage 1: The epidermis is intact but the area is reddened (hyperemic) and indurated. The reddened area blanches when touched, then returns to red. This stage is reversible.

Stage 2: The epidermis and dermis are broken, resulting in a shallow skin ulcer with distinct edges. The surrounding area is reddened, warm, and indurated. Drainage, usually serous, may be present. This stage is also reversible.

Stage 3: Breakdown extends through the dermis into subcutaneous tissues. The skin edges appear rolled and pigmented, clearly outlining the wound, which may have a necrotic base that has caused undermining. Drainage, usually serous or purulent, is present. This stage may be life threatening.

Stage 4: Breakdown extends beyond the subcutaneous tissue, through the fascia, and into the muscle or bone. Drainage, usually serous or purulent, is present. Sinus tracts and widely undermined areas may be present. Osteomyelitis or septic arthritis in contiguous joints may prove fatal.

Laboratory Findings

Wound cultures: Routine culturing of pressure sores in the absence of clinical symptoms and signs of infection (elevated temperature, inflamed wound margins, malodorous exudate) is of questionable value. Growth of common pathogens (eg, *Staphylococcus* sp, *Escherichia coli*) in such cultures does not necessarily imply the presence of infection requiring antibiotic therapy. If, however, there are symptoms and signs of bacteremia or systemic infection, or if healing of the pressure sore is delayed, a wound culture and sensitivity test is indicated. Bacterial counts of 100,000 organisms/gm of tissue (determined by biopsy in special situations) represent a critical value for wound infection, correlating with the inability of the wound to heal normally.

If the wound is untreated, cellulitis or a chronic infection may develop. A diagnosis of osteomyelitis in the bone underlying the pressure sore must then also be considered. This complication is frequently overlooked, yet it carries a high degree of associated morbidity and mortality. Although more commonly accompanying pressure sores of long duration, osteomyelitis may be seen with those present for as little as 2 wk. A **technetium 99m medronate scan,** alone or in combination with an x-ray, is recommended to detect osteomyelitis. If either test is abnormal, a biopsy of the bone underlying the pressure sore should be obtained and antibiotic therapy initiated according to the results.

Other laboratory values that may be abnormal in patients at risk for or with pressure sores are a low Hb ($<$ 12 gm/dL), a low total lymphocyte count ($<$ 1200 μL), and a low serum albumin level ($\leq$ 3.3 gm/dL).

Prevention and Modification of Risk Factors

Identification of risk factors, which may occur in combination, and at least daily examination of the patient's skin, are essential, especially over bony prominences (see FIG. 13–1). Once risk factors have been identified and the degree of limitation determined, a preventive regimen should be initiated and documented in the patient's record.

1. **Institute a turning schedule,** adapting it to the patient's activity level and daily routine. The patient's position should be changed q 2 h.

2. **Limit the time the patient is sitting up in a chair** to no longer than 1 ½ to 2 h. This position creates intense pressure on the ischial tuberosities. Select a chair in which the patient will not slide down, to avoid friction and shearing forces. **A seat cushion should be used** to reduce pressure against bony prominences (eg, 4 in. high-density, convoluted "egg-crate" foam gel pads made of plastic or silicone). However, no cushion uniformly distributes and relieves pressure entirely. *Devices that should not be used* because they may cause compression and decrease blood supply to the area include pillows and rubber rings ("donuts").

3. **Avoid elevating the head more than 30°** when the patient is in bed (unless the patient is eating) to reduce shearing forces. For the same reason, a pull sheet should be used to help move the patient up in bed.

4. **If possible, teach the patient to change position and to make frequent small body shifts** to help redistribute body weight and promote blood flow to the tissues. **Range-of-motion exercises and ambulation** (if possible) should be performed at least q 8 h to prevent contractures, and to maintain joint integrity, mobility, and muscle mass, as well as to improve circulation.

5. **Select the appropriate bed surface.** The following bed surfaces are listed in order of effectiveness, from minimal to maximal pressure relief.

Convoluted polyurethane egg-crate foam mattress: A high-density foam is less likely to "bottom out" or be compressed by the patient's weight. **Advantages:** It is (1) inexpensive, (2) lightweight, and (3) provides a comfortable surface. **Disadvantages:** It (1) provides minimal pressure relief and, therefore, limited protection, (2) may cause retention of body

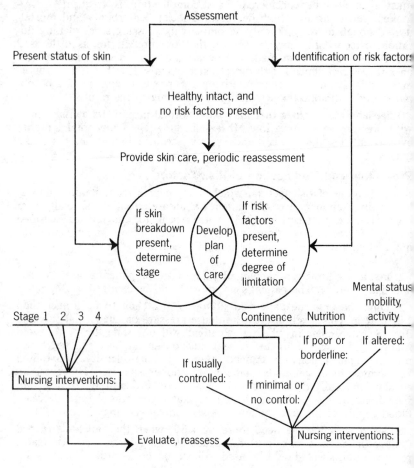

Fig. 13–1. Pressure sore decision tree.

heat, thereby increasing perspiration and potential maceration, and (3) is a fire hazard (may emit lethal fumes if ignited). **Indications** include patients whose activity is limited for a short duration; eg, postoperative surgical patients and those in the operating room undergoing lengthy surgical procedures.

Alternating pressure mattress: A vinyl, air-filled mattress is designed to inflate and deflate small air cells at regular intervals via an electric pump. Some models also have vents that allow air to circulate between the mattress and the patient. **Advantages:** It (1) mechanically alters the points of pressure against the body, (2) provides a moderate degree of protection against pressure, (3) decreases maceration (models with air vents), (4) is lightweight, and (5) is easy to clean if wet or soiled. **Disadvantages:** It (1) minimizes but does not totally prevent pressure, (2) may be uncomfortable because it feels "lumpy," and (3) is more costly because an electric pump is needed. **Indications** include patients who are at high risk for skin breakdown or who already have Stage 1 or 2 pressure sores.

Water mattress: A heavy, vinyl mattress filled with water (via a hose) is placed on top of the bed mattress. **Advantages:** It (1) distributes the patient's weight evenly over the greatest possible surface, (2) provides a moderately high degree of protection against pressure, (3) is comfortable, (4) is easy to maintain (no pumps required), and (5) is easy to clean if wet or soiled. **Disadvantages:** It (1) minimizes but does not prevent pressure, (2) is heavy (130 to 150 lb when filled), and (3) costs about the same as an air mattress. **Indications** include patients at high risk for or who already have Stage 1, 2, or 3 pressure sores.

Air-fluidized bed (eg, Clinitron® bed): A mattress filled with ultrafine silicone-coated beads has warm air flowing through a compressor. A loose polyester sheet separates the patient from the beads, allowing air to circulate around the skin and body fluids to drain into the bed. When the compressor is turned off, the beads firmly mold around the patient, facilitating positioning for dressing changes, transfers, or CPR.

Advantages: It (1) supports the patient at subcapillary closing pressures (< 15 to 33 mm Hg); (2) provides a high degree of protection against pressure, friction, shearing, and maceration; and (3) is usually considered very comfortable by patients. **Disadvantages:** Its (1) fixed height and immovable head make it difficult to get patients in and out of the bed; (2) inability to maintain the patient in semi-Fowler's and Fowler's position is a problem when eating and for patients with pulmonary problems; (3) weight is approximately 1500 lb; (4) circulating warm air may have a dehydrating effect on the patient and the wound; (5) motion or molding make turning the patient difficult (although the manufacturer claims the patient needs to be turned less often, turning and range-of-motion exercises should be performed to prevent pulmonary and renal complications, as well as to prevent formation of flexion contractures); (6) rental fee is expensive ($65 to $85/day); and (7) complexities make it unadaptable for home use. **Indications** include (1) patients with any stage of skin breakdown, particularly Stages 3 and 4 pressure sores and (2) those undergoing graft or flap surgery.

6. Select the appropriate adjunctive devices. Sheepskin is not thick or dense enough to reduce pressure but may be useful if the patient is predisposed to skin breakdown secondary to friction. For example, a sheepskin may be used at the foot of the bed to decrease friction against the heels in patients with vascular disease.

Heel and elbow protectors (pads made of sheepskin or a synthetic equivalent) are primarily effective in decreasing friction. Some models offer protection from pressure as well.

A trapeze enables the patient to move or shift weight while in bed.

7. Evaluate and manage alterations in continence. An assessment of the patient's patterns of continence and incontinence should be followed by an appropriate medical evaluation to elucidate remediable factors (eg, UTI, side effects of medication). A bowel and bladder management program involving the patient and family should be developed.

8. Keep the skin clean and dry. The following is a suggested regimen:

Gently wash the area with plain water or a minimal amount of mild soap and water. Soap removes the skin's natural protective oils, and cleansing the residue may mean massaging already damaged tissues. After cleansing, apply a thin layer of moisturizing lotion, taking care to massage gently around, rather than over, the reddened area. Vigorous massage may increase tissue damage by creating shearing forces.

Apply a thin layer of a petroleum-based product after the area has been moisturized. Petroleum products are water resistant and provide a protective barrier against urine and feces. Heavier agents, eg, zinc oxide and aluminum paste are not recommended; although protective, they are difficult to remove.

Do not use plastic-lined paper bed pads directly against the patient's skin, since they can be drying and irritating. Use only the number of pads necessary to protect the bedding, and cover them with a draw sheet or pillowcase. Use a light dusting of a noncaking body powder (eg, commercially prepared cornstarch baby powder) in skin folds to reduce friction and shearing as well as to absorb moisture. Household cornstarch is not recommended, since it clumps and may support the growth of bacteria.

Use absorbent incontinence briefs, indwelling bladder catheters, or condom catheters judiciously. These may be indicated in some patients but should not be substituted for efforts to help the patient regain bowel or bladder control through continency management programs.

9. Monitor alterations in nutrition. Nutrition should be monitored at least twice a month. A nutrition consultation is recommended for patients who have a borderline or poor nutritional status. Anthropomorphic measurements and laboratory data (serum albumin level and total lymphocyte count) should be obtained. If the serum albumin is < 3.3 gm/dL and the total lymphocyte count is < 1200 μL, oral supplements should be given. Canned oral supplements, which are relatively inexpensive, provide additional protein, calories, essential fatty acids, and trace elements necessary for wound healing.

Functional disabilities affecting intake should be identified and modified whenever possible (eg, poor dentition, poorly fitting dentures). If a patient's nutritional requirements cannot be met through oral supplementation, alternative methods must be considered (eg, nasogastric, gastrostomy feedings, or total parenteral nutrition).

Treatment

Following are the most commonly used dressings and topical agents in the treatment of pressure sores:

Liquid barriers (eg, United Skin Prep®, Bard Protective Barrier Film®) that contain plasticizing agents and alcohol provide a protective waterproof coating over affected areas, reducing maceration and shearing. These may be applied via a spray, wipe, or roll-on method and generally are nonirritating and not affected by urine, perspiration, or digestive acids. Although insoluble in water, they can be dissolved by a soap solution. **NOTE:** Use of tincture of benzoin on reddened areas is not recommended. It has a high alcohol content and becomes sticky when dry, which can pull fragile skin.

Transparent vapor-permeable dressings (eg, Bioclusive Tegaderm®, Op-Site®): Polyurethane dressings are permeable to gases and vapors but not to fluids, allowing O_2 to reach the healing tissues while preventing the entrance of fluids that would contaminate the wound. These dressings work on the principle that healing occurs more quickly in a moist environment. The dressing, which is usually left in place 5 to 7 days, keeps the wound exudate against the wound surface, promoting migration of epithelial cells across the wound defect.

The exudate that collects under the dressing varies in color and consistency from thin, clear, and serous to thick and cloudy brown. This is considered normal, and the exudate should not be drained. The dressing may need to be changed if exudate leaks from its edges. If wound infection is suspected, the dressing should be changed daily. As the amount of exudate decreases, it becomes darker and begins to dry. When healing is complete, the dressing may be removed or may continue to be used to protect the new skin by reducing shearing, friction, and maceration.

Points of emphasis: (1) The wound should be cleansed and the surrounding skin must be completely dry for the dressing to adhere. (2) The dressing should cover at least a 1-in. margin around the wound. (3) The dressing should not be stretched tightly over the wound, since this will exert shearing forces against the tissues. (4) Dressings may be cut or overlapped without reducing effectiveness. (5) If excessive exudate threatens to loosen and pull off the dressing, the drainage may be aspirated through the dressing with a small-bore needle. The dressing may seal itself or may need to be patched with another piece of dressing.

Opaque hydrocolloid occlusive barriers (eg, DuoDerm®, Comfeel Ulcus®) are occlusive dressings consisting of inert hydrophobic polymers containing fluid-absorbent hydrocolloid particles. When these particles come in contact with the wound exudate, they swell to form a moist gel that promotes cell migration and cleansing, debridement, and granulation. The products work on the principle that optimal wound healing occurs in a closed, moist environment. The lack of atmospheric O_2 is not believed to prevent healing when wounds are superficial.

Points of emphasis: (1) The wound and surrounding skin should b cleansed prior to application. The surrounding skin should be com pletely dry for the dressing to adhere. (2) The dressing should con pletely cover the wound and extend at least 1 ½ in. beyond the woun edges. (3) The dressing may be left in place up to 7 days unless leakag of exudate occurs, necessitating a change. (4) The dressing is not recom mended for wounds that show clinical signs of infection (elevated tem perature, purulent malodorous exudate, inflamed borders).

Debriding enzymes (eg, Travase®, Elase®, Granulex®) are proteolyti or fibrinolytic agents that act against devitalized tissue. They are mos useful on superficial wound layers and are ineffective on dense, dry es char (the product must be in contact with the substrate of the wound These agents should be used as an adjunct to mechanical or surgical de bridement.

Points of emphasis: (1) All hardened or dry eschar should be remove or crosshatched so the enzyme can come in contact with the wound. (2 Antibacterials and antiseptics (povidone-iodine, hexachlorophene, silve nitrate, hydrogen peroxide, benzalkonium chloride) may inhibit the ac tion of some enzymes (sutilains ointment). (3) Since some preparation become inactive in 24 h, they must be freshly reconstituted with eac use to be optimally effective. They may also require refrigeration (fibr nolysin and desoxyribonuclease, combined [bovine]). (4) Enzymati sprays (eg, 0.1 mg trypsin, 72.5 mg Peruvian balsam, 650.0 mg casto oil) are easy-to-use, economical products for home use on superficia wounds.

Absorption dressings (eg, Debrisan®, Bard Absorption Dressing®, Hy draGran®) are hydrophilic beads, grains, or flakes designed to absor excess wound exudate and necrotic debris that may inhibit tissue reger eration. At the same time, they keep the wound moist enough to en courage healing. These dressings also deodorize the wound.

Points of emphasis: (1) The dressings usually require changing once o twice a day. (2) The products, reconstituted according to manufacture instructions, are gently packed into the wound and covered with a dr outer dressing.

Suggested **local treatment** for pressure sores Stage 1 through 4 is a follows. Reduction of risk factors and related interventions are essentia for all stages.

Stage 1 (local care): Cleansing with normal saline solution alone i safe and effective. Mild antibacterial solution (eg, hexachlorophene 3% ½ strength povidone-iodine) may also be used and should be followe by a normal saline rinse. **Selection of the dressing** may be dictated b location of the wound: Either a transparent vapor-permeable dressing, liquid barrier, or an opaque hydrocolloid occlusive barrier may be usec All decrease friction, shearing, and maceration.

NOTE: *Heat lamps are not recommended for this or any other stage c breakdown.* In addition to being a source of potential injury to the pa tient, heat lamps dry and dehydrate wounds, inhibiting the healing process.

Stage 2 (local care): Cleansing—same as Stage 1; dressing—transparent vapor-permeable, opaque hydrocolloid occlusive barrier, or enzymatic spray, which has a mild debriding action and improves epithelialization by stimulating the vascular bed. Wet-to-dry dressings may also be used, although they require more frequent changes, tend to be less comfortable, and inhibit inspection of the wound. Dry sterile dressings are not recommended, since they dry out a wound at this stage and retard healing.

Stage 3: Assess and modify risk factors. At this stage, one may become so focused on the local care that risk factors are overlooked. For healing to occur, the wound must be free of infection and necrotic tissue. If signs of infection are present (elevated temperature, malodorous exudate, inflamed tissue surrounding the wound), cultures and sensitivity studies should be done to determine what the organism is sensitive to. In addition, wound and skin precautions should be taken until the results are known.

Debridement by 1 of 3 methods may be performed to attain a clean wound. For **mechanical debridement**, ½ strength hydrogen peroxide (1 part hydrogen peroxide:1 part normal saline) is used as an irrigation to enhance cleansing a wound that has purulent drainage or necrotic debris. This should be followed by a normal saline rinse, since hydrogen peroxide can be irritating to the tissues after prolonged contact. A wet-to-dry dressing, consisting of plain gauze moistened with normal saline or a dilute antiseptic solution (¼ strength povidone-iodine or ¼ strength chlorinated lime), is then gently packed into the wound. Loose necrotic tissue and wound drainage are absorbed into the dressing and removed with each dressing change (usually q 8 h). Mechanical debridement is minimally effective on eschar.

Surgical debridement is the quickest way to remove necrotic tissue and the only effective method of removing eschar. Although effective, surgical debridement may add to the risk of hemmorhage, infection, increased wound size, and pain. **Chemical debridement** (using enzymatic agents) is most effective when used in combination with mechanical or surgical debridement (see above).

Local care of a wound that is clean and free of necrotic material consists of 3 basic components: irrigation, packing, and an outer dressing. For **irrigation,** normal saline is recommended in clean wounds. With aseptic technic, a catheter-tipped syringe may be used to direct the flow of irrigant into the wound. Alternatively, a high-pressure dental irrigation device provides a pulsating stream of irrigant that both aids in debridement and stimulates circulation.

Packing material should be appropriate to the wound size and depth. If wet-to-dry technic is used, the dressing should be plain gauze without cotton filling, since this is more absorbent. With aseptic technic, the dressing should be gently packed to conform to the wound without extending onto the intact skin, since this may cause tissue irritation or maceration. Care must be taken not to pack the wound too tightly, since this inhibits the absorptive capability of the dressing and applies pressure on the area. Other packing materials include the absorptive dressings described above.

An **outer dressing** should be applied over the packed wound to prevent contamination from the external environment. This dry, sterile dressing should be of an appropriate size for the wound and should be secured with hypoallergenic tape or other methods (eg, Montgomery straps, stockinette). Care must be taken to protect the intact surrounding skin.

Care of a Stage 3 pressure sore is costly and labor-intensive. Although many such sores heal slowly by secondary intention, surgical closure is often used to shorten hospitalization and rehabilitation time.

Stage 4: Procedures for care are similar to those for Stage 3. Variations may be indicated in the presence of sinus tracts or exposed bone. **Irrigation** should be performed, using aseptic technic, as described for Stage 3. If sinus tracts are present, an appropriately sized red rubber catheter attached to an irrigating syringe may be used to direct the flow of irrigant. All exudate and necrotic debris must be removed from narrowed pathways.

Packing should be done loosely, directed into all crevices and sinuses of the wound. Gauze, if used, should be kept in one piece to permit easy removal and to avoid the possibility of dressing material being left in the wound. Rolled gauze is available in various widths. If more than one roll is needed, the rolls should be tied together. Exposed bone should be covered with a wet, normal saline dressing and changed q 4 h to avoid drying and to maintain viability of the bone tissue.

An **outer dressing** should be applied, as in Stage 3. **Osteomyelitis** must be considered a potential complication at this stage.

Stage 4 pressure sores are associated with high morbidity and mortality. Surgical debridement to thoroughly excise infected or necrotic tissue usually is followed by a musculocutaneous flap procedure. Postoperative care includes monitoring the patient for infection and keeping pressure off the flap site.

§2. SPECIFIC APPROACHES

14. HISTORY AND PHYSICAL EXAMINATION

Perry J. Starer and *Leslie S. Libow*

Assessment of the elderly patient may be difficult when a complete history cannot be obtained. Since the physician may need to make decisions before all data are available, greater emphasis is placed on the physical examination, while efforts are made to obtain historical data from other sources.

THE HISTORY

Challenges in Obtaining History

Elderly patients may suffer from sensory deficits such as hearing or vision loss, or from aphasia, all of which interfere with the interview process. The interview must be modified for the individual patient. Certain standard questions may not be applicable to patients with functional limitations; eg, the complaint of dyspnea or chest pain with exertion will not be elicited from a patient whose mobility is severely limited by arthritis. If the patient's history is incomplete because of memory disturbances, an alternative source for the data is required (eg, a family member, home health aide, or previous medical history obtained from a physician or institution). However, the patient's chief complaint may differ from what the family views as the main problem.

Older patients may present with multiple, nonspecific symptoms, making it difficult to focus the interview. In addition, clinical features of diseases may differ from those seen in younger patients. Further complicating the process, older patients may underreport symptoms because they consider their illness part of normal aging; eg, they may not volunteer symptoms of dyspnea, hearing loss, vision loss, incontinence, gait disturbances, constipation, dizziness, or falls. No illness should be attributed to normal aging. Nevertheless, a knowledge of which diseases *can* occur in the elderly is essential for diagnosis. For example, although fever, abdominal pain, and diarrhea may be seen with infectious gastroenteritis or diverticulitis, malignancy or Crohn's disease also need to be considered.

Although most elderly patients have a lengthy medical history, they may have difficulty recalling all illnesses, hospitalizations, operations, and drugs used during a lifetime. Further, terms such as "stroke," "heart attack," "constipation," and "dizziness" may require interpretation. For example, "constipation" could mean infrequent bowel movements, hard stool, small stool, or the sensation of incomplete evacuation of stool. Physicians should be prepared to spend increased time in evaluating elderly patients.

Interview Technics

Before the interview, medical records and a list of currently used drugs should be made available. The physician should greet the patient, introduce himself and his staff, and identify any other individuals present. It is essential to determine historical reliability. This may require a mental status evaluation early in the interview, tactfully performed so the patient will not be offended or become defensive. Usually, an explanation for the mental status examination should be given. Some patients may be embarrassed to have a relative present during such an examination. If another person is present, he should be told not to assist the patient in answering questions unless asked to do so by the physician.

If the patient is unable to provide a reliable history, a relative or other person may have to do so. Some patients may even prefer to have a relative present. However, if the patient's mental status is not impaired, he should be interviewed alone to avoid inhibiting him from discussing personal matters. Having a relative present without asking the patient's approval implies that the patient is incapable of telling the entire history. Similarly, asking the patient to wait outside while a relative or friend is interviewed is detrimental to the physician-patient relationship.

To overcome communication problems involving auditory or visual deficit, the physician should move close to the patient, face him directly, and speak slowly. The room should be well lighted and free of extraneous noise. If appropriate, the patient should wear his dentures, eyeglasses, or hearing aid to facilitate communication. If the patient has difficulty hearing the interviewer, an early examination of the auditory canals should be made for the presence of cerumen.

The patient may require additional time to respond to questions, undress, and transfer to the examining table and should not be rushed. If there is a language barrier, an interpreter should be present. An elderly patient may not be able to tolerate a long session; thus, the initial evaluation may need to be divided into 2 sessions.

MEDICAL HISTORY

The review of past medical illnesses should include diseases that, although not common today, may have afflicted patients in the past (eg, rheumatic fever, poliomyelitis). Treatments have changed over the years, and some may not be known to younger physicians (eg, pneumothorax therapy for tuberculosis and mercury for syphilis). A history of previous immunizations (tetanus, influenza, pneumococcus) should be obtained, along with any adverse reactions to them. Results of previous skin tests for tuberculosis should also be obtained.

Although the patient may recall having had surgery in the past, he may not remember the nature of the procedure or the reason for it. If the patient knows where and when he was hospitalized, surgical records can be sought.

A history of blood transfusions should be obtained. Acquired immunodeficiency syndrome **(AIDS)** has been reported in elderly patients but is more likely to be attributed to blood transfusions than to homosexual activity or IV drug use. Similarly, acute hepatitis in elderly patients is usually secondary to blood transfusions.

DRUG HISTORY

All drugs should be reviewed by the physician to identify possible adverse effects. Cognitive dysfunction has been associated with many drugs, including nonsteroidal anti-inflammatory drugs **(NSAIDs)** and cimetidine. NSAIDs may also be associated with upper GI tract bleeding, and digitalis intoxication may be manifested by depressive symptoms or cognitive dysfunction. In the diabetic patient treated with oral agents, symptoms of hypoglycemia may be masked by β-blockers. Topical drugs should also be reviewed. Eye drops, frequently used in the treatment of glaucoma, can be absorbed systemically, with cardiovascular, pulmonary, or central nervous system effects.

A special review should be made of nonprescription medications, since the patient may neglect to mention them. Abuse of OTC drugs can have serious consequences; eg, abuse of laxatives can result in constipation, and aspirin abuse may lead to salicylism.

Simply because a patient produces medication vials does not guarantee that he is complying with treatment. It may be necessary to count the number of tablets in each vial on the initial and subsequent visits. If drugs are administered by someone other than the patient, this person also must be interviewed. The method of storing drugs needs to be assessed. Some patients combine all tablets in 1 vial, making it difficult to differentiate among the drugs. In other cases, a patient may have difficulty opening bottles, especially child-resistant containers. This can be demonstrated in the office by asking the patient to open the vial. A patient may have problems reading the label if the print is small. Further, the actual nature of any drug "allergies" reported must be determined.

SOCIAL HISTORY
(See also Ch. 97)

The social history should include assessment of the patient's living arrangements: number of rooms, availability of elevators, heat, air conditioning, etc. A home visit is the optimal way to assess the home situation. In addition, valuable information can be gained from having the patient describe a typical day.

Support groups available to the patient should be identified. The family's ability to assist the patient should be determined; a full-time job, traveling time to the patient's home, and the health of the family members all play a role. The patient's attitude toward the family and the family's attitude toward the patient need to be probed. The patient's social network (friends or a religious or senior citizens' group) and status (single, married, widowed, or living in a relationship without marriage) should be explored. A pet may play an important role in the patient's life.

An elderly individual suffers many losses that may have an impact on health and well-being. The patient may have experienced the loss of a spouse, a sibling, a child, a friend, or a pet. He may have lost a job and income through retirement; he could also lose his home, status, or independence because of financial or health reasons. He may have lost a longtime physician, either because the physician died or retired or because the patient moved to a new residence.

The social history should include questions about tobacco and alcohol use. Although alcoholism is a serious problem in the elderly, it is often not diagnosed. Signs of alcoholism may include confusion, anger, hostility, alcohol odor on the breath, and tremors.

The physician should discuss and document the patient's wishes and attitudes regarding medical approaches to the prolongation of life in acute or chronic settings.

NUTRITIONAL HISTORY
(See also Chs. 2 and 43)

The patient should be asked what, how much, and how frequently he eats. The number of hot meals eaten weekly should be documented. A diet prescribed by another physician (eg, low salt or low carbohydrate) should be noted, as should a self-prescribed fad diet. Information about the intake of dietary fiber, OTC vitamin preparations, and alcohol, as well as the types of snacks consumed, is useful.

The patient's ability to consume food should be addressed; eg, he should be asked how well he can chew and swallow. The pleasure of eating may be reduced by a decreased sense of taste or smell. The amount of money spent on food and the accessibility of food stores are important issues. A patient may not be able to prepare meals if proper kitchen facilities are not available. Some patients are unable to prepare meals because of visual limitations, arthritis, immobility, or tremors.

PSYCHIATRIC HISTORY
(See also Ch. 85)

Psychiatric problems in the elderly may not be detected as frequently as those in younger patients. Insomnia, constipation, changes in cognition, or somatic complaints may be the first signs. The patient should be asked about feelings of sadness, depression, and hopelessness. Episodes of crying may indicate depression. The earlier suicidal thoughts are uncovered, the more likely suicide can be prevented. The recent loss of a loved one should be discussed. A history of psychiatric care, including psychotherapy, institutionalization, ECT, and the use of psychotropic drugs or antidepressants, should be elicited.

FUNCTIONAL STATUS

(See also Ch. 15)

The functional assessment should include an evaluation of mobility, continence, mentation, and self-sufficiency. The patient may ambulate independently or may require the assistance of a cane, walker, or another person. His ability to transfer and toilet himself should be assessed, as should the need for assistance with cooking, cleaning, or shopping.

THE PHYSICAL EXAMINATION

The physical examination takes on greater importance in older than in younger patients, since a complete medical history may not initially be available. The examination should be conducted in a pleasant, non-threatening environment; temperature should be comfortable and lighting adequate. If an examining table is used, it should be lowered to a height that allows easy access by the patient. The patient should not be left alone on the table. Privacy is essential; if the examination is conducted in the patient's room and a roommate is present, the curtains must be drawn. The patient should be asked if he wants a relative or aide in the room during the examination.

APPEARANCE

Observation may quickly indicate whether the patient appears uncomfortable, restless, malnourished, inattentive, pale, or cyanotic. Preliminary assessment of the patient's functioning can be made early. The patient's clothing and hygiene can be observed. If the patient is examined at the bedside, the use of a water mattress, a sheepskin, or restraints should be noted, as should the use of a urinary catheter or adult diaper.

Skin

In addition to seeking evidence of premalignant or malignant lesions, examination of the skin should include a search for areas of **tissue ischemia** or **pressure ulcers**. Increased pressure over a bony prominence leads to a cone-shaped pressure gradient with the base of the cone on the bone. For this reason, the size of the ulceration seen on the skin surface underestimates the size of the soft tissue lesion (see also Ch. 13).

Unexplained bruises may be the only clue to abuse of an elderly person. The lesions of **herpes zoster** occur in a dermatomal distribution. **Postherpetic neuralgia** is pain in a dermatomal distribution that can persist $\geq$ 1 mo after herpes zoster. The pain is aggravated by even light touch.

Since the dermis becomes thinner with age, **ecchymoses** may occur easily in traumatized areas of the skin, such as the forearm. Venous stasis may lead to eczematoid eruptions over the lower legs (stasis dermatitis). **Seborrheic keratoses** commonly occur; these elevated, well-demarcated, dark lesions with a verrucous surface appear to be "stuck on" the skin (see also Ch. 92).

VITAL SIGNS

Compared with younger patients, febrile elderly individuals in an ambulatory setting are more likely to have a serious disease than a benign illness, such as a viral syndrome, otitis media, or pharyngitis. Subjected to the appropriate stresses, the elderly patient can present with hypo- or hyperthermia. The diagnosis can be made by recording his temperature. Measurements should not be made immediately after the patient has consumed cold liquids. The diagnosis of hypothermia can be missed if the thermometer used does not measure low temperatures (see also Ch. 5).

BP can be altered by anxiety, bladder distention, pain, meals, tobacco, changes of environmental temperature, or exertion. Since BP may fluctuate, multiple measurements under resting conditions should be made. BP may be overestimated in elderly patients because of arterial stiffness. This **pseudohypertension** should be suspected if the brachial or radial artery is still palpable after the BP cuff has been inflated to a point greater than the systolic pressure (Osler's sign) (see also Ch. 30).

Although some authorities have reported that an **orthostatic fall in BP** increases with age, others have observed no effect of age on the prevalence of **postural hypotension.** To determine whether changes in BP are associated with changes in posture, the patient must be observed for at least 3 min in the standing position. Postural hypotension with an unchanging pulse rate can be seen in **Shy-Drager syndrome. A postprandial decrease in BP** with virtually no compensatory increase in pulse rate has been demonstrated in elderly institutionalized patients (see also Ch. 31).

Pulses and BP should be checked in both arms. Respiratory rate can also be a clue to acute illness. The normal rate in elderly patients is 16 to 25 breaths/min. A respiratory rate > 25 breaths/min suggests the possibility of a lower respiratory tract infection prior to the appearance of other clinical signs.

REVIEW OF SYSTEMS
(See TABLE 14–1)

Head

Face: With aging, the eyebrows steadily decline below the superior orbital rim, the chin descends, the angle between the submandibular line and the neck is lost, and the skin wrinkles and becomes drier.

Nose: There is a progressive descent of the nasal tip with age, which causes the upper and lower lateral cartilages to separate. This enlarges and lengthens the nose. Although olfaction declines with age, an asymmetric loss is abnormal.

Eyes: (See also NEUROLOGIC ASSESSMENT, below, and Ch. 93.) With aging, there is a loss of orbital fat, gradually displacing the eye backward into the orbit **(enophthalmos).** Thus, sunken eyes are not a reliable sign of dehydration in the elderly. This recession is accompanied by a deepening of the upper lid fold and a slight obstructive reduction in peripheral vision. A decrease in pupil size and in aperture of the eyelids **(pseudoptosis),** a turning in of the lower lid margins **(senile entropion),** or an eversion of the lower lid **(senile ectropion)** can occur. In senile entropion, the eyelashes may irritate and damage the cornea, and tear drainage may be inefficient, with an overflow of tears.

Acute angle-closure glaucoma is easy to detect because of the associated intense pain; redness; a mid-dilated, fixed cloudy pupil; and loss of vision. However, open-angle glaucoma might not be recognized, since loss of vision is gradual, there is no pain, and the eye appears normal. Findings in glaucoma include an elevated intraocular pressure, damage to the optic disk, and visual-field defects. Tonometry is an important screening tool.

Acute angle-closure glaucoma may be induced by a mydriatic if the anterior chamber is narrowed. (NOTE: Fibrosis of the iris causes a reduced response to mydriatics with age.) Prior to dilating the pupil, the depth of the anterior chamber can be estimated by shining a light from the temporal side of the eye across the plane of the iris. If the entire plane is illuminated, anterior chamber depth is adequate. If the nasal aspect of the iris is shadowed, the anterior chamber is narrowed.

Cataracts cause a gradual, progressive loss of vision. A syndrome has been described in which elderly people with decreased visual acuity experience visual hallucinations despite normal mental function.

Because the lens yellows with age, older patients may not be able to distinguish blue from green. Although hypertension or diabetes may be evidenced on funduscopic examination, there are no significant age-specific changes in the appearance of the retina. Prior to testing vision in the patient who wears glasses, one should check to see that the glasses are properly centered and the lenses clean.

Ears: (See also Ch. 94.) The patient should be assessed for hearing loss. Tophi may be noted during inspection of the pinna. The external auditory canal should be examined for cerumen. If the patient wears a hearing aid, it should be removed and examined; the ear mold and plastic tubing can become plugged with wax. If the battery is dead, a whistle (feedback) will not be heard when the volume is turned up.

Temporomandibular joint: (See also Ch. 95.) Degeneration of the temporomandibular joint (osteoarthrosis) occurs as teeth are lost and excessive compressive forces occur in the joint. Crepitus may be felt at the head of the condyle as the patient opens and closes his jaw. Jaw movements may be painful.

Mouth: (See also Ch. 44.) Dentures should be removed prior to examination of the mouth. Denture wearers are at risk for resorption of the alveolar ridges and for oral candidiasis. Inflammation of the palatal mucosa and ulcers of the alveolar ridges are also associated with improperly fitting dentures. Painful, inflamed, fissured lesions at the commissures of the lip (angular cheilitis) may occur in edentulous patients who do not wear dentures. Inadequate support of the facial musculature accentuates the grooves at lip commissures, creating a moist, protected area conducive to fungal growth.

TABLE 14-1. REVIEW OF SYSTEMS

System	Symptom	Problem
Head	Headaches	Temporal arteritis, depression, anxiety, cervical osteoarthritis, subdural hematoma
Eyes	Loss of near vision (presbyopia)	Normal with age
	Loss of peripheral vision	Glaucoma, stroke
	Loss of central vision	Macular degeneration
	Pain	Glaucoma, temporal arteritis
	Glare from lights at night	Cataracts
Ears	Hearing loss	Acoustic neuroma, tumor of the cerebellar pontine angle, presbycusis, cerumen, Paget's disease, noise trauma, ototoxicity from drugs (aminoglycosides, furosemide, aspirin)
	Loss of high-frequency range	Common with age
Mouth	Loss of taste	Infection of mouth or nose, adrenal insufficiency, nasopharyngeal neoplasm, drugs (antihistamines, antidepressants), radiation therapy, smoking
	Limitation of tongue motion	Oral cancer
	Burning tongue	Pernicious anemia
	Pain caused by dentures	Poorly fitting dentures, oral cancer
	Dry mouth	Drugs (diuretics, antihypertensives, psychotropics, antihistamines), salivary gland damage (infection, radiation therapy), autoimmune disorders (rheumatoid arthritis, systemic lupus erythematosus, Sjögren's syndrome)
Throat	Voice changes	Tumor on vocal cord, hypothyroidism
	Dysphagia	Foreign body, Zenker's diverticulum, esophageal stricture, Schatzki's ring, carcinoma
Neck	Pain	Cervical arthritis, polymyalgia rheumatica
Chest	Pain	Angina pectoris, anxiety, herpes zoster, gastroesophageal reflux, esophageal motility disorders, costochondritis

(Continued)

TABLE 14–1. REVIEW OF SYSTEMS *(Cont'd)*

System	Symptom	Problem
Cardio-vascular	Difficulty in eating or sleeping	Heart failure
	Paroxysmal nocturnal dyspnea	Heart failure, gastroesophageal reflux
Gastro-intestinal	1 bowel movement q 2–3 days	Normal
	Change in bowel habits	Colon carcinoma
	Constipation	Hypothyroidism, hyperparathyroidism, dehydration, hypokalemia, anorectal disease, low-fiber diet, drugs (aluminum-containing antacids, anticholinergics), laxative abuse
	Pain, constipation, vomiting, diarrhea	Fecal impaction
	Rectal bleeding	Colon angiodysplasia, ischemic colitis, diverticulosis, colonic carcinoma, hemorrhoids
	Fecal incontinence	Cerebral dysfunction, spinal cord lesions, rectal carcinoma, fecal impaction
	Lower abdominal pain (crampy, sudden onset)	Ischemic colitis
	Postprandial abdominal pain (15–30 min after eating, lasting 1–3 h)	Chronic intestinal ischemia
Genito-urinary	Frequency, dysuria, hesitancy	Benign prostatic hypertrophy, prostate carcinoma
	Dysuria	Urinary tract infection
Musculo-skeletal	Proximal muscle pain	Polymyalgia rheumatica
	Back pain	Osteoarthritis, compression fractures, Paget's disease, metastatic cancer, infection (tuberculous spondylitis)
Neurologic	Syncope	Postural hypotension, seizure, cardiac dysrhythmia, aortic stenosis, hypoglycemia
	Fall without loss of consciousness	Transient ischemic attack, "drop attack"
	Transient interference with speech, muscle strength, or sensation	Transient ischemic attack
	Numbness, tingling in fingers	Cervical spondylotic myelopathy
	Clumsiness in tasks requiring fine motor coordination (eg, buttoning shirt)	Cervical spondylotic myelopathy, arthritis

(Continued)

TABLE 14–1. REVIEW OF SYSTEMS *(Cont'd)*

System	Symptom	Problem
Endocrine	Constipation, confusion, lethargy	Hypothyroidism, hyperparathyroidism (↑Ca)
	History of thyroidectomy, treatment with radioactive iodine	Hypothyroidism
	Fainting, dizziness, chest pain	Hypoglycemia
	Frequency of urination, fungal infections	Hyperglycemia
Extremities	Swollen ankles	Heart failure (bilateral swelling), venous insufficiency, hypoalbuminemia
	Leg pain	Osteoarthritis, radiculopathy (lumbar stenosis, disk herniation), intermittent claudication, night cramps
Skin	Itching	Dry skin, jaundice, uremia, carcinoma, hyperthyroidism, allergic reaction, lice, scabies

The mouth should be examined for bleeding or swollen gums, loose and broken teeth, fungal infections, and signs of oral cancer (leukoplakia, erythroplasia, ulceration, and tumor mass). Darkening of the teeth may occur with age, as a result of extrinsic stains and a decrease in the translucency of the enamel.

Tongue: Both the dorsal and ventral surfaces of the tongue should be examined. Varicose veins on the ventral surface of the tongue are common. Erythema migrans (geographic tongue) is also considered a normal age-related change.

The tongue may increase in size in an edentulous patient to meet masticatory demands. Tongue enlargement may also be a sign of amyloidosis or hypothyroidism. A smooth, painful tongue may indicate vitamin B_{12} deficiency.

Neck

The significance of asymptomatic carotid bruits is unclear. In patients with asymptomatic carotid bruits and stenosis, MIs occur more frequently than do cerebral infarctions. Parotitis may occur in dehydrated elderly patients. The parotid gland is swollen, firm, and tender; pus may be expressed from Stensen's duct.

Back

A direct relationship between **scoliosis** and back pain has not been demonstrated. **Spontaneous osteoporotic fractures** of the sacrum (characterized by severe low back, hip, and leg pain and by marked sacral tenderness) may occur in elderly patients. **Tuberculous spondylitis** presents as pain over the affected vertebrae and is often associated with malaise, fever, and weight loss.

Chest

Heart: (See also Ch. 29.) The most common **systolic murmur** in the elderly is due to aortic sclerosis, which lacks hemodynamic significance. Aortic stenosis, mitral regurgitation, and hypertrophic obstructive cardiomyopathy also produce systolic murmurs. The murmur of hypertrophic obstructive cardiomyopathy is intensified when the patient performs Valsalva's maneuver. **Mitral valve prolapse** may cause symptomatic heart disease in the elderly, including chest pain, arrhythmias, mitral regurgitation, and heart failure.

Fourth heart sounds are common findings in persons who have no evidence of cardiovascular disease. Heart rates as low as 30 to 40 beats/min may be normal in the elderly. The presence of an unexplained **sinus bradycardia** in apparently healthy persons does not adversely influence long-term cardiovascular morbidity or mortality, although it is associated with abnormalities of atrioventricular or intraventricular conduction.

The pacemaker syndrome refers to the symptoms and signs related to adverse hemodynamic and electrophysiologic consequences of ventricular pacing. It should be considered in older patients with implanted ventricular pacemakers who develop new neurologic or cardiovascular symptoms, especially if those symptoms correlate with the onset of pacing. Physical examination may reveal hypotension, heart failure, cannon waves in the neck veins, or variability of heart sounds, murmurs, or pulses.

Abdomen

Patients with **ischemic colitis** may have abdominal tenderness, possibly associated with distention. The abdomen is soft and only mildly tender in patients with ischemia of the small intestine, unless there is perforation or peritonitis. Although most **abdominal aortic aneurysms** are palpable, only the lateral extent of the aneurysm can be assessed on physical examination.

Rectum

The anorectal area should be examined for fissures, hemorrhoids, and strictures, as well as sensation and anal winks as part of the neurologic examination. A digital examination may reveal a mass or fecal impaction.

Estimation of prostate size by digital examination lacks accuracy and correlation with urethral resistance. In acute prostatitis, the prostate gland is tender, swollen, and indurated.

Musculoskeletal Assessment (see also Ch. 62)

The joints should be examined for tenderness, swelling, subluxation, crepitus, warmth, and redness. **Heberden's nodes** are bony overgrowths at the distal interphalangeal **(DIP)** joints, whereas **Bouchard's nodes** are bony overgrowths at the proximal interphalangeal **(PIP)** joints. Either can occur in patients with osteoarthritis. Patients with chronic rheumatoid arthritis may exhibit subluxation of the metacarpophalangeal joints with ulnar deviation of the fingers. Hyperextension of the PIP joint and flexion of the DIP joint result in a swan-neck deformity. Hyperextension of the DIP joint and flexion of the PIP joint result in a boutonnire deformity.

Both the active and the passive range of motion of the joints should be determined. The presence of contractures should be noted and muscle strength tested. Muscle atrophy should be sought and noted.

Polymyalgia rheumatica (see also Ch. 63) is relatively common in middle-aged and older persons. It is characterized by aching and stiffness in the muscles of the limb girdles.

Feet: (See also Ch. 67.) **Onychomycosis,** fungal infection of the toenail, causes the nail to appear thickened and yellow. The ingrown nail **(onychocryptosis)** has borders that curve inward and down toward the midline and plantar aspect of the digit. Psoriatic nails are whitish, scale easily, and may have a pitted surface.

The **bunion deformity** consists of a medial prominence of the head of the first metatarsal and lateral deviation (hallux valgus) and rotation of the big toe. The **bunionette deformity** is a lateral prominence of the fifth metatarsal head.

Hyperflexion of the PIP results in a **hammer toe.** Hyperflexion of both the PIP and DIP toe joints results in a **claw toe.**

Neurologic Assessment

Compression of the upper arm against the armrest of a wheelchair can cause **injury to the radial nerve,** resulting in weakness of the extensor muscles of the wrist, fingers, and thumb and loss of sensation over portions of the dorsum of the forearm.

In **Paget's disease,** random remodeling of bone and a marked increase in skeletal blood flow occur, which can lead to neurologic complications. Neurologic disturbances can involve the cranial nerves, brainstem, spinal cord, or spinal roots and nerves. In **carpal tunnel syndrome,** percussion over the median nerve at the wrist produces a tingling sensation in the hand along the distribution of this nerve (Tinel's sign). While vibratory sensation in the legs decreases with aging, sensation to light touch and pinprick do not change.

A decline in extraocular muscle function often results in a loss of ability to rotate the eye upward $> 15°$ from the horizontal plane by age 70. In the elderly, the light reflex and accommodation are sluggish, a defect in ocular convergence occurs, and pupil size decreases. However, these findings do not represent disease.

Postural control, reflexes, and gait: Postural reflex impairment occurs with aging, and this loss of postural control may contribute to falling. Postural sway (movement in the anterior-posterior plane when the patient remains stationary and upright) also increases with age.

Generally, the **deep tendon reflexes** do not change with aging. Although some authorities claim that the ankle jerk is lost with normal aging, it can be elicited with skillful technic in most elderly patients. Primitive reflexes, eg, the snout and the glabellar blink reflexes, may reemerge with aging. The significance of these abnormal signs depends on the total clinical picture.

Although a **senile gait disorder** has been reported, its characteristics have been poorly defined. However, several different diseases can produce gait disturbances in elderly patients. In **normal pressure hydrocephalus,** initiating the gait is difficult and step height is reduced, resulting in a shuffling gait in which the feet appear to be stuck to the floor. Gait abnormalities may be present without bladder symptoms or mental changes.

In **Parkinson's disease,** the associated movements of the upper limbs are more consistently disturbed during walking compared to normal pressure hydrocephalus. In fact, Parkinson's disease has 2 clinical subgroups; in 1, the dominant features are postural instability and gait abnormalities and in the other, tremor is the dominant feature. (See also Ch. 84.) The parkinsonian tremor occurs at rest, disappears during sleep, and may reappear during the rapid-eye-movement **(REM)** phase of sleep. It is most pronounced distally in the extremities, beginning asymmetrically in the fingers and thumb and progressing to pronation-supination of the forearm and flexion-extension of the wrist or foot. Involuntary movements of the upper-airway musculature may limit airflow.

Spondylotic cervical myelopathy can also cause a gait disturbance that may be spastic and shuffling. This myelopathy often interferes with complex processes (eg, climbing stairs) before it affects walking on a level surface. Neck flexion and extension are limited and may produce pain that radiates into the extremities or down the back. Deep tendon reflexes are facilitated below the level of compression, and muscle tone is increased.

Mental Status

Assessment of mental status, a key component of the history and physical examination, is discussed in Ch. 80.

Speech and Language

Assessment of mental status in a patient who has a disorder of speech or language is difficult. Such disorders include dysarthria, aphasia, and speech apraxia. **Dysarthria** is *an inability to articulate because of an abnormality of the speech mechanism.* **Aphasia** is *an impairment of language function secondary to cerebral damage.* **Speech apraxia** is *an inability to produce speech, although the speech mechanism is not dysfunctional and language function is not impaired;* the individual movements necessary to produce speech are intact, but the patient appears to have forgotten how to speak.

The dysarthric patient may experience weakness or poor coordination of the lips, tongue, palate, vocal cords, or respiratory muscles, interfering with speech production. Dysarthria may occur in patients with neurologic diseases or mechanical lesions affecting the speech mechanism, such as vocal cord tumors. The rhythm of the speech and articulation of the words should be noted when assessing the patient (TABLE 14–2).

Although the patient with speech apraxia is able to move the muscles involved in speech and understands what needs to be done, he has difficulty speaking. He can perform overlearned acts (eg, counting) and write sentences without a problem. In contrast, the aphasic patient has difficulty speaking or writing. Previously acquired language ability has been lost.

TABLE 14–2. ASSESSMENT OF THE DYSARTHRIC PATIENT

Type of Dysarthria	Area Damaged	Etiology	Speech Pattern
Dysarthria of pseudobulbar palsy	Upper motor neurons	Cerebrovascular accident, amyotrophic lateral sclerosis	Slow, great effort required; prolonged, hardly intelligible words
Ataxic dysarthria	Cerebellum	Degenerative disease, alcohol, multiple sclerosis, vascular episodes	Slow, staccato, blurred, jerky
Hypokinetic dysarthria	Extrapyramidal system	Parkinson's disease	Hesitation, loss of vocal inflection, blurred articulation, stoppages and bursts of speed, sentence often ends in a mumble
Flaccid dysarthria	Lower motor neurons or disorders of neuro-muscular transmission (weakness and hypotonia of respiratory and speech musculature)	Myasthenia gravis	Shortness of breath with resulting short phrases, difficulty in producing loud tones, harsh voice

(From "Speech and Language Disorders," by F. T. Sherman, S. M. Meisells, E. Margolis, and L. S. Libow, in *The Core of Geriatric Medicine,* edited by L. S. Libow and F. T. Sherman. Published 1981 by The C. V. Mosby Company. Copyright 1986 by L. S. Libow and F. T. Sherman. Used with permission.)

Evaluation of language function includes assessment of spontaneous speech, comprehension of spoken language (performance of verbal commands, yes or no answers to questions, pointing to objects), repetition of words and phrases, word-finding ability, comprehension of written material, and writing. In assessing spontaneous speech, attention should be given to the rate of verbal output, the effort involved in initiating speech, and the length of phrases (TABLE 14–3). In testing word-finding ability, the patient should be asked to name objects and parts of objects.

TABLE 14–3. ASSESSMENT OF THE APHASIC PATIENT

Spontaneous speech
  Nonfluent aphasia: Lesion anterior to central sulcus (eg, Broca's aphasia); < 50 words/min; considerable effort required to initiate speech; 1- or 2-word phrases
  Fluent aphasia: Lesion posterior to central sulcus (eg, Wernicke's aphasia); 100 to 200 words/min; easy initiation of speech; uses incorrect words and grammar; makes little sense

Word-finding difficulty
  Circumlocutory phrase (eg, *what you use to tell time* for *clock*)
  Nonspecific words (eg, *thing*)
  Incorrect words (paraphasia)
      Literal paraphasia (eg, *pone* for *phone*)
      Verbal paraphasia (eg, *spoon* for *knife*)
      Jargon (*googooga joob* for *egg*)

(From "Speech and Language Disorders," by F. T. Sherman, S. M. Meisells, E. Margolis, and L. S. Libow, in *The Core of Geriatric Medicine,* edited by L. S. Libow and F. T. Sherman. Published 1981 by The C. V. Mosby Company. Copyright 1986 by L. S. Libow and F. T. Sherman. Used with permission.)

Emotional Status (see Ch. 85)

Nutritional Assessment (see also Chs. 2 and 43)

Many of the measurements commonly performed in nutritional assessment may be unreliable in the elderly. Accurate measurements of height, weight, and body composition (lean body mass and fat content) can be altered by the aging process. Thus, measurement of the long bones of the arm may be more useful than a measurement of height, and use of multiple sites instead of only the triceps may provide more reliable skinfold measurements. (See TABLE 14–4.)

UNUSUAL PRESENTATIONS OF ILLNESS

Thyroid Disease (see also HYPERTHYROIDISM in Ch. 69)

Symptoms and signs of **hyperthyroidism** may be subtle in very old patients, and classic eye findings and an enlarged thyroid gland may not

TABLE 14–4. SIGNS OF NUTRITIONAL DEFICIENCIES

Vitamin C deficiency
"Sheet" hemorrhages along the lower extremities in the bedridden patient
Corkscrew hairs
Gingival hemorrhages
Perifollicular hemorrhages

Vitamin A deficiency
Loss of visual acuity in dim light
Follicular hyperkeratosis

Protein deficiency
Increased ease with which hair can be pulled out
Transverse white band across the nail or a pearly opacity of the nail (leukonychia)

Iron deficiency
Atrophy of filiform papillae of tongue
Hypertrophy of fungiform papillae of tongue
Spooning of the nails (koilonychia)
Cheilosis
Angular stomatitis

Folic acid deficiency
Aphthous ulcers (mouth)
Atrophy of filiform papillae of tongue
Hypertrophy of fungiform papillae of tongue

Vitamin B_{12} deficiency
Loss of vibration sense in lower extremities
Paresthesia in lower extremities
Hyperactive lower-limb reflexes
Spastic ataxic gait
Atrophy of filiform papillae of tongue
Hypertrophy of fungiform papillae of tongue

Magnesium deficiency
Tremor
Carpopedal spasms
Choreoathetoid movements

(From "Clinical Aspects of Nutrition," by C. J. Foley, L. S. Libow, and F. T. Sherman, in *The Core of Geriatric Medicine,* edited by L. S. Libow and F. T. Sherman. Published 1981 by The C. V. Mosby Company. Copyright 1986 by L. S. Libow and F. T. Sherman. Used with permission.)

be present. Presenting symptoms include weight loss, palpitations, and weakness; clinical signs include fine skin, tremor, atrial fibrillation, and tachycardia. Elderly patients with hyperthyroidism may have an apathetic rather than a hyperkinetic appearance. **Hypothyroidism** may present with weight loss rather than gain.

Appendicitis (see also DISEASES OF THE APPENDIX in Ch. 53)

Older patients may complain of diffuse abdominal pain that is not followed by localization to the right lower quadrant. However, tenderness in this quadrant is a significant early physical sign.

Hyperparathyroidism (see also HYPERCALCEMIA in Ch. 71)

The clinical picture can include fatigue, decreased intellectual capacity, emotional instability, anorexia, constipation, and hypertension. Patients often do not have any characteristic symptoms.

Myocardial Infarction (see also Ch. 32)

MI may present as dyspnea, syncope, weakness, vomiting, or confusion, rather than as chest pain. MI is often silent in elderly persons.

Heart Failure (see also Ch. 35)

Instead of complaining of dyspnea, an elderly patient with heart failure may present with confusion, agitation, weakness, insomnia, or lethargy.

Bacteremia

Elderly patients with bacteremia may not be febrile; rather, they may demonstrate nonspecific findings, such as general malaise or an unexplained alteration in mental status.

Systemic Lupus Erythematosus (see also Ch. 62)

Elderly patients have a lower incidence of Raynaud's phenomenon, malar rash, nephritis, and neuropsychiatric disease than do younger patients. However, the incidence of pneumonitis, interstitial fibrosis, subcutaneous nodules, and discoid lupus is higher in the elderly. Older patients may present with the symptoms of a systemic illness (fever, weight loss, arthritis).

Sarcoidosis

The clinical manifestations of sarcoidosis in the elderly are variable. Presenting symptoms include shortness of breath, blurred vision, myopathy, adenopathy, and fatigue.

Pneumonia and Tuberculosis (see also Ch. 39)

The older patient with pneumonia may present with malaise or confusion. Although tachycardia and tachypnea are common, fever may be absent. Coughing may be mild and without copious, purulent sputum. Concomitant illnesses may alter the presentation of tuberculosis. Symptoms may be nonspecific (eg, fever, weakness, confusion, anorexia).

Biliary Disease

Elderly patients with biliary disease may present with nonspecific mental and physical deterioration (malaise, confusion, loss of mobility) without jaundice, fever, or abdominal pain. Abnormal liver function tests may be the only indication that biliary disease is present.

(References for this chapter are available from the authors upon request.)

15.   COMPREHENSIVE FUNCTIONAL ASSESSMENT

(See also Ch. 103)

Marsha D. Fretwell

The practical application of functional measures in the clinical evaluation and care of the older patient.

Gradual and variable declines in functional capacity are a normal part of aging. Around age 75, a distinct loss in functional reserve evolves that varies tremendously from one body organ to another and among individuals. Superimposed on this decline is the impact of disease. *In the elderly, disease can present first or solely as functional loss.* The physician's role is to minimize this decline by preventing and treating disease and by restoring optimal levels of function after acute illness.

Function may refer to activity at the cellular level (eg, the membrane's function is to pump sodium out of the cell), at a more complex tissue and organ level (eg, the cardiac output), or at the even more complex level of the class of organism (eg, the ability of an individual to file income tax returns appropriately). Caring for older patients involves all of these levels but particularly higher level functions, such as the ability to remember to take drugs, to perform toileting activities, to ambulate, to eat, to socialize, and to get around outside of the home. Because acutely ill older patients usually experience loss of functions in several organs simultaneously as well as in several areas (mental, physical, and social), patient assessment must include a broad set of measurements at several levels.

The medical diagnosis and the description of a patient's function provide the most accurate assessment of that particular patient. A diagnosis alone does not indicate how sick an individual is or how much care that person needs. For example, the diagnosis of diabetes mellitus has a broad range of medical and functional implications, ranging from being completely functional and controlled by diet alone to being hospitalized and requiring intensive care for hyperosmolar coma.

Loss of functional ability is the most sensitive indicator for identifying new disease and monitoring progress of treatment. Loss of functional reserve in older individuals frequently is not manifested until the person is under stress, either emotional or physical. Most older persons have "a most-vulnerable function"; eg, cognition, memory, ability to remain continent, or walk. Because of this most-vulnerable-function phenomenon, such disorders as pneumonia, UTI, MI, and heart failure all may present initially as confusion or incontinence in certain older patients. Knowledge of a person's baseline functional status allows early detection of disease; improvement is a sensitive indication of recovery.

Rates and direction of change in measures of mental, physical, and social function are the most accurate means of predicting outcome of illness in older patients. The overall prognosis of an acutely ill individual provides important information to help determine how aggressively medical technology should be used. This prognosis is best estimated by considering not only the patient's age and severity of illness but also the premorbid level of function and the rate at which change has occurred with this acute illness. The higher the level of function before illness and the steeper the downward curve resulting from a reversible illness, the better the prognosis for recovery.

Comprehensive Patient Assessment

In the traditional **biomedical model** of care, assessment focuses on the biologic pathophysiologic changes in organ systems. Attempts to apply this assessment model to the frail older patient are thwarted by the nonspecific presentations of current illness, extensive and interacting past medical illnesses, multiple positives in review of systems, and multiple abnormalities on physical and laboratory evaluation. Cognitive and communication deficits further impair the collection of accurate information. Additionally, problems outside the biomedical realm must be assessed; ie, social, cognitive, emotional, physical, functional, and economic losses that influence health outcomes. Not including these items in an accurate data base enhances the potential for missed diagnosis, inappropriate medications, and adverse effects from treatment.

An approach that includes an assessment of all of these descriptive variables and takes into account the interaction among them is referred to as **comprehensive functional assessment (CFA)**, a **biopsychosocial** functional model. In CFA, functional measures are used to systematically collect data from this broadened, complex base *and* to focus the care plan on issues of greatest concern to patients and families. Instruments to aid in this type of evaluation and document the patient's status over time are discussed in Ch. 103.

The patient data base is divided into the 3 major domains of the biopsychosocial (biomedical, psychologic, and social) model and the 2 functional scales of basic and instrumental **activities of daily living (ADLs).** The biopsychosocial domains provide discrete units of information, while the ADLs provide summaries of their interactive impact on the patient's everyday life. Subsets of data in each of the major domains are particularly relevant to health outcomes in older patients (see TABLE 15–1). Additionally, information is reviewed about the patient's values and attitudes toward health, the possible use of extraordinary means to preserve life, and institutional placement. An outline of patient strengths, identified through the data base, acknowledges that health outcomes result from a balance between the strengths and weaknesses of the patient and family as they face the emotional and physical stress of disease.

TABLE 15–1. COMPREHENSIVE FUNCTIONAL ASSESSMENT:
THE DATA BASE

Biomedical data
  Medical diagnoses, present and past, with statement of duration and impact on
    overall patient function
  Nutritional data (albumin, cholesterol, actual weight changes, appetite)
  Medications, including duration of use and adverse reactions; calculation of
    creatinine clearance

Psychologic data
  Cognitive function, using Folstein Mini-Mental State Examination and preserving
    subcategories (orientation, registration, short-term memory, attention, language
    use, comprehension)
  Emotional function, including screening for depression, paranoia, hallucinations,
    personality types, coping style and ability
  Perceptive function, including hearing, speech, vision

Social data
  Individual social skills, including marital history, acceptance of help, presence of
    confidant
  Support system, including quantity and quality of the system, use of formal
    supports

Summary scales
  Basic ADLs: feeding, bathing, dressing, use of toilet, transfer, mobility, continence
  Instrumental ADLs: use of transport, shopping, finance, telephone, medications,
    housework
Patient values/strengths

The summary scales of patient function in TABLE 15–1 and baseline cognitive function may be used to describe succinctly the patient's functional status at several key stages: prior to illness, at beginning of treatment, and following therapeutic interventions. Comparison of these stages allows the tracing of a trajectory of patient functions that increases understanding of the patient's problems and the effects of interventions. Thus, trials of adding or reducing medications can be evaluated by comparing pre- and posttreatment function. The desired improvement in a patient's function and what loss of function is risked can be defined *before* therapies are initiated.

The ADLs help focus this assessment on functional issues relevant to both the physician and the patient in the development of a **care plan.** For the physician, noting changes in patient function is important for achieving accurate diagnosis and prognosis, as well as appropriate treatment. For the patient, sustaining the ability to function physically and mentally is critical for maintaining independence and dignity. TABLE 15–2 illustrates how the information collected by CFA is used in the development of a care plan.

TABLE 15-2. THE CARE PLAN
(EXAMPLE: 85-yr-old woman with UTI and new-onset confusion)

Areas of Concern	Recommendations
1. Accurate medical diagnosis:	
UTI	Culture urine/blood
Acute confusional state	Evaluate mental status and repeat when acute confusion clears
Hypertension	Check postural BP; if normal, continue current medication
2. Nutrition: Previously intact	Measure initial weight/albumin; monitor oral intake and bowel function during period of confusion
3. Medications: Previously receiving hydrochlorothiazide only	Calculate creatinine clearance; adjust antibiotic dosage; avoid sedative-hypnotics; monitor antibiotic blood levels, BUN, and creatinine
4. Mobility: Previously independent	Mobilize with nursing assistance until mental status improves; expect full recovery
5. Continence: Previously continent	Anticipate incontinence in confusional state; anticipate voiding; educate patient and family as to transient nature; evaluate if persistent after mental status clears
6. Cognitive function: Previously intact	Evaluate (see No. 1); orient patient frequently; educate family; expect slow recovery; encourage family to support patient during this time
7. Emotional function: Previously intact	Patient at high risk for depression secondary to medical illness and confusion; monitor for mood, appetite, sleep, energy, and hallucinations
8. Social support system; Living alone with support only from daughter	Obtain social service consultation; orient family to issues concerning confusional state; evaluate prior and planned use of formal services
9. Appropriate use of resources	When patient's acute confusion clears, initiate discussion of patient and family values concerning use of gastrostomy tubes, extraordinary means, and nursing home placement.

Performance of CFA provides not only a systematic approach to patient care but also a framework for scientific inquiry into the human characteristics and behaviors that influence health outcomes. By applying CFA to every patient, the multiple, complex biopsychosocial variables become predictable patterns rather than isolated events. By focusing the care plan on everyday patient function, *and* by routinely establishing the improvement of function as a therapeutic goal, greater patient and doctor satisfaction is achieved. If available, a computer-assisted patient-information management system can facilitate the collection, storage, and use of this expanded data base, as well as the observation of changes in function over time or in response to particular interventions.

Cost-Effectiveness of CFA

The CFA is the basis for a multidisciplinary team approach to the function of a geriatric assessment unit **(GAU)**, an approach with proven benefits to health care outcomes. Among the benefits reported are more accurate diagnoses, better treatment planning, more appropriate placement decisions with fewer referrals to nursing homes, improved patient functional and mental status, longer patient survival, and lower overall use of costly institutional care services.

Not every older patient has access to a formal GAU evaluation, but a similar approach can be incorporated into any physician's patient-assessment process. Thus, cognitive functions, basic and instrumental ADLs, and social circumstances may be routinely evaluated and considered along with medical diagnoses.

With practice, a physician can fit such a CFA into an initial visit of 45 to 60 min. Follow-up visits require rechecking only variables that change with time or in response to treatment.

---

16.   ESTABLISHING THERAPEUTIC OBJECTIVES: QUALITY OF LIFE ISSUES

Richard W. Besdine

In one sense, a discussion of quality of life issues and their influence on establishing therapeutic objectives specific to older persons is not appropriate for this manual. The very title of this chapter reeks of ageism, with the implication that ill older persons have different quality of life concerns, which require alteration of the traditional therapeutic objectives in medicine. But the goals of medical treatment have remained the same since Hippocrates, and the age of the patient should not be relevant to considering them. Medicine and its practitioners cure when possible, while always caring and relieving suffering. Active termination of life, by definition, is forbidden.

Although age should not, per se, become part of the equation for deriving treatment goals, several phenomena that affect medical treatment goals become more prevalent with increasing age and intrude upon this discussion. Chronic physical disability, cognitive impairment, institutional confinement, diminished life expectancy, and heavy health care utilization, although not unique to old age, are more commonly associated with it and demand attention when considering ways to enhance quality of life for persons receiving medical care.

Assessing the quality of human life is a thorny concept, in some ways more suited to philosophy than to medicine. In the context of health care, the focus on quality of life should be narrow, referring to the experience of the person being treated. No absolute standards are implied in the use of the phrase "quality of life," since in the absence of disease or medical treatment, consideration of life quality is an intensely subjective and thus variable concept. Most people are comfortable talking about their own quality of life, but when asked to determine that of another person, they become appropriately uncertain and reluctant. Thus, it seems preferable to avoid using the phrase entirely, on the basis of physicians' potential lack of knowledge concerning the personal values and pleasures of their patients, particularly those who are elderly and seriously ill in the hospital setting, where quality of life issues commonly are raised.

It is suggested that more concrete and thus objectively assessable parameters be established as a guide for clinicians treating older patients who have characteristics suggesting that therapeutic objectives might be modified. Examples of useful indicators include the presence and severity of suffering (either mental or physical) or pain, the likelihood of having previous life-style and pleasures restored by treatment, the prognosis for survival, and the prospect that future suffering will be engendered by disease or treatment. The adverse impact on the patient of a proposed diagnostic test or treatment should always be scrutinized and compared with the potential benefit, regardless of the age of the patient. Coexisting conditions may influence the net gain or harm, but in principle, the need to modify therapy remains unchanged by patient age. These and other ethics-based issues are discussed more fully in Ch. 100.

Chronic disease, accompanied by chronic functional impairment (see Ch. 15), is increasingly common with age. Some 50% of noninstitutionalized elderly persons have limitations in activities of daily living and > 75% have at least one chronic disease. More than 33% cannot perform major activities independently, and 5% are homebound. Beyond 75 yr of age, 15% are confined to their homes, and over age 80, the figure rises to 25%. More than 80% of US health care resources are devoted to chronic illnesses, and 80% of deaths over age 65 are attributable to chronic disease. Successful treatment of chronic conditions requires a shift in traditional therapeutic emphasis from cure to continuing care. Management that emphasizes improved function, postponement of deterioration and disability, and prevention of secondary complications characterizes the best of geriatric health care. These principles are merely good common sense applied to therapeutic objectives in the care of older patients.

The presence of cognitive impairment does not by itself require a change in therapeutic objectives but does deserve full evaluation. The severity of loss and its functional impact should be measured before deciding whether treatment plans should be modified. Producing an iatrogenic or treatment-related discomfort, even if only transient, which cannot be explained to or understood by an elderly demented patient may demand a change in the clinical approach and treatment goals. In addition, explanations must be made and consent obtained especially carefully with such a patient.

Diminished life expectancy is another important factor in considering objectives of treatment. A patient who has only months of life remaining should not have to spend them enervated, nauseated, and confined by oppressive chemotherapy. When the prognosis for a specific disease determines a reduced life span, planning treatment in light of life expectancy is reasonable, regardless of patient age. But when life expectancy is based on predictions related to the cohort (eg, 19 yr for a 65-yr-old woman, 14 yr for a man), variability among individuals is so great that calculations based on these data become meaningless. Who is to say that coronary artery bypass surgery should be withheld from an 82-yr-old based on a prediction of "only" 5.3 yr of life remaining if the procedure has a high probability of major pain relief? And despite an average of only 12 yr of life remaining for a 75-yr-old woman, how can one know if an individual will deviate a great deal in either direction from the mean or will fall directly on it? And finally, it could be argued that fewer years of remaining life may increase rather than decrease their value to the person and thus the importance of preserving them through medical intervention, whether heroic or ordinary.

Nursing home residents have a disproportionately high prevalence of the characteristics relevant to consideration for modification of treatment goals, including extreme age, poverty, cognitive loss, physical disability, reduced life expectancy, chronic disease, pain and suffering, accumulated losses, and social isolation. Despite these negative characteristics, quality of life is a very personal, subjective evaluation; therefore, the physician must accurately summarize the treatment issues and present them clearly in terms the patient can understand. Informing the patient and respecting autonomy is crucial, regardless of the patient's age or dwelling place. Only after the patient is an informed participant in the decision can the physician be comfortable in modifying treatment objectives.

In old age, many phenomena occur that may present an argument for altering the usual therapeutic objectives for clinical intervention. But these modifiers demand individual consideration, and age is largely irrelevant. The quality of human life is, for the most part, a concept that each individual must consider, and if it is applied to making health care decisions, it will produce more complexities than solutions. Special attention must be given to the personal characteristics of older patients. Including patients in the process of deciding about treatment plans will most often enhance their quality of life and bring greater satisfaction to the physician.

---

17. PREVENTIVE STRATEGIES

T. Franklin Williams and *Shirley P. Bagley**

Today, far more people than ever before are living into their 70s and beyond in relatively good health, leading vigorous, independent lives. Recent studies indicate that most body organs will function nearly as well in later life as in younger years in individuals without chronic diseases who maintain healthy life-styles. However, chronic diseases and disabilities do tend to accumulate in many persons as they age, posing threats to continued independence.

Thus, there are 2 general objectives of preventive strategies for older persons: (1) the maintenance of good health and functioning through behavioral choices and life-styles, beginning in middle or earlier years and extending through later years, and (2) the minimization of loss of health and function when chronic disabilities do occur. The latter objective is the goal of rehabilitation in the aging and is addressed in Ch. 23.

Preventive life-styles: A number of studies have documented what many have long thought—that a life-style including **regular exercise, sound nutrition, moderate (if any) alcohol intake, involvement in meaningful activities, adequate amounts of sleep** (generally 7 to 8 h/night), and **not smoking** (or stopping smoking, at any age) is associated with a longer and healthier later life.

Exercise, particularly weight-bearing exercise such as walking or bicycling 20 to 30 min several times a week, is associated with improved cardiac capacity, maintenance of muscle strength, and a reduction in the loss of bone mass that tends to occur progressively with age. Individuals, in their 60s and 70s who have taken part in organized fitness programs have not only increased their maximum aerobic capacities almost as much as younger persons in such programs but have demonstrated improvement in glucose tolerance and blood lipid levels. While organized fitness programs may not be of interest to everyone, vigorous walking can be made a regular part of virtually everyone's routine. Stretching exercises, performed regularly, are also important to maintain flexibility of joints.

---

* This article was written by Dr. Williams and Ms. Bagley in their private capacities. No official support or endorsement by the National Institutes of Health is intended or should be inferred.

Good nutrition for older persons has not been clearly defined, because adequate dietary, metabolic, or longitudinal data are not yet available. However, based on what is known from studies in younger adults, it is recommended that older persons have adequate but not excessive amounts of protein (0.6 to 1.0 gm/kg/day); relatively low fat and cholesterol intakes; and the National Research Council's recommended daily allowances of vitamins and minerals, in food or as supplements if needed. The importance of including about 1 gm Ca in the daily diet should be stressed. However, the value of taking more than the recommended daily allowances of food supplements, ie, the "megadoses" advertised and marketed to the general public, has not been proved and in some cases, these doses may be toxic.

In addition, it seems appropriate also to recommend adequate fiber intake (the simplest means of minimizing constipation and gaining such potential benefits as reducing the risk of colon cancer and diverticulosis). The consumption of complex sugars, such as starchy foods, rather than simple sugars may also be recommended, although the value of this substitution, like that of fiber intake, has not been proved conclusively. Salt intake should be modest, ie, little or no salt should be added to foods unless more salt is medically indicated.

A modest amount of alcohol, eg, equivalent to 4 oz table wine daily, appears not to be harmful; in fact, one study reported it to be one of the factors associated with overall better health. Another study, however, suggested that *any* alcohol intake is associated with increased risk of breast cancer in women, but this conculsion is controversial.

Most important, nutritional intake (including alcohol) should be tailored to the individual. It must take into account hereditary tendencies toward hyperlipidemia, history of alcoholism, evidence of diabetes, need to achieve weight reduction, and activity level.

Immunizations: Because most, but not all, older persons have been immunized at some time for tetanus and diphtheria, a person's immunization status should be checked before new vaccines are administered. A **tetanus booster** is recommended every 10 yr. For **influenza immunization,** the current year's vaccine should be given to any older person with an underlying condition favoring reduced immunity or tendency toward pulmonary infections. In fact, many experts recommend yearly influenza immunization for all persons ≥ 65 yr of age. (See also Ch. 78.)

The use of **pneumococcal vaccine** is more controversial. Again, the vaccination of older persons prone to pulmonary infections appears to be appropriate. As more data become available, however, it may become desirable to vaccinate all persons ≥ 65 yr. The pneumococcal vaccines currently available may not be effective for more than 4 yr. However, because more local reactions are reported with second vaccinations than with the first, revaccination may not be avisable, except with overriding indications. More data and further guidance about use of pneumococcal vaccines should be forthcoming.

Skin: Persons of all ages should be advised to avoid extensive sun exposure and to use sunscreen agents to prevent skin cancer. (See also Ch. 92.)

Oral health: As a result of the general fluoridation of water supplies and more frequent regular dental check-ups, most older people today still have their own teeth. Therefore, the continuation of good oral health practices should be stressed, including regular dental prophylactic examinations, early correction of problems, and performance of personal dental care at least twice daily. Good condition of the mouth and teeth are essential for proper nutrition, good appearance, and general enjoyment of life. (See also Ch. 44.)

Foot care: Maintaining the ability to walk comfortably requires properly fitted, supportive shoes; clean feet; and routine care of nails and skin, including attention to calluses. A podiatrist should be consulted for foot problems that affect function or comfort. (See also Ch. 67.)

Accident prevention: Accidents, particularly falls, increase markedly with age. Because falls often result in hip fractures and fear of further falling, they constitute one of the major causes of loss of functional independence. The overall maintenance of good physical condition is a measure for prevention of such accidents. (See also Ch. 7.)

Measures to ensure the safety of the home environment should be stressed, eg, hand rails on stairways both inside and outdoors, good lighting, nonskid rugs, and smoke and fire alarms. The safety of the neighborhood should be assessed and alternative living arrangements should be considered, if needed.

Careful driving is clearly important in preventing accidents, and the willingness to modify practices such as not driving at night if night vision is impaired should be encouraged. The need for precaution in hazardous situations, such as walking or driving in wet or icy conditions, should be emphasized. If any significant decline in mental or physical condition develops because of a disease or condition that might make driving risky for the older person or others, a decision to stop driving altogether should be seriously considered by the affected person and family members in consultation with a physician.

Screening: An essential aspect of preventive strategies in older persons is routine screening of areas in which problems are likely to develop. With early detection, many of these problems may be reversible or correctable. Such screening procedures are usually part of a general medical examination and are discussed in detail elsewhere in this volume, but they deserve emphasis here.

Older persons should routinely undergo review and testing of **hearing, vision, BP, Hb, cholesterol level, and urinalysis.** In addition, the **skin, oral cavity, breasts** (male and female), **prostate, colorectal area** (including tests for occult blood), and **cervix** and **uterus** should be examined regularly for evidence of early cancer. For the latter 2 organs, opinion differs about the frequency of examinations needed after age 65 when one examination is normal; no symptoms, such as bleeding, are present; and the person is not receiving estrogen therapy. Some specialists recommend continued yearly examinations, others only one every 5 yr. Because **hypothyroidism** can develop unexpectedly in older persons, clinical examination should include a specific search for even subtle signs and appropriate laboratory follow-up.

Attention should be given to special characteristics of the individual. If there is a family history of diabetes or a tendency toward obesity, a glucose tolerance test should be considered. A family history of symptomatic osteoporosis, a thin build, or loss of stature suggests that radiologic and laboratory examination for osteoporosis should be done. More frequent pelvic and cytologic examinations are indicated if estrogens are being used.

The older person's **use of medications,** both prescribed and OTC, should be reviewed regularly, with attention to potential interactions and side effects, as well as consistency in following prescribed regimens.

The **general condition** and **vigor** of the older person should be assessed, including height and weight as well as any changes, ability to walk with normal gait and speed, joint flexibility, ability to carry out ordinary daily activities, and history or evidence of urinary incontinence.

Mental and emotional status: Despite recent conclusive evidence to the contrary, many professionals, as well as laypersons, still consider some **loss of cognitive function** to be "just old age." In fact, any significant decline in memory or other mental function that is observed or detected on simple mental status tests calls for a thorough evaluation, because the changes are almost certainly due to some disease process, which may be reversible. These problems are addressed elsewhere in this volume (see Chs. 9, 80, 81, 82, 83, and 84). Similarly, any evidence of **depression** reported by patient or family or observed during a routine review should be investigated and treated appropriately. Although depression is common in older persons, it is *not* a normal part of aging, and early attention can be beneficial.

Psychosocial features: Evidence of **psychosocial stresses**—in family relationships, living environments, or marital and sexual relationships—should also be explored with older persons and family members. Significant stresses can affect immune competence, as well as interact with other chronic medical conditions. An older person's social and supportive network of family and friends and involvement in outside activities also figure in maintaining overall health and enjoyment of life. A goal of preventive strategies is to ensure the effectiveness of support networks through counseling and use of social resources.

Fundamentally, each person, older or younger, is his own best monitor, with assistance from close family members and friends. Thus the preventive strategies described here should be transmitted to and used by older persons themselves, in addition to serving as guides for the physicians and other professionals responsible for their care. (See also Ch. 97.)

18. CLINICAL PHARMACOLOGY

David T. Lowenthal

Understanding the pharmacologic consequences of the physiologic changes associated with aging is critical to safe and effective therapeutics. The most important changes involve cardiovascular, CNS, renal, and hepatic function; body composition; tissue sensitivity to drugs; and reduced baroreceptor reflex sensitivity.

CHANGES IN BODY COMPOSITION AND ORGAN FUNCTION

There is a reduction in body size, with a decrease in lean body mass (primarily muscle mass) and body water content, and an increase in fat per unit of body weight (see TABLE 18–1). Decreased hepatic albumin synthesis results in a lower serum albumin concentration, which may yield more free drug entry to tissues or to elimination mechanisms. A gradual decrease in visceral blood flow reduces drug clearance through the liver or kidney. Consequently, a given dose of a relatively water-soluble drug may result in higher blood concentrations and increased pharmacologic activity. Conversely, a highly lipid-soluble drug might have longer pharmacologic activity; eg, the increase in adipose tissue enhances the storage of lipophilic drugs, such as diazepam; increases the volume of distribution; and delays elimination (ie, increases half-life).

TABLE 18–1. AGE-RELATED CHANGES AFFECTING
PHARMACOKINETICS

Body Component or Function	Direction of Change
Renal function	↓
Hepatic blood flow	↓
Serum albumin	↓
α_1-Acid glycoprotein	↑
Body fat	↑
Lean muscle mass	↓
Body water	↓

Changes in Cardiovascular Function

In fit elderly patients without ischemic heart disease **(IHD)**, no significant change in resting CO occurs. There is, however, less increase in heart rate in response to exercise, possibly as a result of a decrease in β-receptor sensitivity. CO is maintained by increased force of cardiac contraction (Frank-Starling mechanism). (See also Ch. 28.)

Symptomatic and asymptomatic IHD, which is prevalent in older individuals in more developed countries, can result in a reduction in ventricular function without overt heart disease. Episodes of nonischemic cardiomyopathy may also decrease ventricular function. Consequently, in many older individuals there is a gradual and asymptomatic *reduction* in CO, associated with a gradual fall in blood volume. Diuretic therapy, which causes acute volume contraction, may result in orthostatic hypotension and reduced organ perfusion. β-Blockers and Ca entry blockers, given alone or in combination, can produce significant negative inotropic effects, thereby potentiating impaired ventricular function, resulting in heart failure.

Orthostatic hypotension may also result from a decreased preload due to venous pooling and, thereby, a reduction in CO after the administration of α-adrenergic blockers, such as prazosin. Patients need to be instructed to sit up first and proceed slowly when going from a supine to a standing position while taking these drugs.

Tricyclic antidepressants and phenothiazines can have cardiac effects and may induce potentially lethal ventricular arrhythmias, especially in patients with IHD. Reduction in maintenance dose by 50%, monitoring of plasma concentrations of the drug, and use of ambulatory ECG monitoring help avert these effects, which are probably due to altered tissue sensitivity.

Patients receiving chemotherapy for cancer or leukemia may develop drug-related cardiotoxicity. Doxorubicin can cause direct cardiotoxicity, affecting ventricular function and electrical conduction. The likelihood of these effects depends on the patient's age, pretreatment cardiac status, drug dose, and duration of therapy. Patients should have baseline and follow-up radionuclide angiography, with periodic ambulatory ECG monitoring, and clinical assessment for heart failure.

Baroceptor Reflex Activity

As a result of decreased responsiveness and sensitivity of the baroreceptor reflex, patients may develop postural hypotension when taking long- and short-acting nitroglycerin preparations, phenothiazines, diuretics, and other antihypertensive agents.

Changes in CNS Function

Blood supply to the brain may be compromised by atherosclerotic narrowing of the vertebral and carotid systems. Hypothetically, this decrement in blood flow could cause neuronal loss and be responsible for the altered sensitivity to centrally acting drugs. Patients with Alzheimer's disease and similar organic brain syndromes may likewise exhibit altered sensitivity to highly lipid-soluble drugs that penetrate the CNS (eg, some β-blockers, Ca entry blockers, tricyclic antidepressants, barbiturates, long-acting benzodiazepines, opiates).

Although the cardiac and peripheral effects of methyldopa and Ca entry blockers are beneficial, both drugs can produce CNS side effects—depression and paranoia, respectively. The relationship between some β-blockers and depressive reactions remains controversial.

Renin-Angiotensin-Aldosterone System

Plasma renin levels, both at baseline and in response to position and volume changes, decline with age for unknown reasons. Aldosterone concentrations remain essentially unchanged.

However, in individuals with insulin-dependent diabetes and progressive renal insufficiency, there is a decrease in sympathetic tone to the juxtaglomerular apparatus, resulting in falls in renin concentration, angiotensin II, and aldosterone production, which may enhance Na excretion and K retention. Potassium retention (and hyperkalemia) may also result from coadministration of K-sparing diuretics or administration of drugs that suppress the renin-angiotensin system (eg, nonsteroidal antiinflammatory drugs **[NSAIDs]**, β-blockers, angiotensin converting enzyme **[ACE]** inhibitors).

Some have suggested that, because of lowered renin activity, elderly and black hypertensive patients may respond more readily to diuretics and Ca entry blockers than to β-blockers and ACE inhibitors.

Fluid and Electrolyte Balance

As a result of intrinsic and diuretic-induced renal dysfunction, water retention (or loss) may occur, producing hypo- or hypernatremia. In addition, prostatic hypertrophy can result in obstructive uropathy, producing further, postrenal deterioration in kidney function, water conservation, and hyponatremia, which continue until the obstruction has been relieved.

The use of diuretics can induce a vicious circle in which volume contraction stimulates thirst, leading to increased fluid intake. An individual may have access only to water but insufficient solute to replace salt and other electrolyte losses, resulting in *hyponatremia*.

Normal fluid balance depends on an integration of cerebral, cardiopulmonary, excretory, and endocrine functions. Many chronic systemic diseases may produce hyponatremia due to a reduced renal ability to eliminate a water load. The syndrome of inappropriate antidiuretic hormone **(SIADH)** activity has also been associated with a variety of drugs (see TABLE 18–2).

Conversely, the drugs listed in TABLE 18–3 as well as certain cerebrovascular, renal, or adrenal diseases or hypertonic peritoneal dialysis may result in excessive water loss and *hypernatremia*. (See also Ch. 4.)

TABLE 18–2. DRUGS ASSOCIATED WITH SIADH AND/OR HYPONATREMIA

Chlorpropamide
Tolbutamide
Cyclophosphamide
Morphine
Barbiturates
Vincristine
Carbamazepine
Acetaminophen
Indomethacin and other NSAIDs
Chlorothiazide and hydrochlorothiazide
Hormones with mineralocorticoid and/or glucocorticoid
   effects (eg, aldosterone, estrogen, progesterone)

TABLE 18–3. DRUGS ASSOCIATED WITH WATER LOSS RESULTING IN HYPERNATREMIA

Lithium	Glyburide
Alcohol	Propoxyphene
Demeclocyline	Amphotericin B
Phenytoin	Methoxyflurane
Acetohexamide	Povidone-iodine (principally
Tolazamide	H_2O loss from skin)

PHARMACODYNAMIC–PHARMACOKINETIC PRINCIPLES

Absorption

Absorption of food and drugs remains unaltered in elderly patients with an intact gastric mucosa, despite increased gastric pH and reduced GI blood flow. However, absorption may be altered by nutritional deficiencies (eg, of vitamin B_{12} or intrinsic factor), partial gastrectomy, and drug interactions with laxatives, antacids, and agents that decrease gastric emptying (eg, anticholinergics or antihypertensives). Kaolin-pectin, antacids, and iron inhibit the absorption of tetracycline; antacids can decrease the bioavailability of digoxin by 25%.

Distribution

The changes in body composition mentioned above affect drug distribution. Drugs that are highly protein bound will have less albumin for binding, resulting in more free drug available for (1) tissue distribution, (2) pharmacologic activity, and (3) elimination (see TABLE 18–4).

Weakly acid organic compounds, eg, salicylates, barbiturates, warfarin, theophylline, and sulfonamides, bind principally to plasma albumin. α_1-Acid glycoprotein **(AAG)**, on the other hand, binds mostly basic drugs. AAG tends to increase with age, and binding to AAG is increased during acute illnesses such as MI. In the latter instance, lidocaine or propranolol given for prophylaxis against arrhythmias may be more avidly bound to AAG, yielding a decrease in the concentration of free drug. When the acute phase of the illness passes and the patient improves, there is less binding, more free drug available, and more rapid elimination. If elderly patients receiving β-blockers, which decrease CO and hepatic blood flow, concomitantly receive lidocaine, the resulting drug interaction leads to a decrease in lidocaine clearance and an increase in lidocaine distribution. As a result, lidocaine toxicity can occur.

TABLE 18–4. DRUGS WITH POSSIBLY REDUCED
PLASMA PROTEIN BINDING IN THE ELDERLY

Warfarin	Phenylbutazone
Diazepam	Tolbutamide
Lorazepam	Meperidine
Phenytoin	Disopyramide

Metabolism and Changes in Hepatic Function

The ability of the liver to metabolize drugs does not decline similarly for all pharmacologic agents with advancing age. The most frequent changes involve the microsomal mixed-function oxidative system (phase I), but little or no change occurs in the conjugative processes (phase II) (see TABLE 18–5). Changes due to hepatitis or, more commonly, a decrease in hepatic blood flow as a result of heart failure may also impair the liver's ability to metabolize drugs.

Although liver size and blood flow decline with advancing age, routine tests of liver function yield normal results in the absence of disease. This reflects the current inability to quantify hepatic function. As a consequence of reduced metabolism, certain drugs that are cleared by the liver may require administration in lower dosages to avoid accumulation and excessive pharmacologic effects.

Decreased hepatic clearance of the following drugs has been shown: benzodiazepines (diazepam, flurazepam, alprazolam, chlordiazepoxide) and their active metabolites (desmethyl-diazepam, desalkyl-flurazepam), quinidine, propranolol, lidocaine, and nortriptyline.

The clinical effects of a reduction in diazepam clearance would be greater sedation and possibly iatrogenic pseudodementia. Flurazepam accumulation can produce prolonged sleep. This response is age and dose related. Although men clear diazepam and several metabolites more slowly than women do, the difference is not clinically significant.

TABLE 18–5. DRUGS WITH REDUCED HEPATIC METABOLISM

Phase I (Preparative) Reactions
Oxidation
  Hydroxylation
    Alprazolam
    Antipyrine
    Barbiturates
    Carbamazepine
    Imipramine
    Desipramine

    Nortriptyline
    Ibuprofen
    Phenytoin
    Propranolol
    Quinidine
    Warfarin

  Dealkylation
    Amitriptyline
    Chlordiazepoxide
    Diazepam
    Flurazepam
    Diphenhydramine

    Lidocaine
    Meperidine
    Theophylline
    Tolbutamide

Reduction
  Nitroreduction
    Nitrazepam

Phase II (Synthetic) Reactions
(Essentially unchanged in the elderly)
  Conjugation
  Acetylation
  Methylation

Hepatic induction and inhibition have not been studied extensively in the elderly, but TABLE 18–6 lists interactions involving drugs commonly used by elderly patients.

Antibiotics (eg, cloxacillin, nafcillin, ampicillin, oxacillin), and cephalosporins (eg, cefoperazone and ceftriaxone) are excreted unchanged by the biliary system (to be reabsorbed in the small intestine, the so-called enterohepatic circulation). Biliary tract surgery and chronic pancreatic disease may alter biliary excretory and enterohepatic recirculatory functions.

Elimination and Changes in Renal Function

Biotransformation in the liver prepares the drug for elimination by producing metabolites, which are then excreted in the urine (via the **renal system**) or feces (via the **biliary system**).

Drugs such as digoxin, lithium, and aminoglycoside antibiotics, which are minimally metabolized, are eliminated by the **kidney** predominantly unchanged.

Beginning with the fourth decade of life, there is a 6 to 10% reduction in GFR and renal plasma flow every 10 yr. Thus, by age 70 a person may have a 40 to 50% decrease in renal function, even in the absence of kidney disease. Hypertension, common in this population, is associated with nephrosclerosis, which may produce parenchymal disease and an even greater reduction in renal function.

TABLE 18–6. HEPATIC FUNCTION AND DRUG INTERACTION

Primary Drug	Interacting Drug	Mechanism	Clinical Consequence
I. Effect enhanced			
Warfarin	Phenylbutazone	Inhibition of drug metabolism; displacement from albumin binding	Hemorrhage
	Metronidazole	Inhibition of drug metabolism; displacement from albumin binding	Hemorrhage
Sulfonylurea hypoglycemics	Chloramphenicol	Inhibition of drug metabolism; displacement from albumin binding	Hypoglycemia
Benzodiazepines (diazepam, chlordiazepoxide)	Cimetidine	Inhibition of drug metabolism; displacement from albumin binding	Excessive sedation
Theophylline	Cimetidine	Inhibition of drug metabolism	GI upset, arrhythmias, seizures
II. Effect decreased			
Warfarin	Barbiturates, rifampin, disopyramide	Induction of drug metabolism	Loss of anticoagulation
Prednisone	Barbiturates	Induction of drug metabolism	Loss of antiallergic and anti-inflammatory properties
Quinidine	Barbiturates	Induction of drug metabolism	Decreased antiarrhythmic effect
Propranolol	Tobacco (cigarette smoking)	Induction of drug metabolism	Loss of BP and heart rate control
Theophylline	Tobacco (cigarette smoking), phenytoin, rifampin	Induction of drug metabolism	Loss of bronchodilation

Drugs that are eliminated substantially by renal excretion (see TABLE 18-7) should be given in reduced doses or less frequently to avoid accumulation and untoward pharmacologic effects. As an example, the pharmacokinetic parameters of digoxin in older and younger subjects are presented in TABLE 18-8.

TABLE 18-7. COMMON DRUGS ELIMINATED PRIMARILY BY THE KIDNEYS

Digoxin
Aminoglycoside antibiotics
Atenolol, nadolol
Lithium
Diuretics
Procainamide, tocainide, disopyramide
Clonidine
NSAIDs
Ranitidine, famotidine
Captopril, enalapril, lisinopril

Dosage adjustment of renally excreted drugs can be based on an estimate of creatinine clearance, as follows:

$$\frac{\text{Creatinine clearance}}{\text{(mL/min)}} = \frac{(140 - \text{age}) \times \text{body weight (kg)}}{72 \times \text{serum creatinine (mg/dL)}}$$

For women, multiply by 0.85.

Since drugs may compete for the same specific site of renal excretion, elimination of one drug may be impaired by the concurrent administration of another. Examples are presented in TABLE 18-9.

Generally, drug accumulation increases pharmacologic effect. However, although furosemide accumulates as renal function falls, its efficacy is reduced. Because furosemide and other diuretics act on the luminal side of the renal tubule, their access to this site of action is reduced as renal function falls. Thus, more furosemide may be required to produce the desired diuretic response.

Finally, some drugs cause an increase in BUN and serum creatinine. For example, tetracycline inhibits protein synthesis, provoking a catabolic effect, whereas glucocorticoids are directly catabolic; thus, both can elevate BUN and creatinine and aggravate uremia. Cimetidine and trimethoprim have been shown to interfere with creatinine excretion. Aminoglycoside antibiotics can cause reversible nephrotoxicity.

Tissue Responsiveness (Sensitivity)

Elderly patients tend to exhibit enhanced responses to CNS-active drugs, attributed to a greater tissue sensitivity, as well as the altered pharmacokinetics described above. Possible consequences with diaze-

TABLE 18–8. AGE-RELATED DIFFERENCES IN DIGOXIN ELIMINATION

Subjects	Age (yr)	Creatinine (mg/dL)	% Absorbed	$t_{1/2}$ Oral (h)	V_D AUC (L)	CL_r (mL/min)
Young (n = 6)	47 ± 4.6	0.88 ± 0.15	84.3 ± 6.5	36.8 ± 4.5	338.7 ± 35.0	106.2 ± 13.6
Elderly (n = 7)	81 ± 2.4	0.95 ± 0.12	76.0 ± 10.0	69.6 ± 13.1	193.8 ± 24.0	37.4 ± 5.9

V_D = volume of distribution, CL_r = renal clearance, AUC = area under the curve.
(Adapted from B. Cusack et al: "Digoxin in the elderly: Pharmacokinetic consequences of old age," in *Clinical Pharmacology and Therapeutics*, Vol. 25, pp. 772-776, 1979. Used with permission of The C. V. Mosby Company.)

TABLE 18–9. RENAL FUNCTION AND DRUG INTERACTION

Primary Drug	Interacting Drug	Mechanism	Clinical Effect
Digoxin	Quinidine	Inhibition of renal and nonrenal clearance; volume of distribution	Digoxin toxicity
	Verapamil	Inhibition of renal and nonrenal clearance	Digoxin toxicity
	Spironolactone	Inhibition of renal and nonrenal clearance; volume of distribution	Digoxin toxicity
Methotrexate	Aspirin	Inhibition of renal excretion	Bone marrow depression
Penicillin	Probenecid	Inhibition of renal excretion	Penicillin accumulation
Quinidine	Sodium bicarbonate	Inhibition of renal excretion	Quinidine intoxication producing wide QRS complex

pam, opiates, and nifedipine are ataxia, respiratory depression, and changes in mentation, respectively. Similarly, haloperidol and metoclopramide are more likely to cause extrapyramidal syndromes, and meperidine may produce respiratory depression. Some studies have shown an increase in sensitivity to oral anticoagulants. Thus, dosage reduction may be required for warfarin and similar drugs. Dosage of heparin is not significantly affected by age.

In some instances, patients may exhibit a decreased rather than exaggerated response at the tissue level. Such is the case with β-blockers; *increased* dosage may be required to achieve therapeutic effect.

Specifically, β-receptors exhibit diminished responses to both agonists and antagonists; eg, a 65-year-old requires 5 times the dose of isoproterenol needed by a 25-year-old to increase the heart rate by 25 beats/min. Similarly, propranolol efficacy decreases with age, not because of a reduction in the number of β-receptors but probably as a result of reduced receptor sensitivity.

Adverse Drug Reactions

Generally, adverse drug reactions (ADRs) are categorized as allergic (eg, penicillin rash), nonallergic (eg, methyldopa-induced hemolysis), and idiosyncratic (eg, chloramphenicol-caused aplastic anemia). ADRs are more prevalent in the elderly because of their greater use of drugs, and the consequences of ADRs may be more severe.

The risk factors for ADRs are age, gender, race (occurring most frequently in elderly white women), number of drugs, dosage, duration of treatment, patient noncompliance (eg, excessive dosage), and underlying conditions (eg, hepatic or renal insufficiency).

A thorough pretreatment history may reveal symptoms that might otherwise be attributed incorrectly to a drug prescribed later. The history is critical in differentiating possible ADRs from underlying disease. A symptom appearing 1 to 2 mo after a medication regimen has been started may indicate a new (or previously dormant) disease process, rather than an ADR.

Elderly patients may develop ADRs that are clearly different from those seen in younger patients. Thus, the unorthodox or bizarre reaction may be the rule rather than the exception. Some common expressions of ADRs in older patients are listed in TABLE 18–10.

TABLE 18–10. COMMON SYMPTOMS AND SIGNS OF ADVERSE DRUG REACTIONS (ADRs) IN THE ELDERLY

Restlessness
Falls
Depression
Confusion
Loss of memory
Constipation
Incontinence
Extrapyramidal syndromes (eg, parkinsonism, akathisia,
    tardive dyskinesia)

The decision to administer a drug must take into consideration the potential benefits and risks to the patient. A serious ventricular arrhythmia must be treated despite the potential toxicity of antiarrhythmic agents. The benefits incurred by reducing BP and preventing stroke or heart failure usually outweigh the risks of ADRs associated with many antihypertensive agents, but the special needs of the patient should be considered in selection of therapy.

The drugs most commonly associated with ADRs in the elderly are analgesics, antibiotics, anticoagulants, antidepressants, antihypertensives, antiparkinsonian drugs, antipsychotics, bronchodilators, digitalis, diuretics, NSAIDs, oral hypoglycemics, and sedative-hypnotics. The distribution of ADRs within these categories varies with the site of care (see TABLE 18–11). Principles of safe prescribing are listed in TABLE 18–12.

Patient Compliance

The use of fewer drugs at lower doses and in convenient combinations will usually enhance compliance as well as decrease the incidence of ADRs. Once the therapeutic goal has been achieved, dosage should be reduced or the drug discontinued as soon as possible. The dosage sched-

TABLE 18-11. RELATIONSHIP BETWEEN ADVERSE DRUG REACTIONS (ADRs) AND SITE OF CARE

Most Common Causes of Hospital-Acquired ADRs	Most Common Causes of Nursing Home–Acquired ADRs
1. Digoxin	1. Tranquilizers (phenothiazines)
2. Aminoglycoside antibiotic	2. Sedative-hypnotics
3. Anticoagulants (heparin and warfarin)	3. Warfarin
4. Insulin overdose	4. Antacids
5. Steroid-induced GI bleeding	5. Oral hypoglycemics
6. Aspirin	6. Digoxin
	7. Aspirin

TABLE 18-12. PRINCIPLES OF SAFE PRESCRIBING

All patients can benefit from these principles of safe geriatric prescribing:

1. Diagnosis of the illness and knowledge of the individual's personal and social status must precede treatment.

2. A detailed medication history obtained from the patient or the patient's family and friends is an important aid to avoiding adverse drug interactions.

3. It is important to know the clinical pharmacology of drugs prescribed; a few drugs should be used well rather than many poorly.

4. It is better to begin with a low dose of a drug and titrate up to achieve the desired response.

5. The regimen should be kept as simple as possible.

6. Medications should be reviewed regularly, and those not needed should be discontinued.

7. It should be remembered that new symptoms (and illness) may be caused by a drug as well as by a new illness.

(Modified from "Geriatric Clinical Pharmacology: An Overview," by R. E. Vestal, in *Drug Treatment in the Elderly,* edited by R.E. Vestal, pp. 24-26. Copyright 1984 by ADIS Health Science Press. Used with permission of ADIS Health Science Press and the author.)

ule must be kept simple, and multiple-drug regimens must, if at all possible, be minimized. If the patient cannot read or comprehend directions, family members must be given simple written instructions. Containers must be provided that can be easily opened so the drug can be readily dispensed. Other solutions to noncompliance may be the use of liquid formulations (when swallowing difficulty is experienced) or a transdermal preparation (when multiple-drug regimens are required or visual impairment exists).

---

19. THE ROLE OF THE PHARMACIST

Bruce M. Schechter, W. Gary Erwin, and Philip P. Gerbino

Geriatrics has emerged as a model of multidisciplinary cooperation in providing patient care, and pharmacists are increasingly involved as team members. Although knowledge is limited concerning altered pharmacokinetics and pharmacodynamics in the population $\geq$ 65 yr of age, it is relatively substantial when compared to the near-total lack of similar information in individuals $\geq$ 85 yr of age.

The most important determinant of drug use in the elderly is health status, and most seniors are healthy. In a 1984 survey, 67% of community-dwelling elderly viewed their health as excellent, very good, or good; the perceived health status of those > 85 yr of age is similar. In contrast, 1.2 million disabled elderly living in the community and 1.5 million elderly living in long-term care facilities use a disproportionately large percentage of available health care resources, including drugs. The population $\geq$ 65 yr of age accounts for about 30% of prescription and 40% of nonprescription drug use. The most frequent symptoms and diagnoses based on physician office visits by persons $\geq$ 75 yr of age are listed in TABLES 19–1 and 19–2.

Drug utilization increases with advancing age. Forty percent of office visits to physicians by individuals $\geq$ 65 yr of age involve therapy with $\geq$ 2 drugs, compared with 27% of office visits by all individuals. Multiple drugs are prescribed to 44% of patients $\geq$ 75 yr of age. The therapeutic classes of drugs most often used in the elderly are shown in TABLE 19–3. Polypharmacy in the elderly is associated with adverse drug reactions, drug interactions, noncompliance, and increased cost.

TABLE 19–1. MOST FREQUENT SYMPTOMS IN INDIVIDUALS
$\geq$ 75 YR OF AGE*

Rank	Symptom	Rank	Symptom
1	Dizziness	6	Chest pain
2	Vision dysfunction	7	Shortness of breath
3	Back pain	8	General weakness
4	Leg pain	9	Knee pain
5	Cough	10	Skin lesion

* Based on number of mentions/1000 physician office visits.

TABLE 19–2. MOST FREQUENT DIAGNOSES IN INDIVIDUALS
≥ 75 YR OF AGE*

Rank	Diagnosis	Rank	Diagnosis
1	Essential hypertension	6	Heart failure
2	Chronic ischemic heart disease	7	Cardiac dysrhythmias
3	Diabetes mellitus	8	Arthropathies, other and unspecified
4	Osteoarthritis and allied disorders	9	Glaucoma
5	Cataract	10	Hypertensive heart disease

* Based on number of mentions/1000 physician office visits.

TABLE 19–3. TOP DRUGS GROUPED BY THERAPEUTIC CLASS
FROM PENNSYLVANIA'S PACE PRESCRIPTION DRUG PROGRAM*

Rank	Therapeutic Class
1	Cardiovascular agents
2	Diuretics
3	Analgesics
4	GI agents
5	Antidiabetics
6	K supplement/replacement

* PACE = Pharmaceutical Assistance Contract for the Elderly, the nation's largest state-level pharmaceutical program for the elderly.

Of a series of 740 ambulatory patients visiting a clinic at Johns Hopkins Medical Center, 25% experienced ≥ 1 **adverse effects** associated with their drug use (see TABLE 19–4). The elderly are more likely to be hospitalized as a result of adverse drug reactions than are younger individuals. In a study of 293 admissions to a family medicine inpatient service over a 1-yr period, 15.4% were identified as drug related and almost 10% were primarily drug related. At highest risk for drug-related admissions were persons in their 50s and 70s. In pharmacoepidemiologic studies, common age-associated complications of drug therapy include upper GI bleeding with nonsteroidal anti-inflammatory drug use and hip fracture with psychotropic drug use.

Polypharmacy also potentially increases the number of **drug-drug, drug-disease,** and **drug-nutrient interactions.** While there are few data to document the incidence of clinically significant interactions, a number of factors clearly point to an increased risk: ≥ 1 chronic illnesses, altered pharmacodynamics, and age-related changes in pharmacokinetics (see Ch. 18).

TABLE 19–4. ADVERSE DRUG EFFECTS REPORTED MOST FREQUENTLY BY 740 AMBULATORY ELDERLY PATIENTS AT JOHNS HOPKINS MEDICAL CENTER

Adverse Effect	% of Patients Reporting
Urinary frequency	8.3
Very dry mouth	7.6
Indigestion or nausea	3.3
Dizziness	3.0
Rashes, itching, bruising	1.8
Diarrhea	1.6
Depression, tiredness	1.5

Another complication of polypharmacy is **noncompliance,** *a patient's deviation from a prescriber's planned drug therapy regimen.* The elderly are no more noncompliant than other age groups, but they are a high-risk group. Major contributing factors include multiple physicians, diseases, medications, dose-administration times, and pharmacies. Consequences include inadequate treatment, relapse, drug toxicity, increased incidence of adverse effects, unnecessary hospitalizations, and increased medical expenses. However, noncompliance should not always be viewed negatively; refusal to take medications as prescribed may signal the necessity to alter a planned regimen, and each instance of noncompliance should be evaluated carefully by the physician and pharmacist.

Polypharmacy can also be costly. In 2 studies conducted in long-term care facilities, widespread use of H_2-receptor antagonists at prolonged, full-dose therapy was noted for undocumented, inappropriate, and poorly supported diagnoses. Also demonstrated was concurrent use with other antiulcer and ulcerogenic medications. The prevalence of this polypharmacy (use of a drug without a specific indication, at unnecessarily high doses, to prevent the potential adverse consequences of another drug, or in combination with another when 1 is sufficient) and the cost of these agents consumes large amounts of limited financial resources available to long-term care patients.

When choosing the most appropriate drug for the older patient, several factors should be considered. Preferred drugs have a high ratio of efficacy to toxicity, a simple mechanism of action targeted to a single specific site, and minimal effects on other sites. Also preferred are drugs that are reliably absorbed when taken orally, minimally bound to plasma protein, and predictably metabolized and excreted, even in the presence of liver or kidney impairment. Drugs should not have significant interactions with other drugs, disease states, laboratory tests, or nutrients.

Containers should be simple, storable, and portable, with readable labels. Optimally, the prescription should encourage compliance and not allow the drug to interfere with or cause a change in the dosage of other prescribed medications.

A pharmacist's expertise can help determine the suitability and acceptability of a drug. In consultation with physicians, pharmacists can help choose appropriate agents or recommend alternatives, advise and monitor patients, improve compliance, minimize adverse effects, and improve the therapeutic outcome. No longer solely the dispenser of a product, the pharmacist today acts as a consultant, educator, counselor, and researcher in geriatric medicine.

Long-Term Care Pharmacy

Since January 1974, federal regulations have required pharmacists in long-term care facilities to provide consultant services and to conduct monthly drug regimen reviews for each patient, so that skilled nursing facilities can qualify for Medicare and Medicaid reimbursement. These regulations were expanded in 1987 to include intermediate care facilities. Accordingly, pharmacy professional organizations have developed standards of practice and defined the pharmacist's role in developing, coordinating, and supervising pharmaceutical services in long-term care facilities. Drug delivery, inventory control, and clinical services (eg, IV admixture preparation, nutrition support) are coordinated by pharmacists. In addition, pharmacists have become involved in investigational programs; eg, postmarketing surveillance, clinical trials, and other patient-related services such as individualized medication dosing, consultation, and drug-holiday programs.

Monthly drug regimen reviews identify and report potential problems with medications (eg, duplication, polypharmacy, drug interactions, inappropriate prescribing or dosing, and adverse drug reactions). A written report of all findings is given to the administration, the director of nursing, and the primary physician for appropriate actions. The US Department of Health and Human Services has published guidelines for use by federal and state surveyors in assessing a facility's drug regimen review process (TABLE 19–5). These reviews have helped decrease polypharmacy, minimized duplication of drugs, prevented significant drug interactions, and reduced inappropriate use of drugs. A review of the literature published between 1975 and 1987 shows an estimated total savings to Medicare during this period of > $220 million.

Hospital Pharmacy

Many hospital pharmacies commonly provide a number of programs, including comprehensive drug information centers, pharmacokinetic dosing advice, and nutrition support services. In addition, pharmacists are members of multidisciplinary teams in the medical and surgical services of many hospitals and have developed or participate in specialized programs to meet the needs of geriatric patients. For example, as a member

TABLE 19–5. INDICATORS FOR ASSESSING DRUG REGIMEN REVIEWS

Apparent Irregularities

1. Multiple orders for the same drug for the same patient by the same route of administration
2. Administration of drugs without regard for established stop-order policies
3. Administration of as needed (prn) drugs as directed every day for > 30 days
4. Administration of ≥ 3 laxatives concurrently
5. Continuous use of hypnotic drugs for > 30 days
6. Use of ≥ 2 hypnotic drugs at the same time
7. Administration of hypnotic drugs in excess of the listed maximal doses
8. Use of antipsychotics or antidepressants for < 3 days
9. Use of ≥ 2 antipsychotic drugs at the same time
10. Use of antipsychotic drugs in excess of the recommended maximal daily dose
11. Use of anxiolytic drugs in excess of recommended maximal dosages
12. More than 2 changes of an antidepressant within a 7-day period
13. Use of antidepressants in excess of the recommended maximal daily dose
14. Use of anticholinergics with antipsychotic drugs in the absence of recorded extrapyramidal side effects
15. Repeated loss of seizure control in a patient taking anticonvulsants
16. Administration of thyroid drugs without an assessment of thyroid function
17. Administration of anticoagulant therapy without some assessment of blood clotting function at least every month
18. Administration of antihypertensive drugs without BP checks at least weekly
19. Administration of cardioactive drugs without recording a pulse rate daily in the first month of therapy and weekly thereafter, or when the chart shows a pulse consistently < 60 or > 100 beats/min
20. Administration of diuretics without a serum K level determination within 30 days after initiation of therapy
21. Administration of diuretics and cardiotonics (eg, digoxin), without a serum K determination within 30 days after initiation of the cardiotonic therapy and q 6 mo thereafter
22. Use of cardiotonics (eg, digoxin) in the absence of documentation of 1 of the following diagnoses: heart failure, atrial fibrillation, paroxysmal supraventricular tachycardia, or atrial flutter
23. Administration of insulin or oral hypoglycemics without a urine glucose test at least daily or a blood glucose test at least q 60 days
24. Administration of iron preparations, folic acid, or vitamin B_{12} without an RBC assessment during the first month of therapy
25. Use of methenamine mandelate, methenamine hippurate, sulfamethoxazole-trimethoprim, or nitrofurantoin in patients with chronic UTIs if a urinalysis has not been performed at least once 30 days after therapy was initiated or if therapy is continued when urine pH is continually > 6
26. Use of nitrofurantoin for conditions other than treatment or prophylaxis of UTIs or when BUN or serum creatinine levels are not recorded on the patient's chart
27. Orders for ≥ 3 analgesics at the same time
28. Administration of phenylbutazone or oxyphenbutazone continuously without at least 1 CBC determination 30 days after initiation of therapy
29. Continuous use of antibiotic/steroidal topical ophthalmic preparation for periods of > 14 days

(Continued)

TABLE 19–5. INDICATORS FOR ASSESSING DRUG REGIMEN
REVIEWS *(Cont'd)*

30. Use of aminoglycosides in the absence of a baseline serum creatinine determination when therapy was initiated
31. Orders for drugs for which there is a known allergy documented in the patient's record
32. Crushing of solid dose forms when the likely result causes patient discomfort or undesired blood levels

of an interdisciplinary geriatric assessment unit, the pharmacist obtains a medication history for each patient that includes patterns of use of all prescribed and OTC medications, compliance with previously prescribed regimens, therapeutic effectiveness, duplication of drugs, adverse drug reactions, and drug interactions. Recommendations are then made to optimize drug use (eg, counseling and educating the patient and family, recommending alternative therapy, or adjusting the current regimen). Similar activities are conducted in hospital-based geriatrics clinics and in community-outreach programs, in which patients are seen in satellite clinics, congregate housing facilities, or at home. Major additional objectives are to maintain the older person's active ambulatory life-style and to decrease the use of institutional services.

Outpatient clinics in which patients are seen and followed up by pharmacists provide refill authorization and medication and compliance monitoring for those with chronic diseases. Published reports have documented better control of chronic diseases, improved compliance, and overall cost reduction with such a program.

Community Pharmacy

The community pharmacist is often the first health care professional to have contact with the elderly patient, providing advice and counseling on OTC drug use and referring patients to physicians. This pharmacist can maintain up-to-date medication profiles and monitor drug use to decrease adverse reactions, drug interactions, and duplicate drugs for patients under the care of multiple physicians.

The OTC market accounts for > $3 billion in annual expenditures. The elderly purchase more OTC drugs, especially analgesics, cough and cold preparations, vitamins, antacids, and laxatives, than any other segment of the population. Pharmacist counseling and monitoring of OTC drug use can decrease the potential for adverse reactions or drug interactions. Some pharmacists offer screening services (eg, blood pressure, cholesterol) and, as more home laboratory tests become available, pharmacists will become more involved in assisting patients with these products.

Many large community pharmacies are also involved in the provision of home health care products (eg, the preparation and dispensing of nutritional products and IV medications, and the sale and rental of durable medical goods).

Pharmacy Education in Geriatrics

The number of pharmacists trained to deal with geriatric problems depends on the access of pharmacy students and practicing pharmacists to adequate professional training, which is currently limited. However, more educators are being trained in geriatrics, and the number of pharmacy colleges offering courses in this area is increasing. The American Society of Hospital Pharmacists and the American Society of Consultant Pharmacists recognize and accredit residencies in geriatrics, and several research-oriented fellowship programs in pharmacy are available.

---

20. SITE-SPECIFIC CARE

Mary Jane Koren

Because old age is a time of impairment and disability for many, physicians must be familiar with institutional and community-based services so they can counsel patients and families and use resources wisely. This chapter focuses on the formal structures that exist to help the elderly cope with declining function, highlights the need for ongoing physician involvement with patients in these programs, and presents factors that influence placement decisions.

NURSING HOMES

Approximately 5% of persons > 65 yr of age reside in nursing homes at any one time, although about 20% spend time in a nursing home at some point in their lives. Nursing home residence is strongly age associated: < 2% of residents are age 65 to 74 yr, 10% are age 75 to 84 yr, and > 20% are over age 85 yr. Half the patients admitted to nursing homes die there, leading many persons to regard institutionalization as a prelude to death.

Increased demographic demand means a need for more nursing home beds. Prospective payment systems, such as Diagnosis Related Groups **(DRGs),** are producing admissions from hospitals of patients who are more acutely ill or unstable and who have greater rehabilitative potential. Such patients probably will be in the nursing home for short stays (< 3 mo), rather than permanently, but they require more costly care than the traditional custodial-care patient.

Payment methodologies are being reevaluated to provide for the patient who needs a higher level of care. Case mix, which ties payment to the care needs of the patient population in the nursing home, is one approach being tested. Most states trying case mix systems place patients in hierarchically arranged categories that depend on the amount of resources consumed (eg, staff time spent attending to patients for rehabilitation and nursing care needs). One of the longest running demonstrations of this reimbursement methodology, New York State's Resource

Utilization Groups system, has 5 levels: the Rehabilitation Level for patients with restorative goals; the Special Care Level for patients who are comatose or require nasogastric feedings and similar care; the Clinically Complex Level for patients receiving O_2 therapy, chemotherapy, or transfusions, or who are terminally ill; the Severe Behavioral Level for patients who are physically aggressive or disruptive; and the Physical Care Level for patients whose primary problem is related to reduced physical functioning. Further stratification within each of these categories is achieved by ranking patients according to the sum total of ADL deficits.

This type of system provides financial incentives for nursing home operators to develop facilities for patients who require more complex care. There is, of course, an inherent danger that nursing homes will foster dependence or maintain the need for high levels of care to maximize reimbursement. It is therefore necessary that quality assurance systems be closely tied into any case mix reimbursement system.

CARE IN THE NURSING HOME

Although nursing homes function as part of the medical continuum of care, the hospital model should not be applied. Nursing homes are not hospitals; they are people's residences—their homes. Too often, nursing home residents are deprived of rights because institutional needs for routines and efficiency dominate planning. Quality of life may be lost when clinical care needs are given precedence. To protect residents from such abuses, the new Federal Nursing Home Requirements for Participation in Medicare or Medicaid have an entire section on resident rights and another on quality of life.

Because of the complexity of problems in the typical nursing facility resident, an interdisciplinary team approach is required. The team must work together to perform 4 major activities. First, each discipline thoroughly assesses the resident. Second, a comprehensive care plan must then be developed. Third, the care plan must be implemented, and finally the success of the care plan should be evaluated and modifications made when appropriate. Whether the team consists of core members such as the physician, nurse, and social worker or incorporates nutritionists, pharmacists, physical and occupational therapists, and others, each discipline has a responsibility to perform the 4 steps above so that all aspects of resident well-being may be planned.

Levels of care: Because of widespread public dissatisfaction with the quality of services being provided to nursing home residents, the Department of Health and Human Services contracted with the Institute of Medicine in 1983 to study the problem. Their report, issued in 1986 and entitled "Improving the Quality of Care in Nursing Homes," contained a number of provisions that were incorporated into the Omnibus Reconciliation Act of 1987 (Public Law 100-203, Subsection C: the Nursing Home Reform Law). One of the most significant changes made by this statute is the elimination of the 2 levels of care currently provided under

Medicaid—the Skilled Nursing Facility level and the Intermediate Care Facility level. Beginning in October, 1990 all Medicare or Medicaid certified facilities will be required to provide a wide range of services including 24-hour nursing coverage. This will eliminate the need for level of care reviews and the possibility that residents must be moved from one facility to another to access services.

Cost: Long-term care is expensive, primarily because of its duration. With costs often > $23,000/yr, few individuals or families are able to afford ongoing care. Historically, Medicare has not paid a meaningful proportion of nursing home costs; however, the Medicare Catastrophic Coverage Bill (under reconsideration by Congress at press time) extended coverage to up to 150 days of nursing home care per year without a prior hospital stay requirement. This still includes a copayment or coinsurance charge and requires that the 3 elements for eligibility to skilled nursing facility **(SNF)** level of care be met: (1) skilled services are required, (2) these services are required on a daily basis, and (3) as a practical matter, they must be furnished in a nursing facility. Most people who require long-term nursing home care must "spend down" their own resources before becoming eligible for Medicaid coverage, the largest third-party payor for nursing home services in the USA.

The spend-down requirement has 3 dire consequences for nursing home residents: (1) For couples, depletion of joint assets may jeopardize the welfare of the spouse remaining in the community. (2) Carefully accumulated savings intended to be passed on as inheritances are used up. (3) No assets remain for the patient's future return to the community, if that becomes clinically feasible. Thus nursing home placement becomes permanent. (See also FINANCING HEALTH CARE in Ch. 97 and Ch. 104.)

Medical coverage: Physicians providing care to nursing home residents assume a complex responsibility that requires time, energy, and a longstanding relationship with each patient to assess problems and advocate appropriate interventions. Assessing the need for long-term rehabilitation therapy is a particularly important function. Medicare mandates that patients be seen and orders rewritten every 60 days for those in an SNF and every 90 days for those in an ICF after being seen every 30 days for the first 3 mo after admission. This does not exonerate a physician from failing to see patients more frequently if active medical problems are present. Visits, even if routine, should not be perfunctory; patients should be examined, medication status assessed, and laboratory tests ordered as needed. Findings should be documented in the chart to inform other staff members about any problems. To ensure continuity, the same physician should monitor chronic problems and care for acute illnesses, both in the nursing home and in the hospital.

Caring for nursing home patients often involves considerable work with the family. Rapport can be established at the outset if the patient and family are made to feel that someone in authority is listening to them and trying to address their concerns. If nursing home physicians

engage in positive discussions of what can be done, even if only palliative, instead of stressing withholding or cessation of treatment, fears of
abandonment can be assuaged. Relatives are often perceptive about subtle instances of abuse and neglect—eg, unwise use of pharmacologic or
physical restraints for managing disruptive behavior, use of nasogastric
tubes for nutritional support in lieu of feeding, and use of indwelling
bladder catheters and diapers instead of rigorous toileting programs. An
interdisciplinary team can more easily address such problems and advocate good geriatric care, particularly if they include patients and families
in the decision-making process.

Two trends in patient care may help solve the problems of medical
coverage in nursing homes. One is that some physicians are limiting
their practice to long-term care facilities. This allows them to spend
enough time in the nursing home to participate in team activities and be
readily available for consultation with other staff members when
changes in patients that may presage the onset of serious illness are observed. Full-time practice in long-term care facilities is enhanced if it is
combined with teaching medical students and house staff, and providing
patient care in hospitals—activities that help the nursing home physician remain current with patient care practices.

The second trend is that many nursing homes are hiring nurse practitioners **(NPs)** or physician assistants **(PAs),** who improve care by seeing
patients when needed, alerting the physician to serious problems, reviewing old medical records, interviewing families, and performing other
important tasks. However, all tasks may not be delegated and federal
requirements continue to mandate periodic physician visits and involvement with patient care.

Similarly, medical students and house staff can provide valuable services in long-term care facilities while refining skills not taught elsewhere; eg, how to perform a functional assessment examination or use a
cognitive-screening instrument. This exposure also makes them aware
that not all nursing home residents are obtunded, dehydrated, and febrile, a misconception often held when the only contact with such patients is in the emergency room of a hospital.

The medical director is the key to maintaining excellent medical services in nursing facilities and can be the primary care physician's closest
ally, since the director can influence care at a policy-making level and
institute staff training programs concerning geriatric issues. The medical
director provides leadership in developing and implementing policies
and procedures and serves as liaison between the nonphysician staff, the
patients, and the rest of the medical staff. If students are present, the
medical director can contribute to their education by participating in
curriculum development and acting as preceptor.

QUALITY-CARE ASSESSMENT

The Federal government, through the Health Care Financing Administration, requires states to maintain surveillance agencies. These agencies

inspect nursing homes for adherence to specific requirements that must be met for participation in Medicare and Medicaid as well as for compliance with state regulation. A copy of the survey report for a particular facility, including any deficiencies cited, may be useful for families or physicians in selecting a nursing home, but nothing is better than a personal visit.

Methods for assessing quality of care in nursing homes are under scrutiny. Since the decision by the 10th Federal Circuit Court of Appeals in Smith vs. Heckler that the government is responsible for assuring that a facility is actually **giving** good care, not merely **capable** of providing adequate care, outcome measures of quality have replaced many of the more structural aspects of quality assessment. Using physical findings or events that are objective and easily measured (such as falls, contractures, use of nasogastric feeding tubes, development of UTIs or decubitus ulcers, etc.) as triggers or indicators that poor care may be present, the survey, through a system of observation, interview, and record review, attempts to ascertain a facility's performance. Surveyors weigh findings for severity and scope to see if such problems in facilities reflect inadequate care and represent deficiencies.

HOME HEALTH CARE

Home care is a rapidly growing area of health care and may be one of the few safety nets for older people who wish to remain in the community. Although a few insurance companies provided limited coverage early on (eg, that begun by the Metropolitan Life Insurance Co in 1909), home health care received its biggest boost in financing with the advent of Medicare and Medicaid in 1965, which provided funding for home care services. At that time, only 250 agencies met the standards outlined in the Medicare conditions of participation. Today, > 6000 home health agencies are Medicare-certified and probably an equal number exist without certification. In 1985, these agencies sponsored > 4.5 million visits to Medicare recipients alone. Medicare is the largest third-party payor of home health benefits, and currently accounts for > $9 billion of the nation's health care expenditures; it is projected to grow at a rate of 15 to 20%/yr.

Several other factors have also contributed to the growth of home health care: (1) The increase in life expectancy and burdens of dependency have created many potential users. (2) Most people prefer to be cared for at home, especially if such care replaces or delays nursing home care. (3) Technologic advances have made treatments easily available at home that were once available only in hospitals (eg, IV therapy, dialysis, parenteral and enteral nutrition, and ventilator support). In addition, the development of the mobile laboratory that can provide portable x-rays, ECGs, and blood testing has further diminished the need for institutional care.

Home health care agencies may be either proprietary (for profit) or voluntary (not for profit), or may be run by a public or government agency. They may be freestanding (community based) or may function as part of a hospital or nursing home. Whatever their organization or affiliation, home health care agencies can be classified according to major types of programs: certified home health agencies, long-term care programs, and hospices.

CERTIFIED HOME HEALTH AGENCIES

The Certified Home Health Agency **(CHHA)** has been the prototype for most programs, reflecting the major influence of Medicare. To be certified, an agency must meet state licensing requirements as well as the federal conditions of participation for payment in the Medicare program. Agencies so designated may then be reimbursed by either Medicare, Medicaid, or other private third-party insurers.

Several requirements must be met for patients to be considered eligible for home health care benefits under Medicare (See TABLE 20–1). One is that the patient must be homebound (ie, a considerable effort would have to be made or health risked for the patient to leave the home). Usually, visits to a physician's office or clinic are excepted. Another requirement is that the patient needs skilled care from 1 of 3 trigger services: nursing, physical therapy, or speech therapy. (These may be expanded to include occupational therapy.) Once it has been determined that the requirement for **skilled care** has been met (see TABLE 20–2), the patient is eligible to receive ancillary services (see TABLE 20–3).

Although aides are an important element of home health care programs, their services are being increasingly limited by third-party payors in efforts to control costs. The number of hours of aide services that will be reimbursed varies but is usually < 2 h/day, 5 days/wk. Patients typically stay in CHHA programs for several weeks to months, but the duration of services they are entitled to is usually linked to the prognosis and rate of achievement of predetermined therapeutic goals.

TABLE 20–1. GENERAL MEDICARE REQUIREMENTS FOR
HOME HEALTH CARE BENEFITS

Beneficiary must be homebound
Beneficiary must need ≥ 1 of the following:
    Skilled nursing
    Physical therapy
    Speech therapy
Service must be:
    Reasonable and necessary
    Provided in the patient's place of residence
    Ordered by the physician
    On an intermittent basis

TABLE 20-2. SKILLED-CARE SERVICES*

Nursing
Teaching: Use of medications, diet, use of prosthetic or other devices, safety and accident prevention, bowel and bladder training, behavior modification
Assessment: Physical examination, environment, functional support systems, health knowledge, nutrition
Monitoring: Self-care by patient, wound status, medication use and side effects, coping ability
Case Management: Arranging referrals, ordering supplies and equipment, making appointments, obtaining transportation, conferring with and coordinating services of other care providers, supervising aides
Treatment: Chronic wound care, parenteral feeding, tracheostomy/ostomy care, range-of-motion exercises, pain management, venipuncture, injections, fecal disimpaction

Physical therapy
Evaluation and functional assessment
Exercises: Passive, active, resistive, therapeutic, stretching
Training: Gait, prosthetic device, transfers
Therapy: Chest physiotherapy, ultrasound, hot or cold packs, whirlpool

Occupational therapy
Evaluation and activities-of-daily-living (ADL) assessment
Training—Adaptive devices, ADLs
Teaching—Muscle reeducation, adaptation of therapy or condition to home environment

Speech therapy
Evaluation and assessment
Training: Alaryngeal speech, language processing, speech/voice
Aural rehabilitation

Medical social work
Assessment: Social support network, emotional factors
Counseling
Assistance with placement, housing, financial problems

* This is a partial list.

TABLE 20-3. ANCILLARY SERVICES*

Occupational therapy

Medical social services

Home health aide services

Medical intern or resident services

Medical supplies

Durable medical equipment

Prosthetic devices

* Available once patient meets general Medicare eligibility criteria.

LONG-TERM HOME HEALTH CARE

Long-term home health care programs, which are funded by Medicaid, are unavailable in many states and differ substantially from the Medicare model. Eligibility criteria and program offerings vary by state; information or availability can usually be obtained from state offices for the aging, departments of social service, or health departments.

A prototype for such programs is New York's Nursing Home Without Walls, which is modeled after nursing home programs. This program is primarily for nursing home patients and substitutes home health aides, care management, and limited skills services for nursing home placement. Patients are served on a long-term basis as long as they meet state placement criteria for nursing home care and the cost does not exceed 75% of expenditure for a comparable level of nursing home care. Attainment of a therapeutic goal or the continued need for skilled services is not required as it is for Medicare patients in a Certified Home Health Agency Program.

Although such long-term health care programs are popular with patients and families, they have not proved effective in forestalling or replacing institutionalization. Accordingly, many legislators consider them supplementary rather than substitutive programs and hence are eager to restrict their growth.

HOSPICE CARE
(See also Ch. 97)

Well over 1000 hospice programs throughout the USA provide care to terminally ill patients and support to their families. Initially philanthropic, they are now included in Medicare coverage, and some states are considering including them in Medicaid programs (as is currently done in Kentucky, Michigan, Florida, and New York).

Most hospice programs are home based, and Medicare and Medicaid regulations require that at least 80% of hospice care be provided in the patient's home. Requirements for hospice reimbursement include Medicare eligibility and certification by a physician of terminal illness (≤ 6 mo of life left). Patients must sign a statement indicating their willingness to waive Medicare benefits for curative services, so they can receive benefits for hospice care. Core services that must be provided include nursing, medical, and social services and bereavement counseling. Noncore services include physical and occupational therapy, home health care aide services, medical supplies, general counseling, and short inpatient stays.

The hospice employs multidisciplinary teams, consisting of a physician, a registered nurse, a social worker, and a counselor. This is the only Medicare home health care program in which the conditions of participation specify that a physician must be a salaried member of the team.

The reimbursement formula has both prospective and retrospective features; although a cap is specified (approximately $7500), intensity of services can fluctuate, depending on the patient's needs.

The requirement that physicians certify the patient's life expectancy is ≤ 6 mo has proved a major stumbling block. Most physicians do not believe they can predict death accurately, and hospices are unwilling to accept the financial risk of having patients outlive predictions, since they may not discharge patients nor be paid for continuing service. The average length of hospice care is, therefore, only about 6 wk, which tends to nullify the goal of the program—ie, to help the patient and family prepare for death by improving the physical, mental, and spiritual quality of the remaining life.

A hospice patient's own physician need not relinquish primary medical responsibility to the hospice physician. However, most primary care physicians have neither the expertise in pain management and symptom control that hospice physicians have nor the ability to be as accessible to other team members for home visiting and problem solving. (See also Chs. 26 and 97.)

THE ROLE OF THE PHYSICIAN IN HOME CARE

Initially, Medicare legislation was based on the presumption that the physician would act as the gatekeeper for home health care, referring patients to more intensive care programs when that was reasonable and necessary, and writing orders for home care services when appropriate. To guard against fraud and abuse, no physician was permitted to refer a patient to or write orders for a patient participating in any home health agency program in which that physician had a > 5% financial interest. No provision was made, however, for reimbursement for case management by the referring physician or for telephone consultation or conferences with the home health care staff. Moreover, no incentive was provided for agencies to hire their own physicians, as was later done in hospices. For these reasons, physicians have become removed from the day-to-day process of developing plans of care. The physician's role has become limited to signing already developed plans and validating orders written by the agency's own staff.

A major benefit of home health care is that skilled professionals can observe changes in the patient at home and quickly apprise the physician of problems. The home care staff can function as the physician's eyes and ears by monitoring the progress of an active medical problem. In addition, they can vigorously treat chronic problems, and individualize rehabilitation to the patient's home environment. Even minor deterioration can be detected early, thus avoiding frequent visits to emergency departments and repeated hospitalizations. Although ideally, physicians should make home visits, this is an unrealistic expectation for many. However, by maintaining close telephone contact with agency staff, the physician can provide adequate support for patients.

CONGREGATE OUTPATIENT SERVICES

Congregate programs include day care, adult day health care, day hos pital, aftercare, and medical day care. These outpatient programs hav certain similarities. Patients with medical, physical, cognitive, or socia disabilities are transported to a center for several hours a day, severa days a week, for group activities designed to forestall institutionalizatio and to improve well-being. In this discussion, the generic term "da care" is used.

Most day-care programs conform to 1 of 3 models, although all, wit rare exceptions, are built around a group of core services that includes meal, transportation, and recreational activities. (See TABLE 20–4). Th **day hospital model** emphasizes rehabilitation therapy or intensive medi cal/nursing care, along with medical monitoring and recreational an social activities to improve functional independence or recuperation. It i designed for individuals recovering from acute events such as stroke amputation, or fractures. These programs are usually time-limited, rang ing from 6 wk to 6 mo. The ratio of professional staff to patients i high, which makes these programs costly to operate. Some of them bil Medicaid or Medicare for a clinic visit, which provides a higher reim bursement rate than billing for each service separately or billing at day-care rate.

The **maintenance model** of day care combines some medical car (largely preventive) with social work and recreational services and is de signed to help maintain and enhance an existing level of function for a long as possible. Because the ratio of professional staff to patients i lower, this type of program is less costly to operate. It is most benefi cial if provided for long periods; however, the balance between deman and available resources often limits duration.

The **social model** may resemble a typical senior citizen center program in which participation may be for an unspecified period, or it may b geared to serving patients with dementing or mental illnesses, wit shorter periods of participation. Admission criteria vary, but most pro grams require that patients be ambulatory or able to get about i wheelchairs, continent, and not socially disruptive. Unfortunately, thes criteria may discriminate against those with dementia, who might deriv a great deal of benefit from participation and whose care givers woul get a few hours of respite.

On the other hand, some day-care centers specialize in serving thos with dementia. Services include family support activities; therapy; recre ation activities designed to maintain stability and orientation; and at tempts to modify disruptive behavior by providing positive, consisten reinforcement for efforts of self-control and social appropriateness. Al though these services cannot halt the inexorable progression o dementia, temporary improvements in functional capacity that enhanc the quality of life have been noted in many instances.

TABLE 20-4. MODEL OF CONGREGATE OUTPATIENT PROGRAMS

	Restorative/Rehabilitative (Day Hospital)	Maintenance	Psychosocial/Mental Health
Program duration	Time limited	Long term	May be time limited
Target population	Patients with major disabilities or serious illnesses (strokes, fractures, etc)	Frail elderly, chronically ill, or disabled	Patients with: Fewer physical disabilities Cognitive impairment Affective disorders Social impairment
Services	Core services (transportation, nutrition, activity programs), plus: Rehabilitation (PT, OT, ST) Nursing	Core services, plus: Screening/monitoring chronic illnesses Social, recreational, educational activities (health promotion, disease prevention) Physical exercises	Core services, plus: Counseling Group therapy
Goals	Rehabilitation Restoration of function Improvement of clinical status	Improve quality of life Delay or prevent institutionalization Improve patient self-image Prevent loneliness, isolation, and withdrawal Eliminate monotony of daily existence	Improve mental health Manage medication Modify behavior Encourage self-expression Develop coping technics

PT = physical therapy; OT = occupational therapy; ST = speech therapy.

One of the most difficult issues faced by time-limited programs is that of developing discharge criteria. Patients become dependent and resist discharge, or they may become depressed when it is imminent. Discharge planning, therefore, needs to begin even before admission, with the potential for ultimate discharge a part of enrollment criteria. The staff, as a team, needs to define goals and track progress.

Because many patients require some formal support after leaving the day-care program, assessment of posttreatment needs is important. Conferences with patients and families to identify outside community agencies that may be helpful will ensure continuity of care and prevent families from feeling abandoned. A gradual decrease in the number of days per week spent at the day-care center, periodic evaluation of patient readiness for discharge, and parties or ceremonies at the end of the course, with follow-up contacts after discharge, may help to lessen some of the anxiety patients experience when leaving a program.

Transportation is a major barrier to day-care participation for non-Medicaid patients. Medicare does not cover the costs associated with travel to and from day-care centers, so unless a patient is entitled to Medicaid benefits or is able to pay the costs out of pocket, the program is inaccessible. Day-care centers may use donated funds to help subsidize transportation, and many use a means test and a sliding-fee scale to accommodate patients. Yet, many who would benefit from these services are underserved. (See also Ch. 97.)

RESPITE CARE

Some 60 to 80% of the care the disabled elderly receive in their own homes is provided by friends and relatives, usually a spouse. This often unremitting responsibility drains the physical, financial, and emotional resources of care providers. Respite care is a generic term applied to programs designed to provide temporary relief to family care givers, in contrast to those designed to directly benefit the patient. In Great Britain, respite care is recognized as an important component of a vertically integrated system of geriatric services and is widely used. Very few respite programs are available in the USA, and they vary in organization and approach.

Most respite programs offer services in the patient's home, usually in blocks of several hours on a regular basis. For example, 1 evening or 1 or 2 afternoons a week, the caregiver is free to run errands or engage in social or recreational activities. Full days of respite care may allow the care giver a crucial vacation or other benefit.

Respite care is distinguished from the hiring of part-time help by families on their own, because respite-care workers are usually provided through a structured program that incorporates quality-assurance measures.

Some respite programs provide services in an institutional setting for periods of several days to a few weeks for persons whose needs vary from custodial to total care. Inpatient services are harder to provide because of the volume of paperwork involved, the lack of reimbursement available, and the disruption of the institution's normal routine.

ASSESSMENT OF THE NEED FOR INSTITUTIONALIZATION

Accurate assessment of the need for institutional placement involves 4 areas of consideration: (1) medical needs, (2) social support network, (3) cognitive or intellectual function, and (4) physical function status.

Medical problems: The burden of chronic illness increases with age; exacerbations of underlying conditions and acute episodic illnesses become superimposed. Depending on the amount of physiologic reserve a patient has, an acute illness in one who is already compromised may necessitate some form of institutional care, even if only on a temporary basis. Illnesses that may respond completely to treatment (eg, acute infections or fractures) may leave a frail older individual weak and debilitated. The individual may require skilled care available only in a nursing home or in an aggressive home health care program for an extended period before complete independence is regained.

Social factors: Consideration must be given to whether potential care givers are willing and able to perform the tasks necessary to keep the older person in the home. Strongly motivated families often can perform elaborate and detailed care, but ascertainment is needed to ensure that the care givers are not indifferent or angry about assuming such responsibility. Home health care is often a long-term commitment and may prove an unremitting burden to a family. Physicians should watch for and be ready to intervene if elder abuse is suspected. As the patient ages, so do the spouse and children. Their own frailty or impairment may prohibit their providing necessary care, regardless of how much they may wish to do so.

Cognitive function: Intellectual impairment alone can provoke institutionalization. Bizarre or antisocial behavior can endanger both the patient and those around him. Even with a supportive family, the manifestations of advanced dementia may be intolerable; if 24-h custodial care is required, a nursing home is usually preferable. But mildly demented patients can function quite well in their own familiar environment with some assistance in managing funds and guidance when traveling to an unfamiliar place.

Physical function: The ability to perform the activities of daily living **(ADLs)**—bathing, ambulating, toileting, eating, dressing, and grooming—and instrumental activies of daily living **(IADLs)**—shopping, cooking, cleaning, managing of finances, and telephone use—is crucial in deciding whether nursing home placement is necessary. (See also Ch. 15 and Ch. 103.) The single most important factor for someone who lives alone is mobility. Varying levels of functional impairment may be less of a handicap with adaptive devices, and skillful assessment of a

person in his home (eg, by an occupational therapist) is extremely useful.

Placement decisions, whether made during hospital discharge planning
or on an outpatient basis, will more likely be appropriate if the
strengths and weaknesses of the patient are considered in these 4 areas
No single factor should be considered alone; rather, their interplay determines the care plan.

---

21.   DIAGNOSTIC AND THERAPEUTIC TECHNOLOGY

Paul A. L. Haber

The explosive growth of technology has given the elderly the possibility of having a longer life and improved quality of life, but it has also
brought potential disadvantages. **Adverse effects** of invasive technology
include trauma, infection, and problems associated with drugs and radioisotopes. This technology has been criticized, particularly when applied
in the elderly, because of concerns that it may increase the cost of
health care and replace personal medical attention with machine-driven,
dehumanizing care. However, technology that provides better health
care is usually cost-effective, and no technology should be permitted to
diminish personal care. Relative costs of new technologies and their relative value in imaging different organ systems are shown in TABLES
21–1 and 21–2, respectively.

The risk of dehumanized care arises because new procedures sometimes
require a great deal of attention from subspecialized personnel, some of
whom may be more comfortable attending the equipment than the patient. Furthermore, the multiplicity of required personnel tends to make
each individual assume that others are meeting the patient's personal
needs. For example, when a patient is sedated, intubated, and connected
to a respirator, several people and a high level of skill are needed to
monitor the patient and manipulate the drugs and equipment, as well as
to perform associated procedures (eg, maintaining IVs and fluid balance,
checking blood gas levels). To do all this well and also communicate
with the patient on a personal basis requires a highly trained, well-motivated, and compassionate staff.

Other problems arise because of the detailed and sophisticated information that new technology can provide, particularly when these data
are accepted despite conflicting clinical data. Worse yet is the tendency
to take less adequate histories, to perform less thorough physical examinations, or not to attempt to learn something about the patient as a
person—all on the assumption that the new technologies will provide all

TABLE 21-1. RELATIVE COSTS OF NEW TECHNOLOGIES

	CT	MRI	PET	US	Gamma Camera
Equipment	$650,000–$1.2 M	$800,000–$1.2 M	$800,000	$40,000–$130,000	$150,000–$500,000
Installation and site preparation	$50,000	$1.5 M–$2.2 M	$700,000	NA	$50,000
Accessories			cyclotron $2.5 M		
Cost per procedure	$200–$400	$700–$800	$500–$700	$45–$60	$45–$50

CT = computed tomography; MRI = magnetic resonance imaging; PET = positron emission tomography; US = ultrasound.

TABLE 21-2. RELATIVE VALUE OF NEW TECHNOLOGIES IN FINDING PATHOLOGY

	CT	MRI	PET	US and Echography	Radionuclide
Head and CNS					
Brain	+++	+++	++	0	++
Brainstem	++	+++	++	0	0
Spinal cord	++	+++	++	0	0
Spine	++	++	0	0	0
Neck	+++	++	0	++	0
Thorax					
Lungs	+++	++	0	0	++
Heart	++	++	0	+++	++
Mediastinum	+++	+++	0	+	0
Breast	++	++	0	++	0
Abdomen					
Liver	+++	++	0	++	++
Pancreas	+++	+++	0	++	0
Spleen	++	++	0	+	+
Gallbladder	++	++	0	+++	++

Stomach	++	+	0	+	0
Bowel	+	+	0	0	0
GU system					
Kidneys	+++	+++	0	++	++
Ureters	+	+	0	+	+
Bladder	++	++	0	++	+
Prostate	++	++	0	++	0
Extremities					
Vasculature	+	+	0	++	++

CT = computed tomography; MRI = magnetic resonance imaging; PET = positron emission tomography; US = ultrasound.

0 = No value
+ = Marginal value
+ + = Considerable value
+ + + = Great value

the answers. These problems should not be blamed on technolog
rather, they result from poor medical practice and misuse of technolog

During the 20th century, hospitals have become the primary loci
new technology. However, trends indicate that some of the technolog
will be decentralized and find its place in the doctor's office, the is
lated laboratory, and even (with the appropriate biotelemetry) the p
tient's home or the nursing home. Thus, the need for hospitalizatic
(which entails some associated morbidity) may be averted. Further, i
vasive procedures are giving way to noninvasive procedures, a
demonstrated by the disappearance of pneumoencephalography in fav
of computed tomography (CT) scanning, positron emission tomograph
(PET) scanning, or magnetic resonance imaging (MRI) technologies an
the increasing substitution of MRI for myelography in studies involvir
the spinal cord.

DIAGNOSTIC TECHNOLOGIES

COMPUTED TOMOGRAPHY (CT)

CT scanning has rendered many invasive procedures obsolete, notab
pneumoencephalography, and altered the indications for many oth
types of studies (eg, angiography of the brain).

Classic x-ray imaging and CT depend on the differential absorption
x-rays by body structures to create images. Standard x-ray images repr
sent a superimposition of all shadows of all structures through whic
the beam passes. CT scans present "slices" of structures that are not s
perimposed on one another. CT also is more sensitive to differences
density and is able to distinguish densities of 0.5%.

Recent advances in CT reflect refinements of image manipulation tec
nics. Complex 3-dimensional (3-D) representations of body parts can l
made, which are particularly useful in imaging bone deformities. Con
puter-assisted manufacturing technics can use the 3-D images for pro
thesis design. Reconstructive surgery can be planned more precisel
and surgical approaches may be modified. However, while CT appea
to be a mature technology, MRI supersedes CT scanning in many situa
tions.

CT Examination of the Head

While the CT scanner delineates normal and diseased areas of tl
brain, images of supratentorial structures are clearer than those of i
fratentorial regions because of the artifact produced between the petro
pyramids. Clear distinction between white and gray matter is general
possible (eg, the cerebral cortex, basal ganglia, ventricular system, an
basal cisterns are clearly defined).

CT scans of the brain usually consist of 12 to 15 slices, each about
to 10 mm thick. Locations of the slices are referred to as supraventricu
lar, high ventricular, low ventricular, and intraventricular.

Bones as well as soft tissues can be visualized very precisely, and **intracranial tumors** are diagnosed with 95 to 99% accuracy. Meningiomas, gliomas, glioblastomas, astrocytomas, and metastases are well visualized. CT scanning is also useful in staging tumors and in planning and evaluating therapy.

The diagnosis of stroke with CT scan has been enormously successful. CT enables one to distinguish between intracerebral and subarachnoid hemorrhage, as well as between primary, intracerebral hematoma and ischemic infarction on the basis of differences in density. **Subdural** and **extradural hematomas** and **linear skull fractures,** commonly suspected following a fall in an older patient, are readily detected.

CT is less sensitive than MRI but more sensitive and specific than angiography or nuclear studies. However, cost and availability may favor CT. **Blood clots** often have a dramatic appearance on CT, because their density is greater than brain density. However, angiography (either a standard or a digital subtraction technic) is more accurate than CT for evaluating blood vessels. Angiography may be necessary to detect cervical and intracranial atherosclerosis, some aneurysms, and arteriovenous **(A-V)** malformations. Visualization of **aneurysms** $\leq$ 2.5 cm with CT usually requires contrast enhancement, which is also used to visualize vascular malformations, including hemangiomas. Rupture of an aneurysm along with subarachnoid hemorrhage can be detected in 75 to 85% of patients if CT is performed early.

Intracranial infections (eg, brain abscesses, tubercular abscess, luetic pathology, and opportunistic infections) can be detected and characterized by CT; however, specific etiologic diagnoses cannot be made.

Cerebral atrophy can be detected, but its clinical significance may be unclear. CT is useful in diagnosing Alzheimer-type dementia, mainly by ruling out other diseases.

Finally, **obstructions of the free flow of CSF** can be detected, which may unmask obstructive or communicating hydrocephalus.

CT Examination of the Heart and Mediastinum

CT scanning of the heart is useful in certain pathologic conditions affecting aging patients, but it has not yet lived up to expectations. The pericardium is easily visualized and effusions can be defined, but demonstration of hemopericardium, which may be isodense with myocardium, is not always possible. CT also helps differentiate restrictive cardiomyopathy from constrictive pericarditis. A new use of CT scanning is the demonstration of bypass graft patency. CT is particularly useful when graft location, number, and size are known in advance.

Lesions of the thyroid, especially substernal thyroid, are better visualized by CT than by radioactive iodine (^{131}I) scanning. An important consideration in examining the mediastinum is the demonstration of abnormal lymph nodes and differentiation of these from lipomas or mediastinal cysts. The 3 most common causes of mediastinal adenopathy are Hodgkin's and non-Hodgkin's lymphomas and metastases. Posterior mediastinal lesions (eg, metastatic disease) can be distinguished from locally invasive carcinoma (eg, bronchogenic and esophageal carcinomas). CT may be the 1 means of differentiating between involvement of the hilum and that of lung parenchyma, which helps in staging of disease and planning therapy.

CT Examination of the Lungs and Chest Wall

CT scanning of the lungs and chest wall has been limited, because conventional radiography and tomography are inexpensive, widely available, and very useful. However, in selected cases, CT gives otherwise unobtainable information and may help identify the nature of the problem.

CT is most useful in defining small metastatic nodules not visible on standard x-rays and lesions located peripherally, retrosternally, behind the heart, in the costophrenic angles, and high in the apices. Surprisingly, however, linear tomography is more sensitive than CT for very small calcified nodules. Cavities are well imaged on CT, as are fatty masses and cysts, especially in the right cardiophrenic angle. Atelectasis is also well visualized, as are abnormalities of the chest wall, including the sternum. The diagnosis of pleural effusions and determination of their extent and location are greatly facilitated.

CT Examination of the Abdomen

Lesions of the liver and biliary tract: Although hepatic arteriography, cholangiography, and radionuclide imaging all have a major role in visualizing the liver, CT is valuable when used for problem solving rather than for diagnostic screening. It is superior to radionuclide imaging in evaluating jaundice by visualizing dilated intrahepatic bile ducts, which indicate surgical jaundice; the absence of dilation suggests nonobstructive jaundice. Lesions of the gallbladder are probably best visualized by ultrasonography.

CT is most useful in clarifying the nature of solitary space-occupying lesions seen on radionuclide studies (eg, primary and metastatic neoplasms, abscesses, cysts, and hematomas). Diffuse disease of the liver is ordinarily not well visualized by CT, but ascites and large collateral veins are commonly seen.

CT examination of the pancreas is a valuable addition to other modalities (eg, radionuclide imaging, arteriography, retrograde cholangiopancreatography, and ultrasonography). All of these have serious limitations in diagnosing pancreatic disease (see also NEOPLASMS OF THE PANCREAS in Ch. 52 and DISORDERS OF THE PANCREAS in Ch. 53).

Diagnosis of carcinoma is based on identification of a change in the shape, size, configuration, or density of the pancreas, or obliteration of the peripancreatic fat plane. Differentiation of pancreatitis from carcinoma is difficult, although more diffuse involvement or the presence of calcification suggests pancreatitis rather than cancer. Dilation of the common bile duct or the presence of liver metastases or retroperitoneal lymphadenopathy also points to a diagnosis of malignancy when associated with a mass in the pancreas. Cysts and abscesses are readily defined.

CT Examination of the Spine

CT can visualize malignancies, infections, traumatic lesions, herniated disks, and displacement and compression of the spinal cord. In addition, it can establish certain specific diagnoses (eg, abscesses that contain gas, lipomas, and intramedullary hematomas). CT is especially useful in following the course of a lesion, particularly one associated with trauma, because it can differentiate among edema, hemorrhage, and soft tissue masses.

Myelography using metrizamide and high-resolution CT is indicated when diffuse abnormalities or small, widespread lesions are present; in certain cases of chronic and subacute spinal cord injury and in some tumors; and when angulation of the spine in scoliosis is significant.

CT Examination of the Kidneys and Urinary Tract

CT scanning is helpful in cases involving an indeterminate excretory urogram, when other findings suggest a renal neoplasm, when a mass is incidentally discovered, and when metastasis from unknown primary tumors is suspected. CT is useful in determining the extent and location of invasion and the number of metastases. In addition, it can be used to guide needle biopsy or aspiration.

Ordinarily, opaque **kidney stones** are better evaluated by excretory urography, ultrasound, and plain-film tomography. Occasionally, however, stones are detected incidentally on CT scans performed for other indications. The location and size of the stones can be determined accurately before surgery. Adrenal masses also can frequently be evaluated by CT.

Negative contrast (gas-filled bladder) is used for staging **bladder cancers,** permitting noninvasive visualization of the tumor and showing the size and area of invasion. Repeat scans can be used to evaluate response to therapy. However, there are pitfalls in the staging of bladder cancer (eg, failure to recognize normal structures, to demonstrate pelvic mobility, or to recognize fibrosis from prior surgery or radiation therapy).

Benign prostatic hypertrophy, which is of special importance in the older patient, is visualized as an intravesical mass on the floor of the bladder.

MAGNETIC RESONANCE IMAGING (MRI)

MRI (previously called **nuclear magnetic resonance**) has enormous advantages as a noninvasive, nonionizing-radiation imaging technic. It enables one to differentiate between biologic fluids (eg, blood and CSF) and solid tissue (eg, fat, muscle, brain white and gray matter, and bone), all of which have different proton contents. MRI affords the opportunity to achieve superb tomography with excellent spatial resolution, like that achieved with CT; tissue information like that provided by ultrasound; and information about metabolic processes like that provided by nuclear medicine. The contrast resolution of MRI is > 500% in soft tissue, and there are no known biologic ill effects. Pharmaceuticals labeled with magnetic isotopes can extend the capability of MRI studies by providing specific image enhancement.

CT scans reflect the density of tissues visualized, whereas MRI defines anatomic structures with differing water content. For example, gray matter in the brain has about 15% more water than white matter and can be differentiated on MRI. Thus, MRI is useful in visualizing cerebral infarcts, tumors, hemorrhages, and vascular abnormalities and may have potential in diagnosing Alzheimer's disease. It is better than CT for visualizing the posterior fossa and upper spinal cord. MRI has greater contrast than CT for visualizing the brain, spine, pelvis, head and neck, and the extremities (particularly the knee) but is less useful for the lungs and is deficient in detecting calcifications and differentiating tumor types.

MRI has largely replaced myelography for visualizing certain lesions of the spine, especially in older patients who may have spondylosis in the cervical region or stenosis in the lumbar region.

The ability of MRI to monitor metabolism in vivo is equaled only by some of the high-resolution aspects of positron emission tomography (PET) and single photon emission computed tomography (SPECT).

MRI is being used increasingly in **cardiac evaluation,** in which moving blood effectively acts as MRI contrast, identifying the relative positions and orientation of the cardiac chambers, valves, and great vessels. The use of MRI for diagnosis of **thoracic lesions,** particularly ectopic thyroid tissue, and the evaluation of extravascular pulmonary water is being explored. MRI can detect **abdominal disease** and is beginning to be used in imaging the liver and the pancreas, which had been resistant to other imaging technics. **Rhabdomyosarcoma** can be differentiated from normal muscle because of the longer relaxation time that characterizes malignant tissue, a quality that has been extended to identification of some breast carcinomas and liver metastases. MRI has great potential for detecting **pelvic and urogenital lesions. Bone marrow** and **joint disorders** will be better analyzed in the future by MRI than by any other noninvasive diagnostic method.

Disadvantages of MRI include slow scanning that degrades images of organs moving in several directions. The strong magnetic field of a superconducting imager creates potential hazards with loose metallic objects that can cause injury. The optimal magnetic-field strength has not yet been determined. Location of MRI devices presents major problems at every facility because of the potential for mutual interference with other equipment. Their installation, maintenance, and operation require prodigious expenditures, raising the cost of an individual MRI scan to $700 to $800.

ULTRASONOGRAPHY (US)

US uses ultra-high-frequency sound waves that can be passed through biologic tissues and reflected back to the generating source, permitting a graphic representation of differences in tissue density. The sound waves are generated and received by a transducer. US is a rapid, noninvasive diagnostic technic, usually taking 15 to 45 min, and is relatively inexpensive.

Brain imaging (echoencephalography): US can be used to detect midline deviations, measure the transverse diameter of the lateral ventricles in certain instances of hydrocephalus (more appropriate in infants than in older adults), and diagnose subdural or epidural masses (eg, hematomas and, under favorable conditions, intracerebral tumors). Generally, however, CT and PET scanning and MRI are more useful in diagnosing lesions within the skull.

Heart: Echocardiography is useful in diagnosing valvular lesions, often obviating the need for cardiac catheterization. With Doppler US, laminar flow can be differentiated from turbulent flow, thus providing information about valvular kinetics (eg, detection and evaluation of aortic and mitral valvular regurgitation and insufficiency). Aortic outflow tract obstruction, fairly common in older patients, can be detected with the Doppler technic.

Abdomen: Lesions of the liver are equally well visualized by US and nuclear imaging; both have about 75% diagnostic accuracy. Usually, US cannot visualize areas of the liver obscured by the ribs, and radionuclide scans are more effective in screening for space-occupying lesions. However, US can be used to determined whether such lesions are cystic or solid. In diagnosing cirrhosis, US has a sensitivity of 81% but a specificity of only 76%.

Biliary tract: Both nuclear and US technics are useful in visualizing the biliary system. Biliary calculi are probably best visualized by US; gallstones are identified by both their sonic density and change in position when the patient's position is changed. Biliary scanning can also be used to detect biliary tract constriction, to assess patency of the cystic duct, and to measure dilation of the extrahepatic biliary ducts. Gallbladder inflammation can be detected by a thickening of its wall or finding contraction or failure of contraction associated with eating.

Spleen: The spleen is better visualized by nuclear scanning because the ribs interfere in US.

Pancreas: CT is better for visualizing the head and tail of the pancreas, but US is better for lesions in the body. Inflammation of the pancreas results in edema, which decreases the internal echogenicity. Dense echoes suggest calcification. The pancreatic duct can often be visualized as a small channel < 2 mm in diameter.

Urinary tract: US provides information about the size and shape of the kidneys, the consistency of mass lesions, and the presence of hydronephrosis and polycystic disease. In renal transplantation, the renal pyramids can be used as landmarks to check for swelling as an early sign of rejection.

Bladder distention permits visualization of mass lesions that protrude into the lumen, and the prostate can be visualized transrectally or through the filled bladder. In the former technic, a rotating transducer enclosed in a water-filled balloon is inserted into the rectum; close inspection of the prostate echo pattern often helps distinguish benign from malignant enlargement.

RADIONUCLIDE DIAGNOSTICS

There are 2 major subdivisions of radionuclide diagnostics: (1) **non-imaging technics,** including in vitro (eg, radiommunoassays) and in vivo (eg, RBC and plasma volume calculations, thyroid uptake studies, and the Schilling test) and (2) gamma-emission **imaging technics.** This discussion will deal mostly with the latter, which are useful in the study of bone, brain, lungs, heart, liver, spleen, biliary tree, kidneys, the genitourinary system, and inflammatory processes.

Brain scanning, performed with ^{99m}Tc chelates, has been largely replaced by CT, PET, and MRI, although it is still useful for **determining the integrity of the blood-brain barrier and the vascularity of lesions that have been identified by other means** and in **head trauma** (to identify epidural or subdural hematomas when CT is normal or equivocal). **Other indications** include diagnosis of benign, malignant, or metastatic neoplasms; brain abscesses; vascular abnormalities; and, especially, cysts. Some studies can be performed more precisely together with other imaging procedures (eg, radionuclide cisternography in conjunction with CT is used to assess hydrocephalus, particularly that in which pressure is normal). CT with contrast enhancement also is more accurate in diagnosing dementia, with or without hydrocephalus.

Radionuclide study of the heart permits noninvasive investigation that previously required cardiac catheterization. The radioisotopes most frequently used are ^{201}Tl and ^{99m}Tc. Thallium provides a **pattern of myocardial perfusion** with and without stress; coronary vasculature per se is *not* visualized. It is particularly useful for determining the patency of vasculature after cardiac surgery. Thallium has properties similar to those of K, and its distribution in the myocardium is proportional to regional myocardial blood flow and cellular viability. However, ^{99m}Tc pyrophosphate is more commonly used for **imaging acute MIs** and for **determining ventricular function.**

The lungs are ideally suited for radionuclide imaging. Radioactive xenon is used for evaluating ventilation and ^{99m}Tc macroaggregated albumin **(MAA)** for evaluating perfusion. These noninvasive procedures are valuable in the elderly when pulmonary vascular impairment (eg, pulmonary embolism), acute obstructive lung disease, bronchogenic carcinoma, or bronchiectasis is suspected.

In pancreas visualization, radionuclide imaging currently has *no* role; US and CT are superior. **The liver and spleen** may be visualized with ^{99m}Tc, a simple, inexpensive, noninvasive modality widely used for evaluating size, morphology, and presence of focal lesions; it compares favorably with CT in sensitivity and specificity. This technic is an important aid in diagnosing splenic trauma and is extremely useful in evaluating diffuse liver disease. However, it is not useful for differentiating primary from metastatic neoplasms.

Both perfusion and static images of **the kidney** are possible, allowing comprehensive evaluation of renal blood flow, individual kidney function, patency of collecting systems, and morphologic assessment.

Other radionuclide procedures include bone imaging, biliary imaging with ^{99m}Tc-labeled imino diacetic acid **(IDA)** derivatives to evaluate the patency of the biliary tract, imaging tumors and sites of inflammation or abscess with ^{67}Ga citrate or ^{111}In-labeled WBCs (for abscess), thyroid scanning, and testicular imaging for differentiation between testicular torsion and epididymitis.

Single Photon Emission Computed Tomography (SPECT)

SPECT is another technic based on activity of radiotracers and, using 2 or 3 gamma cameras, it allows the patient's radiation dose to be lowered by $1/3$. It is useful in visualizing diseases of the liver, including diffuse hepatocellular disease, cirrhosis, and chronic hepatitis. SPECT is much less expensive than PET or MRI, but it is also less accurate and versatile than either. However, improvements are being made.

Bone Absorptiometry (see Ch. 64)

THERAPEUTIC TECHNOLOGIES

EXTRACORPOREAL SHOCK WAVE LITHOTRIPSY (ESWL)

ESWL is used for treating urinary tract stones, greatly reducing the need for surgery. The cost of a lithotriptor and associated equipment is about $1.8 million, and annual maintenance typically costs about $100,000; nevertheless, it is cost-effective in many patients with kidney and ureteral stones. ESWL can also be used to fracture biliary stones but results are still preliminary.

In ESWL, a shock wave is generated in a tub of water by a spark gap at the focal point of a metallic reflector. (Newer technology substitutes a fluid-filled pillow for the water tub.) The patient is positioned and monitored by biplanar fluoroscopy. Anesthesia (epidural or general) is required to prevent excessive movement by the patient (who is usually anxious) and to minimize the pain and unpleasant sensation caused by shock wave therapy. Firing of the spark plug is triggered by ECG monitoring, and typically, 1000 to 1500 shocks are given in series of 100 in a course of treatment. Patients who weigh > 136 kg or whose height is > 2.13 m or < 1.2 m are unsuited to such treatment.

Overall effectiveness rates indicate at least partial disintegration of renal stones in 98% of patients, and 75% of patients are free of stones 90 days after the procedure. Very large stones (> 2 cm), staghorn calculi, or those associated with UTI are less susceptible to shock wave fracture. Cystine stones are less amenable to ESWL than are calcium oxalate stones. Pure monohydrate stones are refractory, while calcium phosphate stones are often initially resistant. More frequent, higher voltage waves are needed to disintegrate uric acid stones.

Stones in the proximal ureter usually are easier to dislodge, and younger patients pass them more readily than do older patients. Stone passage depends on adequate hydration and absence of other complications. Treatment of complex stones (large renal pelvic, multiple and large renal, partial and complete staghorns, and cystine) includes a combination of percutaneous surgery and ESWL.

RADIATION THERAPY

There have been no dramatic breakthroughs in radiation therapy in the last 10 yr, although incremental progress has been made in its use for diagnosing and treating malignancies. Radiation therapy may use implants placed in the tumor or external beam sources.

Radiocurability depends on the histologic type and grade of the cancer, tumor size, site of origin, and potential pattern of spread. New methods of predicting radiocurability are available (eg, in vitro assays of cellular radiosensitivity, morphologic or biochemical estimates of radiation cell survival, assessment of tumor oxygenation, measurement of tumor cell kinetics, and quantitative estimates of tumor cell markers).

Once a radiation dose has been determined, it is usually divided into treatment fractions (eg, treatment of 5 days/wk with each fraction consisting of 180 rads for a total of 3000 to 7000 rads). Greater doses tend to damage local tissue and are not well tolerated.

Seminomas and lymphomas are the most radiosensitive tumors. Moderately radiosensitive tumors include squamous cell carcinomas and adenocarcinomas. The least radiosensitive tumors are sarcomas and melanomas. Commonly treated neoplasms include carcinoma of the lung, prostate, bladder, and breast; Hodgkin's disease, Stages I and II; and carcinomatous metastases.

Certain brain tumors, including solitary metastases, glioblastomas, and astrocytomas, should be treated with radiation postoperatively. More than 50% of colon tumors are operable, and a few of these should also be treated with postoperative radiation.

Fast-neutron teletherapy for head and neck cancer and sarcomas of soft tissue and bone is controversial; theoretical advantages include increased killing effect for hypoxic tumor cells.

AIDS FOR THE VISUALLY HANDICAPPED

(See also Ch. 93)

About 1.56 million people are blind or severely visually impaired, and > 50% are > 65 yr of age. The major causes are macular degeneration, cataracts, glaucoma, and diabetes. A number of devices can help these people in the activities of daily living **(ADL)** and in vocational and avocational pursuits.

Assistance for visually handicapped persons involves 3 strategies: (1) enhance the visual stimuli, (2) substitute other senses for the visual stimulus to perform critical elements of the task, and (3) supplement the visual stimulus with other sensory input. The potential need for a visual aid should be established first (ie, whether the person has problems with near, intermediate, or distant vision), because different devices resolve different problems.

Closed-circuit television with lenses to enlarge the image on a cathode ray tube can aid in reading. Another device is a wide-angle mobility light **(WAMO)** that helps people with retinitis pigmentosa or those who for other reasons have difficulty with night vision. In personal grooming, magnifying mirrors and a source of intense illumination are helpful.

A number of computers, calculators, thermometers, clocks, and rheostats have voice output using synthesized speech. Also available are devices that will translate braille print to voice output. The Kurzweil reader, which has been under development for a number of years, scans a printed page and provides synthesized speech output. It is fairly reliable for certain kinds of standard printing.

A number of devices are under development that aid ambulation by preventing a person from bumping into objects and preventing falls. For example, a laser cane sends out a laser beam and returns a vibratory stimulus, but its use in the elderly is limited to those who are physically active and highly motivated.

---

22. SURGERY: PREOPERATIVE EVALUATION AND INTRAOPERATIVE AND POSTOPERATIVE CARE

Ronald G. Tompkins and *Claude E. Welch*

Indications for surgery in older patients often differ from those in younger persons. Since life expectancy in the elderly is measured in months or years rather than in decades, prophylactic surgery is of less importance. Treatment of serious illness is essential whenever cure or alleviation of pain or disability is possible. Because elective procedures for older patients are given more consideration before they are performed, emergency procedures are more common.

Among the common emergency operations performed on elderly patients are those for a fractured hip, strangulated hernia, complications of gallbladder disease, intestinal obstruction, and intra-abdominal catastrophies, such as ruptured aortic aneurysm or mesenteric thrombosis. Elective operations likely to be performed include those for cancer (chiefly involving the colorectal area, breast, and uterus), cataract, inguinal hernia, urinary incontinence, rectal prolapse, aortic aneurysm, and diseases of the peripheral arteries (particularly those of the lower extremities and internal carotid arteries).

Other operations that might be justified in younger patients are not indicated in the very old except in unusual circumstances. Such procedures include cosmetic surgery, extensive reconstructive dental procedures, renal transplantation, joint replacement in the absence of severe pain, and cholecystectomy for asymptomatic gallstones. *It must be stressed, however, that chronologic and physiologic ages are not necessarily equivalent.* The indications for surgery in an older patient who is fit and "younger than his years" are essentially the same as those in the younger patient. This is especially true of heart surgery, which may be beneficial and associated with low risk in carefully chosen elderly patients. The characteristic heterogeneity of the older population requires that each person be assessed individually and that judgments be based on the individual's problem and physiologic status rather than on age alone.

In the USA in 1985, 36% of all hospitalized patients ≥ 65 yr of age underwent a surgical procedure. Some 3,816,000 operations (or 24% of all procedures) were performed on patients in that age group. Since the geriatric population is expected to increase in future decades, the implications for hospitals and physicians are significant.

Postoperative complications are more common and mortality is higher in the elderly. An initial complication is much more likely to lead to other complications; failure of one organ to function adequately is more likely to lead to failure of other organs. In one study, the mortality rate for patients ≥ 70 yr of age undergoing elective cholecystectomy was nearly 10 times higher than that for younger patients. In another study of abdominal operations performed on older patients, the mortality rate for those aged 80 to 84 yr was 3%; for those aged 85 to 89 yr, 9%; and for those aged ≥ 90 yr, 25%.

Emergency operations carry a greater risk than elective ones in all age groups, particularly the elderly. For example, in operations for massive bleeding peptic ulcer at Massachusetts General Hospital in the past decade, the mortality rate was 10.6% in patients ≤ 70 yr; in contrast, the mortality rate was 41.9% in patients ≥ 70 yr. A corollary observation is that certain indicated surgical procedures should be treated electively; eg, inguinal hernia and abdominal aortic aneurysms are associated with a low mortality rate when handled as elective procedures and a high mortality rate when complicated by strangulation or rupture.

PREOPERATIVE EVALUATION

The preoperative evaluation of a geriatric patient scheduled for elective surgery should include the determination of additional risks related to age. Such risks result from compromised physiologic systems including cardiovascular, respiratory, renal, and immunologic, which may not necessarily be related to the primary diagnosis. In elective operations, such system deficits can be identified and attempts can be made to correct them. In emergency operations, complete evaluation or correction is impossible; therefore, system failure is much more common. Nevertheless, whenever possible, a preoperative evaluation should be conducted that includes the following:

History: The history can furnish important clues, but many older patients suffer from deafness, memory deficits, or confusion, and are unable to identify important symptoms. Further, they tend to deny having any disabilities. Thus, obtaining a history can require a great deal of time and patience. Often, a patient may have multiple disabilities. For example, in one study of patients > 65 yr of age, an average of > 3 disabilities were found per patient; in a study of more than 2000 autopsies, an average of 7 significant lesions were found.

A complete history of drug use is especially important. A study of 178 chronically ill patients, for instance, showed that 59% made medication errors; in 26% of these patients, the errors were potentially serious. Therefore, patients should be instructed to bring all of their medications to the doctor's office or hospital and to describe exactly how they are using the drugs.

Because nutritional deficiencies are common in the elderly and not necessarily limited to the poor, nutritional status should be determined. Low levels of serum potassium or albumin are fairly common and potentially serious.

Physical examination: The skin, oral mucosa, and tongue can provide important information concerning hydration and nutrition. The neck should be examined for lymph nodes, thyroid masses, carotid pulsations, and bruits. Blood pressure should be measured, and a complete examination of the heart, lungs, and breasts should be performed. The abdominal examination must include a search for asymptomatic lesions such as hernias, aortic aneurysms, or masses. Rectal examinations are mandatory, as are pelvic examinations in women. In examination of the lower extremities, pulses in the femoral, popliteal, and pedal regions should be noted. Any evidence of venous disease, such as varicose veins, postphlebitic ulcers, or edema, should also be identified.

Laboratory examinations: Urinalysis, peripheral blood count, a limited blood chemistry profile, and measurement of coagulation factors are necessary. Periodic serum electrolyte studies are useful for patients who take diuretics. A chest x-ray and an ECG must be obtained before patients undergo surgery.

Evaluation of surgical risk: The physician must estimate the patient's ability to withstand an operation. The prognosis may be good for many older patients who have survived the ages in which ischemic heart disease and strokes have claimed the lives of numerous peers. Other excellent prognostic factors are the patient's general mood and mental status, which provide valuable clues as to how well the patient will withstand the surgical procedure.

The operative risk is increased by many concomitant conditions, including coronary artery occlusive disease, carotid artery occlusive disease, chronic obstructive or bronchospastic lung disease, chronic renal insufficiency, cirrhosis, arterial or venous disease of the lower extremities, and severe malnutrition.

Cardiac problems: The presence of certain cardiac conditions contraindicates elective noncardiac procedures. Recent myocardial infarction **(MI)** dramatically increases the risk of surgery. One study reported a mortality rate of 40% for individuals who had surgery within 3 mo of an acute MI, compared with a 14% mortality rate for those who had a healed infarction. A series from the Mayo Clinic indicated the patients who were operated on within 3 mo of an MI had a 37% reinfarction rate. This rate decreased to 16% between 3 and 6 mo after MI and to 4 to 5% after 6 mo following MI.

A patient who has heart failure **(HF)** is not a candidate for elective surgery. Patients whose HF is still evident preoperatively are more likely to develop postoperative failure and pulmonary edema than those who are no longer in failure or who have no history of heart failure. Patients with jugular venous distention and a third heart sound are considered at increased risk.

Judicious use of digitalis, diuretics, and vasodilators can improve cardiac performance preoperatively and reduce the risks of surgery. Digitalis is recommended preoperatively for patients who have a history of previous HF or cardiac dysfunction, as evidenced by signs of impaired ventricular response, nocturnal angina, atrial fibrillation or flutter with rapid ventricular response, or frequent episodes of paroxysmal atrial or junctional tachycardia. Patients receiving digitalis therapy should be carefully monitored because of the potential for digitalis toxicity in the perioperative period.

The exercise tolerance of patients with cardiac disease should be assessed by questioning them about usual daily activity and how easily they tire. Nonspecific T wave and ST segment changes in the stable ECG are relatively unimportant when the history is unremarkable and a thorough physical examination has been performed. New ischemic patterns, however, should be assessed with serial tracings before an elective procedure is performed.

Atrial premature contractions are a benign finding unless they occur frequently, in which case they may indicate impending atrial fibrillation or supraventricular tachycardia. ECG abnormalities that correlate with postoperative cardiac deaths include the occurrence of 5 premature ventricular contractions **(PVCs)** per min documented at any time preoperatively and a rhythm other than sinus on the preoperative ECG. Occasional solitary PVCs do not require preoperative treatment.

In general, no drug commonly used to treat heart disease should be withdrawn before surgery, including β-blockers. In fact, withdrawing these drugs suddenly could be dangerous. If the patient has been stabilized on a regimen of Ca channel blockers preoperatively, administration of these drugs also should be continued. However, if a β-blocker is used concomitantly, with verapamil or nifedipine, myocardial depression may be enhanced, increasing the risk of heart failure. The anesthesiologist should be informed of the use of these agents, since they alter the body's response to anesthetics and other vasoactive drugs. The presence of antiarrhythmics such as lidocaine, procainamide, phenytoin, and quinidine is a concern for the anesthesiologist primarily as an indicator of an underlying organic lesion.

Hypertension should be controlled prior to surgery, and antihypertensive drugs should not be withdrawn. Patients with untreated or inadequately controlled hypertension have larger absolute reductions in BP during anesthesia than those who are adequately controlled. If a patient has been receiving thiazide diuretics, the anesthesiologist should be informed and the patient's serum potassium levels should be checked to be sure they are not below the danger level of 3.5 mEq/L. If the serum potassium level is lower, elective surgery should be postponed until adequate potassium supplementation has been provided.

Carotid artery occlusive disease: The influence of this disease upon perioperative mortality and stroke is more controversial. The presence of carotid occlusive disease in patients undergoing myocardial revascularization appears to increase the perioperative stroke rate, thereby increasing operative risk. In other types of operative procedures, however, an increased rate of perioperative strokes may be limited to patients who have had previous transient ischemic attacks **(TIAs)** or to those who have severe occlusive disease involving both internal carotid arteries and the vertebral arterial system.

Pulmonary disease: Chronic obstructive or bronchospastic lung disease also increases the risk of an operative procedure, mainly for patients with severe disease who have a forced expiratory volume of < 1 L at 1 sec **(FEV₁)**. Preoperatively, the bronchospastic component may improve with bronchodilator therapy. In addition, the patient should refrain from smoking in the preoperative period and would likely benefit from a few days of active physical therapy, including the use of broncholytic agents and percussion.

Liver disease: Evidence of impaired liver function before surgery is especially ominous. Attempts to improve liver function preoperatively are limited to correction of coagulation abnormalities with vitamin K or protein blood products, such as fresh frozen plasma or coagulation concentrates.

Renal disease: Renal function must be assessed by measuring BUN and creatinine levels. Dehydration may lead to prerenal azotemia, which can be corrected by administration of fluids. If elevations of these levels persist, peritoneal dialysis or hemodialysis may reverse the uremia and reduce the high risk of operation.

Malnutrition: Since malnutrition is common in the elderly, symptoms and signs must be noted in the preoperative evaluation. About half the patients > 65 yr of age who require surgery for serious disease have had a recent weight loss ranging from 5 to 50 lb, according to one study. Since weight loss may lead to certain complications, such as delayed wound healing, preoperative nutritional supplements should be provided when possible. This supplementation can include high-caloric foods, vitamins, enteral feedings (continuous or intermittent), or if necessary, total parenteral nutrition.

Anesthetic risk: Most anesthesiologists use the following classification recommended by the American Society of Anesthesiologists to assess anesthetic risk: **Class 1:** a normally healthy patient, **Class 2:** a patient who has mild systemic disease, **Class 3:** a patient who has severe systemic disease that is not incapacitating, **Class 4:** a patient who has incapacitating systemic disease that is a constant threat to life, and **Class 5:** a moribund patient who is not expected to survive for 24 h, with or without surgery.

Although age is not a factor in this classification, a greater proportion of older patients obviously will fall into the higher classes of risk. One study has demonstrated that although patients > 50 yr of age accounted for only 35% of the surgical population, they had a disproportionately high rate (45%) of deaths from anesthetics.

Pharmacology: Responses to drugs are often altered in the elderly as a result of differences in pharmacokinetics and tissue responses. The use of multiple drugs leads to the risk of drug interactions as discussed in Ch. 18.

Trauma: Assessment and management of trauma in the elderly is similar to that in younger patients. Upon initial presentation of a patient with severe injury, immediate life-threatening conditions should be identified. This is done by following the ABCs of trauma management: *A*irway, *B*reathing, and *C*irculation. An adequate airway is maintained with neck extension, oropharyngeal airway (if the patient is unconscious but breathing), or the use of endotracheal or nasotracheal tubes (if the patient has an obstructed airway or inadequate ventilation). Once airway and ventilation are assured, attention should be given to maintaining an adequate BP. Hypotension from hemorrhage can usually be controlled by applying pressure directly to the bleeding site and replacing blood volume. Exploration of wounds and placement of clamps are inadvisable except in cases of thoracic vascular injuries. Intra-abdominal hemorrhage is best managed in the operating room following a brief evaluation in the trauma area.

Adequate BP generally can be achieved by vigorous blood volume replacement, usually with crystaloids, such as lactated Ringer's solution or normal saline, followed as soon as possible by appropriate replacement blood products. Vasopressors rarely are needed to maintain BP in the trauma patient. Among the goals of BP management are the achievement of a normal mental status when possible, and maintenance of normal coronary artery and renal perfusion. A urine output of at least 1 mL/kg/h is a reasonable goal; output should not drop below 0.5 mL/kg/h.

Once the ABCs are addressed, other life-threatening conditions are evaluated by physical examination. A chest examination and x-ray will identify penetrating injury as well as pneumothorax, hemothorax, or a widened mediastinum, all of which require further evaluation. Abdominal examination will identify penetrating abdominal injury as well as tenderness in the conscious patient. A rectal examination will identify intestinal bleeding from contusion or perforation injuries and prostatic injuries. Pelvic instability should be examined to identify pelvic fractures, which can be lethal. Examination of the urethra is important before placement of a urinary catheter to identify blood at the meatus. The presence of blood requires cystourethrography to rule out urethral injuries. In the presence of urethral injury, catheterization should be suprapubic rather than transuretheral. Extremities should be examined for fractures and dislocations of long bones.

Diagnostic infraumbilical peritoneal lavage should be performed in the unconscious patient in whom significant blunt abdominal trauma is suspected as well as in the conscious patient in whom intraperitoneal hemorrhage is suspected. The peritoneal lavage fluid should be examined for RBC and WBC counts and measured for bilirubin content and amylase activity. An RBC of $> 100,000/\mu L$ strongly suggests intraperitoneal hemorrhage; an RBC of 50,000 to $100,000/\mu L$ is borderline and should be further evaluated by repeated abdominal examinations, peritoneal lavage, CT imaging, or other diagnostic procedures. A WBC count $> 500/\mu L$ suggests an injury to a viscus. The presence of bile or amylase suggests injury to the pancreas, intestine, or biliary system.

Additional imaging procedures may be carried out in a stable patient. An IV urogram (previously referred to as "IV pyelogram") should be performed to identify urinary tract injuries in patients who have hematuria. When necessary, renal trauma may be evaluated with abdominal CT and vascular contrast. Abdominal or chest CT imaging and arteriography can be carried out in stable patients to evaluate a widened mediastinum or to identify intraperitoneal hemorrhage. The diagnostic accuracy of CT in this setting has only recently begun to be fully evaluated. Ultrasound is not diagnostically useful in the trauma patient.

INTRAOPERATIVE CARE

Selection of the proper operative procedure depends upon a number of factors, including the patient's ability to withstand an operation, the surgeon's skill, and the operating conditions. In general, the simpler the operation that will produce the desired result, the better. For example, separate procedures for purely prophylactic purposes rarely should be performed. Thus, a routine appendectomy is very seldom indicated during the course of an operation for acute cholecystitis in an elderly patient. If, however, a large gallstone is found during the performance of a right colectomy for cancer, and adequate exposure has already been achieved, the stone should be removed either by cholecystectomy or cholecystostomy to reduce the risk of early postoperative acute cholecystitis.

Choice of anesthetic agents and technics: Regional anesthesia should be used when feasible in elderly patients who are fair-to-poor risks. For example, a brachial block using the axillary approach is excellent for operations on the arm. Most inguinal hernia operations can be performed wih local anesthesia. **Spinal anesthesia** is usually preferred to peridural anesthesia or individual nerve block for extraperitoneal operations below the umbilicus; it is frequently used for inguinal hernia repairs, anorectal operations, prostatic resections, hip pinnings, and leg amputations.

General anesthesia in an elderly patient nearly always requires intratracheal intubation to maintain an adequate airway. This type of anesthesia is preferred for abdominal operations because extensive exploration is generally necessary and spinal anesthesia is rarely satisfactory. Induction of general anesthesia requires an agent such as thiobarbiturate. Anesthesia is usually maintained by gases that are eliminated mainly through the lungs. In many cases, preliminary insertion of a nasogastric tube may be necessary to prevent aspiration of gastric contents.

Patients with clinically significant heart disease or advanced respiratory disease should receive oxygen by mouth before and during barbiturate induction. The **usual inhalation agents** are nitrous oxide, halothane, enflurane, isoflurane, and methoxyflurane. These agents may be supplemented by IV morphine or meperidine. Some anesthesiologists prefer fentanyl because of its short duration of action, which allows the dosage to be closely controlled.

The **dissociative agent** ketamine, a potent analgesic that can be administered IV or IM, is useful in geriatric patients. Hallucination on emergence from ketamine anesthesia is unusual in these patients. Ketamine may be the sole anesthetic agent used for burn debridements and dressing changes or for positioning the patient in the bed for hip pinning before induction of spinal anesthesia. Relatively small doses, such as 25 to 75 mg, provide analgesia while maintaining BP at adequate levels.

Muscle relaxants, such as succinylcholine, tubocurarine, and pancuronium, are well tolerated by older patients when used judiciously. Overdosage occurs, however, if the anesthesiologist uses the same dosage as that used in younger patients, because skeletal muscle is usually decreased in size and vigor in the elderly. A peripheral nerve stimulator may be used to determine the proper dosage for the individual patient.

Intraoperative monitoring: Pulse, cuff BP, and ECG should be monitored in all patients undergoing surgery. If the procedure is lengthy, a urinary catheter is usually needed for monitoring urine output. If the operative field involves the pelvis, drainage of the bladder often aids operative exposure.

Temperature should be measured and recorded in all major operations, since significant hypothermia is a common sequela of a long procedure, particularly when the viscera are exposed. At the end of a complicated operation, a rectal temperature of 32.2 to 35.0 C (90 to 95 F) or lower is common. Even this degree of hypothermia can lead to death secondary to ventricular fibrillation, which is thought to occur at 31.6 C (89 F). Thus, measures should be taken to maintain reasonable body temperature, including warming of all fluids, maintaining a reasonable operating room temperature, keeping the abdominal viscera in the abdominal cavity as long as possible, and using warm, normal saline lavage.

Central venous pressures (CVPs) should be monitored with the catheter tip in an intrathoracic vein, such as the superior vena cava. Such pressures reflect intravascular volume and are particularly valuable when blood loss has occurred. The normal pressure is usually 8 to 10 mm Hg. Lower pressures generally indicate the need for blood or fluid replacement; elevated pressures may occur in the presence of right or biventricular heart failure. Pulmonary arterial hypertension secondary to pulmonary disease, high bronchial airway pressure, and right ventricular failure may elevate CVP out of proportion to the left ventricular end diastolic pressure. Such an elevation would suggest adequate blood volume when, in fact, blood volume is inadequate.

To monitor left ventricular filling pressure, a **balloon-tipped pulmonary artery (Swan-Ganz®) catheter** must be passed through the right ventricle into the pulmonary artery, and pulmonary capillary wedge pressures must be obtained; normally, 4 to 12 mm Hg indicates adequate blood volume. In the presence of left ventricular failure, the wedge pressures may rise to ≥ 40 mm Hg. These measurements are particularly valuable as guides to intraoperative management of replacement fluid therapy, and management of cardiac inotropic activity and peripheral vascular resistance when vasopressor support is used in patients with cardiac dysfunction.

Continuous peripheral arterial BP measurement is essential for complicated operative procedures, particularly vascular surgery. Measurements may be taken by placing an intra-arterial catheter in the radial artery and connecting it to a transducer for continuous monitoring. This is especially useful in carotid artery surgery, in which brief periods of hypotension are poorly tolerated and may result in intraoperative cerebral infarction.

Complications can occur after any of these invasive procedures. For example, pulmonary artery catheters can cause pulmonary hemorrhage and, although rare, intra-arterial catheters have produced thrombosis and gangrene of fingers. This has led to the recent development of such methods as **transcutaneous monitoring of tissue oxygen tension,** which is extremely safe and beneficial for elderly patients with pulmonary disorders.

Choice of abdominal incision: Exposure of the operative field must be the foremost consideration in the choice of an incision. Generally, when wide exposure is needed, as for resection of an abdominal aortic aneurysm, a long vertical midline incision is best. However, the patient's body habitus should also be considered. For example, a cholecystectomy in a patient with a very narrow costal margin usually can be undertaken more readily through a vertical incision than through the usual subcostal incision. In very obese patients with a pendulous apron, a supraumbilical transverse incision usually can be substituted for a vertical one; this may avoid the deep-fat apron and prevent a subsequent wound seroma. Because chronic obstructive GI disease is common in geriatric patients, upper abdominal incisions should be selected carefully. Generally, vertical incisions in the epigastrium are less painful postoperatively and more effective in clearing postoperative pulmonary secretions.

POSTOPERATIVE CARE

Most postoperative patients are treated in intensive care units **(ICUs)** overnight or up to 72 h before they are returned to the surgical floor. Geriatric patients are especially likely to require this pattern of care. Although postoperative complications cannot be definitively divided into those that occur within the first few days after surgery and those that occur later, the 2 phases of postoperative care do demonstrate different problems and are carried out by different personnel.

Certain preventive considerations are important in the care of convalescing older patients, even when the convalescence is uncomplicated. Thromboembolism is more likely to occur in patients who do not ambulate early after operation. One study showed an increase of 10% of pulmonary embolism following repair of a fractured hip compared with an incidence of 0.2% for the general surgical population > 40 yr of age. Elderly patients are at risk for developing acute confusional states, particularly at night ("sundowning"). Thus, they must be protected, especially at night, from such dangers as dislodging their catheters and tubes and falling from bed. To prevent decubitus ulcers on the sacrum, trochanters, and heels, careful washing and lubrication of skin, frequent position changes, and, when necessary, application of alternating airpressure mattresses, sheepskins, and foam pads are necessary. Ambulation should be started soon after surgery; often, two assistants will be needed for several days. In brief, the older patient requires more nursing care than the younger patient.

Feeding tubes, nasogastric tubes, IV lines, and drains are all essential for postoperative care but are potential sources of sepsis unless handled with care. Sterile technic must be used in handling surgical drains. Profuse drainage (eg, from the biliary tree or an intestinal fistula) requires the use of sterile adherent collection bags.

Intestinal stomas require meticulous skin care and attention to intestinal output. Skin sutures are usually removed after a week, but if the patient is malnourished or is being treated with corticosteroids, they must be left in place for a longer time.

INTENSIVE CARE

Monitoring of all physiologic functions is essential during the entire time spent in the ICU. Pulse, BP, temperature, respiratory rate and depth, and state of consciousness must be measured and recorded on flow charts. Hourly urine output should also be noted. CVP must be monitored when oligemia or fluid depletion requires the administration of large amounts of fluid, particularly when cardiac or pulmonary reserve is limited. In addition, a postoperative ECG should be taken and repeated later if necessary. Chest x-rays should also be taken immediately after the operation and then daily. The usual laboratory studies of blood and blood chemistry must be supplemented by arterial blood gas determinations whenever cardiorespiratory problems are present.

At times, additional monitoring may be required. For example, arterial catheters that may remain in place for days or weeks for the direct measurement of BP must be observed frequently to ascertain that they are not dislodged and that circulation to the fingers is not compromised. Pulmonary artery (Swan-Ganz®) catheters inserted in the operating room or in the ICU must be maintained when the right ventricular pressure reading obtained by CVP monitoring does not adequately reflect left ventricular pressure. Such a situation may occur with severe pulmonary disease, severe left ventricular failure related to ischemia, or other diseases associated with significant pulmonary hypertension. The data obtained by the pulmonary catheter assist in maintaining adequate blood volume and in determining physiologic treatment of the patient's cardiac inotropic state and peripheral vascular resistance.

Early Postoperative Complications

Many postoperative problems occur within the first 2 or 3 days following surgery. Following are some of the most common ones:

1. Hypotension: Hypovolemia, the most common cause of hypotension in the early postoperative period, results from inadequate replacement of intraoperative fluid losses, inordinate postoperative bleeding, or internal losses of fluid such as reaccumulation of ascites or third-space losses. Third-space losses represent intravascular fluid losses by tissue edema, especially in the operative site. After abdominal surgery, considerable intraperitoneal hemorrhage can occur, despite relatively few physical findings. The usual test for this occult hemorrhage is to administer large amounts of blood or fluids; if BP immediately rises to normal levels, followed by rapid recurrence of hypotension, abdominal reexploration for bleeding is usually indicated.

The patient's course during the operative procedure must be reviewed covering the anesthetics used, the estimated fluid loss, and fluid replacements administered during the procedure. The patient's **respiratory status** must be assessed. If the intratracheal tube is still in place, the chest is examined to be certain that the tube has not blocked a main-stem bronchus or that a pneumothorax is not present. If the tube has been removed, the rate and depth of respirations must be determined, since reintubation may be necessary.

Drains and catheters should be examined for escaping blood. Laboratory tests, including arterial blood gas studies, ECG, peripheral Hct and, if necessary, a chest x-ray should be performed. Vasopressors should not be given for postoperative hypotension unless the condition is severe and thought to be compromising coronary or cerebral blood flow, or found to be caused by cardiogenic or neurogenic shock.

A major concern is postoperative hypotension caused by shock from cardiac failure. This may be either left ventricular failure resulting from **myocardial ischemia** or **infarction** in coronary artery disease, or right ventricular failure related to pulmonary arterial hypertension secondary to an acute **pulmonary embolus.** These causes of failure are rare, however, in the immediate postoperative state. If myocardial ischemia is suspected, the ECG tracing should be closely compared with the preoperative tracing. Hypovolemia must be avoided if myocardial ischemia is present. Even if blood volume is adequate, the ischemia may be exacerbated by tachycardias. Other details of management include the use of vasodilators, such as transdermal or IV nitrates, and serial ECGs to assess the drugs' efficacy. In addition, β- and Ca channel blockers in expert hands can be used to diminish cardiac ischemia, taking due note of the negative inotropic properties of these agents. Blood should be drawn for measuring cardiac isoenzyme levels, which can be used subsequently to distinguish between myocardial ischemia and infarction.

Other causes of apparent hypotension are unusual in the early postoperative period. Septic shock can develop postoperatively in a patient who had preoperative signs of **sepsis,** eg, a patient with massive burns or severe intra-abdominal sepsis. **Factitious causes** should also be considered, especially if the history and physical examination do not correlate with the degree of hypotension. Pressure monitors must be inspected to be certain they are functioning properly. Since arteriosclerotic peripheral vascular disease is common in the elderly, one should look for discrepancies in BP between the right and left brachial arteries, which could indicate obstructive lesions in the brachiocephalic and subclavian arterial systems. It is important that both brachial artery pressures be checked for symmetry.

2. Hypothermia: Temperatures in the 32.2 to 34.4 C (90 to 94 F) range are often seen immediately after extensive operative procedures. Further lowering should be prevented because bradycardia, cardiac irregularity, and cardiac arrest could occur in the 31.1 to 31.6 C (88 to 89 F) range. Hypothermia can be treated by warming all IV or other fluids and by increasing the ambient temperature around the patient with several blankets and covers to raise the patient's core temperature.

3. Respiratory problems: In the early postoperative period, respiratory problems are particularly important. The usual signs of shallow, ineffective respirations and cyanosis are not always present, so other symptoms (eg, extreme restlessness or hypotension) should be noted. Problems can be confirmed by arterial blood gas determinations.

Treatment will depend upon detection of the underlying cause and may include relatively simple measures, such as reintubation, repositioning an indwelling endotracheal tube, or applying positive end-expiratory pressure **(PEEP)**. Inadequate reversal of muscle relaxants or narcotics may be the cause of the respiratory problem. In any questionable case, O_2 should be administered immediately and diagnostic arterial blood gas determinations should be obtained.

Respiratory difficulty in the immediate postoperative period is usually treated successfully in the course of a few days; in some instances, however, protracted ventilatory support may be necessary. Mechanical ventilation may, in turn, introduce various other complications.

When prolonged **ventilatory assistance** is required, volume-controlled ventilators usually ensure adequate tidal volume despite changes in pulmonary compliance. Oxygen should be delivered at the lowest concentration that maintains Pa_{O_2} at an acceptable level. Inspired O_2 concentrations of 40% or less are usually well tolerated indefinitely; with higher concentrations, however, one runs the risk of causing O_2 toxicity with alveolar collapse, interstitial edema, and hyaline membrane formation.

When increased Pa_{O_2} is required, PEEP may be used to maintain positive airway pressure throughout the ventilatory cycle. This does not allow airway pressure to return to the level of atmospheric pressure, but it does allow a minimum of the designated PEEP pressure to be maintained. PEEP is believed to open collapsed alveoli, thus permitting ventilation of perfused alveoli, and to cause ventilation at a higher functional residual capacity. If PEEP is used in the face of hypovolemia, however, it may produce hypotension by blocking blood return to the left side of the heart. Under these circumstances, volume replacement must be carried out before significant PEEP is instituted.

Mechanical ventilation usually requires the use of **endotracheal tubes,** which may be left in place for at least 5 days with few complications. If longer intubation is required, a low-pressure cuff-type tube should be used to prevent tracheal erosion, which could result in such later complications as fatal hemorrhage or late tracheal stenosis. Meticulous care of endotracheal tubes is essential to prevent contamination of the lung. For instance, sterile gloves should be worn when trachea and bronchi are suctioned. Tracheal specimens for culture should be drawn periodically. Severe tracheobronchial bacterial infection or pneumonia requires appropriate antibiotic therapy. Sufficient humidity should be delivered by the ventilator to prevent inspissation of bronchial secretions. Highly viscous, thick bronchial secretions and bronchospasm are treated with mucolytic and bronchodilating agents, respectively.

When a patient is extubated, every effort should be made to maintain good pulmonary cleansing; deep breathing and coughing at regular intervals should be encouraged. Nasogastric suctioning may be necessary to stimulate coughing. Occasionally, bedside bronchoscopy may be necessary to remove secretions from specific lobes or from the peripheral bronchial tree. Early ambulation helps to stimulate breathing, and an upright position increases lung capacity by 15 to 25%.

Other supportive measures include prevention of abdominal distention by using a nasogastric tube and avoiding tight abdominal binders and dressings. Pain medications should be used sparingly (only for severe pain), to avoid narcosis, which would prevent adequate pulmonary cleansing.

Elderly patients who have marginal pulmonary reserve are likely to develop major areas of collapse, atelectasis, or heart failure **(HF)**. Mortality is common if the exact cause of the pulmonary failure is not determined and corrected immediately. The most common causes include pneumonia, pulmonary edema, pulmonary embolus, fat embolus, and adult respiratory distress syndrome **(ARDS)**.

ARDS can be defined as *a respiratory failure with life-threatening respiratory distress and hypoxemia, associated with various acute pulmonary injuries.* It is difficult to recognize in the early phase because the chest x-ray is normal. The patient is in obvious respiratory distress, however, exhibiting agitation, cyanosis, and grunting with respiratory effort. Frequently, arterial blood gas studies demonstrate surprisingly low Pa_{O_2} values, often in the 30 or 40 mm Hg range, and respiratory alkalosis with a low Pa_{CO_2}. The latter will eventually begin to rise, with the development of respiratory acidosis and further respiratory failure. On x-ray, perihilar and diffuse parenchymal infiltrates will appear.

The treatment of ARDS includes fluid restriction (usually to 1000 to 1500 mL/day), diuresis (induced with agents such as furosemide or ethacrynic acid), and mechanical ventilation. Relatively high tidal volumes (12 to 15 mL/kg) are used along with PEEP, and appropriate antibiotics are administered, depending upon results of sputum cultures.

4. Postoperative delirium: Geriatric patients often develop a degree of delirium in the ICU, ranging from mild confusion to total psychotic disorientation. Many factors, including environmental and physiologic derangements, are responsible. Preexisting dementia, fluid and electrolyte imbalance, drugs, loss of sleep, frequent interruptions for nursing care, and loss of ability to keep track of time all contribute to disorientation. The condition will clear, however, as recovery progresses (see also Ch. 9).

5. Fluid and electrolyte maintenance: Management of fluids and electrolytes in the elderly is difficult because these patients have a reduced capacity to maintain homeostasis. There is a relatively narrow margin between too little and too much fluid in the treatment of these patients. Proper **fluid replacement** can be determined only by careful monitoring. Initially, a rough estimate can be made, but it should be followed by a definitive plan, which can then be modified to optimize BP, pulse, and urinary output.

For several days after an operation, the body normally retains water and Na in response to increased aldosterone and ADH. For this reason, excessive fluid administration should be avoided in the elderly patient whose cardiovascular function is reduced. Enough fluid should be given to provide for urine output of 0.5 mL/kg/h or about 30 mL/h, to replace insensible fluid losses, and to replace other measured or estimated external losses. All of these fluids are usually given IV in the early postoperative period.

When external losses are not great, fluid requirements for 24 h usually range from 1500 to 2500 mL. Considerably more fluid may be required, however, if excessive third-space sequestration of fluids occurs, eg, as with distended bowel or inflamed subcutaneous tissues that occur with burns. Precautions should be observed with these cases, because the sequestered fluid usually is mobilized on the 3rd to 5th postoperative days. CVP, pulmonary wedge pressure, and urine output provide further guidance for fluid management.

The amount of insensible fluid loss is relatively constant, and usually averages 600 to 900 mL daily. This amount may increase up to 1500 mL daily with hypermetabolism, hyperventilation, or fever. Insensible loss usually is replaced with 5% D/W. After the first few postoperative days, fluid overload is no longer a danger; then approximately 1 L of fluid daily is needed to replace the urine volume required to excrete the catabolic end products of metabolism. The urine volume usually is *not* replaced on an mL-for-mL basis, because a urine output of 2 to 3 L on a given day could represent diuresis of fluids that were given during the surgical procedure or excessive fluid administration. GI losses usually are isotonic or slightly hypotonic; they are replaced with isotonic salt solution. When the estimated loss is slightly above or below isotonicity, appropriate corrections can be made in the daily water intake. Maintenance fluids should be administered at a steady rate over 24 h.

Electrolyte replacement must include 40 mEq/L daily of potassium (K) to replace urine losses, in addition to about 20 mEq/L to replace GI losses. Inadequate K replacement may prolong postoperative ileus and, if not corrected, may lead to a resistant metabolic alkalosis. Ca and Mg also may be replaced, if serum values warrant.

Excessive administration of isotonic solutions results in overexpansion of the extracellular fluid spaces. This is well tolerated in normal individuals, but it may be dangerous in geriatric patients because of their limited cardiopulmonary reserves. Theoretically, Na and Cl requirements in the immediate postoperative period are minimal. If little or no NaCl is given at this time, however, a prolonged hyponatremia and hypochloremia will persist after normal salt retention. Therefore, 75 mEq Na/day usually will maintain a normal serum osmolality and serum Na level. If external losses occur, as from nasogastric suction or diarrhea, additional salt should be given.

Hyponatremia, *a decrease in the serum Na concentration below the normal range of 136 to 145 mEq/L,* is a particularly perplexing but relatively common problem in the geriatric patient. The first clinical indication may be confusion or a seizure occurring a few days after an operation. The Na level may drop from a norm of 140 mEq/L to as low as 115 mEq/L, with symptoms likely to appear when it falls below 130 mEq/L.

It must be determined whether the patient's total body Na content is increased, normal, or diminished. The presence of pulmonary edema, excessive peripheral edema, or evidence of major third-space losses suggest increased total body Na content. The relationship between total body water **(TBW)** and total body Na content must also be determined. Total body free-water content may be elevated because of excessive administration of 5% D/W solutions during the postoperative period, or because the body's response to surgery is altered, resulting in excessive antidiuretic hormone. After evaluating the patient's TBW and total body Na content, the physician should decide whether to administer or withhold free water or Na in subsequent fluids.

6. Acid-base derangements. Acid-base abnormalities occur frequently in the postoperative period. The major ones are respiratory acidosis, respiratory alkalosis, metabolic acidosis, and metabolic alkalosis. Diagnosis may be suspected on clinical grounds, but confirmation requires determination of blood gas levels and interpretation by nomograms.

Respiratory acidosis *is a primary increase in Pa_{CO_2}; pH is low and CO_2 content increases if renal function is intact.* It is produced by many factors that reduce pulmonary function, including inadequate ventilation with airway obstruction, atelectasis, pneumonia, pleural effusion, hypoventilation, and abdominal distention. It is particularly serious in patients with chronic obstructive lung disease and chronic compensated respiratory acidosis, because it may be markedly accentuated in the postoperative period. Although restlessness, hypertension, and tachycardia are indicative of inadequate ventilation with hypercapnia, these signs may also be caused by pain.

Respiratory alkalosis *is a primary decrease in Pa_{CO_2}; pH is raised and CO_2 content reduced.* It is caused by excessive elimination of CO_2, which may occur from hyperventilation induced by apprehension or pain, or by excessive mechanical ventilation. Mild respiratory alkalosis is of little consequence, and most patients require no therapy. Moderate hypocapnia, however, may result in cerebral vasoconstriction, further compromising blood flow in patients whose cerebral blood flow is already compromised because of extracranial arterial disease. This could result in irreparable cerebral damage.

Metabolic acidosis *is a primary fall in extracellular fluid bicarbonate concentration; pH and CO_2 content are reduced.* It has many potential causes, but in the postoperative patient, the cause is usually renal dysfunction. The kidneys normally maintain acid-base balance by excreting nitrogenous waste products and acid metabolites and by reabsorbing sodium bicarbonate in the renal tubule. When renal damage causes these functions to be lost, or when an excessive loss of alkaline GI fluids from the pancreas or the lower GI tract occurs, metabolic acidosis may ensue. Administration of IV fluids that have an appropriate chloride-to-bicarbonate ratio, such as is found in lactated Ringer's injection, is indicated for therapy.

Other situations that can lead to metabolic acidosis include diabetic acidosis, which is treated with insulin, and cardiac arrest, which requires the administration of large amounts of IV sodium bicarbonate. This lactic acidosis also occurs with poor tissue perfusion resulting from severe soft tissue damage or any state of diminished O_2 delivery to tissues.

Severe acidosis further impairs the circulation by decreasing the responsiveness of smooth muscle to vasopressors such as epinephrine. Attempts to correct the acidosis by administering large amounts of sodium bicarbonate are futile, unless blood volume or circulation is restored. When adequate tissue perfusion is restored, lactic acid is quickly metabolized and the pH returns to normal. The use of lactated Ringer's injection to replace the extracellular fluid deficit accompanying hemorrhagic shock concomitant with the administration of whole blood does not accentuate lactic acidosis; instead, lactate rapidly decreases and pH returns to normal.

Metabolic alkalosis *is a primary increase in blood bicarbonate; pH and CO_2 content are elevated.* It results from uncompensated losses of acid and retention of bases. In most instances, the patient has some degree of hypokalemia. Depletion of cellular K results in an exit of K from within the cell and a corresponding entry of H and Na ions; as a result, intracellular pH is lowered and extracellular alkalosis develops.

Metabolic alkalosis may follow an aldosterone-stimulated exchange of Na and H ions for K, resulting in a **paradoxic aciduria.** Clinically, this syndrome may be seen with prolonged nasogastric suctioning or repeated vomiting. The dangers of metabolic alkalosis are related to K depletion and may include cardiac arrhythmias, tetany, sensitivity to digitalis, and paralytic ileus. Less serious symptoms include irritability and neuromuscular excitation.

7. Nutritional management: Three important questions must be addressed in the nutritional management of the geriatric surgical patient: (1) Which patients should receive nutritional support in the postoperative period? (2) What level of caloric intake will enable the patient to respond adequately to the operation? (3) Which mixture of substrates, proteins, carbohydrates, and fats will adequately meet the patient's metabolic needs without incurring a negative nitrogen balance?

First, patients who should receive early, aggressive nutritional support include those with primary malnutrition; those with complications such as sepsis or associated injuries; and those admitted late in the course of their disease who have lost > 10% of their premorbid weight. This support should be in the form of supplemental oral feedings, tube feedings, or total parenteral nutrition, depending upon the patient's condition. If anorexia or dysphagia makes oral feeding difficult or impossible but gastric motility and absorption are normal, enteral feedings may be given by continuous drip. The enteral route is preferable to the parenteral route because it involves fewer complications and costs less. Total parenteral nutrition is used in the absence of normal intestinal motility or absorption.

Second, to determine caloric requirement, it should be noted that a brief increase in metabolism as measured by O_2 consumption occurs in the postoperative period, unless a complication such as sepsis is part of the clinical picture. The metabolic rate in the early postoperative period, however, does not exceed twice the normal basal metabolic rate **(BMR)** as calculated by the Harris-Benedict equation, ie, for males:

$$BMR = 66 + (13.7 \times W) + (5.0 \times H) - (6.8 \times A);$$

for females:

$$BMR = 665 + (9.6 \times W) + (1.7 \times H) - (4.7 \times A).$$

In this equation, BMR is the normal basal metabolic rate in kcal, W is the ideal body weight in kg, H is the height in cm, and A is the age in years. It should be noted that age, sex, height, and weight are considered in determining basal caloric requirement, but body temperature, protein losses through wounds, and the patient's muscular work related to physical activity, such as ambulation, are ignored. Thus, an adequate estimate for total daily caloric requirement is 2 times the BMR as determined above.

Finally, determining what mixture will adequately meet metabolic needs is more complex. The total caloric requirement is met with carbohydrate, fat, and protein. Carbohydrate infused at a rate of 5 mg/kg/min provides enough calories to prevent amino acid breakdown as an energy source and suppresses endogenous glucose production via hepatic gluconeogenesis, which requires mobilization of amino acids as gluconeogenic precursors.

This glucose infusion rate also approximates the maximum rate of glucose oxidation for a patient on strict bed rest. Any additional glucose in such a patient is not used for ATP production but is simply converted to fat. At this infusion rate, the respiratory quotient is just below unity, indicating that the glucose is oxidized to CO_2, water, and energy and is not being stored as fat.

Protein is infused at 1.5 to 2.5 gm/kg/day. In most patients, the lower rate may be used. Nitrogen **(N)** balance analysis and kinetic amino acid turnover studies have shown that this rate of administration maintains positive N balance in adults as well as in injured children. Although it has not been studied in the elderly patient, this protein infusion rate represents a reasonable first approximation.

The patient's total caloric requirement is not met with glucose given at 5 mg/kg/min and protein at 1.5 gm/kg/day. Therefore, fats must be given either parenterally or enterally to meet the remaining caloric requirement. Fats furnish enough calories to minimize the need for mobilization of endogenous proteins for energy and gluconeogenesis, and they supply essential fatty acids.

Other Postoperative Complications

The following common complications can occur either in the ICU or later during convalescence.

1. Cardiorespiratory arrest: Primary respiratory arrest may be caused by airway obstruction or respiratory depression, or it may be secondary to cardiac arrest. Airway obstruction may be caused by blockage of an endotracheal tube or tracheobronchial tree by mucus, blood, or a foreign body or by blockage of the larynx from an aspirated bolus of food or vocal cord spasm. **Respiratory depression** may occur from primary pulmonary disease, such as bacterial pneumonia; pneumonia from aspiration of vomited gastric contents; or pulmonary embolus; or it may occur as a side effect of narcotics. In the postoperative patient, **cardiac arrest** is associated with fibrillation or asystole, which initially are treated identically.

Cardiac or respiratory arrest requires immediate attention and treatment. Complete lack of ventilation for 3 min is usually fatal. If the patient does not die, brain damage may occur. Treatment is based upon the ABCD mnemonic of resuscitation: *A*irway, *B*reathing, *C*irculation, and *D*efinitive treatment. Reestablishment of an airway and the establishment of adequate breathing or ventilation are necessary, either by performing mouth-to-mouth resuscitation, by using a bag-valve-mask device, or by using an endotracheal tube and manual or mechanical ventilation. A reasonable breathing rate for adults is 12 breaths/min while using 100% O_2.

Primary cardiac arrest also leads immediately to cerebral anoxia and loss of respiratory exchange. Thus, circulation must be reestablished. In the postoperative period, the arrest usually occurs when the patient is not being monitored and the endotracheal tube has been removed. A few chest compressions can determine whether the airway is open. Then ventilation must be maintained either by intermittent chest compression or by intubation and mechanical ventilation, if necessary. A hard blow with the fist to the sternum will sometimes produce a return of cardiac rhythm, but if it does not, external cardiac compression is necessary. Thoracotomy and cardiac massage may be possible in some cases.

For further treatment of the cardiac arrest, drugs and an ECG are necessary. In 85% of cases, sudden cardiac arrest is caused by ventricular fibrillation. Further treatment depends upon whether **asystole, fibrillation,** or **bradycardia** (or idioventricular rhythm) is present on ECG. Bradycardia is treated with atropine sulfate 0.5 to 1.0 mg IV or isoproterenol 1 to $\geq$ 5 μg/min IV to obtain a reasonable ventricular rate.

Fibrillation is treated by cardioversion (defibrillation), initially with 200 to 300 joules. If this is unsuccessful, epinephrine (5 to 10 mL of a 1:10,000 solution) should be administered IV—by intracardiac injection, or transtracheally—and followed by another cardioversion. If these treatments fail, other factors, such as arterial oxygenation or acidosis, should be considered. Oxygenation may be quickly ascertained by obtaining arterial blood gas determinations and should be treated accordingly. During cardiopulmonary resuscitation (CPR), acidosis occurs rapidly. Sodium bicarbonate, 1 or 2 ampules (7.5%, 44.6 mEq), may be injected rapidly IV and repeated every 5 to 10 min.

If fibrillation persists, repeated cardioversion, continuous epinephrine IV infusions, and possibly antiarrhythmics, such as lidocaine, procainamide, or bretylium tosylate may be used. In critical situations, when cardiac inotropy is weak and digitalis toxicity is not suspected, calcium chloride (10 mL in a 10% solution) may be given IV as a cardiac inotrope.

Asystole usually must be converted to fibrillation before it can be cardioverted. Cardioversion may be attempted, but early use of epinephrine and sodium bicarbonate usually is necessary to convert asystole to fibrillation.

Preventive measures may be taken to avoid cardiac arrest. Patients known to be at increased risk include those who have had previous cardiac disease, infection, or anemia that makes further work demands upon the heart, serious electrolyte or acid-base abnormalities, severe hypo- or hypervolemia and severe pulmonary edema, arrhythmias, or excessive digitalization. From a practical point of view, patients at risk should be placed on cardiac monitors. If the monitor shows the recent onset of more than 3 PVCs/min, particularly if they are multifocal or appear early in the diastolic phase (near the T wave), lidocaine should be given as a bolus of 50 to 100 mg, followed by a continuous infusion of 1 to 4 mg/min.

Older patients in cardiac arrest, especially those whose illness is terminal, present serious ethical and social considerations. Resuscitation may not be in the patient's best interest if expectations for his health after resuscitation are not at least as good as they were before arrest (see Ch. 45 and 47).

2. Thromboembolism may be either peripheral thrombophlebitis, pulmonary embolism, or both. Patients who have had previous thromboembolism, prolonged operations, and prolonged postoperative immobilization, as well as those who are obese, are at increased risk for developing thromboembolism. Most fatal pulmonary emboli originate in the lower extremities from peripheral thrombophlebitis.

Many prophylactic measures are available to reduce the incidence of thrombophlebitis, with appropriate anesthesia, expeditious operations, and early ambulation the most important. Other methods include postoperative use of elastic stockings, pneumatic compression devices, and anticoagulants. Disagreement exists about the choice and amount of anticoagulant agent to be used. Because prophylactic heparin, even in small doses, often leads to hemorrhage, many surgeons hesitate to use it routinely, restricting application to high-risk patients. Heparin can be replaced by oral warfarin sodium within a few days. The antiplatelet drug aspirin also has been used prophylactically for thromboembolism but does not appear to be as satisfactory as heparin.

Anticoagulation is generally considered to be the therapy of choice for established thromboembolism. In adults, a loading dose of IV heparin (5,000 to 10,000 u.) is given initially, followed in 2 to 3 h by a continuous IV infusion of 1,000 u./h. The heparin is adjusted to increase partial thromboplastin time **(PTT)** to twice normal. After 7 days, heparin is replaced by warfarin, which is usually adjusted to elevate prothrombin time **(PT)** to 1.5 times normal. This treatment is generally successful.

If embolization recurs despite anticoagulation or if contraindications to anticoagulation are present, a vena cava filter may be inserted either directly or percutaneously through the right internal jugular vein. If this is done accurately and expeditiously, recurrent embolization is substantially eliminated.

Venous interruptions of the superficial femoral vein are rarely necessary today, although in the past, ligation of these veins, and in later years, vena cava ligation, was common. The latter procedure was discontinued because of lack of competent anastomotic veins about the ligature and immediate hyperdistention of distal veins, and later because of excessive edema of lower extremities. Vena cava clips, which allowed for the passage of blood but strained out nearly all emboli, were also used frequently in the past. These devices have been replaced by the vena cava filter described above. Pulmonary embolectomy is still used successfully in selected cases of life-threatening cardiogenic shock resulting from massive pulmonary emboli.

3. Acute renal failure (ARF) is more common in older than in younger patients following surgery because of the compromise in renal reserve resulting from coexistent diseases such as atherosclerosis and diabetes. ARF is associated with a rapidly increasing azotemia and, usually, oliguria (< 500 mL/day).

Causes of postoperative ARF fall into 3 diagnostic categories: **prerenal, renal,** and **postrenal.** The most common **prerenal causes** are severe dehydration and a severely diminished blood volume, cardiac failure, hepatorenal syndrome, and septicemia. The most common **renal causes** of ARF result from a direct injury to the kidneys and include the following: (1) acute tubular necrosis, which follows episodes of renal ischemia resulting from hypotension during or after an operation, or which is associated with renal injury from toxins such as hemoglobin or myoglobin; (2) acute renal artery or vein occlusion resulting from the operation; and (3) acute nephritis, which is associated with potentially nephrotoxic drugs such as the aminoglycosides, arteriography contrast dyes, or papillary necrosis in diabetes. The most common **postrenal causes** of ARF are obstructive and are related to blockage of the ureters or the prostatic urethra.

A progressive rise in serum creatinine is diagnostic of ARF, but the urinary sediment also should be examined. Red cell casts and red cells suggest a vascular, neoplastic, or glomerulonephritic etiology. Eosinophils in urine suggest that nephrotoxic drugs may be the cause. Renal ultrasound has proved useful in detecting postrenal obstructive causes of ARF.

Prophylaxis is concerned chiefly with preventing hypotension and maintaining adequate urinary flow during the postoperative period. Because renal injury from nephrotoxic drugs may be dose related, drug levels of agents such as aminoglycosides should be monitored closely. Potential renal injury from myoglobin should be anticipated in clinical circumstances such as extremity crush injuries in trauma or acute severe arterial occlusive disease and profound extremity ischemia. Maintenance of a high glomerular filtration flow rate and alkalinization of urine with sodium bicarbonate are helpful.

Treatment of the patient with failing kidneys is very difficult. An adequate blood volume must be maintained in the early stages. Meticulous intake and output measurements and daily weights are necessary to monitor fluid and electrolyte therapy. Dosages of drugs excreted by the kidney, such as digoxin and many antibiotics, must be adjusted. Acid-base balance and nutrition must be closely monitored.

Dialysis may be necessary in patients with concomitant oliguria, increasing acidosis, and heart failure **(HF). The indications for dialysis** (either hemodialysis or peritoneal dialysis) are retention of nitrogenous solutes (urea and creatinine) and uremic encephalopathy or serositis, overexpansion of the blood volume and HF, hyperkalemia (serum $K > 6$ mEq/L), and metabolic acidosis (pH < 7.20).

4. Stress ulcers *are superficial mucosal erosions of the stomach that occur after stressful conditions, eg, trauma, burns, sepsis, or operations.* They are manifested by upper GI bleeding that may vary from minimal to life-threatening. This may be vomiting of bright red blood, or a "coffee-grounds" bleeding identified in the nasogastric tube aspirates. Stress ulcers may develop at any time during convalescence but usually occur when oral intake has not been resumed postoperatively, the abdomen is distended, and concomitant pulmonary complications are present. Diagnosis is best made by upper GI endoscopy.

Prophylaxis, which involves treatment of any pulmonary complications, prevention of gastric distention by decompression via a nasogastric tube or gastrostomy, and maintenance of a neutral or alkaline pH in the stomach, is very successful. Gastric acidity may be controlled by either of 2 methods: Antacids may be delivered via nasogastric tube to maintain gastric pH above 5.5, or IV histamine H_2-receptor antagonists (eg, cimetidine) may be administered. Administration of antacids requires additional nursing time to monitor pH and to deliver antacids hourly, making this method more expensive. Thus, most institutions currently use histamine antagonists for prophylaxis for stress ulcers. Care must be taken, however, to avoid the CNS, dose-related side effects of cimetidine, which are thought to occur more frequently in elderly patients. These effects include confusion, delirium, slurred speech, and hallucinations. One disadvantage of substances that elevate gastric pH is that they allow colonization of the stomach with gram-negative bacteria that may lead to pulmonary aspiration and pneumonia. However, recent evidence shows that sucralfate, a mucosa-coating drug, avoids this problem and is just as effective in preventing hemorrhage.

If stress bleeding does occur, conservative treatment by endoscopic coagulation or angiographic embolization may be effective. Very serious cases may require surgery, either a high gastrectomy plus vagotomy or a total gastrectomy, to control the hemorrhage. Because these operations are associated with a high perioperative mortality, prevention of stress ulcers is extremely important (see also Ch. 53).

5. Antibiotic-associated pseudomembranous colitis should be considered when diarrhea, which is common after abdominal operations, occurs postoperatively in a patient who has received antibiotics. This inflammatory disorder is generally limited to the colon and is characterized by membrane-like plaques of exudate that replace necrotic colonic mucosa. The pseudomembranous plaques consist of fibrin, mucin, leukocytes, and sloughed necrotic cells. The underlying mucosa shows varying degrees of superficial necrosis, edema, and inflammation. Strains of *Clostridium difficile* and its toxin, which may be identified in the stools of these patients, usually lead to this diagnosis.

Previous exposure to antibiotics is thought to alter the balance in normal gut flora, allowing overgrowth of *C. difficile*. The diarrhea usually develops within 3 to 4 wk following exposure to antibiotics. Clindamycin and lincomycin are the antibiotics most frequently associated with pseudomembranous colitis, although ampicillin, cephalosporins, penicillin, amoxicillin, tetracycline, chloramphenicol, and trimethoprim-sulfamethoxazole have also been implicated. Diagnosis is usually made by bacterial stool culture, stool examination for *C. difficile* toxin, and sigmoidoscopy. Both oral vancomycin (500 mg q 6 h) and metronidazole (7.5 mg/kg q 6 h or 500 mg q 6 h) are considered safe and effective treatments. This disease is usually self-limited, but in extremely severe cases, treatment with IV steroids and emergency colectomy may be necessary.

If diarrhea does occur in a postoperative geriatric patient, stool specimens for bacterial culture and toxin analysis should be taken immediately. When watery diarrhea was found in postoperative patients at the Hartford Hospital, *C. difficile* assays were performed in 691 patients; 75 of them had confirmed *C. difficile* infections. The average age of the involved patients was 68 yr. The average time from the initial administration of antibiotics to onset of the diarrhea was 2.7 days. Many of these patients were immunosuppressed because of cancer, sepsis, or diabetes. In 30% of them, the diarrhea disappeared after the antibiotics were discontinued. The others required specific therapy with vancomycin, bacitracin, or metronidazole. Two deaths occurred in this series as a direct result of this type of colitis.

6. Hemorrhagic complications result from the massive bleeding encountered during long operations in which large amounts of blood have been transfused and hypothermia and coagulopathy are present. They also may occur during convalescence when a secondary operation is required for a complication. The standard treatment for all such episodes includes discontinuing anticoagulant therapy, reversing the effects of heparin with protamine, and transfusing fresh frozen plasma, cryoprecipitate, and platelets.

In cases in which the bleeding is intolerable during an operative procedure, the surgeon may have no alternative but to stop the procedure, insert large packs, and close the abdomen. The abdomen may then be reopened after 48 h. During this interval, correction of the coagulopathy should be vigorously conducted, using fresh frozen plasma, cryoprecipitate, fresh whole blood, and platelets as necessary. After 48 h, the capillary bleeding usually will have stopped, the packs may be removed, and the operation may be completed.

7. Other complications after abdominal surgery: In general, the incidence of **wound infections** increases with age, possibly because elderly patients are more likely to undergo operations with a high potential for wound infections. Such procedures include cholecystectomy, herniorrhaphy, colon or other bowel resection, amputations, hysterectomy, total hip replacement, and total knee replacement. For these operations, prophylactic antibiotics should be given.

Wound infections are usually suggested by fever that appears 3 to 5 days after an operative procedure. Physical examination of the wound may elicit more tenderness than is usually expected. Warmth and redness near the wound suggest an infection or early cellulitis. Any superficial wound fullness or swelling, which is suggestive of a collection of fluid, should be closely examined and may be drained. Fluid obtained should be gram-stained and cultured for aerobic and anaerobic bacteria. Drainage does not mean that the wound must be opened extensively. Rather, adequate drainage can usually be obtained by opening only a small portion of the incision and inserting either a rubber or cloth drain to ensure a persistent opening or tract for complete drainage.

Intra-abdominal abscesses are not within the wound but are deep to the fascia. These abscesses are also suggested by persistent fever and, in many cases, by localized abdominal or flank tenderness. Intra-abdominal abscesses include subphrenic, subhepatic, pelvic, and intraloop abscesses, all of which may be difficult to localize. The CT scan has proved extremely useful in the diagnosis and localization of such abscesses. Ultrasound is also a valuable adjunctive imaging modality. Using these imaging technics, percutaneous placement of catheters for drainage has been successful in many cases. Surgery (including operative drainage of the abscess), however, remains the final method of therapy.

Anastomotic suture leakage may occur during the course of healing, when the anastomosis dehisces, allowing leakage of GI contents, feces, bile, pancreatic secretions, or urine into the peritoneal or retroperitoneal spaces. These rare complications are exceedingly dangerous if not treated promptly. They occur in the first 10 days postoperatively, and are marked by acute onset of an unusual degree of abdominal pain and tenderness.

Treatment consists of immediate reexploration. When possible, the suture line is exteriorized from the abdomen. In cases such as perforation of a duodenal stump, the only possible course is to place drains close to the perforation. In perforations of low colonic anastomoses, drainage and a proximal colostomy are necessary.

Dehiscence means *disruption of either the skin or fascia closure.* **Skin dehiscence** is of minimal significance and leads to delay in complete skin healing. **Fascial dehiscence,** the disruption of the fascial closure, however, is usually associated with evisceration or herniation of intraperitoneal organs and is a life-threatening condition.

Dehiscence of an abdominal incision often is heralded by profuse discharge of clear fluid from the incision. In nearly all cases of fascial dehiscence, resuture of the incision is necessary. The only treatment for evisceration is placing sterile towels over the exposed bowel and immediately returning the patient to the operating room for fascial closure. In fascial dehiscence, late hernia formation is common.

---

23. REHABILITATION

Mathew H. M. Lee and *Masayoshi Itoh*

GENERAL CONCEPTS OF GERIATRIC REHABILITATION

The most important goal of geriatric rehabilitation is to reattain independence in activities of daily living **(ADLs)** after loss by a medical or surgical event. Progress may be slow. The elderly, especially those with neuromuscular and skeletal disabilities, fatigue more rapidly than younger people, and therapy must be geared to the patient endurance.

Disuse atrophy of the muscles, osteoporosis, poor coordination, slow reaction times, memory impairment, use of certain medications, lack of motivation, anger, frustration, and depression may further complicate the rehabilitative process.

A relatively unrecognized syndrome is that of the "good day and bad day." On a good day, the patient feels full of energy and may make great progress, while on a bad day he performs as on his first day of the program. This syndrome appears to be more physical than psychological, but its exact cause is unknown.

Rehabilitative modalities are administered by various allied health professionals **(AHPs).** A physician issues a "referral," which (like a drug prescription) is considered a legal document, and contains instructions to an AHP who usually cannot otherwise treat the patient.

The physician is responsible for the efficacy and side effects of treatment, so the referral should be reasonably detailed. However, it is often written as "Rx: Physical therapy." Strictly, this is invalid, since physical therapy is not a modality. Such an order is analogous to a drug prescription that states "Rx: Antibiotics." Some therapists may accept such a prescription because it allows them freedom in choosing modalities. However, the physician would share responsibility for any untoward results.

THERAPEUTIC APPROACHES
THERAPEUTIC EXERCISES

Before prescribing any exercise program, the physician should evaluate cardiopulmonary, metabolic, and neuromusculoskeletal status, including muscle power and range of motion of the affected joints.

Range of motion (ROM) exercises. Normal ROM values are shown in TABLE 23–1. Goniometric ROM evaluation should be recorded before therapy and regularly thereafter.

TABLE 23–1. NORMAL VALUES OF RANGE OF MOTION OF JOINTS

Joint	Motion	Range
Hip	Flexion	0° to 115°–125°
	Extension	115°–125° to 0°
	Hyperextension*	0° to 10°–15°
	Abduction	0° to 45°
	Adduction	45° to 0°
	Lateral rotation	0° to 45°
	Medial rotation	0° to 45°
Knee	Flexion	0° to 120°–130°
	Extension	120°–130° to 0°
Ankle	Plantar flexion	0° to 40°–50°
	Dorsiflexion	0° to 20°
Foot	Inversion	0° to 35°
	Eversion	0° to 25°
Toes		
(MP joints)	Flexion	0° to 20°–30°
	Extension	0° to 80°
(IP joints)	Flexion	0° to 50°
	Extension	50° to 0°
Shoulder	Flexion to 90°	0° to 90°
	Extension	0° to 50°
	Abduction to 90°	0° to 90°
	Adduction	90° to 0°
	Lateral rotation	0° to 90°
	Medial rotation	0° to 90°

(Continued)

* Extension beyond midline.

TABLE 23–1. NORMAL VALUES OF RANGE OF MOTION OF JOINTS
(Cont'd)

Joint	Motion	Range
Elbow	Flexion	0° to 145°–160°
	Extension	145°–160 ° to 0°
	Pronation	0° to 90°
	Supination	0° to 90°
Wrist	Flexion	0° to 90°
	Extension	0° to 70°
	Abduction	0° to 25°
	Adduction	0° to 55°–65°
Fingers (MP joints)	Flexion	0° to 90°
	Extension	0° to 20°–30°
(IP joints)	Flexion	0° to 120°
	Extension	120° to 0°
(IP distal joints)	Flexion	0° to 80°
	Extension	80° to 0°
Fingers	Abduction	0° to 20°–25°
	Adduction	20°–25° to 0°
Thumb (MP joints)	Flexion	0° to 60°–70°
	Extension	60°–70° to 0°
(IP joints)	Flexion	0° to 90°
	Extension	90° to 0°
Thumb	Abduction	0° to 40°–50°
	Adduction	40°–60° to 0°

Physiologically normal ROM must be differentiated from functional ROM. Typically, the ROM values of an elderly person who is functioning independently in all activities of daily living **(ADLs)** will be lower than in younger individuals for certain joints. Functional ROM allows a person to perform ADLs without assistance, and without need to increase ROM to the "normal" range.

Exercises to maintain ROM. Moving a given joint within its full range will maintain the current ROM. **Active ROM exercise** is used when a patient is able to perform this exercise alone. **Active assistive ROM** is used when muscle power is too weak (requiring additional strengthening exercises), or joint movement produces discomfort and the patient needs assistance. **Passive ROM exercise** is used whenever a patient cannot actively participate.

Assistive or passive ROM exercise must be carried out *very gently,* as osteoporosis increases the risk of fracture. The joint should be moved within its full range with the least possible pain. Movements producing severe pain should be avoided, as this may damage the joint and lead to refusal of the patient to participate further. Passive ROM exercise should never be applied to joints adjacent to a fracture.

Exercise to increase ROM. Limitation of ROM is caused primarily by pain, bony ankylosis, and soft tissue ankylosis and contracture. Exercise is effective only in soft tissue contracture (caused by a tight muscle or joint). If there is no pain, a tight muscle can be stretched more vigorously than a tight joint, but caution is required with osteoporosis, long-standing paralysis, or an anesthetic limb.

The joint must be moved beyond the point of pain, but without any residual pain. Momentary forceful stretching is not as effective as sustained moderate stretching, which is usually applied by weights from 5 to 50 lb with pulleys for a duration of 20 min/day. Manual stretching is time-consuming and requires enormous force for major joints.

When tissue temperature is raised to about 43 C (109 F), stretching exercise is more effective, with less pain. Various forms of heat may be applied immediately before or concurrently with exercise (see HEAT/COLD THERAPY, below).

Exercise to increase muscle strength. Muscle strength is usually tested by a physical therapist, and is expressed in 5 grades (see TABLE 23–2). There are many technics for increasing muscle strength, but 2 basic principles: **resistance** (applied manually or mechanically) and its **progressiveness,** eg, progressive resistive exercise **(PRE).** Gravity may be used as resistance in grades of "poor" or less. Mechanical resistance is easy to measure. Strength need be increased only until the patient can easily perform a target function. Applying resistance to a spastic muscle is not recommended, as the increase in tone can be more troublesome than the prior weakness.

Exercise to increase endurance involves the reciprocal use of several large groups of muscles and is vigorous, often requiring special equipment. Cardiovascular and respiratory capacities should not be compromised.

Proprioceptive neuromuscular facilitation (PNF) promotes useful neuromuscular activity through stimulation of proprioceptors in affected muscles. PNF is used exclusively in a patient with upper motor neuron damage, with resulting spasticity, by stimulation of the reflex arc; eg, if strong resistance is applied to the left elbow flexor (biceps) of a right hemiplegic patient, the right elbow begins to flex through contraction of the hemiplegic biceps. Various technics (eg, Brunnstrom, Rood, and Bobath) are widely practiced.

Exercise to improve coordination involves the repetition of a meaningful movement. This is not simple movement of a body segment, such as flexing an elbow, but is task-oriented, eg, touching the nose with the hand, which combines flexing the elbow with other coordinated joint activity. Successful outcome depends on the patient's rational state, cooperation, and ability to learn, as well as on intact proprioception to monitor muscular activity and a pain-free arc of joint motion.

TABLE 23-2. GRADES OF MUSCLE STRENGTH

Grade	Description
5 or N or Normal	Full range against gravity and full resistance for the patient's size, age, and sex
N − Normal minus	Slight weakness
G+ or Good plus	Moderate weakness
4 or G or Good	Movement against gravity and moderate resistance at least 10 times without fatigue
F+ or Fair plus	Movement against gravity several times or once with mild resistance
3 or F or Fair	Full range against gravity
F− or Fair minus	Movement against gravity and complete range once
P+ or Poor plus	Beginning motion against gravity of range ≤ 95%
2 or P or Poor	Full range with gravity eliminated
P− or Poor minus	Incomplete range of motion with gravity eliminated
1 or T or Trace	Evidence of contracture (visible or palpable) but no joint movement
0 or Zero	No palpable or visible contracture and no motion of joint

Using the tilt table to reestablish hemodynamic balance. The tilt table has a padded top with a footboard. The patient is strapped to the table in a supine position, and tilted manually or electrically. A goniometer measures the angle, which is increased very slowly to an 85° upright position, as tolerated by the patient.

This modality is used mainly for reestablishing the hemodynamic balance, eg, in early paraplegia or quadriplegia, following prolonged bedrest or immobilization, or in total debilitation.

The general conditioning exercise is a combination of various programs (described above) to reestablish hemodynamic balance, increase cardiorespiratory capacity, and maintain ROM and muscle strength. The indications are debilitation, prolonged bedrest, or immobilization.

Ambulation Exercise, Elevation Exercise, and Gait Training

Ambulation exercise improves walking on level surfaces. Before starting, functional ROM and muscle strengthening exercises, such as PRE, may be indicated. If some muscles remain less functional, an orthotic device, eg, a brace, may be used. The patient must be able to balance on standing. Falls should be avoided. The patient trains initially on parallel bars and progresses to walking with aids, eg, walker, crutches, or cane. Independent ambulation (without an aid) is not an essential goal in most geriatric rehabilitation programs.

Elevation exercise (training to ascend or descend steps) should be started next, using the hand rail and a crutch or cane. This exercise is not recommended for a patient who requires a walker.

Ascent starts with the noninvolved leg and descent with the involved leg (ie, "good is up and bad is down"). One step at a time is safer when ascending or descending stairs than using both legs alternately. If a patient is expected to walk outdoors, he should be taught how to cross the sidewalk curb.

Gait is the pattern, style, and cadence of walking. Independent ambulation is necessary for gait training, since gait is always abnormal with any aid. A lower extremity prosthesis causing gait variation should be adjusted by a prosthetist.

Activities of Daily Living (ADLs) Training

ADLs encompass many activities, eg, personal hygiene, grooming, dressing, feeding, transfers, and homemaking (cooking, cleaning, recreational activities, etc). The patient's physical and social responsibilities at home determine training needs. Even in an institution, ADL training is crucial to dignity and physical independence (see Ch. 24).

The patient's functional status should first be evaluated. This may indicate a need for a self-help device (see below). Training should be conducted in an actual or simulated environment. The therapist must be very patient and repeat each activity until it can be performed independently, without supervision.

Transfer activity describes movement between a wheelchair and stationary objects such as a bed, toilet seat, or furniture.

RELIEF OF PAIN AND INFLAMMATION

HEAT/COLD THERAPY

Heat increases blood flow and the extensibility of connective tissue, decreases joint stiffness, pain, and muscle spasm, and helps resolve inflammatory infiltrates, edema, and exudates.

There are 2 modes of heat application: superficial and deep. The intensity and duration of the physiologic effects are determined mainly by tissue temperature, rate of temperature elevation, and volume of the treated site.

Indications for heat therapy are acute and chronic traumatic and inflammatory conditions such as sprains, strains, fibrositis, tenosynovitis, muscle spasm, myositis, painful back, whiplash injuries 48 h after onset, various forms of arthritis, arthralgia, and neuralgia.

Superficial Heat

Infrared: Site of application, frequency, and duration of treatment should be specified. Contraindications include advanced heart disease, peripheral vascular disease, impaired skin sensation (particularly of temperature and pain), and hepatic and/or renal insufficiency.

Hotpacks: Most commercially available hotpacks consist of cotton cloth containers filled with silicate gel, applied to a prescribed location over several layers of towels to protect the skin from burns. Contraindications are as for infrared heat, above.

Paraffin wax is melted to remain liquid at 49 C (120 F). It should not be used above 54.4 C (130 F). Since the heating effect is relatively short-lived, even if the area is wrapped with towels, radiant heat may be applied immediately afterwards.

Paraffin can be applied by dipping, immersion, painting, or wrapping; eg, a hand is very easy to dip or immerse whereas a knee or elbow is best treated by painting.

Indications include those listed above, and particularly, conditions associated with skin contracture. Contraindications include an open wound or allergy to paraffin.

Hydrotherapy may be utilized as heat therapy, for ROM exercise or increasing muscle strength, or (when water is agitated with a turbine) to cleanse wounds.

Indications for the Hubbard tank at 35.5 to 37.7 C (96 to 100 F) include extensive burn wounds, large decubitus ulcers, arthritis, and conditions in which the buoyancy of the water allows weak muscles to function. Total immersion at temperatures of 37.7 to 40 C (100 to 104 F) may be used for sedation, relief of pain, or raising body temperature. The whirlpool and lowboy are used for more localized areas.

While there are no specific **contraindications,** the patient may become fatigued and caution is necessary if a patient is debilitated or has cardiac disease.

Deep Heat

Shortwave diathermy appears to be less efficacious than previously thought. **Indications** include those listed above, pain of urinary calculus, pelvic infections, and acute and chronic sinusitis. **Contraindications** include malignancy, hemorrhagic conditions, peripheral vascular disease, loss of sensation, or the presence of fixed prostheses, pacemakers, or electrophysiologic braces. Shortwave diathermy cannot be used with metallic implants (eg, bars, screws, plates) since the heated metal may cause a burn. Implanted devices may also malfunction or be destroyed. Similarly, to avoid burns, no metallic substance should be in contact with the skin.

Microwave diathermy: The advantages of microwave over shortwave diathermy are simplicity of application, accuracy of output measurement, adequate deep heating without undue heating of the skin, and maximum comfort for the patient. Microwaves are selectively absorbed in tissues with high water content, such as muscles. Despite its advantages, microwave diathermy is not used as widely as shortwave diathermy or ultrasound.

Indications are similar to those for shortwave (see above). **Contraindications** include ischemic or edematous tissues, hemorrhagic areas, malignant tissue, anesthetic areas, early stages of trauma, treatment over wet dressing, metallic implants (including pacemakers), healing bones, testes and ovaries, and treatment of the frail and debilitated.

Ultrasound: Indications include a limitation of ROM due to muscle shortening and fibrosis, scarring of skin or subcutaneous tissues, calcific bursitis and tendinitis, pain due to postoperative neurofibromas (especially when embedded in scar tissue), phantom pain, reflex dystrophies such as shoulder-hand syndrome, Sudeck's atrophy and causalgia, bursitis, myositis, tenosynovitis, epicondylitis, spondylitis, contusions, and neuritis. Additional possible indications are sciatica and other forms of radiculitis, myofascial pain syndrome, and chronic skin ulceration.

Contraindications include ischemic tissue, hemorrhagic diathesis, malignancies, anesthetic areas over areas of acute infection, and treatment over the eyes, brain, spinal cord, ears, heart, reproductive organs, brachial plexus, or healing bone.

Ultraviolet (UV): No significant penetration of UV occurs beyond the epidermis. The biologic effects of UV on the skin include erythema, tanning, vitamin D production, and an acceleration of the superficial wound healing process. The bactericidal effects of UV have long been used for therapeutic and industrial purposes. However, UV is not effective against bacterial spores; therefore, it must be used daily on infected wounds and ulcers.

The most commonly used device is the cold quartz lamp, which produces erythema with minimal pigmentation and blistering, and has a high rate of bactericidal activity.

Precautions include prevention of burns (third- and fourth-degree erythema) and protection of the eyes of both patient and therapist, by using protective goggles. Since UV does not penetrate deeply, the treated area must be free of any covering material, including creams or ointments. UV is therefore often applied to wounds or ulcers immediately after hydrotherapy.

Contraindications include photosensitivity (natural or drug-induced), cardiac or renal failure, hyperthyroidism, diabetic peripheral neuropathy, and certain dermatologic conditions; eg, acute onset of psoriasis, acute eczema, lupus erythematosus, herpes simplex, or xeroderma pigmentosa.

Cryotherapy

The spread of cold on the skin depends on the thickness of the epidermis, its underlying fat and muscle, the water content of the tissue, and the rate of blood flow. Cold can be applied locally as an ice bag or cold pack. Local cooling may also be produced by evaporation of volatile fluids, eg, ethyl chloride.

Indications include muscle spasm, pain of myofascial or traumatic origin, acute low back pain, acute inflammatory lesions, and induction of local anesthesia. **Precautions** include the avoidance of tissue damage (ie, frostbite) and general hypothermia. **Contraindications** include healing wounds and extreme cold sensitivity.

ELECTRIC THERAPY

Electricity is used to stimulate denervated skeletal muscle and innervated muscle that a patient is unable to contract voluntarily or involuntarily to avoid disuse atrophy, and to reduce muscle spasticity. The **unipolar technic** uses a large dispersive electrode at a distant part of the body and a smaller active electrode on the muscle to be treated. The **bipolar technic** uses 2 small electrodes of about the same size, placed over each end of the muscle.

The unipolar technic uses a lower current, and if the desired contractile response is obtained, is the method of choice. The bipolar method is well suited for severely degenerated muscles due to gross anatomic or physiologic interruption of nerve supply, and for unusually high skin impedance; eg, when there is massive edema in the treatment area.

Indications include hemiplegia due to cerebrovascular accident, traumatic paraplegia and quadriplegia, and peripheral nerve injuries. Ten to 20 muscle contractions per session are usually sufficient. Overstimulation may cause muscle fatigue, which may eventually result in damage. Electrode burns may be caused by inadequate skin contact or use of too high a current. **Contraindications** include advanced cardiac disease, any type of pacemaker, and application over the eyes.

Transcutaneous electrical nerve and muscle stimulation (TENS) is a low-frequency variation of electric therapy. The patient feels a gentle tingling sensation without increase in muscle tension. Stimulation may be applied several times daily, each session ranging from 20 min to several hours, depending on pain severity. **Indications** include chronic pain; eg, back pain, rheumatoid arthritis, sprained ankle, contusion, postherpetic neuralgia, causalgia, phantom limb syndrome, and trigger points. TENS has also been said to assist in the callus formation of a nonunited fracture. When the electrodes are placed on the skin improperly, erythema may develop. **Contraindications** include advanced cardiac disease (risk of arrhythmia), any type of pacemaker, and application over the eyes.

TRACTION

Spinal traction is used to facilitate rest by immobilization, to overcome extrinsic muscle spasm, and to separate bony surfaces. A weight and pulley system, the body weight of the patient, and manual or motorized force can be used. The force may be applied continuously or intermittently.

For **cervical traction,** the force must exceed the weight of the patient's head, which is about 5 to 10 lb. Whereas sustained traction with > 20 lb is poorly tolerated by a patient for more than a few minutes, motorized intermittent rhythmic traction can be tolerated very well. **Indications** include pain from cervical spondylosis, disk prolapse, whiplash of the neck, or torticollis.

Although **lumbar traction** may be administered in a vertical position, a horizontal position is more often used. **Indications** include pain of lumbar osteoarthritis or spondylolisthesis. Its value in treating acute discogenic pain is debatable.

Contraindications include infections of the spinal vertebrae, advanced osteoporosis, vertebral malignancy, spinal cord compression, hypertensive cardiovascular disease, rheumatoid arthritis, or *frail and debilitated persons.*

MASSAGE

Massage is sedating, relaxing, and pleasurable. It should not produce discomfort or pain.

Indications include relief of pain, reduction of swelling and induration associated with trauma (eg, fracture, joint injury, sprain, strain, bruise, or peripheral nerve injury), and mobilization of contracted tissues. Massage should also be considered for low back pain, arthritis, periarthritis, bursitis, neuritis, fibrositis, hemiplegia, paraplegia, quadriplegia, multiple sclerosis, or cerebral palsy.

Contraindications include infection of the area to be treated, malignancy, debilitation, burns, and thrombophlebitis.

ACUPUNCTURE

Acupuncture involves skin penetration with a series of very thin needles made of stainless steel, gold, or platinum at specific body sites, frequently quite remote from the site of pain. The needle is twirled rapidly and intermittently for a few minutes, or a low electrical current is applied. Increases in circulating endorphins are believed to be responsible for its analgesic effect.

Caution must be exercised to prevent cross-infection, pneumothorax, or hemorrhage. **Indications** include chronic pain of various origins. **Contraindications** include severe debilitation, advanced cardiac disease, and acute infectious processes.

ORTHOTIC DEVICES

Shoes: Safe ambulation by a physically disabled person requires soundly constructed orthopedic shoes. These have steel shanks and low rubber heels shaped to increase ankle or foot stability. The height of the shoes (oxford or high top) and closing system (shoelace, strap, buckle, or Velcro®) depend on the patient's needs. If there is leg shortening, a lift, made of light material, eg, cork, may be added.

Canes, crutches, and **walkers** can assist with ambulation, both after injury or surgery and in chronic disability. Walkers provide a movable, stable platform that protects against falling, but offer little protection against weight-bearing forces, cause considerable slowing of gait, and are not suitable for use on stairs. Ordinary crutches are usually inappropriate for the elderly, who often lack the necessary upper-body strength and motor coordination. Canadian crutches with forearm supports and hand grips require less upper-body strength and are useful for the chronically disabled. Canes assist with balance and reduce the weight-bearing forces across the hip; correct length requires that the patient's elbow is only slightly bent when maximal force is being applied. A cane should be held in the contralateral hand for hip injuries and in the hand of preference for knee, ankle, and foot injuries.

Leg brace: A short leg brace, which stops just below the knee, is used for ankle disability. A knee brace, extending from the mid-thigh to the mid-calf, may be used for disability confined to the knee (eg, inability to lock the knee due to extensor weakness). A long leg brace, reaching the mid-thigh, is indicated for disabilities in both ankle and knee. A long leg brace with a pelvic band and hip joint is used for disability in the ankle, knee, and hip. However, such a brace is seldom practical for a geriatric patient since walking with it requires considerable energy.

A weight-bearing brace, where the weight is borne at the tibial condyle or ischeal tuberosity, may be prescribed for a patient (eg, with a non-united fracture—see also REHABILITATION AFTER HIP FRACTURE, below) who cannot bear body weight on an affected leg.

Neck brace: A neck brace is used for immobilization or minimization of weight bearing of the head. It can be attached to a rigid corset, and is not usually worn in bed.

Corset: A corset is used for immobilization of the thoracic or lumbar spine, or for weight bearing as described above under "neck brace." The prolonged use of a corset may result in the weakening of abdominal and spinal muscles.

Upper extremity orthotic devices: The **static splint** is for maintenance of current ROM of wrist and finger joints and prevention of contracture. It is often used for hemiplegic hands. The **dynamic splint** allows movement of the wrist and fingers to perform such tasks as pinch or grasp and is often used for quadriplegic hands. Splints help a patient maintain personal hygiene.

Wheelchair: There are 2 types: indoor (large wheels in the rear) and outdoor (large wheels in the front). Most patients use the indoor model. A **one-arm-drive wheelchair** may be suitable for a hemiplegic patient with good coordination. (See also discussion under REHABILITATION AFTER LOWER EXTREMITY AMPUTATION, below.) A **motorized wheelchair**, which requires little strength, is prescribed for a patient who has little or no function in the upper extremities. Since the wheelchair may reach 5 mph, the user should have good coordination, vision, and judgment.

SELF-HELP DEVICES IN THE HOME

Kitchen Work

Prolonged standing while working in the kitchen is stressful and tiring; a high stool to provide comfort while working at countertop level should have a backrest for trunk stability. A rolling cart can be used to transport heavy or cumbersome articles, and decrease trips between kitchen and dining table. The oven section of the regular gas or electric stove is often too low for comfort; a relatively inexpensive table top electric broiler oven eliminates this stressful body position. If a gas range is not equipped with a pilot light or electric ignition, an older person should use long fireplace matches to prevent burns. Pot holders or padded mitts should always be used. An ironing board with an electric outlet prevents tripping on the iron cord. Since an uncoordinated person tends to drop articles on the floor, plastic dishes can be used to prevent breakage of chinaware. Tools with long handles for housekeeping (dustpan, duster) or gardening (weed puller, pruner) also help avoid stooping. A long-handled reacher to retrieve items from high shelves can avoid the hazard of climbing a kitchen ladder. Other useful items include an electric can opener, a jar opener installed on the wall, and a rubber door lever that can be slipped on the door knob.

The Bathroom

A hand-held shower with an extension hose connected to the regular shower outlet may be easier to use, particularly with a shower chair. Soap-on-a-rope can be hung from the neck to avoid losing or slipping on the soap during bathing or showering. A regular cake of soap placed in a small bag made of a dishcloth with a loop of soft string attached, or a mitten with a pocket for soap can serve the same purpose. Similarly, a shower caddy may be used to store necessary articles. When bathing, a child's pool raft or a small air mattress can be floated in the tub and the necessary items placed on it. A raised toilet seat, available in medical and surgical supply stores, can be easily installed. Storage shelves should be adjusted to a convenient height.

Dressing Aids

A long-handled shoe horn, hairbrush, comb, toothbrush, or bath sponge can be useful. A ring, or a cord about 18 in. long with a metal hook at the end, can be attached to a zipper. A boot jack, elastic shoelaces, front closure bra, and button hooks are examples of other useful objects for patients with limited ROM of hand or arm joints.

Low Vision Aids (see also Chs. 21 and 93)

Many persons with low vision tend toward depression and avoidance of reading or writing. However, the continuing use of the eyes helps prevent further deterioration of vision.

Hand-held magnifiers (with or without a light attachment) are often used by mildly or moderately impaired individuals, and a concave magnifying mirror may be useful for grooming. Eyeglasses and telescopic lenses, which may be permanently attached to the upper part of the eyeglasses, are available to supplement poor vision. Large-print newspapers, magazines, and books (eg, the *New York Times* and *Reader's Digest*) are also available. Talking books are stocked by public libraries. Radio reading services and closed circuit television for those with visual impairment are also available.

Although moderate illumination is helpful for low vision, too much causes a white-out, and too little a black-out, effect. A strong contrast of light and dark on a flat floor, as in a long corridor of a hospital, may create the illusion of a step. Even lighting is important for safety. The selection of colors for a hospital or institution should consider the low vision population (pastels may please the medical staff, but be invisible to those with low vision). A door or the protruding corner of a wall should be painted with a high contrast color for easy recognition.

Blindness

Rehabilitation involves (1) training the other senses; (2) training in skills and the use of devices; (3) restoring psychologic security; and (4) assistance in meeting and influencing the attitudes of others.

The patient must learn to develop skill, confidence, and grace in walking and traveling, become familiar with a new means of spatial orientation, read and write in braille, and develop conversational skills to overcome mannerisms in facial and physical expression. During rehabilitation training, group discussions are extremely useful to share experiences, difficulties, frustrations, fears, and other feelings.

Family members or friends who are very close to the blind individual should receive training in how to live with a blind person. Sighted persons should speak to the blind person directly rather than to a third person; while walking, they should not hold the blind person, but let him hold onto their forearm so that he can feel the environment through this touch.

SPEECH THERAPY

Speech pattern of the healthy elderly includes a shift to lower frequencies in vocal pitch, voice tremor, laryngeal tension, air loss, imprecise consonant production, and slow rate of articulation. Apparently healthy elderly may show a reduced amount of vocabulary, disturbance of prosody, and a tendency to make semantic errors.

Aphasia

An impairment in interpretation or formulation of language symbols. Speech and language functions are mediated by the left brain hemisphere in about 93% of the general population and aphasia occurs in about 40% of patients with strokes in the left hemisphere. Aphasia may be fluent, nonfluent, or global.

Prognosis and treatment: Recovery from aphasia generally continues for 1 to 2 yr after stroke onset. The goal of speech therapy is to establish the most effective individual means of communication. While direct treatment with drills and repetitive practice is not effective for severely involved patients, a communication book with photographs and pictures can be very useful. A moderately severe to mildly aphasic patient may benefit by the stimulation approach (repetitive presentation of linguistic stimuli) and the programmed approach (a learning process for reacquisition of language behavior). A context-centered approach that emphasizes ideas and thoughts rather than words is very effective for mildly aphasic patients.

Home treatment: The patient's family and close friends can provide indispensable therapy at home, although they may experience enormous stress, frustration, and even anger. The physician and speech pathologist should, therefore, provide the following guidance:

(1) Recognize that the patient is not mentally ill.

(2) Be extremely patient at all times.

(3) Use simple sentences; verbal stimulation is the best treatment.

(4) Treat the patient as an adult, with respect and understanding; do not use baby language.

(5) Do not leave the patient alone.

(6) Avoid stressful situations.

(7) Use gestures and point to objects as a supplement to speaking.

(8) Phrase questions so that the patient can answer "yes" or "no," by nodding or shaking the head.

(9) No matter how long it takes, do not cut the patient off or interject.

Dysarthria

A group of speech abnormalities resulting from disturbances in muscular control due to damage of the central or peripheral nervous system, resulting in weakness, slowness in response, or incoordination of the speech mechanism. Dysarthria is the second most common communication disorder in elderly patients. It may be flaccid, spastic, ataxic, hypokinetic, hyperkinetic, or mixed, and may involve several or all of the basic mechanical processes of speech (respiration, phonation, resonance, articulation, and prosody).

Treatment: Patients recovering from an acute neurologic episode (eg, stroke, head trauma, or surgery) must first develop the motor skills necessary for speech production under the guidance of a speech pathologist.

The treatment strategy for dysarthria due to progressive neurologic disease is quiet different. During the early phase of the disease, the patient is encouraged to maintain premorbid function as long as possible. As the disease progresses, the patient will begin to experience various dysarthric speech patterns and must modify his speech to control rate, consonant emphasis, and articulation. Some patients may acquire such adjustment without practice. In very advanced cases, an augmentative communication system may be required.

Apraxia

A disorder of articulation due to impairment in the sequencing of muscle movements for the volitional production of phonemes. There is no significant muscle weakness, slowness, or incoordination in reflex and automatic acts. Prosodic alterations may occur. Apraxia may occur in patients with brain damage due to stroke, head injury, or surgery.

Treatment: Melodic intonation therapy (the use of natural melody patterns to facilitate speech) may be used when a patient has a nonfluent aphasia with apraxia. However, if the patient has poor auditory comprehension and error recognition, this therapy cannot be used. Intensive practice of sound patterns and speech is an alternative approach.

Rehabilitation After Laryngectomy

While a patient with a partial laryngectomy may have only an alteration in voice quality, a total laryngectomy results in a patient who is barely able to whisper. Such a patient has 3 options: reconstructive surgery (pseudoglottis or shunt), esophageal speech, or electrolarynx. Esophageal speech requires the patient to take air into the esophagus and expel it forcefully, causing a vibration in the upper narrow portion of the esophagus. The articulation technics are the same as those for normal speech. However, not every patient can master esophageal speech. While some may be candidates for an electrolarynx, others may object to its artificial sound. The Lost Chord Club, sponsored by the American Cancer Society, and other groups provide invaluable emotional support.

CARDIOVASCULAR REHABILITATION

(See also Ch. 25)

The ultimate goal of cardiac rehabilitation is restoring the patient to an independent life-style within his physical capability.

Physical activity is proportional to O_2 used, and can be expressed in metabolic equivalents **(METs)**. One MET is the metabolic O_2 consumption under basal conditions (about 3.5 mL O_2/kg/min). Under normal conditions of working and living, excluding recreation, metabolic demand rarely exceeds 6 METs. Various daily activities can be classified according to MET requirement (see TABLE 25-5 in Ch. 25).

For those in poor physical condition due to physical inactivity, prolonged bed rest, or illness, the maximum working capacity of the heart is greatly reduced. Restoring cardiac reserve is especially important following acute MI (see also Ch. 32), and is just as essential in elderly as in younger patients. Activity should be minimal immediately after MI onset, then increased gradually. Although mortality and morbidity are greater, most older patients are able to resume their previous physical activities.

Each patient responds differently to the stress of a severe illness, and the rehabilitation program must therefore be individualized. Typical programs begin with light activities of 1 to 2 METs' intensity and progress during the course of hospitalization to moderate activities of 4 to 5 METs' intensity under the supervision of a physical therapist or occupational therapist. A 2-METs exercise test may be performed about 1 week after an uncomplicated MI to evaluate progress; an exercise test of 4 to 5 METs prior to discharge helps guide physical activities at home.

The maximum allowable workload for each functional class of cardiac patient (New York Heart Association classification) is shown in TABLE 23-3. During hospitalization, all physical activities should be controlled to keep the heart rate below 60% of maximum for the patient's age and, during the home recovery period, below 70% of maximum for age (eg, at age 60, the maximum heart rate is about 160/min).

Absolute contraindications for exercise include any condition associated with increased risk for sudden death; eg, unstable angina pectoris,

TABLE 23-3. NEW YORK HEART ASSOCIATION CLASSIFICATION OF SUSTAINED AND INTERMITTENT WORK LOADS

Functional Classification	Physiologic Symptoms	Maximal Cal/Min		Maximal METs
		Sustained	Intermittent	
I	Patients with cardiac disease but without resulting limitations of physical activity: ordinary physical activity does not cause undue fatigue, palpitation, dyspnea, or anginal pain.	5.0	6.5	6.5
II	Patients with cardiac disease resulting in slight limitation of physical activity: they are comfortable at rest; ordinary physical activity results in fatigue, palpitation, dyspnea, or anginal pain.	2.5	4.0	4.5

(Continued)

TABLE 23-3. NEW YORK HEART ASSOCIATION CLASSIFICATION OF
SUSTAINED AND INTERMITTENT WORK LOADS *(Cont'd)*

Functional Classification	Physiologic Symptoms	Maximal Cal/Min		Maximal METs
		Sustained	Intermittent	
III	Patients with cardiac disease resulting in marked limitation of physical activity: they are comfortable at rest; less than ordinary physical activity causes fatigue, palpitation, dyspnea, or anginal pain.	2.0	2.7	3.0
IV	Patients with cardiac disease resulting in inability to carry on any physical activity without discomfort; symptoms of cardiac insufficiency or of the anginal syndrome may be present even at rest; if any physical activity is undertaken, discomfort is increased.	1.5	2.0	1.5

(From "Cardiac Rehabilitation," by S. S. Karwal, in *Current Therapy in Physiatry. Physical Medicine and Rehabilitation,* edited by A. P. Ruskin. Copyright 1984 by W. B. Saunders Company. Used with permission of W. B. Saunders Company.)

ventricular arrhythmias, or heart failure. Relative contraindications include moderate aortic stenosis or uncontrolled supraventricular arrhythmia.

To assess endurance, the patient can undergo a standardized test using the hand or bicycle ergometer or treadmill. MET requirements should be closely regulated by changing the ergometer load or treadmill speed and grade. Test duration should be 6 min and heart rate should not exceed 70% of maximum for the patient's age; continuous ECG monitoring should be done during the entire course of the test.

If a patient demonstrates any significant symptoms or signs of cardio-respiratory decompensation during exercise, the exercise should be stopped immediately; reassessment of cardiac status and modification or temporary suspension of the exercise program is indicated.

A patient who can tolerate a 5-METs exercise test for 6 min can safely perform all sedentary activities at home, but must have sufficient rest between activities. After discharge, he should be given a detailed home activity program.

Common problems during the home recovery period include emotional stress and an overly cautious patient and family. The result may be physical inactivity, which is detrimental to recovery. It is therefore important for the physician and other health care workers to provide sufficient psychologic support.

Although geriatric patients seldom mention sexual relations, the physician should give appropriate advice. As a guide, young couples expend 5 to 6 METs during active intercourse (see also Ch. 58).

REHABILITATION AFTER STROKE

Recovery of function: There are 2 distinct recovery processes after cerebrovascular accident **(CVA).** The neurologic or natural recovery occurs in varying degrees, depending on the mechanism of the stroke (ie, thrombotic, embolic, or hemorrhagic) and the location and size of the lesion. In general, the smaller the lesion, the better the recovery. About 90% of recovery usually occurs within 3 mo. The remaining 10% occurs much more slowly. Recovery from a hemorrhagic CVA is particularly slow, and often a complete neurologic recovery cannot be expected.

The second type of recovery is improvement in functional performance, irrespective of neurologic recovery, through the application of various therapeutic modalities. Some modalities, eg, proprioceptive neuromuscular facilitation (see above), may assist in neurologic recovery.

Rehabilitation potential depends on general condition, joint range of motion, muscle strength of both the affected and sound side of the body, bowel and bladder function, premorbid functional ability, social situation (including prospects of returning to the community), ability to participate in a rehabilitation regimen under the supervision of nurses and therapists, learning ability, motivation, and coping skills.

Efficient assessment depends on a rehabilitation team that, with the physician, formulates goals and target completion dates for the patient and family. It is common, even after careful explanation, for the patient and family to have unrealistic goals. The physician should not raise false hope, but should explain the patient's prospects as gently and positively as possible to avoid undue depression.

Early care: The rehabilitation program should be started as early as possible, even before assessment can be completed. This may prevent secondary disabilities and help avoid depression.

Passive ROM exercise should be applied to affected joints (see below). With hemiplegia, 1 or 2 pillows should be placed under the affected upper extremity to prevent dislocation of the shoulder joint. A posterior foot splint, in a 90° ankle dorsiflexed position, should be applied to prevent an equinus deformity and foot drop. The patient may be incontinent and have sensory paralysis at this stage, with high risk of decubitus ulcers *that must be prevented* (see Ch. 13).

Sitting up: A patient can safely begin sitting up when fully conscious and without further progression of neurologic deficits, usually within 48 h of the stroke. If there is upper limb involvement, while the limb remains flaccid, a well-constructed sling should be provided so that the weight of the arm and hand does not overstretch the deltoid muscle with subluxation of the shoulder joint.

Transfer activity: Regaining the ability to get out of bed and transfer to a chair or wheelchair independently has a very positive psychologic impact. However, in addition to motor and sensory paralysis, the patient may also have incoordination, dyspraxia, visual field defect, and impaired judgment and planning, making this activity very difficult. Patience and close supervision by the therapist are mandatory until the patient can transfer safely.

Therapeutic exercise: During the initial rehabilitation period when the involved extremities are still flaccid, passive ROM is given, through the normal range, 3 to 4 times in each joint once/day, at the patient's bedside.

After 1 wk, if progress is good, reeducation and coordination exercises of the involved upper and lower extremities should be added. Active exercise without fatigue of the extremities on the sound side must also be encouraged. Various ADLs can be performed; eg, movement in bed—turning, changing position, or sitting up.

After another week, active and assistive exercise of the involved extremities should be started to maintain ROM and, if indicated, to increase muscle strength. In hemiplegics, the most important muscle for ambulation is the quadriceps on the sound side. If weak, this muscle should be strengthened to the level of good or better.

Resistive exercise for hemiplegic extremities is controversial, as it may encourage an increase in spasticity. The therapist should observe muscle activity carefully since the appearance of spasticity is insidious; *if present, resistive exercise should not be given.*

Standing exercise is safest using the parallel bars. If an elderly hemiplegic cannot stand after 3 or 4 days of attempts with assistance, the height of the chair or wheelchair seat should be increased (eg, using firm cushions). Once the patient can stand from an elevated seat, its height may be gradually decreased. The distance between the patient's feet should be 6 in. or more, while holding onto the bar with the sound hand. If the hemiplegic upper extremity is flaccid, a sling must be worn (see above). To correct bad posture, the patient must stand with hips and knees fully extended, leaning slightly forward and toward the sound side. Hemiplegic patients are subject to vertigo and must change body position slowly when standing up or turning. After standing, there should be a pause before walking.

Ambulation exercise: Once the patient can stand up and balance safely, ambulation exercise can be started. It is safest to begin on the parallel bars, even if hemiplegia is mild. The patient must first stand up straight, lean toward the sound side, and take a step with the bad leg. The therapist should always be on the patient's hemiplegic side so that if balance is lost, assistance will be available.

The patient should be reminded to take a shorter step with the hemiplegic leg and a longer step with the sound leg. When the patient first begins to walk outside the confines of the parallel bars, the therapist must physically assist and later supervise ambulation. The cane should be heavy to provide proprioceptive feedback through the hand. During the training period, a weight of 2 to 5 lb may be attached to a tripod or quadripod cane, then gradually decreased. The cane handle should be large enough in diameter to accommodate an osteoarthritic hand.

Most hemiplegics exhibit some abnormality of gait (eg, the intermittent double-step gait, which may sometimes be desirable since it is safer than the alternate gait). If the patient can ambulate safely, there should not be much gait pattern correction. The hemiplegic patient should walk with the affected side close to a wall, which can provide support and prevent a fall.

The patient may drag the hemiplegic leg during the swing phase because of weakness in the hip flexors or foot drop caused by weak ankle dorsiflexors or spastic plantar flexors. In the last case, an equinus deformity may develop, producing a circumduction or abduction gait on the hemiplegic side. A strengthening exercise to the hip flexors may be indicated. Foot drop can be corrected with a short leg brace.

Spasticity may or may not be beneficial for ambulation. Slightly spastic knee extensors can lock the knee during the stance phase but spastic knee extensors cause hyperextension or genu recurvatum; a knee brace with an extension stop may be necessary. When resistance is applied to spastic plantar flexors, ankle clonus is seen; a short leg brace *without* a spring mechanism should minimize this.

Stair-climbing: The basic principle of elevation exercise, "good is up and bad is down," can also be applied to the stroke patient. The railing or banister should ideally be on the patient's sound side while ascending the stairs so that he can guide himself with the sound hand on the railing. The patient should not look up the staircase since this may cause vertigo. While descending, the hemiplegic side should be against the railing and a cane used.

Preventing falls: The most common accident is a fall, usually explained by the patient as "my knees gave way." If muscle strength, particularly of the trunk and lower extremity, shows deficiency, initial strengthening exercises must be performed. Other common causes of falls at this phase include vertigo on standing or orthostatic hypotension. Use of the tilt table or increasing the length of time the patient should sit on the edge of the bed with feet dangling will help restore normal hemodynamics. Since the patient's balance when sitting may be poor, a therapist or nurse must be present. Slipping is another common cause of falls. The floor of the patient's room should be dry and not highly waxed. The patient should wear shoes with rubber soles and heels (women's heels no higher than 3/4 in.).

Other Problems

Hemianopsia: The patient should be made aware of his deficit and receive a clear explanation. He must be taught to move his head toward the hemiplegic side when scanning.

Hemiplegic upper extremity: While even minimal motor recovery of the lower extremity allows ambulation, upper extremity function requires considerable motor and sensory capacity for fine coordination.

Although bilateral activities are used commonly, their effectiveness is controversial. Neuromuscular reeducation, including electric stimulation (see above), has been applied with variable success. Proprioceptive neuromuscular facilitation may also be useful (see above).

Heat or cold can temporarily decrease spasticity and allow stretching of the muscles or the application of strengthening antagonists (see above). Drugs (eg, diazepam or methocarbamol) are of limited value.

Most hemiplegic hands and wrists exhibit flexor spasticity. Unless frequent passive ROM exercises are given several times a day, flexion contracture may develop rapidly, resulting in pain and difficulty in maintaining personal hygiene. Any discomfort, pain in the hand, or even emotional upset can increase muscle tone or spasticity in the lower extremity and thus interfere with ambulation. A hand or wrist splint may also be useful, but should be easy to apply and to clean.

REHABILITATION AFTER HIP FRACTURE

(See also Chs. 8 and 24)

Postsurgical Rehabilitation

Appropriate therapeutic exercise for the noninvolved extremities, eg, PRE or stretching (see above), should be started as soon after surgery as possible if there is any muscle weakness or less than functional ROM, to allow weight bearing and support when using parallel bars, crutches, or canes. At first, the patient should be allowed only isometric exercise for the involved limb, keeping it in a fully extended position. At no time should a pillow be placed under the knee, as it may cause flexion contracture of the hip and knee. Later, gradual mobilization of the affected limb should lead to full ambulation. Prosthetic replacement usually requires less rehabilitation and has a better functional outcome than nail- or pin-and-plate fixation. As a guide, ambulatory exercises should begin between 6 and 10 days postoperatively, and stair climbing after about 11 days.

When the patient rises to stand from a sitting position, he exerts considerable stress on the head of the femur, and so should hold onto the arm of a chair or a table.

An occupational therapist should analyze the patient's home needs and offer training in special activities; eg, the transfer of a heavy pot from the kitchen to the dining table. If a cane is used, the pot cannot be carried with both hands. Placing the pot on a utility cart allows the patient to push it like a walker and dispense with the cane.

Before returning home, the patient should learn how to perform daily exercises to strengthen the trunk muscles and quadriceps of the involved leg. Any prolonged lifting or pushing of heavy items, or stooping, reaching, or jumping can be harmful. Sitting on a chair (particularly a low one) for a prolonged period should be avoided, and the chair arm should be used for support when standing up. While sitting, the patient should keep the legs uncrossed, as this can also be harmful. When walking, the mechanical stress does not differ greatly with the use of 2 canes as compared to 1 and may interfere with certain ADLs.

Rehabilitation When Surgery Is Contraindicated

Nonsurgical treatment is generally associated with poor functional prognosis. During immobilization (usually at least 6 to 8 wk), it is important to prevent secondary disabilities; eg, decubitus ulcers, disuse atrophy of muscles, joint contractures, and general deconditioning.

On mobilization, the patient should undergo a restorative process similar to that following surgery, but much slower and preceded by general conditioning exercises.

Approaches to weight bearing: (1) Some physicians advocate that no weight bearing should be permitted unless there is x-ray evidence of bony union. However, union is rarely detected within 8 wk, and usually cannot be detected for at least 10 to 12 wk after injury. (2) Others suggest comparison of x-ray findings under nonweight- and weight-bearing conditions. If no change is found, weight bearing can proceed. (3) The patient often begins weight bearing, even if told not to, as soon as there is no discomfort. Relying on the patient's perception seems more reasonable than basing a decision solely on x-ray findings.

REHABILITATION AFTER LOWER EXTREMITY AMPUTATION

Preoperative preparation: The physician must explain the prosthesis, the rehabilitation program, and the functional prognosis to the patient. Psychologic counseling may be indicated. An elderly amputee, walking with a prosthesis after successful rehabilitation, can visit the preoperative patient to share experiences. A similar visit by a wheelchair-bound amputee may be arranged for the patient who is not a candidate for prosthetic training.

Postoperative care: The most important aim during the immediate and late postoperative period is to prevent secondary disabilities, especially contractures. Flexion contracture of hip or knee may develop rapidly after surgery and would make prosthetic fitting difficult, if not impossible, and the amputee would have poor control of the prosthesis. Exercises for general conditioning, stretching of the hip and knee, and strengthening of all extremities are important. Endurance exercises may also be prescribed.

The elderly amputee should begin standing and balancing exercises on parallel bars as early as possible.

Preprosthetic care: Stump conditioning assists the natural process of shrinking. All stumps must be formed into a conical shape, and an elastic stump shrinker or ACE™ bandages are applied and maintained on a 24-h basis. While an elastic stump shrinker is easy to apply, ACE™ bandages may be preferred because the amount and location of pressure can be controlled. The disadvantage of the ACE™ bandage is the frequent need to reapply it whenever it becomes loose. After a few days of stump conditioning, rapid shrinkage may be seen. It is essential to avoid edema in the stump.

Early ambulation with a pylon or temporary prosthesis not only makes the amputee active, but also accelerates stump shrinkage, prevents development of flexion contracture, and reduces phantom pain. The socket of the pylon is made of plaster of Paris and should fit the stump snugly. Various temporary prostheses with adjustable sockets are commercially available. Ambulation can start on the parallel bars and the patient can progress to walking with crutches or canes until a permanent prosthesis becomes available. It is useful to observe the patient's cardiac and respiratory responses to prosthetic ambulation.

The prosthesis must be lightweight and meet the needs and safety requirements of the amputee. Providing a perfect prosthetic fit is an art. If the prosthesis is made too soon, the stump may have shrunk beyond the size initially measured, and adjustments may be required to satisfy the patient and produce a good gait pattern. For most geriatric below-the-knee (BK) amputees, the patella tendon bearing (PTB) prosthesis with a solid ankle cushion heel **(SACH)** foot and suprapatellar cuff suspension is best. Unless there is a special reason, a standard BK prosthesis with thigh corset and waist belt is not prescribed because of its weight and bulkiness.

Stump care and prosthesis maintenance: While a PTB prosthesis wearer has the fewest problems with ambulation, a number of gait variations have been recognized in above-the-knee (AK) prosthesis wearers. The causes may be medical, surgical, prosthetic, psychologic, or related to inadequate training. The examiner must observe ambulation carefully and repeatedly, since there is often more than one variation.

Especially when ascending or descending stairs, an elderly amputee should always use an ambulation aid, eg, crutches or a cane.

The most common complaint is pain in the stump. When phantom pain (see below) and other conditions can be ruled out, an ill-fitting socket is usually the cause. The socket may be too small, the stump may be edematous, or the patient may have gained weight.

The patient should be instructed in **stump hygiene.** Since a lower extremity prosthesis is a device only for ambulation, an amputee should never wear it while sleeping; otherwise severe dermatitis may develop and result in prolonged loss of use of the prosthesis. Before the patient goes to bed, the stump should be inspected thoroughly (with a mirror, if the patient is inspecting it alone), washed with a mild soap and warm water, and dried thoroughly, using talcum powder. If the skin is too dry, lanolin or petrolatum may be used. If the stump perspires excessively, a commercially available antiperspirant may be applied. Any skin inflammation must be treated immediately. If there is an opening on the skin, the prosthesis should not be used until the wound has healed. The stump sock and ACE™ bandage should be changed daily, washed with mild soap, and dried completely before wearing.

A prosthesis is neither waterproof nor water resistant. Therefore, if even a part of it becomes wet, it must be dried immediately and thoroughly; however, heat should not be used.

The prosthesis, especially the socket, should be cleaned daily, first with a slightly moist cloth to remove any dust, then with a dry cloth. To prevent fungal growth and subsequent infection of the stump, mild soap may be used for cleaning the inside of the socket. When an AK prosthesis is not in use, it should be placed on the floor to avoid breakage.

Wheelchairs: *An elderly amputee should have an "amputee wheelchair."* During the night, it is too bothersome to put on a prosthesis, and the use of crutches without a prosthesis may be unsafe. At other times (eg, due to the condition of the stump) the patient may not be able to use the prosthesis. Moreover, even if he is independent in ambulation for ADL purposes, walking long distances may be too difficult, or inadvisable. Finally, most patients undergoing unilateral lower extremity amputation due to peripheral vascular insufficiency become bilateral amputees within 5 yr.

The **amputee wheelchair** compensates for the loss of lower extremity weight, with a longer distance between the wheel axes to prevent tilting. With proper maintenance, such a wheelchair will probably last 5 to 10 yr.

Phantom Limb, Phantom Pain, and Painful Stump

Phantom limb, *a painless awareness of the amputated part possibly accompanied by mild tingling,* is experienced by almost every new amputee. The sensation can be so vivid that some amputees can describe the position of the foot, which is often very closely related to its position at the time of amputation. This sensation may last from several months to several years, but will eventually disappear without treatment. The sensation is frequently incomplete, as many patients sense only the foot, which also is the last phantom sensation to disappear. The phantom limb sensation is not harmful, unless an amputee, without thinking, attempts to stand up with both legs and falls.

Phantom pain in the lost part is very disagreeable. A painful condition prior to amputation carries a greater risk of phantom pain. Various treatments, such as simultaneous bilateral "exercise" of the phantom and of the contralateral normal limb, massage of the stump, percussion of the stump with fingers, use of mechanical devices (eg, a vibrator), and ultrasound have been reported effective.

A **painful stump** involves mild to severe pain on palpation, or when the use of a pylon or prosthesis is introduced. This pain is localized and totally different from phantom pain. The most common causes of painful stump are either a painful amputation neuroma or spur formation at the amputated end of the bone. An amputation neuroma is usually palpable, but this is extremely painful for the patient. Spur formation may be diagnosed by palpation and x-ray examination. **Treatments** include injection of corticosteroids or analgesics to the neuroma or in the surrounding area, application of cryotherapy, or continuous 24-h tight bandaging of the stump. The most effective modality is daily ultrasound treatment for 5 to 10 sessions. The results of surgical resection of the neuroma are often disappointing. The only effective treatment of spur formation is surgical resection.

Follow-up Care

A patient who successfully completes the program of prosthetic rehabilitation and returns to the community should be followed q 3 to 6 mo for the first 2 yr. The stump usually continues to shrink with use. Eventually (usually within the first 2 yr) the stump will become too small and a new socket will be necessary. Because of continuous use, various components of the prosthesis may deteriorate, possibly resulting in a gait variation. The circulatory status of the sound leg should be examined at follow-up, as this leg should be kept intact as long as possible. If it eventually requires amputation, ideally this should be a **BK** amputation.

Bilateral Amputation

The functional prognosis for a bilateral lower extremity amputee will depend on cardiopulmonary capacity and the level of the amputation. A bilateral BK amputee, even if elderly, usually can manage 2 prostheses fairly well. In contrast, almost all bilateral AK geriatric amputees are unable to ambulate with prostheses because they cannot meet the energy and strength requirements. The functional prognosis for those with a combination of AK and BK amputations differs greatly. When such an amputee walks with prostheses, the BK side becomes the functional leg and a manual knee lock may sometimes be required on the AK prosthesis. A pair of canes or crutches must be provided for a bilateral amputee during ambulation, and even with 2 prostheses, the walking distance is limited. A wheelchair must be used outdoors or for walking a long distance.

24. OCCUPATIONAL THERAPY

Gail Hills Maguire

Occupational therapy **(OT)** is concerned primarily with effecting a change in "occupational" behavior, defined as *a person's autonomous decision making, use of time, energy, attention, habits, and skills in self-care, rest, play, and work activities.* An imbalance or problem in performing ≥ 1 of these tasks, or occupations, is seen as a dysfunction needing remediation through OT.

Services offered by OT include the following: (1) training in activities of daily living **(ADLs)** (eg, eating, bathing, grooming, dressing, homemaking); (2) application of therapeutically designed or adapted activities (eg, crafts or games); (3) application of sensorimotor activities; (4) design, fabrication, and application of splints, braces, and other devices intended to improve function; (5) selected applications of exercise; (6) analysis, selection, and use of adaptive equipment; (7) cognitive retraining; (8) individual and group psychosocial intervention; and (9) adaptation of the psychosocial and physical environment, including architectural barriers.

The occupational therapist analyzes, designs, and adapts specific occupational tasks or performance methods for individual needs. Depending on the problem, the patient might need only 1 or 2 OT sessions, or might need to be seen over a period of months. For example, an elderly patient with RA might be seen for evaluation and training in dressing and grooming and for advice on adaptive equipment. In homemaking activities, the patient might be shown joint conservation technics (eg, optimal ways to hold heavy objects, how to use 2 hands rather than 1 to relieve joint strain, and how to minimize movement that causes ulnar drift of the hands). The patient might be fitted with static hand splints to wear while sleeping and wrist support splints to wear during the day. An elderly mentally ill patient scheduled for transfer to a group home following hospitalization might attend a life-skills program to practice socially acceptable behavior.

Factors such as age, sex, and culture are considered in designing occupational tasks, since these variables affect specific activities. For example, a quadriplegic patient who is a student might require a writing splint to take lecture notes, while a retired individual might be more concerned about learning a skill to occupy free time. Unlike physical or mental tasks that are done as isolated exercises or passively performed by a therapist for a patient, a therapeutically designed activity integrates mental and physical functioning. A patient may practice the separate components of transfer from a bed to a chair by doing a standing transfer, but actually moving to the edge of the bed, leaning forward, standing, pivoting, grasping the chair, and easing himself into the chair as one activity, requires much more coordination and motor planning.

Patients must collaborate in setting treatment goals, ultimately aiming to achieve autonomy of self-management. Therapists provide guidance in how to make the best use of patients' remaining abilities, thereby enabling them to achieve their personal goals.

Education and Training of Therapists

The professional education of the occupational therapist, registered **(OTR)**, covers theories of OT, kinesiology, basic sciences (eg, human anatomy, physiology), pathology, neurology, psychiatry, human development (including gerontology), self-care, adaptive homemaking, and therapeutic technics (eg, splinting). Evaluation of a patient's functional level and analysis and modification of occupational tasks to individual needs are emphasized. This education is documented by a certification examination, followed by state licensure, where required.

Certified OT assistants **(COTAs)** evaluate, plan, and implement OT programs under the direct supervision of an OTR. Assistants may supervise activity program personnel with lesser training (eg, arts and crafts instructors or activity aides). COTAs who have graduated from an accredited program must pass a certification exam, and licensures where required.

Occupational Therapy and the Elderly

The goals of OT for elderly individuals are similar to those for younger patients. However, the elderly need assistance in adapting to aging processes such as reduced vision, hearing, and physical endurance, as well as to specific disabilities (eg, stroke or hip fracture). Furthermore, elderly patients are more likely to have ≥ 1 chronic conditions in addition to the illness or disability that precipitated the need for the current therapy.

The therapist evaluates the impact of aging, disease, and social change on all the activities of the elderly patient before designing a specific program to modify behavior, environment, or both. Teaching a hemiplegic patient who has high muscle tone and limited motion in the affected extremities to dress from a seated position, with the affected upper extremity extended and the affected lower extremity flexed in order to reduce tone, is an example of adapted behavior. Recommending use of equipment such as a long-handled shoehorn and elastic shoe laces is an example of modifying both behavior and the environment. Recommending installation of grab bars at the toilet and bathtub areas and the removal of scatter rugs, without changing the way a person transfers or ambulates, are examples of modifying the environment.

Care in an institution: Hospitals and other institutions are traditional areas of OT service and offer the most sophisticated OT practice in geriatrics. The need for services to the frail elderly in long-term care facilities is increasing. OTs may provide direct services or consultation. In the role of consultant, the therapist makes recommendations but does not give direct supervision or treatment. The patient can accept or reject the recommendations.

Services in institutions include treatment to increase strength, range of motion, cognitive-perceptual-motor skills, constructive use of time through meaningful activities, and independence in ADLs. Treatment is programmed according to the goals established for individual patients or groups.

Treatment goals for terminally ill patients are similar to those for other patients, except that the former may need assistance in relinquishing particular tasks and roles for which they no longer have sufficient strength and energy.

Treatment for psychosocial dysfunction may include resocialization and occupational skills training as needed to reenter the community or function in an institution. Such training includes performing worker or volunteer role activities, maintaining good hygiene and grooming, practicing sound financial management, being on time, and maintaining safety.

Example: A rehabilitative OT approach in a hospital for an 87-yr-old woman with osteoarthritis, who suffered a fracture of the neck of the femur treated by a total joint replacement, might include the following plan. She would be evaluated in performance of ADLs, including grooming, dressing, and a review of her role as a home manager. To prevent falling, the patient would be taught to dress herself while sitting in a chair, rather than on the edge of the bed. She would be taught how to put on stockings and shoes with the assistance of a sock aide and a long-handled shoehorn. After transfer to an extended-care facility to continue her rehabilitation, OT would recommend installation of grab bars and training in toilet and tub transfers and would provide training in homemaking skills, using an ambulation aid such as a walker recommended by PT and joint-conservation technics for her arthritis.

Prior to the patient's discharge, the therapist would make a home visit and recommend the following changes: Remove scatter rugs from living and dining rooms, bathroom, and kitchen. Install grab bars in the bathroom. Provide a dining cart with a handle and large wheels to transport items from the kitchen to the dining table. Provide a stool with a back to use at the stove or kitchen counter. Remove storage items from the small table in the kitchen and relocate the table so it could be used as a sitting work area. Rearrange items in kitchen cabinets so they are within easy reach.

Hip fractures are common in the elderly and constitute a significant health hazard. While the acute care phase of treatment is generally good, therapy may be discontinued before patients reach their highest level of independence, leading to further and unnecessary deterioration. Because of declining abilities and fear that they may be "failing," older patients often generalize their sense of dependency to include areas of life not directly affected by the current medical problem (eg, limitation in ambulation may be extended to decision making in financial affairs).

In the example described above, maintenance OT activities in the extended-care facility would include working on an activity independently and preparing to resume previously important roles, such as home manager and church member. Prior to her fall, this patient was agitated and depressed over the death of her daughter and had ceased all activities except watching television and overeating. The occupational therapist helped the patient begin a needlepoint project, which the patient then worked on independently. She also was taught to plan low-calorie menus, using the diet designed for her by the dietitian. The patient then independently planned meals, which she prepared during her homemaking sessions, using methods and equipment adapted during therapy sessions in the kitchen, where she would also practice using her walker. She was encouraged to contact her church to arrange a ride to services and to a weekly work session.

Home health care: Occupational therapists who see older persons in their homes usually require a physician referral and plan the treatment in conjunction with other health team members. Because of health care coverage regulations, many referrals are for continued rehabilitation following hospitalization for an acute condition or a new episode of an existing condition. A system of referral, evaluation, goal setting, treatment, and documentation, similar to that in an institution, is used. Areas of concentration include evaluation and treatment of dysfunction in self-care, cognition, sensorimotor abilities, strength, range of motion, and endurance. Working in the patient's home rather than the OT department is often less efficient or convenient but has the advantage of providing a more realistic assessment of needs. The therapist usually visits 1 to 3 times/wk, and the effectiveness of treatment often depends on the patient's ability and motivation as well as the cooperation of family members or the available social support system.

Occupational therapy for the well elderly in the community is less well structured than direct service to the impaired elderly, mainly because of a lack of sources for reimbursement for OT services and a lack of recognition of need by the general public. Services to this population focus on the functional abilities of older individuals and the supportive services that will enable them to remain in the community. They include consultation to improve safety in the home and increased ease of functioning and referral for equipment or appropriate specific services. The occupational therapist working in this capacity usually does not require a physician's referral but accepts referrals from the patient, family, friends, social workers, or similar sources. This type of OT can have a profound impact on a large number of individuals and their families at minimal financial cost to society. An assessment often can determine dysfunctions that can be substantially improved by occasional, limited intervention by an occupational therapist. Training can be provided for energy conservation, joint protection, compensation for visual and hearing losses, reduction of safety hazards, and removal of architectural barriers. Such assistance can help people stay in their own home and maintain the highest possible quality of life.

Indirect service to older persons is also less well developed than therapy for the impaired elderly but is growing steadily. Occupational therapists can make unique contributions through consultation, education, and political action on the federal, state, and local levels on such issues as maintaining a balance between work and play, enhancing the environment in the community and the home, and maintaining maximum autonomy and functional independence.

The "human occupation" frame of reference for OT provides a holistic approach to consultation, assessment, and training in broad policy issues in such areas as housing, activity programs, physical and mental health care needs, preretirement and retirement planning, time management, and work specification technics.

When to Refer a Patient for Occupational Therapy

If a physician, health care worker, family member, or an elderly person himself determines or even questions whether he is as independent as possible in self-care, work, recreation, or leisure, a referral for an OT evaluation may be indicated. The occupational therapist will request a physician referral if necessary, perform an initial assessment, determine if treatment is indicated, document the findings, and recommend appropriate intervention.

---

25. EXERCISE

Mary E. Wheat and *David T. Lowenthal*

BENEFITS OF EXERCISE

IMPROVEMENTS IN FUNCTIONAL CAPACITY

Approximately 35% of noninstitutionalized persons > 65 describe themselves as having limitations in some type of activity. Some of this limitation results from chronic disabling conditions or from the aging process itself, but a substantial portion results from disuse of muscles and joints. Yet the physiologic changes associated with exercise translate into practical benefits.

Only 29% of those > 65 yr of age report doing any regular exercise, including walking. Aerobic capacity (usually limited by cardiovascular more than respiratory decline) is so low that even in normal seniors ($\geq$ 65), activities such as making beds, shopping with a light load, or dressing and undressing may use $\geq$ 50% of the average individual's maximal capacity. Since working at this intensity for several hours causes significant fatigue in persons who are not physically fit, even a small (10 to 15%) improvement in work capacity can facilitate improved functional ability, quality of life, and continued independence. The very sedentary (ie, those who do not walk outside the house or exercise), achieve greater benefit from a small increment in physical activity than do their more active counterparts.

Goals of exercise differ among subgroups of the older population as well as from those of younger populations. In those > 75 yr of age, emphasis is placed on maintenance of flexibility, strength, coordination, and balance but not on aerobic training. Walking and range-of-motion exercises are appropriate activities for previously sedentary members of this age group. In those 65 through 74 yr of age, and those ≥ 75 who have remained physically active, exercise may also include moderate aerobic conditioning. Physicians should provide individualized activity prescriptions based on a patient's previous exercise experience, current activity, general physical condition, and medical history.

OTHER BENEFITS

Exercise enhances **weight control** by increasing caloric expenditure and suppressing appetite. When exercise accompanies negative caloric balance, fat is lost and lean body mass is preserved as long as protein intake exceeds 1.2 gm/kg body weight/day. **BP declines** independently of weight reduction. Persons with diabetes mellitus, particularly type II (noninsulin-dependent), may benefit from **increased insulin sensitivity** associated with exercise-facilitated uptake of glucose by muscle.

Physical activity retards the progression of osteoporosis by **slowing the rate of bone loss,** but adequate dietary Ca (1 to 1.5 gm/day) is needed for healthy bone remodeling. **Increased muscle strength** may protect vulnerable joints (eg, quadriceps exercises improve knee function), thus enhancing overall physical ability.

Studies also suggest that **perceived well-being** and **self-image improve** with regular exercise, probably resulting from both social interaction and physical conditioning. An improvement in symptoms of depression and aspects of cognitive function, including reaction time, has also been reported. Anxiety decreases (particularly its somatic manifestations), and sleep patterns and bowel function may improve.

RISKS OF EXERCISE

The most serious adverse effects of exercise are cardiovascular, including sudden death. Although such sequelae are rare, they usually occur in persons with decreased left ventricular function and myocardial ischemia. A survey of cardiac arrests that occurred in cardiac rehabilitation centers showed a nonfatal arrest rate of 1/34,673 patient-exercise hours, with a fatal arrest rate of 1/116,402 patient-exercise hours. No comparable data exist for arrests among community-dwelling elderly excercising in nonsupervised settings. The risk of sudden death increases severalfold during vigorous exercise, but when exertion is comparable between those who exercise regularly and those who are sedentary, the former are at lower risk. Since inactivity produces its own medical complications, (eg, loss of bone mass and muscle strength), relative risks and benefits must be assessed for each individual.

The dangers of **injury from falls** and other musculoskeletal complications should be considered. Shock-absorbing shoes with traction soles (eg, running or walking shoes) are indicated for all active older persons. Proper warm-up, gentle stretching, and gradual onset of activity help reduce the incidence of injury. Most community-dwelling elderly are able to walk, however, and walking, coupled with stretching exercises, is an excellent way to maintain function and reduce the risks associated with extreme inactivity.

EVALUATION FOR EXERCISE

Preexercise screening facilitates the placement of individuals in an appropriate activity program, excluding those very few for whom any physical exertion is an unwarranted risk.

Cardiovascular training should not be an automatic goal of exercise for all older persons but is appropriate for many young-old and for those > 75 yr of age who have continued to be physically active. Assessment should include previous and current activity; cardiovascular, mental, and metabolic status; balance; and gait stability. The practitioner must be aware of subtle cognitive decline that might limit a person's ability to follow an exercise prescription, as well as sensory impairment or balance problems that could predispose one to falls.

The pertinent **history** should include the above areas, as well as respiratory symptoms, musculoskeletal complaints, and drug history (all medications plus alcohol and tobacco use). **Physical examination** should focus on visual and mental status and on the cardiovascular, pulmonary, and musculoskeletal systems, including range of motion and gait stability. The patient's walk should be observed and current physical capacity should be assessed, using either a reliable history or direct observation. Nutritional status and weight should also be evaluated. **Laboratory tests** should include a resting ECG, Hct and blood glucose studies, and urinalysis, as well as any tests indicated by the history and physical examination.

TABLE 25–1 lists common drugs having side effects that may affect an exercise program. Patients taking drugs that can cause volume depletion or orthostatic hypotension should have BP and pulse checked while both reclining and standing. Patients taking diuretics should have K levels measured. β-Adrenergic blockers do not preclude the ability to participate in or achieve the benefits of regular exercise, but the blunting of exercise-induced tachycardia must be considered in the prescription.

Persons with diabetes mellitus need to be evaluated for metabolic control, particularly for risk of hypoglycemia; those taking insulin or oral hypoglycemics should be monitored for possible dosage decreases as they increase their level of exercise. Insulin-dependent diabetics must be cautioned not to inject their insulin directly into muscle groups used in exercise, since the increased blood flow may increase insulin uptake and precipitate hypoglycemia.

TABLE 25–1. COMMON DRUGS THAT MAY AFFECT AN EXERCISE
PROGRAM

Drugs	Effects
Hypnotics	
Tranquilizers	Orthostasis and falls
Antihypertensives	
Diuretics	Hypokalemia → arrhythmias, muscle cramps
	Dehydration → orthostasis and falls, thermoregulatory disturbance
Antidepressants	Orthostasis and falls, arrhythmias
Insulin, oral hypoglycemics	Hypoglycemia
β-Adrenergic blockers	Decreased heart rate, fatigue, masking of hypoglycemic symptoms

EXERCISE STRESS TESTING

The purpose of stress testing is to identify a safe range for heart rate
(HR) during exercise, regardless of the presence or absence of coronary
artery disease. *Patients without evidence of coronary artery or other car-*
diovascular disease do not require stress testing if the planned exercise
program consists only of walking. For those who plan to do more intense
exercise or those with a history of significant cardiovascular disease,
stress testing is recommended. Some 10 to 43% of community-dwelling
persons who volunteer to participate in unsupervised exercise programs
of moderate intensity (ie, 70 to 85% of maximal heart rate) are excluded
from those programs on the basis of medical evaluation. Reasons for exclusion include active coronary artery disease or clear presence of risk
factors, severe arthritis or other musculoskeletal disability, and uncontrolled hypertension or diabetes. Of those exclusions, 70 to 80% occur
prior to stress testing.

Maximal stress testing is not required, although protocols should allow subjects to reach at least 85% of age-predicted maximal HR. Either
a treadmill or a bicycle ergometer provides a satisfactorily graded stress
under continuous electrocardiographic monitoring. Although treadmills
use walking, which is a familiar activity, many older persons experience
problems with balance, particularly as speed and grade increase. The
Balke or Naughton protocols are better tolerated than the Bruce protocol. Bicycle ergometers offer the advantage of being able to sit with
handlebar support and are an appropriate alternative for individuals
with gait or visual disorders. However, because cycling is a less common activity than walking, local muscle fatigue may impede perfor-

mance before an adequate HR is reached. Patients should continue taking their usual medications, including digitalis or β-adrenergic blockers, at the time of testing.

True **maximal stress testing** is defined as *reaching a plateau of O_2 consumption*. Predictions of maximal capacity from submaximal treadmill tests show a systematic underestimation (15 to 25%) in elderly patients. This may be partly because of reduced mechanical efficiency in sedentary elderly. Patients must be habituated to the treadmill or bicycle ergometer prior to testing, and, if possible, mechanical efficiency should be measured directly. If it cannot be measured, a lower value should be assumed in older than in younger persons (21.5 vs. 23%). Maximal HRs in North American elderly populations may exceed those assumed in common V_{O2MAX} prediction nomograms, possibly because these groups are in poorer condition than the European populations in whom the nomograms were developed.

Precise assessment of maximal capacity would increase the accuracy of the exercise prescription. However, $\geq$ 1/3 of elderly patients will not be able to meet the criterion for maximal stress testing. Furthermore, maximal tests increase the risks of testing, particularly in individuals with cardiovascular or musculoskeletal impairments. Testing to 85% of age-predicted maximal HR equals or exceeds the level of exertion recommended for exercise programs for the elderly. Electrocardiographic abnormalities (TABLE 25–2) occurring at less than 85% of age-predicted maximal HR identify those who should not exercise or who require medically supervised exercise. Indications for terminating an exercise stress test are listed in TABLE 25–2.

The Borg rating scale of perceived exertion may be used during exercise testing and fitness evaluation (see TABLE 25–3). The individual rates his perception of overall effort according to the scale. Perceived exertion and HR together predict maximal capacity more accurately than HR alone, aiding fitness evaluation and the subsequent exercise prescription.

Submaximal values (eg, HR, BP) achieved at a given work load can also be used to assess fitness and monitor the effect of exercise. As fitness improves, the HR required to reach a given level of exertion falls. Some researchers have used ratings of perceived exertion to regulate exercise intensity; however, these ratings have not proved accurate in guiding HR range at the lower work levels appropriate for older persons. One practical guideline: If a person is unable to talk comfortably while exercising, he is probably exceeding the anaerobic threshold (approximately 50% of V_{O2MAX}); ie, the person is building an O_2 debt. The pulse should be checked promptly to ascertain that it is within the training range (see below).

ST segment abnormalities during exercise stress testing are most indicative of coronary disease when they occur with angina, arrhythmias, or an abnormal BP response or at very low exertion. A high pretest likelihood of disease (history of symptoms or risk factors) also increases the test's positive predictive value. Patients who develop hypotension or sig-

TABLE 25–2. CRITERIA FOR STRESS TEST TERMINATION

Premature ventricular contractions
  Multifocal
  In pairs, with increasing frequency
  Ventricular tachycardia ($\geq$ 3 in a row)
Blood pressure
  Fall in systolic $\geq$ 10 mm Hg
  Systolic > 250 mm Hg
  Diastolic > 115 mm Hg
New-onset atrial tachycardia, fibrillation, or flutter
Second- or third-degree heart block
Angina, faintness, marked fatigue, dyspnea, nausea, pallor, confusion
Claudication or significant musculoskeletal pain
Significant ST segment depression (> 1 mm of horizontal or down-sloping ST segment
  depression at 80 msec from J point, or > 2 mm or up-sloping ST segment
  depression at 80 msec from J point)
ST segment elevation
Achievement of 85% of age-predicted maximal heart rate

(Adapted from J.D. Posner et al: "Exercise capacity in the elderly," in *American Journal of Cardiology*, Vol. 57, p. 56c, 1986. Copyright © 1986 by Cahners Publishing Company. Used with permission.)

TABLE 25–3. BORG SCALE OF PERCEIVED EXERTION

6	
7	Very, very light
8	
9	Very light
10	
11	Fairly light
12	
13	Somewhat hard
14	
15	Hard
16	
17	Very hard
18	
19	Very, very hard

(Adapted from G. Borg: "Perceived exertion as an indicator of somatic stress," *Scandinavian Journal of Rehabilitation Medicine*, Vol. 2, pp. 92-98, 1970. Used with permission of Alnqvist and Wiksell Periodical Co.)

nificant ST segment depression during the first 3 min of exercise have a substantial risk of high-level (triple-vessel or left-main) coronary disease and require prompt diagnostic follow-up. Exercise is contraindicated in such individuals until a definitive diagnosis is made and appropriately treated.

Symptoms and electrocardiographic changes occurring near maximal exertion are relative contraindications to an exercise program. Activity may still be prescribed at a lower HR, generally 75% of that at which abnormalities occurred. However, in these cases, individuals should participate initially in a medically supervised program.

Elderly persons who develop significant ST segment depression *without* chest pain or other symptoms, particularly at higher levels of exertion, constitute the most difficult diagnostic category. A substantial number of abnormal exercise stress tests (25 to 50%) occur in asymptomatic older persons, particularly women; however, 25 to 45% of these abnormal test results are normal on repeat testing, or the ST segment depression resolves with conditioning. TABLE 25–4 lists causes of false-positive stress tests.

TABLE 25–4. CAUSES OF FALSE-POSITIVE ST SEGMENT CHANGES DURING EXERCISE STRESS TESTING

Hyperventilation
Abnormal ventricular depolarization-repolarization
    Left ventricular hypertrophy
    Left-sided intraventricular conduction delays
    Wolff-Parkinson-White syndrome
Other cardiac abnormalities (valvular disease,
   asymmetric septal hypertrophy)
Vasoregulatory abnormalities
Cardiac glycosides
Hypokalemia
ST segment depression at rest

(Adapted from R.J. Shepard: "Prognostic value of exercise testing for ischemic heart disease," in *British Journal of Sports Medicine,* Vol. 16, pp. 220-229, 1982. Used with permission of the *Journal.*)

Unless the medical and family history suggests a high risk of coronary artery disease, exercise may be prescribed at an HR not to exceed 75% of that at which asymptomatic abnormalities occurred. Men and high-risk women should begin exercising in a supervised setting; low- or average-risk women may not require supervision. All should be instructed in the danger signs of ischemia (see below) and told to stop exercising and return for further evaluation if such signs occur. If the history suggests a high-risk patient or if abnormalities occur with moderate exertion, noninvasive tests, such as exercise thallium scintigraphy or exercise echocardiography, may clarify the diagnosis.

THE EXERCISE PRESCRIPTION

Exercise programs should always be individualized. For aerobic conditioning, a program that produces a training benefit in sedentary elderly persons is based on **HR reserve**, which is calculated as **maximal HR (MHR)** (220 minus age in years) minus **resting heart rate (RHR)**. A training response occurs when **30 to 45%** of the HR reserve is added to the RHR. This is the **target HR range**, approximately 65 to 80% of predicted MHR, somewhat lower than the 70 to 85% of MHR recommended by the American Heart Association for aerobic conditioning.

The target HR range for a 70-yr-old with an RHR of 84 is calculated as follows:

1. 220 − age (years) = MHR: 220 − 70 = 150

2. MHR − RHR = HR reserve: 150 − 84 = 66

3. Take 30% and 45% of HR reserve

    30% × 66 = 20   45% × 66 = 30

4. Add to RHR: 84 + (20 to 30) = 104 to 114

    Target HR range = 104 to 114

This method allows for variability in RHR. Persons who are not physically fit, who generally have a higher RHR and thus smaller HR reserve, require a smaller increment to achieve training benefit.

Individuals should palpate the radial pulse in the first 10 sec after ceasing activity (exercise HRs fall off very rapidly) and multiply by 6 to calculate their exercise HR. This should be within the target range calculated for that individual. Each person should be taught to adjust, or titrate, the intensity of exercise. If palpation indicates an HR below the training range, intensity should be increased; eg, a person who is walking should adopt a brisker pace. Conversely, if palpation indicates an HR above the target range, intensity should be reduced.

Initially, participants' calculations of their actual HR should be checked by a monitor or other trained individual. Because the pulse is checked for only a fraction of a minute, an error of a single beat is multiplied significantly.

All exercise sessions should begin with 5 to 10 min of gentle stretching and flexibility exercises of the neck, trunk, and limbs. Sitting stretches to reach the toes; neck rotation; and hamstring, quadriceps, and lateral trunk stretches are all appropriate. The person should hold the stretch for 10 sec (just beyond what is comfortable) and *refrain from bouncing;* bouncing increases muscle tension by stimulating antagonist muscles. Light limb exercises should follow. Such warm-up periods decrease musculoskeletal complications and reduce myocardial ischemia during exercise. Cool-down and flexibility exercises should be repeated at the end of the session; muscles tend to shorten during more vigorous exertion, and stretching after the workout decreases the incidence of muscle cramps. When aerobic conditioning is contraindicated, stretching and range-of-motion activities can be prescribed either alone or before and after walking.

Most studies show that an optimal training effect results from a 30-min period of increased HR 3 to 4 times/wk. Lower-intensity exercise (50 to 60% MHR) may produce a training effect if duration is extended. However, less frequent exercise is unlikely to improve fitness. Exercising > 5 times/wk increases the incidence of musculoskeletal injury; high-intensity exercise increases both musculoskeletal and cardiovascular risk.

Initially, most sedentary persons will be unable to sustain a training HR for 30 min. One should begin gradually, eg, by alternating 2 to 3 min of exercise with 2 to 3 min of recovery time over a span of 15 min. The total activity period should be increased by 2 to 3 min/wk until a total of 30 min is reached. Then the exercise interval should be increased by 1 to 2 min/wk until the target HR can be sustained for 30 min. For previously inactive persons > 75 yr of age, lower-intensity and more frequent but shorter periods of activity are advised. An appropriate goal would be 15 to 20 min of walking 6 times/wk.

The previously inactive or frail patient > 75 yr should be advised to use shorter intervals to build endurance (eg, alternate 30 sec of activity with 30 sec of rest) and to increase the activity intervals by 30 to 60 sec/wk as endurance improves. In those who are physically unfit, work capacity may be so low that aerobic conditioning occurs as the by-product of a program that would produce no training benefit in those who are more fit. Clinical signs of improved aerobic capacity include a lower RHR and decreased perceived exertion. The distance walked in 6 min can also be used to assess fitness: The patient is asked to walk a measured course (eg, up and down a 100-ft hall) for 6 min. As fitness improves, the patient is able to walk farther during the 6-min period.

Activity intensity is often expressed in **METs** *(1 MET is the O_2 expenditure at rest, about 3.5 mL/kg body weight/min)*. Maximal O_2 uptake **(MET capacity)** can be derived from stress test data. When the HR response is normal, 80% MHR corresponds to 70% of MET capacity. TABLE 25–5 shows the MET level of some common activities.

A *written* exercise prescription should detail the activity recommended for each patient, including initial intensity, duration, and frequency, and ways in which the activity should be increased as fitness improves. The prescription should include instructions to stop exercising promptly and see a physician if ischemia-related symptoms develop (eg, chest pain, marked dyspnea, dizziness, claudication, or extreme fatigue). Patients should also be told to drink ample amounts of fluid and to refrain from vigorous activity in extreme heat and cold.

Generally, jogging is inappropriate for older persons not already accustomed to this activity. Walking, cycling, dancing, and swimming all provide excellent conditioning (aerobic or otherwise), with less stress on the lower back and lower extremity joints. Physical activity should also be incorporated into a person's daily routine. For example, use of a

TABLE 25-5. METABOLIC REQUIREMENT OF COMMON ACTIVITIES

Activity	METs	kcal/h
Walking at 2–3 mph Cycling (level) at 6 mph Light stretching exercises Swimming (with float board) Light to moderate housework	2–4	180–300
Walking at 4 mph Cycling at 8 mph Golf (walking, pulling cart) Light calisthenics Swimming (treading water) Heavy housework or yard work	5–6	300–360
Walking-jogging at 5 mph Swimming (½ mile in 30 min) Cycling at 11–12 mph Recreational tennis Hiking	7–8	420–480

(Adapted from P.G. Hanson et al: "Clinical guidelines for exercise training," in *Postgraduate Medicine*, Vol. 67, No. 1, pp. 120–138, January 1980. Copyright © McGraw-Hill, Inc. Used with permission.)

shopping cart may enable a person to walk to stores rather than drive or ride, and stairs can be used rather than the elevator. James Mason, former Director of the Centers for Disease Control, has said that "marathons are not for everybody, but walking around the block probably is."

Medically supervised exercise programs can be found through hospital or cardiac rehabilitation programs, the American Heart Association, or senior-citizen groups. Persons with a history of cardiac disease and those with abnormal stress test results who still are allowed to exercise should begin programs more vigorous than walking only in a supervised setting. If no adverse effects occur, such persons may continue independently at the same intensity level after 3 to 6 mo of supervised exercise.

Very frail elderly persons, those who cannot walk several blocks without difficulty, and those with cognitive impairment precluding reliable self-monitoring also should increase activity only under supervision. If musculoskeletal symptoms of overuse occur, the activity should be stopped or changed (eg, swimming instead of jogging) until the person is pain free. If injury or illness causes a cessation of exercise for more than 1 wk, activity should be resumed at a lower intensity.

Exercise may be performed alone or with a group. Except for individuals who require supervision (generally provided in a group setting), either is appropriate. The social interaction of a group may produce psychologic gains as well as facilitate adherence to the exercise program.

Selecting an activity the individual likes, setting attainable goals, and providing encouragement and reinforcement during training and at follow-up visits also foster adherence.

With appropriate screening and individualized exercise prescription, regular physical activity can and should be incorporated into the lifestyle of older persons. Increased activity has the potential to bring major benefits in functional capacity, sense of well-being, and other improvements in health.

---

26. CARE OF THE DYING PATIENT
(See also Ch. 20)

Barbara J. Carroll and *Joanne Lynn*

Dying is not a "disease" calling for medical intervention, yet the care of the dying often is entrusted to professionals who focus on physiologic care when spiritual care is needed more. Dying is the ending of a human life, and its significance to the patient and to others is unlike that of any other experience. Finding and creating meaning in this experience is generally more important than adhering to medical routines or correcting physiologic abnormalities. The physician has at least 2 responsibilities to a dying patient: (1) to allow the patient and family to maintain control whenever possible, and (2) to provide optimal prevention and relief of symptoms.

People differ in what they consider important, especially when facing death. Some people find spiritual reward in enduring pain or disfigurement, while others consider such stressful experiences to be worse than death. Some find an appropriate time and way to bring a satisfying life to a close, while others never really make peace with their mortality. Thus, the patient's preferences and values take priority, and it is essential to know these in planning the care.

The goal of care should be to achieve the best possible future for the patient, from the patient's perspective. This means that the patient who fears dementia more than death should be treated differently from one who cherishes every moment of life, regardless of its quality. A knowledge of local law and institutional policy governing *living wills, durable powers of attorney,* and *orders against resuscitation* or hospitalization is also important to ensure that the patient's wishes are followed when he is no longer able to direct his own care (see also Chs. 99 and 100).

The goal of medical care varies in different contexts and may be (1) prevention, (2) cure, (3) rehabilitation, or (4) support. For dying patients, supportive care may be the only realistic goal. Yet, *to say that a patient's care has changed from cure to care, or from treatment to palliation, is an oversimplification of a complex situation.* Dying people often benefit from curative, rehabilitative, or preventive services, just as persons not near death may benefit from supportive care such as symptom control and psychologic intervention.

In fact, labeling specific individuals as "dying" can be considered arrogant in that everyone is dying. Little moral distinction should be made between those who are expected to die soon and those who will die later. All significant medical interventions require careful decision making, regardless of whether a patient appears to be near death. Similarly, access to health care should not be limited because of the nearness of death. Certain symptoms are more common when death is close, however, and for these, treatment should be shaped by the length of time the patient is expected to live.

SYMPTOM CONTROL

Both physical and mental distress are common in the terminal phase of many illnesses. Relief of this discomfort improves the quality of the remaining life and allows the patient to focus on living as fully as possible, as well as on the unique issues presented by approaching death. Patients need control of symptoms for comfort, and they need reassurance to allay the common fears that suffering could be prolonged and that no one will care. For dying patients, the physician's role is broader than merely diagnosing and treating disease.

Optimal control of symptoms usually involves **determining their causes** in order to identify appropriate therapy. For example, treatment of vomiting caused by hypercalcemia differs from that caused by elevated intracranial pressure.

The appropriateness of **diagnostic investigations** varies, however, depending on how burdensome the test and how useful the information it would provide might be. When expected survival is brief, the severity of symptoms frequently dictates initial treatment choices. Often, the fear that a symptom will worsen is more crippling than the symptom itself, and reassurance that effective treatment is available may be all that is needed. At other times, a symptom is so severe and the diagnostic alternatives so poor that an immediate trial of therapy is warranted.

Since one symptom can have many causes and may respond differently to therapy as the patient's condition deteriorates, effective treatments must be closely monitored and continuously reevaluated. *Special care must be taken to avoid inadvertent overdosage of medications during periods of altered drug disposition.*

Pain (see also Ch. 11)

Among dying patients, those with cancer are most likely to have severe pain. Although only 50% of cancer patients have substantial pain, as many as ½ of those that do may never obtain adequate relief. Often it is not well controlled because both patients and physicians have misconceptions about pain and about the drugs, especially narcotics, that are used to control it. Pain in other terminal conditions is less common but is treated virtually the same way.

Patients differ in their perception of pain, depending on such factors as fatigue, insomnia, anxiety, depression, and nausea. Treatment must therefore include attention to these factors. Often, a supportive environment is all that is needed to control pain.

The **cause of pain** should be considered when choosing an analgesic, since some types of pain will respond to specific types of treatment. For example, salicylates and nonsteroidal anti-inflammatory drugs **(NSAIDs)** are helpful for bone pain from metastases, while amitriptyline is effective for dysesthesias from nerve compression.

The most important concept in pain control is the maintenance of the analgesic level by scheduled dosing. Controlling pain after it recurs is more difficult, since repeated pain requires more analgesic over time, partly because it generates patient anxiety about recurrence. Thus, analgesics should be prescribed on a regular schedule and the patient closely monitored for overdosage, underdosage, and adverse effects. In hospice units, nurses or patients can make the necessary dosing or scheduling adjustments.

When no specific treatment is available, the choice of analgesic depends largely on the **intensity of the pain.** The assessment of pain intensity is subjective and can be done only by talking with and observing the patient. Almost all pain can be relieved with an appropriately potent drug. Commonly used drugs are aspirin or acetaminophen for mild pain, codeine or oxycodone for moderate pain, and morphine or hydromorphone for severe pain.

Morphine is the most commonly used narcotic in terminal illness. Possible adverse effects include nausea, drowsiness, and confusion. Constipation should be anticipated and treated prophylactically (see below). The patient usually develops tolerance to the respiratory depressant and sedative effects of morphine but not as much to the analgesic effect. The usual starting dose of morphine is 10 mg orally q 4 h, but this may need to be lowered in elderly and very sick patients to decrease initial drowsiness. The maximum dosage is whatever is necessary to relieve pain, preferably without adverse effects. The oral route is preferred, but when it is not feasible, continuous IV infusions or intermittent IM or s.c. injections may be used. Morphine is now available in suppository form (5, 10, 20, or 30 mg). Estimated equianalgesic doses for conversion are shown in TABLE 26–1.

Hydromorphone is also available in a suppository form that is especially convenient for patients at home. Because hydromorphone is more soluble than morphine, it can be injected in smaller volumes. A pharmacist can prepare hydromorphone for high-dose therapy at up to 100 mg/mL from commercially available powder for IV use. **Heroin** is also more soluble than morphine but has no other proven advantage and cannot legally be prescribed in the USA.

Useful longer-acting alternatives to morphine include **levorphanol** and **methadone.** Pentazocine and other mixed agonist/antagonist drugs are not recommended because of low potency, erratic oral or IM absorp-

TABLE 26–1. EQUIANALGESIC DOSES OF NARCOTICS USED FOR
CHRONIC PAIN

Drug	Oral Dose (mg)	IM or s.c. Dose (mg)	Usual Effective Interval (h)
Codeine	200	130	4–6 po; 3–4 IM and s.c.
Morphine	40	10	4–6 po; 3–4 IM and s.c.
Hydromorphone	7.5	1.5	4–6 po; 3–4 IM and s.c.
Methadone	20	10	4–8
Levorphanol	4	2	4–8

(Adapted from D. J. Lynn: "Supportive care for dying patients: An introduction for
health care professionals," in President's Commission for the Study of Ethical Problems
in Medicine and Biomedical and Behavioral Research: *Deciding to Forgo Life-Sustaining
Treatment,* US Government Printing Office, 1983.)

tion, and greater incidence of adverse effects, especially psychosis. Furthermore, mixed agonist/antagonist drugs are contraindicated in combination with pure agonist narcotics. Meperidine is also not recommended
because of its short duration of action and production of toxic metabolites (causing psychosis) at relatively low doses.

If a narcotic alone produces adverse side effects, a lower dose may be
effective if potentiated by the addition of a tricyclic antidepressant, steroid, or hydroxyzine. Also helpful are **pain-modification technics,** such as
hypnosis, guided mental imagery, counseling for stress and anxiety, and
relaxation methods. In extreme cases, a pain tract may need to be eliminated through neurosurgery or anesthesia.

Dyspnea

Dyspnea is one of the most feared and probably the most distressing
symptom in a dying patient. It has multiple causes and should be
treated by correcting its cause whenever possible. For example, a chest
x-ray might show a pleural effusion, which could be evacuated by thoracentesis. In some instances, elevating the head of the bed and administering O_2 may be sufficient to alleviate respiratory distress.

The respiratory depressant effect of a narcotic can be used to slow respirations when a patient's blood gas levels deteriorate. Often, the body's
response to CO_2 retention or O_2 decline is severe, although the levels are
still adequate. In these circumstances, blunting the medullary response
may obliterate symptoms without producing adverse effects. Bronchial
secretions can be dried up with atropine (for acute episodes) or furosemide (for episodes of longer duration).

Anorexia

Anorexia is common in dying patients. It is usually more distressing to the family than to the patient, so counseling may be needed to help them accept it. If the patient is overwhelmed by a full meal tray, small amounts of food served more frequently may help. Also, giving a favorite alcoholic beverage ½ h before meals may help. Foods that have stronger flavors or smells sometimes stimulate appetite. Giving low-dose steroids (dexamethasone 1 mg or prednisone 5 mg tid) may also improve appetite and sense of taste.

Nausea and Vomiting

Seriously ill patients usually experience nausea, frequently without vomiting. If the cause is easily treatable (eg, hypercalcemia), then specific treatment may be warranted, provided it makes the patient more comfortable. Nonspecific treatment is always indicated, however, and **phenothiazine therapy** is the most effective because of its action on the chemoreceptor zone in the medulla.

Prochlorperazine can be given prophylactically in a dose of 10 mg orally before each meal. If vomiting precludes using the oral route, the drug can be given in suppository form (25 mg qid) or 5 to 10 mg qid by IM injection. **Metoclopramide** is useful for nausea and vomiting caused by decreased gut motility, because it increases peristalsis and relaxes the pyloric sphincter. Other helpful antiemetics are antihistamines (eg, **hydroxyzine** and **dimenhydrinate**), which act centrally. As with analgesics for pain control, antiemetics must be given regularly to prevent nausea and improve patient comfort.

If vomiting is caused by obstruction and the patient is near death, serious consideration should be given to conservative treatment without relieving the obstruction. Sometimes, paralyzing the gut with morphine and treating dry mouth with ice chips is better than constant gastric suction or surgery.

Constipation

Most dying patients experience constipation because of inactivity, decreased fiber in the diet, dehydration, narcotics, and anticholinergic drugs. Therefore, laxatives should be given prophylactically to prevent fecal impaction. A stool softener (soluble or insoluble fiber or docusate sodium) should be tried first. Stimulants (eg, casanthranol, senna, cascara sagrada, or bisacodyl) should be added as needed. Most patients require both types of laxatives, and some prefer an osmotic agent such as milk of magnesia or lactulose.

If the patient has not had a bowel movement in 3 days and stool is present on rectal examination, a glycerin or bisacodyl suppository should be administered. If still no bowel movement occurs, an enema should be administered. The importance of a regular bowel regimen in keeping a dying patient comfortable is too often underestimated by physicians.

Confusion

Mental changes that may accompany the terminal stage of illness are often more distressing to the family than to the patient, since the patient is usually unaware of them. Confusion is common and may have multiple causes, including drugs, metabolic disturbances, and intrinsic CNS disease. If the cause can be determined and is easily remediable, then treatment may be worthwhile, provided it enables the patient to communicate in a more meaningful way with family and friends. In other cases, if a patient is comfortable and less aware of the surroundings, it may be better to leave the patient in that state. The physician must carefully assess the relative merits in each case.

Nonspecific therapy may include tranquilizers (phenothiazines and related drugs or antihistamines) if the patient is agitated. Also, low doses of haloperidol may help the patient who has vivid dreams or threatening hallucinations.

Depression

Almost all dying patients experience some degree of depression. One patient may have many regrets about his life, while another may be preoccupied with legal, social, or financial problems. Providing **psychologic support** and allowing the patient to express his concerns and feelings is the best and simplest course of action. Assisting the patient and family to settle any unresolved matters may decrease his level of anxiety. A skilled social worker, physician, or nurse can help with conflicts that distance the patient from his family.

Antidepressants should be reserved for those patients who have persistent, clinically significant depression or whose depression is a side effect of needed bedtime sedation or narcotic potentiation. In this circumstance, dying patients may be helped with a low dose of a tricyclic antidepressant (eg, desipramine or amitriptyline 10 to 25 mg) once a day at bedtime. If the depression is associated with anxiety, then hydroxyzine or a phenothiazine may be beneficial. Benzodiazepines and alcohol usually induce depression, so they should be avoided in general unless the patient has a history of long-term use or has benefited from either in the past.

Stress

Approaching death is most stressful when it is unexpected or when interpersonal conflicts keep patient and family from sharing their last moments together. The latter situation can lead to excessive guilt or inability to grieve among survivors and can cause anguish for the patient. Stress in dying patients and families is generally best treated with compassion, information, counseling, and even time-limited psychotherapy. Tranquilizers should be used sparingly and only for a brief time.

When the dominant or especially skilled partner in a marriage dies, the spouse may find decision-making about legal or financial matters or managing the household overwhelming. With an elderly couple, the death of one partner may reveal in the survivor cognitive impairment that had been compensated for by the deceased spouse. Stress is even greater if there is no support from friends or other family members. Obviously, physicians must learn to identify such high-risk situations in order to mobilize the resources necessary to prevent undue suffering and dysfunction.

Not everyone is at ease with dying patients, but those who choose to work with them often find rewards in providing support to the family and comfort to the patient. Nurses who work in a hospice setting do not seem to experience the same degree of burnout that frequently occurs in such settings as an oncology ward or an intensive care unit. However, staff members are at risk of becoming so involved with the patient or family that they grieve with them. This stressful involvement can be mitigated by a staff support group that meets regularly to share responses to dying patients and their families. Physicians and others who work in less supportive environments may need to form similar support groups and sources of guidance.

Bereavement

Grieving is a normal process that usually begins before an anticipated death. For the patient, it often starts with denial caused by fears about loss of control, separation, and the unknown future, as well as the notion that death is necessarily painful. The staff can assist the patient in accepting the prognosis by listening to his expression of concerns and helping the patient to see meaning in the life that remains.

The family may also need support in expressing grief. A staff member who has come to know the patient and family may be best suited to help the family through this process and direct them to professional services if needed. Physicians, hospitals, and others responsible for the care of dying persons need to develop regular procedures that ensure follow-up of those persons who are grieving.

SOCIETAL CONCERNS
(See also Chs. 99 and 100)

Homicide, Suicide, and Assisting With Suicide

In some cases, the care of a dying patient may seem to be directed more toward hastening the patient's death than toward prolonging life. Whether such a plan should be construed as good medical care or as the criminal taking of life (homicide or assisting with suicide) is an increasingly troubling issue. This problem arises with patients who request discontinuance of parenteral hydration and nutrition; with those who choose to forgo treatment that would be expected to yield long, disease-free remissions; and with those who develop suffocating dyspnea that can be relieved with sedation, a treatment that accelerates dying.

Rarely are such cases recognized as having potential criminal involvement. Most cases involving medical actions that accelerate death are intended to relieve pain or other suffering. In such cases, the forgone life would have been so brief and the alternative so anguished that no need is perceived to question whether treatment to prolong life should have been carried out. **Once the question is raised, however, the issue of what constitutes wrongful death does arise.**

Criminal law does not differentiate between intentional and unintentional crime, although motivation may mitigate the penalty. Thus the patient whose pain is relieved only by doses of narcotics that cause deep sedation and who expectedly dies from the effects of treatment could be considered the victim of wrongful death.

Why are these cases virtually never brought to court? There are several reasons: (1) Most people, including prosecutors, judges, and jurors, do in fact consider motivation in their assessments and usually find no element of willful destruction, only the pathos of a situation that has no better outcome. (2) The means used to bring about the death are those ordinarily used in treatment (analgesics, sedatives, or anesthetics), and are not those associated with crime (poisons, guns, or knives). (3) The means by which the death was caused are not as certain to result in death as are those in clearly criminal cases. Of course, none of these explanations is definitive in demarcating criminal from meritorious behavior.

Acts that are usually considered punishable (eg, poisoning a patient to avoid time-consuming care) are only a little different from those that are usually considered meritorious (eg, narcotizing a patient to avoid overwhelming pain). In most aspects of life, the gulf between felonious acts and meritorious ones is large and filled with intermediate actions that regress from felonies to misdemeanors to unprofessional practices to adequate practices. But here there is no such clarification. Instead, society must craft a working distinction for the management of dying that increases satisfying aspects of death, reduces suffering while allowing no outright killing, and affirms that living has value.

As patients become more accepting of death, they must receive appropriate support and symptom relief, encouragement to persevere and continue to live, and vigorous treatment of any reversible aspects of depression and cognitive dysfunction. When the patient or surrogate proposes an action that seems seriously contrary to the patient's interests, mechanisms should be available within institutions and agencies to ensure that the response is defensible.

Assisting with suicide remains criminal under most states' laws, but the laws vary substantially and are rarely invoked. Directly providing lethal drugs to a dying patient, along with instructions for using them, might be grounds for prosecution in some states but not in others. Physicians confronted with such situations should seek legal guidance before acting.

Charges of homicide rather than of assisting with suicide are more likely to be filed if the patient's interests are not carefully advocated, if documentation is sparse, and if the prosecutor's electoral base is expected to approve. *The best defenses are good decision-making practices and careful documentation of the reasoning that led to forgoing life-sustaining treatment.* This should be further supported by documented consultation with professional colleagues, the patient, family, and friends.

Finally, the health care provider should not use any treatment modality that is conventionally construed as a means of homicide. Even though the provider may maintain that such a treatment was intended to provide comfort, the claim may be doubted when the patient dies. Then the provider could be charged with committing a felony, which might be difficult to disprove.

Managing the Death

For many people, death follows an extended course of illness that has come to be recognized as fatal. **The procedures to be performed after an expected death** must accomplish various goals for the family and society while still being unobtrusive and efficient:

1. The determination that death has occurred should be prompt and accurate. An accurate determination always takes at least a few minutes.

2. The care system should facilitate actions comforting to the bereaved family. For example, some families need time alone, others need an appropriate place to grieve, and still others want to assist in dressing and cleaning the body.

3. Society needs to ensure that the death did not result from wrongdoing. Although procedures vary, physicians are obliged to notify a medical examiner, coroner, or police department of any deaths that could be categorized as potentially suspicious.

4. Society and the family need an accurate death certificate for managing the estate and for epidemiologic reasons.

5. The body must not pose a risk to public health. Usually, this means the body must be handled in prescribed ways and by authorized persons.

Since physicians bear some responsibility for creating good health care systems, they should know how death is managed in their practice area and seek to make the practices comply with principles of good care. *Specifically, the physician should be able to determine that death has occurred.* The most serious errors here are misdiagnosing severe hypothermia or making too brief an examination. Also, the physician should have considered in advance the needs of family and friends and should have sought to meet these needs whenever possible.

Often, skillful management of death consists of the following: (1) making sure that someone (eg, a nurse or volunteer) is with the body when the family visits after death; (2) offering to assist in notifying clergy or funeral directors; (3) providing reassurance that the patient was comfortable and that family and care givers did all that could be done; and (4) making a follow-up phone call a few weeks later to the most affected survivor to answer questions and ascertain that reasonably healthy adjustment is taking place. Families should usually be offered the option of having an autopsy performed. Inquiry regarding organ donation, if made, should occur prior to death when reasonably possible.

Financing Terminal Care

Financial coverage for the care of dying persons is problematic. Medicare regulations exclude supportive care except in a hospice setting. However, not all patients qualify for hospice care, and physicians are often reluctant to make the 6-mo prognosis required for coverage. Even a certified need for a "skilled nursing" level of care may not gain admission to a nursing home for a short-term, terminally ill patient.

§3. ORGAN SYSTEMS

§3. ORGAN SYSTEMS: INTRODUCTION

Contents for CARDIOVASCULAR DISORDERS begin on page 309.

---

27. AGING PROCESSES

John W. Rowe and *Edward L. Schneider*

In many disciplines, the existing number of theories is inversely proportional to the extent of knowledge. Since biologic gerontology is a relatively new discipline (receiving intensive research support only within the past 10 yr), it is not surprising that many theories have been proposed to explain aging. We consider it naive to view all aging processes as explicable by one theory. Just as increasing knowledge in oncology indicates there are multiple mechanisms for the origin of cancers, it is reasonable to suppose multiple aging mechanisms at the molecular, cellular, organ, and organism levels.

The major current theories of aging can be divided into 2 types: those that suppose aging events occur randomly and accumulate with time (stochastic theories) and those that suppose aging is predetermined (nonstochastic theories).

STOCHASTIC THEORIES

Error Catastrophe Theory

This elegant theory proposes that, with time, an accumulation of errors in protein synthesis ultimately results in impaired cellular function. No biologic process is 100% accurate and errors do occur in the processes of transcription and translation. Since these errors could lead to abnormalities in the proteins involved in transcription and translation, further errors could accumulate with aging. However, most research indicates that transcription and translation continue to function well with advancing age. Other findings that do *not* support the error catastrophe theory include evidence that there is (1) no change in amino acid sequence in proteins from young and old animals, (2) no increase in defective tRNAs with age, and (3) no age-related differences in the accuracy of poly(U)-directed protein synthesis.

Cross-Linking Theory

This theory proposes that the cross-linking of proteins and other cellular macromolecules leads to aging and the development of age-dependent diseases and disorders. While this theory cannot explain all the changes associated with aging, it may account for some. One consistent observation is that extracellular collagen becomes increasingly cross-linked in humans as well as in experimental animals. While this cross-linking decreases mobility of certain tissues, it does not appear to have a major clinical impact. However, glycosylation of proteins and their subsequent cross-linking may play an important role in the age-dependent development of increasing opacification in crystalline lens protein and the eventual development of cataracts. Cross-linking between glycosylated immunoglobulins and glomerular basement membrane proteins and between glycosylated lipoproteins and arterial wall proteins have also been proposed as important in the development of age-dependent glomerular and arterial diseases in humans and experimental animals.

Wear and Tear Theory

This theory proposes that the body is composed of irreplaceable components and the accumulation of damage to vital parts leads to death of cells, tissues, organs, and finally the organism. Cellular DNA is cited as an example of a crucial cellular macromolecule. Throughout life, DNA is constantly damaged. Should DNA repair be incomplete and/or age-related impairments in the repair mechanisms occur, then progressive age-dependent declines in cellular function might occur. DNA repair capacity has been positively correlated with species lifespan, suggesting a possible role of efficient DNA repair in the evolution of longevity. However, studies of DNA repair during the aging of experimental animals have not shown a consistent decline with aging (some studies show a decline while others demonstrate no change). Studies in this area are complicated by the presence of multiple DNA repair mechanisms and uncertainty regarding which mechanisms might be critical to aging and which are less important. Further refinement of the technics for detecting DNA damage may permit a clearer picture of whether DNA damage does accumulate with aging.

Free Radical Theory

Free radicals are highly reactive molecules that can damage membrane proteins, enzymes, and DNA. The most important source of free radicals is the metabolism of O_2, which yields the superoxide radical O_2. Proponents of this theory believe that low-level free radical damage accumulates over time, resulting in the findings associated with aging. Studies in which various antioxidants were fed to animals found an apparent increase in life expectancy, but in many of these studies antioxidant administration was accompanied by significant weight loss, which is known to produce a significant increase in life expectancy independently. However, levels of the cellular antioxidant superoxide dismutase correlate well with lifespan in primates, while in some lower forms of life, mutations leading to defects in production of free-radical–quenching enzymes are associated with a shorter lifespan.

NONSTOCHASTIC THEORIES

Pacemaker Theories

Certain organs or organ systems (eg, the immune and neuroendocrine systems, notably the hypothalamus) are thought to be intrinsic "pacemakers" of the aging process, being genetically programmed to involute at specific times in the lifespan of an organism.

With aging, there are declines in both B- and T-cell functions. T-cell functions are more significantly impaired, the decline paralleling the involution of the thymus gland that begins during adolescence. The importance of these changes in the aging process is supported by studies of mice identical except for the major histocompatibility complex **(MHC)**, which show a close relation between MHC and lifespan. The age-related increase in malignancies also may be related to the age-dependent decline in immune surveillance.

Adrenergic activity increases with age, and β-mediated vasodilation is reduced. These changes have been considered to be possibly linked to age-related increases in BP, impaired carbohydrate tolerance, and new sleep patterns.

Studies of hypophysectomized animals receiving hormone replacement therapy suggested that aging is diminished in these animals, and prompted a search for the presence of a "death hormone" that increases with age or a "Methuselah hormone" that decreases with age. However, no data support these notions.

All of these theories are flawed. For example, they fail to explain the origin of the changes in the pacemaker system itself, and fail to take into account that not all organisms have well-developed immune or neuroendocrine systems.

Genetic Theories

Genetic factors are clearly important determinants of aging, although the mechanisms involved are unknown. There is a remarkable species specificity to lifespan, and, in humans, the life expectancy of identical twins is more similar than that of siblings. Mutant varieties of *C. elegans,* a nematode, have been produced with lifespans increased by 50%; the increase appears to be due to a single gene in some of these strains.

Some biologic changes noted in the elderly are related to aging alone, while others are the result of disease. In evaluating and managing health and disease in the elderly, it is important, although not always possible, to understand and recognize the differences. Some changes are clearly physiologic; eg, growth and development, characterized by rapid increases in many physiologic functions, peaking in the late 20s or early 30s. From that point on, some functions are known to begin a progressive linear decline.

However, there is great variability in the rate of age-related declines in organ function, with the result that people become less alike as they age. There also is substantial variability in a given individual in the rate of decline of various organs such as kidneys, lungs, heart, or immune system.

Age-adjusted criteria have been established for several clinically important functions; eg, spirometric measures of pulmonary function, which are commonly expressed as "percent of expected" for age and body size, and cardiac exercise tolerance tests to detect ischemic heart disease with age-adjusted criteria for maximum heart rate. In the case of renal function, there are age-related changes in GFR and declines in creatinine clearance (about 10 mL/min/decade). The latter is affected by similar reductions in endogenous creatinine production, so that serum creatinine levels are unchanged. Thus, while normal levels of serum creatinine are the same in young and old, the serum creatinine level reflects substantially less GFR in the older patient. Familiarity with these changes is important in prescribing drug therapy in the elderly.

"SUCCESSFUL" (NORMAL) VS. "USUAL" (ABNORMAL) AGING

It has recently been recognized that delineating disease from aging provides only a partial view of "normal" aging processes. The variability of age-related physiologic changes and the capacity of many factors to modify the effects of the intrinsic aging process have led to stratification of "normal aging" into 2 categories.

"Successful aging" refers to *those individuals demonstrating only physiologic decrements with age and in whom age-determined changes are uncomplicated by disease, environmental exposures, and lifestyle factors (eg, diet, exercise).* It represents greater physiologic capacity and lesser risk of disease and implies that there are preventable or reversible components to what was previously considered to be normal aging. **"Usual aging"** refers to *changes seen in the elderly that are determined by the combined effects of the aging process and the effects of disease and adverse environmental and lifestyle factors.* For example, O_2 consumption increases in elderly people who regularly perform aerobic exercises; instead of showing the significant decline in maximal O_2 consumption usually seen in the elderly, these individuals can achieve higher levels than most normal young adults. Therefore, it should not be assumed that the differences between elderly patients' clinical status and that of healthy younger individuals represent only the effects of aging. These differences are a mixture of interdependent age-dependent and disease-related effects, which range from a lack of interaction at one extreme to age changes simulating "disease" at the other.

Most often, a disability or an abnormal physical or laboratory finding is the result of a specified disease or disorder that occurs more commonly at older ages. For example, older individuals with low Hcts are all too often incorrectly diagnosed as having an "anemia of old age" without further diagnostic evaluation or treatment. However, there is no age-dependent change in Hct in healthy community-dwelling older persons, and a low Hct always requires prompt investigation and treatment. Most common clinical laboratory measures are not significantly influenced by age. There are a few exceptions; eg, oral glucose tolerance diminishes, but fasting blood glucose levels are unchanged.

A key distinction must be made between test results that reflect adequate homeostasis and studies that show reduced physiologic reserve. Many age-dependent reductions in biologic functions reduce compensatory reserve capability, increasing the risk of clinical symptoms and illness. This is particularly the case when aging effects are aggravated by lifestyle or environmental factors to induce usual rather than successful aging. Thus, commonly seen reductions in immune, renal, cardiac, and pulmonary function, and the declines in glucose tolerance seen during physiologic stress place many elderly at risk for disease or a more serious clinical course of illness. For example, many healthy nonagenarians have pulmonary function only $1/2$ that of the average 30-yr-old. Additionally, age-dependent decreases in immune functions result in greater susceptibility to infection. Therefore, an acute bacterial pneumonia is more likely to occur and to be a dangerous illness in the elderly.

Since renal function in the typical older person is about 40% less than that in healthy younger adults, the loss of one kidney for any reason will result in a clinically significant reduction in overall renal function. Severe burns result in increased mortality with advancing age throughout adulthood (see FIG. 27–1), probably reflecting multiple reductions in

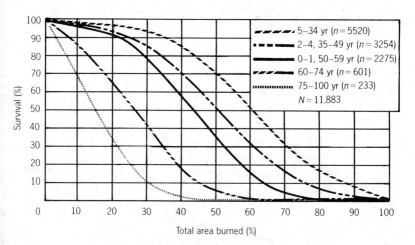

FIG. 27–1: Survival of patients as a function of the total percentage of body surface burned and age. (From J. W. Rowe, in *Cecil Textbook of Medicine,* ed. 18, edited by R. L. Cecil, J. B. Wyngaarden, L. H. Smith. Philadelphia, W. B. Saunders Company, 1988, p. 25. Reprinted by permission of W. B. Saunders Company and the author.)

physiologic functions during middle age and early senescence, since this increased risk is apparent well before diseases become highly prevalent.

Aside from the increasing vulnerability to disease, age also affects disease presentation in that many diseases have different clinical presentations and natural histories depending on the age of the affected individual. For example, while uncontrolled diabetes generally results in diabetic ketoacidosis in children and young adults, it frequently produces hyperosmolar nonketotic coma, with much higher blood glucose levels and little or no circulating ketones, in the eldery. Instead of presenting with severe metabolic acidosis, polyuria, and volume depletion, the elderly will be obtunded or in coma secondary to high blood osmolality.

Throughout this section of THE MANUAL, the known interactions of normal and successful biologic aging, and diseases of major organ systems will be discussed in greater detail.

§3. ORGAN SYSTEMS: CARDIOVASCULAR DISORDERS

28. NORMAL CHANGES OF AGING

Edward G. Lakatta

It is assumed that age-related alterations in cardiovascular structure and function enhance the probability of disease occurrence, decrease the threshold at which symptoms and signs arise, and affect the clinical course and ultimate prognosis of disease. Conversely, the widespread presence of disease complicates gerontologic study. In particular, occult forms of disease can exaggerate functional declines assumed to be due to aging, leading to an erroneous perspective of the age effect. For example, the prevalence of occult coronary artery disease **(CAD)** is strikingly high in elderly individuals. Approximately 1 of every 2 individuals $\geq$ 60 yr of age may have severe coronary artery narrowing, yet only 50% of those afflicted have clinical symptoms or signs.

The functional decline in cardiovascular performance found during stress testing may be due, at least in part, to this disease or to its interaction with age-related changes. Unfortunately, the methodology for screening research subjects vigorously for occult CAD was developed only recently and is still not widely used. This partly explains the large variability in cardiovascular reserve reported among elderly individuals in different studies.

Other variables include level of physical activity, nutritional status, smoking behavior, educational and socioeconomic status, and even personality traits. These life-style variables are difficult to quantify at a single point in time (eg, as in a cross-sectional study) or repeatedly over a longer time (eg, as in a longitudinal study), and probably account for the diversity of results and opinions in the scientific literature (see FIG. 28–1).

The increasingly sedentary behavior of community-dwelling older individuals has also led to erroneous conclusions regarding the impact of aging on cardiac functional reserve capacity. In older individuals who remain physically fit, maximal work capacity can be twice that of those who are sedentary, and the percent body fat does not increase as it does in sedentary individuals. Indeed, recent studies suggest that in some instances, disease and life-style may have a far greater impact on cardio-

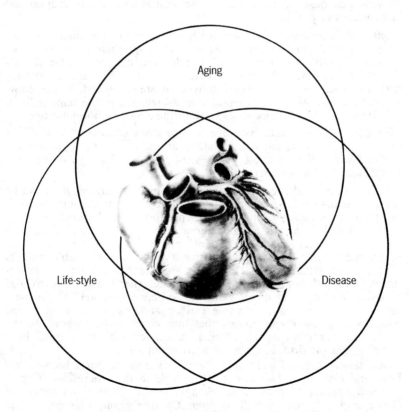

FIG. 28–1. **Age-related changes in cardiac structure and function alter presentation of cardiovascular disease in the elderly.** (Adapted from E. G. Lakatta: "Health, disease and cardiovascular aging," in Institute of Medicine and National Research Council, Committee on an Aging Society: *Health in an Older Society,* © 1985 by the National Academy of Sciences, Washington, DC. Used with permission.)

vascular function than aging. This suggests that older patients should be thoroughly evaluated both for proper diagnosis and appropriate treatment.

Cardiovascular Structure

Heart: The aging heart can atrophy, remain unchanged, or exhibit moderate or marked hypertrophy. Cardiac atrophy has been described in studies from chronic-care hospitals; it usually coincides with various wasting diseases and does not represent normative aging. The same can be said for the extreme ventricular thickening found in some (usually hypertensive) women. While several studies, both post- and antemortem (by echocardiography), have defined a modest increase in left ventricular wall thickness with advancing age (see Ch. 30), this is within the clinically normal range in normotensive individuals and is only exaggerated in hypertensive patients.

Left atrium dimension increases with age, even in individuals who are rigorously screened to exclude disease. Left ventricular cavity size may increase slightly, but this is not usually statistically significant. Although the cardiac silhouette on chest x-ray does not appear to vary with age when those of different individuals are compared, it does show a slight increase with age in repeated measurements in the same individual. However, this increase is also within the clinically normal range.

Fibrous tissue increases with age but does not contribute appreciably to the increase in cardiac mass. Rather, an increase in myocyte size underlies heart wall thickening. While some myocytes enlarge, others may be replaced by fibrous tissue.

With sensitive and specific histologic staining methods, amyloid can be detected in the cardiovascular system in nearly 50% of patients > 70 yr of age, and the incidence increases sharply thereafter. Approximately $1/2$ of the involved hearts have only minor quantities of amyloid, confined to the atria. Whether cardiac amyloid can be considered characteristic of normal aging is debatable, because it is not an invariable finding, even in centenarians. "Senile" cardiac amyloid has 2 immunologically distinct forms, 1 limited to the atria and the other found in ventricular deposits and, often, in minor extracardiac deposits as well. Cardiomegaly is not characteristic of senile cardiac amyloidosis, as it is in the much rarer primary amyloidosis that may occur in the elderly. In the senile form, amyloid accumulation is associated with myocardial fiber atrophy, and the firm, large, waxy heart is not seen.

Vasculature: Arterial walls stiffen with age, and the aorta becomes dilated and elongated. This is not attributable to the atherosclerotic process but appears to result from changes in the amount and nature of elastin and collagen as well as from Ca deposition. Changes in the cross-linking of collagen, in particular, may render it less elastic. Atherosclerosis also increases markedly in incidence and severity with advancing age. Whether age-related changes occur in vascular permeability, smooth muscle function, or the inflammatory response to injury is not known.

Cardiovascular Function

Cardiovascular function is determined by the interaction of several variables, each of which is ultimately dependent on biophysical mechanisms that regulate cardiac muscle and ventricular function (see FIG. 28–2).

Determinants of Cardiac Output

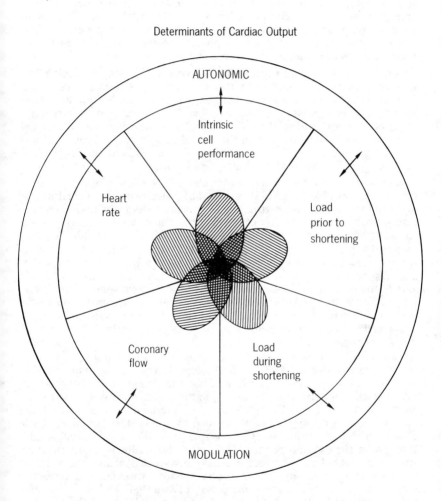

FIG. 28–2. **Factors that govern CO.** The overlap at the center indicates the interdependence of these determinants of function. The bidirectional arrows indicate that each function is not only modulated by autonomic tone but also is governed by a negative feedback on modulation. (Adapted with permission from *Journal of Chronic Diseases,* Vol. 36, E. G. Lakatta, "Age-related changes in the heart," copyright 1983, Pergamon Press PLC.)

Cardiac filling and preload: Factors that determine the ventricular volume (ie, fiber stretch, end-diastolic blood volume, and filling pressure) are sometimes referred to as preload. Preload is related to the filling volume and degree of myocardial stretch prior to excitation; hence, it is a determinant of myocardial function and pump performance. Left ventricular compliance (inverse of stiffness) affects the atrioventricular pressure gradient, which determines left ventricular filling rate. While ventricular compliance is thought to slacken with advancing age, this has not been proven in man, since its precise measurement requires the simultaneous determination of pressure and volume.

However, a substantial (up to 50%) slowing in the **early diastolic filling rate** between ages 20 and 80 yr (see FIG. 28–3) has been demonstrated by echocardiography, radionuclide angiography, and Doppler ultrasound. This reduction in filling rate has been attributed to structural changes (fibrous) within the left ventricular myocardium or to residual myofilament Ca activation from the preceding systole (ie, prolonged isometric relaxation), which occurs in nearly every animal species, including man, and is discussed in greater detail below.

Despite the reduction in left ventricular filling early in diastole, a reduction in end-diastolic volume does not usually occur in healthy elderly individuals. Because stroke volume at rest does not decline appreciably with age (see below), the at-rest filling volume during each cardiac cycle is roughly the same in younger and older individuals. Thus in healthy persons, more filling occurs later in diastole to compensate for the reduction in early filling. Recent studies have shown that this later response is due to a more vigorous atrial contraction (see FIG. 28–3) and is manifested on auscultation as a fourth heart sound (atrial gallop). Loss of this atrial kick occurs with acute atrial fibrillation in elderly individuals whose ventricular function is compromised for other reasons. The end result may be heart failure, particularly if the ventricular rate is rapid.

Afterload: The extent to which all muscle shortens during the contracted state varies inversely with the load borne by the individual fibers. Forces that resist myocardial fiber shortening after the onset of myofilament Ca activation (ie, during systole) are collectively referred to as **afterload.** There are 2 major sources of afterload: cardiac and vascular. **The cardiac component** is determined by the ventricular radius, both at the onset and during the Ca-activated state (ie, at end diastole and throughout the ejection period). The ventricular radius is an afterload as well as a preload factor, since it affects myocardial wall stress via Laplace's law; ie, at a constant ventricular pressure, vascular wall stress increases as ventricular radius increases. Myocardial wall stress is the force generated by the myofilaments/cross-sectional area of the myocardial wall. Thus, wall thickness (see above and below) is also related to afterload.

The **vascular component** of afterload is determined by vascular input impedance. Vascular impedance has steady and pulsatile components: the steady component is commonly referred to as **peripheral vascular re-**

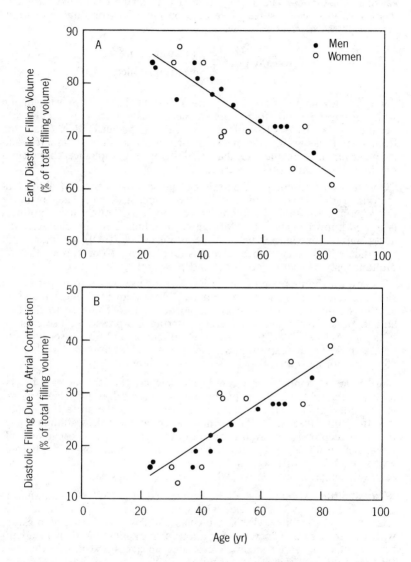

FIG. 28–3. **Age-associated decrease in early diastolic filling rate is compensated for by an increase in filling due to the atrial contraction.** (Based on data from C. J. Swinne et al: "Age-related changes in left ventricular performance during isometric exercise" [abst]. In *Journal of the American College of Cardiology*, Vol. 13 [suppl A], p. 56A, 1989.)

sistance **(PVR),** while the pulsatile flow is referred to as **characteristic vascular impedance.** The average total PVR can be calculated indirectly from steady-state measures of cardiac output **(CO),** or flow, and mean arterial pressure via Ohm's law:

$$\text{Steady flow} = \frac{\text{mean pressure}}{\text{mean resistance}}$$

Some studies have reported an increase in the basal PVR with aging, while others have not found this to be so. Characteristic vascular impedance is usually $< 10\%$ of total vascular impedance. It is calculated from instantaneous measurements of pressure and flow harmonics, and its determinants are the vascular circumference, compliance characteristics, and transmural pressure gradient.

One index of vascular stiffness is the **pulse wave velocity (PWV).** Numerous studies have found that the PWV increases with age, owing to the arterial structural alterations noted above. Although aortic stiffness is a well-known concomitant of aging, an increase in the characteristic aortic input impedance, the aortic component of (total) vascular input impedance, has recently been demonstrated in man (via probes that simultaneously measure blood flow and pressure).

Because of the increase in aortic PWV, pressure waves from peripheral sites are returned to the heart sooner in older than in younger individuals. This causes the pressure in the aortic root to continue to increase and to peak later in systole, thereby altering the pressure pulse contour with aging (see FIG. 28–4). Arterial stiffening and the associated increase in PWV appear to cause the increase in systolic BP within the clinically normal range that is associated with aging.

On the other hand, some physiologists suggest that the increase in systolic BP reflects a resetting of the baroreceptor reflex to a higher level in the elderly. The same structural changes within the aorta that render it stiffer and cause the PWV to increase could mean less stimulation of the baroreceptor for a given change in aortic pressure. Alternatively, afferent neural impulses that result from a *given* stimulation of the baroreceptor may vary with age and explain the blunted baroreflex response, as may changes in efferent signals to the arterial system.

Cross-cultural studies suggest that increased vascular stiffening and arterial pressure may not be inevitable concomitants of aging but may be related in part to life-style. The increase in PWV and arterial pressure with age in a rural Chinese population is markedly less than in an urban population, whose members consume an average 6 times more Na. Further studies of this sort are needed.

Current medical practice is to *not* treat patients whose increases in systolic BP fall within the clinically normal range. Epidemiologic studies have shown, however, that even these elderly individuals are at increased risk for cardiovascular events. The magnitude of the excess risk

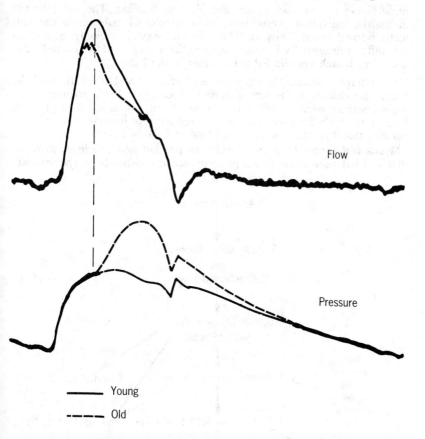

FIG. 28–4. **Ascending aortic blood flow velocity and pressure wave forms from a young and an old subject.** Not only does peak pressure become elevated with aging, it also peaks later during the cardiac cycle. (Adapted from W. W. Nichols, M. F. O'Rourke, A. P. Avolio, et al: "Effects of age on ventricular-vascular coupling," in *American Journal of Cardiology*, Vol. 55, pp. 1179-1184, 1985. Copyright © 1985 by Cahners Publishing Company. Used with permission.)

is a function of the magnitude of the rise in systolic BP. An increase in systolic pressure greater than what has been defined as normal is referred to as **isolated systolic hypertension** (see Ch. 30).

Regardless of whether the increase in systolic pressure is a risk factor for atherosclerosis or is simply inevitable, it increases left ventricular afterload. This chronic increase may cause the left ventricle to empty incompletely during each cardiac cycle, leading to a reduced ejection fraction and ventricular dilatation. Alternatively, left ventricular wall thickness can increase sufficiently to normalize wall stress (see above), thus maintaining normal cavity size and ejection fraction. The latter occurs in healthy individuals whose increase in systolic BP falls within the clinically normal range. Thus, end-diastolic and -systolic volumes at rest do not differ substantially in otherwise healthy younger and older individuals, even though systolic BP is increased in the latter.

The interplay among the age-associated changes and adaptations of the heart and vasculature is summarized in FIG. 28–5. These changes strikingly resemble what occurs in hypertension, but are of lesser magnitude, leading to the belief that aging is a muted form of hypertension, or conversely, that hypertension is an accelerated form of aging.

Myocardial contractility: In addition to preload and afterload, myocardial and left ventricular pump performance also depends on the myocar-

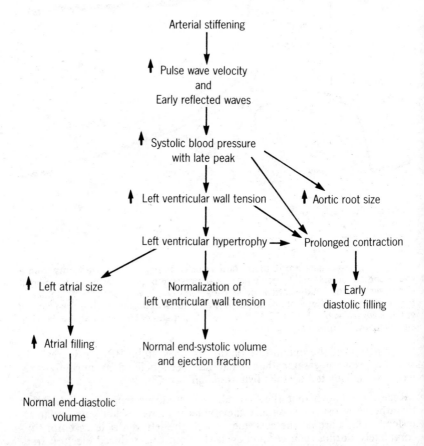

FIG. 28–5. The interplay of vascular and adaptive cardiac changes that occur to varying degrees with aging in otherwise healthy individuals.

dial contractile state (also referred to as intrinsic myocardial cell performance, contractility, inotropic state, or excitation-contraction coupling) (see FIG. 28–2). Recent studies of isolated myocardial cells and tissue indicate that the extent to which myofilaments become Ca activated during systole is determined by the extent of diastolic stretch (preload), and that myofilament shortening during contraction (afterload) affects the extent to which Ca remains bound to the myofilaments throughout systole. Thus myocardial fiber length both prior to and during shortening is a modulatory factor of the strength of the heartbeat. These effects of preload and afterload to alter the extent of myofilament Ca activation thus mimic inotropic stimulants, which also act by altering the extent of myofilament Ca activation before or during contraction.

While various indexes of myocardial contractility have been suggested, none has been fully satisfactory. One explanation is that preload, afterload, and contractility are not *independent* determinants of cardiac muscle performance. Rather, because they are *interdependent* (FIG. 28–2), it is difficult to measure contractility in situ and thus to determine whether or how myocardial performance changes with age.

Data from animal models have demonstrated a constellation of age-associated changes in the mechanisms that govern excitation-contraction coupling. Studies in rats show that contractile force production, at low stimulation at least, is preserved in advanced age. While there is no clear-cut indication that passive stiffness in isolated cardiac muscle increases with age, stiffness measured during contraction does increase. The affinity of the myofibrils for Ca is preserved in senescent muscle, and the increase in myoplasmic Ca following excitation is not age related.

Contraction is prolonged in senescent cardiac muscle, probably because Ca is released more slowly into the myoplasm during systole than in younger hearts. A major cause of this appears to be a reduced rate of Ca sequestration by the sarcoplasmic reticulum. While the action-potential duration is also longer in senescent than in younger cardiac muscle, its role in prolonged contraction is unclear. Action-potential changes could reflect age-related changes in sarcolemmal ionic conductance or could result from the prolonged myoplasmic Ca transient elicited by excitation. In the older heart, myosin isoenzymes shift to slower forms and adenosine triphosphatase activity declines. The latter changes appear to underlie the decline in shortening velocity observed when isolated senescent cardiac muscle contracts isotonically.

These interrelated alterations in excitation-contraction mechanisms and myofibrillar biochemistry can be viewed as adaptive rather than degenerative, in that they serve to maintain the contractile function of the senescent heart. Furthermore, the same constellation of changes occurs in the myocardium of younger rats when myocardial hypertrophy is induced by chronic hypertension or aortic banding. Some of these changes (eg, the prolonged contraction) can be reversed by chronic exercise in senescent animals. Inotropic responses to cardiac glycosides and to β-adrenergic stimulation (see below) are reduced in senescence.

Coronary flow: Another determinant of myocardial performance at rest is the adequacy of coronary flow (see FIG. 28–2). Measurements of coronary flow in individuals of various ages without CAD are not available. Nonetheless, there is no indication that coronary flow is reduced in the absence of disease; therefore, it is assumed that this factor does not limit myocardial performance in healthy elderly individuals.

Ejection fraction and stroke volume: There is no reason for stroke volume or ejection fraction to decline with aging. The resting ejection fraction is not reduced in elderly persons whose resting end-diastolic and -systolic volumes are comparable to those of younger persons. This has been verified in most studies.

Stroke volume can be calculated from measurements of CO and heart rate in the steady state. Many studies have found that stroke volume remains constant with age, even in elderly persons whose systolic BP has increased within the normal clinical range. Other studies have found that resting stroke volume decreases with age, although the hemodynamic mechanisms for this could not be determined, since neither cardiac end-diastolic nor systolic volume was measured. A modest decline in stroke volume at rest occurs in some elderly hypertensive patients.

Heart rate: Resting heart rate does not change with age. It is modulated by the individual's relative sympathetic and, more important, parasympathetic tone. **Spontaneous variations in heart rate** over a 24-h period in men without CAD decrease with age. **Variations in the sinus rate** with respiration are also diminished with advancing age. In contrast to resting heart rate, **intrinsic sinus rate** (ie, that measured in the presence of both sympathetic and parasympathetic blockade) is significantly diminished with age. For example, at 20 yr of age, the average intrinsic heart rate is 104 beats/min compared with 92 beats/min between ages 45 and 55 yr. Studies in older individuals are lacking.

Cardiac output: The interplay of stroke volume (preload, afterload, myocardial contractility, and coronary flow) and heart rate determines the CO (see FIG. 28–2). Data show that as people age, CO at rest is unchanged or decreased, depending on the methods used to screen individuals for study (see FIG. 28–6). While CO need not decline with age, it does so in many elderly individuals. This decline can be due to cardiac or noncardiac factors (eg, severe coronary disease, hypertension, or a reduced demand for flow as a result of a decrease in basal metabolism from a reduction in lean body mass).

Cardiovascular Reserve

In general, homeostatic adjustments enhance both the heart's pumping action and peripheral blood flow. Because these determinants are highly integrated, a change in 1 factor is compensated for by adjustments in others to maintain overall cardiovascular performance within a narrow range. The functional level of each factor is determined by basic cellular and extracellular biophysical mechanisms, each subject to autonomic

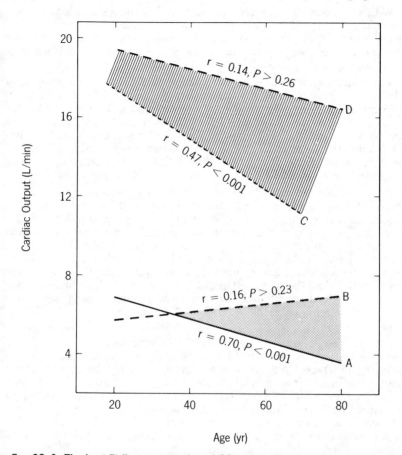

Fɪɢ. **28–6. The best-fit linear regression of CO and age, both at rest (lines A, B) and during bicycle exercise (lines C, D).** Note that regression lines B and D, derived from healthy, active, community-dwelling volunteers screened to exclude CAD by exercise ECG and thallium scintigraphy, are not significantly correlated with age. In contrast, subjects depicted by line A (hospitalized patients recuperating from noncardiac illness) and those depicted by line C (ambulatory volunteers who did not undergo screening to exclude CAD) showed clear reductions with age. (Adapted, with permission, from Lakatta EG: Age-related changes in the heart. *Geriatric Medicine Today* 4(7):86, 1985.)

modulation (see Fɪɢ. 28–2). For example, with a change in position from supine to upright or performance of routine daily activities or exercise, cholinergic modulation decreases while adrenergic modulation increases. Enhanced adrenergic function during activity is documented by increased levels of plasma catecholamines.

With advancing age, the average basal level of norepinephrine increases in many (but not all) populations studied; in response to stress, the average plasma epinephrine and norepinephrine levels increase more in the elderly than in younger persons. However, there is substantial heterogeneity among elderly individuals.

The regulation of cardiovascular function is efficient: In the absence of disease, an increase in CO is matched to the demand for enhanced peripheral blood flow. Maximal work capacity and CO vary considerably in exercise stress tests among elderly persons (see FIG. 28–6), depending on whether cardiovascular or noncardiovascular (eg, psychologic, orthopedic, muscular) factors limited exercise. Age-associated decreases in CO at exhaustion (ie, the maximal measured CO) do not necessarily equate with declines in cardiovascular reserve, as in younger individuals.

Maximum aerobic capacity, ie, the whole body O_2 consumption at exhaustion **(V_{O2MAX}),** is relatively easy to measure and, along with simultaneous heart rate data, has been evaluated in younger and older individuals. Concomitant with a decline in the maximal work capacity, maximal O_2 consumption declines with age and to a variable extent among different individuals. Elderly people in good physical condition can match or exceed the work capacity of nonconditioned younger people. This indicates either that the measured decline in some older individuals is due to physiologic deconditioning or that physical conditioning can retard the effect of aging on cardiorespiratory performance.

Maximal CO and stroke volume are often extrapolated from measurements of V_{O2MAX} and heart rate via the Fick principle (see FIG. 28–7). Specific but variable age-related changes in stroke volume and arteriovenous O_2 difference **(A-V_{O2})** essentially preclude extrapolation of the precise maximal CO from measurements of V_{O2MAX} and maximal heart rate. An assumption that A-V_{O2} remains constant with aging attributes a measured decline in V_{O2MAX} to the central circulation (heart) rather than to peripheral factors. This assumption may not be valid, because during vigorous exercise stress tests, 90% of the CO is directed to working muscles. Lean body mass can decrease 10 to 12% with aging in sedentary individuals. A reduction in A-V_{O2} could occur on this basis and thereby account for the reduction in V_{O2MAX}. Other factors include the efficiency by which blood flow is redistributed to muscles and O_2 is extracted by working muscles. Studies in middle-aged men, and more recent data from elderly individuals, indicate that improved O_2 consumption with physical conditioning is achieved by enhanced A-V_{O2} during vigorous exercise rather than to improvements in maximal CO.

Autonomic modulation of cardiovascular function: A reduction in heart rate during vigorous exercise does not indicate a reduction in CO. For example, β-adrenergic blockade, while lowering the exercise heart rate in younger subjects to a degree observed in most elderly individuals, does not depress CO. This is because cardiac dilatation occurs, and the increase in end-diastolic volume augments stroke volume.

A hemodynamic profile during stress similar to that effected by β-adrenergic blockade in younger individuals has been observed in healthy

Determinants of O$_2$ Consumption

Total body O$_2$
consumption (V$_{O_2}$)   =   Cardiac output (CO)*   ×   Arteriovenous O$_2$
                                                          difference (A-V$_{O_2}$)

Possible limiting factors:

Blood volume	Pulmonary function
Circulation time	Hb
Contractile state	Muscle mass
Afterload	% Extraction

* Cardiac output = stroke volume × heart rate; stroke volume = end-diastolic volume minus end-systolic volume.

FIG. 28–7. **Total body O$_2$ consumption (V$_{O_2}$) during physical work is determined by central, i.e. cardiopulmonary, and peripheral circulation factors and by tissue O$_2$ extraction, i.e. arteriovenous oxygen difference (the Fick principle).** The decline in maximal work capacity and V$_{O_2MAX}$ associated with aging does not appear to be solely attributable to cardiac output. See text for detail.

elderly individuals: CO is maintained during vigorous exercise by an enhanced stroke volume in the presence of a reduced heart rate (see FIG. 28–8). As is the case during exercise in the presence of β-adrenergic blockade, the end-diastolic volume increases and the reduction in end-systolic volume is less in exercising elderly vs younger individuals. This observation suggests that elderly individuals experience less β-adrenergic modulation of cardiovascular function during exercise. Furthermore, increased plasma levels of catecholamines are consistent with the hypothesis that this defect is primarily postsynaptic.

A possible explanation for the increased end-systolic volume and decreased ejection fraction at peak exercise in some elderly vs. younger adults is the large end-diastolic dimension that enhances ventricular afterload (Laplace's law; see above). Another factor may be an age-related deficiency in maximal myocardial contractile function. This could result from a deficit in intrinsic myocardial excitation-contraction mechanisms (FIG. 28–2). While the effectiveness of these mechanisms cannot be measured precisely in man, animal models provide little support that *intrinsic* contractile reserve (measured as peak force or pressure, or peak rates of force or pressure development) decreases with age, even in the senes-

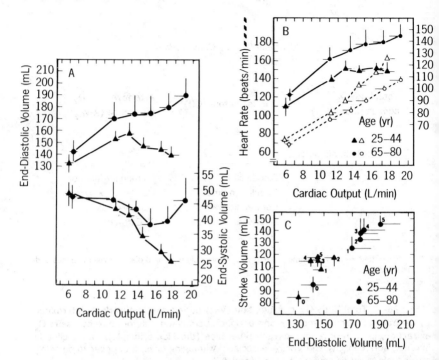

FIG. 28–8. The relationship of end-diastolic volume and end-systolic volume (A) and stroke volume and heart rate (B) to a given CO at rest and during graded upright bicycle exercise in rigorously screened volunteers. During vigorous exercise, older subjects (○ ●) experience a diminution in heart rate (open symbols) but increased stroke volume (closed symbols) to a greater extent than younger subjects (△▲) (Panel B); this is not accomplished by a greater reduction in end-systolic volume but rather by an increase (as much as 30%) in end-diastolic volume (Panel A). Exercise level is represented by CO on the abscissas of Panels A and B. This hemodynamic profile (Panel C) is an example of Starling's law of the heart and resembles that observed during beta-adrenergic blockade. The numbers 0 to 5 indicate progressive exercise work loads from rest (work load 0). (Adapted from R. J. Rodeheffer, G. Gerstenblith, L. C. Becker: "Exercise cardiac output is maintained with advancing age in healthy human subjects: Cardiac dilation in increased stroke volume compensates for a diminished heart rate," in *Circulation*, Vol.69, p. 203, 1984. Used by permission of the American Heart Association, Inc. and the authors.)

cent myocardium. In contrast, β-adrenergic modulation of mechanisms that govern myocardial excitation-contraction coupling decreases with advanced age, and thus contractile reserve can decrease in part on this basis.

β-Adrenergic stimulation has 2 effects on myocardial contraction: The strength is enhanced and the duration is decreased. The latter effect is necessary, because heart rate increases dramatically in response to β-

adrenergic stimulation, and the contraction must be briefer to permit myocardial relaxation and proper filling of the ventricle during a shorter diastole.

In addition to structural changes that may occur within the large vessels a deficiency in arterial dilatation during exercise may contribute to altered vascular impedance and cause alterations in the ventricular ejection pattern with age (FIG. 28–8). Studies of isolated aortic smooth muscle cells from young adult and senescent animals demonstrate that the latter relax less in response to β-adrenergic agonists but not in response to nonadrenergic relaxants.

More recently, it has been demonstrated that elderly men exhibit less forearm vascular dilatation in response to intra-arterial infusion of isoproterenol than younger ones. Catecholamines also modulate venous tone and thus its capacitance during stress. α-Adrenergic-mediated venoconstriction during exercise is not impaired with aging and is a major factor facilitating the return of blood to the heart. The effect of β-adrenergic stimulation to relax veins decreases with age.

β-Adrenergic modulation of pacemaker cells accounts in part for the increase in heart rate during exercise. Bolus infusions of β-adrenergic agonists (eg, isoproterenol) have demonstrated a diminished HR response with advancing age in many studies.

In summary, overall cardiovascular function at rest in most healthy elderly individuals is adequate to meet the body's requests for pressure and flow. The resting heart rate is unchanged. Heart size is essentially similar in younger and older adults, although heart-wall thickness increases modestly with age. This is mainly because of an increase in myocyte size. While the early diastole filling rate is reduced, an enhanced atrial contribution to ventricular filling maintains filling at a normal volume in elderly individuals. Although systolic BP at rest increases with age, the end-systolic volume and ejection fraction are not altered, partly because of the increase in left ventricular thickness.

Physical work capacity declines with advancing age, but the extent to which this can be attributed to a decrement in cardiac reserve is not certain. Part of the age-related decline in maximal O_2 consumption appears to be caused by peripheral rather than central circulatory factors (eg, to a decrease in body muscle mass with age rather than loss of cardiac function). Some elderly individuals exhibit cardiac dilatation, which then increases stroke volume sufficiently to counter the well-known age-related decrease in exercise heart rate; as a result, high levels of CO can be maintained during exercise. This same effect occurs in individuals of any age who exercise while subject to β-adrenergic blockade. When data covering the cardiovascular reserve in intact man to the subcellular biochemistry in animal models are integrated, a diminished responsiveness to β-adrenergic modulation is among the most notable changes that occur in the aging cardiovascular system. In contrast, α-adrenergic responsiveness appears to remain intact.

29.   DIAGNOSTIC EVALUATION

Jerome L. Fleg

New technology, while enhancing accuracy of cardiologic diagnosis, may be relied on excessively. For example, an evaluation for coronary artery disease **(CAD)** could include a chest x-ray, standard exercise ECG, exercise thallium scintigraphy, M-mode and 2-dimensional echo-cardiography, rest- and exercise-gated radionuclide ventriculography, CT, ambulatory ECG monitoring, an invasive electrophysiologic study, and cardiac catheterization. Which of these tests are necessary? Is the same diagnostic approach warranted in an 80-yr-old as in a 50-yr-old?

History

Overall health and level of functioning help determine a realistic diagnostic approach and therapeutic goal. The elderly patient is only as strong as his weakest link, and typically is more concerned with quality than with quantity of remaining years. Thus, an 80-yr-old with severe osteoarthritis and occasional episodes of exertional angina is unlikely to benefit significantly from extensive CAD evaluation until the arthritic symptoms are ameliorated.

Age-related life-style changes frequently mask important symptoms (eg, the patient may deny exertional angina pectoris and dyspnea because he never walks far or fast enough to experience them). Furthermore, the symptom itself may be atypical and therefore misleading. Thus, the age-associated decrease in left ventricular **(LV)** compliance may produce exertional dyspnea rather than angina pectoris. Multisystem disease often decreases the specificity of cardiac symptoms (eg, orthopnea may result from gastroesophageal reflux, and syncope may be due to orthostatic hypotension, carotid sinus hypersensitivity, vertebral artery compression, or inner ear disorders).

The drug history may explain sudden decompensation. Thus, addition of a nonsteroidal anti-inflammatory drug **(NSAID)** may exacerbate heart failure as a result of sodium retention; addition of quinidine to a stable regimen of digitalis and a diuretic may precipitate digitalis toxicity in the elderly; smaller body size and diminished renal function increase susceptibility to digitalis toxicity. Conversely, noncompliance or mis-compliance is common, often resulting in the necessity for hospitalization. In a study of 220 ambulatory patients $\geq$ 60 yr of age, 60% made medication errors averaging 2.6 mistakes per patient; 40% of these were potentially serious.

Physical Examination

In the elderly, arterial BP should be measured in both arms to exclude significant stenosis distal to the origin of the subclavian artery. Systolic BP should first be estimated by palpation, because an auscultatory gap (disappearance and later reappearance of the Korotkoff sounds) increases in prevalence with age and may lead to a sizable systolic under-estimation. A sclerotic noncompressible brachial or radial arterial wall that remains palpable at suprasystolic cuff pressure suggests generalized arteriosclerosis and may cause a falsely high measurement of systolic BP (ie, pseudohypertension, which should be suspected when very high cuff BP is seen without apparent target-organ damage). Intra-arterial pressure measurement confirms the diagnosis. BP should be measured in the supine or sitting position and after 2 min of quiet standing. An orthostatic decline > 20 mm Hg is seen in ≤ 20% of individuals > 65 yr of age; lack of compensatory pulse rate increase suggests autonomic insufficiency, venous varicosities, or drug effect.

Central venous pressure should be estimated from the right internal jugular vein rather than the left innominate vein, which is often compressed by the aortic arch or the left external jugular vein; the latter is frequently kinked near its junction with the left subclavian vein.

Kyphoscoliosis and other chest-wall deformities complicate interpretation of the apical impulse and other precordial movements. Heart sounds are usually softer in older individuals than in the young, probably because of the larger volume of lung tissue between the heart and the chest wall. Audible splitting of the second heart sound (S₂) occurs in only about 30 to 40% of elderly patients. Easily audible splitting that increases with inspiration suggests right bundle branch block. An S₄ is a normal finding in the elderly (as a result of greater reliance on atrial contraction to compensate for diminished early LV filling), whereas an S₃ is always abnormal. This situation is reversed in younger persons.

Systolic ejection murmurs (most often aortic) are present in ≤ 55% of unselected elderly patients. Short duration, low intensity (usually Grade 1 or 2), and failure to radiate distinguish these benign murmurs from those of significant aortic valvular stenosis or hypertrophic obstructive cardiomyopathy. The age-related stiffening of the arterial tree may result in a brisk upstroke of the carotid artery pulse tracing, even when severe aortic stenosis is present. Pulmonary valve murmurs are much less common in the elderly.

In an older person, pulmonary rales are more likely to represent atelectasis, pulmonary fibrosis, or an acute inflammatory process than in a younger individual. Factitious hepatomegaly can be produced by emphysematous lungs displacing the liver inferiorly. Furthermore, peripheral edema in older patients may be secondary to venous varicosities, lymphatic obstruction, or low serum albumin, rather than to right heart failure.

Standard Electrocardiography (see also Ch. 34)

Despite the tendency for heart size to increase with age (see Ch. 28), limb lead and precordial QRS voltages decrease with age. No *age-specific* criteria for ECG diagnosis of LV hypertrophy (LVH) have been developed. In a study of > 500 institutionalized elderly patients in sinus rhythm, a terminal P-wave deflection of > 0.04 mm in lead V₁ had a sensitivity of 32%, specificity of 94%, and positive predictive value of 31% for left atrial enlargement. The well-documented age-related increases in ectopic beats, PR and QT intervals, left axis deviation, and bundle branch block have no prognostic significance in older individuals without clinical heart disease.

An ECG pattern of MI may be the initial manifestation of significant CAD. In the Framingham study, > 25% of all MIs presented silently with a prognosis similar to those with clinical manifestations. However, an ECG pattern of poor R-wave progression in leads V_1 to V_4 has low specificity or predictive value for anterior MI in the elderly, probably because of age-related increases in resting lung volume and anteroposterior chest diameter. The most common ECG abnormality in the elderly is nonspecific change in ST segments and/or T waves, often secondary to digitalis, diuretics, antiarrhythmic or psychotropic drugs, with little independent prognostic significance. When associated with voltage criteria for LVH, however, in the absence of the above drugs, these ST-T–wave changes presage increased cardiovascular morbidity and mortality.

Ambulatory ECG Monitoring (see also Ch. 34)

Given the relatively common occurrence of complex arrhythmias on ambulatory monitoring in healthy elderly subjects, the mere presence of such an arrhythmia does not necessarily indicate that it is the source of the patient's complaints. An accurate diary allows correlation of symptoms with ECG rhythm disturbances. When symptoms are infrequent and nondisabling, an ECG event recorder is economical and allows up to 2 wk of intermittent monitoring. Alternatively, the patient can use a small device to transmit an ECG via telephone to a central recording facility when symptoms occur. Ambulatory ECG monitoring is useful for detecting asymptomatic episodes of myocardial ischemia (usually defined as $\geq$ 60 secs of flat or down-sloping ST-segment depression $\geq$ 0.1 mV.

Electrophysiologic Testing

This includes recording of His bundle activity, atrial pacing, programmed atrial or ventricular stimulation, and mapping of tachyarrhythmias. However, ambulatory ECG recording is generally more sensitive than atrial-pacing–determined sinus node recovery time in detecting the sick sinus syndrome. Similarly, the HV interval *(conduction time from the His deflection to ventricular activation)* has little independent prognostic significance unless extremely prolonged. Programmed ventricular stimulation has been used in predominantly older populations with life-threatening ventricular arrhythmias and shows the same low morbidity and overall favorable results as in younger groups (see also Ch. 34).

Exercise Testing

The safety and diagnostic yield of exercise testing in the elderly are similar to those in younger patients. Sensitivity has been shown to increase and specificity to decrease modestly with age (see TABLE 29–1), consistent with the higher prevalence and severity of CAD in the elderly. Several investigators have found exercise-induced ST-segment depression to have significant diagnostic and prognostic value in older individuals with chest pain. Furthermore, in postinfarction patients > 65 to 70 yr of age, a blunted increase in heart rate–BP product and the occurrence of major ventricular arrhythmias identify patient subsets with a high risk of cardiac death.

TABLE 29–1. DIAGNOSTIC VALUE OF EXERCISE ECG VS. AGE FOR DETECTION OF CORONARY ARTERY DISEASE

Age (yr)	Sensitivity (%)	Specificity (%)
< 40	56	84
40–49	65	85
50–59	74	88
≥ 60	84	70

(Adapted from M. A. Hlatky, D. B. Pryor, F. E. Harrell, et al: "Factors affecting sensitivity and specificity of exercise electrocardiography. Multivariable analysis," in *The American Journal of Medicine,* Vol. 77, pp. 64–71, 1984. Used with permission of the *Journal* and the author.)

Several physiologic and nonphysiologic factors must be considered in applying diagnostic testing to the elderly:

1. The lower maximal aerobic capacity requires a protocol that begins at low energy expenditures and advances in small increments (eg, the Naughton, Sheffield, or modified Balke protocols).

2. Maximal heart rate declines progressively by about 1 beat/min/yr through at least the 80s.

3. Systolic BP at rest and at any given external work load is higher in older persons, although age-related differences are less prominent at maximal effort.

4. The ability to exercise is often limited by noncardiac factors (eg, arthritis, neurologic disorders, or peripheral vascular disease).

5. Older persons often fail to exercise maximally because of psychologic factors (eg, unfamiliarity with vigorous exercise, fear, or insufficient motivation).

The following alternatives to treadmill exercise testing should be considered: (1) bicycle ergometry, for subjects with gait disturbances but good lower-extremity strength; (2) arm ergometry with a hand-cranked ergometer, for those incapable of leg exercise; (3) atrial or esophageal pacing, to increase heart rate in those individuals incapable of exercise but without A-V conduction disease; (4) use of IV or oral dipyridamole to maximize coronary flow heterogeneity.

Phonocardiography and Pulse-Wave Recording

These procedures are used primarily for research and for teaching cardiac physical diagnosis. The phonocardiogram is useful to differentiate between an S_4 and a split S_1 or ejection click and between a delayed pulmonic closure sound, an opening snap, and an S_3. In contrast to younger patients, older persons with severe aortic valvular stenosis may misleadingly show a rapidly rising carotid arterial pulse.

IMAGING TECHNICS

Chest X-ray

Cardiomegaly may be simulated by kyphoscoliosis, other chest-wall deformities, or age-related aortic elongation and unfolding. Even without such changes, the cardiothoracic ratio increases modestly with age but rarely exceeds 50% in normal subjects.

Aortic knob calcification is visible in about 30% of the elderly but has no pathologic significance. In contrast, intracardiac calcification is almost always pathologic; the most common sites are the aortic valve (signifying valvular stenosis) and the mitral anulus. Occasionally, a calcified pericardium (constrictive pericarditis) or a calcified LV wall (old MI) may be seen. Calcification in a coronary artery, best seen on fluoroscopy, does not necessarily imply a major stenosis, as it does in younger patients.

Echocardiography

Technically adequate echocardiograms cannot be obtained in about 25% of elderly patients, partly because of chest-wall abnormalities and pulmonary hyperinflation. M-mode studies, although less useful than 2-D echograms for detailed assessment of cardiac anatomy (eg, segmental LV-wall motion abnormalities, severity of mitral stenosis, and detection of intracardiac masses), are easier to quantify. Age-related changes seen on M-mode echocardiography include modest increases in aortic root and left atrial dimensions, increase in LV-wall thickness with unchanged cavity size, and a diminution of mitral valve E-F closure slope (see TABLE 29–2). These changes rarely fall outside normal limits for any parameter except perhaps E-F slope (see FIG. 29–1). Fractional shortening and velocity of circumferential fiber shortening (measures of global LV function) are not significantly affected by age.

Echocardiography can detect thickened aortic or mitral valve leaflets in the elderly or a calcified mitral anulus, the most common sources of systolic murmurs in this age group. Pericardial effusions, atrial myxomas, LV thrombi, and valvular vegetations are also best detected by echocardiography, particulary 2-D.

TABLE 29–2. M-MODE ECHOCARDIOGRAPHIC PARAMETERS IN NORMAL SUBJECTS

	Group 1 (Age 25–44 yr)	Group 2 (Age 45–64 yr)	Group 3 (Age 65–84 yr)
Mitral valve E-F slope (mm/sec)	102.3 ± 3.7	79.0 ± 3.8*	67.1 ± 5.2[†]
Aortic root dimension (mm)	30.9 ± 0.6	32.0 ± 0.6	32.9 ± 0.8 [‡]
LV-wall thickness (mm)			
Systolic	15.4 ± 0.5	17.6 ± 0.7	18.8 ± 0.6*
Diastolic	8.7 ± 0.3	9.8 ± 0.5	10.7 ± 0.5*
Systolic/m^2	7.6 ± 0.3	9.2 ± 0.3	10.0 ± 0.4[†]
Diastolic/m^2	4.3 ± 0.1	5.0 ± 0.2*	5.7 ± 0.2[†§]
LV dimension (mm)			
Systolic	34.4 ± 1.1	32.1 ± 0.9	32.1 ± 1.4
Diastolic	51.8 ± 1.0	50.8 ± 1.3	51.2 ± 1.4
Systolic/m^2	17.3 ± 0.5	16.7 ± 0.5	16.8 ± 0.6
Diastolic/m^2	26.0 ± 0.5	26.4 ± 0.6	27.0 ± 0.7
Fractional shortening of minor semiaxis	0.34 ± 0.01	0.36 ± 0.01	0.37 ± 0.02
V (circ/sec)	1.17 ± 0.04	1.23 ± 0.04	1.30 ± 0.08

± = Mean standard error; LV = left ventricle; V = velocity of circumferential fiber shortening; circ = circumference.
* $P < 0.01$.
[†] $P < 0.0001$.
[‡] $P < 0.05$ vs. Group 1.
[§] $P < 0.05$ vs. Group 2.
(Adapted from G. Gerstenblith, J. Fredericksen, F. C. P. Yin, et al: "Echocardiographic assessment of a normal adult aging population," in *Circulation*, Vol. 56, pp. 273-278, 1977. Used by permission of the American Heart Association, Inc. and the authors.)

Cardiac Doppler testing, combined with echocardiography, in the elderly is used to quantify aortic valvular stenosis. The transvalvular pressure gradient (roughly 4 × [Doppler blood flow velocity]²) correlated closely ($r > 0.9$) with the catheter-measured gradient in 100 consecutively studied older patients. Similar correlations have been found for mitral stenosis, which is now increasingly recognized in the elderly. A more widespread application is in assessment of diastolic dysfunction. The rate of early diastolic LV filling declines with age (analogous to the decrease in E-F slope seen on M-mode echocardiography). To compen-

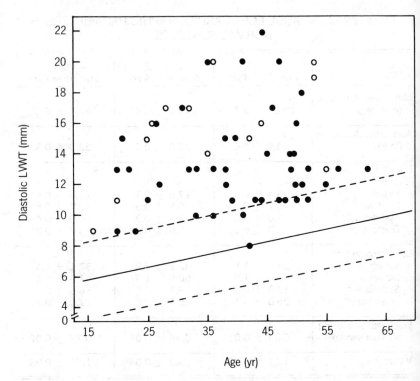

FIG. 29–1. Comparison of the increase in diastolic LV-wall thickness (LVWT) with aging vs. that induced by aortic valvular disease. The solid line represents the age regression in normal subjects, and the dashed lines indicate the 95% tolerance limits in this population. The closed circles denote patients with aortic stenosis, and the open circles, patients with aortic regurgitation. The wall thickness in the majority of the patient group lies well above the age-adjusted normal limit. (Adapted from A. L. Sjögren: "Left ventricular wall thickness in patients with circulatory overload of the left ventricle," in *Annals of Clinical Research*, Vol. 4, pp. 310-318, 1972. Used with permission of *Annals of Clinical Research*.)

sate, the atrial contribution to ventricular filling in late diastole increases with age (see Ch. 28). The contribution of newer Doppler technics, such as color flow mapping, has not yet been assessed in the elderly.

Radioisotope Studies

Although radioisotope technics lack the high spatial resolution of echocardiography, they are particularly well suited for quantifying ventricular function and for detecting heterogeneities in myocardial perfusion.

Radionuclide ventriculography is the most accurate tool for assessing global LV and right ventricular **(RV)** function, especially in the elderly (given the limitations of echocardiography). Two methods are in use: (1) The **first-pass technic** records the initial passage of a peripheral bolus injection of technetium-99m through the cardiac chambers, usually with a highly sensitive multicrystal camera. First-pass studies afford the most accurate assessment of RV ejection fraction, since they avoid the problem of chamber overlap intrinsic to the equilibrium technic.

(2) The more commonly used **equilibrium-gated blood-pool technic** allows the tracer to equilibrate within the blood, followed by the determination of intracardiac counts gated to the ECG, over many cardiac cycles. Gated imaging allows multiple measurements of LV function up to several hours after injection of isotope. Both technics can accurately measure global and regional LV function as well as changes in the LV volumes. Several studies using radionuclide ventriculography have shown no age-related changes in LV ejection fraction at rest.

Both first-pass and gated radionuclide technics have been used to measure LV ejection fraction during bicycle exercise. Although younger subjects normally increase ejection fraction by $\geq$ 5 points on exercise, about 25% of normal subjects > 60 yr of age have a blunted response. Thus, a normal exercise response in elderly subjects should probably be defined as *any increase in ejection fraction from the resting value*. In a large study of patients with chest pain who underwent exercise radionuclide ventriculography, the sensitivity for CAD was unaffected by age or gender, although specificity was decreased in women, particularly those > 60 yr of age (see TABLE 29–3).

Myocardial perfusion imaging with thallium-201 at rest and particularly during exercise is generally considered the most accurate noninvasive test for detecting CAD in all age groups. Thallium-201 concentrates in

TABLE 29–3. USEFULNESS OF RADIONUCLIDE
VENTRICULOGRAPHY IN DIAGNOSIS OF CORONARY ARTERY
DISEASE

Group (age)	% Sensitivity*	% Specificity*	Disease Prevalence (%)
Men (< 60 Yr)	88 (449)	53 (94)	82
Women (< 60 Yr)	91 (82)	27 (107)	43
Men (> 60 Yr)	96 (101)	46 (13)	88
Women (> 60 Yr)	92 (38)	7 (14)	70

* Numbers in parentheses are numbers of patients studied.

(Reprinted by permission of the publisher from "Diagnosis of Coronary Disease in the Elderly," by F. R. Cobb, M. Higgenbotham, D. Mark, in *Coronary Heart Disease in the Elderly* edited by N. K. Wenger, C. D. Furberg, E. Pitt, pp. 303-319. Copyright © 1986 by Elsevier Science Publishing Co., Inc.)

normally perfused cardiac muscle by substituting for K during Na-K exchange. Perfusion defects at rest generally indicate prior MI. Exercise-induced segmental defects that resolve or improve within 3 to 4 h signify exercise-induced ischemia. Specificity of the exercise ECG declines with age, probably because of the higher prevalence of resting ST-segment abnormalities (see above). Thus, a large percentage of older patients with LVH or bundle branch block or who are receiving digitalis are optimal candidates for thallium exercise studies if a noninvasive diagnosis of CAD is desired.

In a series of patients undergoing exercise thallium testing, sensitivity for CAD detection was nearly identical in subjects > 60 yr of age with that in younger individuals, 90 vs. 86%. Specificity was also similar, although the number of older subjects without CAD was small.

Positron emission tomography (PET) assesses both myocardial blood flow and metabolism after IV injection of a radiolabeled fatty acid. It has shown excellent sensitivity, but patient numbers are small, with minimal data in the elderly. The high cost of the tomographic camera and the need for an on-site cyclotron for isotope generation have thus far limited widespread application of this technic.

Promising New Noninvasive Imaging Modalities

Computed tomography (CT) of the heart is useful in diagnosing cardiac masses and pericardial effusions (although echocardiography is the initial procedure of choice). In elderly subjects, cardiac CT may be particularly helpful in distinguishing pericardial fat from effusion, a distinction that is often impossible with echocardiography. Echo-free pericardial spaces, indicative of either fat or effusion, increase in prevalence with age and are demonstrable in about 10% of women > 80 yr of age.

CT is the procedure of choice for defining pericardial thickening, a necessary component of constrictive pericarditis. It is also highly efficacious in the detection of lipomatous hypertrophy of the intra-atrial septum, an abnormality limited to the elderly that has been associated with supraventricular arrhythmias and sudden death. Recent refinements in fast CT have been used to assess the patency of coronary artery bypass grafts, thus avoiding routine postbypass cardiac catheterization. A drawback of this technic is the need for IV injection of iodinated contrast medium.

Magnetic resonance imaging (MRI) can characterize both cardiac anatomy and metabolism without ionizing radiation. It can assess myocardial viability postinfarction, in chronic heart failure, and in numerous other conditions. It provides an alternative to echocardiography for measuring chamber size and thickness. Gating the image acquisition to the ECG allows assessment of ventricular function. Its high cost and substantial overlap with echocardiography are major limitations of its use.

Cardiac Catheterization

Cardiac catheterization with coronary arteriography remains the gold standard of diagnosis. No alternative procedure measures intracardiac pressures or defines the coronary artery anatomy. Percutaneous balloon dilatation of the coronary arteries and cardiac valves has broadened the indications for catheterization beyond elderly patients considered for cardiac surgery.

TABLE 29–4. COMPLICATIONS OF CORONARY ARTERIOGRAPHY IN PATIENTS ≥ 65 YR OF AGE VS. THOSE < 65

Complication	Age < 65 yr (n = 17,165)	Age ≥ 65 yr (n = 2144)	P
Death	0.6	1.9	0.038
Nonfatal MI	2.9	7.9	0.001
Vascular	8.4	8.4	NS
Arterial embolism	0.5	1.9	0.025
Neurologic	1.0	3.7	0.001
Ventricular fibrillation	3.8	4.2	NS

Numbers represent incidence per 1000 cases.
NS = not significant.
(Adapted from B. J. Gersh, R. A. Kronmal, R. L. Frye, et al: "Coronary arteriography and coronary artery bypass surgery: Morbidity and mortality in patients ages 65 years or older. A report from the Coronary Artery Surgery Study," in *Circulation*, Vol. 67, pp. 483–490, 1983. Used by permission of the American Heart Association, Inc. and the authors.)

TABLE 29–5. COMPARISON OF COMMONLY USED TESTS IN DIAGNOSIS OF CORONARY ARTERY DISEASE IN THE ELDERLY

Test	Sensitivity	Specificity	Technical Difficulty	Complication
Echocardiogram	ND	ND	↑	None
Resting ECG	ND	↓	↔	None
Exercise ECG	↑	Mild	↑	↔
Exercise thallium	↔	↔	↔ *	↔
Rest and exercise RNV	↔	↓	↔ *	↔
Catheterization	NM	NM	↑	↑

ND = No data available; NM = Not meaningful; RNV = radionuclide ventriculography.

Direction of arrow denotes whether parameter is increased (↑) or decreased (↓) in older compared to younger patients.

* Although thallium scintigraphy and RNV per se are not more difficult to perform in the elderly, when combined with exercise testing, they inherit the age-related difficulties in performing maximal aerobic exercise tests.

In the multicenter Coronary Artery Surgery Study **(CASS),** the incidence of death and other major complications of coronary arteriography in patients $\geq$ 65 yr of age was low but still significantly higher than in younger subjects (see TABLE 29–4). This may be partially explained by the higher prevalence of cardiomegaly and LV dysfunction in the elderly and the greater difficulty often encountered in obtaining vascular access. Coronary arteriography is nonetheless applicable in a large segment of geriatric patients with heart disease (a comparison with the commonly used noninvasive modalities for the diagnosis of CAD is shown in TABLE 29–5).

Digital subtraction angiography (a computer-enhanced imaging technic) may offer greater safety by allowing a 75% reduction in the amount of contrast medium.

30.   HYPERTENSION

Edward D. Frohlich

A persistent elevation of systolic and/or diastolic arterial pressure of primary (essential hypertension) or secondary basis, both of which may impair heart, brain, or kidney function if uncontrolled.

In acculturated societies, both systolic and diastolic BP tend to rise, until about age 60. Beyond that age, systolic pressure may continue to rise, whereas the diastolic pressure tends to stabilize or decline. In contrast, in some primitive societies, neither systolic nor diastolic BP increases with age; hypertension is practically nonexistent. This has been attributed to the lesser amounts of dietary sodium ($<$ 60 mEq per day) of these populations. In the USA, over 50% of individuals who are $\geq$ 65 yr of age have abnormally elevated systolic or diastolic pressures.

According to the Joint National Committee's 1988 Report on the Detection, Evaluation, and Treatment of High Blood Pressure, systolic pressure elevation is defined as $\geq$ 140 mm Hg and diastolic pressure elevation as $\geq$ 90 mm Hg (see TABLE 30–1). Patients whose diastolic pressures are $<$ 90 mm Hg with systolic pressures between 140 and 159 mm Hg have **borderline systolic hypertension.** By definition, **isolated systolic hypertension (ISH)** is a systolic pressure of $\geq$ 160 mm Hg. When the diastolic pressure is $>$ 89 mm Hg, the condition is called **systemic arterial hypertension.**

The prevalence of elevated arterial pressures in the USA has led many to believe that a rising arterial pressure associated with aging is normal and innocuous. To the contrary, several multicenter prospective studies have shown that the higher the systolic or diastolic pressure, the greater are the cardiovascular and total morbidity and mortality rates. More-

TABLE 30-1. CLASSIFICATION OF ARTERIAL HYPERTENSION BY ARTERIAL PRESSURE LEVELS

	Pressure (mm Hg)	Class
Systolic (when diastolic pressure < 90)	< 140	Normal BP
	140–159	Borderline isolated systolic hypertension
	≥ 160	Isolated systolic hypertension
Diastolic	< 85	Normal BP
	85–89	High normal BP
	90–104	Mild hypertension
	105–114	Moderate hypertension
	≥ 115	Severe hypertension

(Modified from the Joint National Committee on the Detection, Evaluation, and Treatment of High Blood Pressure, *The 1988 Report of the Joint National Committee on Detection, Evaluation, and Treatment of High Blood Pressure*, in *Archives of Internal Medicine*, Vol. 148, pp. 1023-1038, 1988. Used with permission.)

over, these studies have also shown that an elevated systolic pressure is a better predictor of cardiovascular complications than is an elevated diastolic pressure. An isolated systolic pressure elevation imparts a two- to five-fold excess risk of cardiovascular death, a risk of stroke that is 2.5 times greater than that for individuals without ISH, and a 51% excess overall mortality as compared with age-, race-, and sex-matched normotensive individuals.

In general, hypertension predisposes the affected individual to heart failure, stroke, renal failure, coronary heart disease, and peripheral vascular disease. Antihypertensive therapy reduces the risk of developing many of these catastrophic complications. For example, treatment of hypertension has helped importantly to reduce the incidence of fatal stroke in the USA by 50%, and deaths from myocardial infarction **(MI)** have been reduced by 35%, no doubt significantly affected by antihypertensive therapy. Similar treatment benefits have been reported by the European Working Party on Hypertension in the Elderly, which demonstrated a 60% reduction in fatal MI.

Etiology

The etiologies of arterial hypertension are no different in elderly than in younger patients (see TABLE 30–2). **Primary (essential) hypertension,** afflicting at least 85% of approximately 60 million hypertensive Americans, may develop from changes in any or all of the pressor and depressor mechanisms responsible for maintaining normal arterial pressure levels.

The list of possible mechanisms underlying hypertension is long. Among the more important **pressor** mechanisms are increased participation of the adrenergic nervous system and/or catecholamines; increased activity of the renopressor (renin-angiotensin) system (systemically or in autocrine systems of arteries, heart, brain, or other organs); reduced distensibility of the great vessels (eg, from atherosclerosis) with impaired left ventricular impedance; and altered regulation of fluid and electrolyte balance. The latter may be associated with either subclinical renal parenchymal disease or the hormonal and humoral factors that directly affect fluid and electrolyte balance. Underactivity of various **depressor** systems, including the kallikrein-kinin system, the prostaglandins, atrial natriuretic hormone, and others, may also play a role.

TABLE 30–2. CLASSIFICATION OF THE VARIOUS FORMS OF SYSTEMIC ARTERIAL HYPERTENSION BASED ON ETIOLOGY

Primary (essential) hypertension (hypertension of undetermined cause)
 Borderline (labile) essential hypertension
 Established essential hypertension
  Mild
  Moderate
  Severe
 Isolated systolic hypertension

Secondary hypertension (hypertension of attributable cause)
 Renovascular hypertension
  Atherosclerotic renal arterial disease
  Nonatherosclerotic (fibrosing) renal arterial disease
  Renal arterial aneurysm
  Embolic renal arterial disease
  Extravascular compression (eg, tumors, fibrosis)
 Renal parenchymal diseases
  Chronic pyelonephritis
  Chronic glomerulonephritis
  Polycystic disease
  Diabetic glomerulosclerosis
  Others: amyloid, obstructive disease, etc
 Hormonal diseases
  Thyroid diseases
   Hyperthyroidism
   Hypothyroidism
  Adrenal diseases
   Cushing's disease or syndrome
   Primary hyperaldosteronism
    Adenoma
    Bilateral hyperplasia
   Adrenal enzyme abnormalities
  Pheochromocytoma
  Others: ectopic production of pressor hormones in metastatic tumors, growth hormone, hypercalcemic diseases, and hyperparathyroidism

(Continued)

TABLE 30-2. CLASSIFICATION OF THE VARIOUS FORMS OF
SYSTEMIC ARTERIAL HYPERTENSION BASED ON ETIOLOGY
(Cont'd)

Secondary hypertension (cont'd)
    Coarctation of the aorta
    Drugs, chemicals, and foods*
        Excessive alcohol ingestion
        Excessive dietary sodium intake
        Steroidal compounds: steroids for malignancies, asthma, oral estrogens
        Cold preparations (OTCs): nasal decongestants, phenylpropanolamine
        Milk-alkali syndrome, hypervitaminosis D
        Others: licorice, snuff, etc
    Secondary to specific therapy
        Antidepressant therapy (tricyclics, MAO inhibitors)
        Chronic steroid administration
        β-adrenergic receptor agonists
        Radiation nephritis or arteritis
        Cyclosporine (transplantation immunosuppressive therapy)

* (From F. H. Messerli and E. D. Frohlich: "High blood pressure: A side effect of drugs, poisons, and food," in *Archives of Internal Medicine*, Vol. 139, pp. 682–687, 1979. Copyright 1979, American Medical Association. Used with permission of the American Medical Association and the authors.)

Each of the foregoing pressor and depressor mechanisms contributes to the control of arterial pressure in normotensive or hypertensive individuals at any age. Catecholamine levels, particularly norepinephrine, have been found to be elevated with increased age; and β-adrenergic receptor responsiveness suggests these receptors are down-regulated. However, α-adrenergic receptors seem to be unchanged. Plasma renin activity and angiotensin II levels are suppressed in elderly individuals with hypertension, but this has not been associated with expansion of intravascular volume. Thus, participation of the foregoing pressor and depressor mechanisms seems to be as variable and unresolved in elderly hypertensive patients as they are in younger patients.

Because atherosclerosis is common in the elderly, the presence of an atherosclerotic renal arterial lesion is a major secondary etiologic consideration. Such a lesion may produce an elevated arterial pressure de novo or aggravate prior essential hypertension. Underlying endocrine diseases (eg, thyroid diseases, hypercalcemic diseases, release of humoral agents from malignant tumors, primary aldosteronism, and pheochromocytoma) also may account for recent-onset hypertension in the elderly.

Because older patients frequently have multiple diseases, medications (including OTC preparations) should be carefully considered when identifying the etiology of recent onset, aggravation, or complication of hypertension (see TABLE 30-2).

Some of these medications and diseases may predispose hypertensive patients to complications. For example, use of digitalis and a diuretic may cause hypokalemia-related cardiac dysrhythmias; chronic diarrhea and laxative abuse may also predispose to hypokalemia; corticosteroids may produce a hypokalemic form of hypertension; cyclosporine, tricyclic antidepressants, monoamine oxidase **(MAO)** inhibitors, and phenyl-propanolamine or other vasoconstrictors contained in OTC cold preparations may also elevate arterial pressure.

Pathogenesis and Pathophysiology

The hemodynamic characteristics of elderly hypertensives are similar to those of younger patients. Thus, arterial pressure is the product of 2 hemodynamic variables: cardiac output **(CO)** and vascular resistance to the forward flow of blood through the systemic circulation (total peripheral resistance). The CO, in turn, is the product of 2 variables, heart rate and stroke volume; and the latter may be increased by enhanced myocardial contractility or venous return. Vascular resistance may be increased by adrenergic stimulation, increased renopressor activity, and many circulating hormonal or humoral substances. The many factors that can increase arteriolar smooth muscle tone and total peripheral resistance are presented in TABLE 30–3. All of these factors act interdependently in the normal as well as the hypertensive individual.

Since recent studies strongly indicate the presence of a local renin-angiotensin system within the vascular myocyte, it is reasonable to conclude, even if tentative, that the system may contribute to the tone of vascular smooth muscle. This may explain the effectiveness of the angiotensin converting enzyme **(ACE)** inhibitors in patients with low plasma renin activity, including the elderly.

Atherosclerotic disease, so common in the elderly, reduces large artery distensibility, resulting in elevated systolic pressure as the left ventricle ejects its stroke volume into a more rigid and less compliant aorta. This **reduced distensibility of the aorta** and other large arteries is a major factor in the pathophysiology of ISH and also impairs left ventricular impedance. Other pathologic conditions that can contribute to systolic hypertension in the elderly are hyperthyroidism, aortic insufficiency, malnutrition (with clinical or subclinical beriberi), diseases with arteriovenous fistulae, and fever.

As **vascular resistance increases,** so do systolic and diastolic pressures. The heart adapts to this progressively increasing afterload by a process of concentric hypertrophy. Because of the frequent coexistence of pressure-overload left ventricular hypertrophy with myocardial ischemia, blood supply to the myocardium may be insufficient–even if the arterial pressure is not dramatically elevated. The complexity of these alterations is compounded by cardiac enlargement; a reduced β-adrenergic responsiveness; and possible deposition of collagen, amyloid, and other substances in the aging myocardium, even if hypertension is not present (TABLE 30–4).

TABLE 30–3. MECHANISMS OF ALTERING VASCULAR RESISTANCE

Constriction
 Active
  Adrenergic stimulation
  Catecholamines: norepinephrine, epinephrine
  Renopressor: angiotensin II
  Cations: Ca, K (high levels)
  Hormonal and humoral substances: vasopressin, serotonin, certain prostaglandins
 Passive
  Edema: extravascular
  Vessel wall water-logging
  Increased blood or plasma viscosity
  Obstruction (proximal): thrombosis, embolus
  Cold

Dilation
 Active
  Prostaglandins (certain)
  Kinins: bradykinin, kallidin
  Histamines
  Peptides: atrial natriuretic factor, insulin, vasoactive intestinal polypeptide,
    calcitonin gene-related peptide, parathormone, endorphins, enkephalins, renal
    medullary, phospholipid
  Cations: K (low levels), Mg
 Passive
  Reduced blood or plasma viscosity
  Increased tonicity
  Heat

Each of the above factors may **reduce myocardial contractility of the
left ventricle** that may eventually lead to cardiac failure. This process
may be aggravated further if exogenous obesity coexists. Obesity is associated with expanded intravascular volume, increased venous return to
the heart, and elevated CO. This volume overload provides an eccentric
component to the left ventricular hypertrophy, offering an explanation
for the facilitated cardiac failure observed in obesity-associated hypertension.

TABLE 30–4. PATHOPHYSIOLOGY OF CARDIAC ENLARGEMENT IN
              THE ELDERLY

  Increasing afterload associated with hypertensive vascular disease

  Absolute or relative myocardial ischemia

  Collagen tissue deposition

  Reduced number of adrenergic receptor sites

In contrast to the plasma volume expansion that occurs with obesity, **intravascular volume contracts** as arterial pressure and total peripheral resistance rise in most patients with essential hypertension. Because **activity of the renopressor system seems to be reduced** and less sensitive in elderly patients with primary hypertension, an attenuated relationship between intravascular volume and the renopressor system results. This may explain the enhanced responsiveness to diuretics and Ca channel blocking drugs that occurs in some elderly hypertensive patients (particularly those with ISH). The superiority of Ca channel blockers over other agents, however, has yet to be proved.

The Laplace relationship is another important hemodynamic consideration in elderly hypertensive patients. Myocardial O_2 consumption is directly related to left ventricular wall tension. This factor, in turn, is directly related to the product of the left ventricular diameter and the systolic pressure generated within this chamber during contraction.

In hypertensive patients (and even in elderly normotensive individuals), left ventricular and systolic vascular pressures are increased. Both of these tension-dependent factors further increase left ventricular demand for O_2, which explains the development of coronary insufficiency and angina pectoris and provides a rationale for reducing arterial pressure in patients who have only mild diastolic hypertension or ISH.

Hypertension may also impair **brain and kidney function.** Impaired brain function is evidenced by reduced sensory, motor, and intellectual function, the result of transient ischemic attacks **(TIAs)** and strokes.

Hypertension diminishes **renal parenchymal function** in a manner similar to the aging process. Histologic evidence of nephrosclerosis in hypertensive and aging patients demonstrates the altered structure associated with impaired parenchymal function. Thus, renal blood flow decreases in proportion to the reduction of CO; there is consequent increased intrarenal vascular resistance, reduced GFR, and decreased ability to concentrate urine. Hypertension and aging synergistically exacerbate these changes. In patients with untreated essential hypertension, the lower the renal blood flow, the higher the serum uric acid concentration, explaining the high incidence of hyperuricemia in these patients.

Symptoms and Signs

Hypertension, when uncomplicated and not associated with target organ involvement, is usually a **silent disease.** The medical literature suggests hypertension is associated with **headaches, epistaxis,** and **tinnitus.** But these complaints are nonspecific. Young patients with borderline or mild essential hypertension and no target organ involvement may have symptoms of **cardiac awareness** (rapid heart rate, palpitations, or ectopic beats) associated with physiologic findings that confirm a **hyperdynamic circulation.** These changes may also occur in older individuals and in patients with more severe hypertension.

Symptoms and signs occur more often in hypertensive patients with **secondary forms of hypertension.** Thus, **pheochromocytoma** may be associated with headache, flushing, BP lability, and hypermetabolism. **Occlusive renal arterial disease** may produce sudden onset or worsening of BP elevation, headaches, and renal arterial bruits that are systolic and (more significantly) diastolic in timing. Patients with **renal parenchymal disease** may experience recurrent UTI and symptoms of frequency, nocturia, impaired urinary concentratability, microscopic or gross hematuria, and anemia (with advanced disease). The coexistence of hypertension and anemia in younger patients indicates renal parenchymal disease (if hemoglobinopathy is excluded); however, in the elderly, it suggests the possibility of coexistent **neoplasm.**

Patients with **thyroid disease** show the characteristic symptoms of hyper- or hypothyroidism. Those with **primary aldosteronism** exhibit muscle weakness, nocturia, isosthenuria, altered carbohydrate metabolism, and hypokalemic alkalosis. **Cushing's disease** is also suggested by the presence of hypokalemic alkalosis and the typical facies, hirsutism, purplish abdominal striae, buffalo hump, and new appearance of acneiform lesions.

In patients with essential hypertension, the presence of symptoms or signs suggests **target organ involvement.** With **cardiac involvement,** the earliest complaints are easy fatigability, palpitations, and atrial or ventricular ectopic cardiac beats. Chest pain in patients without occlusive coronary disease reflects increased myocardial O_2 demand, with persistently elevated arterial pressures and cardiomegaly (left ventricular hypertrophy). More advanced stages of cardiac involvement are marked by symptoms and signs of heart failure: exertional dyspnea, orthopnea, peripheral edema, and increased ventricular irritability. Edema in the absence of cardiac failure suggests a secondary form of hypertension.

A 3rd heart sound (ventricular gallop rhythm) may develop, usually in association with a 4th heart sound (atrial gallop), which reflects the reduced distensibility and compliance of the hypertrophying left ventricle. Sudden onset of back pain and hypertension suggest aortic dissection.

The earliest symptom of **renal involvement** is nocturia; later symptoms and signs are those of functional impairment: frequency, proteinuria, anemia, and edema. Sensory or motor deficits signal **involvement of the brain;** subtle symptoms of TIAs include transient speech impediments, numbness of fingers and extremities, or unusual weakness. Sudden onset of a severe vertical headache and hypertension suggests a subarachnoid hemorrhage.

All patients should be examined for hypertensive retinopathy. In elderly patients, this should not be confused with the sclerotic changes of increased arteriolar light-striping, arteriovenous nicking, and tortuosity. Arteriolar (and venular) constriction and the appearance of hemorrhages, exudates, and papilledema suggest advancing and more severe degrees of hypertensive vascular disease.

The physician should listen for renal, carotid, aortic, brachial, and femoral arterial bruits. For example, the presence of a carotid bruit with symptoms of TIA suggests embolic phenomena from that vessel.

Laboratory Data

Laboratory studies in patients with hypertension should include: a **blood count** (with Hb, Hct, and WBC); an **ECG** (to identify early evidence of left ventricular hypertrophy, left atrial abnormality, and dysrhythmias); selected **blood chemistries** such as fasting blood glucose and serum levels of creatinine, uric acid, potassium, and lipids (including high- and low-density cholesterol fractions); and a **urinalysis.** A slightly elevated Hct or Hb suggests hypertension-induced hemoconcentration; this may be confirmed by a proportionately higher plasma protein concentration. Hyperuricemia may indicate that the patient is taking a diuretic; has the inborn potential for gout; or, in the untreated hypertensive patient, that renal blood flow is reduced.

The **chest x-ray** is less sensitive than the **ECG** for detecting cardiac enlargement. ECG evidence of left atrial enlargement provides an early clue to left ventricular hypertrophy, before it can be detected by the usual criteria of increased voltage, delayed intrinsicoid deflection of the QRS complex, or left ventricular hypertrophy and strain pattern. The enlarged left atrium does not indicate atrial disease per se. Rather, it indicates reduced left ventricular distensibility associated with development of hypertrophy of the left ventricle.

Even more sensitive than the ECG is the **echocardiogram,** which can clearly demonstrate ventricular hypertrophy in patients whose ECG shows left atrial abnormality only. Moreover, before systolic functional changes occur as a result of left ventricular hypertrophy, diastolic functional changes are revealed by echocardiographic or radionuclide studies showing a reduced left atrial filling rate. Echocardiographic evidence of left ventricular hypertrophy usually precedes early evidence of **renal functional impairment,** which includes slightly reduced renal blood flow in proportion to the height of serum uric acid concentration. Later evidence of renal impairment includes rising serum creatinine or BUN concentrations, as well as reduced creatinine clearance (GFR) and urine concentratability.

Hypercalcemic states are frequently associated with hypertension, and when they are present, the clinician should think first of hyperparathyroidism in younger persons but metastatic bone disease in older patients. Because hypercalcemia is frequently associated with diuretic therapy, this possibility should be carefully explored in the history taking.

Proteinuria occurs infrequently in patients with uncomplicated essential hypertension. When daily urinary protein excretion exceeds 400 mg, nephrosclerosis (associated with essential hypertension or aging) is not likely to be the cause; the entire differential diagnosis of renal parenchymal disease should be considered. A fresh urine sample with an alkaline pH suggests hypokalemia or primary aldosteronism.

Diagnosis

The diagnosis of hypertension depends on demonstration of elevated arterial pressure at levels defined in TABLE 30–1. The elevated pressure should be documented on at least 3 separate occasions, with at least 2 separate BP measurements taken on each occasion.

Proper technic in BP measurement is especially important in the elderly patient. BP should be measured in both arms during the initial examination and periodically thereafter. Frequently, occlusive atherosclerotic disease of the subclavian or brachial arteries reduces systolic pressure in one arm, as evidenced by an abrupt, unexplainable decline. Measurements should be obtained in supine or sitting and standing positions, because postural (orthostatic) hypotension is common in elderly patients, particularly after meals.

If pressures are persistently and strikingly elevated but cardiac size is normal according to chest x-ray and ECG criteria, the physician should suspect "pseudohypertension." This finding occurs when the sphygmomanometer cuff is unable to compress a sclerotic brachial artery. To verify the phenomenon, a direct arterial pressure measurement may be needed. Once actual hypertension is diagnosed, the physician must determine whether the condition is of primary or secondary origin.

Treatment

Nonpharmacologic treatment includes maintaining an ideal body weight, moderating alcohol intake ($\leq$ 1 oz of ethanol-equivalent), controlling dietary sodium ($\leq$ 100 mEq/day), and avoiding smoking. (Studies show that smokers who take certain antihypertensive drugs, such as propranolol, have more complications of hypertension than smokers who receive other treatment, such as thiazide diuretics.) These therapeutic measures may not control arterial pressure completely, but they may be adequate to control pressure in some patients or reduce the number and dosages of antihypertensive drugs in others.

Isolated systolic hypertension (ISH): The efficacy of reducing systolic arterial pressure in patients with ISH has not yet been adequately demonstrated in clinical studies. However, it is known that ISH patients are at greater risk than nonhypertensive individuals; the elevated pressure and larger heart of the elderly ISH patient increases myocardial O_2 demand. The feasibility study for a large multicenter study of systolic hypertension in the elderly **(SHEP)** strongly suggests that elevated systolic pressure can be controlled by diuretics (eg, hydrochlorothiazide, starting with 25 mg and increasing, if necessary, to 50 mg). Alternatively, β-adrenergic receptor blocking agents or Ca entry antagonists may be effective. If one of these agents alone is unable to control the elevated pressure, a second drug may be added (eg, a diuretic and a β-blocker).

Mild hypertension: Patients whose diastolic pressure falls between 90 and 104 mm Hg, and whose pressures are not controlled by nonpharmacologic means, may respond to a diuretic, β-adrenergic receptor blocker, an angiotensin converting enzyme **(ACE)** inhibitor, or a Ca entry antagonist in submaximal doses (see TABLE 30–5). If the initial dose fails to control pressure, the dose may be increased. This concept is consistent with the currently advocated "individualized stepped care" approach to treatment (see TABLE 30–6).

TABLE 30–5. ANTIHYPERTENSIVE AGENTS

Agent	Usual Initial Daily Dose	Maximal Daily Dose
Diuretics (selected agents are compiled in equal dosage forms)		
Chlorothiazide	250 mg qd	500 mg
Hydrochlorothiazide	25 mg qd	200 mg
Furosemide	40 mg qd	2.0 gm
Spironolactone	25 mg bid	100 mg
Adrenergic inhibitors		
Rauwolfia derivatives		
Reserpine (typical of this group)	0.05 mg qd	0.25 mg qd
Methyldopa	250 mg bid	3.0 gm
Guanethidine	10 mg qd	150 mg
Guanadrel	10 mg qd	100 mg
Clonidine	0.1 mg bid	1.2 mg
Guanabenz	4.0 mg bid	32 mg
Trimethaphan	1 mg/mL IV	—
α_1-Adrenergic-receptor antagonists		
Prazosin	1.0 mg bid–tid	20 mg
β-Adrenergic-receptor antagonists		
Acebutolol	100 mg qd	1200 mg
Atenolol	25 mg qd	150 mg
Metoprolol	50 mg qd	300 mg
Nadolol	40 mg qd	320 mg
Pindolol	20 mg qd	60 mg
Propranolol	40 mg qd	480 mg
Timolol maleate	10 mg bid	80 mg
Combined α/β-inhibitor		
Labetalol	100 mg bid	2400 mg
Vasodilators		
Hydralazine	10 mg bid	200 mg
Slow-channel Ca entry-blocking agents		
Diltiazem	30 mg tid	360 mg
Nifedipine	10 mg tid	180 mg
Verapamil	80 mg tid	480 mg
Angiotensin converting enzyme inhibitors		
Captopril	12.5 mg qd	150 mg
Enalapril	5 mg qd	40 mg
Lisinopril	10 mg qd	40 mg

(Adapted from E. D. Frohlich: "Practical management of hypertension," in *Current Problems in Cardiology,* Vol. 10, No. 7, p. 50, 1985. Copyright © 1985 by Year Book Medical Publishers. Reproduced with permission.)

TABLE 30–6. STEPPED-CARE APPROACH TO DRUG THERAPY

Step 1	Begin with less than a full dose of

Thiazide-type *or* diuretic	β-Adrenergic *or* receptor blocker	Angiotensin *or* converting enzyme inhibitor	Ca antagonist

Step 2	Proceed to full dose of Step 1 choice *or* Add a second agent from Step 1 choices *or* Use an alternative agent

Step 3 Add a third agent or proceed with full doses of the two Step 2 choices or select an alternative Step 1 agent

A second agent may be added to low-dose drug administration to prevent development of side effects from full doses of the first agent. Thus, adding a β-blocker to hydrochlorothiazide 25 mg daily may prevent hypokalemia and hyperuricemia. In general, elderly patients respond to diuretics. Ca entry antagonists are also effective with these patients, as well as with blacks and with patients who have not responded to lower doses of β-blocking drugs prescribed for concomitant angina pectoris.

More severe stages of hypertension: In patients with moderate or severe hypertension, any of the first-step agents may be prescribed. If this does not control BP adequately, however, a second or third agent may be necessary. These can be added sequentially, using lower doses first, then increasing doses or adding different agents.

Tailoring therapy rationally by selecting pharmacologic agents most appropriate to the pressor mechanisms of specific patients is possible. For example, the black or obese patient, who is more volume-dependent and has lower plasma renin activity, may respond well to a diuretic or Ca channel antagonist. These agents, therefore, would be wise selections. Elderly hypertensive patients respond well to these and other drugs. The patient with renal arterial disease (unilateral but not in a solitary kidney) or with heart failure may be more responsive to an ACE inhibitor.

Therapy with β-blockers may be appropriate for patients with a previous MI, angina pectoris, migraine headaches, or glaucoma. For a glaucoma patient, an oral β-blocker prescribed for hypertension will usually not be adequate for the glaucoma as well. If the patient has not experienced side effects from prolonged therapy with a topical β-blocker, he probably will not have adverse effects from the addition of an oral agent.

If the patient is already using digitalis, a diuretic should be prescribed with care. Serum potassium levels should be closely followed to obviate cardiac dysrhythmias associated with hypokalemia. Impotence may result in patients treated with diuretics, adrenergic inhibitors, and β-blockers; the ACE inhibitors and Ca entry antagonists have been reported to produce fewer side effects.

Although elderly hypertensive patients have no more side effects from prolonged treatment than younger patients, they are more likely to have postural (orthostatic) hypotension from agents that inhibit adrenergic function. Also, agents with central actions may be more likely to cause depression, forgetfulness, vivid dreams or hallucinations, and sleep problems.

Patients with chronic obstructive lung disease, asthma, or heart block (greater than 1st degree) should not be treated with β-blocking drugs; Ca entry antagonists may be more appropriate. Patients with low heart rates may be good candidates for Ca entry antagonists that do not markedly reduce heart rate.

All hypertensive patients should continue therapy after BP is controlled, because pressure is likely to rise if therapy is discontinued.

---

31. HYPOTENSION

Lewis A. Lipsitz

Many physiologic changes that occur with aging affect BP. Numerous studies in Western countries have shown not only an association between age and BP elevation but also between age, BP elevation, and the risk of hypotension.

Baroreflex mechanisms regulate systemic BP by resisting transient decreases and damping transient increases in arterial pressure. With age, baroreflex response to both hypertensive and hypotensive stimuli progressively declines. At the same time, baroreflex response is reduced by hypertension. Thus the baroreflex function is most impaired in patients who are elderly and hypertensive. Clinical manifestations of this impairment include increased lability of BP in response to daily activities and an increased response to hypotensive stimuli, particularly medications.

Attenuation of baroreflex response may be caused partly by related arterial stiffening that results in a damping of baroreceptor stretch and relaxation during changes in arterial pressure. Reduced adrenergic responsiveness by the aged heart may result in diminished baroreflex-mediated cardioacceleration during hypotensive stimuli. These changes in baroreflex response become clinically significant when common hypotensive stresses, eg, posture change, can no longer be offset by compensatory homeostatic mechanisms.

A progressive decline in cerebral blood flow occurs with advancing age and is enhanced by risk factors for cerebrovascular disease (eg, hypertension, heart disease, diabetes mellitus, and hyperlipidemia). Thus, since elderly patients with such risk factors have reduced cerebral flow, relatively small reductions in BP may produce cerebral ischemia.

Cerebral autoregulatory mechanisms usually compensate for acute reductions in BP. Current data suggest that autoregulation of cerebral blood flow is generally maintained with age, except in certain individuals who have symptomatic orthostatic hypotension (see below). Chronic hypertension, however, raises the threshold for cerebral autoregulation. Although *acute* reductions in BP might not be tolerated well by hypertensive elderly patients, *gradual* reduction, using a variety of agents, can be accomplished without compromising cerebral blood flow.

ORTHOSTATIC HYPOTENSION

A reduction ≥ 20 mm Hg in systolic BP upon standing upright.

Orthostatic hypotension is a common clinical manifestation of impaired BP homeostasis occurring in 20 to 30% of noninstitutionalized elderly persons; its prevalence increases with advanced age and elevation in basal BP. Many healthy elderly people have wide variations in postural BP. A strong relationship exists between postural BP change and basal supine BP; when basal supine BP is highest, the decline in postural BP is greatest.

Etiology

Orthostatic hypotension in the elderly has 2 distinct clinical presentations: (1) physiologic, attributable to normal aging, and (2) pathologic, attributable to disease.

Physiologic orthostatic hypotension in healthy elderly persons varies dramatically from day to day, is related to BP elevation, and is associated with the exaggerated plasma norepinephrine response to postural change that is characteristic of aging. Although generally asymptomatic and labile, transient orthostatic hypotension may become clinically significant when it occurs with other hypotensive stresses; eg, volume depletion, ingestion of hypotensive drugs, or performance of Valsalva's maneuver during voiding. Prolonged bed rest may further compromise physiologic mechanisms, resulting in severe postural hypotension. Postural systolic BP reductions ≥ 20 mm Hg have been shown to be significant risk factors for syncope and falls in elderly patients without other evidence of autonomic nervous system dysfunction.

Pathologic orthostatic hypotension is usually symptomatic and is associated with postural dizziness, syncope, and symptoms of autonomic dysfunction; eg, a fixed heart rate, incontinence, constipation, inability to sweat, heat intolerance, impotence, and fatigability. In young patients, the absence of cardioacceleration upon standing is considered a distinguishing feature of autonomic dysfunction (rather than hypovolemia) as the cause of orthostatic hypotension. However, since this response is often blunted in normal elderly persons because of baroreflex impairment, it is not useful in the diagnosis of pathologic orthostatic hypotension in the geriatric population.

Pathologic orthostatic hypotension may be secondary to any of numerous diseases or to drugs commonly taken by elderly patients. Neuropathic causes of secondary orthostatic hypotension may be classified as central or peripheral (see TABLE 31-1).

TABLE 31-1. CAUSES OF ORTHOSTATIC HYPOTENSION

Drugs
Phenothiazines and other neuroleptics
Monoamine oxidase inhibitors
Tricyclic antidepressants
Antihypertensives
Levodopa
Vasodilators
β-Blockers
Ca channel blockers

Central nervous system disorders
Shy-Drager syndrome
Brainstem lesions
Parkinson's disease
Myelopathy
Multiple cerebral infarcts

Peripheral and autonomic neuropathies
Diabetes mellitus
Amyloidosis
Tabes dorsalis
Paraneoplastic syndromes
Alcoholic and nutritional diseases

Idiopathic orthostatic hypotension

In the absence of another cause, orthostatic hypotension may be primary or "idiopathic." **Idiopathic orthostatic hypotension** is characterized by lower basal plasma norepinephrine levels in the supine position, no increase in norepinephrine level upon standing, a lower threshold for the pressor response to infused norepinephrine, and a greater pressor response to tyramine, despite release of less norepinephrine at the sympathetic nerve ending. These findings suggest that norepinephrine is depleted from sympathetic nerve endings, resulting in postsynaptic denervation supersensitivity.

Patients with the **Shy-Drager syndrome** have normal levels of circulating norepinephrine and a normal response to infused norepinephrine and tyramine, but they also have no increase in plasma norepinephrine levels upon standing. This syndrome is associated with the degeneration of neurons in several areas of the CNS, including the corticobulbar, corticospinal, extrapyramidal, and cerebellar systems of the brain, as well as intermediolateral columns of the spinal cord. Thus the Shy-Drager syndrome is a central disorder of sympathetic BP control, usually associated with extrapyramidal and cerebellar symptoms.

Disorders of the peripheral autonomic nervous system are other major causes of pathologic orthostatic hypotension. These disorders include insulin-dependent diabetes mellitus, in which severe peripheral neuropathy and other end-organ damage is evident, as well as less common entities such as amyloidosis, vitamin deficiencies, and the neuropathies associated with malignancies, particularly cancers of the lung and the pancreas.

Perhaps the most common cause of orthostatic hypotension is the **use of medications,** such as phenothiazines, tricyclic antidepressants, antianxiety agents, and antihypertensive drugs, including both those with central effects (eg, methyldopa and clonidine) and those with peripheral effects (eg, prazosin, hydralazine, and guanethidine). Orthostatic hypotension may occur even from doses within the therapeutic range, which poses a dilemma, in that a positive therapeutic effect is achieved at the expense of this adverse effect.

Diagnosis and Treatment

The proper management of orthostatic hypotension begins with a clear demonstration of a clinically significant symptomatic reduction in BP upon standing. The clinician should not assume that an elderly person who complains of postural dizziness and light-headedness is actually suffering from reduction in BP. Rather, BP and pulse rate should be measured after the patient has been recumbent for at least 5 min and again at 1 and 3 min after the patient has been standing quietly. These measurements should be obtained on several occasions to confirm that reduction of BP is consistent before any therapy is begun. The goal of therapy should be reduction or elimination of symptoms, which often can be achieved without complete correction of orthostatic hypotension. Regardless of the cause of orthostatic hypotension, symptomatic postural reductions in BP should be treated in the stepwise fashion described below.

Initial therapeutic considerations include correction of hypovolemia and evaluation of all prescribed and OTC medications the patient is taking in order to identify a possible offending agent. The patient with chronic orthostatic hypotension should be instructed to rise slowly from bed or chair after a long period of recumbency or sitting. Dorsiflexing the feet before standing often promotes venous return to the heart, accelerates the pulse, and increases BP. Initiating a high salt intake program may produce modest weight gain but also will significantly blunt symptoms of orthostatic hypotension in many individuals. The use of elastic stockings that cover the thigh as well as the calf and, in some cases, the use of abdominal binders may be effective. Elevating the head of the bed 5 to 20° prevents the nocturnal diuresis and supine hypertension caused by nocturnal shifts of interstitial fluid from the legs to the rest of the circulation.

If the patient remains symptomatic after the above measures have been taken, medications may be necessary. Various drug regimens have been attempted, but most of them either have been ineffective or require further study. One agent that appears to be helpful in most types of orthostatic hypotension, however, is **fludrocortisone acetate**. This mineralocorticoid, given in daily doses of 0.1 to 1.0 mg orally until mild peripheral edema develops, produces an increase in extracellular fluid and plasma volume, and sensitizes blood vessels to the vasoconstrictive effect of norepinephrine. These physiologic changes appear to offset the homeostatic defect that occurs on arising in most persons with mild or moderately severe orthostatic hypotension. Except for the occasional development of supine hypertension or heart failure, complications of treatment are rare. Although hypokalemia can develop with large doses of mineralocorticoids, it is unlikely to be a problem.

Other drugs currently under study in the management of pathologic orthostatic hypotension include NSAIDs, such as indomethacin, the central α_2-antagonist yohimbine, the α_2-agonist clonidine, and β-blockers that block β_2-vasodilator receptors or have intrinsic sympathomimetic activity, such as pindolol. Central α_2-antagonists increase central sympathetic nervous system outflow, but in the absence of such outflow (as in Shy-Drager syndrome), α_2-agonists promote venoconstriction peripherally, thereby increasing venous return. Various sympathomimetic agents have yielded inconsistent results. On the other hand, 250 mg caffeine each morning attenuates orthostatic hypotension in younger patients and can be used safely in the elderly. Ergot alkaloids, including oral ergotamine tartrate and dihydroergotamine s.c. with caffeine have also been helpful in some patients. In very severe cases of orthostatic hypotension that resist traditional approaches, atrial pacing may be of value.

POSTPRANDIAL HYPOTENSION

The decline in BP that occurs after a meal.

Postprandial hypotension is another recently recognized clinical abnormality of BP homeostasis in the elderly. Recent studies of clinically stable, unmedicated elderly patients, both institutionalized and noninstitutionalized, showed significant reduction in BP after morning and noon meals, which does not occur in younger persons or in the absence of a meal in the elderly. About $1/3$ of healthy elderly persons have a postprandial BP decline $\geq$ 20 mm Hg within 1 h of eating a meal. This decline can be even greater when hypotensive medications are given before a meal. The incidence of postprandial hypotension is greatest in hypertensive elderly persons and in patients who have postprandial syncope or autonomic dysfunction. This phenomenon is probably a common cause of syncope and falls in the elderly.

Etiology, Symptoms, Signs, and Diagnosis

The mechanism of postprandial hypotension is unknown but is thought to be related to impaired baroreflex compensation for splanchnic blood pooling during digestion. Postprandial hypotension has 2 clinical presentations: (1) a physiologic, age-related phenomenon that is rarely symptomatic unless exacerbated by other hypotensive stresses and (2) a more severe pathologic syndrome related to autonomic insufficiency in which more profound hypotension is accompanied by syncope.

BP should be evaluated before and after meals in geriatric patients who experience postprandial dizziness, falls, syncope, or other cerebral or cardiac ischemic symptoms.

Treatment

In the absence of clinical trials to evaluate treatment of postprandial hypotension, management relies on common sense. Symptomatic patients should avoid taking hypotensive medications before meals and should lie down after eating. Reduction in dosage of hypotensive medications and ingestion of small, frequent meals may also be helpful.

Recent studies of patients with autonomic insufficiency suggest that indomethacin (50 mg q 6 h), caffeine (250 mg) with or without subcutaneous dihydroergotamine (6 to 10 μg/kg), or parenteral somatostatin given by experimental protocol (12 to 16 μg s.c.) before a meal may ameliorate postprandial hypotension. Caffeine (with dihydroergotamine) should be given only in the morning so the caffeine effect wears off by evening, allowing sleep and preventing tolerance to the drug. Other agents given $\frac{1}{2}$ h or so before the meal last for only a few hours.

---

32. CORONARY ARTERY DISEASE (CAD)

Gary Gerstenblith

A condition in which one or more of the coronary arteries is narrowed by atherosclerotic plaque and/or vascular spasm. CAD reflects an imbalance between myocardial O_2 supply and demand, which is expressed clinically as myocardial ischemia, angina, and myocardial infarction.

Incidence

Autopsy studies have demonstrated a dramatic age-related increase in the prevalence of CAD, which is seen in $\geq$ 50% of men $\geq$ 60 yr of age who die of miscellaneous causes; yet a history of symptomatic disease has been noted in only 10 to 20% of this population. This discrepancy may be due to (1) decreased activity levels in the elderly, so work loads that would ordinarily trigger ischemic symptoms are not encountered; (2) increasing likelihood of a neuropathy that alters pain sensation; and (3) age-associated myocardial and possibly pericardial changes, making dyspnea more likely to occur than chest pain when ischemia is present.

Diagnosis

CAD should be strongly suspected in persons with known coronary risk factors and in those with signs of noncoronary atherosclerosis such as cerebrovascular or peripheral vascular disease. Noninvasive ECG stress testing is useful in diagnosing CAD and in predicting subsequent coronary mortality in middle-aged populations with $\geq$ 2 risk factors. It is probably equally useful in the elderly.

ECG stress testing can also be used to evaluate the severity of CAD. Left-main or triple-vessel obstructions typically produce systolic hypotension (a fall in systolic BP of > 15 mm Hg from 1 exercise level to the next), and several types of ECG changes, including global changes (ie, those occurring in both the anterior and inferior leads); marked changes (> 2 mm of ST segment shift); prolonged changes (those remaining positive for > 8 min following exercise); early changes (those occurring during Stage 1 or Stage 2 of the standard Bruce treadmill test) and the appearance of malignant ventricular arrhythmias.

Several points should be considered when evaluating these results: First, ECG changes cannot be interpreted in the presence of left bundle branch block, left ventricular hypertrophy, or digitalis ingestion, all of which occur more frequently in the elderly than in the younger population. Under these circumstances, thallium stress testing is an excellent alternative. Second, the older patient often cannot exercise to 90% of predicted maximum heart rate because of respiratory or musculoskeletal disease. Here, thallium testing following the IV or oral administration of dipyridamole may be very useful. Third, the incidence of false-negative results is increased in a population with a high prevalence of disease, such as the elderly.

Persons with angina pectoris should be carefully evaluated for factors that precipitate increased myocardial O_2 demand and decreased myocardial O_2 supply (eg, anemia, infection, "masked" hyperthyroidism, heart failure, arrhythmias, and hypertension).

Prevention

The principles of CAD management are similar for all patients, and **risk factor modification** may be as important in older patients as in younger ones. Measures should be taken to decrease the progression of coronary atherosclerosis in both symptomatic and asymptomatic elderly individuals.

Data from the Framingham Heart Study indicate that **systolic BP** is the most potent discriminator of CAD risk in men > 45 yr old; more recent studies indicate that treatment of hypertension decreases the risk of cerebrovascular and cardiac mortality in the elderly. A double-blind study to determine the value of treatment of isolated systolic hypertension (defined as a systolic pressure $\geq$ 160 mm Hg in the absence of diastolic hypertension) in the elderly is currently in progress. Until the results are known, the Joint National Committee on the Detection, Evaluation, and Treatment of High Blood Pressure recommends that therapy be instituted in this age group.

Framingham data also indicate that total cholesterol levels are not related to unfavorable cardiovascular outcomes in the elderly. However, data on the fractionated components indicate a significant positive relationship between low-density lipoprotein **(LDL) cholesterol** levels and cardiovascular disease, and a striking negative relationship between high-density lipoprotein **(HDL) cholesterol** levels and cardiovascular disease. Drug and dietary interventions to reduce LDL levels have been shown to reduce cardiovascular risk in middle-aged populations. Although similar data have not been reported for the elderly, it is prudent to recommend dietary and pharmacologic therapy for those older individuals with markedly abnormal lipid levels.

Although Framingham data fail to correlate **cigarette smoking** with increased cardiovascular risk in the elderly, other studies indicate a positive relationship. Studies also show that cessation of smoking for even 1 to 5 yr is associated with a marked reduction in risk.

Antianginal Treatment

In elderly patients with angina, the primary drug options are the same as those in younger patients: nitrates, β-blockers, and Ca antagonists. **Nitrates** act primarily by lowering preload through venous dilation, which decreases venous return and hence ventricular cavity size, and to a lesser extent by reducing afterload through arteriolar dilation. They may also produce coronary vasodilation. Nitroglycerin given sublingually (0.3 to 0.6 mg) or as a lingual aerosol spray (0.4 mg) provides excellent relief during an acute ischemic episode and is useful for prophylaxis. Unfortunately, there is a significant attenuation of the anti-ischemic effect during continuous therapy with both oral (20 to 40 mg qid) and topical (5 to 20 mg/24 h) nitrate preparations. This can be avoided by intermittent dosing. Preliminary reports indicate that removing the transdermal patch overnight and using oral preparations bid or tid may prevent the development of nitrate tolerance. However, this may leave the patient insufficiently protected between doses.

Preexisting diminished intravascular volume, impaired venous valves, and a diminished baroreceptor reflex make older patients more susceptible to the hypotensive effects of nitrates. Thus, it is important to begin with a low dose, increase the dose slowly, and instruct the patients to be in a supine position when they first take any nitrate preparation.

β-**Blockers** work primarily by reducing myocardial O_2 demand; they decrease heart rate, myocardial contractility, and BP. Secondarily, they increase myocardial O_2 supply through the reduction in heart rate (since most of the coronary flow occurs during diastole). Propranolol has been demonstrated to produce a rightward shift of the oxygen-hemoglobin dissociation curve.

Since all available β-adrenoceptor blocking agents block the cardiac β_1-receptors, the choice of a β-blocker in an elderly patient should be based on the drug's associated properties. Low doses of relatively cardioselective drugs (atenolol 50 mg/day or metoprolol 100 mg/day) may be used when blockade of β_2-receptors is undesirable. However, the selectivity is only relative, with blockade of β_2-receptors occurring at moderate to high doses. Hydrophilic β-blockers (atenolol 50 to 200 mg/day or nadolol 40 to 80 mg/day) should be considered when treating patients with concomitant hepatic disease or when it is necessary to minimize CNS side effects. Lipophilic β-blockers, such as propranolol 80 to 240 mg/day, metoprolol 50 to 100 mg bid, or timolol 10 to 20 mg bid, may be preferable in patients with concomitant renal disease.

Secondary prevention is an important additional benefit of some β-blockers; studies have shown that some decrease the risk of subsequent infarction and death when given after MI. These are timolol 20 mg/day, propranolol 160 to 240 mg/day, and metoprolol 100 to 200 mg/day.

Precautions regarding β-blockers in the elderly include the potential pharmacokinetic changes described in Ch. 18 and altered pharmacodynamics, ie, the β-blocking properties of these agents are diminished in these patients. The age-related reduction in cardiovascular responsiveness to β-agonist stimulation (see Chs. 18 and 28) results in a decreased reliance on catecholamines and an increased dependence on the Frank-Starling mechanism to increase cardiac work during times of stress. This suggests that β-blockers may be less effective anti-ischemic agents in the elderly than in younger patients.

Preexisting disease, such as bronchospastic pulmonary disease, claudication, insulin-dependent diabetes, impaired ventricular function, and conduction system disease, may render the elderly more sensitive to the side effects of β-blockers. Prolonged therapy may result in up-regulation of cardiac β-receptors and hence produce an increased sensitivity to endogenous catecholamines following abrupt withdrawal. Thus, when therapy is discontinued in angina patients, *β-blockers should be withdrawn slowly, if possible.*

Ca antagonists are useful in the management of stable and unstable angina, including nifedipine (40 to 120 mg/day), diltiazem (90 to 360 mg/day), and verapamil (120 to 480 mg/day).

Ca antagonists act primarily by decreasing coronary and peripheral vascular resistance, although verapamil (and to a considerably lesser extent, diltiazem) has negative inotropic and chronotropic effects. These agents exert an anti-ischemic effect by decreasing coronary artery resistance and preventing spasm, which increases myocardial O_2 supply, and by inducing peripheral vasodilation, which decreases myocardial O_2 demand. They also have antiplatelet properties, and an antihypertensive effect, which makes them useful in patients with concomitant hypertension.

Concerns regarding the use of Ca antagonists in the elderly are related to their peripheral vasodilating and negative inotropic, chronotropic, and dromotropic effects. In addition to the hypotensive effects associated with peripheral vasodilation, which occur most often in patients who are volume depleted, a sympathetic reflex-induced increase in cardiac work may also occur. This effect can be prevented by the concomitant administration of a relatively small dose of β-blocker. The other cardiac side effects of the Ca antagonists occur primarily in individuals with preexisting impaired ventricular function or conduction system disease or in those who are taking fairly high doses of β-blockers. There does not appear to be any significant rebound phenomenon on withdrawal of Ca antagonists.

Aspirin (325 mg/day) has been shown to reduce by 50% the rate of MI and death following unstable angina; it is also approved for prevention of reinfarction following MI. Although studies have focused on middle-aged populations, it is reasonable and prudent to use the drug in the elderly.

If drug therapy fails to control symptoms, or if noninvasive studies (eg, the treadmill test) or the clinical setting (eg, recurrent ischemia in the postinfarction period) indicate that the patient is at high risk despite medical therapy, **cardiac catheterization** should be considered to evaluate the patient's suitability for **angioplasty** or **bypass surgery**. Some reports indicate that angioplasty in the elderly is associated with a lower success rate and an increased complication rate. More recent studies, however, indicate that the success rate in older patients (83%) is comparable to the success rate in younger patients (86%) and that the complication rate in the elderly (9%) is only slightly higher than that seen in younger patients (6%).

If a patient's coronary artery anatomy is not suitable for angioplasty, bypass surgery should be considered. Although mortality may be 2 to 3 times higher in the older than in the younger age groups, this is primarily related to associated medical conditions such as hypertension, impaired ventricular function, and extensive CAD. The procedure's overall mortality rate of 5 to 6% in the elderly is low enough for surgery to be recommended if the standard indications are present. Although morbidity and hospitalization time and costs are greater in the elderly, the risk of complications is decreasing. In addition, the long-term pain relief and survival rates associated with surgery compare favorably with those of drug therapy.

MYOCARDIAL INFARCTION (MI)

Necrosis of myocardial tissue resulting from obstruction of a coronary artery.

The incidences of mortality, heart failure, pulmonary edema, and ventricular rupture are significantly higher in older patients, possibly in part because of damage from prior MI and/or because hypertension is more prevalent. The elderly also tend to have larger infarctions and lower contractile reserve in noninfarcted regions, possibly related to diminished β-agonist responsiveness. Important topographic changes related to advancing age also occur during the first few hours or days following MI. They may include regional dilation and thinning in the infarcted area and compensatory hypertrophy in the noninfarcted tissue.

Medically supervised rehabilitation following MI results in an increase in conditioning status similar to that observed in younger patient groups.

Treatment

Because of the higher complication rate in the elderly, these individuals benefit at least as much as younger patients from close monitoring in a coronary care unit.

Catheterization studies in 1980 indicated a high prevalence of coronary thrombosis in patients presenting within the first 6 h of transmural infarction. Several randomized studies have subsequently been conducted to assess the effectiveness of early thrombolysis on survival and left ventricular function in patients with known and suspected infarction; they have shown, overall, that early thrombolysis decreases mortality and improves ventricular function. A recent study indicates that the addition of aspirin 160 mg/day provides benefit over and above that achieved with thrombolysis alone.

Some of these studies have reported analyses of patient subsets of different ages. These studies also indicate, in the placebo groups, a striking, several-fold increased mortality in older patients. The benefit of thrombolysis appears to increase with age up to 75 yr, probably because of the age-related increase in mortality in the control groups. Beyond 75 yr, the benefit is less, and the risk of cerebral hemorrhage is increased. Additionally, older individuals have an increased incidence of severe hypertension and history of cerebrovascular accidents, which are *absolute* contraindications for thrombolysis. For those without these conditions, age > 75 yr is a *relative* contraindication to thrombolytic therapy.

In assessing the benefit/risk ratio to decide whether to use thrombolytic therapy in older patients, one should remember that the benefit is increased in those who are treated early and in those who have extensive anterior infarctions.

Drug therapy is otherwise the same as that employed in younger patients. However, there is a marked heterogeneity of response in the elderly, with no strict age-related rules. Therefore, *therapy must be individualized.* The routine dose of **lidocaine** is usually reduced in older patients (to an infusion rate of 10 to 25 µg/kg/min) because of an age-related decrease in hepatic metabolism and an increased predisposition to CNS side effects. **Anticoagulants** should be used with care for 2 major reasons: Heparin is associated with an increased risk of bleeding in older women, and the hazards of chronic warfarin therapy are compounded by the increased risk of falls in older patients. As in younger patients, **β-blockers** may be used for their secondary preventive effects (see above). Such therapy is particularly beneficial for those who are at increased risk for recurrent MI.

33. VALVULAR HEART DISEASE

Nanette K. Wenger

In elderly patients, the predominant causes of valvular heart disease are degenerative calcification, myxomatous degeneration, papillary muscle dysfunction, and infective endocarditis; rheumatic and syphilitic disease are less frequent. Noninvasive imaging technics are important in establishing the diagnosis. Although medical management is appropriate for most older patients, surgery is appropriate when symptoms interfere with daily activities or when hemodynamically important valvular disease occurs acutely.

AORTIC VALVULAR DISEASE

AORTIC STENOSIS

An abnormal narrowing of the aortic valve orifice.

Prevalence and Etiology

Aortic stenosis, the most clinically significant valvular lesion in the elderly, increases in frequency with age. The severity of the stenosis is often underestimated because its progression is so gradual. Calcific aortic stenosis predominates, with calcification of a congenital bicuspid aortic valve seen in the "young elderly" and calcification on the aortic aspect of a tricuspid aortic valve typical in patients > 75 yr of age. The 20% of elderly patients with rheumatic aortic stenosis often have associated mitral valve disease.

Symptoms and Signs

For the minority of patients who are symptomatic, the prognosis is extremely poor. Chest pain is an early symptom. Presyncope (transient alteration of consciousness) progresses to effort syncope, which occurs in about ⅓ of symptomatic patients. Exertional dyspnea may progress to pulmonary edema. About ½ of aged patients with severe aortic stenosis have heart failure **(HF)**, often heralded by atrial fibrillation. Activity-precipitated symptoms may not occur in sedentary elderly patients.

Physical findings include a narrow pulse pressure and a slowly rising, small-volume carotid pulse, with a systolic thrill present at times. However, the poorly compliant arterial wall may mask these abnormalities, rendering the carotid pulse relatively normal. The cardiac apex impulse is sustained. The 1st heart sound is soft; the aortic component of the 2nd heart sound is soft or, when stenosis is critical (ie, severe and life threatening), may be inaudible. Reverse splitting of the 2nd sound may occur with left ventricular failure. A 4th heart sound is common, but disappears in the ¼ of elderly patients who develop atrial fibrillation. Ejection sounds are rare because the valve cusps are immobile.

A harsh, loud crescendo/decrescendo systolic murmur, often associated with a thrill, is maximal at the upper-right sternal border. The murmur peaks in mid- to late systole and often radiates throughout the precordium and into the neck. Transmission of the high-frequency components of the murmur to the lower-left sternal border and toward the cardiac apex is common during most of systole and may mimic the transmission of the murmur of mitral regurgitation. The intensity of the murmur does *not* correlate with the severity of the obstruction. With the decreased cardiac output of critical stenosis, the basal systolic murmur may soften or be absent. Basal diastolic murmurs of aortic regurgitation are heard in $> \frac{1}{2}$ of patients with aortic stenosis.

Laboratory Data

Electrocardiographic evidence of left ventricular hypertrophy is present, although hyperinflated lungs may mask left ventricular voltage elevation. Cardiac enlargement on chest x-ray is evident when HF supervenes. Poststenotic aortic dilatation is a frequent finding. Dense calcification of the aortic valve is best seen on the lateral chest x-ray. Lack of calcification on chest x-ray virtually excludes the diagnosis of critical aortic stenosis.

Two-dimensional echocardiography is used to assess cardiac chamber size, wall thickness, wall motion, valve leaflet motion, and valve orifice size. Valvular calcification can also be identified. Doppler measurement of intracardiac blood velocity permits calculation of the severity of valvular regurgitation or obstruction. Such studies are helpful in identifying appropriate candidates for cardiac catheterization. Exercise testing is *contraindicated* when critical stenosis is suspected because it is associated with an increased risk of syncope and death.

Diagnosis

Aortic stenosis must be differentiated from the benign aortic sclerosis that is present in $\frac{1}{3}$ to $\frac{1}{2}$ of elderly persons. The latter is typically asymptomatic and without hemodynamic significance; the basal systolic murmur is short and peaks early, and the carotid pulse is normal. Echocardiography and Doppler studies help differentiate the 2 conditions.

The chest pain associated with aortic stenosis must be differentiated from that of coronary disease. Likewise, the syncope must be distinguished from that due to atrioventricular block or tachyarrhythmias, 2 conditions that occur frequently in older patients. The dyspnea must be differentiated from that of chronic obstructive pulmonary disease or cardiomyopathy, and the murmur, from that of hypertrophic cardiomyopathy, mitral annular calcification, papillary muscle dysfunction, and aortic sclerosis. Cardiac catheterization, which is sometimes required to make these differential determinations, is warranted in patients with critical aortic stenosis to identify concurrent coronary atherosclerotic disease.

Treatment

Aortic valve replacement is indicated for hemodynamically significant symptomatic aortic stenosis, because only $1/2$ of medically treated elderly patients survive > 5 yr following onset of angina, HF, and/or syncope. In many instances, patients die suddenly.

Aortic valve replacement, even in patients of advanced age, improves survival and quality of life. The procedure can be performed in elderly patients who meet the criteria for Class 3 and 4 of the New York Heart Association Classification. Recent reports cite perioperative mortality as low as 4 to 5% in elderly patients with surgical mortality of 5 to 10%, even after the onset of HF. There is 70% survival at 5 yr, and long-term maintenance of improved function. Concurrent coronary bypass surgery may increase postoperative complications and mortality, primarily because it requires increased pump time.

Porcine heterograft valves have an advantage over mechanical valves in that anticoagulation is not needed with the former, but their durability is less certain. The efficacy and role of catheter balloon valvuloplasty for aortic stenosis are under investigation (see PERCUTANEOUS BALLOON VALVULOPLASTY in Ch. 37).

Elderly patients with noncritical aortic stenosis require serial surveillance because the stenosis progresses in severity, although at an unpredictable pace.

ACUTE AORTIC REGURGITATION

Sudden development of retrograde flow of blood, during ventricular diastole, through an incompetent aortic valve into the left ventricle.

Etiology and Pathophysiology

Trauma, infective endocarditis, or aortic dissection may be causal. Acute severe heart failure **(HF)** is precipitated by abrupt volume overload of a ventricle without compensatory hypertrophy or dilatation.

Symptoms, Signs, and Laboratory Data

Sudden, severe HF occurs with tachycardia and often with hypotension. The HF may mask the anticipated brisk arterial upstroke, wide pulse pressure, and collapsing pulse contour. The pulse pressure may be narrowed because of elevated left ventricular diastolic pressure. The 1st heart sound is soft, and the left sternal border decrescendo diastolic murmur is harsh and shortened by the raised ventricular filling pressure.

The ECG may be normal initially. Echocardiography helps confirm the diagnosis and often shows early mitral valve closure.

Diagnosis and Treatment

Acute aortic regurgitation must be differentiated from other causes of sudden severe HF (eg, papillary muscle or chordal rupture, septal rupture). The pulmonary edema may be erroneously attributed to MI. Urgent valve replacement is generally indicated for acute severe HF.

CHRONIC AORTIC REGURGITATION

Long-standing retrograde flow of blood during ventricular diastole through an incompetent aortic valve into the left ventricle.

Etiology and Pathophysiology

Chronic aortic regurgitation may be produced by valve leaflet disease (congenital, rheumatic, or secondary to endocarditis) or by aortic annular root dilatation (eg, as in syphilis, rheumatoid spondylitis, Marfan's syndrome). Mild to moderate aortic regurgitation is often symptomless for many years because of the sizable stroke volume of the dilated, hypertrophied ventricle and the lowered peripheral vascular resistance.

Symptoms and Signs

Rheumatic aortic regurgitation occurs predominantly in men and is often asymptomatic, even in old age. It is characterized by a soft, short basal diastolic murmur and may be accentuated by hypertension. Syphilitic aortic regurgitation is more severe and has a poorer prognosis, often because of an associated aortic aneurysm. A long, loud, decrescendo basal diastolic murmur, often with a short basal systolic murmur, is characteristic.

In symptomatic patients, effort intolerance and dyspnea may progress to HF. Chest pain is often due to associated coronary atherosclerosis. Palpitations usually reflect the forceful ejection of blood rather than arrhythmias.

The findings of severe regurgitation include bounding peripheral arterial pulses, a wide pulse pressure, occasionally a bisferiens pulse, and a hyperactive precordium with a rocking motion. The high-pitched diastolic murmur is heard best at the cardiac base. It is louder at the right-upper sternal border in aortic root disease and more prominent along the left sternal border in aortic leaflet disease. There may be an associated diastolic thrill and a spindle-shaped systolic murmur of increased aortic outflow. Both 3rd and 4th heart sounds are common, as is an apical diastolic **(Austin Flint)** rumble.

Laboratory Data

Cardiac enlargement with a dilated aorta, and occasionally with an aortic aneurysm, is a characteristic chest x-ray finding. Linear calcification of the ascending aorta is typical in syphilitic aortic regurgitation. This contrasts with the x-ray findings of benign aortic calcification. The ECG shows left ventricular hypertrophy. On echocardiography, the left ventricular cavity is enlarged, often with early diastolic fluttering of the anterior mitral valve leaflet. Enlarging ventricular dimensions and evidence of ventricular dysfunction in the symptomatic patient are indications for surgery.

Treatment

Medical management is the same as that for HF and includes Na restriction, diuretic and vasodilator therapy, and at times, digitalis. Valve replacement should be considered for patients who remain symptomatic on optimal medical therapy, even though the results are less satisfactory than in patients with aortic stenosis because of frequent underlying ventricular dysfunction. Bioprosthetic valves are favored because they do not require anticoagulant therapy, which is associated with an increased risk of bleeding in elderly patients (see Treatment under MITRAL STENOSIS, below).

MITRAL VALVULAR DISEASE

MITRAL STENOSIS

An abnormal narrowing of the orifice of the mitral valve.

Mitral stenosis, due predominantly to rheumatic heart disease, accounts for about ⅓ of mitral valve disease in the elderly. This incidence, however, may decrease because of the reduced incidence of rheumatic fever in developed countries. There is commissural fusion and fibrosis and calcification of the leaflets and chordae. Less often, progressive extension of mitral annular calcification may produce moderately severe mitral stenosis.

Symptoms, Signs, and Laboratory Data

The clinical features of mitral stenosis in the elderly are comparable to those in younger individuals and include a loud 1st heart sound, an apical diastolic rumble with presystolic accentuation, and an opening snap. The latter may soften or disappear with valvular calcification and the diastolic murmur may become softer. A right ventricular parasternal impulse is often palpable, and the venous pressure may be elevated. Atrial fibrillation is more common in elderly patients, as is complicating arterial embolism.

Left atrial enlargement is frequently seen on chest x-ray. Electrocardiographic evidence of right ventricular hypertrophy is uncommon. Echocardiography with Doppler flow studies can document mitral stenosis and help in estimating its severity.

Diagnosis and Treatment

Left atrial myxoma may mimic mitral stenosis and can be differentiated by echocardiography. Most elderly patients with mild to moderate mitral stenosis are in sinus rhythm, have few or no symptoms, and respond well to medical therapy. Although atrial fibrillation often precipitates clinical deterioration, therapy with digitalis, verapamil, and/or β-blockers can slow the ventricular response. Pharmacologic or electrical cardioversion to sinus rhythm may restore compensation.

Although elderly patients with mitral valvular disease and atrial fibrillation are at increased risk for bleeding, anticoagulation is recommended because of the high risk of valve thrombosis and embolism. Brain hemorrhage occurs in 1% of such anticoagulant-treated patients annually, an eight-fold increase in risk compared with the risk in patients who have not received anticoagulant therapy, and major hemorrhage is reported in 3%. Anticoagulation is nevertheless recommended, in the absence of specific contraindications, because of the high risk of embolism in patients with valvular disease and atrial fibrillation. The lower levels of anticoagulation therapy currently recommended, with prolongation of the prothrombin time to 1.5 to 2.0 times control values, may lessen the risk of bleeding complications.

Valve replacement is warranted for progressively severe symptomatic mitral stenosis, since the calcified valve is rarely amenable to commissurotomy. Embolization per se is not an indication for valve surgery. The high risk of thrombosis associated with prosthetic heart valves mandates anticoagulant therapy. Evidence demonstrating the efficacy of catheter balloon valvuloplasty remains inconclusive.

ACUTE MITRAL REGURGITATION

Sudden development of retrograde flow of blood, during systole, from the left ventricle into the left atrium through an incompetent mitral valve.

Etiology and Pathophysiology

Acute, often massive, mitral regurgitation in elderly patients is commonly due to chordal rupture or the development of a flail mitral leaflet. The underlying disorder may be MI, papillary muscle rupture, infective endocarditis, or mucoid degeneration of the valve cusps. The murmur ends early, when the noncompliant left atrium can no longer accept additional volume. Idiopathic chordal rupture also occurs. Pulmonary venous congestion and often pulmonary edema develop rapidly.

Symptoms, Signs, and Laboratory Data

The characteristic findings include sinus tachycardia and a new, harsh, early systolic apical murmur, often with a thrill. The 1st heart sound is soft, and the accentuated pulmonic component of the 2nd heart sound reflects the acute pulmonary hypertension. A ventricular diastolic sound (S_3) is characteristic, and an atrial gallop may be present. Pulmonary venous congestion or pulmonary edema demonstrates hemodynamic significance.

Both the ECG and the chest x-ray may be normal initially, but pulmonary venous congestion soon supervenes. Echocardiography confirms the diagnosis and often suggests the etiology; left ventricular hyperkinetic function is usually seen.

Diagnosis and Treatment

Echocardiography can differentiate between septal rupture and acute mitral regurgitation. Valvular vegetations of infective endocarditis may also be demonstrated.

The management of acute mitral regurgitation is the same as that of acute pulmonary edema. Hemodynamic instability often requires intra-aortic balloon counterpulsation to permit cardiac catheterization and the subsequent induction of anesthesia for surgery. Clinical deterioration is an urgent indication for valve replacement, although operative mortality is increased with emergency surgery. Mortality is also increased when MI is the cause, since concomitant coronary bypass surgery, which increases pump time, may be required.

CHRONIC MITRAL REGURGITATION

Longstanding retrograde flow of blood during ventricular systole from the left ventricle into the left atrium through an incompetent mitral valve.

Etiology and Prevalence

Chronic mitral regurgitation accounts for ⅔ of mitral valve disease in the elderly. About ½ of affected patients have a history of rheumatic fever and about ½ have associate aortic valve disease, usually aortic regurgitation. Isolated mitral regurgitation often results from papillary muscle dysfunction following myocardial infarction. Calcification of the mitral annulus and myxomatous valve degeneration causing mitral prolapse are discussed separately as causes of chronic mitral regurgitation.

Symptoms, Signs, and Laboratory Data

The usual presentation includes atrial fibrillation; an apical holosystolic murmur, often with a soft 1st heart sound; and heart failure **(HF)**. There may be complicating systemic embolism of both rheumatic and MI origin. When mitral regurgitation is due to papillary muscle dysfunction, the apical murmur is spindle-shaped and is heard during midsystole. Electrocardiographic abnormalities and echocardiographic evidence of regional wall motion abnormalities may suggest coexisting coronary disease. Echocardiography can also delineate overall ventricular function.

Treatment

Medical management of atrial fibrillation is the same as that of mitral stenosis, and HF is treated in the standard manner. Surgery is indicated when medical therapy fails to control the HF and ventricular function deteriorates. Surgical plication or valvuloplasty may be effective for myxomatous degeneration. When valve replacement is needed, mechanical valves are typically chosen because the enlarged left atrium, or atrial fibrillation, or both are preexisting indications for anticoagulation. Mitral valve replacement is associated with less satisfactory results and greater mortality than aortic valve replacement, primarily because of significantly greater ventricular dysfunction.

MITRAL REGURGITATION: CALCIFIED MITRAL ANNULUS

Mitral regurgitation due to calcification of the mitral valve ring.

Etiology and Pathophysiology

About 6% of individuals > 60 yr old have mitral annular calcification, and the condition predominates in elderly women. Calcification prevents annular systolic contraction and may limit valve leaflet closure. Although the mitral regurgitation is rarely hemodynamically significant, conduction disturbances may result from extension of the calcification.

Symptoms, Signs, and Laboratory Data

Patients are often asymptomatic. An apical systolic murmur that radiates widely, occasionally to the back, is associated with a soft 1st heart sound. Characteristic radiographic findings and/or dense horseshoe-shaped calcifications on echocardiography define the condition.

Treatment

Patients rarely require therapy other than that needed to control the ventricular response to atrial fibrillation.

MITRAL REGURGITATION: MITRAL VALVE PROLAPSE

Mitral regurgitation associated with bulging of one or both mitral valve leaflets into the left atrium during ventricular systole.

Etiology

Myxomatous valvular degeneration, which increases in frequency with increasing age, is the major cause of mitral valve prolapse in the elderly. The associated dissolution of collagen in the elongated chordae tendineae may explain the high incidence of chordal rupture that often produces life-threatening HF in these patients.

Symptoms, Signs, and Laboratory Data

Presenting symptoms may include disabling chest pain inconsistent with myocardial ischemia, palpitations or syncope due to arrhythmia, and HF secondary to mitral regurgitation. Arrhythmias are common, even in patients with normal ventricular function. Although patients often have a long history of cardiac murmur, there may be a progressive worsening of the mitral regurgitation. Systemic embolization and sudden death may occur. A midsystolic click or clicks and a late systolic or holosystolic murmur with characteristic postural variations are present. These comprise an earlier, louder murmur and earlier and more multiple clicks on assumption of the upright position. Associated evidence of HF appears to be more common in men. The onset of atrial fibrillation may accentuate both mitral and tricuspid valve prolapse and often precipitates hemodynamic deterioration.

Electrocardiographic abnormalities are frequently present. Left ventricular enlargement may be present, although the ejection fraction remains normal.

Diagnosis

The chest pain of mitral valve prolapse must be differentiated from that due to coronary atherosclerotic disease. In mitral valve prolapse, ventricular function is often preserved when chest pain is the predominant finding, but coronary arteriography is needed for differentiation. Palpitations may be due to both ventricular and supraventricular arrhythmias, and an ambulatory ECG is helpful in documenting the etiology. Echocardiography may differentiate mitral prolapse from other causes of mitral regurgitation and can help assess ventricular chamber size and function.

Treatment

Anticoagulants are given to prevent systemic emboli, which occur predominantly with atrial fibrillation and HF. Digitalis is used to control the ventricular response to atrial fibrillation. HF is managed with digitalis, diuretics, and vasodilators. Mitral valve replacement may be indicated for progressive ventricular dilation. For this subgroup of elderly patients, predominantly men, the surgical risk is acceptable because ventricular function is usually preserved.

HYPERTROPHIC CARDIOMYOPATHY (HC)
(Idiopathic Hypertrophic Subaortic Stenosis [IHSS])

Myocardial hypertrophy (increased myocardial mass) of unknown cause.

Prevalence, Pathology, and Pathophysiology

IHHS, which occurs relatively frequently in the elderly, refers to the form of HC associated with a left ventricular outflow gradient. It is due to a disproportionate septal thickening that narrows the left ventricular outflow tract. Abnormal ventricular compliance causes an elevation of ventricular diastolic pressure, with a resultant increase in left atrial volume and pressure and pulmonary venous congestion. It occurs more frequently in women and has a more favorable prognosis in older patients than in younger ones.

Symptoms and Signs

Patients may present with chest pain, dyspnea, dizziness, palpitations, and syncope (caused by tachyarrhythmias or a decrease in CO from outflow obstruction). Ventricular tachycardia is common and increases the likelihood of sudden death. Supraventricular tachyarrhythmias are also frequent. Because brisk carotid pulses, basal systolic murmurs, and 4th heart sounds are common in elderly persons without heart disease, IHSS is often not suspected.

There is a characteristic late systolic murmur from the lower left sternal border to the apex that terminates before the 2nd heart sound. The characteristic bisferiens carotid pulse has a rapid upstroke and a subsequent percussion wave. A prominent 4th heart sound is typical, but disappears at the onset of atrial fibrillation. Provocative maneuvers (eg, the Valsalva) accentuate the systolic murmur, which decreases or disappears on squatting. The murmur may also disappear as systolic dysfunction and cavity dilatation occur.

Laboratory Data

There is evidence of left atrial abnormality and left ventricular hypertrophy on the ECG, with left anterior fascicular block present in about 20% of patients. Septal hypertrophy may also produce nonspecific inferior and apical Q waves; the ECG is rarely normal. The cardiac silhouette enlarges when ventricular systolic function deteriorates. Two-dimensional echocardiography is diagnostic, although systolic cavity obliteration and the outflow gradient may lessen with aging, rendering the systolic anterior motion of the mitral valve more important. An ambulatory ECG to document arrhythmias should probably be obtained annually, since serious arrhythmias are often asymptomatic.

Diagnosis

Differentiating IHSS from valvular aortic stenosis or coronary heart disease with papillary muscle dysfunction is important because the therapies differ. Nitroglycerin, diuretics, and digitalis often exacerbate outflow obstruction and symptoms, which are best treated by β-blockers or verapamil. The murmur must also be differentiated from murmurs due to aortic sclerosis, mitral regurgitation, and mitral valve prolapse, all of which are common in the elderly. The chest pain of IHSS does not necessarily reflect coronary disease, although ischemic infarction may occur even in patients with normal coronary arteries.

Treatment

Therapy with amiodarone (200 to 300 mg daily) has been reported to reduce the risk of sudden death from ventricular tachycardia. This has not been shown with β-blocker or verapamil therapy. Supraventricular tachyarrhythmias also respond to amiodarone. Anticoagulation to prevent embolization in patients with atrial fibrillation or frequent supraventricular tachyarrhythmias is indicated. Propranolol provides the best symptomatic relief for both the dyspnea and the chest pain, because of the predominant diastolic dysfunction. Nifedipine may be given with propranolol, or verapamil may be given alone. Amiodarone has little effect on chest pain or dyspnea.

In the late stage of the disease, when systolic function deteriorates, digitalis and diuretics may be used safely to improve function. Reduced dosages of digitalis and warfarin are indicated when they are given concomitantly with amiodarone, since it potentiates the effects of both drugs. Myomectomy is rarely indicated, except in symptomatic patients who are refractory to medical therapy. If mitral valve replacement is indicated for mitral regurgitation, a low-profile valve should be used.

TRICUSPID VALVE DISEASE
TRICUSPID REGURGITATION

The retrograde flow of blood from the right ventricle into the right atrium during ventricular systole because of inadequate closure of the tricuspid valve orifice.

Tricuspid regurgitation is most often due to a dilated valve ring secondary to right ventricular failure. Infective endocarditis (see below) is a less common cause. The holosystolic murmur (maximal along the lower-left sternal border) is accentuated on inspiration. A large positive systolic wave in the jugular venous pulse is also present. Medical management of heart failure lessens the regurgitation.

TRICUSPID STENOSIS

An abnormal narrowing of the tricuspid valve orifice.

Tricuspid stenosis is rare except in patients with multivalvular rheumatic heart disease or with the carcinoid syndrome. The lower-left sternal border diastolic rumble increases on inspiration. There is a diastolic elevation of the jugular venous pulse—with poor or absent Y descent—and hepatomegaly, without other evidence of heart failure. Medical therapy is indicated for mild disease. Surgical repair is rarely required.

PULMONIC VALVE DISEASE

Pulmonic valve disease is extremely rare in the elderly. When present, it is characterized by the murmur of pulmonic insufficiency, usually due to pulmonary hypertension secondary to chronic pulmonary disease or left ventricular failure. Treatment of the underlying disorders is appropriate.

INFECTIVE ENDOCARDITIS

Patients with all forms of valvular disease are at risk for infective endocarditis, and the proportion of elderly patients who develop this condition is increasing. In addition to the usual organisms seen in younger patients, *Streptococcus bovis* is increasingly identified as a causative organism in older patients, presumably because GI disease, especially of the gallbladder and colon, is common. Similarly, the incidence of enterococcal endocarditis is higher in elderly men, primarily because they frequently undergo genitourinary procedures. These organisms rarely cause infective endocarditis in younger patients.

Symptoms and signs: Because of its atypical presentation, often without fever, infective endocarditis in the elderly is frequently not recognized and treated until it has progressed to a late stage. Thus it has an extremely poor prognosis. Although the clinical manifestations of infective endocarditis in some elderly patients are comparable to those seen in younger individuals, nonspecific presenting manifestations are common. These include anorexia, nausea or vomiting, disorientation, a neurologic deficit secondary to an infected embolus, and progressive anemia and azotemia. These symptoms and signs are often attributed to "aging" or to another illness. Culture-negative endocarditis may occur following antimicrobial therapy given for another presumed illness.

Diagnosis and treatment: Demonstration by echocardiography of a valvular vegetation may aid in diagnosis. A subclavian venous line is advisable for antibiotic administration. This limits the problem associated with repeated IV or IM injections of antimicrobial drugs. Peak and trough antibiotic levels should be ascertained to ensure that blood levels are appropriate for elderly patients, since their excretory and metabolic functions are often impaired.

Antibiotic prophylaxis is indicated in older patients with valvular disease, particularly those with calcified and prosthetic heart valves, who are at especially high risk for developing endocarditis. The prevention of infective endocarditis will assume even greater importance as the percentage of elderly persons in the population increases, and more have prosthetic valves implanted, undergo invasive diagnostic and therapeutic procedures with a potential for bacteremia, and retain their native dentition.

34.   ARRHYTHMIAS AND CONDUCTION DISORDERS

Jerome L. Fleg

An unparalleled number of new antiarrhythmic drugs have been developed in recent years. Similarly, the development of new types of pacemakers has expanded the therapeutic capabilities of cardiac pacing. The roles of these newer agents and devices in the treatment of cardiac arrhythmias and their effects on long-term prognosis for all groups are largely undefined.

ECTOPIC BEATS AND TACHYARRHYTHMIAS

Incidence

Ectopic beats, whether supraventricular or ventricular, simple or complex, detected at rest or during routine activity or exercise, increase in frequency with advancing age, even in individuals carefully screened to exclude latent coronary artery disease **(CAD)**. ECG data from a study of randomly selected patients > 70 yr of age revealed supraventricular ectopic beats **(SVEBs)** in 10% and ventricular ectopic beats **(VEBs)** in 8%. Those with SVEBs showed no increase in risk of sudden death over follow-up periods of 6 to 18 yr. The prognostic significance of VEBs present on resting ECG is not as clear-cut. Some studies found no increase in age-adjusted risk of sudden death while others found a two- to three-fold increase in cardiac mortality.

In a study of healthy subjects, aged 60 to 85 yr, who were carefully screened to exclude the presence of CAD, 24-hr ambulatory ECG monitoring disclosed isolated VEBs in 80%. Frequent SVEBs and VEBs (> 100 in 24 hr) were noted in 26% and 17%, respectively. Short asymptomatic episodes of paroxysmal supraventricular tachycardia occurred in 13%, ventricular couplets in 11%, and nonsustained ventricular tachycardia (VT) in 4%. Other studies have found that the incidence of these arrhythmias is much lower in younger healthy subjects. In contrast, arrhythmias such as atrial flutter and fibrillation, sinus bradycardia < 40 beats/min, sinus pauses > 1.6 sec, and high-degree A-V block were rare or nonexistent in these older healthy subjects who had been noninvasively screened for CAD. The long-term prognostic significance of arrhythmias noted on ambulatory ECG recordings in normal elderly subjects is unknown.

In apparently healthy adults undergoing treadmill exercise testing (those with no overt evidence of heart disease but in some cases exhibiting "positive" exercise ECGs), the incidence of both SVEBs and VEBs has been shown to increase with age. In one study, the incidence of isolated SVEBs increased from 8 to 76% and that of isolated VEBs from 11 to 57% between the 3rd and 9th decades. Asymptomatic runs of VT, none > 6 beats in duration, were seen in nearly 4% of apparently healthy subjects aged 65 yr or older, a prevalence 25 times that in younger subjects. Over a mean follow-up of 2 yr, none of these elderly individuals with nonsustained exercise-induced VT experienced angina, MI, syncope, or cardiac death.

Another study evaluated 80 apparently healthy volunteers, aged 51 to 77 yr, with frequent or repetitive exercise-induced VEBs; only 1 cardiac death occurred over a 4.6-yr mean follow-up period. In geriatric patients, the mere presence of SVEBs and VEBs, even if frequent, complex, or symptomatic, is not an accurate marker for organic heart disease or increased cardiac mortality. Such ectopic activity, therefore, may require no specific therapy.

In contrast, atrial flutter or fibrillation usually signifies organic heart disease. Established atrial fibrillation (AF) in otherwise normal subjects ("lone" AF) appears to substantially increase the risk of cardiovascular morbidity and mortality. In studies, such mortality was increased two- to thirteenfold and stroke more than fivefold in men aged 40 to 65 yr. Thus AF, even in the absence of apparent organic heart disease, should never be considered benign. Because chronic (and even lone) AF is associated with a substantially increased risk of cerebral embolism, anticoagulation should be strongly considered in any elderly patient with this arrhythmia (see also Mitral Stenosis in Ch. 33).

The apparently benign nature of both supraventricular and ventricular arrhythmias in healthy elderly subjects does not mean that these arrhythmias are similarly benign in patients with heart disease. *Regardless of a patient's age, the nature and severity of underlying heart disease are of much greater prognostic significance than the arrhythmia itself.* Because of the paucity of data regarding the significance of specific arrhythmias in old age, most of the information below will focus on standard diagnostic and therapeutic measures.

SPECIFIC TACHYARRHYTHMIAS
(See TABLE 34–1)

SUPRAVENTRICULAR ECTOPIC BEATS (SVEBs)

Isolated SVEBs are common in the elderly and are probably related in part to the increase in atrial pressure or volume associated with aging per se and with the development of organic heart disease. Even when

TABLE 34–1. SPECIFIC TACHYARRHYTHMIAS IN THE ELDERLY: RELATIONSHIP TO AGE AND MORTALITY

Arrhythmia	Independent Effect of Age on Prevalence	Effect on Mortality in Normals	Therapy
SVEBs	↑	None	None
PSVT	↑	?	Digoxin, β-blocker, or Ca channel blocker
AF (chronic)	↑	↑	Above drugs; attempt at cardioversion; ? Anticoagulation
VEBs	↑	Probably none	None in normals; ? antiarrhythmic drugs if heart disease is present
VT	↑	Probably none	? Antiarrhythmic drugs in normals; antiarrhythmic drugs, AICD, or endocardial resection if CAD is present

SVEB = supraventricular ectopic beats, PSVT = paroxysmal supraventricular tachycardia, AF = atrial fibrillation, VEB = ventricular ectopic beats, VT = ventricular tachycardia, AICD = automatic implantable cardioverter-defibrillator they occur frequently, SVEBs rarely require specific treatment. However, they may indicate that a patient has a propensity for sustained supraventricular tachyarrhythmia.

ATRIAL (SUPRAVENTRICULAR) TACHYCARDIA

Paroxysmal supraventricular tachycardia **(PSVT)** is characterized by a regular narrow QRS complex morphology at 150 to 200 beats/min. It is usually due to a reentrant mechanism and can often be terminated by vagal maneuvers; eg, Valsalva, gagging, or carotid sinus massage. *The latter maneuver should not be performed in elderly patients until significant carotid stenosis has been excluded by physical examination.* Carotid sinus massage should not be conducted in any patient with a bruit. If vagal stimuli are unsuccessful, and hypotension is absent, verapamil 5 to 10 mg IV should be given over 2½ to 5 min. If hypotension, cerebral ischemic symptoms, angina, or heart failure is precipitated by the arrhythmia, immediate cardioversion is indicated, starting at 25 to 50 joules. Digoxin is the preferred prophylactic therapy for PSVT because of its documented efficacy and once-daily dosage. β-Adrenergic blockers or Ca channel blockers are alternative choices.

Atrial tachycardia with block is usually caused by digitalis toxicity. Treatment consists of withholding digitalis and correcting hypokalemia.

Multifocal atrial tachycardia is common in elderly patients with obstructive lung disease. Here, the P-wave morphology, P-R interval, and cycle length vary from beat to beat. Although treatment should be directed toward correcting the underlying condition, verapamil has proved efficacious as short-term therapy.

Accelerated junctional rhythm, although not usually a cause of hemodynamic impairment, may be a sign of a serious underlying disorder. It is characterized by a heart rate of 70 to 130 beats/min; the P wave is usually inverted and may precede, follow, or fall within the QRS complex. In the elderly, digitalis toxicity and acute inferior myocardial infarction are the most common causes. Sudden regularization of the ventricular rate in a geriatric patient receiving digitalis for chronic atrial fibrillation should suggest this diagnosis. Treatment is directed at the underlying disorder, eg, digitalis intoxication, myocardial infarction, heart failure, etc.

Atrial flutter should be suspected when a regular tachycardia at a ventricular rate close to 150 beats/min occurs. Carotid massage, causing an abrupt slowing of the ventricular response and the emergence of "sawtooth" flutter waves at about 300/min, confirms the diagnosis (but see warning under PSVT above). CAD and obstructive lung disease are common etiologies in the elderly. Digoxin is the drug of choice if the patient's hemodynamic status is stable. Otherwise, low-level DC cardioversion (25 to 50 joules) converts flutter to sinus rhythm in nearly all cases.

Atrial fibrillation (AF) is recognized by the absence of organized atrial activity and the totally irregular timing of the QRS complexes. In contrast to the other atrial tachyarrhythmias mentioned, AF is much more likely to be chronic than acute. Hypertension, CAD, and mitral valve disease are the most common predisposing conditions in elderly and middle-aged patients. Additional considerations in the elderly include amyloidosis, sick sinus syndrome **(SSS),** and thyrotoxicosis.

As in younger patients, initial treatment is directed toward slowing the ventricular response to 60 to 100 beats/min with digoxin, verapamil, or propranolol given IV. Long-term control of ventricular rate is also achieved with these agents, which are sometimes given in combination. Digoxin and verapamil are contraindicated in the Wolff-Parkinson-White **(WPW)** syndrome, but WPW is rare in the elderly. Because of the associated A-V nodal disease, about ¹/₃ of geriatric patients with AF present with a controlled ventricular response and require no specific therapy. The decision to attempt electrical cardioversion for chronic AF requires that the etiology and duration of AF, atrial size, and the risk of alternative therapy with anticoagulants be considered (see also Ch. 33). Given the poor prognosis in patients with chronic AF, an early attempt at cardioversion is probably warranted in most elderly patients.

VENTRICULAR ECTOPIC BEATS (VEBs)

Although the presence of VEBs—whether isolated or frequent and complex—does not appear to adversely affect the prognosis in clinically healthy elderly individuals, even simple VEBs are associated with increased long-term cardiovascular mortality in patients with documented CAD. Nevertheless, it has yet to be shown that treatment of isolated VEBs in these patients reduces risk of death in the long term.

The generally higher risk of reactions to antiarrhythmic drugs in the elderly should dictate a conservative approach, using low starting doses and titrating cautiously until VEB density is reduced by 75% and VT is eliminated. The combination of low-dose quinidine and tocainide was generally effective and well tolerated in a pilot study of elderly patients with CAD and frequent VEBs. Such low-dose combination therapy with various agents probably warrants investigation in the elderly to minimize the risks of adverse effects from any single drug. As with SVEBs, treatment should be directed toward resolving underlying or exacerbating factors, such as electrolyte disturbances, hypoxia, or heart failure **(HF).**

Ventricular tachycardia (VT) is usually a regular tachycardia with broad QRS complexes and a rate of 100 to 200 beats/min. Although a distinction from PSVT often may be difficult, the presence of A-V dissociation, fusion beats, and QRS duration > 0.14 sec or a QRS axis between $-90°$ and $-180°$ strongly favors a diagnosis of VT. In contrast to the relatively benign nature of isolated VEBs, *sustained VT requires immediate attention.* Common precipitants of VT in the elderly are severe myocardial ischemia, acute MI, digitalis intoxication, or HF.

If VT is well tolerated hemodynamically, a bolus of 50 to 75 mg lidocaine, followed by another 50 mg 2 min later, may be given initially. Recurrent VT or VT that is resistant to lidocaine may be treated successfully with IV procainamide or β-blocking drugs. Current data, derived largely from studies of younger patients, suggest that bretylium is the most effective drug for VT that is refractory to lidocaine. In the elderly, as in younger patients, *VT associated with hypotension or syncope requires immediate electrical cardioversion.*

VT precipitated by an acute event, such as MI or digitalis toxicity, has a low recurrence rate and does not require chronic prophylaxis. However, when VT occurs without an obvious precipitant, it is known as **primary VT**; it has a 1-yr recurrence rate of about 35% in the overall patient population and requires aggressive prophylaxis. In a recent series, the mean age of patients with out-of-hospital cardiac arrest due to a primary arrhythmic event was 68.5 yr, and these patients had a 1-yr mortality of 29%.

The most promising approach to patients with primary recurrent symptomatic VT appears to be intracardiac programmed electrophysiologic stimulation, a technic in which the malignant arrhythmia is induced and the efficacy of various antiarrhythmic agents in preventing it is assessed in a special catheterization laboratory. In a recent randomized trial of 57 patients (mean age 59 yr, and 86% men), invasively determined antiarrhythmic therapy resulted in a lower rate of symptomatic ventricular tachyarrhythmia than did the noninvasive approach. Studies have also shown marked reduction in 1- to 2-yr mortality when drug therapy for recurrent VT was determined by this technic as compared with empirical treatment. A less-invasive alternative (but similarly labor-intensive) approach employing ambulatory ECG monitoring and exercise testing has also been used successfully.

The recent availability of amiodarone and several other new antiarrhythmic drugs increases the likelihood that a successful medical regimen can be found for a given elderly individual. Elderly patients in whom neither of the above approaches is successful should be considered candidates for an automatic implantable cardioverter-defibrillator **(AICD)** or endocardial resection guided by intraoperative mapping. In a recent large series of patients with recurrent VT or ventricular fibrillation, about ½ were treated by these latter invasive approaches; long-term survival was similar in elderly and younger patients, although surgical mortality was higher in the elderly.

Age-Related Pharmacology of Antiarrhythmic Drugs
(See also Ch. 18)

The half-life ($t_{1/2}$) of **digoxin** is prolonged in the elderly because of their reduced GFR; this reduction and a generally smaller body size result in a serum digoxin level for a given dose that is higher in older than in younger persons. Despite the widespread availability of serum drug-level testing, digitalis toxicity continues to be a relatively common occurrence in the elderly, primarily because the drug is frequently used in this age group to treat HF and atrial arrhythmias. In persons 60 to 69 yr of age compared with those 23 to 29 yr of age, **quinidine** clearance is reduced by 34% and elimination $t_{1/2}$ prolonged (from 7.3 h to 9.7 h). Recent findings that quinidine therapy increases serum digoxin levels by about 100% may be particularly significant in the elderly, in whom a combination of these 2 drugs is frequently prescribed.

Because hepatic flow decreases with age, the infusion rate of **lidocaine** should be reduced in the elderly to avoid the CNS toxicity so commonly seen. Similar dosage adjustments are necessary with **propranolol** and other **β-blockers** that undergo first-pass hepatic metabolism. The pharmacodynamic significance of age-related decreases in the binding of propranolol to β-adrenergic receptors is unknown.

BRADYARRHYTHMIAS

HISTOLOGIC CHANGES IN THE CONDUCTION SYSTEM

Widespread histologic changes that occur in the conduction system with advancing age may help explain why there is a striking age-related increase in bradyarrhythmias and conduction disturbances. A progressive decrease in the number of pacemaker cells in the sinoatrial **(S-A)** node begins by age 60 yr; only about 10% of the cells found in young adults are still present at age 75 yr. The S-A node becomes enveloped by fat, which may cause a partial or complete separation of the node from the atrial musculature.

Age-associated changes in the His bundle include loss of cells, increase in fibrous and adipose tissue, and amyloid infiltration. The left side of the cardiac skeleton, which includes the central fibrous body, the mitral and aortic annuli, and the proximal interventricular septum, undergoes some degree of fibrosis in senescence. The A-V node, His bundle, and proximal left and right bundle branches may be involved in this process because of their proximity to these structures. In extreme cases, the resultant "idiopathic" fibrosis may cause A-V block; it is the most common cause of chronic A-V block in the elderly.

AGE-RELATED CHANGES IN THE ECG

Several manifestations of age-related histologic alterations in the conduction system (see above) are apparent on the standard 12-lead ECG. Although resting heart rate does not change with age, the respiratory variation in resting sinus rate (known as sinus arrhythmia) decreases with increasing age. Small age-associated prolongations of the P-R and Q-T intervals also occur, but QRS duration is unchanged. High-resolution surface electrocardiography in healthy volunteers has localized the increase in P-R interval to a delay that is proximal to the His bundle; conduction time from the His bundle to the ventricle appears to be unrelated to age.

The QRS frontal plane axis shifts leftward over time, probably reflecting the combined effects of fibrosis in the anterior fascicle of the left bundle branch and mild age-related left ventricular hypertrophy. Such left axis deviation was the most common abnormality found in a review of a large number of ECGs from elderly subjects, occurring in 51%. Neither first-degree A-V block nor axis deviation leftward of $-30°$ is associated with increased cardiac morbidity or mortality if organic heart disease is absent.

The prevalence of bundle branch block increases with advancing age. Although left bundle branch block **(LBBB)** is usually associated with ischemic or hypertensive cardiac disease, complete right bundle branch block **(RBBB)** is frequently seen in apparently healthy older men and these subjects appear to have a satisfactory prognosis. A recent analysis of the predominantly male, multicenter Coronary Artery Surgery Study population confirmed an independent adverse effect of LBBB, but not RBBB, on mortality over the subsequent 5 yr. *In women, however, RBBB and LBBB are highly—and equally—indicative of underlying cardiac disease.*

Because of the higher prevalence of intrinsic conduction system disease as well as acute processes, such as MI and digitalis intoxication, bradyarrhythmias are more common in the elderly. However, sinus bradycardia < 40 beats/min, sinus pauses > 1.6 sec, and high-degree A-V block are rare or nonexistent in healthy persons > 60 yr old. These conduction disturbances are frequently associated with ischemic, hypertensive, or amyloid heart disease.

SPECIFIC BRADYARRHYTHMIAS
(See TABLE 34–2)

Sinus bradycardia, defined by a sinus rate of < 60 beats/min, may represent excellent physical conditioning, but in the elderly it frequently indicates intrinsic sinus node disease. Inferior MI, hypothermia, myxedema, or increased intracranial pressure may cause this arrhythmia. A longitudinal study of apparently normal subjects between 40 and 80 yr of age with sinus rates < 50 beats/min on standard ECG found no increase in cardiovascular morbidity or mortality over a 5-yr mean follow-up period.

Sinoatrial block occurs when sinus node impulses fail to depolarize the atria. Such block is often 2:1, resulting in a ventricular rate that is exactly ½ the sinus rate. Common causes in the elderly are intrinsic conduction system disease, ischemia, and digitalis toxicity.

First-degree atrioventricular (A-V) block is defined by a prolongation of the P-R interval ≥ 0.22 sec. It may be seen in healthy subjects with high vagal tone or may be caused by intrinsic conduction system disease or by various medications, eg, digitalis, β-blockers, Ca antagonists, and Type 1A antiarrhythmic drugs. No therapy is required.

TABLE 34–2. SPECIFIC BRADYARRHYTHMIAS AND CONDUCTION
DISTURBANCES IN THE ELDERLY

Abnormality	Independent Effect of Age on Prevalence	Independent Effect on Mortality	Therapy
First-degree A-V block	↑	None	None
Complete A-V block	↑	↑	Pacemaker
Sick sinus syndrome	↑	None	Pacemaker for *symptomatic* brady-cardia only
Left axis deviation	↑ ↑	None	None
Left bundle branch block	↑	↑	None known
Right bundle branch block	↑	None	None

Second-degree A-V block (intermittent A-V block) may present as 2 different patterns. **Mobitz Type I,** also called **Wenckebach,** can be recognized by a progressive prolongation of the P-R interval until a ventricular complex is dropped. Because this type of block is usually proximal to the His-Purkinje system, the QRS complex is typically normal in appearance. Digitalis intoxication and acute inferior MI are common precipitating factors. This conduction disturbance is usually transient and rarely requires specific therapy.

In **Mobitz Type II** block, the P-R interval is fixed but QRS complexes are dropped. Because the site of block is at or below the His bundle, the QRS complex is often wide. Mobitz Type II is most frequently associated with acute anterior MI, myocarditis, or advanced sclerodegenerative conduction system disease. Patients with this arrhythmia are usually symptomatic and often present with syncope due to inadequate cerebral perfusion **(Stokes-Adams attack).** Because of its symptomatic presentation and frequent progression to complete heart block, Mobitz Type II block is usually treated by the insertion of a permanent cardiac pacemaker.

Third-degree A-V block (complete A-V block) is characterized by the inability of any atrial depolarizations to activate the ventricle. Block within the A-V node is usually associated with normal QRS complexes and an escape rate close to 60 beats/min. Common etiologies are acute inferior MI and digitalis toxicity. In most instances, block within the A-V node is transient. However, block within the ventricles is accompanied by wide QRS complexes and a slow escape rate, often < 40 beats/min. Such block may occur in patients with severe sclerodegenerative conduction system disease or extensive acute anterior MI. Because these patients usually respond poorly to atropine and isoproterenol, pacemaker insertion is necessary.

Sick sinus syndrome (SSS) encompasses a variety of rhythm disturbances that reflect dysfunction of the sinoatrial **(S-A)** node and are often associated with dysfunction elsewhere in the conduction system. Although SSS may be associated with many cardiac diseases, CAD or a primary sclerodegenerative process is most often responsible. Patients may present with bradyarrhythmias (sinus bradycardia, sinus pauses or arrest, S-A exit block, or AF with a slow ventricular response) or with the so-called bradycardia-tachycardia syndrome, in which a supraventricular tachycardia terminates in a long period of asystole. Symptoms therefore may consist of palpitations or chest pain during tachycardia, and dizziness or syncope during bradycardia. The tachycardia—PSVT, atrial flutter, or atrial fibrillation—is treated with digoxin, other agents, or cardioversion (as outlined above); bradycardia associated with syncope should be treated by permanent pacing.

Acute Therapy for Bradyarrhythmias

Acute therapy for bradyarrhythmias is required in the presence of hypotension, cerebral or cardiac ischemia, HF, and, in the case of acute MI, frequent VEBs. Placing the patient in the supine position, with the legs elevated, often ameliorates hypotensive sequelae acutely. Atropine in a 0.5 mg IV bolus may be repeated at 3- to 5-min intervals until a total dose of 0.04 mg/kg has been given. If atropine is ineffective or causes intolerable side effects, an isoproterenol drip can be started at 1 to 4 μg/min and then titrated to produce a ventricular rate of 60 beats/min. When neither drug is successful, or if isoproterenol is *contraindicated* because of ischemia or infarction, temporary transvenous pacing should be used.

CARDIAC PACEMAKERS

Of the modalities available to treat cardiovascular disorders, cardiac pacing is probably the one most strongly associated with the elderly. In one series, it was found that ⅔ of pacemakers were implanted in patients > 70 yr old; about 50% of these were implanted for complete heart block, and the other 50%, for SSS. Recent data show that SSS now accounts for 48% of all pacemaker implants. Permanent ventricular pacing has eliminated the accelerated mortality formerly associated with complete heart block. However, the long-term prognosis for patients with SSS is determined by the presence and severity of underlying heart disease and is unaffected by pacemaker insertion. Permanent pacing for SSS should therefore be based on ECG documentation of symptomatic bradyarrhythmia.

Pacemaker insertion is not warranted in asymptomatic elderly patients with chronic bifascicular block, with or without P-R interval prolongation, because they rarely progress to complete heart block. Recent advances in pacemaker technology (eg, rate programmability, dual-chamber A-V synchronous pacing, and activity-mediated rate responsiveness) may be extremely useful in selected elderly patients, but their merits in the general population may be overstated. Although not conclusively documented, the greater dependence on the atrial contribution to ventricular filling with advancing age predicts an enhanced benefit of A-V synchronous pacing in the elderly.

Pacemaker Complications

Insertion of a permanent pacemaker is associated with a low but significant rate of pacemaker-induced complications. Abrupt loss of pacing—due to battery failure, fibrosis around the catheter site, myocardial perforation, lead fracture, or electrode dislodgment—may result in marked bradycardia or asystole. Catheter perforation of the right ventricle may cause a pericardial friction rub or, rarely, tamponade. Geriatric patients with little overlying subcutaneous tissue may experience extrusion of the pulse generator or erosion of the pacing wire through the skin. Occasionally, a patient will experience difficulty in adjusting psychologically to pacemaker implantation. All pacemaker patients should be scheduled for regular follow-up physical and ECG examinations.

---

35. HEART FAILURE (HF)

Jeanne Y. Wei

HF occurs when CO is insufficient to meet metabolic demands. A precise numeric definition of HF, stated in terms of CO or ejection fraction, is not expressible because metabolic demands vary from patient to patient.

HF is common in patients > 65 yr of age. Its prevalence rises exponentially with age from the 6th decade. It may result from compromised systolic or diastolic ventricular function, or both, resulting in elevated ventricular end-diastolic pressure. While isolated left or right HF is not rare, combined left and right HF is more frequently observed. The underlying cause may involve the myocardium or other cardiac structures that impede cardiac filling or forward ejection. Appropriate therapy for HF can probably benefit the elderly patient more than can treatment for any other age-related condition of equal severity.

Etiology

The principal causes of HF (see TABLE 35–1) can be divided into 4 categories: impediments to forward ejection, impaired cardiac filling, volume overload, and myocardial failure. Systemic arterial hypertension, which impedes forward ejection, and coronary artery disease (CAD), which leads to primary myocardial failure, are encountered most frequently in the elderly. However, autopsies on elderly persons who died from HF disclosed that about ⅓ to ½ had no significant CAD. High output failure (due to conditions such as thyrotoxicosis, anemia, arteriovenous fistulas, fever, and some dermatologic diseases, such as Kaposi's sarcoma and psoriasis) occurs less frequently in elderly patients.

Pathophysiology

The heart adapts to an increased work load through one or more of the following mechanisms: increased sympathetic stimulation; myocardial hypertrophy; and the Frank-Starling mechanism. Since myocardial and vascular responsiveness to β-adrenergic stimulation is decreased with increasing age and recent data suggest that the myocardial hypertrophic response to a given increase in afterload is impaired, there is greater dependence on the Frank-Starling mechanism in the elderly.

Diastolic Dysfunction

The age-related prolongation in myocardial relaxation time with an increase in myocardial stiffness, which decreases filling, causes elevated

TABLE 35–1. PRINCIPAL CAUSES OF HEART FAILURE IN THE ELDERLY

I. Impediments to forward ejection
  A. Systemic arterial hypertension or elevated systemic vascular resistance
  B. Aortic valve stenosis
  C. Supravalvular stenosis (coarctation)
  D. Subaortic stenosis (left ventricular outflow tract membrane)
  E. Obstructive hypertrophic cardiomyopathy
  F. Pulmonary hypertension

II. Impaired cardiac filling
  A. Ventricular hypertrophy (symmetric or asymmetric)
  B. Myocardial diastolic dysfunction
  C. Pericardial disease (constriction or tamponade)
  D. Restrictive heart disease (endocardial or myocardial)
  E. Ventricular aneurysm

III. Volume overload
  A. Valvular regurgitation
  B. Increased intravascular volume
  C. Increased metabolic demands (thyrotoxicosis, anemia, certain dermatologic disorders)
  D. Arteriovenous shunts or fistulae

IV. Myocardial failure
  A. Primary
    1. Loss of functioning cardiac muscle (myocardial infarction/myocardial ischemia)
    2. Cardiomyopathy
    3. Myocarditis
  B. Secondary
    1. Drug-induced
    2. Systemic disease (hypothyroidism)
    3. Chronic overload

left ventricular diastolic pressures at rest and during exercise. Thus, pulmonary and systemic venous congestion may occur and produce symptoms of HF even in the presence of nearly normal or excellent systolic function.

Several studies have documented the high prevalence of diastolic dysfunction with preserved systolic function in elderly patients with HF. Between 50 and 60% of older patients with HF have adequate ventricular contractile function, with normal or only slightly reduced ejection fractions. Differentiating patients with impaired systolic function from those with impaired diastolic function is important in selecting appropriate treatment.

Symptoms, Signs, and Diagnosis

The usual symptoms and signs of HF are similar in all patients, but atypical presentations are more common in the elderly. Nonspecific signs of illness (eg, somnolence, confusion, disorientation, weakness, fatigue, and failure to thrive) may be presenting features. *Cognitive impairment may confound the difficulties involved in obtaining a reliable history.* A history of dyspnea may be *absent*.

Patients with systolic dysfunction tend to exhibit a gradual, progressive course of decline, while those with diastolic dysfunction often experience acute onset of symptoms and abrupt clinical deterioration. Patients with diastolic dysfunction frequently have underlying hypertension or coronary heart disease, and often present in acute decompensation related to acute ischemia or hypertension. The presence of systemic congestion with a normal ejection fraction does not necessarily imply diastolic dysfunction, however. Other pathologic entities that need to be considered include volume overload, valvular regurgitation, hypertrophic cardiomyopathy, pericardial constriction (acute tamponade or chronic pericarditis), restrictive cardiomyopathy, and high-output states.

Unlike jugular venous distention and hepatojugular reflux, peripheral edema is *not* a reliable sign of HF. While the presence of an S_4 gallop in an elderly person does not necessarily indicate clinically significant heart disease, an S_3 or early diastolic gallop usually does signify HF. Inspiratory rales in the lower half of the lung fields may or may not be present. Signs of right HF may accompany systolic dysfunction but are less frequently observed in patients with predominantly diastolic dysfunction. Presence of a big, baggy heart (laterally displaced point of maximal impulse **[PMI]**) would be compatible with systolic dysfunction, while a forceful, minimally displaced apical impulse with an S_4 and no S_3 gallop would be compatible with diastolic dysfunction.

It must be recognized, however, that clinical distinction between HF due mainly to systolic dysfunction and that due to diastolic dysfunction usually *cannot* be made at the bedside. An objective measure of left ventricular systolic function is often needed.

Noninvasive studies of left ventricular diastolic motion and studies of ventricular diastolic filling using Doppler echocardiographic and radionuclide scintigraphic technics are useful in distinguishing between diastolic and systolic dysfunction, as well as in diagnosing other diseases mentioned above. Patients with diastolic dysfunction typically have good or preserved systolic function (ejection fraction or fractional shortening) but impaired diastolic filling or ventricular relaxation. Those with systolic dysfunction generally have good ventricular filling but decreased ejection fraction and impaired systolic wall motion.

Prognosis

The prognosis for both elderly and younger patients with HF depends on the underlying etiology and the presence of associated diseases. While treatment may not increase long-term survival in patients with chronic severe HF, it may enhance short-term survival. Improved quality of life, rather than prolonged survival, may have to be the ultimate goal of HF management in the elderly.

Treatment

Impaired diastolic function: Elderly patients with impaired diastolic function are often erroneously treated for systolic HF with large doses of potent diuretics, digitalis, and vasodilators that may exacerbate the condition rather than improve it. It is therefore important to administer therapy appropriate for the pathophysiology (see TABLE 35–2).

When systolic function is preserved, therapy should be aimed at improving ventricular filling and relaxation, rather than at decreasing preload, which may exacerbate the already impaired ventricular filling. Agents that may be beneficial in enhancing ventricular diastolic filling include Ca entry blockers and β-adrenergic blockers. If the patient's left ventricular end-diastolic pressure is on the steep portion of the pressure-volume curve, a tiny dose of an angiotensin-converting enzyme (**ACE**) inhibitor or a mild diuretic may be helpful. Therapy, however, must be individualized.

Major emphasis should be on avoiding preload reduction and digitalis, if possible. The primary goals are to optimize ventricular early diastolic filling and reduce ventricular end diastolic pressure. The atrial contribution to ventricular filling should be restored or augmented in patients with atrial arrhythmias by converting to and maintaining normal sinus rhythm (either pharmacologically or electrically). Elderly persons in particular depend on the atrial "kick" to attain adequate ventricular filling.

Systolic dysfunction: The mainstays of therapy are bed rest, digitalis, diuretics, and vasodilators, with reduction of preload and afterload. Because prolonged bed rest in the elderly is dangerous but often necessary, an effective compromise is to have the patient sit in a chair with legs elevated. Bed or chair rest enhances diuresis, as does O_2 supplementation. Improved oxygenation of peripheral tissues increases renal perfusion, decreases vascular tone, and consequently decreases preload and afterload.

The value of long-term **digitalis therapy** in elderly patients has recently been questioned. Digitalis is useful in managing acute and chronic severe HF in patients with sinus rhythm or atrial fibrillation. It may be less useful in patients with *mild* chronic HF and sinus rhythm. While the inotropic response to cardiac glycosides may be diminished in the elderly, the toxic effects, usually due to elevated plasma levels, are not reduced with age. Higher steady state plasma levels and prolonged plasma half-life of digoxin are due in part to the age-related decline in renal excretory capacity. Decreased renal clearance, together with variability in distribution and extrarenal clearance, further reduces the predictability of serum digoxin levels in the elderly (see also Ch. 18).

Fortunately, efficacious diuretics, vasodilators, antihypertensive agents, and new inotropic agents are available to treat acute and chronic severe HF. **Vasodilator therapy** reduces afterload, thereby enhancing myocardial

TABLE 35-2. DRUGS USED TO TREAT HEART FAILURE

Drug Group	Agent	Dosage	Adverse Effects or Problems	Indications*
Digitalis	Digoxin	.125-.250 mg q day	Arrhythmia	SD
	Digitoxin	.05-.10 mg q day	Arrhythmia	SD
Diuretics	Chlorthalidone	25-100 mg q day	Hypotension	SD
	Furosemide	20-1000 mg q day	Hypokalemia	SD
Vasodilators	Nitroglycerin (oral)	6.5-19.5 mg q 6 h	Headache, drug tolerance	SD
	Nitroglycerin (ointment)	0.5-2 in. q 6 h	Headache, drug tolerance	SD
	Nitroglycerin (transdermal patch)	5-30 mg q 12-24 h	Headache, drug tolerance	SD
	Isosorbide dinitrate	10-60 mg q 4-6 h	Headache, drug tolerance	SD
	Nitroprusside	0.5-10 μg/kg/min IV	Hypotension, thiocyanate toxicity	SD
	Hydralazine	25-75 mg q 6-8 h	Fluid retention	SD
	Minoxidil	5-100 mg/day	Fluid retention tachycardia, hirsutism	SD
	Prazosin	1-7 mg q 8 h	Postural hypotension, drug tolerance	SD
ACE inhibitors	Captopril	6.25-100 mg q 8 h	Hypotension, azotemia,	SD
	Enalapril	10-40 mg/day	↓regional blood flow	SD

(Continued)

* SD = Systolic dysfunction; DD = diastolic dysfunction.

TABLE 35–2. DRUGS USED TO TREAT HEART FAILURE *(Cont'd)*

Drug Group	Agent	Dosage	Adverse Effects or Problems	Indications*
Ca entry blockers	Verapamil	40–120 mg q 12 h	Negative inotropy, heart block	DD
	Nifedipine	10–40 mg q 8 h	Negative inotrophy, hypotension, reflex tachycardia	DD
	Diltiazem	30–90 mg q 8 h	Negative, inotropy, heart block	DD
β-Blocker	Metoprolol	6.25–100 mg q day	Negative inotropy, bradycardia	DD/SD
Nonglycoside inotropes				
Sympatho-mimetic amines	Dopamine	1–5 μg/kg/min IV	Tachycardia arrhythmia	SD
	Dobutamine	1–10 μg/kg/min IV	Tachycardia arrhythmia	SD
Phosphodies-terase inhibitor	Amrinone	1–10 μg/kg/min IV	Fever, GI intolerance, thrombo-cytopenia	SD

shortening and increasing stroke volume. The most frequently used vasodilators for HF are the ACE inhibitors, which alone or in combination with nitrates, hydralazine, and diuretics may be effective in reducing filling pressures, increasing CO, increasing renal blood flow, and improving exercise tolerance.

Adverse effects of nitrates or hydralazine, such as tachycardia, rarely occur in the elderly because of an age-related reduction in cardioacceleratory capacity. Limitation of oral sodium intake may be useful in patients with significant reductions in renal sodium excretion, due to renal dysfunction and/or decreased CO.

Although smaller doses of diuretics may be effective in some elderly persons, others may require doses equal to those for younger persons. Caution should be exercised when administering any diuretic to an elderly person for the first time. Initial doses should be lower, with increments in smaller steps, over longer intervals.

Newer agents: In some patients who do not respond adequately to therapy with digitalis, diuretics, and vasodilators, **amrinone** (available only for IV use) and its analog, **milrinone,** have been shown to be effective. These 2 new agents produce a marked improvement in the stroke-work index and a decrease in pulmonary artery pressure. Milrinone has direct inotropic effects on cardiac muscle and, at high doses, has a direct vasodilatory effect.

Another relatively new class of agents, the **ACE inhibitors,** eg, **captopril** and **enalapril,** appear to work predominantly on the peripheral vasculature. ACE inhibitors have also been shown to be very effective in patients who are refractory to digitalis, diuretics, and other vasodilators. **Prazosin,** an arterial and venous system vasodilator, effectively reduces systemic and pulmonary venous pressure and may increase CO, but its effectiveness or propensity for tachyphylaxis in elderly patients has not been extensively documented.

It is likely that a combination of these newer drugs and the more traditional agents will produce synergistic effects. Exactly which agent or combination is best suited for the very old patient (age $\geq$ 76 yr) remains to be established. Currently, it appears that nitrates, hydralazine, diuretics, and ACE inhibitors may all be quite effective at doses that cause relatively few untoward side effects.

---

36. PERIPHERAL VASCULAR DISEASES

Sandor A. Friedman

Peripheral circulatory problems, both arterial and venous, increase in frequency with age and have major deleterious effects on functional capacity and life-style. Physicians often inappropriately ascribe nonspecific complaints to peripheral vascular disease, without objective criteria. Indeed, asymptomatic vascular lesions may coexist with unrelated symptoms. Because the peripheral circulation is accessible to direct scrutiny, thorough physical examination is the key to proper evaluation and treatment. Laboratory tests are useful in confirming the diagnosis and quantifying the extent of disease.

ARTERIOSCLEROSIS OBLITERANS OF THE EXTREMITIES

Occlusion of blood supply to the extremities by atherosclerotic plaques (atheroma).

Progressive arterial disease in the extremities is a very common, age-related process that parallels the development of atherosclerosis in the coronary and cerebral vessels. Although clinical findings usually appear later in life, they result from a slow, insidious pathologic process beginning many years earlier. Almost 70% of the lumen of a vessel must be occluded before the disease can be clinically recognized. Atherosclerosis involves the lower extremities much more extensively than the upper extremities, and symptoms are usually confined to the former.

Etiology and Pathophysiology

The **risk factors** for peripheral arterial disease, similar to those for atherosclerosis elsewhere, include diabetes mellitus, hyperlipidemia, hypertension, cigarette smoking, polycythemia, a family history, homocystinuria, and in women, early hysterectomy or ovariectomy. Diabetes and smoking are particularly important.

The pathogenesis of arterial damage from smoking is still unclear but probably includes a toxic effect on the intima from carbon monoxide and metabolites of smoke components. Because nicotine is a direct arterial vasoconstrictor, damage may be heightened by restriction of distal blood flow. Even after peripheral arterial disease becomes clinically evident, continuation of smoking accelerates arterial deterioration. The incidence of limb amputation is 10 times higher in those who continue to smoke after developing arterial occlusion than in those who quit.

A recently discovered risk factor, homocystinuria, involves impaired renal clearance of homocystine, a vasculotoxic amino acid. Deficiency of the enzyme cystathionine synthetase results in a rise in blood and urinary homocystine and methionine levels and may be a major factor in the development of premature peripheral atherosclerosis before age 50 yr. Its role in arterial occlusions that occur after this age is unknown. Animal studies have shown that high blood levels of homocystine cause intimal damage and consequent platelet aggregation that can be prevented with dipyridamole.

Symptoms and Signs

There are 2 circulations at the small blood vessel level: One supplies skin and subcutaneous tissue; the other supplies skeletal muscle. Because the former is under strong α-adrenergic control, blood flow varies considerably in healthy persons, depending on the degree of vasoconstriction. Vasodilation is mostly due to reduction of α-adrenergic stimulation. Skin generally requires little blood flow for adequate nutrition. On the other hand, muscle requires little blood flow at rest, but needs 500 to 1000 times as much for ordinary walking. In the muscle circulation, there is relatively little α-adrenergic control. β-Adrenergic receptors play a role in increasing muscle blood flow during exercise. Vasospasm in the muscle circulation is not a documented clinical problem.

The cardinal and only specific symptom of peripheral arterial disease is **intermittent claudication.** Its pathogenesis is not known, but it is clearly the result of muscle hypoxia, its coronary counterpart being angina pectoris. Claudication is *pain, tightness, or weakness in an exercising muscle that occurs on walking and is relieved promptly by rest.* The pain is most often described as "squeezing," almost always occurring in the calf in cases of femoropopliteal artery occlusion or in the hip and buttock area in aortoiliac disease. Claudication never occurs while sitting or standing still and is relieved in < 5 min by the latter. Most important, claudication forces the person to halt; continued walking is either too painful or results in loss of muscle function and falling.

The distance at which claudication occurs may change over time but tends to be remarkably constant from day to day if external conditions are unchanged. Cold, windy weather, inclines, and walking more rapidly will shorten the distance at which claudication occurs. Use of canes or crutches will not increase walking distance, since muscle function is normal until hypoxia occurs. With mild claudication, a person may walk up to 6 blocks without stopping, but the usual distance is < 3 blocks and in severe cases may be only a few yards. Unlike angina, claudication does not have atypical variants.

Less specific symptoms of peripheral arterial disease relate to the cutaneous circulation of the foot: numbness, paresthesias, coldness, and pain on rest. **Numbness** may be caused by concomitant diabetic neuropathy. Foot or toe numbness that occurs on walking is more specific for arterial disease and is a claudication equivalent. It results from maximal vasodilatation of muscle arterioles, with "stealing" of blood flow from the skin.

A **sense of coldness** may be secondary to vasoconstriction rather than to arterial occlusion. A recent increase in coldness, unilateral coldness, and coldness that persists after a night's sleep suggest arterial insufficiency. **Foot pain at rest,** when caused by arterial insufficiency, is a dire symptom, indicating that blood flow capacity is reduced to < 10% of normal. The pain is paresthetic, burning in nature, most severe distally, and typically worse at night, preventing the patient from sleeping. Often, it is partially relieved when the foot is in the dependent position. Pain at rest resulting from ischemic neuropathy must be distinguished from other causes of foot pain (eg, diabetic neuropathy may cause similar pain but is generally bilateral and extends above the feet).

Presenting symptoms vary with age and level of physical activity. Claudication is the earliest symptom in a patient accustomed to walking, because exercising muscle requires markedly increased blood flow. However, many elderly people are relatively sedentary and never walk far enough to have claudication; therefore, they present later with pain at rest or even gangrene. Since peripheral sensation decreases with age, particularly in diabetics, dependent rubor and subsequent gangrene may occur without pain.

Because older people usually have multiple areas of occlusion, they are unlikely to present with **Leriche syndrome** *(localized aortoiliac occlusion)*, in which the distal vessels are usually patent and the feet are healthy. Patients with Leriche syndrome have **hip claudication** and **impotence** secondary to hypotension in the internal iliac arteries. Elderly patients with aortoiliac disease generally also have femoropopliteal and tibial occlusions, so distal flow may be seriously impaired. While patients with Leriche syndrome may be more disturbed by impotence than by claudication, elderly individuals may not be because they may already be impotent from other causes (eg, diabetic neuropathy or use of antihypertensive drugs).

Diagnosis

Examination of the peripheral pulses is key to confirming the diagnosis of peripheral arterial disease. The posterior tibial pulse is always present in healthy individuals, although it may be difficult to feel in the presence of edema or with prominent malleoli. It is best palpated with the patient supine and the examiner on the same side as the pulse. Careful palpation under the medial malleolus is necessary; dorsiflexing and everting the patient's foot slightly may help mobilize the artery into a more superficial position.

The dorsalis pedis artery extends along the dorsomedial aspect of the foot, is frequently subject to vasoconstriction, and its pulse is absent in about 5% of the healthy population. The lateral tarsal pulse occasionally can be felt lateral to the dorsalis pedis artery.

The popliteal artery is often the most difficult to palpate. It is best examined when the patient is supine and relaxed, with the knee slightly flexed. The artery can be located posteriorly in the popliteal space, laterally or medially. In obese individuals, very deep palpation may be necessary.

Measurement of pulse strength is subjective and depends on the pulse pressure, girth of the extremity, and patient age. If an artery remains patent, its pulse tends to become more prominent with aging, as the media loses smooth muscle and elastic tissue, predisposing to ectasia. The upstroke of the pulse wave is more important than the amplitude. Bruits heard over the femoral arteries indicate aortoiliac disease.

When the presence or the strength of a peripheral pulse cannot be determined clinically, Doppler ultrasound can be used to assess arterial patency. However, the presence of a Doppler signal does not prove the existence of a palpable pulse or adequate pulsatile flow; a signal may be perceived when systolic BP in the vessel is as low as 30 mm Hg. To obtain a satisfactory Doppler study, a BP cuff must be used to measure systolic pressure in the artery (pressure above which the signal cannot be detected). This measurement is also useful in evaluating arterial insufficiency in a pulseless limb (eg, by determining the **ankle/brachial index**). Normally, this index should not be < 1, but an index > 0.6 usually indicates adequate resting blood flow to the foot. However, many elderly and diabetic individuals have heavily calcified arteries that are difficult to compress and, therefore, ankle pressure may appear falsely high. Thus, foot viability must never be assessed on the basis of a Doppler recording alone; **examination of the foot is essential**. Other technics, eg, plethysmography and percutaneous oxygen electrode measurements after transient arterial occlusion, can be used to assess the degree of ischemia, but they require a great deal of technical expertise.

Differences in temperature between the toes of each foot and color changes are particularly important. The foot should be elevated above heart level for 20 sec to determine whether pallor develops. A severely ischemic foot may appear pale even in the horizontal position. When the foot is moved to the dependent position, pallor that lasts for > 30 sec or the appearance of dependent rubor developing after 20 sec indicates < 10% of normal blood flow capacity. Rubor is more pronounced in the toes and extends proximally for various distances. Both prolonged pallor and rubor, well correlated with pain on resting, are grim signs. More extensive obliterative disease may compromise tissue viability and lead to skin ulceration or frank gangrene, particularly of the toes, heels, and lateral malleoli.

In some cases of mild arterial disease, the ankle/brachial index may be about 1 because of cuff artifact or peripheral vasoconstriction in the involved leg. Rechecking the BP at the ankle after exercise is helpful. Because of the resulting vasodilatation in muscle, BP will fall in the presence of proximal arterial occlusion. The magnitude and duration of the fall after cessation of exercise correlate with the degree of arterial insufficiency.

Treatment

Management is based on the severity of the disease as determined from history, physical examination, and general condition of the patient. Patients can be classified under 3 broad groups: (1) asymptomatic, (2) intermittent claudication only, and (3) significant foot ischemia, with or without claudication.

The **asymptomatic** group is by far the largest. Most patients with peripheral arterial disease, including the elderly, have no symptoms; their feet are adequately perfused through collateral vessels. A significant proportion of patients > 70 yr of age have weak or missing pedal pulses but have no difficulty with their extremities unless an unusual stress is experienced. However, an infection or traumatic or thermal injury may cause serious consequences because increased tissue metabolic demands cannot be met by a marginal circulation.

Therapy consists primarily of prevention: **(1) Cold:** Patients should avoid extreme cold, dress warmly in winter, and not bathe or swim in cold water. **(2) Heat:** Neither heat nor ice should ever be applied to the feet; feet and legs should not be exposed to the sun. **(3) Position:** Legs should be level with the bed during sleep and should not be crossed while sitting. **(4) Cleanliness:** Feet should be washed with mild soap, using lukewarm water only, and dried carefully, especially between the toes. **(5) Dry scaly skin:** Lanolin or cold cream may be applied to the feet and gently massaged into the dry scaly areas. **(6) Toenails:** A podiatrist or a family member should cut the toenails straight across, being careful to avoid cutting in at the corners or too close to the skin. **(7) Corns and calluses:** A podiatrist should treat these. **(8) Shoes and socks:** Patients should not walk barefoot; they should wear comfortable, properly fitting shoes, preferably with square or round toes, and clean socks every day. Circular garters or hose with elastic tops should be avoided. **(9) Local medication:** Strong antiseptic, tincture of iodine, corn remedies, and corn plasters should be avoided; only medications ordered by the physician should be used. **(10) Exercise:** Patients should walk regularly to improve circulation. **(11) Injuries:** Foot injuries, even minor ones, should be avoided by following the above rules; a physician should be consulted at the first sign of discomfort in the legs or if any injury occurs to the legs or feet. **(12) Self-inspection:** Patients should examine their feet weekly for cracks, cuts, or color changes, consulting the physician if any of these conditions occur, with or without pain.

For patients with intermittent claudication but adequate cutaneous blood flow, medical therapy is somewhat limited. Besides being given foot care instructions, they should be advised to avoid smoking, to lose weight if they are overweight, and to walk as much as possible. At the point of claudication, they should stop to rest and then continue. In a small but significant percentage of patients, the symptoms ameliorate within the first 3 mo; these patients can walk considerably farther. Vasodilators have been ineffective in the treatment of claudication.

Pentoxifylline is the first of a new class of drugs approved for the treatment of claudication. In vitro, this agent decreases blood viscosity and improves RBC flexibility, leading to improved microcirculatory flow through arterioles and capillaries. In a double-blind, controlled study, subjects increased mean walking distance by about 50 m. Most patients do not notice any significant improvement upon taking this agent, but a few believe they can walk several blocks farther before needing to rest. The recommended dosage, 400 mg orally tid, may have to be taken for up to 2 mo before any improvement occurs.

For patients who have both coronary and peripheral arterial disease, questions have been raised about the use of β-adrenergic blocking agents. Except for the β-blockers that have intrinsic sympathomimetic activity, these drugs are mild peripheral vasoconstrictors; thus, their administration could aggravate intermittent claudication. However, because this rarely happens, these drugs should not be withheld from a cardiac patient with claudication. The proven increase in longevity that β-adrenergic blocking agents provide for patients with atherosclerotic coronary artery disease clearly outweighs the theoretical possibility of a slight decrease in the distance at which claudication occurs.

The only clearly effective treatment for intermittent claudication is surgery, either arterial bypass or, in less severe cases, percutaneous transluminal angioplasty **(PTA).** The decision for or against surgery must be based on the patient's age, general health, life-style, presence or absence of heart disease, and location of the lesions, among other factors.

Whether a surgical approach is feasible can be determined only by angiography that allows visualization of the entire peripheral tree from the distal aorta through the tibial vessels. The runoff beyond the obstruction must be evaluated. For surgery to be successful, a major vessel beyond the obstruction must be patent, with good distal flow beyond this patent area. Angiography is an invasive procedure, which should be performed *only* if surgery is being considered.

Bypass surgery: The presence of significant coronary artery disease is a **contraindication** to peripheral arterial surgery for 2 reasons: (1) Heart disease increases operative mortality. (2) An improvement in walking distance may be mitigated or prevented by angina, which becomes the limiting factor after a successful bypass. If walking long distances without stopping is not important to an individual, surgery is not indicated.

The more proximal the lesion, the better are the clinical results of bypass surgery and the longer the graft remains patent. With localized aortoiliac disease, the graft patency rate is > 90% at 5 yr. In femoropopliteal disease, patency rates are probably in the 60 to 70% range at 5 yr. Femorotibial grafts have a 5-yr patency rate well below 50%. With generalized disease, patency rates are even lower. If the patient has bilateral arterial occlusion, a femoropopliteal bypass may result in unmasking of claudication in the contralateral limb, therefore offering only slight clinical improvement. A second operation would then be necessary to achieve a significant increase in claudication-free walking distance.

Percutaneous transluminal angioplasty (PTA) is an alternative to bypass surgery for short stenoses in the aortoiliac and proximal-femoral areas. Although it is a simple procedure that can be performed under local anesthesia, complications (eg, rupture of the artery and distal embolization of ruptured atheromatous plaques) may require emergency surgery. Therefore, a patient undergoing PTA must also be capable of withstanding a full surgical procedure.

Because of these considerations, *very few patients should have surgery for claudication alone,* particularly elderly patients, who usually have significant heart disease, multiple lesions, and no great need to walk long distances without resting. Surgery for impotence should not be offered to the elderly, since the results are poor.

Patients with evidence of severe cutaneous ischemia (eg, pain on resting, dependent rubor, and tissue loss) have a much higher priority for surgery. In this situation, greater risks are justified to relieve disabling pain or prevent amputation. Even here, conservative care is often indicated if the patient is a poor risk for surgery. Ischemic ulcers can heal if the surrounding blood flow is adequate. Patches of dry gangrene, particularly on the toes, should be allowed to demarcate because autoamputation of toes may result in proximal healing. Ischemic ulcers may respond to relief of pressure, use of debriding agents (eg, collagenase), and local antiseptic solutions (eg, povidone-iodine applied bid). Body-temperature wet soaks are also useful in treating infected lesions.

Surgery should be avoided in elderly patients without tissue loss or pain on resting, even in the presence of florid dependent rubor. β-Blockers should be avoided and patients followed closely. If tissue breakdown begins in a foot, arteriography and possible surgery are generally indicated. However, in patients with severe heart disease, amputation occasionally is preferable to the risk of bypass surgery.

Two surgical procedures of relatively low risk can be considered in elderly patients with severe aortoiliac disease and whose feet are threatened with tissue loss or amputation: If iliac disease is unilateral, a **femorofemoral bypass** subcutaneously across the lower pelvic area may be helpful in saving a limb. The patency rate with this procedure is almost as good as that with aortofemoral bypass. When bilateral iliac artery disease is present, a subcutaneous **bypass from an axillary to a femoral artery** may be helpful. These grafts often clot but may be reopened by performing a local thrombectomy within a few days of closure. Perhaps ½ of these grafts will continue to function over the next 5 yr if they are closely followed.

The presence of stenoses in multiple areas is not a contraindication to surgery when a limb is threatened. Bypass of the proximal occlusion often increases collateral flow around more distal occlusions sufficiently to salvage the limb. Angioplasty for a short iliac stenosis may precede a femoropopliteal or femorotibial bypass.

SMALL-VESSEL SYNDROME

Cutaneous ischemia or localized areas of cyanosis or necrosis in a hand or foot in the presence of generally adequate circulation.

Ischemia in a foot or hand with palpable pulses suggests a number of diagnostic possibilities in the elderly: cryoglobulinemia, cryofibrinogenemia, disseminated intravascular coagulopathy, essential thrombocytosis, polycythemia, vasculitis secondary to drug-induced SLE, presence of the lupus anticoagulant, emboli from an arterial aneurysm, cardiac emboli, atheromatous emboli, and scleroderma.

Symptoms, Signs, and Diagnosis

Patients usually present with a cyanotic or gangrenous digit and may have multiple small lesions on several extremities. Occasionally, an entire foot or hand is cyanotic or exhibits dependent rubor. Patients with peripheral atherosclerosis and pulseless limbs must also be evaluated for small-vessel syndrome if they develop sudden, unexplained worsening of cutaneous ischemia or localized areas of cyanosis or necrosis with generally good perfusion of the remainder of the foot or hand. This is particularly important with hand involvement, because severe tissue ischemia is uncommon in the upper extremity, even in the presence of advanced atherosclerosis.

A thorough history is important. The use of drugs (eg, procainamide, hydralazine, and phenytoin) may produce SLE; other findings may include arthralgias and pleural effusion. Weight loss and other symptoms of anorexia may suggest a malignancy responsible for cryofibrinogenemia or disseminated intravascular coagulation (DIC). Back pain may point to multiple myeloma responsible for cryoglobulinemia. An acute history of gangrene with fever may suggest septicemia, leading to cryofibrinogenemia or DIC. Splenomegaly may be a clue to the diagnosis of essential thrombocytosis, a myeloproliferative disease involving megakaryocytes, generally presenting with digital or cerebral ischemia but sometimes with abnormal bleeding. A history of myocardial infarction should prompt suspicion of a ventricular aneurysm.

Physical examination should include a search for abdominal, femoropopliteal, and subclavian aneurysms. Because popliteal aneurysms are most notorious for shedding small emboli, this diagnosis should be strongly considered when ischemic episodes are confined to one foot. Evidence of atrial fibrillation and a dyskinetic left ventricular impulse is also important.

Laboratory evaluation should include a CBC with platelet count, a coagulation screen, and tests for cryoproteins, antinuclear antibodies, and the lupus anticoagulant. An echocardiogram should be performed if mitral valve disease or ventricular aneurysm is suspected, and a sonogram of the aorta and popliteal arteries may be necessary if there is uncertainty about the presence of a pulsatile mass.

"Lupus anticoagulant" (see above) is a misnomer, since it is not an anticoagulant, and most patients with this protein do not have SLE, although the lupus anticoagulant is present in about 10% of patients with SLE. The protein, *an immunoglobulin that interferes with phospholipid-dependent coagulation tests,* binds to phospholipids used to accelerate the activation of prothrombin to thrombin by Factor Xa. This in vitro defect is not corrected by the addition of normal plasma. It may be associated with a biologically false-positive test for syphilis (another antiphospholipid antibody), thrombocytopenia, and a prolonged partial thromboplastin time. Venous and small artery thrombi are common in patients with the lupus anticoagulant. A recent review of the literature suggests a prevalence rate of thrombotic episodes of 27%. Abnormal bleeding is rare, occurring only in the presence of hypoprothrombinemia and thrombocytopenia. The mechanism of thrombosis is not known, but inhibition of prostacyclin synthesis has been suggested as a possible factor.

The diagnosis of **atheromatous emboli** (fracturing of plaques) is reached by exclusion, after all other possibilities have been ruled out. Occasionally, this entity presents with the appearance of livedo reticularis, but a lupus syndrome still must be ruled out.

Treatment

Cardiac embolism is an indication for chronic anticoagulation with warfarin; the prothrombin time should be kept about 50% above control values. Atheromatous emboli are treated with antiplatelet drugs, including aspirin.

Essential thrombocytosis is treated with hydroxyurea or busulfan; most patients require only a few weeks of therapy with close follow-up of their platelet counts. Aneurysms must be surgically repaired. The presence of cryoproteins or DIC indicates assessment for malignancy.

Appropriate therapy for patients with the lupus anticoagulant has not been established, although both antiplatelet drugs and anticoagulation have been advocated.

RAYNAUD'S PHENOMENON

A poorly understood syndrome of peripheral vasospasm with intermittent pallor or cyanosis of the skin.

Symptoms and Signs

In the typical case, exposure to cold first causes blanching and then cyanosis of the hands, feet, and sometimes the ears and the tip of the nose. An erythematous phase follows when the individual enters a warm environment. These episodes can be asymptomatic or associated with varying degrees of pain, numbness, and a sense of coldness. In older individuals, the episodes often are expressed with only a blanching or cyanotic phase and may occur even when the ambient temperature is not very low. Patients tend to have cool hands and feet even in a warm environment. If the problem is severe or of long duration, sclerodactyly may be present.

Diagnosis

The appearance of Raynaud's phenomenon after age 40 is almost always a harbinger of internal disease, unless it is the result of previous frostbite or a thoracic outlet syndrome. In the latter 2 instances, the symptoms are usually unilateral. Secondary causes include hypothyroidism, drug-induced SLE, cryoglobulinemia, cryofibrinogenemia, cold agglutinin disease, scleroderma, and **CREST** syndrome: **C**alcinosis, **R**aynaud's phenomenon, **E**sophageal dysfunction, **S**clerodactyly, **T**elangiectasia.

Raynaud's phenomenon is a helpful clue to the diagnosis of hypothyroidism, which must always be considered, even in the absence of other symptoms. The achilles reflex, when present, often shows a delayed relaxation phase. Many elderly persons become more alert and active when hypothyroidism is treated, even though sluggishness was not noticed before therapy.

Scleroderma, SLE, and cryoproteinemia may also present with digital infarcts. The presence of a cryoprotein mandates evaluation for occult malignancy. Patients with cold agglutinin disease secondary to a cold antibody against RBCs usually have splenomegaly and hemolytic anemia aggravated by a cold environment. A Coombs' test with complement alone is positive. Patients with cold agglutinin disease frequently develop a low-grade lymphoma.

Almost all patients with scleroderma have Raynaud's phenomenon, which can precede all other manifestations by many years. However, the presence of sclerodactyly is not diagnostic of this disorder. Diagnosis requires findings of skin tightening in areas other than the hands and feet or some evidence of visceral involvement. The earliest evidence of visceral involvement is usually abnormal esophageal motility or a decreased pulmonary diffusion capacity. Prognosis depends on whether significant visceral involvement occurs; renal manifestations are the most ominous. Cardiac conduction abnormalities and restrictive cardiomyopathy develop less frequently.

Treatment

In general, treatment of Raynaud's phenomenon per se should be conservative in elderly individuals. Cardiovascular reflexes are often impaired, and subclinical coronary and cerebrovascular disease may be present. Patients are, therefore, very responsive to vasodilators, and can develop orthostatic hypotension with serious consequences. Nifedipine (10 mg orally tid) and griseofulvin (250 mg orally qid) are usually safe and effective. Most patients, however, do well enough by wearing warm clothing, avoiding extreme cold, and not smoking.

Often, patients with scleroderma should be treated more vigorously, because peripheral vasospasm affects internal blood flow. Raynaud attacks have been associated with reversible decreases in renal and cardiac blood flow and with echocardiographic evidence of impaired myocardial contractility. If the patient is also hypertensive, an angiotensin converting enzyme **(ACE)** inhibitor that promotes renal as well as peripheral blood flow is an excellent choice for therapy.

ARTERIAL ANEURYSMS

A localized dilatation of an artery caused by stretching of all layers of the wall.

In the elderly, an aneurysm is a localized exaggeration of generalized ectasia secondary to loss of smooth muscle and elastic tissue in the media of the arterial tree. It is most likely to occur at branching points (eg, the terminal aorta) or at areas of stress (eg, the popliteal artery). Systemic hypertension is also a major risk factor. When a local dilatation develops, forward velocity of blood flow decreases, leading to increased pressure against the arterial wall. This, in turn, results in more dilatation and perpetuates a vicious circle that, in many cases, terminates in rupture of the artery. Saccular aneurysms are more likely to rupture than fusiform aneurysms, because the total wall pressure is applied to a small area. The clinical findings and the prognosis vary with the aneurysm's location.

THORACIC AORTIC ANEURYSM

About 80% of thoracic aortic aneurysms are secondary to arteriosclerosis associated with hypertension. Tertiary syphilis remains responsible for about 14%, always located in the ascending aorta. Other causes include congenital factors, Marfan's syndrome, and blunt trauma to the chest (1%). Aneurysms developing in patients > 65 yr are almost always of arteriosclerotic origin.

Symptoms and Signs

Symptoms and signs are related to the site of the lesion. Dilatation of the ascending aorta rarely causes pain until the aneurysm ruptures. Examination may reveal a loud aortic closing sound and an early decrescendo diastolic murmur of aortic regurgitation secondary to dilatation of the aortic ring. The murmur is usually heard best in the aortic area and may be accompanied by a louder systolic murmur. In a thin person, chest palpation with the patient leaning forward may reveal a pulsation along the right sternal border.

Aneurysms of the transverse thoracic aorta, although asymptomatic when small, may cause symptoms of mediastinal compression as they enlarge. These include hoarseness secondary to compression of the recurrent laryngeal nerve, dysphagia, wheezing, and superior vena cava syndrome. Since these aneurysms may resemble mass lesions on chest x-rays, they can easily be confused with bronchogenic carcinomas and mediastinal neoplasms.

An aneurysm in the descending thoracic aorta is generally asymptomatic until it is very large and can even penetrate the spine without causing pain.

Diagnosis

Diagnosis is usually made coincidentally upon review of routine chest x-rays. Generally, good posteroanterior and lateral views can distinguish the aorta from other mediastinal structures, and tomography can confirm the diagnosis. If the presence of an aneurysm seems likely on chest x-ray, however, contrast CT is recommended to verify its size and location and to distinguish it from a silent aortic dissection. Angiography should be performed only if surgical repair is contemplated.

Treatment

The decision to perform surgery is based on size and location of the aneurysm, presence of symptoms, and general condition of the patient. Rupture is rare in aneurysms < 5 cm in transverse diameter but common in those > 10 cm. Pain or compression symptoms suggest a poor prognosis.

The transverse thoracic aorta is the most critical site for surgery because it requires not only total cardiopulmonary bypass but also reanastomosis of the extracranial arteries into the graft. The descending thoracic aorta is the least critical site because surgery requires only partial cardiopulmonary bypass to protect the kidneys and spinal cord. Most older patients should not be considered for surgery. Rather, they should have chest x-rays every 4 to 6 mo. If the lesion is not expanding and no symptoms occur, a conservative approach is recommended. Hypertension should be treated with drugs that do not increase cardiac stroke volume (which can put stress on the aortic wall). β-Adrenergic blocking agents are the drugs of choice; methyldopa, clonidine, and diuretics can also be used. Vasodilators (eg, hydralazine, prazosin, and ACE inhibitors) should be avoided.

ABDOMINAL AORTIC ANEURYSM

The distal aorta is the site of the most common and most dangerous arteriosclerotic aneurysms. They often involve the proximal common iliac arteries, and rarely (< 2%) extend above the level of the renal arteries. These lesions almost always remain silent until, or close to, the point of rupture. An estimated 1:250 people > 50 yr of age die because of a rupture of an abdominal aortic aneurysm.

Symptoms, Signs, and Diagnosis

Most abdominal aneurysms can be detected by palpation. *Thorough palpation of the abdominal aorta is unquestionably one of the most important components of the physical examination of the elderly.* In individuals of normal girth, the aortic pulse is generally palpable in the epigastrium. Typically, an aneurysm appears as an expansile mass that has both lateral and anterior pulsations. However, often only a strong pulse is felt, making it difficult to distinguish the aneurysm from generalized ectasia and tortuosity. In thin patients, a strong pulse is normal, whereas in obese individuals, any pulsation may signal an aneurysm. About 50% are associated with a bruit. Too often, the lesion is missed or suspected only after an abdominal x-ray taken for another reason. An anteroposterior view may indicate curvilinear calcification of the aorta near the midline, whereas a lateral film may outline the calcified anterior and posterior walls of the aneurysm.

Ultrasonography is the method of choice for confirming the diagnosis. It is virtually 100% accurate, providing precise information on the aneurysm's size, shape, and location. The likelihood of rupture is directly related to the transverse and anteroposterior diameters of the aneurysm and inversely related to its length. Rupture is not likely until diameters exceed 5 cm; thereafter, the rupture rate rises quickly. The rate of expansion is much faster than in the thoracic aorta.

Initially, the rupture is usually a small perforation temporarily tamponaded for hours or even days by a retroperitoneal blood clot. If this is diagnosed rapidly, life-saving surgical repair is possible. Unexplained abdominal or lower back pain in the presence of prominent pulsation should suggest a ruptured aneurysm until proven otherwise. In an older obese individual, sudden pain suggests the diagnosis, even if pulsation is undetectable.

In some cases, immediate exploratory laparotomy should be performed. However, if the index of suspicion is lower and pain was recent, **contrast CT** of the abdomen can be performed. When rupture has already occurred, retroperitoneal swelling can usually be seen. Diagnosis of rupture is the only advantage of a CT scan over ultrasonography.

Other complications of abdominal aortic aneurysms occur infrequently. Mural thrombi may embolize to the lower extremities. Rarely, consumption coagulopathy occurs as well, resulting in thrombocytopenia, elevated thrombin time, fibrin split products in the blood, and a bleeding diathesis. Even more rarely, aneurysms may become infected. The most frequent offending organism is *Salmonella;* a search for arterial aneurysms is indicated in patients with a recurrent *Salmonella* septicemia of unknown origin.

Prognosis

Many studies have confirmed the high mortality associated with un-repaired abdominal aortic aneurysms. The 5-yr survival rate varies from 14 to 37%. In the absence of arteriosclerotic heart disease, most patients die of rupture. In its presence, roughly 50% succumb to the aneurysm. It has been clearly established that surgical repair prolongs life. With an experienced surgical team, elective repair should be associated with < 3% operative mortality, even though most patients have other evidence of arteriosclerotic disease. Contraindications to surgery include recent transient ischemic attacks and unstable angina.

Treatment

Aneurysms > 5 cm in diameter usually should be repaired. In otherwise healthy individuals in the 7th decade, repair of slightly smaller lesions might be considered, particularly if serial ultrasound has shown progressive enlargement. Patients with small aneurysms can be followed clinically and with sonography every 3 to 4 mo.

Treatment of patients with both coronary artery disease and abdominal aneurysms is controversial. Some authorities advocate coronary angiography and bypass surgery as the first intervention in these patients, but most reserve this approach for patients with severe heart disease. Most surgeons forgo coronary angiography in patients with little or no angina and a good ejection fraction (as determined by radionuclide left ventricular cineangiography).

The management of patients with significant stable angina is open to question. One promising technic is the use of thallium scanning of the heart before and after IV injections of dipyridamole. In a study of pre-operative patients, evidence of redistribution of blood flow following dipyridamole was well correlated with postoperative MI. Conventional submaximal stress tests also can help to assess the need for coronary bypass prior to aneurysm repair.

POPLITEAL ARTERIAL ANEURYSM

The popliteal artery is the second most common site of aneurysm formation, because of trauma associated with knee movement and compression of the vessel as it leaves Hunter's canal in the lower thigh. The latter leads to poststenotic dilatation, which is then exacerbated by the development of arteriosclerosis. Most lesions are asymptomatic. Patent aneurysms present as pulsatile masses in the popliteal fossa, but an occluded aneurysm may be mistaken for a cyst. Ultrasonography is diagnostic.

Complications include rupture (about 10% of cases), thromboembolism to the distal extremity, popliteal vein compression and thrombosis, and posterior tibial nerve compression with radiating pain or sensory loss in the calf. Thromboembolism—either acute or a series of small emboli to the foot—is the most common complication and often necessitates amputation. Occasionally, the popliteal pulse disappears and reappears as the thrombus changes position in the aneurysmal sac.

Treatment

Occluded aneurysms do not require specific treatment. Patients should be managed like any others with peripheral arterial occlusion.

Patent lesions, however, are quite dangerous. Surgery is required, unless the patient is very debilitated or expected to die shortly of another cause. Spinal or even local anesthesia can be used, if necessary. The aneurysm is not resected but is bypassed and separated from the circulation by proximal ligation. The presence of other aneurysms should be sought; 35% of patients with popliteal aneurysms have been found to have abdominal aortic aneurysms, and the occurrence of popliteal aneurysm in the contralateral extremity is 50%.

FEMORAL ARTERIAL ANEURYSM

These behave similarly to popliteal aneurysms, can also be confirmed by sonography, and require surgical repair.

CAROTID ARTERIAL ANEURYSM

These are rare, occur in the midneck area and present as pulsatile masses. Rupture is rare, but they are a source of cerebral emboli. A carotid aneurysm must be distinguished from the much more common tortuosity and bending of a carotid artery, which lacks clinical consequence. "Kinking" is common in the elderly and usually presents as a strong pulsation just above the clavicle, more often on the right side. Sonography is useful in distinguishing between kinking and aneurysmal dilatation.

Surgical repair is usually indicated for carotid arterial aneurysm.

AORTIC DISSECTION

A hemorrhage into the media following an initial intimal tear.

Aortic dissection (dissecting hematoma) is often inappropriately called a dissecting aneurysm. The tear occurs because of medial necrosis or severe atrophy. In middle-aged and elderly people, the majority of cases result from chronic, sustained hypertension. Dissection secondary to Marfan's syndrome is rare after age 55.

The initial intimal tear is almost always just distal to the aortic valve **(proximal type)** or just beyond the left subclavian artery **(distal type).** Although proximal dissections have been reported more often than distal types, the prevalence of the latter may be underestimated because clinical findings can be more subtle.

Symptoms and Signs

Symptoms are variable. Pain may be excruciating, with widespread radiation through the chest and back; mild and limited to one small area of the back or chest; or totally absent. The clinical findings reflect what is happening to the hematoma that forms in the media, which may do any of the following: (1) extend distally along the aorta, (2) clot at any point along the aorta, (3) extend distally into any major branch of the aorta and compress the lumen, (4) become the major blood-flow channel in any branch of the aorta, (5) reenter the aorta or a branch through a second, more distal intimal tear, or (6) perforate through the adventitia at any point.

Distal dissection may cause mild back pain; frequently, pain is absent. The presenting complaint is often related to regional ischemia. Patients may have abdominal pain due to mesenteric ischemia, flank pain and hematuria secondary to renal infarction, paraplegia from anterior spinal artery involvement, or peripheral ischemia following occlusion of the iliac arteries. Ischemia may be promptly and spontaneously reversed if the dissecting hematoma reenters the normal lumen; absent femoral pulses, for example, may suddenly reappear. *Multiple regions of acute ischemia should always suggest a possible aortic dissection.*

Healing of a dissection usually involves clotting of the hematoma followed by fibrosis occurring around it. However, the wall of the aorta remains weak, and a true saccular aneurysm can develop almost anywhere in the aorta. Because there is little support, the aneurysm usually expands and ruptures rapidly. During acute dissection, rapid expansion of a saccular aneurysm portends imminent rupture. Expansion occurring weeks or months later is generally less rapid, although the aneurysm may rupture within days. In some instances, a thoracic aortic dissection presents as a sudden abdominal aortic aneurysm.

Perforation of a distal dissection usually occurs near the initial tear, with blood tracking into the left pleural cavity. Frequently, an initial small perforation is sealed off by a clot. A small left pleural effusion on chest x-ray may be the only clue.

Proximal dissection: A dissection beginning just beyond the aortic valve is more dangerous than a distal dissection, since it often also involves the aortic valve ring, the extracranial arteries, and the pericardium. A regurgitation murmur and a loud sound on aortic closure are present in many cases. Less frequently, hemodynamically significant acute aortic regurgitation results in low cardiac output, with pulmonary edema and hypotension. Rarely, silent dissection produces chronic aortic regurgitation, and the patient is discovered to have either an asymptomatic diastolic murmur or a murmur and left ventricular failure.

Neurologic symptoms (eg, hemiplegia and aphasia) are common presenting complaints. Both the innominate and left carotid arteries may be occluded by the dissection. If focal neurolgic signs are present, the corresponding carotid pulse should be either diminished or absent. For example, with left hemiplegia, one expects a lower BP in the right arm, as both the subclavian and carotid arteries should be affected by compression of the innominate artery.

If the false channel is prominent in the transverse aortic wall, **mediastinal compressive findings** can occur. Patients may develop hoarseness, unilateral external jugular venous distention, and a unilateral Horner's syndrome. Death often results from rupture of the dissection into the pericardial cavity.

Aortic dissection can be a great masquerader, with an onset that can be acute or insidious. Since the diagnosis is easily missed, certain constellations of findings should always trigger consideration of this entity. These include (1) chest pain, hypertension, and aortic regurgitation; (2) neurologic symptoms, with a contralateral weak carotid pulse; (3) left hemiplegia and hypotension in the right arm; (4) chest pain radiating to the back; (5) chest pain and either a normal ECG or one showing left ventricular hypertrophy; (6) unilateral jugular venous distention; (7) chest pain and absent femoral or subclavian pulses; (8) multiple areas of ischemia; (9) chest pain and the sudden appearance of a pulsatile abdominal mass; (10) limb embolectomy that fails to recover a thrombus, and (11) sudden pericardial effusion.

Diagnosis

Initially, **chest x-ray** is important for evaluation of the aortic shadow. In almost every case, the aorta appears somewhat prominent, especially in the elderly. It is usually tortuous and uncoiled owing to long-standing hypertension, and sometimes it is very dilated. Aortic calcification not extending to the borders of the shadow suggests a false channel and is specific for dissection only if a lateral view demonstrates a lack of Ca in the anterior or posterior wall.

If, after clinical evaluation and review of chest x-ray, the index of suspicion is *not* very high, echocardiography and contrast CT scanning should be performed. **Echocardiography,** either conventional or two-dimensional, is useful only for proximal dissection. It can usually demonstrate the false channel and detect even subclinical degrees of aortic regurgitation. It may also demonstrate early closure of the mitral valve, which indicates acute aortic regurgitation.

CT scanning can demonstrate the false channel and also accurately delineate the location of aortic calcification. Although an excellent screening tool, CT is not yet as reliable as aortography. If both echocardiography and CT scanning appear unequivocally negative, one can be fairly confident that dissection has not occurred. Trans-esophageal color Doppler is a useful new technic for diagnosing distal dissection, even when the false channel is very thin.

Aortography is performed when the index of suspicion for dissection is very high. It is the definitive test for aortic dissection and is usually performed in retrograde fashion through a femoral artery. The aortogram typically shows the false channel, its compression of major branches, and the site of intimal tear. If the false channel contains unclotted blood, it fills with contrast material. A false channel containing clotted blood does not opacify. This finding has prognostic value, since clotting is the first step in the healing process. One danger of aortography is that the catheter can enter the false channel and subsequent pressure from the injected contrast material can cause perforation.

Treatment

Uncomplicated **distal dissections** can be treated medically. Systemic BP must be normalized with drugs to decrease the rising pressure against the aortic wall. *Immediate control should be obtained with a titratable agent administered by continuous IV infusion.* Either a sympathetic ganglionic blocking agent such as trimethaphan camsylate or labetolol (α- and β-adrenergic blocking agents) can be used. At the same time, oral therapy is begun with a β-blocker and a diuretic. The dosage of oral agents is increased until there is no need for the IV infusion. Direct vasodilators (eg, prazosin, nitroprusside, and hydralazine) and angiotensin blocking agents (eg, captopril and enalapril) should be **avoided** because they increase left ventricular contraction against the aortic wall and may do more harm than good. Centrally acting vasodilators (methyldopa and clonidine) can be used if necessary, since they have little or no effect on cardiac output. Surgery must be considered if pain is not reduced within the first few hours of medical therapy and eliminated within the first 2 days.

After discharge, patients should be followed weekly for the first month and at least every 3 mo afterwards. Chest x-ray should be obtained after 1 mo and 3 to 4 times a year for the first 2 yr to look for development of a saccular aneurysm. Mortality rates after 3 and 5 yr for patients with uncomplicated distal dissections are about the same, whether they are treated medically or surgically.

Proximal dissections are much more treacherous and tend to cause severe complications if treated only medically. Perforation rates are high, with pericardial tamponade being the most common cause of death. First, hypertension should be controlled with IV drugs if the patient is stable, and then surgery should be performed. The introduction of synthetic grafts that can be placed inside the thoracic aorta has simplified surgery and reduced mortality. A graft with an attached aortic valve is also available for patients with severe aortic regurgitation. The false channel can be obliterated after graft insertion into the true lumen. If there is a distal saccular aneurysm or interference with blood flow through any major distal branch of the aorta, repair at the local site is mandatory. Thus, a combined thoracoabdominal approach is often necessary.

DEEP VENOUS THROMBOSIS (DVT)

The presence of a thrombus in a deep vein.

Etiology

The **risk factors** for venous clotting can still be classified under **Virchow's triad:** factors involving the movement of blood, blood itself, and the vessel wall. Since there is no propelling cardiac force that moves venous blood, the emptying of veins in the extremities depends entirely on skeletal muscle pumping and one-way valves in the lumen that prevent retrograde flow. Thus, immobilization or even a relatively sedentary existence favors stasis of blood in the veins and predisposes the patient to thrombosis. Since incompetent valves also lead to this scenario, DVT tends to be a recurring phenomenon. Any factors that increase Hct (eg, the use of diuretics) cause greater blood viscosity and a higher incidence of clotting. In a patient with DVT, it is important to look for risk factors if none is obvious.

The major risk factors are immobilization and decreased physical activity, previously damaged vein, obesity, heart failure, polycythemia, thrombocytosis, diuretic use, malignancy, fractured hip, use of estrogens, and dehydration.

Malignancy is associated with venous thrombosis in several ways. Patients with advanced cancer are often inactive, whereas those with early lesions may experience venous clotting as a paraneoplastic effect. In addition, cancer patients are often in a hypercoagulable state because of thrombocytosis, circulating cryoproteins, or DIC.

Fracture of a hip is an important cause of venous thrombosis in the elderly. Factors include immobilization and injury to the femoral vein and its tributaries. The rate of venous thrombosis (clinical and subclinical) approaches 50%, and pulmonary embolism is probably the leading cause of death in these cases.

Estrogen predisposes to venous thromboembolism by decreasing blood levels of antithrombin III, the most important natural anticoagulant. It can also lead to venous dilatation and stasis. Because of the current interest in preventing postmenopausal osteoporosis, more elderly women are taking oral or transdermal estrogen preparations. In addition to posing the danger of uterine carcinoma, estrogen replacement increases the risk of venous thrombosis and pulmonary embolism. Men receiving estrogen for prostatic cancer are also at high risk for venous thromboembolism.

Other factors relative to age — most important, decreasing activity and gradual weight gain—increase the incidence of venous thrombosis. The onset of cardiovascular and chronic pulmonary disease, chronic arthritic complaints, or cognitive losses often limit walking considerably. Weight gain causes individuals to be less active, and obesity is associated with decreased production of plasminogen activator by venous endothelium. Plasminogen activator is essential for normal thrombolysis of early clots.

Symptoms and Signs

The hallmark of DVT is the rapid onset of unilateral leg swelling in a gravitational pattern. Generally, this swelling is first noted upon awakening. An ambulatory patient has maximal swelling at the ankle and lower leg, usually occurring over the course of 1 or 2 days. Pain may be present but is usually not severe. Physical examination often reveals unilateral pitting edema and a mild-to-moderate increase in skin temperature over the calf or thigh. In patients with heart failure and DVT, both legs are swollen but the phlebitic one more so.

There is always a gap between the level of thrombosis and the location of edema. With popliteal and lower femoral venous occlusion, edema involves only the lower leg and ankle. When the clot reaches the midfemoral vein area, most or all of the leg is swollen. With upper femoral and external iliac vein involvement, the thigh is also swollen. Tenderness, if present, involves the calf for femoropopliteal and the medial thigh for iliofemoral venous thrombosis.

Calf vein thrombosis is often asymptomatic or may present with mild tenderness and little or no edema. Normally, there are 4 to 6 deep calf veins (anterior tibial, posterior tibial, and peroneal); thus, occlusion of 1 or 2 is not likely to impair venous drainage, as all tibial veins drain into the popliteal vein.

Phlegmasia cerulea dolens is a serious form of iliofemoral venous thrombosis. This syndrome is characterized by massive edema of thigh and calf and a cold, mottled foot. Pedal pulses are usually absent, and the leg is quite tender. Findings are secondary to proximal iliac vein thrombosis and associated arteriospasm. The danger of massive pulmonary embolism is great, even with anticoagulation. Gangrene of the foot is also possible but is a less frequent consequence. Phlegmasia is often taken for arterial embolism, but misdiagnosis can be avoided if one remembers that acute arterial occlusion does *not* cause edema. Phlegmasia, which often indicates occult malignancy, calls for a thorough evaluation.

Diagnosis

When a patient gives a typical history of sudden onset of lower leg swelling in a gravitational distribution without trauma, and a precipitating factor is obvious, DVT can be clinically diagnosed by physical examination. However, if the onset of swelling is not clearly acute and the findings are not entirely typical, laboratory confirmation is required. Trauma, for example, is not always obvious. Traumatic edema should be suspected if the patient noted its onset during or shortly after walking. A forceful dorsiflexion of the foot on sudden downward movement can rupture the plantaris tendon or injure the gastrocnemius muscle. The resulting swelling tends to be asymmetric and confined, occurs above the ankle, causes much tenderness, and is often associated with visible ecchymosis.

Palpation of the popliteal fossa is also important. A popliteal cyst, by extension into the calf, can cause upper leg swelling and, later, compress the popliteal vein. Again, this diagnosis should be suspected if the edema develops initially during physical activity. A sonogram can easily confirm or eliminate this possibility.

In an ambulatory patient, DVT can usually be ruled out if no swelling is present. To confirm this, use a tape measure to compare the legs at several levels. The most important measurement is just above the ankles. Calf vein thrombosis without swelling is common only in sedentary or bedridden individuals and is, therefore, an important consideration in the elderly. This diagnosis can be made only through laboratory evaluation.

The gold standard for confirmation of DVT is **radio-contrast venography**. Contrast material is injected through a dorsal foot vein with the leg in the dependent position or with a tourniquet above the ankle, in order to direct the material into the deep rather than superficial veins. The result in a normal study is an anatomic map of the deep venous system, from tibial veins to the common iliac vein. Venous occlusion can be seen as a cutoff of flow or as a filling defect in the vessel, with contrast material streaming around it. In the tibial area, a sparsity of visible veins is diagnostic.

Collateralization between the deep and superficial veins is usually obvious, but this sign alone is not specific for thrombosis. Deep vein incompetence or a technical problem can lead to filling of the superficial veins from the deep system. The length of venous clots is often striking on venography, and it is not surprising that pulmonary emboli often result from them. Many observers believe that a long filling defect separated from the walls of the vein by a thin stream of contrast material (a so-called floating thrombus) is more likely to cause pulmonary embolism.

Contrast venography should be avoided in the presence of significant renal failure (creatinine level > 3 mg/dL) and used with caution when mild azotemia is present. The passage of the material through the renal tubules can aggravate preexisting renal disease.

Impedance plethysmography indirectly demonstrates venous thrombi. This test detects changes in venous volume by the application and removal of a thigh tourniquet. If a proximal vein is occluded, a dampening of the usual rapid and large increase in venous volume would be expected when the tourniquet is applied. Changes in venous volume are measured by applying a very low amperage current to the calf and measuring the voltage necessary to sustain it. Since blood is a good conductor, an increase in venous volume should decrease electrical impedance and, therefore, the required voltage. Failure to decrease impedance with a tourniquet indicates venous thrombosis.

Plethysmography is reliable only for occlusions above the knee and of recent onset. If a week or more has elapsed, venous return through collateral circulation leads to a false-negative result. Although controversial, the accuracy rate of impedance plethysmography is probably about 85% for thrombi above the knee.

Real-time sonography of the thigh is another promising technic for diagnosing femoral vein thrombosis. Often, a diagnostic filling defect can be seen in the inguinal area of the femoral vein or in the popliteal vein. A less reliable sign is inability to compress the vein. However, since obesity or edema from other causes can interfere with external compression, this sign is not specific.

Radionuclide venography can be performed even in patients with severe azotemia or allergy to contrast material. Macroaggregated albumin tagged with technetium is injected into a dorsal foot vein to outline the venous tree and detecting equipment indicates filling defects. This technic is generally accurate when positive but does not provide as much detail as conventional venography. It has the advantage, however, of allowing for perfusion lung scanning and venography with one injection. Although it does not visualize the tibial veins, it can detect thrombi in the inferior vena cava.

In general, if both sonography and radionuclide venography fail to reveal any clot, venous thrombosis above the knee is very unlikely. Therefore, the advent of these technics has relegated contrast venography to a much smaller clinical role.

Isotopes injected IV **for diagnosis of small vein thrombi,** although mainly used in research, have greatly increased understanding of venous thrombosis. Fibrinogen tagged with ^{125}I accumulates in areas of active clotting, providing a "hot spot" in the calf. Its long half-life allows scanning for a week after a single injection. It is accurate only in nonedematous limbs, where it can follow a small clot in the soleal sinusoids until it reaches the upper tibial area. The test is cumbersome because it requires tagging the patient's own fibrinogen to eliminate risk of viral hepatitis. It is also overly sensitive, detecting thrombi that will never become clinically significant. More recently, indium 111-labeled platelets have been similarly used.

Treatment

The objective is to prevent pulmonary embolism and the development of chronic venous insufficiency. **Anticoagulation,** beginning with heparin and continuing with warfarin, is the mainstay of treatment. **Heparin** can be given s.c. q 6 h, IV q 4 h, or by continuous IV infusion. Continuous infusion is associated with the lowest bleeding rate. If this route is used, the patient must first receive a bolus of 5,000 to 10,000 u. The initial infusion rate is usually 1000 u./h; thereafter, the rate is adjusted according to the partial thromboplastin time **(PTT),** which should be kept between 1.5 and 2.5 times the normal control value. The PTT must be measured daily, since the necessary flow rate may change. Some patients require faster initial rates of infusion. The danger of continuous infusion is the possibility of inadequate anticoagulation, which can occur 1 h after infusion stops. If infusion is then restarted, another bolus injection must be given first. The duration of heparinization is debatable. We usually recommend 5 to 7 days for femoropopliteal and 7 to 10 days for iliofemoral thrombosis.

A **syndrome of paradoxical thrombosis** has been reported in recent years in thrombocytopenic patients receiving heparin. About 1% of patients develop some degree of thrombocytopenia, usually between the 5th and 10th days of heparin therapy. A small proportion of them develop arterial and venous thrombi. Although the exact mechanism of this reaction is not clear, these patients have known heparin-dependent platelet antibodies and, in vitro, their serum deposits abnormal amounts of immunoglobulin on endothelial cells. The rate at which serotonin is released from normal platelets increases when platelets are exposed to heparinized plasma from these patients. Thus, periodic platelet counts should be obtained in heparinized patients, particularly between the 5th and 10th days. *Heparin therapy should be discontinued if the patient is consistently thrombocytopenic.*

Warfarin should be started 4 days before heparin is stopped, to avoid discontinuity in anticoagulation. The only clotting factor significantly depressed during the first 2 days of warfarin administration is Factor VII, which is not involved in the intrinsic clotting pathway. The prothrombin time should be adjusted to a level 1.2 to 1.4 times the normal control value. For uncomplicated venous thrombosis, at least 3 mo of therapy is usually recommended, but it may be extended for patients at high risk for recurrent thrombosis.

Problems with warfarin therapy: In anticoagulated patients over age 70, the risk of serious hemorrhage and its consequences are often high. Vascular integrity is impaired, and even a small head injury can lead to intracranial bleeding. A small GI hemorrhage in a patient with atherosclerosis can trigger a myocardial infarction or a stroke. Patients with organic brain syndrome may not follow directions carefully, and they may be taking multiple drugs that modify warfarin's effect. Even influenza vaccine can potentiate the effect of warfarin. Since many older people with arthritic and neurologic problems fall frequently, warfarin should generally be *avoided* in patients over age 80 and feeble individuals over 70.

Patients receiving long-term warfarin therapy must be warned not to take other drugs without first consulting the physician who prescribed the anticoagulant. Many older patients may be seeing more than one physician, making miscommunication a real danger. Because many drugs have either a potentiating or inhibiting effect on warfarin, it is wise to review the known effects of all drugs before prescribing them.

Thrombolysis: Extensive clotting leads to permanent valvular damage in veins and residual venous occlusion. Therefore, patients with severe iliofemoral venous thrombosis and marked edema are at particularly high risk for chronic venous insufficiency. Heparin prevents further clotting but does not lyse preformed thrombi. In severe iliofemoral venous thrombosis with massive edema, thrombolytic therapy should be considered (eg, streptokinase or urokinase).

Since the risk of bleeding is higher with these agents, one must be sure there are no contraindications to their use (eg, a coagulopathy, recent GI bleeding, recent stroke, history of cerebral hemorrhage, uremia, and surgical procedures within the preceding 7 days). The older the patient, the greater the risk of hemorrhage. The risks of serious bleeding must be weighed against the morbidity of chronic, severe leg edema. In a small number of elderly individuals, thrombolytic therapy is advisable.

There are differences between streptokinase and urokinase. Streptokinase forms a complex with plasminogen activator, whereas urokinase directly lyses the clot. Streptokinase is occasionally associated with allergic reactions. Urokinase can be given repeatedly; however, streptokinase cannot be repeated for 6 mo because with each usage, it induces antibodies that cause drug resistance and increase the chance of a serious allergic reaction. Streptokinase may be ineffective following streptococcal infections.

Before starting thrombolytic treatment, heparin's effect must be allowed to abate. The average dosage of streptokinase is 100,000 u./h, administered over 12 h, after a loading dose of 250,000 u. in the first hour. The patient should be monitored closely during infusion and an Hct value should be obtained q 3 to 4 h.

Serial thrombin times are used to monitor the drug's action. *Elevation of the thrombin time (TT) to at least twice normal is necessary.* If the TT cannot be raised, thrombolytic therapy should be stopped and heparin restarted for 2 reasons: (1) A rise in TT occurs if fibrin split-products are being formed. If there are no split-products, no clot lysis is occurring. (2) Without a TT elevation, the patient is not anticoagulated and is at high risk for pulmonary embolism. Thrombolytic therapy is not likely to be effective for clots more than 3 days old.

Alternatives to warfarin include short-term heparin treatment only or following heparin therapy with insertion of an **inferior vena cava filter (umbrella).** The umbrella is usually inserted through the external jugular vein, passed through the right atrium, and placed in the inferior vena cava ust below the renal veins. If this is technically difficult or the patient already has a transvenous cardiac pacemaker, an umbrella should be inserted through a femoral vein into the inferior vena cava. The umbrella acts as a plication, preventing large pulmonary emboli. The complication rate is low, although occasionally an umbrella can loosen and migrate into another vein or even a pulmonary artery. Although pulmonary embolism from the lower extremities after umbrella insertion is uncommon, it can occur through collateral veins after a few months.

The decision to use an umbrella depends on the likelihood of recurrence, the presence or absence of pulmonary emboli, and the location of the venous clot. Tibial vein thromboses rarely embolize and can remain untreated even in patients at high risk for hemorrhage. Iliofemoral thrombi embolize often, and an umbrella is strongly indicated.

Other reasons for umbrella insertion include (1) hemorrhage while receiving anticoagulation, (2) bleeding diathesis preventing anticoagulation, (3) phlegmasia cerulea dolens, (4) survival after a massive pulmonary embolism, and (5) recurrent pulmonary embolism in an adequately anticoagulated patient.

Identification of risk factors: If the risk factor is obvious (eg, confinement to bed or heart failure), no further evaluation is necessary in cases of femoropopliteal and tibial vein thromboses. However, all patients with iliofemoral venous thrombosis should have a diagnostic abdominal study to rule out extrinsic compression by tumor and clot in the inferior vena cava. In most cases, abdominal sonography is adequate. One should be particularly concerned about right iliofemoral venous thrombosis if there is no local problem in the right lower extremity. Because the inferior vena cava is located on the right, iliofemoral venous thrombosis related to abdominal pathology is more likely to occur on that side.

If a risk factor is not obvious, especially in patients with recurrent and migratory DVT, other tests are indicated to look for coagulopathies and tumors. These generally include stool for occult blood (3 specimens); platelet count; tests for antinuclear antibody, cryoproteins, lupus anticoagulant, antithrombin III deficiency, and occasionally, protein C and protein S deficiency; abdominal sonography or CT scanning; and rectal, pelvic, and breast examinations.

One clue to antithrombin III deficiency is relative resistance to heparin. Heparin acts primarily as an antithrombin by forming complexes with antithrombin III. Protein C is a vitamin K-dependent anticoagulant; patients with this deficiency typically develop venous thromboembolism if warfarin therapy is initiated without heparin, before there is time for the vitamin K procoagulant factors to be reduced.

Prophylaxis

Because of the high incidence of DVT (usually asymptomatic) in certain clinical situations, there is considerable interest in prophylaxis. Studies with ^{125}I fibrinogen have shown a 20 to 25% rate of DVT in routine postoperative patients > 40 yr old. Similar results have been found for immobilized medical patients with myocardial infarction or heart failure. After hip surgery, the incidence approaches 50%. Several methods of prophylaxis are available for these high-risk patients.

Low-dose heparin has been the most widely used. The usual dosage is 5000 u. s.c. q 8 to 12 h. Controlled studies have shown significant decreases in both DVT and pulmonary embolism in surgical patients > 40 yr of age. Significant bleeding is rare at this dosage. Heparin is **contraindicated** in patients who have had ophthalmologic or neurosurgical procedures. Low-dose heparin is of limited prophylactic value in patients who have undergone orthopedic procedures involving the extremities. Full-dose heparin or warfarin is effective in these cases, although each carries a significant risk of hemorrhage.

Oscillating boots applied to the calves are another, even safer, method of prophylaxis. A pump rhythmically inflates the boot to between 30 and 40 mm Hg and then deflates it, thus keeping the peripheral veins drained. Results have been comparable to those of low-dose heparin but without risk of bleeding. **Galvanic stimulation** of calf muscles, begun intraoperatively and continued until the patient is ambulatory, is also quite effective.

Low–molecular-weight dextran has been used successfully to prevent venous thrombosis. Its strong antiplatelet effects decrease both aggregation and adhesiveness. However, it is also a volume expander, and expansion can lead to fluid overload in patients with borderline cardiac or renal status. Dextran has also been associated with acute renal failure and allergic reactions. It does not seem suitable for general use but may be helpful in some high-risk patients.

Mobilizing patients as quickly as possible and encouraging them to move their legs frequently while in bed should always be done.

SUPERFICIAL THROMBOPHLEBITIS

Inflammation associated with a thrombosed superficial vein.

Etiology

In > 90% of cases, the risk factor is the presence of varicose veins. Stasis within these incompetent veins leads to clotting, which can be prevented with the use of elastic bandages or stockings.

In a small percentage of cases, phlebitis occurs in the absence of varicose veins or is recurrent and migratory. This must be considered a potential harbinger of internal disease and indicates assessment for occult neoplasm, especially pancreatic cancer; thrombocytosis or polycythemia; antithrombin III deficiency; collagen-vascular disease; cryoprotein; and lupus anticoagulant.

Symptoms, Signs, and Diagnosis

Superficial phlebitis is a more inflammatory process than is DVT. The usual presenting symptom is pain. Physical examination reveals an area of erythema, warmth, and tenderness overlying a palpable venous cord. The cord is easily felt superficially, represents the thrombosed vein, and is always present. Multiple areas of thrombosis are often found along the course of a superficial vein. A long segment of the greater saphenous vein along the medial aspect of the lower extremity or the short saphenous vein in the posterior calf can be involved.

Although superficial phlebitis can propagate, it rarely leads to pulmonary embolism. The one exception is phlebitis of the greater saphenous vein propagating up the thigh toward the inguinal area, where it meets the femoral vein. If the clot propagates into the latter vessel, pulmonary embolism can occur.

Treatment

For superficial phlebitis below the knee, treatment consists of warm soaks, decreased ambulation, and a nonsteroidal anti-inflammatory agent (eg, aspirin 600 mg q 6 h or indomethacin 25 mg tid). The process is self-limiting, and inflammatory signs usually fade within 5 to 10 days. The patient may have no residual findings or a nontender cord, which represents a permanently thrombosed vein. The cord may calcify months or even years later.

For superficial phlebitis in the lower thigh, a short course of heparin is advisable. Treatment can be discontinued as soon as the inflammatory signs are gone, if there is no evidence of further propagation. If the cord reaches the upper thigh, the greater saphenous vein should be ligated at its most proximal point. This minor procedure can be performed under local anesthesia.

CHRONIC DEEP VENOUS INSUFFICIENCY

A syndrome occurring after thrombosis that involves destruction of the deep and communicating valves of the leg and obliteration of the thrombosed veins.

Chronic deep venous insufficiency **(postphlebitic syndrome)** is almost always the result of previous symptomatic or asymptomatic DVT, although most patients cannot recall having had episodes consistent with DVT. Rarely, chronic venous stasis is due to arteriovenous fistula in the leg, causing chronic venous hypertension and eventual valvular incompetence. The fistula is almost always due to trauma in the inguinal area. The trauma may be accidental or iatrogenic (eg, following cardiac catheterization and angioplasty performed via the femoral vein). Since fistulas are associated with continuous bruits, the inguinal and upper femoral areas should be auscultated in patients with chronic venous insufficiency, especially if the findings are unilateral.

Chronic venous insufficiency rarely causes pain. **The symptoms and signs of stasis** are (1) **chronic edema,** which is generally worse at the end of the day; (2) **hyperpigmentation** around the medial malleolus and just above it; (3) **stasis dermatitis** (scaling and pruritus) in the same area; (4) **hyperemic ulcers** in the same area; and (5) **varicose veins.**

If edema is severe and persistent, fibrosis leads to secondary lymphedema and trapped fluid. The calf becomes permanently enlarged and hard. Ulcers then occur more frequently and are more difficult to heal.

Prevention and treatment: Elastic support is important to prevent this vicious circle. Since elderly people often find it difficult to bandage their legs each day, elastic stockings should be prescribed. In most cases, a stocking that exerts 30 mm Hg pressure from the toes to just below the knee is sufficient, especially since significant edema of the thighs is unusual. Patients should also be advised to elevate their legs intermittently during the day and to avoid standing still for extended periods. Ambulation should *not* be limited. If significant swelling persists overnight, patients can be advised to sleep with their legs elevated 3 to 4 in. above heart level. For severe edema, pumps are available to reduce swelling. Earlier models exert a uniform pressure in rhythmic fashion to the edematous extremity, transmitting the pressure through an encircling sheath. More advanced models exert the pressure in a distal-to-proximal direction, providing more efficient venous return.

Ulcerations are also treated by elastic support and frequent leg elevation. Topical antimicrobial therapy (eg, povidone-iodine) and warm soaks are indicated for infected lesions. A plaster boot often heals large, clean ulcers. Although the boot has to be changed every 1 to 2 wk, this is preferable to limiting ambulation, especially in the elderly.

VARICOSE VEINS

Many elderly people have moderate-to-large varicose veins, which are merely *superficial veins with incompetent valves.* Incompetence can be secondary to chronic venous insufficiency but mostly represents primary valvular degeneration, which has strong hereditary predisposition.

Diagnosis

Primary varicose veins are distinguished from **secondary varicosities** by the absence of (1) signs of stasis or (2) evidence of deep and communicating vein competence on a tourniquet test. In the latter case, venous filling time is recorded when the patient rises from Trendelenburg's to a standing position. This measurement is then repeated with a venous tourniquet placed at various levels on the lower extremity. All varicose veins fill rapidly in retrograde fashion. By contrast, compression of the superficial veins impedes retrograde filling when the deep and communicating veins are competent. If the deep veins are totally competent, complete venous filling after tourniquet application requires at least 45 sec.

Treatment

Primary varicose veins represent no danger to the patient, except for possible superficial phlebitis and easy bleeding if they are traumatized. Elastic support is the only treatment necessary.

Venous ligation and stripping procedures have almost no role in the care of the elderly. Surgery for primary varicosities is only cosmetic, and recurrence is common. In chronic venous insufficiency, stripping is useless because the pathogenesis of the syndrome is related to hypertension in the deep venous system.

---

37. CARDIOVASCULAR SURGERY AND PERCUTANEOUS INTERVENTIONAL TECHNICS

Bernard J. Gersh

The growing number of elderly but active patients with symptomatic heart disease has had a major impact upon cardiovascular medicine in the USA. Treatments such as cardiovascular surgery and newer technics including percutaneous transluminal coronary angioplasty **(PTCA)** and balloon valvuloplasty are increasingly being performed on elderly patients. For example, the number of patients undergoing coronary artery bypass surgery increased fivefold between 1975 and 1980, and in 1985 about 36% of these procedures were performed on patients $\geq$ 65 yr of age.

Older patients differ from younger ones in regard to the indications for these procedures, the results of medical therapy, the presence of coexisting disorders, and both short- and long-term morbidity and mortality of surgery. Differences in cardiovascular surgery indications and results are discussed below, as are the clinical and angiographic characteristics that may affect surgical outcome.

While the results of newer procedures (eg, PTCA and balloon valvuloplasty) are also discussed below, the application of these procedures to the elderly is likely to be altered substantially in the next decade. Moreover, existing data on these procedures emanating from a younger patient population should not be extrapolated directly to the growing numbers of older patients undergoing coronary artery bypass surgery or PTCA, because of new drugs and evolving socioeconomic considerations.

CORONARY BYPASS SURGERY

Clinical Profile

Direct comparisons between older and younger patients undergoing coronary bypass or angiography alone are scanty, but the National Heart, Lung, and Blood Institute's Coronary Artery Surgery Study **(CASS)** Registry, limited to patients undergoing angiography between 1974 and 1979, is a valuable resource. Analyses of clinical and angiographic variables suggest that **older patients were "sicker"** than younger ones—a difference that could reflect the longer duration of disease in the elderly or referral patterns that lead to the selection of older patients with more severe disease or symptoms.

Older patients in the CASS study had a greater frequency of unstable angina and histories of heart failure as well as a greater number of associated medical diseases. High-risk coronary artery disease **(CAD)**, as evidenced by left main coronary artery stenosis of $\geq 70\%$ and triple vessel disease, was more common in older patients undergoing coronary bypass and receiving medical treatment. Similary, indexes of **left ventricular dysfunction,** including an impaired left ventricular ejection fraction, abnormal left ventricular wall motion, cardiomegaly, and an elevated left ventricular end-diastolic pressure, were more frequent in elderly patients.

Other studies of older patients undergoing coronary bypass support the CASS Registry data, particularly in regard to the frequency of coexisting conditions such as diabetes, hypertension, cerebrovascular disease, peripheral vascular disease, chronic obstructive pulmonary disease, severe and unstable angina, triple vessel disease, and left ventricular dysfunction in the elderly.

These variations in preoperative status are important and may in part account for differences between older and younger patients in short- and long-term mortality after coronary bypass procedures. Recognition of these factors, particularly the presence and severity of associated medical conditions, is an essential aspect of the assessment of the elderly for coronary artery surgery (see TABLE 37–1).

TABLE 37–1. CONSIDERATIONS IN THE ASSESSMENT OF THE
ELDERLY FOR CARDIAC SURGERY

Evaluation of severity of symptoms and effect on quality of life
Pharmacologic therapy of angina pectoris and heart failure
Efficacy
Toxicity
Psychosocial factors
Patient's desires, motivation, and life-style
Physiologic as opposed to chronologic age
Associated *medical* diseases
Severity and extent of coronary artery and valvular heart disease
Potential for adequate revascularization
Left ventricular function
Coexisting *cardiac* conditions

Peri- and Postoperative Mortality and Morbidity

Analysis of 22 series of coronary bypass surgery performed in patients $\geq$ 65 yr from 1969 to 1983 documented a perioperative mortality ranging from 0 to 21.1%. This wide range reflects different patient selection criteria, the relatively small size of some individual series, changing results over the first 2 decades of coronary bypass surgery, and age (even within an elderly population).

In the CASS study, the early mortality for isolated coronary artery bypass was 5.2% in elderly patients vs. 1.9% in those < 65 yr. *Mortality increased with age even within the elderly group;* it was 4.6% in patients 65 to 69 yr, 6.6% in those aged 70 to 74 yr, and 9.5% in those aged $\geq$ 75 yr. Surgical mortality today is probably lower than it was during the CASS study; a clear trend suggests that *the mortality associated with coronary bypass in the elderly has declined substantially* in the last 5 yr, as it has in other high-risk patient groups.

The reasons for increased perioperative mortality in the elderly are not clear. In part, this is expected in a patient population considered to be at high risk on the basis of many clinical and angiographic features. Indeed, elderly patients considered to be at lower risk because of the presence of stable angina, good left ventricular function, few or no associated medical conditions, and the absence of heart failure and left main CAD had a significantly lower perioperative mortality in the CASS study (see TABLE 37–2).

Furthermore, for the most part, *the technical details of coronary artery bypass are unaltered in elderly patients,* although their tissues may be more friable. Abnormalities of the ascending aorta resulting from aging or severe calcific atherosclerosis (or both) may complicate arterial cannulation or proximal anastomoses in older patients. Increasing experience in current technics has, however, tended to minimize these constraints.

TABLE 37–2. INDEPENDENT ADVERSE PREDICTORS OF SURVIVAL FROM ISOLATED CORONARY BYPASS SURGERY IN PATIENTS ≥ 65 YR OF AGE IN THE CASS REGISTRY*

Predictors of perioperative mortality
Left main coronary artery stenosis ≥ 70% in association with left dominant circulation
Left ventricular end-diastolic pressure
Current cigarette smoking
Pulmonary rales on auscultation
Associated medical diseases

Predictors of 5-yr survival
(in perioperative survivors)
Associated medical diseases
Functional impairment caused by heart failure
Severity of abnormal left ventricular wall motion (determined angiographically)
Left ventricular end-diastolic pressure

* Variables identified using multivariate analysis technics.

Nonetheless, analysis of the CASS data suggests that other unmeasured or as yet unidentified variables intrinsically associated with aging per se adversely influence the outcome of coronary bypass surgery (see TABLE 37–3). In an analysis of 7658 patients undergoing isolated coronary bypass, age ≥ 65 yr was an independent adverse predictor of survival, although not the most powerful. This emphasizes that *the greater the risk of a procedure, the more stringent should be the criteria for its implementation.*

Perioperative morbidity is also increased in the elderly, who have a higher frequency of stroke, supraventricular arrhythmias, transient psychoses, heart block, and pulmonary embolism. In the CASS study, this increased morbidity resulted in prolonged hospital stays, which length-

TABLE 37–3. INDEPENDENT ADVERSE PREDICTORS OF ISOLATED CORONARY BYPASS SURGERY SURVIVAL IN THE CASS REGISTRY (ALL AGES)*

Severity of heart failure
Left main coronary artery stenosis ≥ 70% in association with left dominant circulation
Age ≥ 65 yr
Severity of abnormal left ventricular wall motion
Female sex
Unstable angina pectoris

* Variables identified using multivariate analysis technics.

ened as the ages of patients within the older group increased: The mean duration of hospital stay was 11.4 days in patients < 65 yr, 12.9 days in those aged 65 to 69 yr, 14.0 days in patients aged 70 to 74 yr, and 16.5 days in patients ≥ 75 yr. Since that study, the absolute duration of hospitalization has declined in all age groups, although *the elderly continue to require longer hospitalization.*

Long-Term Surgical Results

Mortality: The cumulative 5-yr survival of patients in the CASS Registry (including perioperative mortality) was 83% in elderly patients and 91% in patients < 65 yr. In patients discharged from hospital, 5-yr survival was 88, 85 and 77%, respectively, in patients aged 65 to 69, 70 to 74, and ≥ 75 yr.

Preoperative left ventricular dysfunction and the presence of associated medical diseases exert a powerful adverse effect on long-term survival (see TABLE 37–2). Five-year survival (including perioperative mortality) in elderly patients with normal left ventricular wall motion was 87%; it was 89% in those who had no associated medical conditions. Thus, a key element in the preoperative assessment of the elderly is an analysis of these clinical and angiographic characteristics that are such important determinants of outcome. The results of the procedure in the individual physician's institution are also an essential factor in estimating the risk-benefit ratio for the surgical candidate.

Functional outcome: Any therapeutic modality in the elderly must focus upon the **quality of life,** particularly in a population that can reasonably expect years of active existence ahead of them. Several studies note that relief of angina is as effective or possibly more effective in older patients than in younger ones, although this may partially reflect reduced activity in the elderly. In older patients, as in younger ones, the symptomatic benefits of coronary artery bypass are superior in men, with a higher recurrence of angina in women. This may relate to anatomic considerations, including the smaller luminal diameter of the coronary vasculature in women, which correlates with reduced body surface area and smaller hearts.

Comparison of surgical and medical therapy: No randomized data are available on the elderly. Information from large, multicenter randomized trials of coronary bypass and medical therapy cannot be extrapolated directly to the elderly, because these trials—designed when perioperative mortality in the elderly was high—excluded patients > 65 yr of age.

A comparison of medical and surgical therapy in 1491 patients with symptomatic angina pectoris in the CASS Registry shows a cumulative survival at 6 yr (after adjustment for major differences in baseline characteristics) of 79% in the surgical group and 64% in the medical group. Relief of chest pain was also significantly greater in patients treated surgically. However, a nonrandomized study such as this is subject to bias and cannot supplant a randomized trial. No amount of statistical adjustment is likely to eliminate some degree of bias, and this could significantly influence conclusions.

Very likely, the improved survival among surgically treated older patients reflects their high-risk preoperative status. In a subset of lower-risk older patients who had mild, stable angina, well-preserved left ventricular function, and no left main CAD, the survival pattern mirrored that seen in randomized trials of younger patients with similar characteristics, ie, there was no difference in survival between those treated medically and those treated surgically.

Assessment for Coronary Bypass Surgery

A careful preoperative assessment with attention to the whole patient as opposed to a specific organ or system is crucial to a successful outcome (see TABLE 37–1). Certain specific characteristics of the elderly should be considered when deciding whether to perform coronary bypass.

Angina pectoris: In older patients, an assessment of the severity of angina pectoris and the effect of its symptoms upon the quality of life may be complicated by vagaries of memory, the masking of symptoms by physical limitations from other causes, the frequency of anginal equivalents such as dyspnea, and the presence of coexisting medical conditions simulating angina, such as cervical spine disease and diaphragmatic hernias.

Medical control of angina pectoris, together with a change in life-style to accommodate a reduced level of activity, is hampered by the severity of symptoms and coronary pathology in many elderly patients. *The attainment of maximal medical therapy is more difficult in the elderly* for many reasons:

1. Alterations in pharmacokinetics, eg, decreased renal function and hepatic perfusion, may result in higher plasma levels for some drugs.

2. The elderly are more likely to experience adverse side effects secondary to age-related changes in cerebral blood flow, impaired reflexes leading to orthostatic hypotension, and the presence of associated diseases.

3. Social factors leading to reduced compliance and comprehension may also limit the efficacy of medical therapy.

Special considerations: In addition to assessing the effect of symptoms on the quality of life, understanding the patient's desires, motivation, and life-style is important in the determination of therapy. In this regard, an evaluation of physiologic as opposed to chronologic age may be helpful. Meticulous attention to the presence and severity of coexisting medical conditions is essential. A careful clinical and social history, physical examination, and routine laboratory investigations should provide solutions to most of these problems.

These clinical data must be reviewed along with **angiographic assessment** of the severity and extent of disease, the potential for adequate revascularization, and the presence and severity of left ventricular dysfunction and other cardiac conditions (eg, aortic stenosis and conduction disease).

Postoperative Management

In the postoperative intensive care unit, prolonged physiologic monitoring and respiratory support require that attention be given to the **prevention and treatment of sepsis.** The higher incidence of postoperative psychoses and a tendency toward reduced mobility in the elderly require that specific attention also be given to chest physiotherapy and wound care. Gradual but steady resumption of normal activity, mobility, and independence are the major objectives during this phase.

PERCUTANEOUS TRANSLUMINAL CORONARY ANGIOPLASTY (PTCA)

PTCA is an increasingly attractive option for treating elderly patients with symptomatic coronary disease, particularly those with other medical diseases that could adversely affect the short- and long-term results of coronary artery bypass. Other constraints imposed by the more prolonged postoperative convalescent period in the elderly and the disadvantages of thoracotomy and general anesthesia have also stimulated interest in alterate forms of therapy such as PTCA. In 1985, approximately 26% of balloon angioplasties carried out in the USA were in elderly patients. A carefully controlled, preferably randomized trial of PTCA vs. coronary bypass surgery is needed, and several such trials are in preparation.

Angiographic Complications

Although the overall risks of coronary angiography in the elderly are low, older patients in the CASS study had an approximately three-fold increase in mortality associated with angiography (0.19%) when compared with patients < 65 yr and a stroke incidence of 0.37% vs. 0.01% in younger patients. An increased incidence of peripheral vascular complications at the site of the femoral arteriotomy in elderly patients undergoing PTCA has also been reported.

Results: The National Heart, Lung, and Blood Institute's PTCA Registry from 1979 to 1981 documented a clinical success rate of 62% in patients < 65 yr vs. 53% in older patients (p < 0.01). The difference was small, and the clinical impact was probably minor. Technical difficulties, eg, tortuous vessels thwarting the crossing of the area of stenosis, were more frequent in the elderly. After passage of the guide wire, however, *the rate of subsequent successful dilatation was similar to that in younger patients.*

The acute mortality in older and younger patients was 2.2 vs. 0.7% (p < 0.01), but these results were obtained in a relatively early "learning phase" of PTCA. Newer developments and increasing experience with PTCA have led to an increased success rate and to lower mortality in the elderly. A primary success rate of about 80 to 90% was recently reported in older patients with stable and unstable angina. In some series, the success rate in older patients was similar to that in younger patients, although selection criteria may differ between the groups.

Because PTCA is a relatively new procedure, data on its long-term results in an elderly population are limited. Since the elderly have a high incidence of multivessel and diffuse disease, the benefits of multilesion and multivessel balloon angioplasty on long-term survival and symptom relief are potentially exciting but await further analysis.

VALVE REPLACEMENT
(See also Ch. 33)

Epidemiology and Etiology

The patient population undergoing valve replacement in the 1980s has changed substantially from that seen in the 1960s and early 1970s; patients currently undergoing surgery are older. In Olmsted County, Minnesota, between 1980 and 1983, the peak incidence of valve replacements in men was in the 75- to 79-yr age group and in women in the 65- to 74-yr age group. At the Mayo Clinic between 1981 and 1985, 50% of stenotic aortic valves replaced were in patients $\geq$ 70 yr, compared with only 21% between 1965 and 1980.

In patients undergoing aortic valve replacement at the Mayo Clinic, degenerative (senile) calcification is currently the most common cause of aortic stenosis seen. The incidence of congenitally bicuspid aortic valves has declined slightly, and the incidence of postinflammatory (primarily rheumatic) disease has declined markedly. This may relate to the increasing age of patients undergoing aortic valve replacement, and to other factors such as referral patterns, changing life expectancy, and the impact of newer noninvasive diagnostic technics. In patients undergoing mitral valve replacement, the incidence of postinflammatory disease has similarly declined, whereas that of degenerative mitral valve disease has increased.

Results of Valve Replacement

The results of valve replacement in elderly patients have improved because of refinement in surgical and myocardial preservation technics and advances in pre- and postoperative care. Although comparable results have been reported in older and younger patients, advanced age, partly through an association with disease of other organs, is generally considered a significant risk factor for early morbidity and mortality.

A review of 14 series that included 818 elderly patients who underwent **isolated aortic valve replacement** revealed an overall mortality of 10.2% (range 0 to 33%). This is higher than in younger patients. In patients operated on since 1970, mortality had fallen to approximately 6.5%. In 10 series including 316 patients aged $\geq$ 65 yr who underwent **mitral valve replacement,** overall mortality was 15.2% (range 9 to 37%), with a mortality of 12.3% in patients operated on since 1970.

Mortality for multiple valve replacements is considerably higher. The wide range of reported results reflects changing surgical technics and differences in patient selection criteria, the valves replaced, and the nature and etiology of the lesions, in addition to the acuity of the clinical presentation.

As expected, *postoperative morbidity is generally greater in the elderly,* with an increased frequency of respiratory distress, bleeding, supraventricular arrhythmias, conduction disturbances, delayed wound healing, psychoses, and stroke.

Whether advanced age alone is associated with a poorer long-term functional result is not clearly established. What is more important, however, is that judiciously timed valve replacement in the symptomatic elderly patient with severe valvular heart disease usually results in excellent long-term survival and symptomatic improvement. Long-term (5 to 10 yr) survival appears far superior to that attainable with medical therapy alone.

The prevalence of CAD in elderly patients with valvular disease raises the question of whether **coronary revascularization** should be carried out at the same time as valve surgery, particularly in patients who do not have angina or prior myocardial infarction. The increased operative mortality entailed by performing concomitant coronary artery bypass has diminished in recent years, but no randomized, controlled data comparing the merits of both approaches are available.

Generally, severely obstructed but operable coronary arteries should be bypassed at the time of valve surgery, even in the absence of angina. However, the decision to do this should be based on the clinical and hemodynamic status of the patient both pre- and intraoperatively.

Assessment for Valvular Surgery

The severity of symptoms, psychosocial factors, the evaluation of concomitant medical diseases, and associated cardiac conditions are as important in the assessment of the patient with valvular heart disease as they are in the patient with primary coronary disease.

Age per se is not a contraindication to valve replacement or repair, and the **indications for the procedure** are similar to those in younger patients: the presence and severity of symptoms, the nature of the valve lesion (whether regurgitant or stenotic), the etiology of the disease, and left ventricular function.

In **aortic stenosis,** poor left ventricular function apparently does not contraindicate surgery, provided the mechanical effects of the valve lesion are the primary cause of the patient's clinical status. In **valvular insufficiency,** prolonged delay in the referral of the elderly for surgery may result in irreversible left ventricular dysfunction, with a markedly adverse impact upon both early and late results.

Coronary angiography to identify significantly stenosed but bypassable lesions is a generally accepted part of the preoperative assessment in the elderly.

The **choice of a valve substitute** in the elderly warrants careful assessment and discussion during the preoperative period. A lower incidence of thromboembolism in patients who have sinus rhythm with **biologic prostheses** (especially in the aortic position) enhances their value in the elderly. This is particularly so in patients $\geq$ 70 yr in whom long-term prosthesis durability is of less importance and the risks of chronic anti-coagulant therapy are higher. In this age group, bioprostheses (eg, Carpentier-Edwards, Hancock) are generally recommended. The favorable hemodynamic characteristics of certain low-profile mechanical valves (eg, Starr-Edwards, St. Jude Medical, Hall) may warrant their use in specific situations; often this decision can only be made with confidence at the time of operation.

In the case of the elderly with senile degenerative calcific valve disease on a tricuspid aortic valve, **aortic valve decalcification** may offer an alternative to valve replacement. Similarly, patients with mitral regurgitation may benefit from the technic of **mitral valve repair,** thus avoiding the need for valve replacement. Current trends strongly emphasize the expanding use and advantages of a mitral valve repair when possible.

PERCUTANEOUS BALLOON VALVULOPLASTY

As an alternative nonsurgical treatment for patients with aortic or mitral stenosis, the technic of percutaneous balloon valvuloplasty is promising, but it remains **investigational.** Although individual responses to balloon valvuloplasty for aortic stenosis may vary substantially, a successful procedure results in a reduction in transvalvar gradient, an increase in valve orifice area and cardiac index, and an improvement in ventricular function. The magnitude of the improvement appears limited and the duration, without restenosis, needs to be established.

Despite the success of aortic valve replacement in the elderly, some patients are **poor candidates for surgery,** eg, because of malignancy, severe chronic lung disease, extreme age, inability to tolerate anticoagulants, or personal preference. In these patients, **balloon valvuloplasty offers the potential for palliation.** Whether percutaneous balloon valvuloplasty will ever achieve the status of primary therapy for **aortic stenosis** in adults will depend upon further evaluation and technical improvements in increasing the valve area.

The role of balloon valvuloplasty as primary or palliative therapy in patients with **mitral stenosis** is as yet undefined. The indications and expectations of the procedure may vary with age, the valve involved, and the severity and pathology of the lesion.

§3.   ORGAN SYSTEMS: PULMONARY DISORDERS

Contents for GASTROINTESTINAL DISORDERS begin on page 461.

---

38.   THE EFFECTS OF AGE ON THE LUNG

Melvyn S. Tockman

Aging affects not only the physiologic functions of the lungs (ventilation and gas exchange) but also the ability of the lungs to defend themselves. The specific biologic mechanisms responsible for these changes are unclear. For example, while many investigators have reported a progressive decline in pulmonary function as measured by serial examinations over the course of increasing age, it is not clear whether aging exerts its effect by prolonging exposure to environmental toxins, by permitting progression of subclinical disease, or by allowing expression of a time-dependent feature of pulmonary pathophysiology after a certain age. It also is unclear whether the increasing rate of ventilatory functional decline with age results from a progressive, lifelong process or occurs abruptly in brief steps, leading to symptomatic airways obstruction **(AO)** over a few years.

The association of AO with age may be partially explained by an accumulation of inflammatory injuries. Repeated disruption of the balance of inflammatory mediators and humoral protection (elastase/antielastase, oxidant/antioxidant), neutrophil recruitment, and tissue repair, which culminates in inflammatory lung destruction and AO, has been well documented in cigarette smokers. Accumulated environmental oxidant injuries could result in similar, although less extensive, lung destruction in nonsmokers.

An understanding of the relationship between aging and AO may explain why the latter (but not chronic bronchitis) is associated with increased age-specific death rates from all causes, most of which are due to cardiovascular disease. In fact, survival parallels preservation of ventilatory function. In addition to increasing the risk of death from chronic obstructive pulmonary disease **(COPD)** and heart disease, AO is associated with increased risk of lung cancer. *Thus, increased risk for 3 of the 5 leading causes of death in men and for 3 of the 7 leading causes of death in women can be identified by impaired pulmonary function on spirometric testing.*

Age-related changes in ventilation and gas distribution are due primarily to simultaneous changes in compliance of both the chest wall and the lungs. Lung volumes (at rest) are determined by the equilibrium between inward elastic tissue forces of the lung and outward forces of the chest wall and muscles of respiration. Through the developmental years, growth of the lungs and chest wall parallels the growth of the body and correlates closely with height (squared). With increasing age, especially after age 55, respiratory muscle strength weakens in both men and women. This weakened outward muscular force and the increased stiffness (decreased compliance) of the chest wall are counterbalanced by a loss of elastic recoil (increased compliance) of the lungs.

Compliance

Lung recoil results from the combined effects of parenchymal elastic fibers and inward-directed surface forces (from the air/fluid interface of the terminal respiratory units). There is no evidence that the surface forces or the opposing surfactant effect is altered with age. Therefore, the age-related loss of lung elastic recoil is probably a function of the elastic fibers. Beyond the early 20s, however, there is no age effect upon the length or diameter of individual elastic fibers. Instead, the age-related increase in lung compliance may be due to damage or lost alveolar attachments to these elastic fibers, resulting in an increase in the proportion of collapsible small airways.

Chest wall compliance gradually falls (becomes stiffer) with increasing age, probably as a result of ossification of cartilage/rib articulations. The increased outward pull of the stiffer chest wall, combined with reduced ability of the lung to pull inward, results in small age-related increases in total lung capacity **(TLC)**, with larger increases in functional residual capacity **(FRC)**, the volume at which the lung comes to rest at the end of a quiet expiration and residual volume **(RV)**, the volume which remains in the lung after a maximal expiration (see TABLES 38–1 and 38–2).

Airflow Rates

During forced expiration, increasing contraction of chest wall voluntary muscles added to the elastic recoil of the lungs increases expiratory airflow until dynamic compression of the airways limits further expiratory flow (after approximately 25% of the vital capacity has been exhaled). Collapse of the airways (at the equal pressure point) is prevented only by intra-alveolar (upstream) pressure, generated by lung elastic recoil. Age-related loss of elastic recoil may result in early collapse of

TABLE 38–1. EFFECTS OF AGE ON NORMAL PULMONARY FUNCTION IN MEN (as Determined by the Age Coefficient Term From Male Reference Value Prediction Equations)

Pulmonary Function*	Equation	95% Confidence Interval†	Loss of Function/ Yr of Age	Reference
TLC	$0.0795 \times$ H‡ $+ 0.0032 \times$ Age $- 7.333$	1.61	(Increase) 3 mL	Morris§
FRC	$0.472 \times$ H $+ 0.0090 \times$ Age $- 5.290$	1.46	(Increase) 9 mL	Morris
RV	$0.0216 \times$ H $+ 0.0207 \times$ Age $- 2.840$	0.76	(Increase) 20 mL	Morris
FVC	$0.3759 \times$ H $- 0.0250 \times$ Age $- 4.241$	1.45	25 mL	Morris
FEV$_1$	$0.2337 \times$ H $- 0.0320 \times$ Age $- 1.260$	1.08	32 mL	Morris
FEV$_1$/FVC	$-0.7920 \times$ H $- 0.2422 \times$ Age $+ 107.12$	15.27	0.24%	Morris
Pao$_2$	$- 0.323 \times$ Age $- 100.10$		0.32 torr	Sorbini**
N$_2$P$_{III}$	$0.4160 \times$ H $+ 0.010 \times$ Age $+ 0.710$	0.84	(Increase) 0.01% N$_2$/L	Buist††
DL$_{COSB}$	$0.4160 \times$ H $- 0.219 \times$ Age $+ 26.34$	8.20	0.2 mL CO/min/mm Hg	Crapo‡‡
$\dot{V}$O$_2$MAX (Cotes)	$0.4100 \times$ H $- 0.210 \times$ Age $- 26.31$	8.20	32 mL O$_2$/min	Crapo
	$- 0.032 \times$ Age $+ 4.2$ (SD $\pm$ 0.4)			Jones§§
expressed per kg	$- 0.550 \times$ Age $+ 60$ (SD $\pm$ 7.5)		0.55 mL/kg/min	Jones

* TLC = total lung capacity, FRC = functional residual capacity, RV = residual volume, FVC = forced vital capacity, FEV$_1$ = forced expiratory volume in the 1st sec, Pao$_2$ = arterial oxygen pressure, N$_2$P$_{III}$ = single-breath nitrogen Phase III, DL$_{COSB}$ = single-breath carbon monoxide diffusing capacity, Hb corr. = hemoglobin correlates, $\dot{V}$O$_2$MAX = maximal oxygen consumption.

† Note: Lower boundary of normal determined by calculating predicted value from equation, then subtracting the 95% confidence interval.

‡ H = Height

§ Morris AM, et al: Clinical Pulmonary Function Testing: A Manual of Uniform Laboratory Procedures, ed 2. Salt Lake City, Intermountain Thoracic Society, 1984.

** Sorbini CA, Brassi V, Solinas E, et al: Arterial oxygen tension in relation to age in healthy subjects. Respiration 1968; 25:3-13.

†† Buist AS, Ross BB: Quantitative analysis of the alveolar plateau in the diagnosis of early airway obstruction. Am Rev Respir Dis 1973; 108:1078-1087.

‡‡ Crapo RO, Morris AH: Standardized single breath normal values for carbon monoxide diffusing capacity. Am Rev Respir Dis 1981; 123:185-189.

§§ Jones NL, Moran Campbell EJ, Edwards RHT, et al: Clinical Exercise Testing. Philadelphia, WB Saunders, 1975.

TABLE 38–2. EFFECTS OF AGE ON NORMAL PULMONARY FUNCTION IN WOMEN
(as Determined by the Age Coefficient Term From Female Reference Value Prediction Equations)

Pulmonary Function*	Equation	95% Confidence Interval†	Loss of Function/ Yr of Age	Reference
TLC	$0.0590 \times H\ddagger + 0.0000 \times Age - 4.537$	1.08	(Increase) 0 mL	Morris§
FRC	$0.0360 \times H + 0.0031 \times Age - 3.182$	1.06	(Increase) 3 mL	Morris
RV	$0.0197 \times H + 0.0201 \times Age - 2.421$	0.78	(Increase) 3 mL	Morris
FVC	$0.2921 \times H - 0.0240 \times Age - 2.852$	1.02	24 mL	Morris
FEV_1	$0.2261 \times H - 0.0250 \times Age - 1.932$	0.92	25 mL	Morris
FEV_1/FVC	$-0.1725 \times H - 0.1815 \times Age + 88.70$	13.41	0.18%	Morris
Pa_{O_2}	$- 0.323 \times Age - 100.10$		0.32 torr	Sorbini**
N_2P_{III} (<60 yr)	$+ 0.009 \times Age + 1.036$	1.12	(Increase) 0.01% N_2/L	Buist††
N_2P_{III} (≥60 yr)	$+ 0.058 \times Age + 1.777$	2.55	(Increase) 0.06% N_2/L	Buist
$DL_{CO_{SB}}$	$0.256 \times H - 0.144 \times Age + 8.36$	6.0	0.1 mL CO/min/mm Hg	Crapo‡‡
Hb corr. (Cotes)	$0.282 \times H - 0.157 \times Age + 10.89$	6.1	0.1 mL CO/min/mm Hg	Crapo
V_{O_2MAX}	$- 0.014 \times Age - 2.6$ (SD ± 0.4)		14 mLO_2/min	Jones§§
expressed per kg	$- 0.370 \times Age - 48$ (SD ± 7.0)		0.37 mL/kg/min	Jones

* TLC = total lung capacity, FRC = functional residual capacity, RV = residual volume, FVC = forced vital capacity, FEV_1 = forced expiratory volume in the 1st sec, Pa_{O_2} = arterial oxygen pressure, N_2P_{III} = single-breath nitrogen Phase III, $DL_{CO_{SB}}$ = single-breath carbon monoxide diffusing capacity, V_{O_2MAX} = maximal oxygen consumption.

† Note: Lower boundary of normal determined by calculating predicted value from equation, then substracting the 95% confidence interval.

‡ H = Height

§ Morris AM, et al: *Clinical Pulmonary Function Testing: A Manual of Uniform Laboratory Procedures*, ed 2. Salt Lake City, Intermountain Thoracic Society, 1984.

** Sorbini CA, Brassi V, Solinas E, et al: Arterial oxygen tension in relation to age in healthy subjects. *Respiration* 1968; 25:3–13.

†† Buist AS, Ross BB: Quantitative analysis of the alveolar plateau in the diagnosis of early airway obstruction. *Am Rev Respir Dis* 1973; 108:1078–1087.

‡‡ Crapo RO, Morris AH: Standardized single breath normal values for carbon monoxide diffusing capacity. *Am Rev Respir Dis* 1981; 123:185–189.

§§ Jones NL, Moran Campbell EJ, Edwards RHT, et al: *Clinical Exercise Testing*. Philadelphia, WB Saunders, 1975.

poorly supported peripheral airways. Dynamic compression of the smaller airways in older lungs, therefore, may lead to a decrease in flow at low lung volumes, similar to the obstruction of small airways produced by chronic cigarette smoking.

Forced expiratory airflows reach a maximum at 20 yr of age in women and at 27 yr in men as a result of growth and increasing chest wall muscle strength. Further aging leads to a progressive decline in lung function, although until 40 yr of age, the age-related decreases in forced vital capacity **(FVC)** and maximal expiratory flow rate are thought to be due to changes in body weight and strength rather than to attrition of tissues. Cross-sectional studies of pulmonary function have identified a constant (linear) decline of 32 mL in the forced expiratory volume in the 1st sec **(FEV$_1$)** and 25 mL in the FVC with each increasing year of age in males (see TABLES 38–1 and 38–2). These observations are based on single examinations of variously aged persons in the general population. However, when individual participants are followed, the annual decline in FEV$_1$ is observed to be small at first and to increase progressively with age. Increasing age is also accompanied by a progressive reduction of flow at low lung volumes, seen on the maximal expiratory flow volume curve.

Although loss of elastic recoil may explain an age-related flow decline in a given person, individual conductance differences are more complex. Airway conductance is related not only to elastic recoil but also to gender and to non-age-dependent differences in lung size, which develop as a result of relatively lesser growth of the conducting airways compared to the parenchyma. The failure of the conducting airways to grow as rapidly as the parenchyma results in relatively narrow airways and slower emptying of larger lungs compared with smaller lungs at any age. Clinically, this is demonstrated by a lower FEV$_1$/FVC ratio observed in taller compared with shorter persons (all healthy nonsmokers) and in men compared with women. Not only do the larger lungs empty more slowly (specific for volume) but there is evidence of a greater heterogeneity of emptying units in nonsmoking men compared with nonsmoking women.

This observation seems to make sense, since lungs do not grow equidimensionally (like a sphere) but enlarge in a cylindric shape, increasing the range of diversity in conducting airways lengths in larger compared with smaller lungs. Furthermore, this increased male heterogeneity of emptying units is enhanced when smokers are examined, since the effect of smoking is greater on the slower emptying units. Whether lung function decline accelerates in men and in those with larger lungs as age increases has not yet been determined, although it is suggested from cross-sectional yearly loss of FEV$_1$ (see TABLES 38–1 and 38–2).

Distribution of Ventilation

The elastic fibers within alveolar walls are tethered to the respiratory and terminal bronchioles, helping to maintain the patency of these small conducting airways at low lung volumes. The loss of these elastic attachments leads to increased compliance of affected alveoli, collapse of the small conducting airways, nonuniformity of alveolar ventilation, and air trapping.

The single-breath nitrogen (SBN₂) washout technic has been used to evaluate the uniformity of alveolar ventilation and the lung volume at which small conducting airways collapse. Nonuniformity of ventilation is shown by an increased slope of the SBN$_2$ Phase III (N$_2$P$_{III}$), or alveolar plateau, while the volume at which terminal respiratory units begin to close is demonstrated by elevations of the SBN$_2$ Phase IV (closing volume). With advancing age, the slope of the N$_2$P$_{III}$ increases (see TABLES 38–1 and 38–2), and the closing capacity (closing volume plus residual volume) may exceed the FRC, indicating that closure of terminal respiratory units occurs at the end of a normal tidal breath. Closing capacity begins to exceed the supine FRC at about 44 yr of age, and the sitting FRC at approximately 65 yr of age. This nonuniformity of ventilation probably underlies the age-related changes observed in arterial P$_{O2}$. It is possible, therefore, that the association observed between AO and mortality may be mediated partly by mechanical limitations of ventilation and a lowered arterial O$_2$ tension.

Diffusing Capacity

After increasing to a maximum in the early 20s, the single breath carbon monoxide diffusing capacity (DL$_{CO}$) gradually undergoes a decline with age, due to both morphologic changes (loss of surface area of the alveolar-capillary membrane) and increasing inhomogeneities in ventilation and/or blood flow. This reduction has been estimated to be approximately 0.5% (0.2 mL CO/min/mm Hg)/yr (see TABLES 38–1 and 38–2), with women having 10% lower diffusion capacity values than men for the same age and height. As was found with measurements of FEV$_1$, the age-related decline in DL$_{CO}$ is not linear, although linear prediction regressions are used.

Pulmonary resistance to gas diffusion comes from 2 sources: the area and thickness of the alveolar-capillary membrane, and the ability of the gas to combine with elements of the blood. Age-related decreases in total pulmonary diffusing capacity are primarily due to loss of membrane diffusing capacity, which is more evident after 40 yr of age than before.

Arterial O₂ Tension

The gradual decline in Pa$_{O2}$ with advancing age parallels the loss of elastic recoil. As described earlier, progressive loss of elastic recoil leads to reduction of airway caliber, early airway closure, and maldistribution of ventilation. While collapse of peripheral airways decreases ventilation to distal gas exchange units, perfusion remains unaffected. Thus, a ventilation-perfusion imbalance is created that accounts for most of the reduction of Pa$_{O2}$. The linear deterioration of arterial O$_2$ tension associated with aging (approximately 0.3% Pa$_{O2}$/yr, see TABLES 38–1 and 38–2) has long been recognized. The ventilation-perfusion imbalance is particularly treacherous in older individuals, since the Pa_{O_2} (and thus O_2 delivery) may be further compromised by age-associated reductions in cardiac output **(CO)**. When ventilation and perfusion are evenly matched, changing CO has no effect on Pa_{O_2}. As ventilation-perfusion inequalities worsen, the Pa_{O_2} at any given CO decreases; further loss of CO magnifies the reduction of O_2 delivery.

Investigators who have observed desaturation in asymptomatic asthmatic patients have proposed that maldistribution of ventilation caused by narrowing of small airways was the mechanism for this hypoxemia. Several studies have shown that cigarette smokers have a lower Pa_{O_2} than do nonsmokers. One study of arterialized earlobe blood from more than 1000 men indicated that smokers had an average of 4 mm Hg lower Pa_{O_2}, with a dose-response correlation between number of cigarettes smoked and reduction in Pa_{O_2}.

Control of Breathing

Ventilatory and heart rate **responses to hypoxia and hypercapnia** diminish with age and may make otherwise healthy older persons more vulnerable to diseases producing lower O_2 levels (eg, pneumonia, COPD) compared with younger persons. The ventilatory response to hypoxia is reduced by 51% in healthy older men (64 to 73 yr of age) compared with young healthy men (22 to 30 yr of age), while the ventilatory response to CO_2 is reduced by 41%. Although the reasons for the suppression of breathing have not been fully explained, it appears that age attenuates chemoreceptor function, either at peripheral chemoreceptors or in the integrating CNS pathways.

It has been confirmed that the reduced ventilatory responses to hypoxia and hypercapnia observed in the elderly are independent of the aging mechanical properties of the lung. The decreased ventilatory responses to hypoxia and hypercapnia noted above are accompanied by a parallel decrease in inspiratory occlusion pressure—a measure of total neuromuscular drive to breathe, which is unaffected by the compliance of the respiratory system. Thus the elderly, who are most likely to be afflicted with chronic pulmonary diseases, are least able to defend against acute hypoxia or hypercapnia because of reductions in both their mechanical ability to ventilate and their neural drive to breathe.

Exercise Capacity

The ability to deliver O_2 to the tissues **(maximal O_2 consumption, or V_{O_2MAX})** is generally accepted as the standard measurement of physical work capacity (fitness) in man. The V_{O_2MAX} measures the integrated performance of the 3 components of the delivery system that transports O_2 from the outside air to the working muscles: pulmonary ventilation, blood circulation, and muscle tissue. At any age, the V_{O_2MAX} is related to the physical dimensions of these components: pulmonary (vital capacity, diffusing capacity), cardiovascular (heart volume, blood volume, RBC mass), and skeletal muscle mass. Since body size is such an important component of V_{O2MAX}, this measure of fitness often takes weight into consideration (and is expressed as maximal O_2 uptake per kilogram of body weight, or V_{O2MAX}/kg). Lean body mass is a more reliable predictor of cardiorespiratory performance than is weight (especially in obese subjects). Lean body mass may be obtained from body weight by correcting for body fat, which can be estimated from skinfold measurements or underwater weighing.

Work capacity (as measured by V_{O2MAX}) increases during childhood, reaches a peak in the late teens, plateaus until the mid-20s, and then gradually declines. The early increase is due to the growth of muscle, heart, and lungs, and the later decline is due in part to the gradual reductions in maximal heart rate and muscle mass observed with advancing years. The gradual decline of O_2 delivery (32 mL/min/yr in men, and 14 mL/min/yr in women) can be described by a prediction equation. However, only body size and age are considered in the prediction regression (see TABLES 38–1 and 38–2).

The age term in the V_{O2MAX} prediction represents the age-related decreases in CO and muscle mass, as noted above. Age-related changes in CO may result from specific alterations in cardiac biochemistry and metabolism, such as maximal myocardial O_2 consumption and substrate oxidation rates, which seem to decline with age. Although pulmonary function measurements (eg, FEV_1) decline with age, reduced ventilation seldom limits exercise in healthy subjects. However, in patients with a ventilatory capacity reduced sufficiently to limit exercise performance, the FEV_1 is a reasonably accurate indicator of maximal ventilation in exercise. More typically, the reduced V_{O2MAX} seen in elderly individuals with mild to moderate AO is due to cardiovascular deconditioning associated with lowered levels of habitual physical activity.

The differences in exercise performance between similarly aged men and women largely disappear when other factors, such as size (lean body mass), Hb level, and levels of structured activity (training), are taken into account. Similarly, there are few race-related differences in exercise performance if allowance is made for these factors. The level of habitual physical activity influences O_2 delivery ability by imposing a degree of regular fitness training. Similarly fit individuals have been compared by assessing their daily physical activity through a simple questionnaire that allows the observer to categorize them into 4 groups: sedentary; sedentary with some daily activity; active, through occupation or recreation activity; and trained athlete.

Regular training can substantially slow the decline in maximal O_2 delivery due to age-related cardiovascular deconditioning. After sedentary subjects underwent a period of exercise training, a study by Yerg and colleagues (*Journal of Applied Physiology*, 1985) concluded that "the increase in V_E/V_{O2} (ventilatory response for a given O_2 uptake) during submaximal exercise observed with aging can be reversed by endurance training, and that after training, previously sedentary older individuals breathe at the same percentage of MVV (maximal voluntary ventilation) during maximal exercise as highly trained (master) athletes of similar age."

Finally, total muscle mass gradually declines with increasing age, mediated by a reduction in the total number of muscle fibers. That old age is accompanied by a decrease in muscle strength consistent with this loss of muscle fibers will come as no surprise. However, since the metabolic capacity, enzymatic profile, and capillary density of the muscle fibers in elderly subjects appear to be the same as those in younger persons, it is clear that the age-related decrease in aerobic exercise capacity is quantitatively linked to attrition of lean muscle mass rather than to functional impairment of the muscles. This decline, too, may be slowed by exercise training.

Defense Mechanisms

Clearance mechanisms: There seems to be an inverse relationship between age and the rate of **mucociliary transport.** While mucociliary transport is capable of removing inhaled particulate matter from the ciliated airways, the importance of mucus transport as a pulmonary defense mechanism has not yet been clearly demonstrated. Nevertheless, clinical observation of patients with Kartagener's syndrome (situs inversus, chronic sinusitis, and bronchiectasis), who also had immotile spermatozoa, suggests that primary ciliary immotility, perhaps the result of deficient microtubular bridges within the ciliary substructure, is responsible for the development of recurrent respiratory tract infections and, eventually, chronic bronchitis and bronchiectasis in these patients. If these observations are correct, the diminished mucociliary clearance seen with increasing age may have clinical significance.

Loss of an effective cough reflex (and subsequent aspiration) also contributes to an increased susceptibility to pneumonia in the elderly. While cough is not essential for normal clearance of the respiratory tract, it is a powerful adjunct when normal mucociliary clearance is overloaded by foreign materials or secretions. An intact cough reflex is a necessary defense, for example, under conditions of dysphagia and impaired esophageal motility, which are more frequently encountered in old age. The elderly are also subject to a variety of conditions associated with reduced consciousness, including sedative use and neurologic diseases, which result in the loss of an effective cough reflex.

Humoral immunity: (See also Ch. 75.) Blood immunoglobulin levels are only a rough guide to humoral immune competence. Despite the lack of age-related changes in IgA and IgG concentrations, the acute antibody response to extrinsic antigens, such as pneumococcal and influenza vaccines, is considerably reduced in old age. It is possible that the maintenance of circulating immunoglobulin levels reflects increased production of antibody to various intrinsic antigens (ie, autoantibodies), which replaces production of antibodies to extrinsic antigens. Interestingly, serum values of IgM decrease with age, although the significance of this observation remains uncertain.

The ability to generate an effective humoral response depends on the interaction among helper T cells, suppressor T cells, macrophages, and B lymphocytes. Age-related reductions in T-cell helper activity, increases in T-cell suppressor activity, and the reduced ability of B cells to produce normal heterogeneous high-affinity antibodies in response to an antigen have all been observed. In contrast, the mucosa-associated IgA secretory antibody production shows no age-related decline in functional capabilities.

Cellular immunity most clearly exhibits an age-related decrease in functional ability. One manifestation of cell-mediated immunity, delayed hypersensitivity, is demonstrated clinically by the number of positive skin reactions to 5 common antigens. The number of positive skin tests declines in those > 60 yr of age; in 1 study, this skin test hyporesponsiveness correlated with increased mortality over 2 yr. A functional depression in lymphocytes from elderly (75- to 96-yr-old) compared with young (25- to 50-yr-old) adults has been demonstrated experimentally by a reduced blastogenic response to plant mitogens (phytohemagglutinin and pokeweed mitogen).

The decline of cell-mediated immunity with increasing age correlates with an increasing frequency of reactivation tuberculosis. However, while reduction in the levels of thymic hormones is clearly age related, the association of thymic involution to increased susceptibility to infection in the elderly remains speculative.

---

39. PNEUMONIA AND TUBERCULOSIS

John G. Bartlett

PNEUMONIA

An inflammatory reaction to microbes or microbial products involving the pulmonary parenchyma.

Infections of the lower respiratory tract, which are the most common lethal infections, are the 5th leading cause of death by disease in the USA. Pneumonias are a frequent and severe problem in the elderly. Sir William Osler referred to the disease as "a special enemy of old age" in the 1st edition of his famous textbook, but he subsequently referred to it as "the friend of the aged" in the 3rd edition. It is perhaps befitting that he eventually had a lingering death due to pneumonia, during which his major regret was that he "would not be able to witness the autopsy."

A review of 44,684 cases of pneumonia that occurred in Massachusetts between 1921 and 1930 showed an incidence of pneumonia approximately fivefold for patients in their 80s compared with those in their

20s. Far more striking was the nearly 100-fold increase in the mortality rate for those in their 8th decade, a rate that increased about 10% for each decade after age 20.

Despite availability of antimicrobial agents, pneumonia is found in 25 to 60% of elderly patients at autopsy; it is still the most common cause of death in centenarians. Hospital-acquired pneumonia, the most frequent lethal nosocomial infection in acute-care facilities, is also a major problem in chronic-care facilities, where its prevalence may be as high as 50 times the rate in age-matched, home-based patients.

Etiology

Valid information concerning the distribution of specific pathogens is limited because the usual specimen source, expectorated sputum, is contaminated during passage through the upper airways. In most studies, no likely pathogen is detected in 30 to 50% of cases; many of the organisms implicated in the remaining cases are a matter of arbitrary judgment. Studies based on more reliable diagnostic specimen sources, such as transtracheal aspirate cultures, blood culture, and specific serologic tests, indicate that the following microorganisms account for most cases of pneumonia in the elderly: *Streptococcus pneumoniae,* anaerobic bacteria, gram-negative bacilli, *Legionella pneumophila,* and the influenza virus. Other less common but well-established pulmonary pathogens in both the young and the aged are *Staphylococcus aureus* and *Hemophilus influenzae.*

The pneumococcus is the most frequent bacterial cause of community-acquired pneumonia in the elderly as well as in younger persons. Studies based on expectorated sputum bacteriology in community-acquired pneumonia indicate that the recovery rate of *H. influenzae* is second only to that of *S. pneumoniae;* however, interpretation is difficult because it is possible that either organism is simply an oropharyngeal contaminant. **Gram-negative bacilli** are relatively infrequent pathogens in patients with community-acquired infection; they are far more frequent in hospitalized patients and in residents of chronic-care facilities.

In institutional settings, *Klebsiella, Pseudomonas aeruginosa, Enterobacter* spp, *Proteus* spp, *Escherichia coli,* and other gram-negative bacilli appear to account for 40 to 60% of all pneumonias. This differing pattern in the distribution of pathogens for community- vs. institutional-acquired pneumonia may reflect the increased rate of colonization of the oral pharynx by gram-negative bacilli in nursing home residents and in hospitalized patients, who are apparently susceptible because of serious associated diseases or reduced capacity for self-care.

Anaerobic bacteria appear to play an important role in both community-acquired and nosocomial pneumonia in the elderly when the appropriate microbiologic studies are done. Expectorated sputum specimens are not valid for meaningful anaerobic culture because of contamination by the normal flora of the upper airways. Transtracheal aspirates obtained prior to antibiotic therapy in the elderly show a high yield of anaerobes, presumably reflecting the propensity of these patients to aspirate because of associated conditions, such as neurologic disorders, and other illnesses involving altered consciousness, and the use of sedatives.

Legionella became the subject of national interest during the 1976 epidemic in Philadelphia, and it was clear that older individuals were uniquely susceptible. A review of 182 cases in the Philadelphia outbreak indicated that 75% of patients infected with *Legionella pneumophila* were > 40 yr of age; the risk of infection among those > 60 yr of age was about twice that for younger persons. Numerous subsequent studies continue to show a direct correlation between the attack rate and patient age.

There are now at least 23 recognized species of *Legionella,* but *L. pneumophila* accounts for approximately 85% of pneumonia cases; *L. micdadei* accounts for most of the remaining 15%. Although the pulmonary infection referred to as **legionnaires' disease** and ascribed to *L. pneumophila* usually occurs sporadically, epidemics often occur and usually are associated with hotels or hospitals. This organism, like anaerobic bacteria, frequently will be missed unless special diagnostic tests are performed—in this case, respiratory secretions for direct fluorescent antibody stain and culture using special media.

Viruses that can cause pneumonia in elderly patients include influenza and parainfluenza viruses, respiratory syncytial virus **(RSV)** and possibly adenovirus. While parainfluenza viruses and RSV represent important pulmonary pathogens in children, they are infrequently encountered in healthy adults; their relative frequency among the elderly presumably reflects waning immunity.

But the most important viral agent of pulmonary infections in adults —and especially in the elderly—is **influenza.** Attack rates are age-related, with the incidence in persons > 70 yr of age about 4 times that in individuals who are < 40 yr old. The increased morbidity and mortality rates associated with influenza in the elderly are far more impressive. In most years, persons > 65 yr old account for about 90% of influenza-associated deaths in the USA. Epidemics—sometimes associated with high mortality rates—are major problems in chronic-care facilities, which is why annual influenza vaccination is recommended for staff and residents.

Influenza A virus is the most frequent cause of severe and even fatal illness, in part because of its propensity for antigenic shift; however, **influenza B,** which is usually a relatively benign pathogen in younger persons, also may be associated with serious infection and high mortality rates in the elderly.

Pathogenesis

The 2 most common routes for potential pathogens to reach the lower airways are by **inhalation** and **aspiration.** Aerosolized organisms inhaled as microparticles into the lower airways include *Mycobacterium tubercu-*

losis, Legionella spp, and the influenza virus. *M. tuberculosis* and the influenza virus are transmitted by infected individuals via aerosolized secretions produced by coughing. *Legionella* organisms are not passed from person to person but are usually aerosolized from a waterborne source, eg, air conditioners or shower heads. Other waterborne organisms may be delivered to the lower airways by small-particle aerosols from reservoir nebulizers used with ventilation equipment, or they may be introduced into the lower airways via instrumentation. The usual pathogens transferred in this fashion are bacteria that survive well in water, including *P. aeruginosa,* other pseudomonads, *Serratia marcescens, Achromobacter, Flavobacterium,* and *Acinetobacter* spp.

Usually, pneumonia pathogens in the elderly are aspirated, but the organisms vary in different circumstances. Large-volume aspiration results in a relatively large inoculum of oropharyngeal bacteria in the lower airways and is associated with conditions that compromise consciousness or cause dysphagia. The usual pathogens in community-acquired aspiration pneumonia are anaerobic bacteria that normally reside in the gingival crevice, eg, peptostreptococci, fusobacteria, and *Bacteroides melaninogenicus.* For aspiration pneumonia acquired in acute- or chronic-care facilities, the usual pathogens are gram-negative bacilli in association with anaerobes. Most cases of pneumococcal pneumonia and gram-negative bacillary pneumonia presumably follow microaspiration, which is an occult event resulting in a fairly small inoculum of more virulent bacteria residing in the posterior pharynx. Some cases of pneumococcal pneumonia probably are also acquired by inhalation, especially those that occur in the occasional epidemic.

The tendency of elderly patients to develop gram-negative bacillary pneumonia appears to reflect the propensity of these organisms to colonize the posterior pharynx of debilitated, seriously ill patients. Throat cultures from various populations have shown that the colonization rate with these organisms correlates directly with the severity of associated disease and the degree of functional impairment. An important message from these studies is that the high incidence of gram-negative bacillary pneumonia in institutionalized patients does not appear to reflect the clustering of patients but simply that severely ill or impaired persons are more likely to be found in institutions. Nevertheless, the epidemiology of organisms within a particular institution dictate bacteriologic patterns of colonization and the antibiotic sensitivity of these organisms.

Numerous factors may contribute to the increased incidence of pneumonia in elderly patients and to the high resultant mortality. **Changes in pulmonary function** that occur with aging may result in a decrease in effective cough, increased residual volume, increased compliance, increased closing volume, decreased diffusing capacity, and reduced O_2 saturation. There is little evidence that these changes in pulmonary physiology constitute a substantial risk for pneumonia, but they markedly increase susceptibility to morbid complications. A similar conclusion applies to chronic obstructive airways disease and to chronic bronchitis, both of which are exceptionally common in older individuals. Other conditions that appear to be associated with increased risk for pneumonia as well as increased morbidity in the elderly patient include severe hypoxia, pulmonary edema, acidosis, alcohol intoxication, and azotemia.

With regard to **host defenses,** invasion by microorganisms involves a complex interplay of the mucociliary elevator, the alveolar macrophages, polymorphonuclear leukocytes, humoral defenses, and cell-mediated immune function. Studies in healthy, aged volunteers indicate that the functional capacity for most of these defense mechanisms remains intact or is only mildly reduced. The most clearly defined and pronounced defect that appears to represent a consequence of aging concerns T-cell function—ie, cell-mediated immunity. This defect is readily demonstrated by the increased rate of anergy noted using common skin test antigens, and it apparently accounts for the increased incidence of TB. Nevertheless, other opportunistic pathogens reflecting defective cell-mediated immunity are relatively uncommon unless there are superimposed modifiers, such as administration of corticosteroids, lymphoma, or cancer chemotherapy.

Humoral defenses measured by serum antibody response to vaccination with tetanus or pneumococcal vaccine show a somewhat blunted response that is nevertheless generally adequate to provide "protective" levels. The response to influenza vaccine is clearly suboptimal in terms of both antibody titers and clinical protection conferred. Another factor in humoral response concerns the duration of protection afforded by antigens confronted during childhood. This loss presumably accounts for the enhanced susceptibility of the elderly to parainfluenza viruses, RSV, and possibly the influenza viruses.

Symptoms and Signs

The classic clinical features of pneumonia are cough, fever, and sputum production. While these are expected in elderly patients with pneumonia, they tend to be deceptively subtle even in cases with an ominous prognosis. The fever pattern may be particularly misleading. Elderly patients have a lower basal temperature and a reduced ability to mount a significant fever in the face of infection. To stress this point, Dr. Louis Weinstein often states, "The older, the colder." The cough associated with pneumonia in older persons may frequently be mistaken as a reflection of chronic lung disease or a URI with bronchitis. The expected findings on physical examination are rales and/or signs of consolidation over the involved area.

The major clinical clues to the etiology of the infection are the tempo of the disease process, changes on chest x-ray, and the epidemiologic setting. Although the onset of pneumococcal pneumonia in the elderly is rarely marked by the typical shaking chill, it is an acute pulmonary infection. Few clinical features distinguish this form of pneumonia from that due to gram-negative bacilli other than the institutional association noted above and the high mortality rate.

Legionnaires' disease also tends to be an acute pulmonary infection, but the initial feature is often fever *without* prominent pulmonary symptomatology. When pulmonary infection occurs during an influenza epidemic, in any setting, the influenza virus should be regarded as the cause, whatever the vaccine status of the host. The major problem is that it may be virtually impossible to distinguish primary influenza pneumonia and influenza associated with a superimposed bacterial infection. One clue favoring the latter is an acute febrile illness followed by clinical improvement and subsequent deterioration with a new infiltrate on chest x-ray.

Chronic pneumonia is more likely to involve a different array of pathogens, primarily *M. tuberculosis*, fungi, or anaerobic bacteria. These infections are associated with fever and symptoms of chronic disease such as weight loss and anemia.

Anaerobic pulmonary infections tend to involve segments of the lung that are dependent when the patient is in the recumbent position, primarily the superior segments of the lower lobes or the posterior segments of the upper lobes. The long-term sequelae of these infections are suppurative complications such as lung abscess and empyema. In most cases, the patient is noted to have putrid sputum or breath, which is considered diagnostic of anaerobic infection.

Another recognized form of what is probably anaerobic pneumonitis is a condition previously referred to as **"hypostatic pneumonia"** or **"nursing home pneumonia,"** which is associated with subtle clinical findings and evidence of pulmonary infiltrates in the lower lobes on chest x-ray. This condition has never been studied bacteriologically with sufficient precision to identify specific microbial probabilities, but the anticipated pathogens are anaerobic bacteria, *S. pneumoniae, H. influenzae,* and gram-negative bacilli.

Laboratory Findings

The most useful laboratory tests in evaluating suspected pneumonia are the CBC, the chest x-ray, and microbiologic studies of respiratory secretions.

Although **the CBC** is helpful in determining the leukocyte count, this is seldom useful unless it is very high ($> 25,000/\mu L$), suggesting overwhelming pneumonia, or very low ($< 3,000/\mu L$), suggesting a viral infection or overwhelming bacterial pneumonia. The hemoglobin is also useful in determining the probability of an associated chronic disease, which may represent a component of the present infection, such as TB, anaerobic pulmonary infection, or another associated underlying condition.

The diagnosis of pneumonia requires demonstration of **an infiltrate on chest x-ray.** Rarely, the chest x-ray will be normal early in the course of the disease, but an infiltrate is almost invariably present 24 h following the onset of symptoms. Cough, fever, and sputum production with a normal chest x-ray are usually ascribed to bronchitis or a noninfectious problem. Thus the chest x-ray becomes pivotal in management decisions, since pneumonia is virtually always treatable with specific antimicrobial agents, whereas data are conflicting regarding the efficacy of antibiotics in the treatment of bronchitis. Chest x-rays showing cavity formation raise the probability of specific causes, primarily TB and anaerobic bacterial infection.

A major goal in patient management is to identify the etiologic agent to guide the selection of antimicrobial agents. **Expectorated sputum specimens** are unreliable when cultured; even when a potential pathogen is recovered, there is no assurance that it is responsible for the pulmonary infection. Exceptions to this are *M. tuberculosis* and *Legionella* spp, all of which require special technics for detection but virtually always represent causative agents when identified. A potential benefit of an expectorated sputum culture is that in patients with infections involving gram-negative bacilli and *S. aureus,* these organisms will usually be detected; the major limitations of these specimens are false-negative cultures for *S. pneumoniae* and *H. influenzae,* and false-positive cultures for gram-negative bacilli and *S. aureus.* **Gram stain of expectorated specimens** may actually provide more useful information than culture, as well as doing so at the time that therapeutic decisions are required.

Alternative, more reliable technics for recovering conventional bacteria and anaerobes include transtracheal aspiration, transthoracic aspiration, and fiberoptic bronchoscopy with the protected brush, but these procedures are rarely used for routine diagnostic evaluation. Blood cultures should be done on febrile patients, and thoracentesis should be done in patients with pleural effusions on chest x-ray to detect empyema.

Specific recommendations for microbiologic studies are as follows:

Conventional bacteria: One expectorated sputum specimen should be obtained for Gram stain and culture prior to antibiotic treatment.

Legionella spp: Two expectorated sputum samples (or other pulmonary specimens) should be obtained for direct fluorescent antibody stain and culture on special media, preferably before erythromycin therapy or after no more than 3 days of such therapy.

Anaerobic bacteria: An uncontaminated specimen should be obtained before antibiotic therapy, via transtracheal aspiration, transthoracic needle aspiration, thoracentesis, or fiberoptic bronchoscopy using the protected brush; Gram stain of expectorated sputum specimen is of limited value, and culture of these in anaerobic conditions is not recommended.

M. tuberculosis: Three expectorated sputum samples are needed for acid-fast bacillus **(AFB)** stain and culture on special media.

Influenza virus: Viral cultures may be obtained on throat washings, and serologic tests using paired serum specimens collected 3 wk apart; in most cases, this is a presumed diagnosis based on typical symptoms that occur during an epidemic in which the epidemic strain is identified in a limited number of concurrently ill individuals.

Diagnosis

The symptoms and signs of the infection, combined with the demonstration of a pulmonary infiltrate on chest x-ray, are diagnostic of pneumonia. The greatest diagnostic problem is not the presence or absence of pneumonia but the enigma of sorting out the etiologic agent. Other conditions that may present similar or identical findings include atelectasis, heart failure, and pulmonary embolism, with or without infarction.

Prevention

Preventive measures include the use of vaccines, judicious use of antibiotics, and intervention during epidemics. Unfortunately, the protection afforded the elderly by influenza vaccine is sharply reduced. Pneumococcal vaccine is even more controversial. Studies of serologic response indicate that elderly patients develop protective titers of antibody following immunization with the commercially available 23-valent vaccine; nevertheless, clinical studies in patients > 45 yr of age and residents of chronic-care facilities indicate minimal reduction in the overall incidence of pneumonia—including pneumococcal pneumonia, and even pneumonia involving the serotypes included in the vaccine. Persons who have received either the 14- or 23-valent pneumococcal vaccine should not be revaccinated.

Patients who are prone to aspiration may benefit from the head-down position, and those who repeatedly aspirate food may benefit from a feeding gastrostomy. Patients who are unconscious and consequently susceptible to aspiration pneumonia do *not* appear to benefit from prophylactic antibiotics. Their use simply seems to predispose such patients to infection involving resistant strains and should be restricted to those who have clinical evidence of pneumonia.

Epidemics in institutions such as hospitals or nursing homes are most often caused by the influenza virus. Unlike bacterial infections, influenza epidemics tend to involve all exposed persons rather than just the debilitated host; acquisition is from an exogenous rather than an endogenous source; and the organisms responsible are usually implicated in concurrent outbreaks in the community. Preventive measures include restriction of visitors and elective admissions, restriction of afflicted health care workers, and respiratory precautions in patients with documented infection. Such outbreaks may be reduced or prevented by immunization with influenza vaccine and the use of amantadine in exposed patients. When amantadine is used prophylactically, the usual dose is 100 mg/day. This may be complicated by changes in mental status.

Eradication of *Legionella* spp, when responsible for outbreaks of pneumonia, requires detection of the waterborne source. An epidemic source of these organisms is found in about $1/2$ of the epidemics, with the primary sources being cooling towers of air-conditioning systems and the potable water leading to contaminated shower heads; once identified, *Legionella* spp must be eradicated using either excessive heat treatment or high concentrations of chlorine. In epidemics of pneumonia involving the previously noted waterborne gram-negative bacilli, the source of the organisms should be sought and is usually found to be contaminated respiratory therapy equipment or instruments such as bronchoscopes.

Treatment

The principal therapeutic modalities are antimicrobial agents, respiratory support and other forms of supportive care, and drainage of empyemas and large pleural collections. A most difficult and important decision concerns the selection of antimicrobial agents, which is simplified if the etiologic agent is identified. Specific recommendations by etiologic agents are as follows:

Streptococcus pneumoniae: Penicillin, cephalothin, or erythromycin.

Hemophilus influenzae: Ampicillin, cefamandole (or cefuroxime), or a 3rd-generation cephalosporin.

Gram-negative bacilli: Sensitivity tests are required, but the usual recommendation is a 3rd-generation cephalosporin, imipenem, or aztreonam; an aminoglycoside is often added.

Pseudomonas aeruginosa: Sensitivity tests are required, but the usual recommendation is an antipseudomonad penicillin plus an aminoglycoside (tobramycin or amikacin).

Anaerobic bacteria: Penicillin or clindamycin.

Legionella spp: Erythromycin.

Staphylococcus aureus: An antistaphylococcal penicillin (nafcillin or oxacillin), cephalothin, cefamandole, or vancomycin.

Influenza A: Amantadine and/or an antibiotic for suspected superinfecting bacteria. (See Ch. 77 for routes of administration and dosages.)

When no likely etiologic agent is identified (**"enigmatic pneumonia"**), the recommendation is a regime that includes erythromycin. This agent alone is usually satisfactory therapy in patients who are not seriously ill with community-acquired pulmonary infections. In patients who are seriously ill, however—especially in those with institution-acquired infection—there is a need to extend the antimicrobial spectrum by using a regimen such as erythromycin combined with a 3rd-generation cephalosporin, with or without the addition of an aminoglycoside.

These recommendations are similar to those for younger patients with pneumonia, *although the elderly require more careful therapeutic monitoring.* Agents with nephrotoxic potential, primarily aminoglycosides, must be used with particular caution, including monitoring of serum levels and frequent measurements of renal function. Intravenous administration of fluids and electrolytes as well as other forms of osmotic loading must be done with care because of the reduced cardiac reserve in older individuals. Hypersensitivity reactions are not more frequent in elderly patients, although an age-related risk of antibiotic-associated diarrhea or colitis is common with ampicillin or clindamycin. Drug interactions may also occur between antibiotics and other therapeutic agents commonly used in the elderly, eg, warfarin sodium.

TUBERCULOSIS

An infectious disease caused by Mycobacterium tuberculosis.

Remarkable progress has been made in the control of TB in the USA and other industrialized countries. At the turn of the century, the mortality rate in patients with this disease was approximately 200:100,000 population, which has steadily declined to approximately 1.5:100,000 in the 1980s. The incidence of active TB has diminished in all age groups, although the elderly have not benefited to the extent that younger individuals have. Women are affected more frequently than men, with a ratio of 2:1. Persons over age 65 now account for 25 to 30% of newly diagnosed cases of TB. The reasons are threefold: (1) Many of these older individuals acquired their infection when the prevalence of TB was substantially higher. (2) The loss of cell-mediated immunity that accompanies aging favors reactivation of dormant foci. (3) The disease has an epidemic or endemic spread in chronic-care facilities; prolonged contact with a large number of susceptible hosts in a closed setting favors person-to-person spread.

Pathophysiology

M. tuberculosis is acquired by inhalation of droplet nuclei containing microorganisms aerosolized from persons who are untreated. The untreated patient poses a threat, since the risk of transmission is remarkably lower once treatment has begun, even during the interval when sputum cultures continue to yield the microbe. Also, the duration of contact is important. The infecting inoculum has been termed a quantum, and, under ordinary circumstances, sustained exposure for at least 2 mo is required to achieve the inoculum necessary for transmission. The inhaled organisms are deposited in the alveoli, most commonly in the lower lobes, which are the best-ventilated portions of the lung. There the organisms replicate slowly, only about once every 24 h. They gain access to lymphatic channels to involve the regional lymph nodes in the chest and then pass through the thoracic duct to the bloodstream, where widespread hematogenous dissemination may occur.

The patient may develop a bronchopneumonia, usually involving the lower lobes and often with regional lymph node involvement, or a unilateral pleural effusion may be present with the initial infection, which is known as **primary TB.** More frequently, the patient remains asymptomatic and the prior infection is detected only with a positive skin test, sometimes associated with x-ray changes that usually consist of a nodule or a nodule accompanied by hilar adenopathy (**Ghon complex**). The nodule is often calcified, which assists in its distinction from carcinoma.

Patients with positive skin tests generally harbor viable organisms within macrophages, and they can retain this balanced host-parasite relationship for decades. Most cases of TB reflect reactivation of organisms in this dormant stage and are referred to as **reactivation TB.**

Reactivation usually occurs when immune defenses are compromised, primarily cell-mediated immunity, which appears to be most important in the balanced host-parasite relationship. Numerous studies have shown that thymic atrophy is a normal consequence of aging. By the 5th decade, minimal thymic tissue is present, although lymphocytes and monocytes capable of antigenic recall continue to circulate for 2 to 3 decades. This accounts for the relatively high rate of anergy with standard skin tests for cell-mediated immunity seen in the elderly. Despite this loss, most elderly patients are not susceptible to the usual pathogens seen in other conditions characterized by anergy, such as immunosuppression from corticosteroid therapy, cancer chemotherapy, lymphomas, or AIDS. TB appears to be the exception.

Reactivation TB tends to occur at sites with relatively high O_2 concentrations, presumably reflecting that the organism is an obligate aerobe. In the lung, the favored anatomic site is the upper lobe, where ventilation-perfusion ratios provide high O_2 concentrations. However, elderly people (especially those in nursing homes) often vary from the expected, exhibiting TB as a pneumonitis in the lower and middle portions of the lungs.

Symptoms and Signs

Because TB in the elderly is often subtle, many of the clinical complaints, including weight loss, cough, weakness, and dyspnea, may be ascribed to associated conditions or even to aging itself. Fever is usually present but is generally low grade and may not be appreciated by the patient unless measured. Night sweats and hemoptysis, which specifically suggest TB, are often not present or not pursued.

Diagnosis

The major diagnostic studies are the skin test, chest x-rays, and sputum cultures. The preferred skin test is performed by intradermally injecting 0.1 mL purified protein derivative **(PPD)** containing 5 tuberculin units **(TU)** in the volar or dorsal surface of the forearm. The test should be read on the 2nd or 3rd day. The size of the reaction correlates with the probability of TB; induration $\geq$ 10 mm is officially classified as significant. A smaller reaction (5 to 10 mm of induration) is recognized as suspect in selected high-risk populations. BCG given in childhood does not account for a positive PPD skin test several decades later.

In elderly patients, a negative test should be followed by a repeat test in 1 wk to achieve the **booster phenomenon** in detecting reactivity that has waned with time. Most patients with active TB have positive tests, although some are anergic to all skin test reagents; a small portion with active disease are selectively anergic only to tuberculin. There is *no role* for the second-strength (250 TU) PPD tuberculin test, and patients with a history of a positive test should not be retested. **The interpretation of a positive test** is that the person harbors viable organisms, although the test will not distinguish those with dormant bacilli from those with active disease. This distinction is made by chest x-rays and cultures.

All patients with a newly detected positive PPD test should have a chest x-ray and clinical evaluation. When a patient's chest x-ray findings are compatible with TB, they should be compared with prior x-rays. TB is considered active if progressive changes on chest x-ray films are ascribed to current infection, if symptoms are ascribed to current infection, or if a culture yields *M. tuberculosis.* All patients suspected of having TB should have 3 morning sputum stains for AFB, as well as 3 morning sputum cultures for mycobacteria. Sputum stains for AFB will detect approximately 50% of patients who subsequently have positive cultures in the absence of cavitary disease; most patients with cavitary disease have a large mycobacterial load and will have positive AFB smears. Patients who cannot produce expectorated sputum should have sputum induced, and if this is not successful, they should undergo bronchoscopy.

Because TB may present atypically on chest x-ray, some authorities recommend that any elderly person requiring hospitalization for pneumonitis should have at least 1 sputum culture for TB. Chronic-care facilities should have standard procedures for routine skin tests and chest x-rays for all new employees and new residents; usually, these should be continued on an annual basis.

Treatment

One type of treatment consists of **preventive therapy** with isoniazid **(INH),** 300 mg daily for 6 to 12 mo in high-risk persons who do not have active disease. This therapy is recommended in household members and other close contacts of potentially infectious persons; in newly infected persons (a tuberculin skin test conversion within the past 2 yr); in persons with positive skin tests and abnormal chest x-rays compatible with previous TB; and in persons with positive skin tests in selected clinical situations, such as those with silicosis, diabetes mellitus, immunosuppression (including that resulting from corticosteroid administration and cancer chemotherapy), positive human immunodeficiency virus **(HIV)** serology, hematologic and reticuloendothelial malignancies, endstage renal disease, and associated conditions characterized by rapid weight loss or chronic malnutrition.

The other type of treatment involves **patients with active TB,** who require at least 2 antituberculous drugs, and 2 regimens are commonly advocated: (1) INH 300 mg daily and rifampin **(RMP)** 600 mg daily for 9 mo or (2) INH, RMP, and pyrazinamide **(PZA)** 2 gm daily for 2 mo followed by INH and RMP for 4 mo.

These recommendations must be modified in patients with resistant strains according to in vitro sensitivity tests. **Resistance is suspect** in patients who have undergone prior courses of treatment, in those with recently acquired disease, in immigrants from areas with a high prevalence of resistant strains, and in persons who acquire the infection from contact with these sources. Since most elderly patients acquired their original strains many decades before, when the rate of resistance was nil, the treatment regimens mentioned above are appropriate.

Monitoring during treatment should include baseline measurements of liver enzymes, bilirubin, and serum creatinine; a CBC; and a platelet count or estimate. Serum uric acid should be measured when PZA is used. *Patients should be monitored clinically for adverse reactions, with specific attention to symptoms suggesting hepatitis, eg, jaundice, fever, anorexia, and dark urine.* This is especially important in elderly patients receiving INH, since the frequency of this side effect shows an age-related correlation. Patients should be seen or contacted at least monthly during treatment and specifically questioned concerning these symptoms.

Routine laboratory testing is not recommended in the absence of symptoms, although some physicians assess liver function tests monthly, especially during the first 6 mo of treatment, when hepatitis is most likely to occur. A threefold or greater increase over normal values in transaminase levels is a contraindication to further administration of INH. For patients with active disease, sputum should be examined at least monthly until the sputum tests convert to negative, which in at least 90% of patients should occur within 3 mo of initiating the recommended regimens. The most common reason for treatment failure is lack of compliance; in such cases, the drugs should be given under observation.

---

40. CHRONIC OBSTRUCTIVE PULMONARY DISEASE (COPD)

Peter B. Terry

A group of diseases, including chronic bronchitis, emphysema, bronchiectasis, asthma, and small airways disease, characterized by chronic airflow obstruction with reversible and/or irreversible components. Airflow obstruction is a reduction in the ratio of forced expiratory volume in the 1st sec to forced vital capacity (**FEV$_1$/FVC**). Although each type of chronic obstructive pulmonary disease (**COPD**) is a distinct clinical entity, it is common to find $\geq$ 2 types in the same patient. In clinical practice, COPD usually refers to various combinations of chronic bronchitis, emphysema, and small airways disease, whereas asthma and bronchiectasis are normally considered separate entities.

A description of each disease follows: **Chronic bronchitis** is characterized by its clinical presentation—a chronic, productive cough occurring most days of the month for 3 mo of the year for 2 consecutive years. Histologically, mucous-gland hyperplasia is seen in the airways. **Emphysema** is characterized by its morphologic abnormalities, which include enlarged alveolar spaces and destructive changes in the alveolar walls, reducing the surface area for exchange of gases. **Asthma** is characterized by an increased responsiveness of the bronchi and bronchioles to various stimuli, manifested by a widespread narrowing of the airways, changing in severity either spontaneously or as a result of therapy. **Bronchiectasis,** a permanent dilatation of ≥ 1 bronchi, is clinically characterized by production of copious sputum, which separates into distinct layers. **Small airways disease** is characterized by physiologic test abnormalities compatible with dysfunction of airways $\cong 2$ mm in diameter.

Prevalence

Of the 10 leading causes of death in the USA, COPD ranks first in rate of increase during the past 15 yr. Approximately 3% of the population of the USA has chronic bronchitis, whereas approximately 1% has emphysema. However, only 5% of patients with chronic bronchitis and approximately 40% with emphysema have clinically significant airways obstruction. COPD ranks second only to coronary arterty disease as a cause of Social Security–compensated disability.

Etiology

COPD results from a combination of a genetic predisposition and contributory environmental exposures. Advancing age is also a risk factor; the relative risk of chronic bronchitis, for instance, ranges from 1.2 to 2.3 in older persons compared with that of younger individuals. Other risk factors for COPD are male sex, lower socioeconomic status, and childhood respiratory illnesses. Cigarette smoking is the most common environmental risk factor and is believed to contribute to COPD in $> 80\%$ of cases. Smoking contributes to airways obstruction **(AO)** by (1) causing an inflammatory reaction, with or without production of mucus in the airways; (2) promoting the influx of polymorphonuclear leukocytes, which release inflammatory mediators and elastases that break down lung elastin, leading to emphysema; and (3) inhibiting the body's endogenous elastases. Pollution, occupational contacts, and other environmental exposures contribute to a lesser degree to the development of AO.

The prototypic example of genetic predisposition to the development of COPD is the rare condition called α_1-**antitrypsin deficiency,** which results in inadequate levels of endogenous antiprotease to counteract the proteolytic enzymes released by inflammation in the lung. Other, as yet undefined, genetically controlled defects may also be present, since COPD frequently occurs in the absence of α_1-antitrypsin deficiency in many families.

Pathophysiology

Cigarette smoke leads to inflammatory changes in the lungs, which present clinically as chronic bronchitis and emphysema. Patients with **chronic bronchitis** invariably have an increased ratio of mucous glands to bronchial wall thickness (the Reid index). This is primarily due to an increase in the number of glands (hyperplasia), rather than an increase in size of existing glands (hypertrophy). Patients with asthma or emphysema also have an increased number of mucous glands. Production of mucus correlates roughly with the Reid index, but there is no strong relationship between the degree of glandular hyperplasia and the degree of AO. This suggests that other factors, perhaps smooth muscle hyperplasia, may be more important in the development of obstruction.

The most common forms of **emphysema** are centrilobular and panacinar. Centrilobular emphysema is proximal acinar emphysema involving the respiratory bronchioles; it is most commonly found in the upper zones of the lung. Panacinar emphysema involves the entire acinus and is more evenly distributed throughout the lungs. Patients with severe emphysema may have large bullous lesions scattered throughout the lungs.

The pathologic transition from normal lung to emphysema is gradual, but may begin with smoking-induced respiratory bronchiolitis. Other changes that may occur in the transitional phase include an increase in peribronchial muscle, fibrosis, goblet cell metaplasia, and increased intraluminal mucus. At autopsy, mild degrees of emphysema are found commonly in older persons with no history of dyspnea or cigarette use. Although correlation between the degree of emphysema and symptoms is not as high as expected in emphysema patients, AO does appear to correlate with the degree of emphysema.

Symptoms and Signs

The most common symptoms of COPD are cough, increased sputum production, dyspnea, and wheezing. Disabling symptoms increase rapidly in patients > 50 yr of age and are more frequent in men than in women. **Cough** associated with sputum production usually begins within several years after starting to smoke. The cough may be mild, or it may be disabling because of posttussive syncope, vomiting, or micturition. The **sputum** is usually opalescent and varies in amount from < 1 tsp to several tbsp. Larger quantities or color variations (eg, green or yellow) suggest bronchiectasis or infection.

Dyspnea, the most disabling of all symptoms, usually begins at about 50 yr of age and progresses thereafter. Some patients associate the onset of dyspnea with a respiratory infection. Day-to-day variation in degree of dyspnea usually indicates bronchospasm. Dyspnea is more severe and frequent in men than in women. **Wheezing,** not present in all COPD patients, is usually first noted when the patient is supine. Later, it may occur while the patient is in any position, and it is usually associated with bronchospasm.

Although not all patients with COPD have signs of severe obstructive disease, when such signs are present they are quite specific. The classic sign of pursed-lipped breathing is seen in patients with severe obstruction. This type of breathing delays airway closure so a larger tidal volume can be maintained. Breathing in the sitting position with elbows resting on the thighs is another commonly observed sign of severe obstruction. This position may fixate the upper thorax and increase the curvature of the diaphragm, making breathing more efficient. Breathing with extrathoracic muscles suggests severe obstruction but does not differentiate emphysema from asthma.

Exacerbations of bronchitis in COPD patients are usually due to viruses, *Mycoplasma pneumoniae, Hemophilus influenzae,* and *Streptococcus pneumoniae.* Fever and leukocytosis may be absent in patients with acute infections. Acute hypoxemia accompanying a respiratory infection may lead to confusion and restlessness, which may be misinterpreted as senility in older patients.

Uncorrected hypoxemia leads to pulmonary hypertension, cor pulmonale, reduced free-water clearance in the kidney, arrhythmias, polycythemia, and altered cognitive function.

Physical Examination

Early or moderate obstructive disease may be associated with no physical signs except prolonged forced expiration. Consequently, it is important to ask patients to inhale as deeply as possible, then exhale as rapidly and fully as possible. Auscultation allows the physician not only to time the length of expiration (which should be < 4 sec) but also to hear wheezing. Obvious inspiratory noises, heard with the unaided ear or by placing a stethoscope over the trachea, are common in patients with bronchitis.

Patients presenting with severe COPD can be stereotyped as either **pink puffers** or **blue bloaters.** In actuality, most patients have features of both stereotypes, but these descriptions help define the extremes of the spectrum of obstructive disease.

The **pink puffer** is typically an asthenic, barrel-chested, emphysematous patient who exhibits pursed-lipped breathing and has no cyanosis or edema. Such a patient is often seen using extrathoracic muscles to breathe and usually has minimal sputum and little fluctuation in the day-to-day level of dyspnea. Diaphragmatic excursions are reduced, and breath and heart sounds are distant. Arterial blood gas levels show only mild to moderate hypoxemia and normal arterial Pa_{CO_2}. The barrel-shaped chest is nonspecific, since older persons commonly have increased lung compliance and larger resting lung volumes.

The **blue bloater** is often overweight, cyanotic, and edematous and exhibits a chronic cough and sputum production (chronic bronchitis). Arterial blood gas levels show hypoxemia and hypercapnia. Nocturnal hypoxemia may be profound. Elderly blue bloaters are uncommon, because this form of disease presents 5 to 10 yr earlier than does the type exhibited by the pink puffer. In addition, blue bloaters often have cor pulmonale, which rapidly leads to mortality when not treated appropriately.

Laboratory Studies

Chest x-rays are not sensitive for early or moderate obstructive disease. Typical findings in emphysema are a flattened diaphragm, a narrow heart, enlarged lungs, a paucity of peripheral vascular markings, and an increased retrosternal air space. These findings may also be seen during acute bronchospasm. Patients with bronchitis may have normal chest x-rays or evidence of increased vascular markings and may show enlarged pulmonary arteries.

Spirometry documents the obstructive component of the disease. Measurement of pulmonary function following administration of an aerosolized bronchodilator suggests the degree of reversibility of airways narrowing. Obstruction is present when the FEV_1 is < 80% of the forced vital capacity **(FVC)**. Patients are usually not dyspneic until the FEV_1 approaches 1.5 L. Determination of lung volume by the helium dilution technic or body box plethysmography shows an increased functional residual capacity **(FRC)** and residual volume **(RV)** in emphysema but may be near normal in bronchitis. Normal aging is also associated with a slight increase in FRC and RV. The diffusing capacity is low in emphysema but near normal in chronic bronchitis. An increased dead space can often be measured in patients with emphysema.

Arterial blood gas levels are typically abnormal in COPD. Hypoxemia, when present, is due to ventilation/perfusion mismatching because of bronchospasm, intrabronchial mucus, or premature airways collapse. True shunting of blood is uncommon in COPD. When hypoventilation is present, reflected by hypercapnia, hypoxemia can be due to reduced alveolar P_{O_2}. Chronic hypercapnia in these instances is confirmed by a near-normal blood pH and a concurrently elevated serum bicarbonate concentration. Care must be taken in the interpretation of hypoxemia in older persons because the normal Pa_{O_2} of a 75-yr-old person is approximately 75 mm Hg.

Prognosis

Intensive rehabilitation programs, including drug therapy, reconditioning through exercise, and close monitoring, can improve the quality of life and reduce the number of hospitalizations for patients with COPD. However, little evidence suggests that longevity can be improved in patients who do not present with hypoxemia. Patients who smoke and are developing COPD lose FEV_1 at the rate of 50 to 60 mL/yr, while nonsmokers have a decline of 25 to 30 mL/yr. Survival rates correlate with FEV_1. An FEV_1 > 1.5 L is usually associated with a normal adjusted life span, while an FEV_1 of 1 L or less is associated with an average survival of ≤ 5 yr. Poor prognostic signs include resting tachycardia, ventricular arrhythmias, and hypercapnia.

Treatment

The therapeutic goal for geriatric patients with COPD is maintenance of functional independence. Respiratory compromise eventually leads to functional impairment and loss of independence, often accompanied by anxiety, lowered self-esteem, depression, role reversal, and possibly sexual dysfunction.

Successful rehabilitation requires a caring family and physician, as well as a positive attitude on the part of the patient. Education concerning exercise, nutrition, avoidance of infections, and appropriate use of drugs improves the quality of life.

Sexual function often improves if the person is rested, schedules sexual activity for the "best-breathing" time of day, uses a bronchodilator 20 to 30 min beforehand, avoids intake of large amounts of food and alcohol, and assumes a position that does not put pressure on the chest or abdomen or require arm support.

Drug therapy is directly primarily at reduction of dyspnea; control of cough and sputum production are additional therapeutic goals. Because treatment is not curative, therapy is considered successful if it produces a favorable balance between symptomatic relief and drug-related side effects. Clear, written directions are important for older patients because their age-adjusted cognitive skills are further impaired by hypoxemia, leading to poor short-term memory and an inability to concentrate.

Infections: Prevention of infections is optimized by annual influenza vaccinations, once-in-a-lifetime polyvalent pneumococcal vaccine immunization, hand washing after contact with persons who have viral syndromes, and avoidance of crowds in poorly ventilated spaces during influenza epidemics. Antibiotics should be started promptly at the first sign of purulent sputum. Tetracycline, ampicillin (0.5 gm qid for 10 days), and trimethoprim-sulfamethoxazole are useful antibacterial agents in these instances. Increased administration of bronchodilators may also be necessary.

Bronchospasm: A reversible component of bronchospasm is documented when spirometry demonstrates an approximately 15% improvement in FEV_1 after a bronchodilator has been inhaled. This should not imply that absence of improvement in FEV_1 means a bronchodilator offers no therapeutic benefit. On the contrary, most bronchodilators (either oral **theophylline preparations** or oral or aerosolized **β_2-sympathomimetics**) improve mucociliary clearance, may delay fatigue of the diaphragm, and may improve myocardial contractility. Additionally, theophylline may be a mild respiratory stimulant and a diuretic. Inhaled β_2-sympathomimetics may be preferable because of a reduced risk of cardiovascular side effects in a patient population with a high incidence of heart disease.

The disadvantage of hand-held, metered-dose, aerosolized bronchodilators is that some older persons may not be able to synchronize inhalation of the drug with inspiration because of musculoskeletal problems such as rheumatoid arthritis. This can be circumvented by using either a spacer, which is attached to the metered-dose inhaler, or a compressor nebulizer, which does not require patient coordination. The half-life of theophylline preparations is prolonged in older patients, and dosage must be reduced appropriately.

An atropine derivative, ipratropium bromide, reverses bronchospasm in COPD. However, adverse effects may occur in patients with glaucoma or prostatic hypertrophy. **Corticosteroids** are beneficial during acute exacerbations of bronchospasm in patients with severe COPD and may reduce the length of stay in intensive care units, as well as the overall duration of hospitalization. Corticosteroids are also beneficial in selected patients with end-stage COPD in whom all other forms of therapy are ineffective. Prolonged or sustained use of high-dose corticosteroids should be avoided because of the propensity of these drugs to cause osteopenia, cataracts, s.c. hemorrhage, and cutaneous fragility.

Cough and sputum: Avoidance of irritants is the most important and effective therapy. Because cough is a natural protective mechanism, it should not be completely suppressed pharmacologically, but neither should it be allowed to be so forceful or frequent as to cause rib fractures or syncope. Over-the-counter drugs containing dextromethorphan are often effective in moderately suppressing cough. When necessary, stronger, narcotic derivatives may be useful for short periods.

Liquefaction and expectoration of sputum may be facilitated by adequate hydration and, occasionally, by use of potassium iodine solutions. Older persons have a tendency to become dehydrated because of altered renal function, so they must be told to drink a specific amount of fluids daily. So-called mucolytic agents have not been documented as being effective when inhaled, nor have expectorants been documented as improving the removal of secretions. Postural drainage after use of an inhaled bronchodilator has been shown to be effective in patients with bronchiectasis.

Dyspnea: Treatment is approached in a multimodal manner. Since dyspnea is thought to be the result of respiratory muscle fatigue caused by an inappropriate amount of work for a given level of ventilation, attempts are made to (1) reduce the amount of work, (2) reduce the propensity for muscle fatigue, and (3) reduce the amount of ventilation. The work of breathing is reduced by decreasing airways narrowing; by using bronchodilators and corticosteroids; and by a regimen of pulmonary care. Diaphragm-strengthening exercises, adequate nutrition, and use of theophylline preparations may reduce the propensity to muscle fatigue. O_2 requirements for a given level of activity can be reduced by conditioning exercises (and theoretically by ingesting a low-carbohydrate, high-fat diet), thereby decreasing the work of breathing. Anxiety associated with dyspnea can often be diminished by showing the patient how pursed-lipped breathing can reduce this unpleasant sensation.

Hypoxemia: The physician should determine the time at which hypoxemia ($Pa_{O_2} < 60$ mm Hg) occurs (ie, at rest, during exercise, or during sleep). If hypoxemia is present at rest, O_2 should be administered continuously. If it is not present at rest, oximetry measurements should be made during exercise and during sleep. If hypoxemia is documented, the lowest O_2 concentration capable of raising the P_{O_2} to approximately 65 mm Hg should be given. This can usually be accomplished with a Venturi mask (24 to 28%) or low-flow O_2 (1 to 2 L/min by nasal cannula). A slight rise in Pa_{CO_2} of 5 to 10 mm Hg is acceptable under these circumstances.

Hypercapnia: This condition, which commonly accompanies severe airways obstruction, is not dangerous when the blood pH is near normal. A rapid rise in P_{CO_2} with a drop in pH suggests fatiguing respiratory muscles and the need for intensive ventilatory support.

Heart failure (HF): Right-sided HF and biventricular failure are the 2 most common forms of cardiac decompensation in older patients with COPD. Right-sided HF, usually due to hypoxemia-induced pulmonary hypertension, is treated with O_2, judicious use of diuretics, and correction of electrolyte imbalances (eg, hypokalemia). Avoid digitalis preparations if there is no evidence of left-sided HF. Pulmonary vasodilators (eg, nifedipine and hydralazine) may be helpful in selected patients with severe pulmonary and systemic hypertension.

Exercise: Patients with COPD are commonly in poor physical condition. The physician should determine whether this state is the result of end-stage lung disease or other causes. If the patient has no respiratory reserve, exercise is unwarranted and an attempt should be made to decrease the work of daily living, thereby reducing O_2 requirements to a minimum. The physician may suggest that the patient live on 1 floor, not wear shoes that require tying, and so on. Graduated exercise programs should be instituted for patients thought to have respiratory reserves. Simultaneous supplemental O_2 may be required to allow patients to exercise long enough to benefit from the program. Exercise should be continued year-round. Activities may include walking outdoors in nice weather, in malls in bad weather, and up and down stairs in the house in winter, as well as using as exercise bicycle, if available.

---

41. PULMONARY EMBOLISM (PE)

John R. Michael

Lodgment of a blood clot in a pulmonary artery with subsequent obstruction of blood supply to the lung parenchyma. A pulmonary embolus occurs when a blood clot or other material traversing the circulatory system occludes a portion of the pulmonary vasculature. Although a blood clot is the most common cause, air, fat, bone marrow, foreign bodies, amniotic fluid, and tumor cells also can embolize the pulmonary vessels.

PE is common and difficult to diagnose correctly, but can be effectively treated. In the USA, the incidence of PE is estimated to be 650,000 cases annually, the primary cause of death of 100,000 persons each year, and a contributory factor in perhaps another 100,000 deaths annually. Because the symptoms and signs are nonspecific, PE may be over- or underdiagnosed. For example, some believe that perhaps 30% of cases are misdiagnosed, while others believe that PE is overdiagnosed in patients with cardiac and other respiratory conditions. Accurate diagnosis minimizes the risk of both untreated PE and unnecessary anticoagulant therapy. Such therapy appears to improve survival in patients with PE; the mortality rate is approximately 8% in those treated vs. an estimated 30% in untreated patients.

Pathophysiology

Approximately 90% of the blood clots that cause PE arise in the lower extremities. The risk that a clot will embolize to the lung is greater if the clot is in the popliteal or iliofemoral vein (approximately 50%) than if it is confined to the calf veins (< 5%). Other, less common sites of thrombosis that may give rise to PE are the right atrium; the right ventricle; and the pelvic, renal, hepatic, subclavian, and jugular veins. The classic risk factors for the development of venous thrombosis are injury to the vessel wall, stasis, and an increase in the tendency of the blood to clot. Common medical conditions, eg, trauma to leg vessels, obesity, heart failure (HF), malignancy, hip fracture, and myeloproliferative disorders, predispose to venous thrombosis, as do immobility, estrogen use, and surgery.

Symptoms and Signs

The degree of pulmonary vascular obstruction caused by the embolus and the patient's prior cardiopulmonary function affect the symptoms and signs. Patients who have small thromboemboli may be asymptomatic. The most common symptoms are shortness of breath (80%), chest pain that may be pleuritic (70%), anxiety (60%), leg pain or swelling (40%), hemoptysis (35%), and syncope (15%). The most common physical findings are tachypnea (90%), tachycardia (50%), fever (40%), leg edema or tenderness (33%), cyanosis (20%), and a pleural friction rub (18%). Although most patients with PE have deep venous thrombosis, only 1/3 have clinical signs of thrombosis; eg, leg swelling, tenderness, increased warmth, or Homans' sign.

Less than 20% of patients have all components of the **classic triad of dyspnea, chest pain, and hemoptysis.** However, most patients have shortness of breath, chest discomfort, and/or tachypnea. The most frequent finding is tachypnea (respiratory rate > 16/min). If tachypnea is absent, PE is unlikely to be the cause of the symptoms.

About 1/3 of patients with PE have a **pleural effusion,** usually unilateral, although bilateral effusions may occur. Two thirds are bloody (> 100,000 RBC/mL). The differential diagnosis of bloody effusion is limited to 3 principal conditions: PE, cancer, and trauma. Patients with PE and a bloody pleural effusion generally have a **pulmonary infiltrate** on chest x-ray, which suggests hemorrhagic consolidation of the lung parenchyma. Most of these patients have only pulmonary hemorrhage, and the infiltrate will resolve over several days. About 10% of patients with pulmonary emboli, especially those with severe HF, will develop pulmonary infarction. Two thirds of nonbloody effusions are exudates, with elevated WBC (up to 75,000/mL), as in infected pleural effusions.

Mechanical obstruction of a portion of the pulmonary circulation may lead to **increased pulmonary vascular resistance,** although vasoconstriction secondary to alveolar capillary hypoxemia and mediator release may contribute. The increased pulmonary vascular resistance causes right ventricular and pulmonary arterial pressures to increase in order to maintain CO. In patients with no prior cardiopulmonary disease, the pulmonary arterial pressure correlates with the percentage of the pulmonary vascular bed occluded by the emboli. Thus, the presence of pulmonary hypertension (> 25 mm Hg) in a patient with previously normal heart and lungs indicates extensive obstruction (> 40 to 50%) of the pulmonary vascular bed. However, in patients with prior cardiopulmonary disease, the pulmonary arterial pressure does not correlate with the percentage of the blocked vascular bed. In these patients, a small clot may be enough to produce a marked hemodynamic effect because of the limited cardiac reserve.

Syncope, a systolic BP < 100 mm Hg, or a marked decrease in the systolic BP in a hypertensive patient suggests the possibility of massive PE or a hemodynamically significant embolus in a patient with marginal cardiopulmonary function. An acute increase in pulmonary vascular resistance to the point at which the right ventricle cannot generate sufficient forward flow causes right ventricular failure, a decrease in CO, and hypotension. The latter is ominous, because the decrease in aortic diastolic pressure may significantly reduce coronary blood flow to the overworked right ventricle, establishing a vicious circle.

A patient who is hypotensive because of PE will have elevated right atrial and ventricular pressures. Consequently, the presence of a normal right atrial or right ventricular pressure in a hypotensive patient excludes PE as the cause of the hypotension.

Laboratory Findings

Chest x-rays in patients with PE may be normal or show nonspecific abnormalities, eg, atelectasis, an elevated hemidiaphragm, pleural effusion, or an infiltrate. Findings such as an enlarged pulmonary artery on one side or hyperlucency of 1 lung because of reduced pulmonary vascular markings are infrequent and are more commonly produced by rotation of the patient than by PE. A pleural-based pyramidal infiltrate that points back toward the hilus (Hampton hump) is infrequent but should suggest PE. Although the chest x-ray cannot make or exclude the diagnosis of PE, it can lead to the diagnosis of other conditions that may explain the patient's symptoms, eg, pneumothorax, rib fracture, or HF.

The electrocardiographic findings in patients with PE are also generally nonspecific, as many as $1/3$ of such patients have a normal ECG. The most common abnormal findings are sinus tachycardia and nonspecific ST- and T-wave changes. Infrequent changes that are highly suggestive of PE indicate strain on the right side of the heart; they include T-wave inversion in the precordial leads V_1 to V_4, transient right bundle branch block, right or left deviation of the QRS axis, sudden onset of atrial fibrillation or other atrial arrhythmia, and development of electrocardiographic signs of right ventricular hypertrophy or right atrial enlargement. The $S_1Q_3T_3$ pattern (deep S wave in limb lead I and a Q wave and inverted T wave in limb lead III) also suggests PE. This pattern of right-sided heart strain is usually accompanied by T-wave inversion in the precordial leads.

Arterial blood gases: PE often results in arterial hypoxemia, because areas with a low ratio of ventilation to perfusion develop secondary to airway closure and bronchoconstriction in lung segments adjacent to the emboli. Intrapulmonary shunting of blood and a reduced mixed venous O_2 tension also contribute to the arterial hypoxemia. A rare cause of right-to-left shunting of blood is the opening of a patent foramen ovale due to right atrial hypertension from massive PE.

Although PE often causes marked hypoxemia, approximately 10% of patients will have a Pa_{O_2} between 80 and 90 mm Hg while breathing room air. Thus, a Pa_{O_2} in this range is uncommon but does not exclude an embolus. Perhaps more helpful is a sudden decrease in Pa_{O_2} that cannot be easily explained by another diagnosis. Because PE generally causes tachypnea and respiratory alkalosis, arterial blood gas values typically show a decrease in Pa_{CO_2}.

A lung scan that shows no perfusion defect excludes PE. One that shows a perfusion defect as large as or larger than a lung segment, *without a matching ventilation defect,* indicates a high probability of PE. In patients with such a scan, the likelihood that PE will be demonstrated on pulmonary angiography is 85 to 90%. In patients with such a scan plus a *matching ventilation defect,* the likelihood of PE is 30 to 45%.

A lung scan with a subsegmental perfusion defect, with or without a matching ventilation defect, is often labeled a low-probability scan; however, such a scan has a 20 to 30% association with PE. The lung scan is termed indeterminate if matching ventilation and perfusion defects correspond with an infiltrate on the chest x-ray. This type of lung scan has a 25 to 40% association with PE.

The pulmonary angiogram is considered the gold standard for the diagnosis of PE. Two findings are pathognomonic of PE: a constant intraluminal filling defect and a sharp cutoff of a vessel. Experimental studies designed to test the sensitivity of pulmonary angiography indicate that single, small emboli may be missed but multiple emboli are rarely missed. Because pulmonary emboli are multiple in a large majority of patients, the incidence of false-negative pulmonary angiograms is believed to be low. Follow-up clinical and laboratory studies in patients with negative pulmonary angiograms also suggest that false-negative angiograms are rare.

Pulmonary angiography is safe in the absence of severe pulmonary hypertension or cardiopulmonary decompensation. The procedure has minimal morbidity and a mortality rate of approximately 0.2% but requires considerable expertise in performance and interpretation. Because the risk of pulmonary angiography is small in experienced hands, a number of authorities believe that the risk of anticoagulation in an elderly patient exceeds the risk of a pulmonary angiogram.

Digital subtraction angiography, fiberoptic angioscopy, and MRI are being evaluated as diagnostic tools.

Venography and impedance plethysmography: Venography is the gold standard for the diagnosis of venous thrombosis, although it may be impossible to perform in patients with significant edema. Side effects, including allergic reactions and the development of thrombophlebitis, occur in 2% of patients.

Impedance plethysmography **(IPG)**, combined with Doppler ultrasound flow studies, is a helpful noninvasive diagnostic test for deep venous thrombosis. Studies correlating the results of IPG with venography indicate that IPG has a sensitivity of 86%, a specificity of 97%, a positive predictive value of 97%, and a negative predictive value of 85%. IPG is excellent for detecting a clot in the popliteal or iliofemoral vein, but it can miss a clot in the calf vein. Fortunately, the risk of PE from clots confined to veins in the calf is small.

Because $1/3$ of negative pulmonary angiograms are associated with deep venous thrombosis, venography or IPG can provide useful therapeutic information in many patients.

Diagnosis

After a history is obtained and a physical examination performed in patients with suspected PE, an ECG, chest x-ray, and arterial blood gas values should be obtained. If PE is still considered likely, the next step is usually to obtain a ventilation-perfusion lung scan. If the presence of deep venous thrombosis is strongly suspected or if there is a high likelihood that the lung scan will be indeterminate (because of underlying lung disease), an alternative approach might be to order an IPG or venogram.

Although the commonly asked diagnostic question is, Does this patient have PE? perhaps a better question would be, Does this patient need therapy for venous thrombosis or for PE? Prospective studies indicate that approximately $1/3$ of patients with a negative pulmonary angiogram have deep venous thrombosis documented by venography. Thus, the best diagnostic approach is to ask, Does this patient have evidence of either a pulmonary emoblus or venous thrombosis?

The likelihood of PE should be estimated, using results of the clinical and laboratory studies, including lung scan. If the lung scan shows no perfusion abnormality, PE can be excluded. If the lung scan shows a perfusion defect smaller than a subsegment of the lung and the clinical likelihood of PE is low, many clinicians would not pursue the diagnosis further. Conversely, if the lung scan reveals a perfusion defect that is segmental or larger, without a matching ventilation defect, and the clinical likelihood of PE is high, most clinicians would treat the patient unless special circumstances require a definitive diagnosis by pulmonary angiography.

Prospective clinical studies indicate that approximately 10% of patients evaluated for PE have both a low-probability lung scan and a clinical assessment that an embolus is unlikely; at the other extreme, about 30% of patients have both a high-probability lung scan and a clinical assessment that an embolus is likely. The management of patients at either extreme is clear, but the appropriate management approach in the other 60% of patients is not. Several approaches are available: Perform a pulmonary angiogram, empirically anticoagulate, obtain an IPG or venogram, or observe.

In patients with a low-probability lung scan, the use of IPG has been suggested to help determine whether the patient should receive anticoagulant therapy. Patients with a positive IPG should be treated with heparin for deep venous thrombosis. In patients with less than a high-probability lung scan, only a moderate clinical probability for PE, an adequate cardiopulmonary reserve, and a negative IPG, observation and serial evaluation may be appropriate. In general, the greater the risk of not treating the patient for PE or the greater the risk of therapy, the greater the need for definitive angiographic diagnosis.

Prognosis

With anticoagulant therapy, the mortality rate from PE is only 8%, compared with 30% in untreated patients. Prognosis is poorest in patients with severe underlying cardiac or pulmonary disease. The greatest risk of death is in the first hours following embolization.

PE is believed to recur in 5 to 10% of patients despite heparin therapy. The likelihood of recurrent emboli is greatest in patients with massive pulmonary embolization or in whom anticoagulant therapy has been inadequate. If recurrence develops in the first few days of heparin or thrombolytic therapy, these treatments are usually continued. If recurrent episodes or massive embolization occurs from clot present in the legs, considerations should be given to interrupting the inferior vena cava.

The long-term prognosis for patients surviving PE is determined by the underlying medical problems and cardiopulmonary status. Recurrent PE leading to chronic pulmonary hypertension and cor pulmonale is uncommon, occurring in < 2% of patients.

Treatment

The general principles of therapy are to provide adequate supplemental O_2 to achieve a Pa_{O_2} of 60 to 70 mm Hg, to relieve pain with morphine or other analgesics, to provide adequate intravascular fluid to maintain CO, to monitor for evidence of bleeding with anticoagulant therapy, and to avoid drugs that adversely affect platelet function (eg, aspirin or other cyclo-oxygenase blockers).

The hypotensive patient with PE should be treated with volume expanders, streptokinase to speed clot lysis, and infusion of norepinephrine in amounts sufficient to increase aortic diastolic pressure and coronary blood flow. Studies in experimental animals indicate that norepinephrine is considerably more effective than volume loading or isoproterenol infusion in reversing shock in PE.

Heparin is generally used to treat deep venous thrombosis or PE; it prevents clot formation and extension but does not lyse clots. Heparin is usually infused IV for 7 to 10 days. A loading dose of 5,000 to 10,000 u. is given initially as a bolus, followed by a constant infusion of 1,000 u./h. The infusion rate may need to be lowered to 700 u./h in patients > 60 yr old, especially females. Heparin can also be infused intermittently, although it is believed that the risk of bleeding is reduced by continuous administration. The dose is adjusted to maintain the activated partial thromboplastin time at 2 to 2.5 times the control value to reduce the risk of bleeding.

The major complications of heparin therapy are reversible thrombocytopenia and bleeding. Five to 15% of patients who receive heparin therapy have bleeding significant enough to require blood transfusion. Factors that increase the risk of bleeding with heparin therapy include uremia, liver disease, surgery within the preceding 2 wk, a history of GI bleeding in the preceding 6 mo, a diastolic BP > 110 mm Hg, and age > 60 yr. The risk of bleeding while receiving heparin appears to be particularly high in women > 60 yr of age.

If major bleeding occurs, the usual approach is to *stop the heparin* and allow the anticoagulant effect to disappear over the next few hours. Blood transfusions do not correct the anticoagulant effect of heparin. Although protamine can inactivate heparin, it is generally not used because of the risk of acute hypotension, dyspnea, and bradycardia.

Heparin can also be administered intermittently s.c. Low-dose heparin, 5000 u. bid s.c., reduces the incidence of deep venous thrombosis, PE, and death from PE in patients undergoing abdominal surgery. The use of heparin s.c. to prevent deep venous thrombosis has been extended to medical patients who have an increased incidence of thrombosis, eg patients who are bedbound or have severe HF, hemiparesis following a stroke, or a previous history of venous thrombosis.

The incidence of deep venous thrombosis following hip fracture or replacement is extremely high (30 to 50%), with 20% of all patients having clot in the iliofemoral vein. Effective therapies to reduce this incidence include external calf compression with a pneumatic cuff, aspirin, heparin s.c., and warfarin. Aspirin 500 mg daily beginning the day of surgery is used most commonly.

Warfarin inhibits the liver's synthesis of the vitamin K-dependent clotting factors II, VII, IX, and X. Therapy is monitored by measuring prothrombin time, which should be prolonged to 1.5 to 2.5 times control. Although warfarin administration for only 24 h may increase the prothrombin time, 3 to 7 days of therapy (5 to 10 mg daily) are generally required before a stable antithrombotic state is reached. Clinical studies indicate that warfarin therapy can be safely begun at the same time that heparin therapy is started and that this substantially decreases length of hospital stay and cost.

Long-term anticoagulation is generally continued after hospital treatment for deep venous thrombosis or PE and is achieved by using either warfarin or heparin s.c. (5000 u. bid). How long chronic anticoagulation should be continued is unclear. In a patient with a temporary predisposing factor who has not had a previous clot, therapy is generally continued for 4 to 8 wk. This approach results in a low risk for recurrent thromboemboli. In a patient who has had previous episodes of thrombosis, anticoagulant therapy is often given for 3 to 6 mo or may be continued indefinitely. The need for continued warfarin therapy should be reassessed periodically because of the 10% risk of serious bleeding.

Thrombolytic therapy should be considered in patients with deep venous thrombosis involving the iliofemoral system and in patients with massive PE who have significant pulmonary hypertension, obstruction of multiple segments of the pulmonary circulation, or systemic hypotension. Thrombolytic therapy is used in patients with severe proximal deep venous thrombosis, because it leads to greater revascularization of the deep venous system in the leg than can be achieved with heparin therapy.

Clot lysis results in a reduced incidence of recurrent thrombi and the postphlebitic syndrome. A controlled clinical trial of thrombolytic vs. heparin therapy indicated that the former causes more rapid lysis of PE and more rapid return of pulmonary arterial pressure to normal than does the latter. However, thrombolytic therapy did not improve survival.

Streptokinase is the thrombolytic agent most commonly used, although **urokinase** is also effective and may be employed in patients who are allergic or resistant to streptokinase. Streptokinase is administered as an initial IV bolus of 250,000 u. over 30 min, followed by a constant infusion of 100,000 u./h for 24 to 72 h. The bolus neutralizes antistreptococcal antibody from previous streptococcal infections. Thrombolytic therapy is generally monitored by the thrombin time, measured before therapy, 4 h after beginning therapy, and then every 12 h. The objective is to increase the thrombin time to 2 to 4 times baseline.

After the course of streptokinase has been completed, heparin is typically infused at the standard dose for 5 to 7 days. When switching from streptokinase to heparin, one generally waits 4 h after stopping the streptokinase and then begins infusing heparin without a loading dose.

If major bleeding occurs, whole blood or fresh frozen plasma will reverse the effect of streptokinase. Tissue plasminogen activators are currently undergoing evaluation as therapy for pulmonary thromboemboli.

Contraindications to thrombolytic therapy include eye or CNS surgery within the preceding 2 wk, intracranial neoplasms or vascular abnormalities, stroke within the preceding 2 mo, active bleeding, severe hypertension, and allergy to thrombolytic agents.

Interruption of the inferior vena cava may be required in a small minority of patients who either (1) have a contraindication to anticoagulation, (2) fail to respond to anticoagulant therapy as demonstrated by recurrent emboli, or (3) have pulmonary emboli from septic thrombophlebitis. The most common technic is to place a filter in the inferior vena cava. The filter is introduced percutaneously into the jugular vein, then advanced into a position below the level of the renal veins. In experienced hands, this technic eliminates the immediate risk of further embolization from clot in the legs. However, the immediate benefit of this procedure must be balanced against possible complications, which include chronic leg edema, thrombosis formation above the filter, recurrent embolization through collateral veins, perforation of the vena cava, and migration of the filter.

An endarterectomy may be helpful in patients who have chronic pulmonary hypertension because of a clot occluding the main or lobar pulmonary arteries.

§3. ORGAN SYSTEMS: GASTROINTESTINAL DISORDERS

42. INFLUENCE OF AGING ON GASTROINTESTINAL DISORDERS

Marvin M. Schuster

The gut throughout life is in a constant and rapid state of change. Epithelial cell turnover occurs as frequently as every 24 to 48 h; absorption and secretion are almost constant; and myoelectric and motor activity are continuous.

The primary functions of the gut are digestion and absorption; the secondary functions that subserve these activities are secretion and motility. In this Section, these 4 GI activities are intensely scrutinized at a number of levels—ranging from the molecular to the physiologic and from the morphologic to the demographic and behavioral.

A major obstacle to the advancement of GI gerontology is our ignorance of the basic science of aging. This handicap is analogous to specialists in infectious disease having to function without the basic science of bacteriology. Nevertheless, progress is being made in understanding the effect of aging on GI physiology and pathophysiology. The fact that aging takes place over a long period of time imposes confounding factors on gerontologic studies and the practice of geriatrics. The passage of time is associated with physiologic and pathophysiologic changes in many organ systems (eg, endocrine, cardiovascular, nervous) that affect GI structure and function and produce many variations in presentation of illness.

Time also allows for the superimposition of altered alimentary function by extraintestinal diseases; if common, this could lead to the false impression that the observed alterations result from the natural process of aging. A prime example is the esophageal motility changes recognized in octogenarians that for decades were assumed to be the result of age-determined esophageal muscle changes. Only recently have they been shown to be due to extraintestinal disorders (eg, diabetes and neurologic and vascular changes that supervene with age). In fact, research has shown that most age-related alterations in GI motility are a result of neurologic rather than muscular changes.

The chapters that follow describe the effects of aging on the gut itself, on the clinical presentation of both common (eg, appendicitis) and unusual (eg, celiac disease) GI disorders, and on the response of the gut to extraintestinal disorders.

Obesity is the most common cause of malnourishment in America. However, our concept of the norm is in a state of flux, with recent statistics suggesting that the ideal weight for longevity may be higher than the previously accepted scale. Although dental and oral disorders are particularly common in the elderly, physicians generally have little expertise in this area. The intricate interaction between stress and physiologic function is especially pertinent in the aging population; the elderly are subject to not only the usual stresses of adulthood but such additional stresses as loss of spouse, family members, friends, and job at a time of increasing mental and physical limitations and isolation. The interplay of anatomic, motor, and secretory changes often leads to GI symptoms.

Although constipation, incontinence, and diverticular disease are the GI problems most commonly recognized in the elderly, each of these disorders has a number of different underlying causes, and the specific pathogenesis dictates treatment. Diagnostic approaches are also influenced by aging. Age may alter the presentation of malabsorption, and chronic diarrhea may affect the aging patient differently and more severely than the young. A number of special factors must be considered in deciding on the advisability of endoscopy in the elderly, as well as in determining the endoscopic preparation and appropriate technics.

There is a paucity of recognized changes in the aging liver. Cancer of various intestinal organs is particularly common in elderly persons and requires special considerations for successful surgical management. Benign lesions in the elderly also require a specialized approach. These and other factors are discussed in the following chapters.

---

43. OBESITY

Ronald D. T. Cape

The most common form of malnutrition in the USA is obesity. If one accepts 20% above the desirable weight as the criterion, recent data suggest 24% of women and 14% of men between the ages of 18 and 74 are obese. The most widely used indexes for determining desirable weight are based on body weight and frame in relation to height. Tables of desirable weight provided by the Metropolitan Life Insurance Company have been the most widely used. Desirable weight is the weight at which the lowest mortality rate occurs among individuals who take out life insurance policies. However, recent data have raised questions about the validity of norms established by this means (see below).

The relationship of weight as a function of height can be expressed in other ways. A commonly used method is the **body mass index,** which is calculated by dividing body weight in kg by the square of barefoot height in meters. Acceptable body mass indexes for women range from 19 to 24 and for men from 20 to 25. Another method of assessing percentage of body fat and, thereby, obesity is to measure **skinfold thickness** from either biceps, triceps, subscapular, or suprailiac areas. Triceps skinfold thickness is the most commonly used, but measurement of skinfold thickness has been mainly of value in research studies.

Etiology

Obviously, too great a caloric intake or too little expenditure of energy result in the accumulation of fat and obesity. However, other factors, such as an individual's genetic makeup, are important determinants in the tendency to develop obesity. There is likely also to be a considerable effect from what might be termed "nervous energy." The mild to moderately obese individual tends to be more relaxed and placid, which may account for the accumulation of some extra pounds. Persons who are less relaxed, more emotionally and intellectually labile, and more physically active, tend to remain lean.

Treatment

Obesity is associated with hypertension and cardiovascular disease, particularly in younger and middle-aged populations. However, in the octogenarian and beyond, the need to treat obesity becomes debatable. In a study involving 7 countries, the minimal mortality rate occurred in 7 of 8 populations whose weight was relatively greater than the norm. Thus, overweight subjects had a *better* prognosis. The highest mortality rate occurred in the leanest quartile of the populations of the USA, Finland, the Netherlands, Italy, Greece, Yugoslavia, and Japan. This implies that being 10 to 20% overweight may be beneficial.

Although other factors are important in determining obesity, people do not become obese unless they eat more than is necessary for their needs; the only effective way to reduce weight is to reduce intake. The extra activities required to lose even a modest amount of weight are considerable, and for an elderly person without a complicating disease who is $\geq$ 20% overweight, there is no need to propose alteration of eating habits.

However, if one is treating an obese 80-yr-old with heart failure due to ischemic heart disease, there are definite advantages to reducing that person's weight. The same applies to a man in his 70s with chronic obstructive airways disease whose activity level is further reduced by obesity. The presence of diseases complicated by obesity warrants an aggressive attempt to help the patient reduce.

---

44. DENTAL AND ORAL DISORDERS

Bruce J. Baum

Two major functions of the oral cavity are to initiate digestion and to allow the production of speech. All of the oral tissues have evolved to permit these activities: The teeth, supporting periodontal tissues, and temporomandibular joint aid in mechanical food processing; the tongue, through its finely coordinated movements, not only mixes and assists in translocating food but also is central to phonation.

Although the mouth is exposed to the outside environment, protection is provided by the oral mucosa. Saliva protects oral tissues through its lubricatory, antimicrobial, and dental-remineralizing proteins. Saliva also participates in the initial breakdown of food and in transforming it to a swallow-ready bolus. The mouth has an intricate sensory control system, including exquisitely developed receptors for taste, touch, pain, texture, and temperature.

The dental and oral disorders encountered by adults affect all of the tissues and functions mentioned above. Most of these problems are not life-threatening but they may be serious, and many have a major impact on the quality of life.

DENTAL CARIES

A disease of the calcified tissues of the teeth resulting from the action of microorganisms on carbohydrates, characterized by decalcification of the inorganic portions of the tooth and accompanied or followed by disintegration of the organic portion.

Previously, older individuals were likely to be edentulous. Because of advances in dental preservation, the elderly are increasingly dentate and dental caries is an increasingly important concern.

Dental caries results from the dissolution of the tooth surface by microbial by-products found in **dental plaque**. The principal type of caries associated with the elderly is found on the root surfaces **(root caries)**. With age, loss of alveolar (supporting) bone around teeth occurs, and root surfaces previously unexposed to the oral milieu are uncovered (see below). **Cementum,** the mineralized substance surrounding the root surface, is an extracellular matrix with about 50% less mineral content than the enamel matrix covering the crown of a tooth. Thus root surfaces in older persons may be increasingly susceptible to abrasion, attrition, and demineralization.

The prevalence of root caries is about 4 times higher in elderly than in younger persons. Among children, adolescents, and young adults, **coronal caries** *(decay on the anatomic crown of the tooth)* is more common. Generally, root caries may be more difficult for the dentist to restore than coronal caries. The rapid and extensive appearance of root caries in an elderly patient is usually a sign of marked salivary dysfunction (see below).

However, older persons are still susceptible to coronal caries. Their frequency is comparable to that in young and middle-aged adults. In the elderly, coronal caries usually recurs around restorations.

Treatment

All forms of caries should be treated by a dental practitioner. Untreated caries will progress; penetrate the dental pulp; cause considerable pain, discomfort, and possibly localized infection; and will require more extensive therapy, (eg, an **exodontic procedure** [extraction] or **end-**

odontic procedure [root canal therapy]). The elderly should be urged to seek regular dental care, including prophylaxis (eg, fluoride rinses, plaque and tartar removal) to limit caries. A regular dental examination once every 6 mo is usually adequate, but a history of rapidly developing carious lesions or conservatively managed periodontal disease may require more frequent visits. Older persons with diminished dexterity may require individually tailored technics for oral hygiene and more frequent dental visits.

PERIODONTAL DISEASE

The periodontium: *the supporting structure of the tooth, including the gingiva, alveolar bone, and periodontal ligament.*

Pathophysiology

Most tooth loss in adults stems from periodontal disease. Degeneration of the attachment apparatus for the tooth results in alveolar bone loss and periodontal ligament destruction. Clinically, this may be associated with gingival recession.

Periodontal disease should no longer be considered a disease of aging. More likely, a person's periodontal status represents the accumulation of lesions over a lifetime rather than increased susceptibility to active disease because of age.

Etiology, Symptoms, and Signs

Like dental caries, periodontal disease is caused by bacterial plaque that accumulates and adheres to the teeth. This results in local immunopathologic destruction of connective tissues; bacterial antigens penetrate periodontal tissues, initiating an inflammatory response. Periodontal disease tends to progress slowly, in an episodic pattern. Initially, gingival tissues bleed, and become edematous—a hallmark sign **(gingivitis).** Later, destruction of alveolar bone and the periodontal ligament **(periodontitis)** results in loss of support for the tooth.

A number of common clinical situations may exacerbate periodontal disease; eg, diabetes mellitus may cause an exaggerated inflammatory reaction with poor tissue response and healing.

Many commonly used drugs can also affect periodontal status. Some (eg, phenytoin and cyclosporine) may irritate the gums, causing **gingival hyperplasia.** Others (eg, antihypertensives, psychoactive drugs, and anticholinergics) can reduce saliva production, thereby diminishing the key endogenous protective mechanism in the mouth (see below).

Prophylaxis and Treatment

Principal prophylactic measures consist of good oral hygiene. A recent significant advance in periodontal prophylaxis is an effective antimicrobial (antiplaque) mouthwash containing chlorhexidine. This is particularly useful for persons who have difficulty with dental hygiene because of diminished dexterity. However, regular use may result in staining of the teeth and composite resin dental restorations. These stains are tenacious but can be removed from the teeth by professional prophylaxis. Unfortunately, stained resin restorations may be permanently discolored.

The use of surgery is restricted because *active* periodontal disease seems to be less common in older persons, and surgery may be contraindicated by confounding systemic factors. The use of nonsteroidal anti-inflammatory drugs **(NSAIDs)** to limit active periodontal disease is under investigation.

ORAL MUCOSAL DISORDERS

Oral mucosal tissues in older individuals have been stereotypically characterized as pale, thin, atrophic, dry, and readily traumatized. However, little hard evidence is available to support this. Despite quantitative histologic evidence of epithelial atrophy with age, there is no indication that this is of clinical significance. Most complaints are probably manifestations of systemic disease (eg, Sjögren's syndrome) or other conditions (eg, side effects of drugs or head and neck irradiation) that diminish salivary gland performance (see below). Other conditions (eg, certain endocrinopathies and nutritional deficiencies) can also adversely affect the oral mucosa.

Most significant concerns are similar to those in younger adults. Many age-related local changes (eg, lingual varicosities, Fordyce's granules) have no clinical significance. In general, the critical barrier function of the oral mucosa is well maintained in healthy adults, regardless of age.

Prosthetic fit: Older edentulous or partially edentulous persons frequently present with traumatic oral mucosal lesions secondary to ill-fitting dental prostheses. These may include **erythematous, hyperplastic, hyperkeratotic,** and **ulcerative lesions.** Patients with such lesions should be referred to a dentist for a new prothesis or repair of the old one.

Palliative, topically applied agents may be helpful, eg, 0.5% dyclonine elixir combined with an equal amount of diphenhydramine elixir. This combination of agents is not commercially available and requires compounding by a pharmacist. It can be applied directly to the intraoral ulcerations if they are few in number, using a cotton-tipped applicator. However, 5 mL of the mixture can be used as an oral rinse prn for pain relief of a generalized stomatitis. Nutritional counseling may also be required temporarily until the mucositis is alleviated. If considerable hyperplastic tissue is present, surgical correction may be necessary to allow normal chewing.

Burning sensations of the oral mucosa have frequently been reported, particularly by postmenopausal women. These symptoms are rare and their etiology is unclear. Patients with so-called **burning mouth syndrome** represent a spectrum of problems; eg, many patients exhibit signs of neurologic dysfunction (frank gustatory disorders). Also, many may undergo complete, apparently spontaneous, remission. Such patients are difficult and frustrating to manage, but they may benefit from referral to an expert in treating chronic pain syndromes.

Oral carcinoma, which represents 3 to 5% of all forms of cancer, is another serious concern. Its prevalence is low until middle age but increases sharply thereafter. White, red, or ulcerated lesions that persist > 3 wk should be evaluated by a dentist. Whether biopsy is indicated will be dictated by the clinical history of the lesion and other oral findings.

NONDENTAL MINERALIZED TISSUE LOSS

Alveolar bone, an important component of the periodontium, provides support for the teeth and is clearly different from the underlying basal jawbone (mandible and maxilla). Although a generalized loss of bone mass occurs with age, resorption of alveolar bone is a result of local factors rather than a part of the aging process. Once the dentition (part or all) is lost, alveolar bone is not needed and atrophy ensues rapidly. This situation is common in the elderly now but will likely decline in the future with better dental preservation.

Widespread alveolar bone loss in edentulous persons presents a considerable management problem. Fabrication of a successful dental prosthesis for patients with severely resorbed alveolar bony ridges is difficult, especially within the mandibular arch. This may adversely affect the patient's dietary selection and nourishment. Alveolar bone loss also results in a loss of facial height and a tendency toward prognathism, which may contribute to a diminished self-image. An osteo-integrated metallic implant can be surgically placed to provide anchorage for dental prostheses and should be considered for these patients.

Temporomandibular joint (TMJ) disorders: The TMJ, located between the glenoid fossa and the condylar process of the mandible, is structurally unique. It is not only essential to all articulated maxillary and mandibular functions but also is involved in many craniofacial pain disorders.

Until recently, many studies suggested that anatomic changes in the TMJ (resulting in dysfunction and discomfort) were age-related and normal. Recent studies dispute this.

"Normal" aging changes are especially difficult to distinguish from osteoarthritic joint changes. Any pathologic alterations can be associated directly with the joint (articular) or with unrelated tissues (nonarticular). The latter are typically of dental (malocclusion), muscular, or psychophysiologic origin. The most common nonarticular disorder is **myofascial pain-dysfunction syndrome,** which is associated with involuntary jaw clenching or tooth grinding as a manifestation of tension.

Clinically, a limited ability to open the jaw (< 40 mm interincisal distance is abnormal) is a sign of TMJ dysfunction that does seem to be age related. Clicking sounds in the joint should be noted, and x-ray studies, tomography, or arthroscopy may help to assess articular pathology. TMJ disorders are difficult to manage. When pain is present, if malocclusion or psychologic etiology is suspected, appropriate referral should be made to a psychiatrist or TMJ specialist.

ORAL MOTOR DYSFUNCTION

The oral motor apparatus is involved in finely coordinated functions, including speaking, chewing, swallowing, and facial posture. Aging, in general, is associated with morphologic and biochemical alterations in neuromuscular systems. Several studies of oral motor function in healthy adults have demonstrated measurable changes in motor performance with age **(eg, reduced masticatory muscle performance and a prolonged oral phase of swallowing)**. The former change is common and appears to lead to an increased willingness to swallow larger food particles than usually accepted at a younger age. This practice could have dangerous consequences if choking or aspiration should result. The lengthened oral phase similarly may interfere with deglutition.

Such motor changes are of greater concern in nonhealthy, elderly patients. Obviously, frank neuropathies may markedly affect performance by the oral-maxillofacial musculature. However, most oral motor dysfunctions are iatrogenic and not necessarily directly related to the neuromuscular apparatus; ie, any treatment that **diminishes salivary gland function** may have important, negative effects on the timing and pattern of the oral swallowing phase. Drugs, (eg, antihypertensives, anticholinergics, antipsychotics, and antidepressants) commonly used by the elderly are reported to affect salivary performance significantly. Similar changes are observed in patients after irradiation (see below) or surgery for neoplasms in the head and neck region. Additionally, some drugs (eg, phenothiazines) are often associated with tardive dyskinesia in the oral and maxillofacial region.

Speech changes: Certain characteristic **changes in voice** and speech production occur with age. However, aging is not normally associated with impaired ability to produce speech and thus is not a general clinical concern.

Many **postural alterations** occur with age. Frequently, a drooping of the lower face and lips is observed in the oral area, resulting from both decreased tone of the circumoral muscles and (in edentulous persons) reduced bone support. This change is not only an aesthetic concern but a potential source of embarrassment, since it can lead to drooling or food spills. Healthy older persons may also have difficulty closing their lips competently while eating, sleeping, or even while at rest. Often, loss of circumoral muscle tone is first recognized when the person complains of excessive saliva.

Management of oral motor dysfunction is best achieved with a multidisciplinary approach. Coordinated referrals to specialists in prosthetic dentistry, rehabilitative medicine, speech pathology, and gastroenterology may be needed.

GUSTATORY DYSFUNCTION

Adequate taste and smell are essential not only for proper food selection but for protection against ingesting spoiled food. Anecdotally, **gus-**

tatory function declines with age. However, recent data suggest that changes in healthy older persons are modest and are specific to the taste quality affected (ie, sweet, sour, salty, or bitter).

Food enjoyment also requires other sensory cues (eg, olfactory and textural). Although few studies of nongustatory oral sensory function have been conducted in older persons, direct measurement of **olfactory function** has shown marked impairment. Thus, an assessment of olfactory function must be included in any evaluation of gustatory or food enjoyment complaints in the elderly.

Hypogeusia, *a decreased ability to taste,* or **dysgeusia,** *the presence of a persistent bad taste in the mouth,* may be associated with neuropathy, URI, drug usage, dental therapy, trauma, menopause, and a host of systemic diseases, but the linkages are weak. Most gustatory complaints by the elderly are likely to be related to dental status and poor oral hygiene, eg, the presence of a dental or periodontal abscess may allow purulent material to distort gustatory signals. Also, many elderly persons have difficulty maintaining good oral hygiene. Poor hygiene, particularly around teeth with extensive restorations or dental prostheses, may result in chronic unpleasant sensations of taste.

Diagnosis

Assessment of gustatory complaints should begin with a thorough history. If the unpleasant taste is usually associated with meals or can be rinsed away with water, suspicion should center on dental disease and dental hygiene. If no local oral cause seems likely, history of head trauma or upper respiratory disease should be checked. Cranial nerve evaluation should include the 1st (olfactory), 7th (facial), 9th (glossopharyngeal), and 10th (vagus) nerves.

Tests for taste: Detailed, meaningful tests of gustatory performance are difficult to administer in a typical clinical setting. If results of screening procedures are inadequate, referral for intensive testing may be necessary.

Tests for olfaction: A useful, reliable, and easy-to-use odor recognition test is the University of Pennsylvania Smell Identification Test. It is a prepackaged, scratch-and-sniff test that requires minimal supervision during administration and is easy to score.

Treatment

There are no good therapies for gustatory dysfunction. Use of zinc preparations appears to have little more than a placebo effect. If olfactory disorders relate to airway obstruction, surgical correction may be possible. Meticulous documentation of complaints and reassurance to patients of the presence of measurable sensory deficits are often helpful and appreciated.

SALIVARY GLAND DISORDERS

Adequate salivary gland function is essential to all aspects of oral function. Resting (basal) salivary production helps protect oral tissues, and stimulated salivary flow is needed for nutrition. Saliva is necessary for proper food bolus formation and translocation, for lubrication and integrity of the oral mucosa, and for prevention of demineralization and promotion of remineralization of teeth. Saliva contains at least 6 antimicrobial proteins that control bacterial colonization patterns in the mouth as well as limit fungal and viral growth. Saliva buffers acids produced by oral bacteria, and mechanically cleanses the mouth. Any situation that affects salivary gland secretion obviously will have broad-ranging negative sequelae.

Many studies have suggested that in older people salivary gland morphology is altered, with parallel reductions in salivary fluid production. Recent studies in carefully defined populations indicate that no general reduction in salivary performance occurs with age; resting and stimulated parotid gland function remains intact throughout the life span. The statistically significant reductions in submandibular/sublingual saliva seen in the well elderly are probably not biologically significant. Most age-related changes in salivary function are attributed to systemic disorders or their treatment.

Etiology

1. Iatrogenic: The most common causes of gland dysfunction are drug related. Xerostomia is a potential side effect of > 400 drugs (see TABLE 44 –1), many of which are used frequently by elderly persons. In addition, head and neck irradiation and cytotoxic chemotherapy for neoplasms have direct, dramatic effects on salivary gland performance.

2. Sjögren's syndrome (SS), *an autoimmune exocrinopathy, primarily affecting postmenopausal women,* is the most common disease affecting salivary glands in older persons. SS may be a primary disorder (affecting only the salivary and lacrimal glands) or a secondary form (glandular effects plus connective tissue disease).

Other, less frequently observed conditions that affect salivary glands include bacterial infections, sialoliths, trauma, and neoplasms.

TABLE 44–1. DRUGS THAT AFFECT SALIVATION

Analgesics	Antipsychotics
Anticholinergics	Other psychotherapeutic drugs
Antidepressants	Diuretics
Antihistaminics	Narcotics
Antihypertensives	Cytotoxic chemotherapeutic drugs

Symptoms and Signs

Xerostomia, *the complaint of oral dryness,* is the most common condition linked with altered salivary performance. It may be associated with reduced salivary output but could result from altered lubricatory factors, defective sensory receptors, or inadequate cortical integration. Patients with true salivary gland dysfunction will present with certain typical symptoms including difficulty swallowing dry foods, the need to take fluids while attempting to swallow, dryness of the mouth and lips during meals, and difficulty in speaking at length. Important signs include an unexpected recent increase in dental caries (especially cervical decay, as noted above) and ulcerated, erythematous, or furrowed mucosa. However, mucosa may appear normal even when gland dysfunction is present.

Diagnosis

Salivary gland status should first be evaluated by careful oral examination. Attempts should be made to assess major gland duct patency and to express saliva from each orifice. Quantitative saliva production should be measured under basal and stimulated conditions. Typically, basal function is severely reduced in affected persons, but many persons will show some stimulated saliva production, indicating the presence of functional gland parenchyma.

Retrograde sialography and **sodium pertechnetate Tc 99m scintigraphy** are useful diagnostic imaging methods. The former is particularly useful when inflammatory or obstructive disorders are suspected; the latter, when objective assessment of acinar function is needed. The radionuclide parallels water movement; both an uptake phase (which shows acinar parenchyma) and an efflux phase (which shows secretion into the mouth) are clearly visualized.

If SS is suspected, biopsy of minor labial salivary glands should be performed, with analysis of several serologic markers of autoimmune disease (eg, ESR, RF, and specific extractable nuclear antigens).

Treatment

Drug-induced gland dysfunction is almost always fully reversible. If the cause is pharmacologic, and action is warranted because of oral complications, either reduction of drug levels or use of alternate drugs may be helpful. In patients with basal secretory deficits who have some stimulated responses, pharmacologic stimulation of salivary glands has been achieved with the cholinergic agent pilocarpine (5 mg orally tid). Patients with autoimmune disorders may also respond to a systemic glucocorticoid (eg, prednisone 30 mg qid).

Patients without functional gland parenchyma have no fluid-transporting cells and will not respond to any directed salivary or systemic therapy. Patients with salivary hypofunction should have frequent, comprehensive, preventive dental care, as noted above.

Salivary substitutes are helpful in limiting hard tissue problems but unsatisfactory for soft tissue complaints. For the latter, only palliative therapy is available. Mouthwashes, including topical analgesics and antimicrobials, are helpful.

---

45. FUNCTIONAL DISORDERS OF THE GASTROINTESTINAL TRACT

Joel E. Richter

Disturbances of gut physiology arising as part of an array of adaptive reactions to life stress. Patients with such complaints account for about 60% of all consultations with physicians for GI symptoms and for approximately 2.4% of all hospital admissions. Although traditionally considered problems of young and middle-aged individuals, functional GI disorders are increasingly encountered in geriatric patients. Loss of a spouse, emotional adjustment to retirement, and frustration resulting from the aging process all contribute to the psychophysiologic stresses faced by elderly patients. The physician must be aware of these behavioral adjustments but not overlook potentially life-threatening organic illnesses presenting with changes in emotions.

Approach to the Patient

A patient-oriented clinical approach, with appreciation of the psychosocial aspects of illness as outlined below, should be followed in patients with possible psychophysiologic complaints.

1. The history should be obtained in an open-ended interview. Questions that encourage the patient to respond spontaneously prevent physician bias from affecting the content of the history. Leading questions or those that elicit yes or no answers should be avoided at first. The historical information should be obtained from the perspective of the patient's understanding of the illness. The symptoms are then likely to be presented by the patient in relation to physiologic and psychologic events that contribute to the illness. At all times, the questions should communicate the physician's willingness to consider all aspects of the illness, whether biologic or psychogenic.

2. The role of psychologic stress factors must be considered. Such information should be sought within the context of the emotional concerns and social setting at the time of onset of symptoms. This is often achieved by having the patient reconstruct the story as it occurred. Rather than asking at the end of the history, "Are you under stress?" a more open-ended request early in the interview, eg, "Tell me what happened and how you felt during your last attack," is less threatening and presents the patient with the opportunity to offer medical and psychologic data concurrently.

3. Decisions must often be made with incomplete or nonspecific information. The tendency to order studies or surgery that is not needed in order to "do something" for the insistent patient with inexplicable complaints should be avoided. When the initial examination and studies are unrevealing and the patient is clinically stable, it is wiser to tolerate the uncertainty in diagnosis and observe the patient for new objective developments over time.

4. A behavioral disorder does not preclude the presence or future development of medical disease. Complete objectivity must guide the approach to even the most vague, dramatic, or bizarre symptom complex. New physical findings or laboratory data suggesting pathologic changes (blood in the stool, fever, anemia) should prompt further evaluation.

5. Removal of the symptoms is not always the goal of treatment. The illness may have such adaptive value to the patient that giving up the so-called benefits of the illness may be a greater loss than the gain achieved from relief of symptoms. When the patient overtly or covertly resists management, the illness can be assumed to fulfill certain needs. In such cases, the illness must be accepted and treatment oriented toward improving function despite the continuation of the symptoms. This approach results in more realistic therapeutic goals, which are more favorable to the patient and less frustrating to the physician.

6. Psychotropic drugs and psychiatric consultations should be used as adjuncts to a good therapeutic relationship between patient and physician. The indications for such treatment should not be based on the severity of complaints but rather on the affective state of the patient. The acutely anxious patient (as evidenced by observation of speech and nonverbal behavior as well as by patient description), whose daily functioning is impaired, can be treated briefly with a benzodiazepine. Tricyclic antidepressants are most helpful in the patient with so-called organic signs of depression (eg, sleep disturbance, weight loss, constipation, loss of libido, and psychomotor retardation), particularly if there is a past or family history of depression. Referrals to a psychiatrist or a psychologist may be viewed as physician abandonment by some patients. Explanations about the reasons for referral, reassurance, and short periodic follow-up visits with the primary physician will do much to ensure the patient's well-being and confidence in his total medical care.

NONCARDIAC CHEST PAIN

Up to 30% of patients with typical or atypical angina-like pain have normal coronary arteries on angiography. Most of them are older women whose chest pain is unrelated to exertion. Coronary artery spasm or small-vessel coronary disease does not appear to be the underlying problem, since the overall clinical course is favorable. Long-term follow-up studies in > 2500 patients revealed that MIs (1.6%) and cardiac death (0.5%) were rare. Nevertheless, these patients suffer real disability if they are not given an alternative diagnosis for their complaints.

They continue to have a limited life-style, frequently are unable to work, and often still believe they have heart disease.

Etiology and Pathophysiology

The most common identifiable causes of noncardiac chest pain are **musculoskeletal** and **esophageal problems.** Other causes include pulmonary embolism, pneumonia, peptic ulcer, biliary tract disease, thoracic pain, and pain from the colon, usually in patients with the irritable bowel syndrome.

Several reports suggest that up to 50% of patients with noncardiac chest pain may have an esophageal cause. More recently, however, ambulatory 24-h pH and pressure monitoring suggests that traditional esophageal causes of noncardiac chest pain may not be as common as previously reported. For example, 2 studies have found that only 30% of chest pain episodes can be directly correlated with acid reflux or motility disorders during prolonged monitoring. Patients with gastroesophageal reflux usually have heartburn, but 5 to 20% may present with only atypical chest pain. Although acid reflux may cause esophageal dysmotility, current data favor stimulation of acid-sensitive chemoreceptors as the cause of chest pain. Theoretically, esophageal motility disorders could stimulate chest pain by high-amplitude, nonperistaltic contractions producing esophageal myoischemia or retarding bolus movement.

The most common esophageal motility disorder associated with noncardiac chest pain is a manometric syndrome characterized by high-amplitude peristaltic contractions confined to the distal esophagus, the **"nutcracker esophagus."** However, esophageal studies have often been inferential because spontaneous chest pain is rarely observed in the manometry laboratory. Therefore, provocative tests, eg, acid perfusion of the esophagus (Bernstein test) and edrophonium (Tensilon® 80 µg/kg IV), have been used to stimulate suspected esophageal chest pain. These tests reproduce suspected esophageal chest pain (positive test) in 20 to 30% of patients, regardless of the presence of a baseline motility disorder.

Psychologic factors and life stresses may contribute to or cause chest pain. Studies suggest that individuals with noncardiac chest pain have more physical complaints than age-matched controls and score higher on psychologic measures of neuroticism and depression. Two studies in patients with noncardiac chest pain and esophageal motility disorders also have confirmed a high frequency of psychiatric diagnoses, primarily depression, anxiety, and somatization. These psychologic profiles are similar to those reported in patients with the irritable bowel syndrome **(IBS).** A recent study reported that > 50% of patients with noncardiac chest pain have intermittent complaints of abdominal pain, diarrhea, or constipation consistent with IBS. Further, these patients have a lower visceral pain threshold to esophageal balloon distention, similar to that observed in patients with IBS after rectal balloon distention. These observations suggest that many patients with noncardiac chest pain may have a form of IBS, ie, **"the irritable esophagus."**

Diagnosis

The differential diagnosis of noncardiac chest pain first demands that cardiac disease be adequately excluded. In older patients, this may require coronary angiography, possibly with ergonovine testing. Occasionally pericarditis and mitral valve prolapse may cause recurrent chest pain.

It is important to find a cause for chest pain in these patients, if for no other reason than to reassure them. After cardiac disease is excluded, emphasis should be placed on the musculoskeletal and upper GI system. Unfortunately, clinical history alone is frequently not helpful in separating diseases of these systems from cardiac problems. A thorough musculoskeletal examination should be performed, with particular attention to locating trigger points that replicate the patient's pain syndrome. Trigger points painful to palpation on the anterior and posterior chest wall can be identified in 10 to 15% of patients with noncardiac chest pain. These musculoskeletal abnormalities may represent part of the **fibromyositis syndrome.** An elevated ESR also supports an inflammatory cause for pain.

Structural lesions of the upper GI tract should be excluded by barium studies or endoscopy. Patients should also undergo a screening evaluation for gallstones, either oral cholecystography or abdominal ultrasound. However, *be aware that many gallstones are silent.* If esophagitis or an ulcer is found, no further testing is required. Further evaluation for an esophageal cause of chest pain may be done with the Bernstein and edrophonium tests. These can be performed in the office, without esophageal manometry. If the tests reproduce the patient's typical chest pain, a diagnosis of an esophageal cause can be made. If the tests are negative, additional studies with manometry and prolonged ambulatory monitoring may be warranted.

Treatment

If a favorable patient-doctor relationship is established, most patients will respond to confident reassurance based on careful diagnostic studies. This supportive approach results in better patient acceptance of symptoms, less limitation of life-style, and frequently, a diminution or even resolution of the chest pain. More specific therapy should be directed at identifiable causes of noncardiac chest pain. Musculoskeletal problems can be treated with nonsteroidal anti-inflammatory drugs **(NSAIDs).** If there is any possibility of gastroesophageal reflux, it should be vigorously treated with life-style modification and histamine H_2 receptor blockers. Esophageal motility disorders may respond to sublingual nitroglycerin, anticholinergics (eg, dicyclomine 20 mg tid), or Ca channel blocking agents (nifedipine 10 to 20 mg tid or diltiazem 60 to 90 mg tid). In patients with clinical evidence of anxiety and/or depression, psychotropic drugs (including amitriptyline 50 to 150 mg/day or trazodone 100 to 150 mg/day) can aid in relieving symptoms. Although not extensively studied, behavior-modification programs and biofeedback may also be beneficial in the long-term management of noncardiac chest pain.

GLOBUS HYSTERICUS

The subjective sensation of a lump in the throat. No specific etiology or physiologic mechanism has been established for this condition. Some studies suggest that elevated upper esophageal sphincter pressure or abnormal hypopharyngeal motility is present when symptoms occur. Other reports suggest an increased incidence of gastroesophageal reflux. Frequent swallowing with aerophagia and drying of the throat associated with emotional states may also contribute to the symptoms.

The term "globus hystericus" is probably a misnomer. In a recent controlled study of 20 patients, nearly all were obsessive, many were depressed, but few were hysterical. The globus sensation resembles the normal reaction of being choked up during events that elicit feelings of grief, pride, or even happiness. Clinically, chronic symptoms may occur during states of unresolved grief and may be relieved by crying.

Diagnosis

Medical disorders that can be confused with globus hystericus include esophageal webs, esophageal motility disorders, gastroesophageal reflux, musculoskeletal disorders (eg, myasthenia gravis, myotonic dystrophy, and polymyositis), or mass lesions in the neck or mediastinum causing esophageal compression. Most often, a careful history and physical examination can exclude these disorders. With globus hystericus, the symptoms occur during certain emotional states and do not worsen during swallowing. Food does not stick in the throat, and the symptoms are occasionally relieved with eating. There is no pain or weight loss. True dysphagia must be ruled out, because it would suggest a structural or motor disorder of the pharynx or esophagus. This can best be done with a cine-esophagogram.

Treatment involves primarily reassurance. No drug has proved beneficial. Underlying depression, anxiety, or other behavioral disturbances should be managed. One older controlled study suggests that such patients significantly benefit from treatment of anxiety with benzodiazepines. At times, providing support and indicating the association of the symptoms with the patient's mood can be beneficial.

NONULCER DYSPEPSIA

A symptom complex, often related to eating, that includes intermittent epigastric pain, bloating, fullness, gaseousness, nausea, and heartburn. These symptoms may suggest peptic ulcer disease; however, between $1/3$ and $1/2$ of patients are found at endoscopy not to have an ulcer. Although a heterogeneous group, these patients have been collectively labeled as having nonulcer dyspepsia. Other terms for this syndrome include nervous stomach, nervous dyspepsia, functional dyspepsia, flatulent dyspepsia, Moynihan's disease, or simply indigestion.

Pathophysiology

The mechanism of symptoms in unexplained dyspepsia is unknown. Older studies have shown that 10 to 40% of patients with normal x-rays and dyspepsia develop peptic ulcer disease. Although endoscopy is a more sensitive technic for excluding ulcer disease, long-term follow-up data are not available to assess the proportion of patients with normal endoscopy and dyspepsia who suffer from unrecognized peptic ulcer disease. This rate would probably be low, because most studies report normal or low basal acid output. Gastritis or duodenitis is found in some patients, but the relationship to symptoms remains uncertain.

Abnormalities in GI motility may contribute to the symptoms of nonulcer dyspepsia. In some patients with flatulent dyspepsia, delayed gastric emptying has been demonstrated by radioisotope scintigraphy. The reflux of alkaline duodenal contents may precipitate symptoms in susceptible patients. Balloon distention studies have shown that epigastric discomfort can be produced by distention of the transverse colon. Fats and many drugs, including NSAIDs, aspirin, alcohol, and tobacco, may also help cause dyspepsia without producing a definite ulcer or gastritis.

Although scientific data are limited, emotional factors generally are thought to play an important role in the genesis of dyspepsia. Several studies confirm a higher prevalence of anxiety, neuroticism, and depression in nonulcer dyspepsia patients than in the general population. These personality characteristics are not related to patients' symptomatic status. Dyspeptic patients are reported to have more negative life stresses associated with the onset of symptoms and to view life as more stressful than controls; they may also have lower pain thresholds.

Diagnosis

Dyspepsia is identified from the patient's history. The pain is epigastric, usually described as burning or gnawing, and intermittent. Generally, the pain is not relieved with meals nor does it awaken the patient at night. Up to 30% of patients report weight loss. If the pain is associated with heartburn, gastroesophageal reflux should be suspected. Pain associated with defecation or with abnormal bowel movements suggests IBS. With nonulcer dyspepsia, physical examination will show no masses or organomegaly and evidence of good nutrition. The presence or absence of epigastric tenderness is not a reliable indicator of peptic ulcer disease. Routine hematologic and biochemical tests produce normal results.

Upper GI endoscopy is the most sensitive and specific method of excluding organic lesions of the esophagus, stomach, and duodenum. Nevertheless, many patients will still be evaluated initially by barium studies, but these may miss 10 to 20% of peptic ulcers and most mucosal lesions. If symptoms persist or are associated with weight loss, endoscopy should be performed. Older persons with severe, persistent pain should also be evaluated by CT scan to exclude pancreatic cancer and by barium enema or colonoscopy to rule out a colonic lesion in the transverse colon.

Treatment

The most important component in treating dyspepsia is reassurance. Many patients have an inordinate fear of cancer that reinforces and magnifies symptoms; this should be eliminated as firmly and quickly as possible.

Three controlled trials have failed to show that either cimetidine or ranitidine is superior to placebo in the treatment of nonulcer dyspepsia. There is no evidence that antacids are effective, but the placebo response rate in most patients with a GI illness is 20 to 80%. One double-blind study showed that nonulcer dyspeptic symptoms responded equally to placebo and an aluminum-containing antacid preparation. Since antacids produce few side effects, they can safely be recommended, as can simethicone tablets in the treatment of flatulence. Metoclopramide (10 mg tid before meals) may also be useful in flatulent patients with delayed gastric emptying; however, side effects are particularly common in the elderly and may be severe (ie, parkinsonism and tardive dyskinesia). The role of sucralfate in nonulcer dyspepsia remains to be tested.

The prognosis depends upon one's point of view. In terms of life expectancy, the outlook is excellent. Peptic ulcer disease will develop in a small percentage of patients. However, the dyspepsia may persist for a lifetime. In a recent study, 70% of patients had intermittent symptoms 2 yr after initial evaluation.

IRRITABLE BOWEL SYNDROME (IBS)

A motility disorder consisting of altered bowel habits, abdominal pain, and the absence of detectable organic pathology.

IBS represents 20 to 50% of all GI complaints in private and institutional care facilities. Symptoms are markedly influenced by psychologic factors and stressful life situations. However, surveys indicate that symptoms justifying the diagnosis of IBS are present in at least 15% of the general population who do not seek medical attention. Female patients outnumber male patients 2:1, and whites have a higher incidence than nonwhites. The preponderance of women with this diagnosis may reflect their greater tendency to seek health care rather than actual incidence.

Symptoms begin before age 35 in $\frac{1}{2}$ of patients, and 40% of patients are 35 to 50 yr of age. IBS is a chronic disorder; symptom severity fluctuates; and, although remission may last several years, recurrence is the rule. Geriatric patients usually have a long history of bowel dysfunction, often beginning in childhood. Initial presentation in the elderly is uncommon and demands a thorough search for organic causes of bowel dysfunction.

Pathophysiology

Although IBS is considered by many to be a disorder of intestinal motility, the motor dysfunctions recorded in the laboratory correlate imperfectly with the clinical pattern and frequently may be simple exaggerations of normal responses. Abdominal pain, which originates in stretch receptors in the distal colon, is caused by distention of the bowel with gas and stool or spastic contractions of the bowel. Under baseline conditions, the colonic motility of IBS patients and that of normals are indistinguishable. However, IBS patients show greater colonic motility in response to emotional arousal, pain, balloon distention, eating, and pharmacologic stimulation by cholecystokinin or pentagastrin. These motility changes differ quantitatively rather than qualitatively from those in normal subjects, suggesting that IBS patients are hyperreactive to a variety of stimuli.

A common myoelectric pattern reported by some groups consists of a greater frequency of slow-wave (3 cycle/min) activity. Other investigators have observed that constipation is related to an increased incidence of short-spike bursts and that diarrhea and postprandial pain are related to a relative absence of long-spike bursts. However, several research groups have failed to support these hypotheses, and they must be regarded as tentative. Finally, balloon distention studies of the rectum suggest that IBS patients may have abnormalities in sensory nerves or in the psychologic processes that mediate pain perception. Therefore, low visceral pain thresholds may characterize IBS patients, but the relationship to colonic motility is unclear.

Psychometric tests reveal that IBS patients are more psychologically disturbed than normal subjects, but they do not reveal any pattern of psychologic traits specific for IBS. Psychiatric diagnoses are noted in 70 to 90% of IBS patients. The most common are depression, anxiety, and somatization (the substitution of bodily complaints for anxiety or depression). Two lines of evidence suggest that psychogenic factors are not a result of the disorder but rather contribute to the onset and exacerbation of symptoms. In 85% of patients, psychologic factors either precede or coincide with the onset of symptoms. Moreover, $\frac{1}{2}$ of patients also note an association between emotional stress and exacerbation of symptoms. Most of the stressors mentioned by patients are everyday concerns about family, work relations, or finances. In the elderly, cancer phobias may predominate and need to be treated.

Symptoms and Signs

Classic IBS symptoms include abdominal pain, erratic bowel habits, and variation in stool consistency. More nonspecific symptoms include bloating, gas, dyspepsia, headache, fatigue, lassitude, and flatulence. **Two major groups of IBS patients are recognized.** In the first group, the **spastic colon type,** most patients have pain over one or more areas of the colon associated with periodic constipation or diarrhea. Most complain of lower abdominal pain or discomfort over the course of the sigmoid colon. The pain is either colicky or a continuous dull ache, commonly triggered by meals, especially breakfast, and may be relieved by a bowel movement. Patients may have either constipation or diarrhea; in some, the 2 alternate. Increased mucus is frequently noted around the stools. The second group of IBS patients complain primarily of **painless diarrhea**. They usually have urgent, precipitous diarrhea that occurs immediately upon arising or, more typically, during or immediately after a meal. Incontinence may occur, but nocturnal diarrhea is unusual.

On physical examination, patients with either type generally appear to be in good health. However, they are frequently tense and anxious, with autonomic lability evidenced by rapid, labile pulse; elevated BP; or sweaty palms. Palpation of the abdomen may reveal tenderness, particularly in the left lower quadrant over the sigmoid colon.

Diagnosis

The diagnosis of IBS is based on a characteristic clinical history and the meticulous exclusion of many other disorders that have similar manifestations. A CBC and ESR should be obtained to rule out anemia and inflammation. Stools must be cultured and examined for occult blood, ova, and parasites. Sigmoidoscopy and barium enema examination are essential in the geriatric patient to rule out more serious underlying disease. Sigmoidoscopy usually reveals normal mucosa except for mild hyperemia and increased mucus. Reproduction of symptoms with air insufflation is a further suggestive finding. Mucosal biopsies may help one exclude early ulcerative colitis or collagenous colitis. A double-contrast barium enema may show exaggerated haustral contractions, particularly in the descending colon or, conversely, effacement and absence of normal haustral markings, often with a lumen of narrowed caliber.

Concomitant diverticulosis may be present, and some authorities suggest that IBS may be the precursor of diverticular disease. If weight loss or obstructive symptoms are present, an abdominal CT scan and small-bowel series should be obtained to exclude malignancy, Crohn's disease, and adhesions. A 3-wk trial of a lactose-free diet is recommended in all patients who complain of distention, bloating, or diarrhea. Transient lactase deficiency, often precipitated by a viral gastroenteritis, may mimic IBS in older persons. *De novo IBS symptoms are distinctly uncommon in the geriatric patient.* Therefore, organic diseases must be excluded before symptomatic therapy is begun. Older IBS patients usually have a long history of bowel problems, but they need to be carefully reevaluated periodically to rule out any intercurrent pathologic process.

Treatment

A firm diagnosis of IBS can usually be established within the first few visits. The patient should be informed and reassured that the necessary tests have been performed to rule out organic disease, particularly cancer. The simple act of applying a name to the disorder may provide comfort. It should be emphasized that the colonic spasm and resulting pain are real and that they are influenced by a number of factors that need to be managed to control the symptoms.

Explanation of the chronic, recurrent nature of the condition will allay some of the alarm caused by persistent or recurrent symptoms. The patient should be assured that IBS does not lead to more serious illness or in any way shorten one's life span. Reassurance and psychologic support are key factors in dealing with the anxiety and stress. It is particularly important to explore with the patient not only possible precipitating factors but also the patient's reaction to them. Frequent but not necessarily prolonged follow-up visits may be required initially and gradually reduced as the patient develops more effective coping mechanisms.

In general, a high-fiber diet should be followed. Psyllium preparations bind water, thus preventing excessive dehydration of stool as well as excess liquidity. They are useful in IBS patients who have either diarrhea or constipation. These hydrophilic colloids should be taken at mealtime so they mix with the stool as it is being formed. Antispasmodics mainly provide relief from painful cramps, but such relief usually is neither dramatic nor permanent. Antispasmodics (eg, dicyclomine 20 mg, propantheline bromide 15 mg, or tincture of belladonna 10 to 20 drops) are given 30 to 45 min before meals to decrease the typical postprandial pain. When diarrhea is severe, frequent small doses of diphenoxylate 2.5 to 5 mg q 4 to 6 h or loperamide 2 mg q 4 to 8 h can be prescribed.

In depressed IBS patients, antidepressant drugs, given either in divided doses or as a single dose at night (eg, amitriptyline 10 to 25 mg tid before meals or 25 to 75 mg at bedtime), have been found to be more helpful than tranquilizing drugs. Relaxation training, provided by a behavioral psychologist or by audiotapes, may also be useful.

PSYCHOGENIC ABDOMINAL PAIN

Very few patients with chronic abdominal pain referred to diagnostic centers are given a specific medical diagnosis. When such patients are studied psychologically, abnormalities of personality and behavior, which presumably explain their symptoms, are often reported. Therefore, psychogenic abdominal pain may commonly be seen by nonpsychiatric physicians.

The true prevalence of psychogenic abdominal pain in unknown. The problem predominates in women over men by 4:1, and most patients are < 50 yr of age. However, geriatric patients may constitute 10 to 20% of this group. Chronic, unrelenting pain, usually of > 6 mo duration and not relieved by bowel movements, characterizes this syndrome. When asked to describe their symptoms, patients initially respond with vague statements, eg, "sharp" or "aching," but when questioned further, descriptions tend to become more personalized and often bizarre, eg, "like blowing out my side" or "a hot poker sticking into my belly." Many patients also have nonspecific symptoms including nausea, bloating, dizziness, fatigue, or musculoskeletal complaints. Up to 30% may have associated symptoms compatible with the IBS.

Diagnosis is difficult because physicians vary in ability to obtain psychologic data, and many patients resist referrals to psychiatrists and psychologists. When carefully and patiently questioned, most patients report antecedent events that were experienced as personal losses, eg, the death of a close family member or events related to childbearing and its disruption. In most cases, symptoms develop soon after the anniversary of the event. Frequently, there is evidence of incomplete grieving, manifested by talking as if the person were still there or by an inability to cry or visit the grave. Depression, hypochondriasis, histrionic or pain-prone personality, or a combination of these disorders may be identified by psychologic testing, but almost 40% of patients have no psychiatric diagnosis.

Treatment

These patients are difficult to manage and often frustrate the physician. They see themselves as medical patients and are reluctant to obtain psychiatric evaluation and treatment. The psychiatric consultant can help the primary care physician confirm the diagnosis and provide treatment guidelines, but general management is best directed by the nonpsychiatric physician. For such patients, a reasonably successful outcome is improvement of psychosocial function (eg, return to work, church, or social activities) despite the pain, rather than complete pain resolution. For some patients with a relatively short duration of symptoms and without evidence of personality disorders, a greater degree of improvement and even pain resolution can be anticipated. Symptoms frequently appear during times of personal stress (eg, the anniversary of the traumatic antecedent event, a meaningful birthday, or the Thanksgiving-Christmas holiday season).

FECAL INCONTINENCE
(See also FECAL INCONTINENCE in Ch. 48)

Instances in which the individual loses stool from the rectum at inappropriate times. For many geriatric patients, this represents a humiliating regression in bodily function, severely impairing activity and socialization. Some 16 to 60% of institutionalized older persons are estimated to have some degree of fecal incontinence. Many also have bladder incontinence.

Etiology

The preservation of continence is complex, and its failure is usually multifactorial. One factor may be impairment of voluntary contraction of the external sphincter as a result of nerve damage from traumatic vaginal childbirth, rectal prolapse (procidentia), prior anal surgery (hemorrhoidectomy, anal dilatation, sphincterotomy), or spinal cord injuries. Diabetes and autonomic neuropathy may produce internal sphincter dysfunction.

Diarrhea of any cause may contribute to incontinence, particularly in the elderly, who frequently have decreased sphincteric pressures and continence for liquids compared with younger persons. Fecal impaction is a common cause of diarrhea in the geriatric population; the stool proximal to the obstructing fecal mass becomes liquefied and oozes around the fecalith. Since such patients usually have long-standing constipation and frequent megacolon, they cannot sense the movement of stool into the rectal vault and the fecal impaction tonically inhibits the internal anal sphincter, leading to fecal incontinence.

Diagnosis and Treatment

Evaluation should begin with consideration of the underlying causes. Although examination of the rectum may show decreased sphincter tone, there is generally a poor correlation between digital examination of rectal tone and objective measurements. Appropriate GI, neurologic, and endocrine studies should be done and treatment individualized. When constipation and fecal impaction are present, the mass must be digitally removed with the help of tap water or Fleet® enemas, and bowel habits should be normalized by administering bulking agents, stool softeners (eg, docusate sodium 50 to 200 mg/day), or mild laxatives (eg, 1 to 2 tbsp milk of magnesia/day or 1 tbsp lactulose or sorbitol bid) to produce 1 to 2 soft bowel movements/day. All these doses can be titrated upward to control constipation.

If diarrhea is a contributing factor, underlying causes should be treated when possible. Nonspecific diarrhea can be treated with bulking agents, antidiarrheal drugs (loperamide or diphenoxylate), and daily sphincter exercises. If sphincter tone is markedly decreased, a regular pattern of enemas may be considered to achieve bowel cleansing. Surgical treatment of incontinence has yielded inconsistent results.

Biofeedback therapy is the most exciting advance in the treatment of fecal incontinence. Successful treatment requires a well-motivated subject who can comprehend and follow directions and who has an external anal sphincter capable of recognizing and responding to rectal distention. Using a 3-balloon rectal system, patients see on the physiologic tracing a normal external anal sphincter contraction during maximal rectal distention and try to reproduce that pattern. The visual picture of the rectal manometric recording provides the biofeedback. Increasing sensitivity is taught using decreasing rectal distending volumes. Because patients frequently improve after a single session, reenforcement sessions are often unnecessary.

Biofeedback has been successful in the treatment of > 70% of patients with incontinence due to sensory or motor impairment. In one study of 18 geriatric patients, 15 improved by at least 50% and 6 were continent after biofeedback training. However, some types of incontinence do not respond to biofeedback, such as severe sensory loss incontinence (eg, diabetes, spinal cord injury) or incontinence resulting from poor rectal compliance (eg, rectal trauma, radiation injury).

46. GASTROINTESTINAL ENDOSCOPY

Jerome D. Waye

Endoscopy is a general term for *the visual inspection of body cavities by instrumentation.* Specific names are derived from the area being examined, so that esophagogastroduodenoscopy **(EGD)** refers to upper GI endoscopy and colonoscopy describes lower GI endoscopy.

Endoscopic fiberoptic technology was developed in the 1950s, and electronic image transmission became clinically useful in the 1980s. Instruments vary in length from 30 to 185 cm, with a special 300-cm enteroscope for inspection of the small intestine. Most endoscopic procedures are performed with the patient under some sedation after appropriate bowel preparation: no food or drink, to render the stomach empty, or a purgative, to cleanse the colon. Although originally considered a complementary procedure to a previous barium x-ray study, many endoscopic examinations are currently performed as the primary evaluation of the GI tract. Neither color changes (eg, gastritis) nor bleeding can be identified radiographically, and both biopsy and therapeutic maneuvers are possible during endoscopic examination.

The flexible instruments have operator-controlled tip deflection capability, which permits guidance through the intestinal lumen. A high-intensity external light source illuminates the field under examination while the image is transmitted through fiberoptic bundles to the operator's eye or via digitized signals (videoendoscope) to a television screen. An internal channel permits the passage of biopsy or grasping forceps, wire snares (for polypectomy), injection needles, and electrocoagulation or laser probes and also allows fluid instillation (for flushing debris from the intestinal wall) or suction aspiration.

GI endoscopy is generally well tolerated by the elderly. However, endoscopic procedures must be performed only for appropriate indications, since complications of invasive investigations are more frequent in this group than in younger persons. Not only are older tissues more fragile and more easily traumatized, but older patients generally have various other medical problems besides the GI complaint.

The older patient is more sensitive to sedative and analgesic drugs; therefore, the doses must be age-adjusted to prevent adverse reactions. Benzodiazepines are among the most frequently used drugs for preendoscopy sedation, and doses may require diminution by 50 to 75% to guard against cardiorespiratory depression. During endoscopy in the sedated elderly patient, attention must frequently be directed to skin color, pulse, and respiration to ensure that the depressant effects of premedication are not overlooked during the pursuit of a diagnosis. Even more important is close monitoring of these factors during emergency endoscopy, since events happen rapidly and the patient's homeostatic mechanisms may be only marginally functioning. Resuscitation of the acutely ill patient takes precedence over the performance of any procedure.

Symptoms in elderly patients may be atypical. Early endoscopy for GI bleeding may aid the physician in selecting patients for whom early surgical intervention is life-saving. The diagnostic accuracy of endoscopic retrograde cholangiopancreatography (ERCP) in the jaundiced patient is unsurpassed, and technics for removal of stones from the bile duct or placement of a stent for biliary decompression through a malignant tumor obstruction may circumvent the need for surgery altogether. The source of unexplained GI bleeding or iron deficiency anemia is frequently determined by colonoscopy, since the blood loss often originates in the colon, an area in which x-ray investigation may be inaccurate.

Transient bacteremia is reported infrequently during endoscopic examination, and patients at high risk for infection should receive antibiotics (usually ampicillin and gentamicin) prior to the examination. High-risk patients are those with valvular heart disease (rheumatic heart disease and valvular prosthesis), neutropenia, and artificial joint implants.

UPPER GASTROINTESTINAL ENDOSCOPY
(Esophagogastroduodenoscopy [EGD])

Visualization of the entire upper GI tract (to the second portion of the duodenum) is the goal during EGD examination.

Indications

Diagnostic indications include exploration of either undiagnosed upper GI symptoms or an abnormality on upper GI x-ray series. An x-ray is not a prerequisite for upper GI endoscopy, since the gastroscope may be passed safely under direct vision even in patients with dysphagia and a possible Zenker's diverticulum. Any pathologic process (ulcer, mass, irregularity) can be characterized by inspection and biopsy. Brush cytology may increase the yield of diagnostic findings in malignant disease.

EGD may be used to monitor the healing rate of gastric ulcer, but endoscopic follow-up in cases of duodenal ulcer is usually unnecessary. Periodic endoscopy and biopsy in Barrett's syndrome, a premalignant process, will detect early evidence of cancer. EGD is the best means of identifying the site of upper GI bleeding and should be performed as soon as the patient is stable; however, whether identification of the bleeding site positively affects the patient's outcome is controversial. The addition of endoscopic therapy for bleeding has markedly enhanced the value of EGD.

Therapeutic indications include dilation of esophageal strictures with a dilator threaded over an endoscopically placed guide wire or under direct vision with a balloon catheter passed through the scope (TTS balloon). An obstructing neoplasm of the esophagus or stomach may be vaporized with a laser wave guide passed through the gastroscope or with a bipolar tumor probe under endoscopic guidance.

Therapy for upper GI bleeding is more readily accomplished with special electrocoagulation equipment (monopolar or bipolar electrodes, heater probe) passed through the scope than with a laser. Sclerotherapy for esophageal varices and injection therapy for actively bleeding vessels may be performed during the initial diagnostic endoscopic examination by passing a long, flexible needle-tipped catheter through the endoscope to inject various medications. An esophageal stent prosthesis can be placed over a guide wire after precise endoscopic localization. Polyps may be resected using a wire snare loop and an electrocoagulation current to prevent bleeding.

Submucosal lesions are not usually amenable to endoscopic resection. Removal of foreign bodies from the esophagus or stomach may require special maneuvers, including affixing to the tip of the endoscope a shield that folds over a sharp object to prevent esophageal injury during extraction. Foreign bodies smaller than the size of a dime frequently pass spontaneously and may not require endoscopic removal. Food bezoars may sometimes be broken apart with the snare, biopsy forceps, or a strong jet of water. Percutaneous endoscopic gastrostomy **(PEG)** is a technic that has largely replaced surgical creation of a feeding gastrostomy and can be accomplished at the bedside with little risk.

Contraindications and Risks

Absolute contraindications are recent MI and acute perforated viscus.

Relative risks: In general, elderly patients tolerate upper GI endoscopy well. Those with cardiorespiratory disease and dyspnea are at special risk; even without sedation, the P_{O_2} is slightly lowered, and with sedation, some patients are particularly vulnerable to respiratory depression. A small-caliber endoscope may be useful in such patients, and additional O_2 should be administered during the procedure.

Application

Upper GI endoscopy requires a minimal amount of premedication and can be performed rapidly. Both diagnostic and therapeutic maneuvers can be performed during the procedure, and specimens can be obtained, including fluid for analysis, cytology, and biopsy.

Procedure

No food or drink for 6 h before the examination is the only preparation required in most patients. Those with either achalasia or gastric outlet obstruction may have retained food for days and require lavage to empty the esophagus or stomach. Sedation is provided with IV narcotics and/or diazepam. Local anesthetic may be applied to the posterior pharynx. The procedure is usually performed with the patient in the left lateral position; the instrument is passed under direct vision through the pharynx to examine the entire esophagus, stomach, and duodenum.

Complications

Perforation occurs in 0.03% of examinations (3/10,000), and death related to complications occurs in about 0.006% of cases (3/50,000). The highest incidence of complications is related to medication and includes arrhythmias, aspiration, and cardiac arrest. Patients at high risk for infection due to endoscopy-related bacteremia require antibiotic prophylaxis.

COLONOSCOPY

Visualization of the entire colon, including the cecal caput, is the goal of colonoscopy. With training and experience, the examiner accomplishes this in > 90% of cases, but the inexperienced examiner may achieve total intubation in < 80% of attempts. Every colonoscopist should be capable of removing polyps during a diagnostic examination, since the patient is placed at additional discomfort and risk when the preparation and examination must be repeated.

Indications

Diagnostic indications: Most colonoscopic examinations are performed to evaluate an abnormality detected on a preceding barium enema x-ray. During colonoscopy, the mucosa and all lesions are inspected directly, biopsies may be performed on tumors, and polyps may be removed. Not all patients require a preceding x-ray. Primary colonoscopy should be considered in patients with a positive fecal occult blood test or iron deficiency anemia and in those who are at high risk for the development of colorectal cancer (previous colonic polyp, previous colon cancer, strong family history of colon cancer, or ulcerative colitis for > 8 yr). Colonoscopy may be difficult during acute, massive lower GI bleeding, but its use in such cases has been advocated by some investigators. Occasionally, elderly patients are unable to retain barium for an x-ray examination but tolerate colonoscopy quite well.

Therapeutic indications: Removal of colonic polyps can be accomplished without surgery in most patients. Bleeding sites (eg, arteriovenous malformations) may be treated with electrocoagulation, and volvulus may be decompressed, as may the dilated colon in **Ogilvie's syndrome** (acute colonic pseudo-obstruction). Laser vaporization of obstructing rectosigmoid neoplasms may afford symptomatic relief. Strictures may be dilated with balloons or bougies.

Contraindications

Absolute contraindications are fulminant colitis, acute diverticulitis, perforated viscus, and recent MI.

Relative contraindications include poor colon preparation. A poor indication is the use of colonoscopy to elucidate the etiology of chronic abdominal pain.

Application

The risk of colorectal cancer increases with age, but the earliest phases are amenable to colonoscopic diagnosis and treatment by removal of polyps. The most straightforward approach to positive fecal occult blood tests and anemia is to investigate the large bowel by colonoscopy, since the colon is the most frequent site of occult bleeding. If colonoscopy is negative, the patient should have an upper GI endoscopic examination. This schema provides answers rapidly and efficiently, thereby decreasing the time needed to make the proper diagnosis and minimizing the inconvenience to the patient.

Procedure

The colon must be clean. One or 2 days of liquid diet and a potent cathartic (castor oil or citrate of magnesia) with enemas on the day of colonoscopy usually suffice; an orally administered electrolyte preparation with polyethylene glycol may cleanse the large bowel without requiring enemas. Sedation is usually accomplished with IV narcotic and/or diazepam. General anesthesia is unnecessary and undesirable.

The flexible instrument is passed to the cecum under direct vision with a combination of dial-control manipulation, advancement and withdrawal of the instrument shaft, and instillation of air. Fluoroscopy, once considered vital for successful colonoscopy, is now rarely necessary. Every centimeter of the colon's surface may be inspected. Care is required to ensure that potentially blind areas just behind acute bends or colon flexures are not missed. Once the cecum is reached, the small bowel frequently may be entered and a biopsy performed.

Therapy is performed as in EGD examinations. Colon polyps are resected by lassoing the base of the polyps with a wire snare loop and then tightening the snare. Electrocautery current passed through the wire loop during polyp removal prevents bleeding.

Complications

Medication complications are similar to those with EGD. The risk of perforation during routine colonoscopy is about 0.1% and the risk of bleeding, nil. Following polypectomy, perforation occurs in 0.3% and bleeding in 1.5% of patients. Antibiotic prophylaxis is recommended in patients at high risk for infectious complications.

ENDOSCOPIC RETROGRADE CHOLANGIOPANCREATOGRAPHY (ERCP)

A lateral-view endoscope is passed orally to the duodenum for visualization of the ampulla of Vater, into which a cannula is placed under direct vision. Under fluoroscopic monitoring, a dye is injected so that it flows counter to the normal flow of secretions for opacification of the common bile or the pancreatic duct and their tributaries. Because of anatomic positions, a cholangiogram (which involves filling of the biliary tree) is more difficult to obtain than a pancreatogram, but an endoscopist with training and experience can visualize the desired duct in > 90% of cases. An ultrathin fiberscope, the size of a cannula, which can be passed through the ERCP instrument directly into the ducts for direct intraductal visualization, is under investigation.

Indications

Diagnostic indications: The etiology of jaundice and the site of obstruction (if any) can be identified with a high degree of accuracy. ERCP is also useful in demonstrating ductal abnormalities in a nonjaundiced patient when the clinical presentation suggests biliary disease, pancreatic malignancy, or pancreatitis and in the preoperative evaluation of chronic pancreatitis or pancreatic pseudocyst. Pressure measurements, performed in medical centers that are highly specialized, assist in diagnosing sphincter of Oddi dysfunction.

Therapeutic indications: In endoscopic sphincterotomy, the muscular fibers at the distal bile duct sphincter are cut to permit egress of stones that cannot pass spontaneously because of the narrow orifice or the stone size. Acute gallstone pancreatitis may be cured by emergency sphincterotomy. Large stones may be crushed by a lithotriptor or dissolved over several days by instillation of chemicals via an indwelling nasobiliary tube placed through the sphincterotomy. Benign strictures may be dilated with balloons, and malignant obstruction may be treated symptomatically with stent placement. Currently, stones in the gallbladder cannot be treated endoscopically.

Contraindications and Risks

Absolute contraindications are recent MI and perforated viscus.

Application

The correct diagnosis of the cause of jaundice and the ability to relieve biliary or pancreatic ductal obstruction without surgery are tremendous advances in dealing with diseases of the hepatobiliary tree and the pancreas. ERCP is not indicated for evaluation of abdominal pain in the absence of symptoms, signs, or laboratory findings that suggest biliary tract or pancreatic disease, nor is it indicated for the evaluation of suspected gallbladder disease without evidence of bile duct disease. ERCP is of little value when pancreatic malignancy has already been demonstrated by ultrasonography or CT scanning.

Procedure

The stomach and duodenum should be empty, requiring a 6-h fast. Barium contrast in the GI tract may overlie the areas of interest; a history of recent barium ingestion should prompt a pre-ERCP x-ray to ensure its absence. Sedation is accomplished with IV narcotic and/or diazepam.

The lateral-view instrument used for this procedure requires blind passage through the esophagus, although visualization of the stomach is adequate. With the endoscope tip at the papilla of Vater, a plastic cannula is inserted into the ductal orifice—a challenging feat, since neither of the ductular lumens may be discernible. A lever on the instrument's control head helps to direct the cannula tip. Fluoroscopic monitoring during retrograde injection of the water-soluble contrast material is essential to ensure cannulation of the desired duct and to prevent overfilling. X-rays should be taken for a permanent record of the examination.

A fine wire may be passed into the biliary tree; when heated with electrocautery current, the wire incises the sphincter of Oddi (sphincterotomy). Stones may be removed by passing a basket or balloon into the bile duct after incision into the papilla of Vater (papillotomy). A lithotriptor may be used to crush large stones entrapped within the basket. Indwelling cannulas or drainage stents may be left in the papilla of Vater for instillation of drugs or drainage of an obstructed duct.

Complications

In addition to perforation (which is rare) and drug reactions, the major complications of ERCP are pancreatitis and infection. Pancreatitis occurs in < 1% of cases and is usually mild. Infection is less frequent, occurring in patients with duct obstruction. Sphincterotomy is associated with a 1.5% mortality rate and an overall complication rate (including bleeding) of < 10%, an incidence less than that of similar procedures performed surgically.

RIGID AND FLEXIBLE SIGMOIDOSCOPY AND ANOSCOPY

These procedures permit examination of the distal portion of the large bowel but do not require extensive preparation or sedation. Disease within the anal canal is best seen with an anoscope—a short, tubular instrument with a sharply angulated bevel that permits direct visualization of the canal and the distal rectum. The rigid sigmoidoscope, when passed to its full length of 25 cm, permits inspection of the rectum and distal sigmoid colon, whereas the 30- or 60-cm flexible sigmoidoscope allows examination of most of the sigmoid or the descending colon, respectively.

Competent use of the flexible sigmoidoscope requires training and experience. More extensive application of the digital rectal examination together with the above procedures allows discovery and removal of precancerous polyps within 6 cm of the anus (the area in which the presence of cancer usually requires removal of the rectum and anus), thereby circumventing the need for colostomy.

Indications

Since ⅔ of neoplasms in the colon are located on the left, the flexible sigmoidoscope may be used to screen for disease in this area. Either rigid or flexible sigmoidoscopy can be used to evaluate the distal colon for suspected disease and complements the barium enema examination of this area. Flexible sigmoidoscopy should not be substituted for total colon examination when indications for colonoscopy (anemia, positive fecal occult blood test, polypectomy) are present. In general, polyps should not be removed during flexible sigmoidoscopy, since more extensive colon preparation is required for safety and because total colon evaluation is recommended whenever 1 colon polyp is identified. Anoscopy is best suited for visualization of perianal problems, eg, fissures, fistulas, or hemorrhoids.

Contraindications and Risks

Recent MI is the only contraindication.

Application

Because of the increased incidence with age of colorectal polyps and cancer and their predominantly left-sided distribution, these procedures are very valuable for early detection. In the absence of symptoms, 2 annual examinations ensure the absence of significant disease in the area examined, and a follow-up sigmoidoscopy every 3 yr allows diagnosis of subsequent tumors at a curable stage.

Procedure

Sedation is not required. One or 2 phosphate enemas preceding the examination usually provide adequate bowel cleansing. The patient usually lies on the left side for flexible sigmoidoscopy but assumes the knee-chest position for rigid sigmoidoscopy. Air insufflation or instrument looping in the colon may cause cramps and discomfort.

Complications

These are extremely rare but may include perforation and infection.

---

47.   UPPER GASTROINTESTINAL TRACT DISORDERS

Donald O. Castell

Most disorders of the upper GI tract seen in the elderly are not unique to this population. However, diseases that are more common in older persons should be carefully considered when these patients present with appropriate symptoms.

DYSPHAGIA SYNDROMES

Dysphagia, or *difficulty in swallowing,* may occur at any age, and can be caused by a variety of conditions. In the elderly, those related to vascular disease, malignancy, and other degenerative conditions are particularly important. **Dysphagia can be divided into 2 distinct syndromes:** (1) that produced by abnormalities affecting the finely tuned neuromuscular mechanism of the pharynx and upper esophageal sphincter **(oropharyn-**

geal dysphagia) and (2) that caused by any of the various disorders affecting the esophagus itself **(esophageal dysphagia).**

OROPHARYNGEAL DYSPHAGIA

Five categories of abnormality are associated with oropharyngeal dysphagia in the elderly (see TABLE 47–1):

TABLE 47–1. LIKELY CAUSES OF OROPHARYNGEAL DYSPHAGIA IN THE ELDERLY

Cerebrovascular accidents (particularly with brainstem involvement)
    Wallenberg's syndrome
    Pseudobulbar palsy
Other neuromuscular disorders
    Parkinson's disease
    Myasthenia gravis
    Hypo- or hyperthyroidism
    Amyotrophic lateral sclerosis
Oropharyngeal tumors
Zenker's diverticulum
Vertebral osteophytes

1. Cerebrovascular accidents: Patients with major strokes will often manifest dysphagia, particularly if the lesion involves critical areas in the brainstem affecting the swallowing center. Dysphagia may occur in **pseudobulbar palsy** or in so-called **Wallenberg's syndrome** *(lesion of the posterior inferior cerebellar artery)*. In patients with these syndromes, dysphagia may be the primary symptom, making the specific diagnosis difficult. Patients with poststroke dysphagia will occasionally respond to retraining technics aimed at rehabilitation of the physical aspects of swallowing. These approaches are best performed during radiologic assessment of effects of different foods (liquid, semisolid, solid) on swallowing.

2. Other neuromuscular disorders: A variety of neurologic or muscular disorders that affect movement of the tongue, pharynx, or upper esophageal sphincter may result in oropharyngeal dysphagia. In the elderly patient, likely candidates include **Parkinson's disease, myasthenia gravis, hypo-** or **hyperthyroidism,** and **amyotrophic lateral sclerosis.** These disorders may present with dysphagia without other symptoms. Each must be searched for, particularly hyperthyroidism, which may not have typical manifestations in the elderly.

3. Oropharyngeal tumors: Head and neck tumors are distinct possibilities in the etiology of oropharyngeal dysphagia, particularly in the elderly. Direct laryngoscopy should be performed to search for these lesions.

4. Zenker's diverticulum: Transient pre-esophageal dysphagia may be the earliest symptom of this outpouching of one or more layers of the esophageal wall located immediately above the upper esophageal sphincter. When the pharyngeal sac becomes large enough to retain food, patients develop the typical symptoms of persistent cough, fullness in the neck, gurgling in the throat, postprandial regurgitation, and aspiration. Some diverticula become so large that patients must perform various maneuvers, such as applying pressure on the neck and coughing repeatedly to empty them. These sacs can become large enough to produce a visible mass in the neck or to obstruct the esophagus by compression.

The pathogenesis of these diverticula is controversial. Both radiographic and manometric studies of patients with Zenker's diverticula have shown evidence of premature closure of the cricopharyngeal muscle. A recent manometric study using more refined technics has failed to show any incoordination between pharyngeal contraction and upper esophageal sphincter relaxation. Preferred therapy is surgical (ie, diverticulectomy). Performance of a myotomy of the cricopharyngeal muscle is controversial.

5. Cervical hypertrophic osteoarthropathy: Dysphagia secondary to compression of the esophagus by hypertrophic spurs of the anterior portion of the cervical vertebrae is unusual, considering the frequency of cervical osteoarthritis. The most common complaint is difficulty swallowing solid foods, but patients also complain of odynophagia, a foreign-body sensation, cough, hoarseness, and an urge to clear the throat. Diagnosis can be made by barium esophagography (lateral views), although endoscopy should be performed to exclude intraluminal pathology.

Diagnostic Approach

Identifying the cause of oropharyngeal dysphagia requires close attention to the history, physical examination, and appropriate diagnostic tests. **Barium x-ray studies** of the pharynx and upper esophageal sphincteric area are often of little help unless **videofluoroscopy** is also performed. Since the sequence of muscular changes occurring in this area requires only about 1 sec for the transfer of ingested material from mouth to upper esophagus, it is essential that rapid-sequence pictures be obtained. **Manometric studies** of the pharynx and upper esophageal sphincter are only occasionally helpful, but improvements in manometric technics, which should provide better diagnostic information, are currently being developed.

Treatment

This depends on the underlying cause. Treatable defects, including Parkinson's disease, myasthenia gravis, and thyroid abnormalities, should receive the appropriate therapy. Tumors should be resected, if possible. For the patient with otherwise untreatable neuromuscular disorders, including strokes, rehabilitation procedures are often effective (eg, altering the diet or eating with the head held in different positions). These approaches should be determined after consultation with a speech pathologist, including radiographic assessment of the patient's ability to swallow various types of food (liquid, semisolid, solid) while maintaining different head positions.

ESOPHAGEAL DYSPHAGIA

A variety of **neuromuscular (motility) defects** or **mechanical obstructing lesions** can cause esophageal dysphagia by interfering with the transport of ingested material down the esophagus. These 2 types of disorders can usually be differentiated by taking a detailed history. Motility disorders are more likely to cause dysphagia for both solids and liquids; obstructing lesions usually produce dysphagia for solids only. TABLE 47–2 lists the relationship of symptom patterns to some of the more common etiologies of esophageal dysphagia in the elderly.

TABLE 47–2. ASSOCIATION OF HISTORY OF DYSPHAGIA WITH DIFFERENTIAL DIAGNOSIS

Intermittent dysphagia
  Solid foods only
    Rings and webs (including vascular lesions)
  Both solids and liquids
    Diffuse esophageal spasm

Progressive dysphagia
  Solid foods only
    Carcinoma
    Peptic stricture
  Both solids and liquids
    Achalasia
    Scleroderma

Associated symptoms
  Chronic heartburn suggests scleroderma or stricture
  Nocturnal aspiration suggests achalasia
  Chest pain suggests esophageal spasm

Achalasia: Most patients with achalasia present between ages 20 and 40, but a second peak occurs in the elderly. An elderly patient may have had symptoms for months or years prior to diagnosis. Pathologically, the disorder is neurologic in origin, with defects of the ganglion cells in Auerbach's plexus of the esophageal wall. Clinically, there is slowly progressive dysphagia for solids and liquids and insidious weight loss. Regurgitation of undigested foods may cause nocturnal coughing and aspiration.

Chest x-ray may show a dilated esophagus with an air-fluid level from retained food and saliva. Approximately 50% of cases will fail to show the normal gastric air bubble. Barium swallow studies reveal a dilated, sometimes tortuous esophagus, with a smooth, "bird-beak" narrowing at the gastroesophageal junction. Esophageal manometry usually provides diagnostic findings of increased lower esophageal sphincter pressure with incomplete sphincteric relaxation during swallowing and an aperistaltic esophagus. These defects result in a major functional obstruction of food passing from the esophagus.

It is particularly important in the elderly to differentiate between **idiopathic achalasia** and so-called **secondary achalasia**, cancer that may rarely produce identical radiographic and manometric findings. Tumors associated with such findings include gastric, pancreatic, and lung cancer. Lymphoma can also present in this manner. Consequently, endoscopy with biopsy of any suspicious area is mandatory in all patients with achalasia. The clinical triad that may suggest secondary achalasia is age > 50 yr, dysphagia for < 1 yr, and weight loss > 15 lb.

Treatment for achalasia can be medical or surgical. Generally, good results can be obtained with either approach, and the choice should be based on the skills of local physicians, the health of the patient, and the patient's preference after adequate education concerning the technics, risks, and expected outcomes. Certainly, medical management may be more suitable for older patients in poor health.

Medical management of achalasia consists of pneumatic dilation via an inflatable bag. The pneumatic dilator is placed in the esophagus so the center of the bag lies within the lower esophageal sphincter. The bag is then inflated while the dilation is monitored fluoroscopically. Surgical management of achalasia consists of a myotomy. When done properly, both procedures have been shown to be successful in alleviating symptoms in most patients.

Occasionally, sufficient relief of dysphagia can be obtained with regular use of a smooth-muscle–relaxing drug given just prior to meals. Either isosorbide dinitrate or nifedipine given sublingually may be effective. The rapid action of these drugs enhances relaxation of the lower esophageal sphincter and may improve dysphagia during the meal. However, most achalasia patients require the more definitive procedures discussed above to open the esophagogastric junction. Because the elderly patient with other serious medical problems may not be a candidate for the potential risk of surgery or pneumatic dilation, treatment with smooth-muscle–relaxing compounds should be considered as possibly definitive therapy.

Scleroderma (progressive systemic sclerosis): Esophageal involvement in scleroderma occurs in > 80% of cases and seems to correlate with the presence of Raynaud's phenomenon. Scleroderma produces a slowly progressive dysphagia for liquids and solids, as in achalasia; heartburn is also a prominent symptom when the esophagus is involved. Up to 40% of these patients develop a peptic esophageal stricture. Manometric findings include decreased peristalsis in the lower esophagus (smooth muscle) in contrast to the upper esophagus (striated muscle), where normal peristalsis continues. In addition, lower esophageal sphincter pressure is very low.

Treatment of esophageal involvement in scleroderma should include intensive management of reflux with elevation of the head of the patient's bed and full doses of histamine H_2 receptor blocking agents to suppress acid secretion.

Diffuse esophageal spasm (DES) and related disorders: DES is an esophageal motility disorder manifested by dysphagia, or chest pain, or, in some cases, both. Dysphagia usually occurs intermittently for both liquids and solids. Both symptoms may be exacerbated by hot or cold foods or drinks and may be induced by stress.

DES may be related to a variety of nonspecific esophageal motility disorders. It may represent part of a spectrum of disorders that can progress to achalasia. The **"nutcracker esophagus"** is another disorder in this spectrum. Patients with a nutcracker esophagus have high-amplitude peristaltic contractions (> 180 mm Hg) and associated symptoms of dysphagia, or chest pain, or both.

Treatment of DES and related conditions consists of nitrates, Ca channel blockers (preferably nifedipine or diltiazem), sedatives, muscle relaxants, or anticholinergics. Esophageal dilation may also be helpful, and in severe, refractory cases, esophageal myotomy may be considered. Often, patients benefit from reassurance that their pain is esophageal, not cardiac, in origin and from learning how to cope better with stress.

Esophageal carcinoma (see also Ch. 52): Patients with this disease are generally older and present with rapidly progressive dysphagia (solids first, then liquids) and weight loss. Typically, they have no history of heartburn, although it may occur. A history of heavy alcohol and tobacco use is common. Barium x-ray studies often suggest the diagnosis, but endoscopy (with biopsy and cytology) is necessary for a more definitive diagnosis. Treatment depends on the extent of disease, with surgical resection, if possible, the treatment of choice. CT scanning may help determine resectability. Radiation therapy, chemotherapy, or both, may be palliative. The prognosis, in general, is grim, with 5-yr survival < 5%.

Peptic stricture: This condition is characterized by progressive dysphagia for solids and usually follows a long history of heartburn or other reflux symptoms. The diagnosis is made by barium radiography, but endoscopy is mandatory to rule out carcinoma. The strictures are smooth, tapered, and of varying lengths. If they are located above the distal esophagus, a **Barrett's esophagus** (ie, metaplastic columnar epithelium lining the distal esophagus) may be present. Patients with this condition, which is related to chronic gastroesophageal reflux, have an increased risk of cancer. Most patients with peptic strictures can be managed with long-term antireflux therapy. Intermittent esophageal dilation is often necessary as well, and occasionally surgery is required.

Rings or webs: These disorders, associated with intermittent dysphagia for solids, are best diagnosed by barium swallow. Endoscopic evaluation is indicated if there is any question about the diagnosis. Because the first episode frequently occurs while the patient is eating steak and bread, the disorder has been termed **"steakhouse syndrome."** The bolus is usually forced down by drinking liquids but occasionally must be regurgitated, and the meal then can usually be finished without difficulty.

The most common type of structural lesion in this category is a **Schatzki's ring,** composed of invaginated mucosa. The ring, located at the gastroesophageal mucosal junction, is seen on barium swallow about 3 to 4 cm above the diaphragm. It most often produces symptoms when the lumen is narrowed to $\leq$ 12 mm. Treatment consists of one-time dilation of the esophagus with a large-caliber bougie. If the symptoms occur infrequently, more careful eating habits may suffice.

Vascular causes: Esophageal dysphagia may also be caused by vascular anomalies that produce compression of the esophagus. The more common lesions are congenital aortic-arch abnormalities, associated with dysphagia presenting early in childhood. Occasionally, symptoms present in adulthood. **Dysphagia aortica** is a disorder of the elderly and is due to compression of the esophagus by either a large thoracic aortic aneurysm or by an atherosclerotic, rigid aorta posteriorly and the heart or esophageal hiatus anteriorly.

DISORDERS OF THE STOMACH AND DUODENUM

Acid/peptic gastric and duodenal disorders are frequently found in the elderly population. There appears to be a tendency toward a *decreasing* incidence of duodenal ulcers with age, which may be related to the diminishing gastric acid secretion. Secretory studies have repeatedly demonstrated decreased acid output with aging and a relative increase in achlorhydria. In association with the decreased acid output, basal serum gastrin concentrations tend to increase with age. Gastric ulcers may actually increase in incidence in the elderly, particularly in those who are chronically taking nonsteroidal anti-inflammatory drugs **(NSAIDs).** In addition, both gastric and duodenal ulcers tend to develop more complications in older patients, making surgical considerations more likely.

ATROPHIC GASTRITIS AND GASTRIC ATROPHY

Atrophic gastritis is characterized by increased numbers of inflammatory cells in the stomach wall and variable degrees of atrophy of the gastric mucosa. It is generally believed that this kind of gastritis tends to be progressive and that it may eventually develop into **gastric atrophy.** The latter is a more diffuse disorder, characterized by a decrease in the number of secretory cells (both chief and parietal) in the mucosa of the gastric body and fundus. Generally, these gastric mucosal changes that occur with age tend to correlate with decreased gastric secretion.

There are 2 types of atrophic gastritis: **Type A** is a more diffuse gastritis that is antral sparing and is usually associated with circulating parietal cell antibodies, as well as with decreased acid output and elevated serum gastric levels. It may evolve into characteristic **pernicious anemia. Type B gastritis** is a more focal, antral condition associated with less reduction in acid secretion, normal serum gastrin levels, and absence of antiparietal cell antibodies.

Patients with these conditions are usually asymptomatic, although benign gastric ulcer may develop. *Of major clinical importance is the potential for malignancy of both atrophic gastritis and gastric atrophy, which share the premalignant status of pernicious anemia.* The management of patients with these conditions, therefore, usually includes periodic surveillance for carcinoma with endoscopic cytology and biopsy. Although the optimal interval for such examinations is not clear, they are generally performed every 1 or 2 yr.

Pernicious anemia is the end-stage condition seen in patients with Type A chronic gastritis. It usually presents as a hematologic abnormality in the elderly, and GI symptoms are unusual. The diagnosis, however, is strongly supported by the finding of characteristic **achlorhydria,** defined as *a total absence of gastric acid secretion in response to maximal stimulation.* Up to 10% of patients with pernicious anemia will eventually be found to have carcinoma of the stomach, which is estimated to occur 3 to 5 times more often in these patients than in the general population of similar age.

HYPERTROPHIC GASTROPATHY

The presence of enlarged gastric rugae involving part or all of the stomach has been termed **Ménétrier's disease.** This is a relatively unusual condition that is not unique to the elderly. A number of conditions that may mimic Ménétrier's disease are more likely to occur in the older population. These include gastric lymphoma; infiltrative carcinoma; granulomatous disorders, such as TB; and other infiltrative conditions, such as amyloidosis. Clinically, these conditions may be associated with vague epigastric pain and weight loss. Of more importance, however, may be the frequent finding of hypoalbuminemia secondary to protein loss across the gastric mucosa.

On barium x-ray studies, all of the conditions described above may show large gastric folds, which may appear as polypoid filling defects along the greater curvature of the stomach. Endoscopy with adequate biopsy will assist in the differential diagnosis. Treatment is dependent upon the final diagnosis. Sometimes, anticholinergics decrease the gastric protein loss in Ménétrier's disease. Occasionally, gastrectomy is required.

PEPTIC ULCER

An ulceration of the mucous membrane penetrating through the muscularis mucosa and occurring in the areas bathed in acid and pepsin.

Although duodenal ulcer is the predominant form of peptic ulceration in younger individuals, gastric ulcer predominates in the elderly and is much more likely to result in mortality. The presentation of peptic ulcer occurring later in life may be more acute, including severe hemorrhage, perforation, and obstruction. These complications are discussed in Ch. 53. Aggressive therapy is often necessary in older patients, and surgical therapy should not be delayed or withheld solely because of advanced age.

Giant duodenal ulcer: Elderly men occasionally present with upper abdominal pain, often radiating into the back, secondary to large duodenal ulcers. These ulcers, which may exceed 2 cm in diameter, may actually involve most of the surface of the duodenal bulb. GI bleeding occurs frequently, and the lesion may involve contiguous organs, such as the pancreas, gallbladder, or liver. A giant duodenal ulcer is diagnosed with barium x-ray studies. Surgery is usually preferable to medical treatment.

Treatment

Therapy for peptic ulcer in the elderly is similar to that in younger patients. However, certain principles require closer attention when treating older patients. (For treatment of complications [hemorrhage, perforation, obstruction], see Ch. 53.)

Anticholingerics: Because of their undesirable side effects, anticholinergic agents are rarely used in the treatment of peptic ulcer disease. Potential problems in the elderly include dry mouth, which may interfere with eating; occurrence of gastric or urinary stasis; or glaucoma, which may be aggravated by dilation of the eye.

Antacids: These medications continue to be used frequently for symptoms of peptic ulcer disease. *In the elderly, one must be aware of the sodium content of antacid preparations to avoid sodium overload.* Riopan® is the antacid with the lowest sodium content. Other possible side effects to be avoided in the elderly are diarrhea and altered absorption of other drugs, including digoxin, quinidine, isoniazid, and broad-spectrum antibiotics.

Histamine H_2 receptor blockers: The major drugs currently used for the treatment of peptic ulcer disease are the H_2 receptor blockers. All of these have the potential for producing mental confusion in the elderly patient, particularly when given parenterally. In addition, cimetidine is associated with a number of important drug interactions and may increase blood levels of diazepam, warfarin, theophylline, and phenytoin.

Sucralfate: By enhancing protective mechanisms of the gastric mucosa, sucralfate provides an effective alternative in the therapy for acute peptic ulcer disease. In the elderly, this drug offers the advantage of being potentially free of the systemic side effects produced by the histamine H_2 receptor blockers.

Gastric irradiation: In the occasional elderly patient with severe peptic ulcer disease who is a poor risk for surgery, acid secretion can be temporarily reduced by gastric irradiation. Treatment can be expected to decrease or abolish gastric secretion in up to 90% of patients. However, the secretory capacity will usually return to pretreatment levels within about 1 yr.

Zollinger-Ellison (ZE) syndrome was initially described by the triad of (1) recurring peptic ulcer disease, (2) marked gastric hypersecretion of acid, and (3) a pancreatic adenoma. It was subsequently found that the adenoma produced high outputs of gastrin, resulting in continuous stimulation of the parietal cells to produce excessive quantities of acid. Approximately ⅓ of patients with this syndrome are over age 60. Therefore, the condition should be considered in any patient with persistent or recurring peptic ulcer disease. A serum gastrin determination should be obtained and, if the diagnosis of ZE syndrome remains a possibility, gastric secretory studies should be performed. Traditionally, patients with ZE syndrome will have a basal acid output > 15 mEq/L, and maximal stimulation will not double the output.

Treatment: The approach to patients with ZE syndrome has changed radically in recent years. Total gastrectomy, once considered *the* essential form of therapy, is no longer used in most patients. With the development of more effective acid-suppressing drugs, particularly the histamine H_2 receptor blockers, many patients can remain pain free, and recurring ulcers can be prevented with medical therapy. To effectively suppress hypersecretion, 10 times the usual dose of an H_2 blocker may be needed, or vagotomy and antrectomy may be considered with lower doses.

BEZOARS

Intragastric masses consisting of extrinsic substances such as hair, fruit and vegetable fibers, or a mixture of both.

Bezoars are seen with increased frequency in the elderly, especially following vagotomy and/or subtotal gastrectomy, and may be related to reduced gastric motility. They occur frequently in the elderly diabetic because of severely abnormal gastric emptying. The edentulous patient may be at risk because of the insufficient breaking up of food fibers. Pulpy fruits or vegetables, especially citrus fruits, but also figs, coconuts, apples, green beans, sauerkraut, berries, potato peels, and brussels sprouts, are the most commonly incriminated foods. Barium x-ray may indicate the presence of a mass lesion in the stomach, which may mimic a cancer. Treatment with endoscopy, including attempts to break up the lesion with a biopsy forceps or a jet spray of water, is often successful.

VOLVULUS OF THE STOMACH

This relatively rare condition is more common in the elderly because of relaxation of the ligaments supporting the stomach. A complete twist of the organ can result in strangulation of the blood supply, which can lead to gangrene. Patients often present with an abrupt onset of severe epigastric pain and a history of early vomiting, followed by retching with inability to vomit or belch.

Two types of gastric volvulus are described. The more common **organoaxial volvulus** involves a rotation of the stomach on its longitudinal axis (from cardia to pylorus), and often presents with an x-ray of an "upside-down stomach" and double air-fluid levels (fundus and antrum). The less common **mesenteroaxial volvulus** results from rotation around a vertical axis passing through the center of the lesser and greater curvatures. Patients usually present with distention of the upper abdomen, which makes passage of a nasogastric tube difficult. An inability to vomit, upper abdominal pain and distention, and an inability to have a nasogastric tube inserted are known as **Borchardt's triad.** Diagnostic clues are usually obtained on x-ray examination, either with a plain film of the abdomen or with contrast material added. *Acute gastric volvulus requires emergency surgical therapy.*

BENIGN TUMORS OF THE STOMACH
(See also NEOPLASMS OF THE STOMACH in Ch. 52)

A variety of nonmalignant tumors may occur in the stomach. They are usually asymptomatic and are found during barium studies or endoscopy being performed for other conditions. If they are symptomatic, the patient is likely to have vague upper GI complaints or may occasionally develop upper GI tract bleeding. Larger tumors in the antrum may rarely cause outlet obstruction. If a decision for active treatment is made, either endoscopic removal (polypoid lesion) or surgical resection should be considered.

Hyperplastic polyps: These epithelial polyps comprise up to 95% of polypoid lesions seen in the stomach. They are small (usually < 1.5 cm in diameter) and are not premalignant. However, the adjacent epithelium may be susceptible to neoplastic transformation, since independent carcinoma has been reported in the adjacent stomach in many cases.

Adenomatous polyps: These polyps are true neoplasms that usually occur as isolated lesions in the gastric antrum. They attain a larger size (frequently > 4 cm in diameter) and are often present in mucosa showing chronic atrophic gastritis with permanent intestinal metaplasia. The incidence of malignancy in adenomatous polyps is greater with large polyps, particularly those with diameters > 2 cm, and in the presence of achlorhydria.

Leiomyomas: These tumors of the gastric smooth muscle usually present as solitary lesions, most often in the antrum. In the elderly patient, very large tumors may occasionally be leiomyoblastomas, which usually require surgical removal.

MALIGNANT TUMORS OF THE STOMACH
(See NEOPLASMS OF THE STOMACH in Ch. 52)

VASCULAR LESIONS OF THE STOMACH

Occult GI bleeding may occur secondary to **arteriovenous malformations** or **angiodysplasia** in the mucosa of the stomach or duodenum. These lesions appear more frequently with advancing age. Occasionally, they can be identified on endoscopy, but often angiographic confirmation is necessary. Choosing appropriate therapy can be a dilemma. Localized lesions may be resected; however, endoscopic therapy with electrocoagulation or laser treatment may be effective.

48. DISORDERS OF THE LOWER BOWEL

John C. Brocklehurst

The most common problems of the colon and rectum are constipation and fecal incontinence. The common diseases are diverticular, inflammatory, neoplastic, and vascular in origin.

Motility

Colonic motility is of 2 types—shuttling and mass peristalsis. Shuttling is continuous, although it diminishes at night and increases after meals. It moves the fecal bolus backward and forward between the haustra ("little bladders"), thus aiding in the absorption of water. Mass peristalsis results from a continuous contraction band, usually starting about the middle of the transverse colon and progressing down toward the rectum. It propels the fecal bolus toward the rectum.

Mass peristalsis usually occurs only bid or tid; it is stimulated by the so-called gastrocolic reflex (ie, the entry of food or fluid into the upper alimentary canal) via a chemically mediated action. Physical mobility also stimulates mass peristalsis. In patients who are immobile, which is common in the elderly, mass peristalsis may not occur, and the urge to defecate, therefore, is infrequent.

Frequency of defecation is no different in active elderly people than in those who are younger (in 98% of normal adults, regardless of age, the range is 3 times/day to 3 times/wk). Although older people tend to take laxatives more often, this may be a cohort effect, reflecting the habits of their younger days rather than real constipation.

Transit time (ie, the length of time taken for markers ingested orally to appear in the feces) in fit and active older people is similar to that in younger individuals. Transit time is longer in inhabitants of industrialized societies than in those of Third World countries because of the low-fiber diets that are typical of the former.

CONSTIPATION

A change in bowel habit, with diminished frequency of defecation, often associated with increased difficulty in defecation. Since frequency of defecation is variable (see above), there is no precise definition of constipation.

Etiology

In old age, constipation commonly is associated with decreased physical mobility and prolonged transit time. The main obstacle is at the rectum and sigmoid. The fecal mass gradually builds up from this distal end of the alimentary canal through the whole colon. Called the **terminal reservoir syndrome,** this is an important cause of overflow fecal incontinence in the elderly (see below). It may also lead to idiopathic megacolon and colonic pseudo-obstruction.

Constipation in the elderly may present as a change in bowel habit or as fecal incontinence. Many older people incorrectly believe that their bowel movements are abnormal, thus, change is important.

Acute constipation may indicate intestinal obstruction, characterized by a distended abdomen, an empty rectum, vomiting, and fluid levels seen on upright abdominal x-ray. Constipation, particularly if associated with intermittent diarrhea, may be a presenting symptom of colonic carcinoma.

Constipation may also be a symptom of certain **systemic diseases** (eg, hypothyroidism, uremia, hypercalcemia, depression) or a presenting symptom of **disease of the colon** (eg, diverticular disease). In addition, it may be caused by **drugs** (eg, anticholinergics, codeine, aluminum hydroxide, or iron).

Treatment

If the rectum is filled with hard or semisolid feces, the problem should be treated first as the terminal reservoir syndrome. This is best managed by giving phosphate enemas or by inserting suppositories. Phosphate enemas must be administered carefully, since the solution is hypertonic and potentially hazardous if the mucosa is damaged by the nozzle of the delivery system. One enema clears the rectum, but 7 to 10 daily enemas may be required to clear the entire large bowel.

To avoid such a prolonged and uncomfortable procedure, alternate methods of emptying the entire colon have been tried (eg, bisacodyl 5 to 10 mg orally at night). Mannitol 200 gm orally, cooled and flavored with fruit juice, is also recommended. It is given as a single dose over 1 h or so, but colic is a prominent side effect.

In the terminal reservoir syndrome, hard fecal masses (scybala) may develop, causing colic and, occasionally, obstruction. They are usually palpable abdominally or rectally and sometimes suggest carcinoma. Treatment may involve softening with a wetting agent (eg, docusate sodium 100 mg tid to qid). If the hard fecal masses are in the rectum, an attempt may be made to soften them with olive oil enemas. Occasionally, impacted masses require manual removal by the physician, who must take great care not to tear the anal mucosa. In the case of obstruction, surgical removal may be necessary.

Once constipation has been successfully treated, steps should be taken to ensure that it does not recur. If the patient remains inactive, recurrence is certain; the most satisfactory way to prevent this is to give an **enema** or **suppository** twice weekly. **Laxatives,** such as standardized senna (Senokot®) 2 tablets at bedtime or lactulose 3.35 gm/5 to 10 mL at night, or 10 mg suppositories in the morning, may also be used but are often less satisfactory. **Dietary fiber** should be increased to a maximum, supplementing it with bran, if necessary, and fluid intake should be maintained. Optimal **physical mobility** must also be encouraged.

Other laxatives (eg, mineral oil and phenolphthalein) are not recommended in elderly persons because of their potential adverse effects.

Once the colon and rectum have been emptied, colonoscopy or sigmoidoscopy and a barium enema must be considered if the history is short, the patient mobile, and other reasons for suspecting carcinoma are present.

Constipation due to systemic diseases resolves as these are successfully treated but may require symptomatic relief in the meantime.

FECAL INCONTINENCE

Continence Mechanisms

The muscles of the anus and anorectal junction that serve as continence mechanisms are the anal sphincters (internal and external) and the puborectal muscle. They constitute part of the pelvic diaphragm. The **internal sphincter** is a continuation of the circular smooth muscle of the rectum. It contributes 80% of anal closing pressure at rest. The **external sphincter** is a continuation of the striated muscle of the pelvic floor (pelvic diaphragm). It contributes only 20% of closing pressure at rest, but this increases to 40% when the rectum is continuously distended and to 65% when it is suddenly distended.

The **puborectal muscle** is also a part of the pelvic diaphragm—that part lying between the levator ani and the external sphincter. It arises from the pubis and is inserted into a raphe on the posterior part of the rectum. Its principal function is to maintain the anorectal angle by its slinglike effect. If the anorectal angle is < 90°, the upper end of the anal canal will be sealed by the distal anal mucosa, performing an important continence mechanism. When the rectum is distended, the anorectal angle increases and is no longer an effective continence mechanism.

All muscles of the pelvic floor, including the external sphincter, receive somatic innervation from the external pudendal nerve. Therefore, they are under voluntary control and can prevent expulsion of rectal contents when coughing occurs or when fluid in the rectum threatens continence.

Other anatomic continence mechanisms include the shape of the anal canal (slitlike in an anteroposterior direction in its upper $\frac{1}{2}$ and Y shaped in its lower $\frac{1}{2}$); it probably has the action of a flutter valve. The hemorrhoidal sinuses also provide cushioning that allows fine sealing of the canal.

Little is known about age-related changes in the anatomic structures described above. The pelvic diaphragm undergoes a loss of motor units. This is presumed to result from pudendal nerve damage occurring in women during prolonged or traumatic childbirth and also in patients who habitually strain at stool. Although motor unit loss increases with age, it does not occur universally and, therefore, is not a basic age change. In a number of people, it leads to the so-called descending perineum that is associated with loss of the anorectal angle, loss of tone in the external sphincter, and possible rectal prolapse and anorectal incontinence.

Etiology, Symptoms, and Signs

Fecal incontinence may be divided into 4 main groups:

Overflow incontinence secondary to constipation, with or without fecal impaction, results from the terminal reservoir syndrome (see above), in which the constantly distended rectum leads to dislocation of the anorectal angle; loss of ability to discriminate between fluid, flatus, and feces; and diminution in anal sphincter tone. As a result, feces tend to leak out, and the condition commonly presents with semisolid fecal soiling many times daily **("paradoxical diarrhea").**

Anorectal incontinence, associated with damage to the external pudendal nerve and consequent weakness in the pelvic floor musculature, is also associated with the so-called descending perineum, loss of the anal reflex, loss of tone in the sphincters (which may be patulous), or even prolapse of the rectum and loss of the anorectal angle. Fecal incontinence commonly occurs several times daily.

Neurogenic incontinence usually follows a gastrocolic reflex in a patient with global cerebral disease (eg, dementia) who is unable to suppress the process of defecation. The incontinence presents with a formed stool once or twice/day.

Symptomatic incontinence, due to colorectal disease, usually presents with diarrhea and fecal incontinence. The stool may be blood stained or may contain mucus, depending upon the underlying pathology.

Treatment

Overflow incontinence: The treatment is the same as that for the terminal reservoir syndrome described above.

Anorectal incontinence: Treatment begins with pelvic-floor exercises, which may be associated with biofeedback to indicate to the patient that muscle power is increasing, or with electrical treatment (faradism or interferential therapy). In many cases, however, surgery is needed. The preferred operation is a postanal repair.

Neurogenic incontinence: Close observation and appropriate timing of breakfast or a hot drink in the morning may allow this to occur when the patient is seated on a commode. Another approach is to alternately induce constipation and planned evacuations by giving a constipating agent in the morning (eg, codeine phosphate 15 to 30 mg or diphenoxylate hydrochloride 2.5 to 5 mg) and a laxative at night (eg, senna). This may allow a controlled bowel movement in the morning and prevent further mass peristalsis during the day. Alternatively, the patient may be constipated with the above preparations bid or tid and the bowel emptied 2 or 3 times/wk with enemas or suppositories.

Symptomatic incontinence demands full investigation to determine its cause. If the patient is constipated, this should be treated first (as described above); if fecal incontinence continues, endoscopy or radiologic investigation is necessary.

DIVERTICULAR DISEASE

A **diverticulum** is a *saclike projection of mucosa and submucosa through the muscular layer of the bowel.* **Diverticulosis** is *the asymptomatic presence of colonic diverticula.* **Diverticulitis** is *infection arising from colonic diverticula.* **Diverticular disease** refers to *painful spasm or other symptoms associated with diverticulosis.*

Diverticula are found throughout the bowel; they are most common in the sigmoid but are rare in the rectum below the peritoneal floor. A recent study of 350 patients requiring surgery for this disease showed that 35% were $\geq$ 70 yr of age. In the geriatric group, women predominated 3 to 1. In 94% of all cases, the primary site was the sigmoid.

Etiology

Diverticulosis is widespread among older people in Western societies (about 50% of 80-yr-olds) and almost unknown in many Third World nations. The reason is thought to relate to the fibrous content of the diet, with a low-fiber, low-residue diet being the causative factor. The generally accepted theory regarding formation of colonic diverticula is that the shuttling motility at the rectosigmoid junction has a functional sphincteric effect. This propels the sigmoid contents away from the rectum, keeping it empty except when a mass peristaltic stripping wave occurs. If the colonic contents are of low bulk because of a low-residue diet, the shuttling motility required to reverse forward movement is greater and the increased contraction of the circular muscle generates higher pressure within the haustra. This higher pressure, in turn, leads to mucosal herniation through vulnerable points in the colonic wall, where arteries perforate the circular muscle.

Diverticula, therefore, may be associated with circular muscle hypertrophy. They generally arise in the rectosigmoid area but may eventually involve the whole colon. Since diverticula develop in close proximity to small arteries, bleeding may be one of the presenting symptoms of diverticular disease.

Symptoms and Signs

Colonic **diverticulosis** is asymptomatic. The most common presenting symptoms of **diverticular disease** are colicky pain in the left iliac fossa (due to the increased circular muscle contraction); a change in bowel habit producing either diarrhea, constipation, or both; and blood in the stool. The latter may be caused by inspissated feces eroding the small artery within the diverticulum. Tenderness is common on palpation of the left iliac fossa, and sometimes the thickened colon is easily felt.

Diverticular disease is often associated with other stigmata, including inguinal hernia, hiatus hernia, varicose veins, hemorrhoids, and gallstones.

If **diverticulitis** develops, symptoms and signs may vary greatly; see Diagnosis, below.

Diagnosis

Diverticulosis is so common in elderly people that caution must be used in attributing symptoms to it when discovered (eg, on barium enema examination). In many cases, additional disease is causing the symptoms. *Any change in bowel habit or blood in the stool requires a full endoscopic or radiologic examination of the lower bowel to exclude other disease, even when colonic diverticula have been demonstrated.* In elderly patients, cancer is the major confounding disease.

The diagnosis of diverticulitis is based on the history and physical examination. Patients with mild diverticulitis complain of lower abdominal pain and have left lower-quadrant tenderness. A low-grade fever, leukocytosis, and variations in normal bowel function—either diarrhea or constipation—often are noted. Confirmation of the diagnosis by barium enema can be made a few days later when the condition has improved. CT scan can help to rule out appendicitis; however, if tenderness is present in the right lower quadrant, a laparotomy should be performed since the appendix may be acutely inflamed.

Findings vary according to associated complications.

Sepsis may result from a pericolic abscess or from localized or generalized peritonitis. A **localized pericolic abscess** may be identified by a palpable mass. Left lower-quadrant tenderness and spasm suggest **localized peritonitis;** an abdominal film, taken in the sitting position, may show subphrenic air.

Intestinal obstruction may arise from small-bowel adhesions, sigmoid colitis, or both. Abdominal x-rays supplement the physical examination.

The bleeding site in hemorrhage may be demonstrated by angiography; in acute hemorrhage, this may be combined with the intra-arterial injection of vasopressin to stop the bleeding.

Fistula formation is discussed separately, below.

Treatment

Diverticular disease may be adequately controlled by increasing dietary fiber, as advised by a dietitian. Intake of vegetables, fruit, and other natural products should be increased. If this is not enough, supplementing the diet with millers' bran or using a bulking agent such as psyllium 3.5 gm in 250 mL water once or twice daily may be helpful. Psyllium may bind coumarin derivatives and should be used with care. Methylcellulose 550 mg daily may also be helpful, although it often produces flatulence. Colonic spasm may be diminished by the use of antispasmodics, eg, propantheline 15 mg bid to tid or dicyclomine hydrochloride

10 mg bid to tid. *These must be used with caution in the presence of possible glaucoma or prostatic hypertrophy.*

Diverticulitis in its early stages may be treated at home with a liquid diet and oral antibiotics. More serious cases require hospitalization; eventually, 20% require surgery. The clinical significance of diverticulitis is reflected by postoperative mortality statistics. In 1 institution, the mortality rate for patients requiring surgery was slightly > 6%; for those ≥ 70 yr of age, it was > 8%.

Bleeding is treated by blood replacement. Vasopressin may be continuously infused under arteriographic control into the artery supplying the bleeding point. Otherwise, surgical excision of all segments of the colon bearing diverticula is necessary.

Sepsis: Patients with pericolic abscess or generalized or localized peritonitis as well as those who fail to improve with conservative measures must be treated surgically. Understandably, one may be reluctant to operate on older patients who have other diseases. *However, generalized peritonitis in elderly patients must be treated immediately by excision of the perforation site; treatment with antibiotics and awaiting resolution of infection leads to an extremely high mortality.*

The choice of antibiotics in patients with severe peritonitis continues to change. Currently, gentamicin and clindamycin IV are preferred.

Obstruction: Small-bowel obstruction is treated by nasogastric intubation, followed by laparotomy and lysis of adhesions. Colonic obstruction is usually treated by proximal colostomy; colon resection, reanastomosis, and colostomy closure are performed later.

Elective surgery for diverticular disease: Operations for complications of diverticulitis have a high mortality. Therefore, surgeons prefer to anticipate complications and perform a 1-stage resection of the affected segment and reanastomosis, without colostomy, *before* complications develop. However, depending on individual considerations, surgery may involve 2 or 3 stages that include a temporary colostomy.

Features of intractable disease that necessitate surgery in the elderly patient include the following: (1) ≥ 2 previous attacks of local inflammation; (2) a persistent, tender mass; (3) narrowing or marked deformity of the sigmoid on x-ray (particularly because of possible cancer); (4) dysuria (which may presage a colovesical fistula); (5) rapid progression of symptoms; and (6) clinical or x-ray signs that are equivocal in ruling out carcinoma. Patients receiving corticosteroids also are at risk for perforation and generalized peritonitis.

COLOVESICAL FISTULA

Fistulas may follow abscess formation or surgical drainage of an abscess, or they may be associated with obstruction. However, many fistulas are simply associated with diverticulitis. In such cases, adhesion and rupture of a single diverticulum probably occurs along a thin-walled, sharply localized tract. The most common form of internal fistula is a colovesical fistula; others occur in the small gut, the vagina, and the left groin. They must be distinguished from fistulas due to Crohn's disease.

Patients with colovesical fistulas usually present because of failure to respond to repeated treatments for UTI. The presence of air in the urine is diagnostic; examination of the urine shows some fecal matter in about ⅓ of such patients. Cystoscopy usually is not helpful, nor is barium enema or sigmoidoscopy, although plain abdominal x-ray in the erect position shows gas in the bladder in about ⅓ of such patients.

COLONIC ANGIODYSPLASIA
(Ectasia)

One or more minute clusters of dilated veins in the mucosa of the colon. A single lesion appears as a small mass of vascular spaces, multiple and often coalescent within the submucosa. In most cases, they are lined only by endothelium, although sometimes smooth muscle may be present. The lesions have a slightly raised, cherry-red center with radiating foot processes. They are generally in the ascending colon or the cecum and are often multiple.

Although first described in 1839, colonic angiodysplasia has been recognized as an important cause of colonic bleeding only in the past 15 yr. It may be the most common cause of lower GI bleeding in later life but can be diagnosed only by colonoscopy or arteriography, which partly explains its tardy recognition. In resected specimens and at autopsy, recognition may be difficult unless the specimen has been injected with a radiopaque substance and the location of the dysplastic lesion identified.

Etiology and Pathogenesis

Although occasionally colonic angiodysplasia is associated with dysplastic lesions elsewhere in the alimentary tract and is probably congenital, it is generally thought to be acquired. There are 2 main theories as to its cause: (1) The effect of intraluminal pressure occurring during peristalsis or straining at stool occludes the mucosal circulation, leading to dilation of the superficial venules and capillaries; (2) lifelong continuing contraction of the circular muscle of the colon tends to obstruct the draining veins, leading to submucosal varices, followed by mucosal varices, and eventually by arteriovenous communication. An association with aortic stenosis has been shown in some surveys, suggesting that low cardiac output may be an additional causative factor.

Symptoms, Signs, and Diagnosis

Apart from bleeding, the condition is symptomless. Patients may present with fresh hemorrhage (bright red blood), intermittent or chronic occult bleeding discovered on investigation for other symptoms, or anemia. Melena is uncommon.

Diagnosis is made by colonoscopy or angiography but is often difficult because the lesions are small and may be in multiple sites. Unless the bleeding is massive and immediate laparotomy is necessary, colonoscopy is usually recommended first. Since the lesions are predominantly situated in the cecum and ascending colon, the colonoscopy should be complete. Advantages of colonoscopy are that electrocoagulation may be used and that it both identifies the lesions and permits biopsy. Since colonoscopy is usually an elective procedure in this condition, adequate bowel preparation is possible and necessary.

Angiography may be used in emergencies and usually identifies the location of the hemorrhage, although diagnosis is occasionally mistaken. Usually, both the superior and inferior mesenteric arteries are catheterized. The criteria for angiographic diagnosis are as follows: (1) abnormal clusters of small veins seen during the arterial phase of the arteriogram along the antimesenteric border of the cecum and the ascending colon, (2) accumulation of contrast material in vascular spaces and intense opacification of the bowel wall during the capillary phase, (3) early opacification of the veins draining the cecum and the ascending colon, and (4) intense opacification of the veins persisting late into the venous phase.

Differential diagnosis presents the common problem in old age of multiple pathology. Colonic diverticulosis is present in 50% of very old people and may be a source of bleeding. Colonic carcinoma and polyps are the second most common finding.

Treatment

Unless bleeding is significant or recurrent, treatment should be conservative. This includes the treatment of iron-deficiency anemia and continued surveillance. If bleeding is severe or recurrent, alternative methods of treatment include electrocoagulation (or laser photocoagulation) and surgical resection. The former is performed by the colonoscopist; the main difficulty is finding the lesion, and the main hazard is perforation of the thin-walled cecum or ascending colon. Several lesions may be treated at once. Results are least satisfactory with cecal lesions.

If bleeding is severe, immediate control is usually possible during arteriography by injection of vasopressin directly into the catheter or into a peripheral vein. If vasopressin control fails or bleeding recurs, segmental colectomy is indicated, although this is sometimes followed by rebleeding from previously unidentified lesions in remaining parts of the colon.

CROHN'S DISEASE

A chronic inflammatory bowel disease involving the small intestine (most commonly the terminal ileum) or the colon, or both, and characterized pathologically by transmural inflammation, deep linear ulceration, and often granulomas.

The onset of Crohn's disease is usually between 20 and 40 yr of age; an increasing proportion of patients now live into old age. In 5 to 20%

of new cases, the disease starts after the age of 60. In old age, the disease is more likely to be confined to the colon, and the prognosis is good compared with the disease in younger patients.

Pathology

The underlying inflammatory process affects all layers of the gut wall and is associated with submucosal fibrosis. In a high proportion of cases, focal granulomas may be identified histologically; these are a major distinguishing feature from ulcerative colitis. Other features distinguishing Crohn's disease from ulcerative colitis are present macroscopically; eg, discrete mucosal ulcers, confluent linear ulcers, fissures, and fistulas. While none of these lesions occurs in ulcerative colitis, ≥ 1 are likely to be seen in most cases of Crohn's disease, although none is universal. Another characteristic of Crohn's disease is the presence of skip lesions in any part of the alimentary tract from the mouth to the anus. Ulcerative colitis is limited to the colon and is confluent. In old age, however, most cases of Crohn's disease are confined to the colon (**granulomatous colitis**), especially the left side, often not affecting the rectum.

Symptoms and Signs

The cardinal presenting features of Crohn's disease of the colon are diarrhea, abdominal pain, and occult lower GI bleeding causing iron-deficiency anemia. Abdominal pain is less frequent and lower GI bleeding more common in older than in younger patients. Weight loss, low-grade pyrexia, fatigue, anemia, and malnutrition are associated symptoms.

Sometimes the disease presents with acute peritonitis due to perforation; in old age, this presentation is often atypical, sometimes painless, and associated with mental confusion. Perforation more commonly results from disease of the ileum than of the colon. Intestinal obstruction and massive lower GI bleeding are further complications. Fistulas, migratory arthritis involving ≥ 1 joints, erythema nodosum, pyoderma gangrenosum, iritis, and renal disease (including nephrolithiasis and amyloidosis) are only occasionally diagnostic features, unlike in younger patients.

Diagnosis

Infectious causes of diarrhea, including *Campylobacter*, must first be excluded by stool culture. The diagnosis then is based on the clinical features, together with findings on sigmoidoscopy or colonoscopy and barium enema; a barium swallow is required to identify lesions in the upper alimentary tract. Interrupted areas of inflammation and ulceration are characteristic, although in about 25% of cases, the disease is continuous. Barium enema identifies skip lesions, fistulas, colonic narrowing, and ulceration. Rectal biopsy should always be performed, even if the rectal mucosa appears grossly normal.

Lennard-Jones' diagnostic criteria for Crohn's disease are discontinuous lesions, terminal ileum affected, deep fissures on x-rays or surgical specimens, enterocutaneous fistulas, chronic anal lesions, normal mucin content of epithelial cells in the presence of mucosal inflammation on biopsy, and lymphoid aggregates in the mucosa and submucosa. If epithelial cell granulomas are identified, 1 other of the above criteria should also be present. If granulomas are not identified, at least 3 other criteria should be present to confirm diagnosis.

Because of the coexistence of colonic diverticula in older patients, the diagnosis is too often delayed, particularly since the disease may be mistaken for diverticulitis (granulomas have been identified within diverticula and the presentation of Crohn's disease may be identical to that of diverticulitis).

Lower GI bleeding in Crohn's disease must be distinguished from bleeding due to diverticular disease. In the latter, bleeding tends to be more occasional and of greater quantity; in the former, it tends to be more frequent and of lesser quantity. Iron-deficiency anemia or the anemia of chronic disease (normochromic anemia) is often present.

Crohn's disease also must be differentiated from ulcerative colitis, carcinoma, and ischemic colitis.

Pseudomembranous enterocolitis (see below) usually can be diagnosed by the pseudomembrane seen on the ulcerated area, although this is not invariably present. Culture of *Clostridium difficile* or demonstration of its toxin in the stool may confirm the diagnosis.

Treatment

Corticosteroids and sulfasalazine are well-established therapeutic agents. The former is more often used in treatment of the acute phase.

Prednisone should be used only for short-term treatment of an acute episode, being gradually reduced as symptoms abate and discontinued completely within weeks. A dose of 0.5 mg/kg is reasonable to begin with. Early side effects are less important than those involved with longer-term use (eg, mental confusion, depression, and peptic ulceration). If relapse occurs, the patient may be maintained on a dosage of 7.5 to 10.0 mg/day after a further short intensive course, or a trial of sulfasalazine may be undertaken.

Sulfasalazine may impair folate absorption and should, therefore, be given with folic acid. Good fluid intake must be maintained to prevent the deposition of crystals in the kidneys. Occasional side effects include hypersensitivity reactions and bone marrow depression, which require immediate withdrawal of the drug. Other side effects include nausea, vomiting, epigastric discomfort, headache, vertigo, and tinnitus. Rare side effects include pancreatitis, polyarteritis nodosa, pulmonary fibrosis, and agranulocytosis. Sulfasalazine is available in 500-mg tablets. In older people, a dosage based on 60 mg/kg/day is a reasonable guide. The full dose should be built up over several days and the tablets given with food in divided doses. Once the acute episode has resolved, the drug should be withdrawn gradually. There is some evidence that sulfasalazine is useful in preventing relapse.

Other therapeutic agents that have been advocated are azathioprine, mercaptopurine, and metronidazole, but none has proved efficacious. Because the immunosuppressives have dangerous adverse effects, particularly in the elderly, advice of a specialist should be sought before they are used. Dietary therapy has been advocated, but no supportive evidence exists for it in old age. The diet should be nutritious.

Surgery is necessary for acute complications; eg, perforation, intestinal obstruction, and abscesses. It may also be required for persistent inflammatory disease in the presence of diverticular disease when medical treatment fails. Surgical therapy includes a variety of procedures. For ileocecal disease, resection and ileotransverse colostomy are the standard. Localized colonic disease may be treated by a limited resection with anastomosis; this may provide relief that lasts for years but will probably be followed by recurrence.

Crohn's colitis involving the entire colon is treated by total proctocolectomy. Duodenal involvement may require gastroenterostomy; since anastomotic ulcer is a frequent sequela, consideration also should be given to concomitant vagotomy. Small rectal fistulas may be excised but usually recur in the presence of active disease in the intestine or colon. Extensive, multiple rectal fistulas require colostomy to relieve sepsis followed later by resection of involved bowel.

Although all of these procedures appear to be only palliative, patients often have remissions lasting $\geq$ 10 yr.

ULCERATIVE COLITIS

An inflammatory disease of the colon of unknown etiology that spreads continuously but rarely penetrates deeper than the mucosa muscularis. Ulcerative colitis can occur at any age, but there seems to be a trough in incidence between the ages of 50 and 60 yr, with a second peak occurring in the 60s. Prevalence rates, on the other hand, are maximal at 50 yr of age. While the initial attack in the older age group has a more sinister prognosis (partly because of delay in making the diagnosis), the course of the disease is generally less severe and the relapse rate lower, provided it is successfully treated in the early stage.

Pathology

Histologically, the first manifestation is dilation and congestion of the mucosal and submucosal blood vessels. This is followed by diffuse ulcerations and epithelial necrosis with depletion of goblet cells and infiltration of polymorphonuclear leukocytes. Crypt abscesses develop, which gradually coalesce, producing a lateral spread. This may undermine the mucosa, sometimes leading to the appearance of pseudocysts on x-ray. Granulation tissue forms, which is highly vascular and friable and bleeds easily.

The disease extends proximally from the dentate line, usually affecting the rectum and the remainder of the colon to a variable extent.

Symptoms and Signs

Ulcerative colitis is generally classified as mild, moderate, or severe. Lower GI bleeding is its major manifestation. In mild cases, intermittent attacks may present with diarrhea, with or without fecal incontinence; anorectal lesions; and few other clinical findings. In severe or fulminating ulcerative colitis, the onset is rapid with additional clinical features, including tenesmus; the passage of blood, pus, and mucus; weakness; cramps; and a distended, tender, and tympanitic abdomen with absence of bowel sounds. There may be rapid weight loss, fever, tachycardia, elevated ESR, and a fall in serum albumin level, together with symptoms of dehydration (due to diarrhea) and anemia (due to bleeding), possibly manifested as mental confusion and postural hypotension.

Complications

Toxic megacolon, possibly precipitated by hypokalemia or inappropriate use of anticholinergic drugs, may have an insidious onset and be complicated by perforation—again, presenting silently. Acute mental confusion, pyrexia, and general deterioration should alert the physician to these possibilities. Plain abdominal x-ray shows colonic dilation and gas under the diaphragm.

Colon carcinoma is a well-recognized, long-term complication of ulcerative colitis, although this usually does not appear for 15 to 20 yr, and, therefore, is less of a hazard in older people.

Complications such as arthralgia, uveitis, erythema nodosum, and pyoderma gangrenosum are less common than in Crohn's disease.

Diagnosis

A diagnosis can usually be made by **sigmoidoscopy** or **proctoscopy.** Disease primarily involves the rectum, and examination shows a granular, friable mucosa. **Colonoscopy** is *not* indicated in acutely ill patients or in those with severe disease because of the danger of perforation. **Radiography** is used as a second-line measure to confirm the disease and define its extent. It may show loss of haustra (now regarded as a relatively nonspecific finding), or it may show ulceration. The double-contrast barium enema may show a granular appearance or the presence of pseudopolyps. **Rectal biopsy** usually establishes the diagnosis.

Establishing the diagnosis is complicated in elderly people because of the possible coexistence of colonic diverticula and the increasing prevalence of ischemic colitis. Irritable colon, probably less common in the elderly than in younger patients, is distinguished by the absence of fever and leukocytosis and the presence of small stools. Acute enteritis must be kept in mind, including *Campylobacter* infection, shigellosis, and amebiasis. The illness is of short duration, and the stool culture is positive. Pseudomembranous colitis should be considered, particularly in patients taking antibiotics (see below). Postradiation proctitis, which may present similarly, is suggested by the history.

Prognosis

In persons > 60 yr of age, the prognosis for the first attack may be poor because of the delayed diagnosis, because of surgery for massive bleeding or perforation, or as a result of pulmonary embolism, heart failure, or superimposed infection elsewhere. If the first attack is mild, subsequent attacks are likely to be mild and 10% of patients have no relapse.

Carcinoma of the colon is 10 times more common in patients with ulcerative colitis than in the general population, although the risk is small in the first 5 to 10 yr of the disease. It is highest with extensive disease, particularly that involving the whole colon. The lesions are those of adenocarcinoma; about 15% are multicentric. Therefore, regular surveillance is necessary, and patients with long-standing disease should be examined using a flexible sigmoidoscope q 6 mo.

Other complications include liver disease, which may be pericholangitis or fatty infiltration (rarely, chronic active hepatitis or cirrhosis). Stenosis of the colon occasionally occurs.

Treatment

In mild cases, sulfasalazine tablets 500 mg bid given with food, gradually increasing to 40 mg/kg/day if necessary, may be used. Alternatively, corticosteroids given rectally may be all that is required. Hydrocortisone succinate 100 mg is administered as an enema bid. It should be retained with the patient supine at first, then lying on the left side, and then on the right side. Antidiarrheal medication is not generally recommended in ulcerative colitis but may be used cautiously in mild cases. A normal diet can be maintained.

In moderate cases, initial treatment is prednisone 40 mg/day, which may be given in a single dose orally. **In severe and fulminant cases,** IV steroids should be used (eg, hydrocortisone 300 to 400 mg/day by constant infusion for 5 to 10 days). Thereafter, prednisone 40 mg/day orally should be substituted and gradually withdrawn (by 5 mg q 5 days). Side effects of prolonged corticosteroid therapy (in addition to confusion, depression, and peptic ulceration) include the onset of hypertension, cardiac failure, diabetes, and candidiasis.

Supportive treatment for moderate and severe cases includes the correction of salt and water depletion and of anemia. In fulminant cases, blood transfusion may be necessary.

Maintenance therapy with corticosteroids generally is not helpful in ulcerative colitis, and significant symptoms persisting or recurring despite a dosage of > 15 mg/day prednisone suggests the need for surgery. However, sulfasalazine in doses of not < 2 gm/day may diminish the frequency of relapse.

Surgery: Elective colectomy is curative in ulcerative colitis and may be performed in 1 or 2 stages. In the elderly, there is a greater risk of perioperative complications, including thromboembolism. Indications for surgery include poor response to medical treatment, the development of strictures, and carcinoma. Emergency surgery may be needed for toxic megacolon or perforation. The latter, as in Crohn's disease, may be relatively silent in its presentation in the elderly and, therefore, diagnosis may be late.

PSEUDOMEMBRANOUS COLITIS

An inflammatory process of the colon in which necrotic epithelium and inflammatory cells form a fragile, easily removed, whitish-yellow slough.

Etiology

The disease most commonly occurs during or after a course of antibiotics, manifesting as an acute illness with guarded prognosis. It is associated in most cases with the presence of *Clostridium difficile*, which produces a toxin thought to be the key etiologic factor. The problem may be more common in patients who develop shock, uremia, or ischemic heart disease. Clindamycin and lincomycin are the antibiotics most commonly associated with pseudomembranous colitis, but ampicillin, amoxicillin, the cephalosporins, penicillin, tetracycline, erythromycin, and trimethoprim may also be associated. The disease may occur up to 4 to 6 wk after discontinuing the antibiotics. Carcinoma of the colon and Crohn's disease are occasionally associated with pseudomembranous colitis.

Symptoms, Signs, and Diagnosis

The disease presents with abdominal pain, tenesmus, and a profuse watery diarrhea, occasionally containing blood. Fever is usually present, with leukocytosis in some cases. The distal colon is involved in most cases, and the diagnosis may be made on flexible sigmoidoscopy, which shows the whitish-yellow pseudomembrane. Colonoscopy can detect cases restricted to the transverse or right colon. Histologically, the pseudomembrane arises from areas of superficial ulceration of the mucosa and is caused by a lesion that, under the microscope, looks much like the eruption of a volcano. Barium enema is *not indicated and may be dangerous because of the risk of perforation.* Plain film of the abdomen may be helpful. Stool culture for *C. difficile* and demonstration of the toxin in the stool are useful tests that are becoming more generally available.

Treatment

The causative antibiotics should be withdrawn, and in mild cases, this may be sufficient treatment. Correction of water and electrolyte loss and use of metronidazole may be effective. Vancomycin has been the specific treatment for this condition and is given orally in a dosage of 125 mg q 6 h, except in fulminant cases, when it may be given IV. It is ototoxic and nephrotoxic. A repeat course of vancomycin may be used for relapses. Bacitracin may also be used.

Cholestyramine, an anion-exchange resin, has also been advocated for treatment of this condition but is less effective. In fulminant cases, surgery (ie, subtotal colectomy or diverting ileostomy) may be lifesaving. Pseudomembranous colitis has a high mortality in the elderly.

ISCHEMIC COLITIS

Inflammation and edema of part of the colon resulting from impairment of its blood supply. Ischemic colitis is generally transient, although it may progress to infarction.

Vascular disease of the alimentary canal is extremely rare in comparison with that of the heart and the brain. This is because of the rich anastomotic circulation provided through the marginal arterial arcade, which distributes blood from the branches of the superior and inferior mesenteric arteries and parallels the course of the colon. The most vulnerable point is usually at the splenic flexure, where there is thought to be a watershed between these 2 arteries (the so-called **Griffith's point**), and 80% of ischemic colitis occurs here. The inferior mesenteric artery is affected to a lesser degree than are the celiac axis and the superior mesenteric artery. In many cases, there is a precipitating factor, particularly one producing hypotension (eg, dehydration, hemorrhage, or low-output heart failure). Polycythemia, diabetes, and the use of digitalis are also occasionally precipitating factors.

Symptoms and Signs

Symptoms usually have a sudden onset, last for a few days, and then resolve. Presenting symptoms are abdominal pain, characteristically in the left hypochondrium or left iliac fossa, and blood-stained, loose stools that may contain blood clots. Vomiting, pyrexia, and leukocytosis may also occur. Examination may disclose abdominal distention and tenderness, with loss of bowel sounds.

A small proportion of patients progress from ischemia to infarction, with a death rate exceeding 50%. However, ischemia alone has a good prognosis, although a stricture develops in a number of cases. This is often asymptomatic, but colicky abdominal pains persisting after the acute stage has subsided suggests that a stricture has formed. In about 15% of cases, further ischemic attacks occur.

Diagnosis

A high index of suspicion is required, particularly when an elderly patient has any of the predisposing or precipitating factors noted above. The diagnosis is made on clinical grounds and confirmed by barium enema, which should be performed promptly. During the first few days, the characteristic sign of thumb printing (or sawtooth pattern) is seen in the affected segment, as a result of hemorrhage and edema in the wall of the colon. These signs, however, are evanescent and often the diagnosis is not confirmed.

A manifestation described as pseudo-obstruction due to secondary spasm with dilation of the gut proximal to the affected segment may occur. If colonoscopy is performed because the diagnosis is uncertain, nodular hemorrhagic areas may be seen early in the disease. The colon is friable, and biopsies must be performed with great precision. Air insufflation should be *avoided*. Patients should be observed for signs of peritonitis, which would indicate a need for surgical intervention.

Treatment

Most cases of ischemic colitis are managed conservatively with correction of dehydration and the use of plasma expanders (eg, low-molecular-weight dextran).

COLORECTAL CANCER
(See in Chs. 52 and 53)

49. DIARRHEA

O. Dhodanand Kowlessar

An increase in the frequency of defecation (> 3 stools/day) associated with increased stool volume (> 300 mL), increased fluidity, and/or abnormal sensations in defecation characterized by urgency and pain.

Diarrhea can be classified on the basis of pathophysiologic processes and disorders. A simple classification entails 6 general processes: **(1) osmotic diarrhea,** secondary to ingestion of osmotically active ingredients in foods and drugs; **(2) toxigenic diarrhea** due to infection by bacteria or viruses, which elaborate toxins that cause the intestinal epithelial cells to secrete water and electrolytes into the gut lumen; **(3) maldigestive diarrhea,** secondary to pancreatic exocrine insufficiency, especially lipase deficiency, and bile acid insufficiency, and bacterial overgrowth syndromes; **(4) malabsorptive diarrhea** encountered in celiac disease, tropical sprue, giardiasis, and Whipple's disease; **(5) diarrhea secondary to the increased secretion of hormones, peptides, and/or biogenic amines from tumors,** including carcinoid tumors, medullary carcinoma of the thyroid, islet-cell tumor of the pancreas (vipoma), gastrinoma (Zollinger-Ellison syndrome), parathyroid adenoma, and small cell carcinoma of the lung; and **(6) colonic diarrhea,** secondary to ulcerative colitis, Crohn's disease of the colon, ischemic colitis, carcinoma of the colon, villous adenoma, radiation colitis, and resection of < 100 cm of the distal ileum (bile-acid–induced diarrhea). Some microorganisms (notably *Shigella, Salmonella, Campylobacter, Clostridium difficile,* and certain pathogenic strains of *Escherichia coli*) can infect the colonic mucosa with ensuing bloody diarrhea.

OSMOTIC DIARRHEA

In the elderly, this type of diarrhea is caused by the ingestion of poorly absorbable solutes, eg, magnesium sulfate, sodium sulfate, citrate-containing laxatives, antacids containing $Mg(OH)_2$ and mannitol, and sorbitol (chewing gum and diet candy). Disaccharidase deficiencies, especially lactase deficiency, can cause osmotic diarrhea. Osmotic diarrhea also occurs postgastrectomy or postvagotomy, in dumping syndrome, in short bowel syndrome, and with chronic small intestinal ischemia. The onset of the diarrhea is abrupt, with an increase in stool volume, and is not associated with blood or fat in the stool. Nausea, vomiting, and crampy abdominal pain are not features of osmotic diarrhea. The diarrhea ceases when the patient fasts or stops ingesting the poorly absorbable solute.

Diagnosis

A complete history is essential. In patients with lactase deficiency, the pH of the stool is usually between 4 and 6 (normal stool pH is > 6.0), with an associated increase in short-chain fatty acids. A lactose-H_2 breath test after lactose ingestion demonstrates an increase in breath hydrogen > 20 ppm within 3 h. Measurement of Mg (normal is < 12 mM), sulfate (normal is < 5 mM), and phosphate (normal is < 12 mM) in stool water may be necessary, especially in cases of surreptitious laxative abuse, a more common problem in elderly women.

Treatment

Stopping the ingestion of the offending solute and explaining to the patient why this is necessary is effective. Lactase deficiency is treated by removing lactose from all food sources and drugs with lactose fillers. Low-lactose milk should be prescribed.

TOXIGENIC DIARRHEAS

These diarrheas are caused by a variety of microorganisms that usually produce an enterotoxin or enterotoxin-like substance. The responsible microorganisms include *Staphylococcus aureus, Vibrio cholerae, Clostridium botulinum, Escherichia coli, Bacillus cereus, Clostridium perfringens, Clostridium difficile,* and *Vibrio parahaemolyticus.*

Staphylococcus aureus FOOD POISONING

Staphylococcus aureus food intoxication is caused by the ingestion of preformed toxin, usually from contaminated food. The onset is explosive, generally within 2 to 6 h following ingestion of the contaminated food. Severe vomiting precedes the passage of loose, foul-smelling stools associated with moderate to diffuse abdominal cramps without tenesmus and fever. The clinical course is self-limited and usually resolves in 12 to 24 h.

Diagnosis is made on the characteristic clinical picture and finding more than 10^5 colony-forming units (CFU) per gram of staphylococci from the incriminated food (eg, cream pastries, coleslaw, potato salad).

Treatment is supportive. Antimicrobial therapy is not indicated.

Bacillus cereus FOOD POISONING

Bacillus cereus, a frequent cause of food poisoning, is usually associated with the ingestion of contaminated refried rice or vegetables. It is characterized by 2 clinical syndromes: **"emesis syndrome"** and **"diarrheal syndrome."** In the emesis syndrome, vomiting begins approximately 6 h after the ingestion of the organisms, is associated with abdominal pain and diarrhea, and mimics *Staphylococcus aureus* intoxication. The diarrheal syndrome mimics *Clostridium perfringens,* occurring 8 to 16 h after ingestion of contaminated food; it is not associated with vomiting, but nausea is occasionally present. It is accompanied by abdominal pain with some tenesmus and profuse, foul-smelling watery diarrhea.

Diagnosis is made by demonstrating 10^5 CFU/gm of the organism in the stool.

Treatment is supportive, and both forms of the illness subside in 12 to 24 h.

Clostridium perfringens FOOD POISONING

Clostridium perfringens is a gram-positive, spore-forming bacillus producing a potent thermolabile exotoxin. It exerts its effect on the proximal small intestine by activating adenyl cyclase, producing increased intestinal fluid secretion and decreased reabsorption. It is associated with the ingestion of contaminated beef, beef products, and poultry. This disorder is characterized by the sudden onset of unusually foul-smelling diarrheal stools without blood or mucus, moderately severe colicky abdominal pain, and no vomiting. It is self-limiting and usually lasts < 24 h.

Diagnosis is established by finding > 10^5 CFU/gm of the organisms in the contaminated food or from stools of ill patients.

Treatment is supportive.

Escherichia coli DIARRHEA

At least 5 types of *E. coli* can cause GI infections, including enteropathogenic **(EPEC),** enterotoxigenic **(ETEC),** enteroinvasive **(EIEC),** enterohemorrhagic **(EHEC),** and enteroadherent **(EAEC)** *E. coli.* Enterotoxigenic *E. coli* comes from contaminated water and is manifested as a subacute illness with a 24- to 72-hour incubation period. It is associated with diffuse, mild abdominal pain; foul-smelling, profuse watery diarrhea; and occasional vomiting. The duration of the illness is < 1 wk.

Diagnosis is clinical.

Treatment is primarily adequate replacement of fluids. Oral tetracycline 250 mg qid for 2 days may be given in severe cases. When toxigenic *E. coli* **(ETEC)** is the causative pathogen in **traveler's diarrhea,** rehydration should be given immediate priority. Bismuth subsalicylate in dosages of 30 to 60 mL (or 2 tablets) qid significantly reduces the diarrhea. In severe cases associated with nausea, vomiting, abdominal cramps, and fever or blood in the stool, antibiotics can reduce the duration of the illness. Trimethoprim/sulfamethoxazole **(TMP/SMX)** 960 mg (TMP 160 mg, SMX 800 mg) or 250 mg TMP should be administered bid for 3 to 5 days. Doxycycline 100 mg bid and ciprofloxacin 500 mg bid are effective.

Elderly patients, especially those in nursing homes, have an increased susceptibility to *E. coli* 0157:H7 infection with high morbidity and mortality rates. The incubation period is approximately 8 days. The clinical picture is hemorrhagic colitis, initially presenting with watery diarrhea; the stool becomes grossly bloody hours to days later. The diarrhea is accompanied by abdominal cramps and vomiting. Fever is not a prominent feature. Potential risk factors include reduced gastric acidity, the use of antacids and H_2 receptor antagonists, and antibiotic therapy. Although rare in adults, hemolytic uremic syndrome has been described in a recent outbreak in a nursing home in southwestern Ontario.

Diagnosis is established by culturing the stools for *E. coli* 0157:H7 within the first 4 days of the illness; stool filtrates should be tested for verotoxin activity.

Treatment is supportive with IV fluid replacement.

INVASIVE DIARRHEA

The principal pathogens include *Salmonella, Shigella, Campylobacter,* and *Yersinia.* The latter 2 are seen predominantly in children and young adults. These invasive pathogens involve the distal ileum and colon, producing mucosal ulceration.

SHIGELLOSIS

Shigellae are a group of gram-negative enteric organisms. There are 4 major subgroups: Group A-serotypes of *Shigella dysenteriae:* Group B-serotypes of *S. flexneri;* Group C-serotypes of *S. boydi,* and Group D-serotypes of *S. sonnei. S. sonnei* is the most common serotype, responsible for 60 to 80% of *Shigella* dysentery in the USA.

Symptoms and Signs

The illness is characterized by lower abdominal pain, rectal burning, tenesmus, and diarrhea. Dysentery stool consisting of blood and mucus is seen in $1/3$ of patients, and fever is present in 40%. Severe disease causes toxicity, and patients are highly febrile. The course is variable, but in adults, the average duration of symptoms is 7 days.

Diagnosis

Microscopic examination of fecal samples reveals multiple polymor-phonuclear leukocytes and RBCs. Stool should be cultured and antibi-otic sensitivity performed. Sigmoidoscopy and biopsy are generally not performed.

Treatment

Therapy consists of rehydration with oral and IV fluids for high-volume diarrhea and excessive vomiting. Narcotic-related drugs are *con-traindicated.* Moderate to severe cases should receive ampicillin 500 mg orally qid or 1 gm IV q 6 h. In communities where isolates are known to be resistant to ampicillin, TMP/SMX at a dosage of 10 mg TMP/kg/day and 50 mg SMX/kg/day for 5 days should be prescribed.

SALMONELLOSIS

Salmonellae are gram-negative, non-spore–forming bacilli that belong to the family of Enterobacteriaceae. There are 3 species: *S. typhi, S. choleraesuis,* and *S. enteritidis. S. enteritidis typhimurium* is the most common serotype, causing infection in humans. It invades mucosal cells and multiplies within them, eliciting a polymorphonuclear leukocyte re-sponse. Fluid accumulation within the intestinal lumen is related to the elaboration of heat-labile and heat-stable enterotoxins.

Symptoms and Signs

The clinical manifestations of *S. enteritidis typhimurium* in the elderly include nausea, vomiting, and an early chill initially, followed by colicky abdominal pain, diarrhea, and vomiting. The diarrhea ranges from a few loose stools to up to 30 bowel movements daily. Characteristically, the stools are watery, green, and malodorous, with variable amounts of mu-cus. Sometimes patients present with high fever and bloody and mucoid diarrhea, suggesting significant colonic involvement. The course is vari-able. It can last for 1 wk or 2 to 3 mo. The average course is 3 wk. The main complications are bleeding, toxic megacolon, and overwhelming sepsis.

Diagnosis

Microscopic examination of methylene blue-stained specimens reveals moderate numbers of polymorphonuclear leukocytes. Stool should be cultured on selective or differential media.

Treatment

Antimicrobial therapy usually is not used in cases of *Salmonella* gas-troenteritis. However, the elderly, especially those with underlying ma-lignancies, lymphoproliferative disorders, cardiovascular diseases, aneu-rysms, and vascular grafts, should be given ampicillin 50 to 100 mg/kg/day in divided doses orally or parenterally for 10 to 14 days.

Alternatively, TMP/SMX is given at a dose of 10 mg/kg/day for TMP and 50 mg/kg/day for SMX to a maximum of 4 tablets/day (320 mg and 1600 mg) for 2 wk.

---

50.   MALABSORPTION SYNDROMES

O. Dhodanand Kowlessar

A spectrum of symptoms and signs usually resulting from excessive fat excretion (steatorrhea) and varying degrees of panmalabsorption of fat- and water-soluble vitamins, electrolytes, and water and maldigestion of carbohydrates and proteins.

The nutritional status of elderly persons is influenced by the effects of age on nutrient digestion and absorption. Aging does not significantly affect the structure and function of the exocrine pancreas, nor does it impair the digestive capacity. Maldigestion and malabsorption occur only when > 90% of pancreatic function is lost. Similarly, the small intestine has a large reserve capacity, and aging has only subtle influences on the digestive and absorptive processes.

The well-nourished elderly person has a reduced mucosal surface area with slight reduction of villus height and normal preservation of enterocyte height, intraepithelial lymphocyte counts, and lamina propria cellularity. Jejunal brush border lactase and alkaline phosphatase decrease with age, while other disaccharidases are relatively stable, declining after the 7th decade. Fat absorption is normal, but absorption of fat-soluble vitamin A and K are increased, while that of vitamin D is reduced.

Carbohydrate absorption measured by breath-H_2 demonstrates excess breath hydrogen excretion in $1/3$ of subjects > 65 yr of age. This abnormality may be multifactorial and is due in part to achlorhydria, abnormal bacterial flora, delayed gastric emptying, and slow intestinal transit. Vitamin B_{12} and folate absorption remain normal, while nonheme iron absorption is reduced. Thus, disorders in absorption and digestion in the elderly are not related to physiologic processes but to disease states.

Malabsorption falls into 3 pathophysiologic categories: **(1) intraluminal maldigestion** secondary to pancreatic insufficiency, intraluminal bacterial overgrowth, and biliary tract disease; **(2) mucosal lesions** resulting from celiac disease, Crohn's disease, and ileal resection > 100 cm; and **(3) lymphatic dysfunction;** eg, retroperitoneal fibrosis, intestinal lymphangiectasia, and retroperitoneal malignancy. In the elderly, there are 3 main causes of malabsorption: celiac disease, bacterial overgrowth syndromes, and pancreatic insufficiency.

CELIAC DISEASE

(Celiac Sprue; Nontropical Sprue; Sprue Syndrome; Idiopathic
Steatorrhea; Gluten-Induced Enteropathy)

*A genetically determined disease of intestinal malabsorption of a wide
variety of nutrients, resulting from characteristic, if not specific, pathologic
alterations of the small intestinal mucosa induced by the ingestion of the
gliadin fraction of gluten.* Gliadin is a mixture of high molecular weight
cereal proteins found in wheat, rye, oats, and barley. Prompt clinical,
biochemical, and histologic improvement follows the withdrawal of
gliadin-containing cereal grains from the diet in most patients.

Celiac disease occurs throughout the world, but its prevalence is not
known. The incidence, which varies considerably in different parts of
the world, is highest in western Ireland (1:300). In recent series, the affected population is older than that previously recorded; many of the
cases are diagnosed in or after the 7th decade. This age-related skew—
seen in the USA, Sweden, Scotland, and Ireland—probably reflects clinicians' greater willingness to consider the diagnosis in the elderly.

Etiology and Pathophysiology

An 80 to 90% incidence of the histocompatibility antigens HLA-B8 or
HLA-DR3 is found among patients with celiac disease. Patients who
lack either of these antigens have the immunoglobulin heavy-chain allo-
type marker G2m(n).

Various mechanisms of etiology and pathogenesis have been proposed.
One theory is that the small intestinal absorptive cell is deficient in one
or more enzymes that normally break down gliadin peptides, and the
residual polypeptides injure the epithelial absorbing cells. Another theory suggests that susceptible patients absorb gliadin, which in turn
causes a humoral and a T-lymphocyte–dependent immune reaction, resulting in lysis and death of absorptive cells with a compensatory increase in crypt cell proliferation and a flat mucosal lesion. A third
proposal is that gluten behaves like a lectin and binds to pathologically
altered carbohydrate structures of the luminal small intestinal cells.

Finally, recent evidence shows that there is an amino acid sequence
homology between the early region Elb protein of the human adenovirus Ad12 and A-gliadin, a major α-gliadin component. This finding
suggests that the immune response to antigenic determinants produced
during a prior intestinal viral infection may be important in the pathogenesis of celiac disease. Immunologic cross-reactivity between Ad12
peptide and gliadin in a murine system, as well as a lack of specific antibodies to the Elb-58kD protein in celiac sera, have not been
demonstrated. Thus, this disease is probably multicausal with genetic,
immunologic, biochemical, and perhaps environmental factors playing a
role.

Symptoms and Signs

The clinical manifestations of celiac disease in the elderly are subtle and variable. The typical features of steatorrhea, diarrhea, weight loss, and malnutrition are present in most patients, but they may be mild or absent. Certain nutritional deficiencies, eg, iron deficiency, bone pain with osteomalacia, hypoprothrombinemia, or fatigue with mild hematologic abnormalities (unexplained macrocytosis, low folate reserve or a peripheral smear showing splenic atrophy—Howell-Jolly bodies, target cells, thrombocytopenia), may obscure the underlying disorder and prevent early diagnosis.

Physical findings vary among patients. Some appear chronically emaciated with pale mucous membranes and dry, scaly skin, which is occasionally hyperpigmented. BP is normal or low and peripheral edema is often present. The hair may be thin and sparse and fingers may show clubbing. Usually, glossitis and cheilosis are present. The striking finding is abdominal distention with hyperactive bowel sounds. Other findings include positive Trousseau's and Chvostek's signs, ecchymoses, hematomas, skeletal deformities secondary to osteoporosis and osteomalacia, loss of height, evidence of peripheral neuropathy, and subacute combined degeneration.

Laboratory Findings

Fat malabsorption can be assessed by microscopic examination of a stool specimen stained with Sudan III, which demonstrates an increase in fat droplets. A 24-h stool collection has increased weight, usually weighing more than the normal 200 gm. Chemical fat determination of a 3- to 6-day stool collection obtained while the patient is ingesting a 100-gm fat diet shows fat excretion of 10 to 40 gm/24 h (normal < 6 gm/24 h). A ^{14}C-triolein breath test that shows an increase in labeled breath CO_2 suggests fat malabsorption.

The 5-h urinary xylose excretion after the ingestion of 25 gm D-xylose is 0.5 to 2.5 gm (normal is > 4.5 gm/5 h), and the blood level of xylose at 1 h is < 30 mg. Both urinary excretion and blood levels of xylose should be obtained in the elderly because of decreased renal function. **Hematologic findings** include iron-deficiency anemia with hypochromia and microcytosis on blood smear. Some patients have a megaloblastic anemia secondary to folic acid or vitamin B_{12} deficiency, or both. Serum folate levels range between 0.7 and 3.5 ng/mL (normal is > 3.5 ng/mL).

In patients with severe ileal damage, **the Schilling test** reveals an excretion of < 8% of ^{57}Co-cyanocobalamin and is not corrected by the addition of intrinsic factor and broad-spectrum antibiotics, thus differentiating celiac disease from pernicious anemia and blind-loop variants, respectively.

Other absorptive defects: The serum carotene is a useful screening test; levels < 50 μg/dL are invariably seen. Low levels of serum albumin, cholesterol, and vitamin A, and low prothrombin time (corrected by administration of vitamin K) may be found. In patients with osteomalacia, the serum Ca is low, with normal or low serum P and elevated bone alkaline phosphatase. A bone biopsy revealing increases in the number of osteoid foci and widening of the osteoid seams confirms the diagnosis of osteomalacia. A generalized deficiency of intestinal disaccharidase activity occurs secondary to brush-border damage. Lactase is most affected. A lactose-H_2 breath test after lactose ingestion shows an increase in breath hydrogen > 20 ppm within 3 h.

Diagnosis

Diagnosis is based upon characteristic histologic changes in a blind or endoscopic peroral jejunal mucosal biopsy. There is loss of villus architecture, markedly elongated intestinal crypts, cuboidal luminal epithelial cells with loss of nuclear polarity, cytoplasmic basophilia, and vacuolization. The brush border is markedly attenuated. There is an apparent increase in intraepithelial cells; in the lamina propia, there is an increased cellularity consisting of immunoglobulin-producing plasma cells (IgM), lymphocytes, and some eosinophils and polymorphonuclear leukocytes.

Characteristically, the abnormal mucosa is confined to the proximal small intestine, but in severe cases, the entire small bowel mucosa is involved. The lesions are not entirely specific for celiac disease, but most patients in the temperate zone with these changes have this disease and respond clinically, biochemically, and histologically to a gluten-free diet. Clinical or biochemical relapse or worsening of the jejunal biopsy with a gluten or gliadin challenge confirms the diagnosis.

Treatment

The treatment of choice is a well-balanced diet containing normal amounts of fat, protein, and carbohydrate, along with strict avoidance of all foods containing wheat, rye, barley, and oats. Lactose-free milk is recommended for patients with lactase deficiency. Most patients show improvement in symptoms and signs within days or weeks, but some may take months.

Patients who do not respond either are not adhering to the diet or have another disease, eg, giardiasis, lymphoma, Whipple's disease, or collagenous sprue. (**Collagenous sprue** is rare; it is characterized by a severe lesion similar to that seen in celiac disease but that also has broad bands of fibrosis and collagen beneath the basement membrane. The prognosis for patients with this disease is generally poor.)

A few patients respond early to gluten withdrawals, but they relapse despite strict adherence to the diet. Some of these refractory or unclassified celiac disease patients may respond to treatment with high doses of corticosteriods (eg, prednisone 60 mg/day) or other immunosuppressive drugs, such as azathioprine or cyclophosphamide. Others, despite such therapy, have a relentless course usually culminating in death.

Supplemental therapy: Patients with iron-deficiency anemia should receive supplemental ferrous sulfate 350 mg tid, while those with folic acid deficiency should receive folic acid 5 mg daily for 1 mo, followed by 1 mg/day as maintenance. B_{12}-deficient patients should receive 100 μg vitamin B_{12} IM daily for 2 wk, then 100 μg monthly. Oral calcium gluconate 5 to 10 gm tid and magnesium gluconate 1 to 4 gm/day correct Ca and Mg deficiencies, respectively.

Patients with radiologic evidence of osteopenic bone disease require 6 to 8 gm calcium gluconate or calcium lactate plus 50,000 u. vitamin D/day. IV vitamin K 10 mg should be given *slowly* to correct prolonged prothrombin time. Therapeutic formula multivitamin preparations containing vitamin A, thiamine, riboflavin, niacin, pyridoxine, vitamin C, and vitamin E should be administered to patients with prolonged and severe malabsorption.

BACTERIAL OVERGROWTH SYNDROME

Intraluminal small intestinal bacterial overgrowth accompanied by nutrient malabsorption secondary to the catabolism of carbohydrates by gram-negative aerobes, deconjugation of bile acids by anaerobes, binding of cobalamin by anaerobes, and patchy damage to small intestinal epithelial cells.

Etiology

In healthy adults, the proximal small intestine lumen contains 0 to 10^4 microorganisms per milliliter, consisting of aerobes and facultative anaerobes, which are largely oral flora. This relative sterility is maintained by normal gastric acid secretion, normal peristalsis of the proximal small intestine, and luminal immunoglobulins. In the elderly $\geq$ 70 yr of age, hypochlorhydria or achlorhydria are common, permitting bacterial overgrowth.

A number of conditions can lead to small intestinal stagnation, including solitary large duodenal diverticulum, multiple jejunal diverticula, afferent loop of Billroth II partial gastrectomy, radiation enteritis, surgical blind loop, stricture, fistulas, and resection of the ileocecal valve. Motor abnormalities secondary to scleroderma, idiopathic intestinal pseudo-obstruction, and diabetic autonomic neuropathy also can lead to small intestinal proliferation of bacteria.

A duodenal diverticulum is present in about 20% of patients > 65 yr of age in whom upper GI series are performed. A similar percentage is found in postmortem studies using plaster casts of the duodenum. Bacterial overgrowth and consequent steatorrhea and nutritional deficiencies may occur in the presence of a duodenal diverticulum.

However, jejunal diverticulosis is uncommon, with an autopsy incidence of 0.5%. Although patients with this disease are usually asymptomatic, they may have multiple large jejunal diverticula, leading to bacterial overgrowth with malabsorption of fat and vitamin B_{12}. Recently, severe malabsorption has been described in patients with duodenal and jejunal diverticulosis, who were found to also have chronic pancreatitis with pancreatic insufficiency; these patients did not respond to broad-spectrum antibiotics alone but did respond when pancreatic enzymes were added.

Symptoms and Signs

The clinical manifestations vary greatly from an asymptomatic state to watery diarrhea secondary to deconjugated bile acids, hydroxy fatty and organic acids, clinically significant steatorrhea resulting in weight loss, bone pain and pathologic fractures, easy bruising (vitamin K deficiency), night blindness (vitamin A deficiency), hypocalcemic tetany, and weakness and easy fatigability secondary to cobalamin deficiency. Occasionally, the patient may present with a dimorphic anemia, both macrocytic and microcytic, the latter due to microulcerations of the stagnant loop with occult blood loss and guaiac-positive stools. Patients with strictures and small intestinal pseudo-obstruction have clinical features of abdominal distention (nausea and crampy periumbilical pain), antedating the onset of diarrhea, steatorrhea, and anemia.

Diagnosis

Increase in stool weight with evidence of excessive fat (on Sudan III stain, 72-h stool fat, or ^{14}C-triolein breath test) should be documented. Upper GI series with small intestine follow-through documents duodenal diverticulum, jejunal diverticula, stricture, gastrojejunocolic fistulas, afferent loop syndrome, intestinal pseudo-obstruction, scleroderma, and Crohn's disease. A small intestine biopsy excludes celiac disease, Whipple's disease, eosinophilic gastroenteritis, and giardiasis. Vitamin B_{12} deficiency should be documented by demonstrating reduced excretion of labeled cobalamin that is not corrected by intrinsic factor but is corrected by broad-spectrum antibiotics. Currently, the 1 gm ^{14}C-xylose breath test to detect bacterial overgrowth is the test of choice; it reveals elevated $^{14}CO_2$ levels in the breath within the first 60 min of the test. Although culture of the small intestinal contents has excellent specificity, it is cumbersome. The ^{14}C-cholylglycine breath test is easy to perform but lacks specificity.

Treatment

The recommended treatment is a 10-day course of cephalexin 250 mg qid and metronidazole 250 mg tid orally. A significant number of patients respond to treatment for 7 to 10 days, but few require repeat therapy and, rarely, continuous therapy for months is needed. Chloramphenicol 50 mg/kg/day orally in 4 divided doses is recommended for patients who fail to respond to cephalexin and metronidazole. Cobalamin deficiency in malabsorption responds to monthly IM injections of 100 μg vitamin B_{12}. Deficiencies of Ca, vitamin D, and vitamin K should be corrected as in celiac disease (see above).

CHRONIC PANCREATITIS WITH PANCREATIC INSUFFICIENCY

Recurrent or persisting abdominal pain secondary to anatomic (calcification, ductal changes, fibrosis) or functional (exocrine and/or endocrine insufficiency) damage to the pancreas. Some patients develop pancreatic exocrine or endocrine insufficiency in the absence of pain; this occurs more frequently in the elderly, many of whom have associated pancreatic calcification.

Etiology

In the elderly, the most common forms of chronic pancreatitis with pancreatic insufficiency are due to heavy alcohol intake for > 15 yr, trauma, vascular disease, abdominal radiation therapy, and carcinoma of the pancreas. Rarely, primary pancreatic atrophy and lipomatosis of the pancreas can cause steatorrhea and diabetes mellitus. A few of these patients are chronic alcoholics without abdominal pain, thus raising the question whether this is a true entity.

Symptoms and Signs

Recurrent attacks of severe abdominal pain are the predominant symptoms in 90% of patients with chronic pancreatitis. In the elderly, the pain is mild or absent except in patients with carcinoma of the pancreas and secondary pancreatic insufficiency. Characteristically, they present with abrupt onset of frequent bowel movements that are bulky and malodorous, greasy, and difficult to flush. Rectal seepage of oil, as well as visible oil in the toilet bowl, may be the presenting complaints. Significant weight loss (6 to 20 kg) occurs secondary to malabsorption and poor oral intake. Polyuria and polydipsia may precede the complaints of abnormal bowel movements. Less common clinical manifestations include subcutaneous fat necrosis, arthritis, and intramedullary fat necrosis with associated bone pain.

Diagnosis

Diffuse, stippled pancreatic calcification on flat plate film of the abdomen is diagnostic. CT scan and ultrasonography should be performed on patients with abdominal pain to rule out pancreatic pseudocyst and carcinoma of the pancreas. Pancreatic insufficiency is documented by the bentiromide urinary excretion test, which demonstrates a cumulative 6-h excretion of p-aminobenzoic acid **(PABA)** < 50% of the ingested synthetic peptide bentiromide. Serum trypsin-like immunoreactivity **(TLI)** reveals a value < 20 ng/mL (normal is 20 to 80 ng/mL) that is characteristic of pancreatic insufficiency, although this test is less sensitive than the bentiromide test.

Endoscopic retrograde cholangiopancreatography **(ERCP)** reveals an irregularly strictured and dilated main pancreatic duct with a beaded appearance that is almost diagnostic of chronic pancreatitis. Steatorrhea can be documented by the Sudan III stain for qualitative fat or by quantitative stool fat or ^{14}C-triolein breath test.

Treatment

Alcohol ingestion should be eliminated. Patients with pain should be given nonaddicting analgesics—salicylates, acetaminophen, and nonsteroidal anti-inflammatory drugs **(NSAIDs).** Large doses of potent pancreatic enzyme preparations high in lipase and proteolytic enzymes are required: 6 to 8 tablets (Ilozyme®, Viokase®) or 6 to 8 capsules (Ku-Zyme HP®, Cotazym®) or 3 enteric-coated tablets (Festal®) or 3 microencapsulated capsules (Pancrease®) with each meal. Gastric acid inactivates lipase; therefore, H_2 receptor antagonists may be prescribed to prevent the inactivation, but this may not be necessary in the elderly, because of their impaired gastric acid secretion. The prognosis is generally good except in patients with carcinoma of the pancreas and in those incapable of completely stopping alcohol consumption.

---

51. THE AGING LIVER

Steven Schenker and *Thomas E. Whigham*

A recurring difficulty in clinical medicine results from the attempt to separate the effects of aging from those of disease. As in many other areas of geriatrics, more questions than answers exist. It may be stated outright that there are no peculiar or characteristic diseases of the aged liver. Furthermore, the liver ages gracefully, without changes of so-called liver function tests. In this context, effects of aging on liver appearance, histology, physiology, and drug metabolism require more detailed comment.

Appearance: Autopsy studies and peritoneoscopy reveal that the liver appears brown and more fibrotic with advanced age. The increased capsular and parenchymal fibrosis should not be confused with the presence of cirrhosis. An age-related decline in hepatic weight occurs in both men and women, and there is some decrease in size of hepatic lobules, with preserved cell number.

Histology: With advancing age, hepatocytes vary in size, with a tendency toward enlargement. Nuclear changes occur with increased nuclear size and polyploidy, and there is an accompanying increase in the quantity of DNA per nucleus. Other organelles show changes, such as increases in mitochondrial size, number of lysosomes, and smooth and rough endoplasmic reticulum, and a decrease in Golgi apparatus surface area. A decline in the phagocytic function of Kupffer's cells has been described.

The brown pigment buildup with aging represents an accumulation of unexcretable metabolic residue acquired over a lifetime and, generally, has no physiologic significance. Much of this pigment is accounted for by an increased number of lipofuscin granules found in hepatocytes. Lipofuscin is a brown pigment resulting from the accumulation of end-stage metabolic products of lipids and proteins.

Some similarities exist between hepatic changes caused by malnutrition and those caused by aging. Both states are associated with a brown, atrophic-appearing liver. However, in malnutrition, the number of hepatocytes is normal, but they are smaller; in aging, there are fewer, but they are larger.

Physiology: A decrease in liver weight is accompanied by a diminished hepatic blood flow (resulting from decreased splanchnic blood flow). The diminished liver mass and blood flow may account for some changes in drug elimination observed in aging patients.

Quantitative and qualitative changes are seen in protein synthesis, with an overall increase of intracellular protein occurring with aging. Whether this protein is functional or, as Hans Popper has said, represents inactive or accumulated "junk" is unknown. Protein accumulation may result from diminished catabolism with accumulation of functionally (but not antigenically) abnormal protein. The accumulation of defective protein with age may be related to the process of hepatocyte aging.

Aging does not produce alteration in so-called liver function tests, which often measure hepatic damage, eg, hepatocellular injury (aminotransferases), selected protein synthesis (alkaline phosphatase), or hepatocyte transport (bilirubin), rather than overall function. Thus, abnormal values for these tests in the elderly reflect disease rather than the effects of aging.

Drug metabolism: Adverse drug reactions are more common in older persons, and a decreased elimination of some drugs has been noted. Available data relative to the liver are primarily from rodent studies and cannot be applied directly to humans. Many factors may influence drug disposition in the elderly (see Ch. 18), including changes in body composition, alterations in serum albumin levels, declining renal function, and individual variability. Thus, discerning the effect of the aging liver per se is difficult. Other physiologic changes, the multitude of drugs taken, poor compliance, and lack of understanding of drug therapy are also common causes of drug reactions in the elderly.

Many of the enzymes responsible for biotransformation of drugs, called microsomal enzymes, are located in the hepatic smooth endoplasmic reticulum. The activity and inducibility of these enzymes vary among individuals because of genetic variations. The biotransformation of drugs by the liver occurs in Phase I and Phase II reactions. Phase I reactions usually involve oxidation, reduction, or hydrolysis and convert the parent drug into more polar metabolites. Phase II reactions involve conjugation of the parent drug or metabolite with an additional substrate (eg, glucuronic acid), achieving the same result. Some Phase I reactions may decrease with aging, but Phase II reactions remain essentially unchanged.

The precise cause of the altered microsomal oxidative function is unknown but has been speculated to be accounted for by the decline in hepatic mass or changes in microsomal isozymes. The role of accumulation of functionally inferior enzymes (possibly because of posttranslational changes, deterioration, and so on) remains unclear. Drugs that exhibit higher first-pass metabolism seem to be particularly affected (eg, propranolol). Dosing changes based on *hepatic* function related to aging are usually not needed. However, age-related changes in renal function require downward dosage adjustments of many drugs excreted by the kidneys (see Ch. 18). Also the doses of certain drugs (eg, sedatives) may need to be adjusted for pharmacodynamic reasons (ie, target-organ sensitivity). The sensitivity of older persons to such agents may depend on receptor alterations, changes in binding of drugs in plasma, drug-drug interactions, presence of intercurrent illnesses, and other unknown factors.

Older organs may not adapt to injury as well as younger organs. Thus, hepatic illnesses (eg, severe hepatitis) may not be tolerated as well by the elderly because of delayed or impaired tissue repair. Further studies in this area are needed.

Since the liver ages without much significant physiologic change, should aging livers be made available for transplants? Many changes seen in the aging liver have little functional significance, and overall the liver is resistant to senescent change. Therefore, the current age limitation of 55 yr for liver donation seems to be unnecessary.

---

52. GASTROINTESTINAL NEOPLASMS

Maxwell Chait and *Sidney J. Winawer*

Cancer is second only to heart disease as the leading cause of death in the elderly, with GI tract malignancy accounting for > 25% of all deaths from cancer. Etiologic factors in GI tract cancer remain elusive, and worldwide variations in incidence of cancer of specific sites are enormous. Environmental factors (eg, dietary content of animal fat, fiber, minerals, and carcinogens) probably play a much greater role than hereditary factors in the elderly.

The more common primary neoplasms of the GI tract in this population are discussed below.

NEOPLASMS OF THE ESOPHAGUS

BENIGN NEOPLASMS

Less than 10% of esophageal neoplasms are benign. **Leiomyoma** is the most common lesion. Rare lesions include inflammatory polyps, squamous papilloma, lymphangioma, and lipoma. These tumors are usually asymptomatic and found incidentally on examination for unrelated complaints or at autopsy. In symptomatic cases, patients may present with dysphagia or upper GI bleeding. Diagnosis is established by barium swallow, followed by esophagoscopy and biopsy. Symptomatic tumors may be resected endoscopically. If the tumor is submucosal or if severe bleeding or obstruction is present, surgical resection is indicated.

MALIGNANT NEOPLASMS

Esophageal cancer accounts for only 4% of all GI cancers in the USA, but is more common in China, Iran, and Russia. A number of carcinogenic factors and disease states have been associated with esophageal cancer, including chronic thermal injury (eg, from drinking very hot tea); poor oral hygiene; esophageal stasis associated with achalasia; intake of exogenous toxins (eg, alcohol, tobacco, silica, nitrates, nitrosamines, and zinc); prior ionizing radiation; lye stricture; severe reflux esophagitis and associated Barrett's epithelium; and the Plummer-Vinson syndrome associated with esophageal webs.

Esophageal cancer occurs predominately in men between the ages of 50 and 70 yr and is more common in smokers and blacks. It usually involves the middle and lower thirds of the esophagus. The tumor may be infiltrative, ulcerative, or polypoid and may cause either a stricture, mass, or plaque.

Squamous cell carcinoma accounts for 95% of all esophageal malignancies. **Primary adenocarcinoma** accounts for < 5%. The remaining types make up < 1% and include primary adenoid cystic carcinoma, carcinosarcoma, melanoma, argyrophil cell carcinoma, and verrucous squamous cell carcinoma.

Symptoms and Signs

The most common symptoms are progressive dysphagia and weight loss. Others include hoarseness, halitosis, recurrent respiratory infections, and hematemesis. Signs appear late in the course of disease, if at all, and include regional lymphadenopathy, vocal cord paralysis, and pulmonary findings (eg, wheezes or rales).

Diagnosis

The diagnosis is usually made with a combination of barium swallow and endoscopy. The upper GI series often shows a stricture or an eccentric or asymmetric mucosal irregularity. Endoscopy provides direct visualization of the lesion and tissue for microscopic examination. The combination of biopsy and brush cytology yields the diagnosis in > 95% of cases. In high-risk areas (eg, Northern China) mass screening using balloon cytologic technics that reveals early lesions seems to result in improved prognosis.

Treatment

Surgical resection is the primary mode of treatment, although lesions in the upper third of the esophagus may not be amenable to such treatment. In high-risk patients, some mid-esophageal cancers can be treated with radiation. Combined radiotherapy and chemotherapy (using, for example, cisplatin and bleomycin) have yielded poor results. This approach is reserved for patients who present with metastatic disease or who are at increased risk, especially those with squamous cell carcinoma. Combinations of surgery, radiotherapy, and chemotherapy remain investigational.

Palliative measures for recurrent luminal obstruction or inoperable cancer may be performed endoscopically (eg, laser fulguration of tumor and placement of an esophageal prosthesis). For further details of surgical treatment, see Ch. 53.

The prognosis is dismal, with 5% overall 5-yr survival, although in carcinoma of the lower portion of the esophagus, selected series show nearly 25% survival. About $\frac{1}{2}$ the patients who have a curative operation in the USA will be $\geq$ 65 yr of age.

NEOPLASMS OF THE STOMACH
(See also BENIGN TUMORS OF THE STOMACH in Ch. 47)

BENIGN NEOPLASMS

Less than 5% of all gastric tumors are benign. Although **leiomyoma** is the most common of these in the general population, hyperplastic and adenomatous polyps are probably more common among the elderly. Other benign neoplasms include fibromas and neural tumors.

Hyperplastic polyps are small, dome-shaped lesions that constitute about 95% of all gastric epithelial polyps. The remaining 5% are predominantly adenomatous polyps, which can attain a diameter > 4 cm. Hyperplastic polyps carry no malignant potential, whereas adenomatous polyps do (usually when they are > 2 cm in diameter).

Gastric polyps most often develop in association with chronic atrophic gastritis and intestinal metaplasia of gastric mucosa, as in pernicious anemia. The **Canada-Cronkhite syndrome,** the only GI polyposis syndrome found in the elderly, includes ectodermal changes, (eg, increased pigmentation, alopecia, and atrophic nails). The polyps consist of dilated, cystic glands and markedly edematous stroma. This nonhereditary syndrome occurs equally in both sexes and, although the lesions are not premalignant, progressive diarrhea commonly leads to cachexia and death in women.

Symptoms and Signs
Most benign gastric tumors are asymptomatic. The most common presenting finding is anemia from chronic occult bleeding. Less commonly, epigastric pain or acute GI bleeding from ulceration of the tumor may occur. If the cardia is involved, dysphagia can occur. If the prepyloric antrum is involved, gastric outlet obstruction may occur.

Diagnosis

An upper GI series using the double-contrast technic provides excellent x-ray definition of small gastric mucosal lesions. Endoscopy provides direct visualization and tissue (from biopsy and cytology) for diagnosis in 90% of patients.

Treatment

Treatment is usually endoscopic excision or fulguration. If the lesion is submucosal or if its size or location prohibits endoscopic resection, surgery may be warranted, particularly if significant blood loss or other symptoms have occurred.

MALIGNANT NEOPLASMS

Adenocarcinoma accounts for 95% of all gastric malignancies. The worldwide incidence varies dramatically with low rates in the USA and high rates in Japan, Chile, and Iceland. However, an unexplained worldwide reduction has been observed, except in black males, over the past 50 yr.

In the USA, about 25,000 new cases and 14,000 deaths occur annually from gastric cancer, and the incidence increases with age. The mean age at the time of diagnosis is 55 yr. Gastric cancer is more common in blacks and among poor socioeconomic groups; the male:female ratio is 2:1.

Lymphoma constitutes about 4% of gastric malignancies. The stomach is the most common site of primary extranodal lymphoma and accounts for up to 75% of all reported cases of primary GI tract lymphoma. Gastric lymphoma generally occurs in the 6th decade of life, mainly in men. Most gastric lymphomas are of the histiocytic variety. Multiple primary malignancies are seen in approximately 25% of patients with gastric lymphoma and include skin cancer and adenocarcinoma in the irradiated gastric pouch.

Other malignancies, including leiomyosarcoma, carcinoid, and Kaposi's sarcoma, account for < 1% of all gastric malignancies.

Gastric abnormalities with malignant potential include adenoma, mucosal atrophy with intestinal metaplasia (with or without associated pernicious anemia), and hypertrophic gastropathy. Gastroduodenal peptic ulcer disease has no firm etiologic association with gastric cancer, although a benign-appearing gastric ulcer can possess a malignant focus.

Pathology

Gastric cancer is generally classified as early or advanced, according to its gross appearance. **Early gastric cancer** is confined to the mucosa or submucosa and is divided into 3 types: (1) protruded, either polypoid or fungating; (2) superficial, either elevated, flat or depressed; and (3) excavated. **Advanced gastric cancer** denotes disease penetrating the muscularis, and the probability of cure is poor. It also is divided into 3 types: (1) a mass lesion, either polypoid or fungating; (2) diffuse or infiltrating;

and (3) ulcerated. Advanced gastric cancer may have more than one of these characteristics. If the tumor infiltration is associated with a fibrous reaction, **linitis plastica** ("leather bottle" stomach) may occur.

Gastric cancer develops predominantly in the distal portion of the stomach and is rarely multicentric, except when it is associated with polyps or partial gastrectomy. Cancer spread is by direct extension and/or metastatic via lymphatics or the bloodstream.

Symptoms and Signs

Symptoms may be insidious in the early stages and dismissed as indigestion. The most common presenting symptom is vague epigastric discomfort, followed by anorexia, early satiety, weight loss, hematemesis, melena, and severe abdominal pain as the tumor progresses. If the cardia is involved, dysphagia may be noted. If the prepyloric antrum is involved, symptoms of partial or complete gastric outlet obstruction (eg, epigastric fullness, nausea, and vomiting) may occur.

In the early stages, there are no specific signs of gastric cancer. In later stages, weight loss; a palpable mass; lymphadenopathy in the left supraclavicular **(Virchow's node)** and left axillary regions; and, on rectal examination, Blumer's shelf may be noted. Liver metastases can present as hepatomegaly, jaundice, and ascites. Dermatologic manifestations of gastric cancer include acanthosis nigricans and dermatomyositis.

The differential diagnosis includes peptic ulcer and pancreaticobiliary tract disease.

Diagnosis

Upper GI x-ray is the initial mode of investigation, but lesions are frequently missed. Improved detection can be achieved by using the double-contrast technic; one may see a mass, an infiltrating ulcer, or only thickened rugae.

Gastroscopy permits visualization of most lesions, provides a means of obtaining tissue for biopsy and cytology, and yields the diagnosis in > 90% of cases.

Other laboratory procedures are of limited help. Elevated levels of carcinoembryonic antigen **(CEA)**, α-fetoprotein, and fetal sulfoglycoprotein and decreased levels of pepsinogen have been noted in approximately 15% of patients with gastric cancer, but these play a minor diagnostic role. However, if CEA is elevated prior to resection and decreases after resection, it may serve as a later predictor of recurrent disease if it rises again. CT scan of the abdomen is helpful in evaluating the extent of disease.

Special consideration should be given to patients who have undergone partial gastrectomy or gastroenterostomy for peptic ulcer disease. Such patients have an increased frequency of gastric polyps, epithelial dysplasia, and carcinoma within the remaining gastric pouch, beginning about 10 to 15 yr after surgery. The only real potential for cure of gastric cancer is early diagnosis and surgical excision.

The patient with **lymphoma of the stomach** presents with symptoms similar to those of gastric carcinoma. The radiographic appearance may also be similar, although the presence of large gastric folds and evidence of infiltration into the duodenum are more typical of lymphoma than of carcinoma. Endoscopy may confirm the diagnosis if multiple directed biopsies combined with brush cytology are positive. Because the lesions are submucosal, this may be unsuccessful and laparotomy may be required for diagnosis.

Treatment

Surgery is widely accepted as initial therapy. **Radiation** alone is ineffective for adenocarcinoma, except for palliation of bone pain due to metastases. Radiation following resection is commonly used with good results in patients with gastric lymphoma. **Chemotherapy,** using either single agents, eg, 5-fluorouracil, or a combination of doxorubicin and mitomycin C has produced initial response rates approaching 25% in adenocarcinoma. However, no definitive cures have been noted. Chemotherapy for gastric lymphoma is much more effective, although it must be used carefully, since free perforation can occur.

Palliation of gastric carcinoma causing distal esophageal or gastric outlet obstruction has been obtained in selected cases using **endoscopic laser photocoagulation.**

The overall 5-yr survival rate for patients with adenocarcinoma is < 10%. In early gastric cancer, 5-yr survival rates of up to 95% have been reported. In primary gastric lymphoma, the 5-yr survival rate approaches 50%. However, prognosis is adversely affected by age; eg, the 5-yr survival for patients < 45 yr of age with gastric lymphoma is 57%; for those > 65 yr of age, it is 32%.

NEOPLASMS OF THE SMALL INTESTINE

BENIGN NEOPLASMS

Benign neoplasms of the small intestine are rare, accounting for only 1 to 5% of all GI tumors. They are usually found in the 5th, 6th, and 7th decades of life. Adenomatous polyps are the most common, followed by leiomyoma, lipoma, and hemangioma; > 80% of lesions occur in the jejunum and ileum. Here, as elsewhere in the GI tract, adenomatous polyps are premalignant lesions.

Lesions most often are asymptomatic, found during investigation for unrelated symptoms or at autopsy. However, patients may present with recurrent abdominal pain, GI hemorrhage, abdominal mass, or intestinal obstruction, often due to intussusception. Diagnosis can be made by small-bowel x-ray. When the duodenum or terminal ileum is involved, small-bowel endoscopy may provide both visualization and tissue for diagnosis. A new, longer enteroscope can be used to explore the lumen of the entire small intestine. Arteriography provides visualization of vascular tumors.

Surgical resection is the treatment of choice. However, endoscopic polypectomy, angiographic embolization, or endoscopic electro- or laser fulguration may be possible in some vascular lesions.

MALIGNANT NEOPLASMS

Less than 3% of all GI tract cancers originate in the small intestine, and usually occur in the 5th and 6th decades. The most common malignancy is carcinoid tumor, followed by adenocarcinoma, lymphoma, and leiomyosarcoma.

Although the appendix is the primary site of the most **carcinoid tumors,** the small intestine ranks second. Only 25 to 30% of those carcinoids are symptomatic. **Adenocarcinoma** more commonly produces symptoms than other small-intestine tumors. Adenocarcinoma is generally found in the proximal small bowel, predominantly in the duodenum. Predisposing factors include adult celiac disease (nontropical sprue), regional enteritis, and the GI polyposis syndromes, such as Gardner's syndrome. Tumors are usually annular and constricting. **Lymphoma** occurs predominantly in the ileum and is usually of the histiocytic type. There is an association between lymphoma and adult celiac disease. **Leiomyosarcoma** is as common as lymphoma.

Symptoms and Signs

Although most small-intestine malignancies are asymptomatic, 60 to 75% of symptomatic small-bowel tumors are malignant. Patients with more advanced disease present with abdominal pain resulting from intestinal obstruction, recurrent intussusception, mesenteric thrombosis, perforation, GI hemorrhage, or a palpable abdominal mass. **The carcinoid syndrome,** characterized by diarrhea and flushing, occurs when hepatic metastases are present. Lymphoma, especially Hodgkin's disease, may present as **malabsorption syndrome,** with weight loss, diarrhea, malaise, weakness, and edema.

Diagnosis

Preoperative diagnosis is generally made by small-bowel x-ray. Endoscopy may provide visualization and tissue, and arteriography may show vascular malignancies. With advanced carcinoid tumors, urinary 5-hydroxyindoleacetic acid **(5-HIAA)** levels may be elevated.

Treatment

Treatment is usually surgical resection. Radiation and chemotherapy are potentially effective only in lymphoma. The 5-yr survival rate of patients with adenocarcinoma is 30%; with lymphoma and leiomyosarcoma, it approaches 50%. The prognosis of patients with carcinoid tumors can be good, with survival commonly exceeding 10 yr.

NEOPLASMS OF THE COLON

BENIGN NEOPLASMS

Benign colonic tumors have a high prevalence in Western Europe and the USA. Most benign tumors are **polyps,** *a clinical term without pathologic significance, referring to any mass of tissue that arises from a mucosal surface and protrudes into the lumen.*

The epidemiology of colonic polyps, eg, their relationship to age, diet, geographic distribution, family history, and prior neoplasms, is similar to that of adenocarcinoma of the colon (see below).

While incidence figures vary from 7 to 75% of the population > 40 yr of age, incidence increases with age, reaching a peak in the 7th decade. However, hamartomas, juvenile polyps, and congenital lesions are not seen in the elderly.

Hyperplastic and **metaplastic polyps** are the most common benign tumors of the colon. They are small, dome-shaped, sessile lesions, often multiple, and have been found in the rectum in up to 75% of persons > 40 yr of age. They have no inherent malignant potential but are found in up to 90% of patients with colorectal malignancy.

Adenomatous polyps, constituting > 65% of all colorectal polyps, are the most common colorectal neoplasm. In autopsy series, they are found in 50 to 60% of patients > 60 yr old. Although they may involve the entire colon, they are more concentrated in the distal colon. Lesions may be sessile or pedunculated. Synchronous lesions occur in about 50% of cases and are classified histologically as tubular, tubulovillous, or villous adenomas, depending upon the type and number of tubular and villous elements noted microscopically. These polyps are true neoplasms with premalignant potential, which varies directly with the size, degree of villous elements, and degree of dysplasia. Although the overall risk for carcinomatous change within an adenomatous polyp is about 5%, carcinoma is present in 25% of villous adenomas > 2 cm in diameter. Further, adenomatous polyps occur synchronously in 50% of patients with colon cancer.

Inflammatory polyps can be seen in patients with no associated disease but are particularly common in those with inflammatory bowel disorders, ischemic colitis, specific infections (eg, amebiasis and tuberculosis), toxic reactions to mineral oil and barium, and colitis cystica profunda. The only multiple polyposis syndrome to affect the elderly is the Canada-Cronkhite syndrome (see NEOPLASMS OF THE STOMACH, above). The average age at diagnosis is 60 yr and lesions resemble juvenile polyps. Although the syndrome has no sex predominance, it runs a relentless course in women, with death occurring in 6 to 18 mo, whereas men tend to have spontaneous remissions.

Lipomas, the second most common benign tumor of the colon, usually occur at or near the ileocecal valve, with a peak incidence in the 7th to 8th decades of life. Colonic **hemangiomas** are predominantly found with

Gastrointestinal Neoplasms 543

advancing age. They may be classified as capillary, cavernous, or mixed type; are frequently multiple; and are a common cause of hemorrhage and a rare cause of intussusception. **Leiomyomas** seem to have a peak incidence in the 6th decade, declining sharply thereafter.

Symptoms and Signs

Most polyps are asymptomatic and are found incidentally during evaluation for symptoms caused by another disorder. The usual symptom is **rectal bleeding,** varying from occult (most common) to massive (quite rare). Rarely, large villous adenomas cause a severe mucoid rectal discharge and diarrhea, which may result in hypokalemia and hyponatremia. Even more unusual are constipation due to large, bulky tumors and rectal prolapse due to distal lesions. In patients with the Canada-Cronkhite syndrome, diarrhea is progressive, leading to inanition and cachexia, especially in females.

Patients with submucosal tumors (eg, lipomas, hemangiomas, and leiomyomas) may present with an abdominal mass or abdominal pain from intussusception.

Diagnosis and Treatment

Polyps are usually detected by a combination of fecal occult blood testing, barium enema, and colonoscopy. Although air-contrast barium enema is far superior to the single-contrast technic, it may miss up to 40% of small polyps. With proctosigmoidoscopy and colonoscopy, tissue can be obtained for diagnosis and treatment by polypectomy. Colonoscopy is usually performed when an adenomatous polyp is found, because of the high frequency of synchronous polyps. Surgical excision may be necessary for submucosal tumors or polyps that cannot be removed endoscopically.

When well-differentiated carcinoma is detected in a polyp and there is no vascular, lymphatic, or stalk invasion, endoscopic polypectomy is usually the only treatment needed if there is a good resection margin. However, if these conditions cannot be met, surgical management may be considered, depending on location of the adenoma and other factors. In patients who are poor surgical risks, partial resection of lesions that cannot be excised may be performed by colonoscopic fulguration.

Periodic follow-up examinations must be scheduled for patients with adenomatous polyps, since metachronous lesions may develop.

MALIGNANT NEOPLASMS

Colorectal cancer is the second most common malignancy (after lung cancer) in both men and women in the USA and Western Europe. In the USA, about 145,000 new cases and 60,000 deaths occur from this disease annually.

The incidence of colorectal carcinoma begins to rise at age 40 yr and doubles every 5 yr thereafter, reaching a peak in the 8th decade. Adenocarcinoma constitutes 95% of all colorectal cancers. No predominance by sex is apparent. In patients followed for > 25 yr, synchronous colon cancers are found in approximately 3.5%, and metachronous lesions, in 5%.

Colorectal carcinoma is more common in higher socioeconomic classes. High-risk populations consume a diet higher in animal fat and refined sugar and lower in fiber than that consumed by low-risk populations.

Predisposing factors include age > 40 yr; history of colonic polyps or cancer of the colon; cancer of the breast or female genital tract; first-degree relative with colon cancer; inflammatory bowel disease (eg, ulcerative colitis, Crohn's disease, or radiation proctocolitis); and chronic parasitic infections (eg, schistosomiasis and amebiasis).

In patients with diffuse ulcerative colitis, the incidence of colon cancer is 25% at 25 yr of disease. Although the risk of cancer is lower in patients with Crohn's disease, right colon lesions are more common. Hereditary disorders (eg, familial polyposis) also are associated with a high incidence of colorectal carcinoma, but they are rare in the elderly.

The degree of tumor spread is graded by a modified Dukes' classification. Dukes' A lesions involve the mucosa, Dukes' B lesions extend through the wall but do not involve lymph nodes, Dukes' C lesions involve lymph nodes, and Dukes' D lesions have distant metastases. There are many modifications of this staging system.

Other colorectal malignancies include lymphoma, leiomyosarcoma, and carcinoid. Lymphomas have been reported in association with ulcerative colitis and various immunosuppressed states. Carcinoids are often multicentric and occur more frequently in the rectum. The carcinoid syndrome occurs only in patients with hepatic metastases, unless the primary tumor is in the bronchus or ovary. Rectal carcinoids are not associated with the syndrome.

Symptoms and Signs

In its early stages, colon cancer is asymptomatic, so diagnosis is made by routine proctosigmoidoscopic examination or stool testing for occult blood. The location of the tumor within the colon influences symptoms. **Right colon lesions** are usually large, fungating, bleeding masses; patients present with iron deficiency anemia, fatigue, and weakness because of the large-caliber, thin-walled right colon containing fluidlike feces. Tumors may grow so large as to be palpable on abdominal examination. **Left colon lesions** are usually "napkin-ring," obstructing tumors that cause rectal bleeding, crampy abdominal pain, or altered bowel habits because of the narrower caliber of the left colon and the semisolid character of feces at that level. Patients with **rectal lesions** generally present with stool streaked or mixed with blood; they may also complain of tenesmus or a sensation of incomplete evacuation. Palpable lymphadenopathy, hepatomegaly, or both, occur only in the late stages and connote a very poor prognosis.

Diagnosis

Diagnosis is made either by x-ray or endoscopy. **Rigid sigmoidoscopy** may not be sufficient to detect colon cancer, since it may not even reach the anticipated 25-cm length of the scope. **The fiberoptic sigmoidoscope** has advanced the ability to detect lesions in the rectum and the sigmoid and distal descending colon region, where > 50% of cancers occur. The more proximal segments of the colon are examined by barium enema x-ray or colonoscopy. **Air-contrast barium enema** is usually superior to the single-contrast technic in detecting colon cancer. **Colonoscopy** provides visualization and tissue for diagnosis and also allows inspection of the remainder of the colon for synchronous polyps or cancers.

Fecal occult blood testing provides for early detection of colonic tumors, both benign and malignant. In 1 study, 2.5% of adults > 40 yr of age had positive stool tests. Colonic neoplasms were detected in 50%, of which 38% were adenomas and 12% cancer. Screening of elderly patients with both fecal occult blood testing using 6 guaiac impregnated slides and sigmoidoscopy allows detection of colon cancer at a potentially curable stage. Both screening tests are strongly age related, with increased yield and better positive predictive value in persons > 60 yr of age. Detected cancers are often early stage and highly curable.

Carcinoembryonic antigen (CEA) may be elevated in patients with cancer of the colon, pancreas, breast, lung, prostate, stomach, or bladder and is, therefore, nonspecific; it is relatively insensitive for early-stage cancer detection and can be associated with other diseases of the liver and lung. However, if an elevated CEA level drops postoperatively and subsequently rises, monitoring CEA may help detect recurrence.

Treatment

Treatment of colorectal cancer consists primarily of anatomic surgical resection and is discussed in Ch. 53.

NEOPLASMS OF THE ANORECTUM
(See also Malignant Neoplasms under NEOPLASMS OF THE COLON, above, and Ch. 53)

Epidermoid carcinoma of the anorectum accounts for 3 to 5% of rectal cancers but 90% of anal cancers. Other malignant neoplasms include basal cell carcinoma, Bowen's disease (chronic squamous cell carcinoma in situ), extramammary Paget's disease, cloacogenic carcinoma, and malignant melanoma. Cloacogenic carcinoma is most prevalent in patients 60 to 70 yr of age. Factors predisposing to anorectal cancer include leukoplakia, lymphogranuloma venereum, chronic fistula formation, and irradiation of the anal skin.

Symptoms and Signs

Bleeding is the most common symptom. Anal discomfort, constipation, and diminished stool caliber are other frequent complaints. The presenting feature may be a mass on digital rectal examination, inguinal adenopathy, or perianal dermatitis, and cancer should be considered in all nonhealing ulcers or fistulas. Biopsy of all suspicious lesions is essential.

Local surgical excision is the treatment of choice preceded by a course of radiation and chemotherapy to debulk the tumor mass. The latter approach may obviate abdominoperineal resection in many patients. Electrofulguration and laser photocoagulation are palliative measures in selected cases.

NEOPLASMS OF THE APPENDIX
(See in Ch. 53)

NEOPLASMS OF THE PANCREAS

EXOCRINE TUMORS

BENIGN NEOPLASMS

The only significant exocrine pancreatic neoplasm is **cystadenoma,** which usually occurs in the body and tail of the pancreas in middle-aged women. Surgical resection is curative.

MALIGNANT NEOPLASMS

Pancreatic cancer is the second most common GI malignancy in the USA, with approximately 26,000 new cases diagnosed annually. The incidence increases with age and is 10 times greater in males > 75 yr of age than in the general population. Risk factors include cigarette smoking, diabetes, and diet high in animal fat, coffee, and nitrosamines.

Ductal cell adenocarcinoma accounts for 75 to 96% of all cancers arising from the pancreas. Others include giant cell carcinoma, adenosquamous carcinoma, and cystadenocarcinoma. **Giant cell carcinoma,** also referred to as carcinosarcoma, is a highly malignant lesion with distant metastases occurring early. **Adenosquamous carcinoma** occurs predominantly in males, often in a patient with a history of prior radiation therapy. **Cystadenocarcinoma,** a low-grade malignancy, has the best prognosis, since only 20% have metastasized at the time of surgery.

Symptoms and Signs

Clinical features of pancreatic cancer often depend upon its location; 80% occur in the head of the pancreas and 20% in the body and tail. Insidious onset of epigastric pain and weight loss are the most common initial symptoms. Lesions of the pancreatic head often present as jaundice, from common duct obstruction, or as nausea and vomiting, from gastric outlet obstruction. Symptoms of lesions of the body and tail are more insidious in onset, amounting to little more than weight loss and vague abdominal or back pain. The duration of symptoms precedes diagnosis by approximately 3 to 6 mo. In ductal cell adenocarcinoma, death often ensues within 6 mo of diagnosis, since metastasis is present in 90% of patients by the time the tumor is discovered.

A number of findings are associated with pancreatic cancer, including depression thromboembolic phenomena associated with Trousseau's syndrome, GI bleeding from gastric varices secondary to splenic vein thrombosis, polyarthritis, diarrhea due to exocrine pancreatic insufficiency, superior vena cava syndrome due to pulmonary metastases, and Horner's syndrome due to thoracic outlet metastasis. Onset of diabetes or worsening of preexisting diabetes warrants evaluation for pancreatic cancer.

Physical examination is negative early in the disease. Later, an epigastric mass, supraclavicular lymphadenopathy, hepatomegaly, or the presence of a large, palpable gallbladder (Courvoisier's sign) may be noted.

Diagnosis

Early diagnosis, when the tumor is still resectable, is rarely possible, occurring only with cancers of the head of the pancreas or at the ampulla of Vater, where jaundice may be an early symptom. Diagnosis may be suggested by upper abdominal sonography. However, a CT scan of the abdomen can better visualize a pancreatic mass. Endoscopic retrograde cholangiopancreatography (ERCP) can detect the tumor, with the characteristic findings of ductal irregularity and cutoff, in up to 90% of cases. Although tissue for diagnosis can usually be obtained by needle biopsy, exploratory laparotomy is often necessary. CEA may be elevated in some cases, but this is rarely useful clinically.

Treatment

Patients who have nonmetastatic, resectable lesions in the pancreatic head may be candidates for Whipple's procedure (pancreaticoduodenectomy). Only 10% of patients with ductal cell carcinoma have localized tumors. In most patients, a palliative bypass (eg, cholecystojejunostomy for distal bile duct obstruction or gastrojejunostomy for gastric outlet obstruction) is the only procedure that can be performed.

Chemotherapy produces some responses but without any long-term benefit. Radiation therapy offers minimal benefit, except for palliation of retroperitoneal pain. Palliative treatment, with a biliary stent placed endoscopically or radiologically, using transhepatic cholangiography may reduce jaundice. However, these measures do not prolong life.

Abdominal pain generally is treated with analgesics, but a neural block may need to be performed for severe, unrelenting pain. Pruritus from jaundice may be relieved with phenothiazines or cholestyramine 4 gm orally 1 to 4 times daily. Pancreatic insufficiency can be managed with pancreatic enzymes (lipase, protease, and amylase). Diabetes can be controlled with diet and insulin therapy.

The overall prognosis is dismal in these patients, with < 10% 1-yr survival and only 2% 5-yr survival. Cystadenocarcinoma, which has a low incidence of metastasis at diagnosis, has a 65% 5-yr survival with aggressive surgery.

ENDOCRINE TUMORS

Endocrine tumors arise from the neuroendocrine cells of the pancreas predominantly in the islets in the body and tail of the pancreas. However, enterochromaffin cells and other neuroendocrine cells can produce tumors in any part of the pancreas. Endocrine tumors are rare in older persons.

These tumors are indistinguishable microscopically without special immunochemical staining. They may be **nonfunctioning** or **functioning** (ie, hormone secreting).

Nonfunctioning tumors may cause obstruction of the biliary tract or duodenum, bleeding into the GI tract, or an abdominal mass. Functioning tumors cause variable syndromes, including hypoglycemia, due to hypersecretion of insulin by an **insulinoma;** Zollinger-Ellison syndrome, due to hypersecretion of gastrin by **gastrinoma; pancreatic cholera,** caused by tumor secretion of vasoactive inhibitory peptide; **carcinoid syndrome,** caused by secretion of serotonin from enterochromaffin cells; diabetes, caused by hypersecretion of glucagon by **glucagonoma;** and **Cushing's syndrome,** caused by hypersecretion of ACTH by various types of tumors. (See also ENDOCRINE TUMORS OF THE PANCREAS in Ch. 53.)

These clinical conditions can sometimes present as multiple endocrine adenomatosis syndromes, in which tumors or hyperplasia occur in 2 or more endocrine glands. Usually, association occurs with tumors or hyperplasia of the parathyroid, pituitary, thyroid, or adrenal glands.

NEOPLASMS OF THE LIVER

BENIGN NEOPLASMS

The **hemangioma,** which is usually clinically silent, is the most common of these. Approximately 5% of autopsies in adults reveal an unsuspected hepatic hemangioma. Other benign tumors include **hepatocellular adenoma** and **focal nodular hyperplasia,** which are most often associated with oral contraceptives and are not usually seen in elderly persons. **Bile duct adenomas** and rare **mesenchymal tumors** have also been reported.

Symptoms, Signs, and Diagnosis

These tumors are usually found incidentally at laparotomy or are detected when investigations such as CT scan, sonography or angiography are performed for unrelated symptoms. Rarely, hemangiomas present with massive hemorrhage from rupture or consumptive coagulopathy **(Kasabach-Merritt syndrome)** resulting from the rich vascular network within the tumor.

Liver function tests are normal or minimally abnormal. The tumors may be detected initially by ultrasound, CT scan of the liver, or arteriography, but the diagnosis can be established by routine liver biopsy in nonvascular lesions, although laparoscopy or laparotomy is often necessary.

Treatment

Therapy is usually segmental resection or hepatic irradiation. Angiographic embolization or arterial occlusion is sometimes effective.

MALIGNANT NEOPLASMS

Metastatic carcinoma is by far the most common form of hepatic tumor. The liver is the most frequent site of metastasis from cancer. Liver metastases are found at autopsy in 30 to 50% of patients with cancer. **Primary malignancy** of the liver is rare in the USA and Western Europe, but very common in Africa and Asia.

About 90% of primary adult hepatic cancers originate from the hepatocyte and are called **hepatocellular carcinoma** or **hepatoma;** 5 to 10% originate from the bile ducts as **cholangiocarcinoma,** or represent a mixed type, **cholangiohepatoma.** Other primary liver cancers are exceedingly rare and include **angiosarcoma** and **hepatoblastoma.** Hepatic malignancies are more common in men than in women and occur between the ages of 50 and 70 yr.

Hepatocellular carcinoma may be nodular, massive, or diffuse. The nodular type is most common and consists of multiple discrete nodules. The massive type, which accounts for essentially the remainder, develops as a large, often necrotic, hemorrhagic mass. The diffuse type is most often associated with cirrhosis and consists of minute lesions scattered throughout the liver.

Symptoms and Signs

About 70% of patients present with right upper quadrant or epigastric pain and weight loss. Deteriorating mental status is noted with progressive liver dysfunction. Pulmonary symptoms and pathologic fractures as a result of metastases have been noted. The rare occurrence of tumor rupture with intra-abdominal hemorrhage and symptoms of an acute abdomen is life-threatening. Physical examination may reveal hepatomegaly, a right upper quadrant mass, or ascites. Splenomegaly is less common.

Paraneoplastic syndromes associated with hepatocellular carcinoma include erythrocytosis, hypercalcemia, hypoglycemia, hyperlipidemia, porphyria cutanea tarda, and dysfibrinoginemia.

Diagnosis

Liver function tests are usually abnormal; elevated serum alkaline phosphatase is common, but elevated serum transaminases and bilirubin are less so. In later stages, prothrombin time may be increased and albumin level decreased.

Diagnosis is often made with a combination of abdominal ultrasound and CT scan, angiography, and biopsy. CT scan may help document lesions but may miss 10% of the tumors. Elevated levels of α-fetoprotein are noted in 90% of patients with hepatocellular carcinoma.

CT scan or ultrasound-guided needle aspiration is a safe, reliable technic. Angiography usually shows a typical capillary blush. Laparoscopy allows inspection of the abdominal cavity for secondary tumor and for directed biopsy.

Treatment

Treatment is unsatisfactory, with a 5-yr survival rate near 0%. Surgical resection of a localized tumor is associated with prolonged survival. Irradiation and chemotherapy have also proved unsatisfactory. Intrahepatic arterial infusion of chemotherapeutic agents and angiographic embolization of vascular tumors prolong survival in some patients.

NEOPLASMS OF THE GALLBLADDER

BENIGN NEOPLASMS

Benign gallbladder tumors are found at cholecystectomy in about 1% of patients, with no increased incidence in the elderly. They include the adenoma, cystadenoma, fibroadenoma, adenomyoma, and hamartoma. Adenomas, which are frequently associated with gallstones and cholecystitis, may have malignant potential.

Symptoms and signs may be nonexistent, vague, or typical of acute or chronic cholecystitis. **Diagnosis** is made by demonstration of a filling defect in the gallbladder. Cholecystectomy is the recommended **treatment** because of the uncertain premalignant nature of some lesions.

MALIGNANT NEOPLASMS

Gallbladder malignancy has been reported in 0.2 to 5% of patients undergoing cholecystectomy, mostly women between the ages of 60 and 70. Adenocarcinoma accounts for 80% of cases; squamous cell carcinoma and adenoacanthoma account for the remaining 20%. Metastasis is present in 75% of cases at the time of diagnosis.

Gallstones are associated with the development of gallbladder carcinoma, and its prevention may be a justification for early cholecystectomy in patients with cholelithiasis.

Symptoms, Signs, and Diagnosis

Symptoms include intermittent pain and dyspepsia, similar to that of chronic cholecystitis. Weight loss and jaundice appear in the late stages. A firm, tender mass is often palpable in the right upper quadrant. Abdominal ultrasonography and CT scan provide visualization of the tumor.

Treatment

Cholecystectomy with resection of the adjacent liver and skeletonization of the bile ducts is the treatment of choice in localized disease. Radiation and chemotherapy are ineffective. The prognosis is dismal, with only a 5% 5-yr survival rate.

NEOPLASMS OF EXTRAHEPATIC BILE DUCTS

BENIGN NEOPLASMS

Papilloma and adenoma are the most common of these, although fibroadenoma, adenomyoma, leiomyoma, granular cell myoblastoma, neurinoma, and hamartoma also occur. Intermittent jaundice and right upper quadrant pain are the most common symptoms. Local excision is the treatment of choice.

MALIGNANT NEOPLASMS

These are rare tumors and often difficult to diagnose. Adenocarcinoma is by far the most common. Bile duct cancer is more frequent in men, with an average age of 60 yr at diagnosis. Tumors of the upper portion of the ducts (50% of all lesions) are intimately related to the liver; those of the middle portion, to the portal vein and hepatic artery; and those of the lower portion, to the pancreas and duodenum. Such localization has both diagnostic and prognostic implications.

Predisposing factors include ulcerative colitis, *C. sinensis* infestation, and industrial exposure (in automobile and rubber manufacturing plant workers).

Symptoms and Signs

Because of their location, malignant tumors usually cause early symptoms. Jaundice occurs in almost all patients. Right upper quadrant pain occurs in > 50% of cases. Weight loss, nausea, vomiting, anorexia, fever, chills, diarrhea, constipation, and clay-colored stools are other associated symptoms.

Signs include hepatomegaly and jaundice. If obstruction occurs below the cystic duct, a distended gallbladder **(Courvoisier's sign)** may be palpated.

Diagnosis

Diagnosis of large tumors is made by ultrasound and CT scan. However, percutaneous transhepatic cholangiography or ERCP is frequently more important in making the diagnosis and localizing the tumor. Liver function tests are consistent with extrahepatic obstruction.

Treatment

Carcinomas in the proximal portion of the bile duct system rarely are operable, requiring complex liver and duct resections with very few long-term survivors. Palliation may be accomplished by dilation and stent insertion, either endoscopically or via transhepatic cholangiography. Resectable tumors of the central portion of the bile ducts may be treated by local en bloc excision. Bile duct drainage is reestablished by hepaticojejunostomy.

In carcinomas of the distal extrahepatic ducts, radical resection and pancreaticoduodenectomy (Whipple's operation) provide some promising benefit, with 5-yr survival rates of 20 to 30% in resectable tumors. In nonresectable tumors, palliation may be accomplished by hepaticojejunostomy or by stent placement followed by internal radiation via percutaneous catheter insertion into the ducts.

NEOPLASMS OF THE MESENTERY

Benign neoplasms are rare but twice as frequent as malignant tumors. Fibromas and lipomas are the most common. They are most often incidental findings during routine examination, frequently growing large before causing symptoms. Symptoms are usually due to compression or traction of adjacent structures; vague abdominal pain and bloating are most common. Intestinal obstruction may occur.

Diagnosis is usually made by x-ray studies that reveal extrinsic compression of large or small bowel. Surgical excision is curative.

Malignant neoplasms are rare tumors, usually fibrosarcoma or leiomyosarcoma. **Symptoms and signs** are similar to those of benign tumors of this region due to traction or compression of adjacent structures and intestinal obstruction. Weight loss, anorexia, and weakness can also occur.

Diagnosis is made by x-ray studies, including upper GI series, barium enema, and CT scan, that reveal extrinsic compression or signs of invasion of the small or large bowel and other local structures. Surgical treatment is the only effective treatment for cure or palliation.

---

53.   SURGERY OF THE DIGESTIVE TRACT

Claude E. Welch and *Ronald G. Tompkins*

INTRODUCTION

In general, mortality increases with age, but calendar age does not necessarily correspond with physiologic age or physical fitness or with the ability to withstand surgical procedures. The decision to operate is influenced by many factors (eg, cure vs. palliation, the presence or absence of coexisting diseases, the patient's quality of life and mental competence, and family attitudes).

In many ways, surgical diseases of the abdomen are different in geriatric patients. Diagnosis, particularly in emergency situations, is more difficult because sensations are not as acute as in the young, and pathophysiologic reactions (eg, pain, tenderness, and response to inflammation) are not as rapid or effective. Thus, for example, minimal symptoms may accompany a potentially fatal bowel perforation, and the first sign may be free subphrenic gas on the plain abdominal x-ray.

Generally, the elderly tolerate a single surgical procedure well, provided the offending lesion is removed. However, complications from second or third operations performed soon after the original one carry a high mortality. If staged procedures are necessary, they should be spaced sufficiently apart to allow complete recovery. These considerations are particularly important in surgical diseases of the digestive tract.

Acute abdominal emergencies result in a high percentage of operations. In the past 12 yr at our institution, surgery for peptic ulcers in patients ≥ 70 yr of age included emergency procedures for massive hemorrhage or acute perforation in 60%, urgent operations in 19%, and elective operations in 11%.

The major indications for **emergency surgery** are perforation of a viscus, appendicitis, intestinal obstruction, and massive hemorrhage. Acute cholecystitis usually requires an urgent operation, whereas most **elective surgery** is for malignant disease. Excluding hernias, surgical procedures involving the colon, the gallbladder, and the stomach as a group generally represent > 90% of abdominal operations, with procedures almost equally divided among these 3 organs.

The acute abdomen should be suspected in patients who complain only of *minimal* abdominal pain. Peritonitis due to perforation of the sigmoid, stomach, or duodenum may be present even if there is only slight abdominal tenderness. Vascular lesions (eg, mesenteric artery thrombosis) also are common. In appendicitis, acute cholecystitis, and cases of strangulated hernias, the interval between onset and gangrene may be only a few hours.

The physical examination is extremely important. Old incisional scars suggest the possibility of intestinal obstruction. Careful examination of potential hernia sites is essential. Absent peristalsis is a serious finding, since auscultatory silence suggests a surgical abdomen. Other diagnostic tests must be carried out expeditiously.

Massive GI hemorrhage is tolerated poorly in older patients. A rapid diagnosis must be made and treatment must be instituted more rapidly than in younger patients, who can better tolerate repeated episodes of bleeding.

Optimal treatment of hernias can be controversial. Obviously, all patients with strangulated inguinal hernias need immediate surgery. Femoral hernias also are prone to strangulation and should be repaired electively, if possible. Many small, direct inguinal hernias, and painless, indirect inguinal hernias with relatively large openings do not represent an immediate threat. However, the *only* hernias that are safe to watch are small, direct, and nonpainful and reduce spontaneously when the patient is recumbent. Otherwise, hernias should be repaired unless surgery is contraindicated. The operation frequently can be done under local anesthesia.

GI hemorrhage and intestinal obstruction are discussed below, followed by a review of major abdominal disorders amenable to surgical therapy.

GASTROINTESTINAL BLEEDING

GI bleeding may be manifested clinically by **hematemesis** *(vomiting of blood)*, **melena** *(passage of black, tarry stools)*, or **hematochezia** *(passage of red blood by rectum)*. Bleeding may be either **occult** *(detectable by chemical means only)* or obvious to the naked eye. Some persons do not recognize overt bleeding; eg, they may not be aware that "coffee-ground" vomitus contains blood altered by gastric juice. Color-blindness also may make it impossible to distinguish red blood. Other ocular diseases (eg, cataracts or presbyopia) that are common in the elderly also limit their power of observation.

There are many potential sites of bleeding in the digestive tract. The most common sources, in descending order of frequency, are the anorectum, stomach, colon, small intestine, and esophagus. Blood that originates from the mouth, the nasopharynx, or the lung can be swallowed and thus mimic gastric bleeding. The liver, pancreas, and aorta are unusual bleeding sites.

While some diseases that cause GI bleeding are common to all age groups, others are much more age-related. Some diseases typically lead to severe bleeding while others result in relatively little blood loss. In the elderly, hemorrhoids and colorectal cancer are the most common causes of *minor bleeding;* peptic ulcer, diverticular disease, and angiodysplasia are the most common causes of *major hemorrhages.*

Diagnosis

Documentation of bleeding is required, as well as identification of the bleeding site. Although diagnosis is often difficult, therapy must nonetheless proceed. The history, physical examination, blood tests, endoscopy, selective arteriography, radionuclide studies, barium-contrast studies, and exploratory laparotomy aid in making the diagnosis.

The history provides important clinical information. Alcoholism and a previous massive upper GI hemorrhage suggest bleeding due to esophageal varices in young adults; however, bleeding is more likely due to peptic ulcer in older patients. If a patient has an aortic aneurysm or an abdominal aortic graft, erosion into the duodenum should be suspected. Massive colonic bleeding is most likely due to diverticular disease or angiodysplasia. Streaks of red blood on the toilet paper usually indicate hemorrhoids, but polyps and cancer must be ruled out.

Physical examination can help one assess the amount of bleeding, as evidenced by syncope or shock. As a rough guide, orthostatic hypotension suggests a 25% loss of blood, shock while recumbent represents at least a 50% loss. Pulse and BP must be monitored closely whenever continued or recurrent bleeding is suspected. Hepatomegaly suggests portal hypertension or metastatic disease. Palpable masses along the course of the colon or in the left hypogastrium suggest colonic or gastric cancer, respectively. Rectal and vaginal (in females) examinations are essential.

Blood tests must include serial Hct or Hb levels, red cell and platelet counts, and smears for RBC, WBC, and platelet morphology. Microcytosis can be an indication of chronic bleeding, even if acute bleeding is superimposed. Prothrombin time and partial thromboplastin time are essential if the patient has been taking anticoagulants or is jaundiced and should be part of routine studies.

Endoscopy includes esophagogastroduodenoscopy, anoscopy, rigid sigmoidoscopy, flexible sigmoidoscopy, and colonoscopy. Both upper and lower endoscopy can be used with exploratory laparotomy. Endoscopy is most valuable if performed when the patient is actually bleeding slowly enough to allow adequate observation.

Selective arteriography is a most important aid in identification of the bleeding site, provided blood loss is ≥ 1 mL/min. It serves to localize lesions in the stomach, small bowel, and colon and may be combined with exploratory laparotomy.

Radionuclide studies of 2 types are generally used in adults. The most common one requires withdrawing about 10 mL of blood, labeling it with a technetium nuclide, and reinjecting it into the patient. The procedure, which takes about an hour, demonstrates a source of bleeding if the loss is ≥ 1 mL/min, even if intermittent. The second method involves the injection of a prepared sulfur colloid nuclide. Identification of a bleeding site is possible within a few minutes if the patient is actively bleeding. Both methods are less useful with upper GI bleeding because of the amount of background scatter. Technetium scans occasionally demonstrate Meckel's diverticulum, since there is selective uptake by gastric mucosa, which may be present in the lesion; however, this is a rare cause of bleeding in geriatric patients.

Exploratory laparotomy is the definitive diagnostic method, although it was used more frequently prior to the development of arteriography. Careful examination of the abdominal viscera, especially the small bowel, identifies many lesions (eg, angiomas, leiomyomas, and diverticula). If a long peroral endoscope is introduced at the time of laparotomy, the whole small-bowel lumen can be examined. Likewise, selective arteriography during exploratory laparotomy has been used to identify bleeding small-bowel lesions, allowing resection of the involved segment.

Treatment

The physician must first decide whether hospital admission is necessary. It is dangerous to treat someone with more than minor rectal bleeding, tarry stools, or hematemesis as an outpatient. Bleeding assumed to be from hemorrhoids or other limited rectal bleeding requiring only diagnostic colonoscopy or barium enema may be managed in an outpatient setting, provided time is not lost making the diagnosis.

The cause of the bleeding may not be in the GI tract. For example, a history of aspirin ingestion may explain GI bleeding. One aspirin tablet can diminish clotting factors for as long as 3 wk, while a larger dose can cause aspirin-induced gastritis. Nevertheless, the physician must not be influenced too heavily by such a history, because many patients take aspirin but bleed from other causes. Other diseases and drugs that may cause GI bleeding should be considered. Alcohol, anticoagulants, anti-inflammatory agents such as ibuprofen or compounds that contain this drug, and coagulopathies such as those associated with metastatic disease or chemotherapy may produce gastritis or, in some instances, lead to bleeding without a demonstrable site of origin as determined either by endoscopy or operation. Hence, the possibility that these lesions may be producing the bleeding should be the primary consideration in determining the source and cause of bleeding.

It often remains difficult to determine whether bleeding originates from the upper or lower GI tract. Therefore, ongoing diagnostic evaluation is essential while bleeding continues. A nasogastric tube should be passed and the gastric contents aspirated. If the aspirate is grossly bloody or guaiac-positive, iced saline solution is used to irrigate the stomach until bleeding slows significantly. At that time, esophagogastroduodenoscopy is performed. However, if the gastric aspirate remains bright red, a choice must be made between selective arteriography and immediate exploratory laparotomy; patients with massive GI bleeding can experience cardiovascular collapse in the angiographic suite.

Essentially the same therapeutic choices are applicable, regardless of whether the bleeding site is in the stomach, duodenum, or colon. The specific choice depends on the patient's age and cardiovascular status, the rate and quantity of blood loss, and the treatment modalities available. Options include expectant treatment by medical measures, by endoscopy using electrocoagulation or laser, by selective arteriography with local or peripheral vasopressin infusion or embolization, or by a definitive surgical procedure.

When selective arteriography has identified the bleeding site, the same catheter may be used to inject vasopressin directly; this can provide immediate control of bleeding in > 80% of cases. Peripheral vasopressin administered at a rate of 0.4 u./min is also an option, although cardiac arrhythmias occur more frequently and caution is necessary. If vasopressin infusion fails, emboli of Gelfoam® or coils may be attempted. However, the danger of postembolic necrosis, arising in either the wall of a viscus or the liver, from a dislodged embolus, must be recognized.

At times, bleeding is so massive that emergency surgery is the only reasonable treatment. In patients who are apparently bleeding from the stomach or the colon, the only recourse is to perform a "blind" gastrectomy or colectomy if the specific location cannot be established and severe blood loss continues. Fortunately, these situations are not as common as they were in the past.

In a recent prospective study of gastroduodenal bleeding, the mortality was extremely low in patients < 60 yr of age who were treated either medically or surgically. Above that age, there was essentially no mortality if patients underwent immediate surgery, vs. a 15% mortality if they were first treated medically and then operated on for persistent or recurrent hemorrhage.

SPECIFIC BLEEDING SITES

Esophagus

Varices secondary to portal hypertension are not common in the aged. When they occur, the primary treatment is sclerotherapy. Recurrent bleeding in a patient who is a reasonable surgical risk is treated by portosystemic shunt.

Esophagitis often is associated with benign ulcers of the distal esophagus and with a sliding hiatus hernia. Slow but persistent bleeding may occur. Treatment with H_2-receptor blockers usually is very helpful because the ulceration is due to acid reflux. However, cancer must be excluded by endoscopy and biopsy. Severe bleeding requiring surgery rarely occurs in the elderly.

Stomach

Mallory-Weiss tears occur in radial direction at or just below the esophagogastric junction. They involve the gastric mucosa and can be identified and often cauterized through the endoscope. If surgical intervention is necessary, suture of the lacerations is required.

Peptic ulcer disease: In the elderly, bleeding is more common from gastric ulcers than from duodenal ulcers, and control of bleeding by conservative measures is less certain in gastric than in duodenal ulcers. The usual operation for intractable gastric ulcer hemorrhage is partial gastrectomy, with or without vagotomy; for duodenal ulcer bleeding, the usual procedure is ligation of the bleeding vessel and either gastric resection or pyloroplasty and vagotomy.

Anastomotic ulcers at the suture line of previous operations for peptic ulcer tend to recur even if bleeding stops after medical measures are initiated. Gastric resection and vagotomy are usually indicated, but the prior operative procedure will determine the subsequent surgical intervention.

Gastritis is troublesome when it involves the mucous membrane of the entire stomach; if bleeding is not controlled by medical measures, only a radical subtotal gastrectomy with vagotomy or total gastrectomy achieves hemostasis. **Stress ulcers** are similar to gastritis but occur after trauma, surgery, burns, or infections. Nasogastric suction, sucralfate, IV H_2-receptor blockers, or oral antacid therapy to control gastric pH, and

IV alimentation are the main components in the medical management of stress bleeding, gastritis, or peptic ulcer disease.

Vascular lesions (cirsoid or racemose aneurysm, or Dieulefoy's disease) are localized arteriovenous malformations and communications in the gastric mucosa. They may be impossible to visualize endoscopically or at surgery unless actively bleeding and are more common in the fundus. If bleeding is active, endoscopic therapy is possible, but high or total gastrectomy has been necessary to achieve hemostasis in some patients.

Tumors may cause any type of bleeding. Slow, persistent bleeding is more typical of malignant than benign tumors. Benign leiomyomas often lead to massive hemorrhage that requires emergency laparotomy.

Small Intestine

Tumors are uncommon in this location but may produce bleeding. Massive bleeding usually is due to large **leiomyomas**. Slow, persistent bleeding is more typical of **angiomas**.

Diverticular disease of the jejunum may be extensive and can lead to massive bleeding as well as malnutrition.

Varices secondary to portal hypertension at times may involve the small intestine and lead to bleeding. **Multiple arteriovenous malformations** usually are discovered in children but also may develop late in life.

Colon

Anemia may be the first indication of carcinoma of the cecum. Many neoplasms are diagnosed on the basis of a positive stool occult blood test. The amount of visible blood in stool due to a cancer or polyp usually is small.

Angiodysplasia and diverticular disease cause massive bleeding with equal frequency. **Angiodysplasia** refers to small (1 to 5 mm in diameter) single or multiple lesions, found chiefly in the cecum or ascending colon, that resemble submucous arteriovenous malformations on microscopy (see Ch. 48). **Bleeding diverticula** are proximal to the splenic flexure in nearly ⅔ of cases, whereas nonbleeding diverticula occur distal to the splenic flexure in > 90% of cases. The average age at diagnosis of both angiodysplasia and bleeding diverticula is 70 yr. Diagnosis of angiodysplasia can be made by colonoscopy in some cases and the lesions destroyed by electrocoagulation. However, if bleeding is profuse, selective arteriography is the best diagnostic modality. The characteristic angiographic finding in angiodysplasia is an early-filling vein in the region of the ileocecal valve. Angiodysplasia can exist concomitantly with other colonic lesions such as cancer.

The exact cause of massive bleeding from the colon cannot be determined in about 10% of cases. The surgeon is bound in these cases to perform a subtotal colectomy; the ileorectal anastomosis is placed within reach of the rigid sigmoidoscope, or < 25 cm from the anal verge.

Liver and Pancreas

In nearly all cases, bleeding from these organs follows trauma. The diagnosis usually is made by selective arteriography, at which time it may be possible to stop the bleeding by embolization. If bleeding continues, surgical intervention and ligation of vessels is necessary.

Bleeding After an Aortic Graft

Older patients may experience relatively sudden onset of massive GI bleeding months or years after an abdominal aortic aneurysm has been excised and replaced with a vascular graft. In such cases, a fistula between the graft and small intestine is the most likely cause. Although aortoduodenal fistulas predominate, there may be erosion into any section of the small bowel.

Endoscopy extending to the distal duodenum usually is diagnostic. CT normally shows a membrane between the graft and the intestine; if this is absent, erosion of the intestinal wall by the graft is certain. Arteriography also may be helpful. Treatment is difficult because infection, which accompanies an established fistula, is a strong deterrent to graft replacement. The usual procedure is to remove the graft and establish an extra-anatomic bypass graft, usually between an axillary artery and the distal aorta; the proximal aorta is suture-ligated.

INTESTINAL OBSTRUCTION

A blockage of the alimentary tract between the ligament of Treitz and the anus, preventing the passage of intestinal contents. The obstruction may be acute or chronic, mechanical or adynamic, simple or strangulated, and present in the small intestine or colon. Certain features are common to all, but the choice of therapy depends on an exact diagnosis.

There are several possible mechanical causes of acute intestinal obstruction. In the elderly, the most common lesions affecting the small bowel are adhesions and hernias; cancer predominates in the colon. Adynamic ileus occurs when absent reflex nerve stimulation precludes peristalsis in an otherwise normal bowel. In simple obstruction, the blood supply to the bowel is not compromised; in strangulated obstruction, the vessels to a segment are occluded by external compression.

Diagnosis

Acute obstruction characteristically presents as rapid onset of abdominal cramps, vomiting, distention, and obstipation. Cramps tend to recur approximately every 3 min and are associated with high-pitched bowel sounds (due to peristalsis) called borborygmi. Although there may be wide individual variation, crampy pain is perceived in the epigastrium with small-bowel obstruction and in the lower abdomen with colonic obstruction; there may be no cramps with high jejunal obstruction. Abdominal distention is usually present and increases with time. *The abdomen is not tender;* when abdominal tenderness is elicited and intermittent cramps change to continuous pain, strangulation almost certainly is present. Simple obstruction can lead to strangulation in as little as 6 h; hence every patient with suspected intestinal obstruction should be hospitalized immediately.

In small-bowel obstruction, vomiting usually occurs early; it may progress to fecal emesis, which can be distinguished from coffee-ground vomitus (due to upper GI hemorrhage) by a guaiac test. Vomiting occurs much later or not at all with large-bowel obstruction, and is usually preceded by distention and cramps. Initially, there may be scanty diarrhea; *complete* obstruction is followed by obstipation.

Symptoms and signs are highly variable and depend chiefly on the site and cause of obstruction, as well as on the time elapsed since its onset.

Physical examination must be complete, with particular emphasis on the cardiorespiratory system, state of consciousness, vital signs, and urine output. The most important portion of the physical examination—that of the abdomen—in addition to inspection for scars of previous abdominal operations and the presence of groin or incisional hernias, includes auscultation for several minutes to detect bowel sounds, palpation to detect tenderness or masses, rectal examination, and vaginal examination in women.

A CBC, blood chemistries, and urinalysis should be performed; determinations of urine output, degree of hydration, and respiratory status are important to establish baselines and the possibility of impending shock. An indwelling bladder catheter and central venous pressure line are usually necessary.

The X-ray examination is extremely important but should be preceded by the passage of a nasogastric tube. Plain abdominal films should be taken in both supine and upright positions. Lateral decubitus films sometimes are helpful, particularly in cases of external hernias.

In typical small-bowel obstruction, a ladderlike pattern of distended intestinal loops is seen. With strangulation, however, a mass rather than distended loops may be visible. Distended loops may also be absent in high jejunal obstruction, particularly if there was a previous gastric resection.

Obstruction of the ascending colon may resemble small-bowel obstruction, provided there is reflux through an incompetent ileocecal valve. Obstruction of the descending colon leads to distention of the entire proximal large bowel with gas. A single large loop of colon filled with gas in the midabdomen or left upper quadrant usually is due to cecal volvulus, and a single loop of distended sigmoid is usually due to sigmoid volvulus. If gas is seen in the intrahepatic bile ducts, gallstone obstruction is likely.

Barium enema is performed when the site of colonic obstruction and the determination of whether the small or large bowel is involved are unclear. Barium may be administered orally to confirm the diagnosis and localize the site of small-intestine obstruction but must be *avoided* in obstruction of the colon. Barium that remains in the ascending colon above a point of obstruction becomes inspissated and forms an almost irremovable concrete-like mass.

Differential Diagnosis

Many abdominal diseases simulate intestinal obstruction (eg, acute appendicitis, acute cholecystitis, diverticulitis, and pancreatitis). In addition, thoracic disease (eg, pneumonia) may cause adynamic ileus.

Treatment

Acute mechanical obstruction calls for surgical treatment. Ideally, this will correct the underlying cause as well as relieve the obstruction. However, in many cases of obstructing carcinoma of the descending colon, precedence must be given to relief of obstruction. Thus, unless the surgeon is extremely skilled and either can perform a subtotal colectomy and ileocolic or ileorectal anastomosis beyond the cancer in nondilated bowel, or can empty the colon and perform a more limited resection, a proximal colostomy is performed first; resection of the tumor is deferred for 1 or 2 wk. Nasogastric intubation and preoperative antibiotics are necessary.

Certain types of intestinal obstruction can be managed by GI intubation and IV alimentation. Besides adynamic ileus, these include early postoperative obstruction and recurrent obstruction due to adhesions from previous intra-abdominal surgery. Although some surgeons believe that simple obstruction often can be treated by intubation, we believe that, with the few exceptions cited, surgery is the treatment of choice for all cases of intestinal obstruction.

In cases of small-bowel obstruction without evidence of strangulation (ie, audible peristalsis and no abdominal tenderness) but with marked dehydration, several hours may be required to rehydrate the patient and establish adequate urinary output. However, some severely dehydrated patients with advanced strangulation who are in shock may require immediate surgery.

SPECIAL TYPES OF INTESTINAL OBSTRUCTION

Adynamic ileus should be suspected in patients with symptoms of obstruction and a history of recent surgery, back injury, severe trauma, or thoracic or renal disease. Peristalsis is absent or infrequent, and abdominal films show gas in scattered areas of the small intestine and colon. Treatment is expectant, with nasogastric suction and IV alimentation. Administration of metoclopramide or vasopressin is not generally helpful.

In colonic ileus, the colon may become enormously distended with gas but because the ileocecal valve is competent, there is no reflux into the small bowel, which remains collapsed. In **Ogilvie's syndrome,** the distention stops at the splenic flexure; inasmuch as no mechanical obstruction is present at this site, the disease also has been called **pseudo-obstruction of the colon.** In such cases, the patient apparently has acute colonic obstruction. The supine film of the abdomen shows a dilated proximal colon with a cutoff at the splenic flexure and nondilated colon distally. However, a barium enema or operation shows no true obstructing lesion. The cause of this phenomenon is not known but is thought to be due to kinking of the colon from proximal distention at the splenic flexure. Advanced cases of colonic ileus were relieved formerly by cecostomy. Currently, colonoscopy is effective but may have to be repeated before complete resolution occurs.

Mechanical obstruction: A few symptom complexes can lead to early diagnosis. For example, a history of gallstone colic prior to the development of intestinal obstruction or tenderness over the gallbladder plus intestinal obstruction probably is due to an impacted **gallstone** in the terminal ileum; the stone may not be seen on x-ray or may appear considerably smaller than it actually is. However, *gas in the intrahepatic biliary tree is diagnostic.*

A patient with false teeth and a previous partial gastrectomy is likely to swallow masses of indigestible fiber, such as orange pulp, that form an **obstructing bezoar** in the small intestine. Bezoars also can produce obstruction in patients who have been treated in the intensive care unit with large doses of antacid to prevent bleeding stress ulcers. Compounds containing laxatives such as magnesium minimize this risk.

Richter's hernia is a nonpalpable, small inguinal hernia involving strangulation of only a portion of the intestinal wall in a small hernial sac.

In the elderly, apparent intestinal obstruction accompanied by shock, a marked leukocytosis, and variable abdominal tenderness is probably due to **mesenteric artery occlusion** from thrombosis or embolism. This condition is not a true mechanical obstruction but an ileus due to lack of peristalsis. At operation, it is usually impossible to carry out any reparative procedure, although in a few cases, thrombectomy may result in survival.

One should suspect **acute appendicitis, diverticulitis,** or **cholecystitis** in elderly patients with signs of intestinal obstruction who also have low-grade fever and slight abdominal tenderness. Patients with a single dilated loop of jejunum or transverse colon (the so-called **sentinel loop**) in the epigastrium may have **pancreatitis.**

Fecal impaction is common and rarely produces complete obstruction. More commonly, repeated attempts to evacuate produce small, diarrheal stools. If the condition is detected early by rectal examination, disimpaction can be achieved digitally or with warm mineral oil retention enemas. In an advanced case, the patient may require sedation to facilitate complete removal. Fecal impaction high in the rectum or in the sigmoid can lead to obstruction, perforation, and fecal peritonitis.

LOWER ESOPHAGEAL DISORDERS
(See also Ch. 47)

The distal 5 cm of the esophagus and the cardia share similar disease patterns and symptoms owing to their proximity.

The normal esophagus is lined with squamous epithelium, but islands of gastric mucosa (columnar epithelium) also can appear above the gastroesophageal junction **(Barrett's esophagus).** The lower esophageal sphincter, lying just above this junction, normally exerts a pressure of approximately 13 cm H_2O, thereby preventing reflux of gastric contents. Squamous epithelium is less resistant than gastric mucosa to the caustic effects of hydrochloric acid, so reflux leads to inflammation, erosion, ulceration, and bleeding and later to scarring and stenosis.

Other than reflux, disorders affecting the esophagus include **obstruction** (which may be due to cancer), **webs** (of which Schatzki's ring is the major example), and **motility disturbances.** Emetic injuries and iatrogenic trauma (chiefly from the endoscope) may lead to perforation. Portal hypertension causes esophageal varices. Large epiphrenic diverticula can form just above the esophageal hiatus.

Symptoms and signs: Dysphagia is the most common symptom of esophageal disease. If it has been present intermittently for many years, a benign cause is probable; if it is of short duration and is characterized by ever smaller food boluses that can be swallowed, cancer is the most likely diagnosis. Regurgitation of gastric contents, heartburn, and aerophagia frequently accompany reflux. Pain deep behind the lower end of the sternum suggests esophagitis.

Diagnosis: Endoscopy and biopsy are the most effective methods of diagnosis. Barium studies help to identify the site and degree of obstruction or the presence of a hiatus hernia or Schatzki's ring. Reflux usually can be documented by the radiologist. Hiatus hernias are demonstrated best by x-ray and may or may not be associated with reflux. If a perforation is suspected, a diatrizoate meglumine swallow usually demonstrates the site.

Differential diagnosis: Coronary heart disease **(CHD)** and esophageal reflux can produce similar symptoms. Esophageal motility studies and 24-h esophageal pH monitoring can help diagnose esophagitis; stress testing and other assessments of cardiac status are important to rule out CHD.

Treatment: Treatment depends on the diagnosis. Dietary modification, dilations with bougies, fracture of webs via endoscopy, and laser sclerotherapy have specific indications. Surgery, which may be either curative or palliative, is emphasized in the following discussion of the various diseases.

Cancer of the Lower Esophagus (see also in Ch. 52)

Many carcinomas that arise in the cardia or in hiatus hernias invade the lower esophagus; they are adenocarcinomas and appear to have a slightly better prognosis than the much more common squamous cell lesions, which account for 95% of esophageal malignancies. It is estimated that 10% of patients with Barrett's esophagus eventually develop cancer.

Metastasis occurs to lymph nodes (including the left gastric as well as thoracic nodes) and to liver, lung, and bone marrow. If scans and x-rays show no metastases, the lesion is approached through a left thoracotomy. At least 5 and preferably 10 cm of apparently normal esophagus above the lesion and 5 cm of stomach below it are resected. Continuity is restored by anastomosing the esophagus to the distal stomach or, occasionally, by using a segment of colon to bridge the gap.

Although the overall cure rate for esophageal cancer is only about 5%, selected series show nearly a 25% survival in patients with cancer of the distal portion. Because the cure rate is so low, experimental protocols have been designed that combine radiation therapy and chemotherapy, using cisplatin and other drugs.

Cancer of the esophagus causes an especially miserable death, chiefly because patients cannot swallow their saliva. Hence, palliative procedures are frequently offered, even when cure is unlikely. Resection and esophagogastrectomy, when possible, is preferred. If the tumor cannot be resected, colon bypass, in which the esophagus is left in place, is favored. Insertion of rubber or plastic tubes (Celestin's or Souttar's) through the tumor have been used, but tend to become displaced and cause perforation, so they are not used frequently. Laser therapy or radiation and chemotherapy can debulk obstructing tumors. Gastrostomy enables feeding but does not alleviate dysphagia.

Esophagitis

Although acid reflux is by far the most common cause of esophagitis, bile reflux frequently occurs after total gastrectomy unless diversion of bile has been accomplished by a Roux-en-Y anastomosis or enteroenterostomy. In individuals who have not had antireflux surgery, symptoms depend on the amount of reflux. Pain is most common when the patient lies flat but also may occur when he bends over. Conservative therapy, effective in the majority of cases, includes weight loss, elevation of the head on at least 2 pillows at night, restricted food intake after 6 PM, and the administration of H_2 blockers or antacids prior to bedtime. More effective control of acid reflux can be secured by full doses of H_2 blockers, such as cimetidine 300 mg 4 times daily or ranitidine 150 mg bid. Intractable esophagitis requires operative relief.

Iatrogenic Injuries

Perforation by an endoscope may occur either in the proximal or the distal esophagus. The perforation is nearly always above the diaphragm rather than below it. It is rare with flexible scopes but not with rigid scopes, which still must be used in many circumstances. Balloon dilation for achalasia, overinflation of Sengstaken-Blakemore tubes, and operations on the upper stomach or esophagus (eg, vagotomy or hiatus hernia repair) are other causes.

Pain and fever are the important clinical findings in a patient with a previously undetected perforation; whenever pain and fever occur after any of the procedures mentioned, esophageal perforation is the probable cause. *This is an emergency.* An x-ray of the chest usually shows mediastinal emphysema, and later there may be extensive subcutaneous emphysemas involving chest, neck, abdomen, and scrotum. A diatrizoate meglumine swallow should be performed immediately; it will nearly always show a perforation if one exists. The perforation must be closed immediately, and the closure reinforced by the stomach, a flap of parietal pleura, or a muscle flap from the chest wall. Drainage is provided by a chest tube.

Emetic Injuries

Vomiting when the stomach is full can significantly increase the pressure in the lower esophagus, particularly if there is a concurrent hiatus hernia and reflux. This can result in rupture of the distal esophagus with either rapid contamination of the left pleural cavity **(Boerhaave's syndrome)** or peritonitis. Complaints of severe pain in the left upper quadrant and/or chest or shoulder after vomiting, or subcutaneous emphysema mandate the same emergency diagnostic and therapeutic measures as taken for iatrogenic perforation.

Motility Disturbances

These are common and are manifested by dysphagia and severe substernal pain secondary to esophageal spasm. **Achalasia,** a condition in which ganglion cells are absent near the esophagogastric junction, leads to failure of smooth muscle to relax. The treatment of early, uncomplicated achalasia is by pneumatic dilation. This can be repeated as required. If it fails, or if achalasia is untreated, enormous distention of the esophagus or an epiphrenic diverticulum may develop. Aspiration of food particles from the lower esophagus or diverticulum may occur. Attempted balloon dilation of the sphincter, in rare cases, has led to rupture. Surgical resection of a diverticulum, if present, and myomotomy of the distal esophagus are the usual procedure. Often, this is combined with an antireflux procedure to prevent later esophagitis.

Disorders of peristalsis can be diagnosed by special technics using multiple ballons. Some motility disorders respond to Ca^{++} channel blockers; others, such as scheroderma, are progressive. In some cases, an antireflux procedure is necessary.

Schatzki's Ring

This is an annular ring of mucosa and submucosa often present at the esophagogastric junction. Since it denotes the proximal end of the stomach, it proves the presence or absence of a hiatus hernia but not of reflux. The ring tends to become smaller with advancing age. When the lumen becomes as small as 15 mm, intermittent dysphagia may occur; a luminal diameter of 11 mm is considered dangerous. When Schatzki's ring is symptomatic, dilation with bougies usually is successful. If surgery is necessary, the ring can be broken with a finger inserted into the esophagus, and any associated hernia repaired.

Epiphrenic Diverticula

These develop just above the diaphragm and are associated with hyperactivity of the lower esophageal sphincter and often with a sliding hiatus hernia. Some may become ≥ 5 cm in diameter; not only are they subject to food retention and infection, but cancer may also arise in the mucosa. If pain or regurgitation occurs, excision is necessary; if the diverticula are asymptomatic, it probably is better to follow them endoscopically. Accompanying distal esophageal spasm is treated with pneumatic dilation.

Esophageal Varices

Very few patients with portal hypertension and esophageal varices reach old age. The initial symptom is usually massive upper GI hemorrhage. Treatment is immediate endoscopic sclerotherapy, or, if this is not available, a Sengstaken-Blakemore tube is used. The balloon is inflated for 24 to 48 h and then deflated. Unless the patient is a good surgical risk, sclerotherapy is then performed; in good surgical risks, if sclerotherapy fails, a portosystemic shunt may be performed.

DISORDERS OF THE STOMACH AND DUODENUM

DIAPHRAGMATIC HERNIA

The stomach is involved in nearly every type of diaphragmatic hernia, except congenital hernias. In the most common type—the **sliding hiatus hernia**—the portion of the stomach just below the esophagogastric junction and the abdominal esophagus ascend into the chest. In **paraesophageal hernia,** the esophagogastric junction remains in place, but the stomach rises alongside the esophagus. There are also combinations of sliding and paraesophageal hernias. In **traumatic esophageal hernia,** the stomach may enter the chest through a rent in the diaphragm.

Sliding Hiatus Hernia

A small hiatus hernia can be detected in most older individuals. Such hernias are almost always asymptomatic unless reflux esophagitis is present. However, mild flatulence or substernal discomfort may occur, and if a Schatzki's ring tightens to a diameter < 11 mm, esophageal obstruction can develop.

The differential diagnosis includes many disorders, such as coronary heart disease, esophageal spasm, gallbladder disease, gastritis, peptic ulcer, and functional complaints for which no organic cause can be found. Symptoms that appear suddenly always suggest malignant disease, not only of the esophagus but of some other abdominal organ. Consequently, an abdominal rather than a thoracic approach is used for repair, since an unexpected tumor may be found.

The diagnosis of a sliding hiatus hernia is based on barium-contrast studies and endoscopy. Asymptomatic hernias should not be repaired; mild complaints are treated by conservative measures, including a bland diet, weight reduction, antacids, and elevation of the head and chest on several pillows at night.

Controversy continues concerning the best surgical procedure for hiatus hernia associated with esophagitis. Each procedure restores a proper length of abdominal esophagus and strengthens the lower esophageal sphincter. In the Nissen repair, the fundus of the stomach is wrapped about the lower esophagus. The Belsey repair creates a valve by suturing the stomach to the anterior surface of the esophagus. The Hill repair anchors that part of the stomach at the gastroesophageal junction to the median arcuate ligament, which lies just anterior to the aorta; a valve is created by anterior sutures through the junction, drawing it back toward the ligament. The abdominal approach is used more frequently, but some surgeons prefer exposure through the chest. The more recently introduced Angelchik procedure uses a plastic collar about the lower esophagus to prevent reflux; migration of the prosthesis and late stenosis have limited the usefulness of this method.

Regardless of procedure, postoperative recurrences are not uncommon after several years because of the negative intrathoracic pressure that occurs with every inspiration. Nevertheless, surgery offers great relief for long periods in properly selected patients. In a few instances, esophagitis is so marked that resection and replacement with a section of jejunum or colon is necessary. In some older patients, recurrent strictures at the gastroesophageal junction can be treated by periodic dilation with bougies.

Paraesophageal Hernias

These can be huge; in advanced cases, the entire stomach may be in the chest. Both the esophagogastric junction and the pylorus may be level with the diaphragm as the gastric fundus rotates upward into either the left or right side of the chest. A large gas bubble can be seen on chest x-ray, and the diagnosis is confirmed by barium-contrast studies.

Paraesophageal hernias can cause complete pyloric obstruction and gastric incarceration, strangulation, and perforation. Unless the patient is a poor surgical risk, these hernias should be repaired.

Traumatic Rupture of the Diaphragm

After injury involving the left side of the chest or left upper abdominal quadrant, the chest x-ray may show a gas bubble above the diaphragm on the left side. The possibility of a diaphragmatic rupture should be suspected, and barium-contrast studies done. The stomach is the usual organ found to be injured but the colon, spleen, and even other viscera can be identified in some cases. Immediate repair is necessary.

PEPTIC ULCER DISEASE

Benign ulcers of the stomach and duodenum are included in this category, although the etiologies may prove different. Peptic ulcer disease includes gastric ulcer, duodenal ulcer, stress ulcer, and anastomotic ulcer.

The adage "no acid, no ulcer" remains true, but the lack of a direct relationship between the amount of acid and severity of the ulcer indicate that other factors are important. Recent studies suggest that duodenal secretion of bicarbonate is deficient in patients with duodenal ulcers and may play a role in ulcerogenesis. Mucosal coating agents (eg, sucralfate) exert beneficial effects on both gastric and duodenal ulcers. Prostaglandins may play an important role that is not yet precisely defined.

The introduction of the **H₂-receptor blockers** has shifted the treatment of uncomplicated ulcers strongly toward pharmacologic control. Today, **peptic ulcer surgery** is performed essentially because of complications or unhealed gastric ulcers. Elderly patients are at particular risk for the major complications: perforation, hemorrhage, and obstruction. In a recent study, 23% of patients who required surgery for peptic ulcer were ≥ 70 yr of age.

Gastric ulcers present special problems since a small percentage appear benign but are malignant. Endoscopic biopsies are not always adequate for differentiation; any persistent ulcer must be regarded with suspicion and treated surgically. Since benign ulcers heal more slowly in the elderly, in the absence of complications at least 6 wk of medical treatment should be allowed before resection (see Ch. 47).

Anastomotic ulcers frequently cause hemorrhage. They are often not revealed by barium studies; endoscopy is the best method of diagnosis. These ulcers respond poorly to conservative therapy. The most effective surgical procedure is gastric resection with vagotomy.

Massive Hemorrhage

This is the most common complication of peptic ulcers in the elderly. In a recent study, 38% of all surgery for massive hemorrhage from ulcers was performed in individuals ≥ 70 yr of age. Methods of diagnosis are discussed in the section on GASTROINTESTINAL BLEEDING, above. Choice of treatment is controversial but we believe that geriatric patients who have lost ≥ 5 u. of blood have a better chance of survival with early operation—ie, gastric resection for gastric ulcer and either gastric resection or vagotomy-pyloroplasty with ligation of the bleeding vessel for duodenal ulcer. Alternative treatments include angiographic control with vasopressin or embolization, which may be hazardous in ulcer disease, and endoscopic thermal coagulation or laser coagulation of the bleeding vessel.

Acute Perforation

Perforation is the second most frequent complication of peptic ulcer disease. Often the typical clinical finding of abdominal rigidity is absent, and the patient may demonstrate only minimal tenderness on examination. This paucity of clinical findings may inordinately delay diagnosis.

Acute ulcer perforation usually is heralded by acute upper abdominal pain followed in a few hours by the rapid progression of shock to cardiovascular collapse. An x-ray taken in the erect position reveals free gas beneath the diaphragm in most patients. In doubtful cases, a diatrizoate meglumine swallow demonstrates extravasation from the stomach or duodenum. Immediate surgery is necessary except in the very few patients so ill from other causes that they probably would not survive laparotomy. For example, a patient who sustains a perforated ulcer a day or 2 after an acute MI can be treated by nasogastric intubation and suction plus antibiotics if the perforation is small or apparently walled off.

The prognosis is poor in older patients. Thirty percent of perforations occur in patients $\geq$ 70 yr of age, and the overall mortality is 20%. Treatment primarily involves closure of the perforation. However, because the incidence of ulcer recurrence is high, if optimal operating conditions prevail, either gastric resection or pyloroplasty combined with vagotomy should also be performed.

Obstruction

Pyloric obstruction occurs from cicatricial stenosis of a chronic duodenal ulcer or from gastric ulcers located near the pylorus. Symptoms include recurring vomiting, weight loss, and metabolic alkalosis, but attempts must be made to rule out a malignant obstructive lesion.

Intractable Pain

Intractable pain is unusual in the older patient with peptic ulcer disease. Conservative therapy is not likely to be successful, and gastric resection is the treatment of choice. Older patients who have been receiving long-term H_2-receptor blocker therapy often develop prolonged postoperative gastric stasis if vagotomy is also performed.

OTHER DISORDERS

Stress Ulcers

Stress ulcers are peptic ulcers, usually gastric, resulting from stress. Grossly, they are typically small (1 to 3 mm) and superficial, being limited to the mucosa. Frequently, they are multiple and associated with gastritis. Many predisposing causes include recent serious operations, trauma, shock, infections, and burns. The important symptom is hemorrhage, which can be massive and life-endangering. It is not surprising that most of these lesions are encountered in intensive care units.

Although the exact etiology is not clear, certain factors other than the predisposing causes enhance the development of these dangerous ulcers; these are gastric dilation and ventilatory insufficiency, as well as reduction in the ability of the mucosa to withstand the effects of hydrochloric acid.

Since treatment is difficult and often unsatisfactory, prophylaxis is extremely important. The stomach should be kept as empty as possible, by means of a sump nasogastric tube placed on suction. Pulmonary function, if not adequate as determined by blood gases, must be aided by intratracheal intubation and assisted ventilation, possibly including PEEP.

Either of 2 methods may be used to reduce the level of gastric acid. The better one, from the viewpoint of acid control, is to give repeated oral doses of an antacid–anti-gas combination drug. A nurse must withdraw acid from the stomach before each administration, measure the pH, and keep it between 5 and 7. This method requires intensive nursing care; thus, IV cimetidine 300 mg q 6 h by constant drip is usually used, even though it is slightly less effective.

If prophylaxis has not been used or if gastric bleeding occurs despite treatment, the possibility of a typical peptic ulcer must be considered. Endoscopy is indicated to determine the exact source. Small bleeding points may be treated by electrocoagulation. If a typical peptic ulcer is found, treatment should be followed as discussed in Ch. 47.

If multiple bleeding points are found and bleeding continues after cauterization, selective arteriography is the next step; if possible, the catheter should be placed in the left gastric artery rather than the celiac axis. This confirms the diagnosis if active bleeding is present; selective vasopressin infusion stops the bleeding in about 80% of cases. If bleeding is not stopped, surgery is required, as a last resort—either total gastrectomy or high subtotal gastrectomy with vagotomy.

During the period when stress bleeding is encountered, a vigilant search for a source of persistent sepsis must be made, and the source should be drained without delay.

Gastritis (see also Ch. 47)

This disease frequently leads to massive upper GI hemorrhage. In most uncomplicated cases, gastritis can be handled medically. All known gastric irritants should be eliminated; the common ones include aspirin, alcohol, ibuprofen, and an excessive intake of caffeine. Smoking is contraindicated. (See also section on GASTROINTESTINAL BLEEDING, above.)

Treatment includes antacids, as well as the H_2 blockers. Sucralfate may be given 1 gm qid; if this drug and H_2 blockers are given together, activity of the latter is reduced. Every attempt should be made to avoid surgery. Selective arteriography and the injection of vasopressin into the left gastric artery usually is effective for massive bleeding. Endoscopy is not likely to be satisfactory, since there often are multiple bleeding points. If surgery is required, distal gastrectomy and vagotomy can be performed if only the distal stomach is involved. However, if gastritis extends throughout the entire stomach, total gastrectomy may be necessary.

Stomach Cancer and Other Tumors (see Ch. 52)

Duodenal Tumors (see also NEOPLASMS OF THE SMALL INTESTINE in Ch. 51)

Cancer of the duodenum is rare; it can be resected by pancreatoduodenectomy, and 5-yr survival is nearly 50%. Diagnosis is established by endoscopy.

Bulky villous adenomas occur occasionally in the duodenum. These large sessile polyps may undergo malignant change. Brunner's gland adenomas occur in the first and second portions of the duodenum. They are benign but may lead to obstruction or bleeding.

Diverticula of the Stomach and Duodenum

In the stomach, these rare lesions tend to occur on the lesser curvature, just below the diaphragm. In the duodenum, they are common and often are found near Oddi's sphincter; at times the common duct empties into a diverticulum. Unless symptoms clearly arise from diverticula, they are best left untreated. Surgical extirpation is difficult and may be dangerous. Food can become impacted in a large duodenal diverticulum; gastric resection with a Roux-en-Y anastomosis probably is safer than excision of the diverticulum.

Other Bleeding Lesions (see GASTROINTESTINAL BLEEDING, above)

DISEASES OF THE JEJUNUM AND ILEUM

Diseases of the jejunum and ileum may exist in isolation or in association with disorders of other viscera (eg, the stomach, duodenum, and colon in gastroenteritis or Crohn's disease). Many of these diseases are treated medically, but some are also treated surgically and must be considered in the differential diagnosis of surgical abdomen.

Diseases of the small intestine may be caused by congenital, acquired, or iatrogenic factors; inflammatory or toxic agents; malabsorption; motility defects; tumors; or they may be functional rather than organic. Special topics are described under GASTROINTESTINAL BLEEDING and INTESTINAL OBSTRUCTION, above, and under CROHN'S DISEASE in Ch. 48.

Congenital Lesions

Meckel's diverticulum, the only common congenital lesion in geriatric patients, is nearly always an incidental finding, and symptoms are rare in the elderly.

Acquired Lesions

The most common of these is **diverticulosis.** In this disease, saclike projections of the mucosa protrude through the muscularis of the bowel. These are most common in the jejunum in patients of advanced age. Diverticulosis may be asymptomatic or may be associated with massive bleeding, malabsorption, or inflammation (diverticulitis). In cases of massive bleeding, it is desirable to locate the exact segment of involved bowel. Selective arteriography, which may be combined with exploratory laparotomy, is the best diagnostic tool. It allows resection of the shortest segment of bowel that may be severely involved. Perforation is uncommon, but if it occurs, resection and reanastomosis are the procedures of choice. (See also Ch. 48.)

Iatrogenic Lesions

The most frequent problems encountered are the following:

Excessive enterectomy: As a general rule, $1/3$ of the jejunum and ileum may be excised without seriously impairing absorption of nutrients. More radical resection is tolerated poorly, and adults who have lost $2/3$ of the small bowel usually develop severe metabolic problems. Total parenteral nutrition has improved survival.

Absorption of vitamin B_{12} and cholesterol is reduced after resection of the distal ileum. A loss of 30 cm usually is well tolerated, but regular supplementation with parenteral vitamin B_{12} (cyanocobalamin) may be necessary after more extensive resection.

Radiation enterocolitis: Radiation therapy is used frequently for cancer of the bladder, prostate, rectum, colon, and female genital organs. The small intestine is damaged by 5000 rad; the colon is slightly more resistant.

The symptoms of radiation enteritis are indistinguishable from those of chronic intestinal obstruction. Radiation colitis is manifested by bleeding and diarrhea. Conservative therapy usually is indicated at the outset, since some acute symptoms may subside with IV alimentation and restriction of oral intake.

Operative intervention is often unsuccessful because radiation diminishes the blood supply to the bowel and all anastomoses tend to heal poorly unless made in normal bowel. Furthermore, since dense pelvic adhesions are likely to be encountered, dissection is arduous; leakage and fistula formation are occasional sequelae. For these reasons, resection may be difficult or impossible, and palliative enteroenterostomy may be required.

Minor degrees of colonic ulceration may be treated with a bland diet and psyllium hydrophilic mucilloid. In severe cases, resection of the involved segment with reanastomosis may be possible; in other cases, a permanent defunctioning colostomy may have to be combined with resection of the involved rectum or colon.

Blind loop syndrome: This arises when surgical procedures create a loop of bowel in which intestinal contents collect and stagnate. Poor drainage leads to secondary infection and, occasionally, to deficiency syndromes. The typical example is a side-to-side anastomosis that "sidetracks" a long segment of small intestine. Similar problems have followed gastrectomy when erroneously the terminal ileum rather than the jejunum was anastomosed to the stomach. Long afferent loops after a gastric resection and gastrojejunostomy have led to major dilation of the afferent loop and, hence, to the **afferent loop syndrome.** Side-to-side small-bowel anastomosis has been followed in some instances by marked dilation of the blind ends of the 2 segments.

Typical symptoms include indigestion, gas, cramps, and diarrhea. Antibiotic therapy (eg, tetracycline) has not been satisfactory. Proper treatment involves reinstating the loop in the intestinal stream if it is long or resecting the loop if it is short.

Inflammatory Lesions

Diseases that can be confused easily with surgical emergencies are common. Acute gastroenteritis, with its typical acute onset, nausea, vomiting, and diarrhea, can mimic a surgical abdomen. Persistent symptoms, localized tenderness, or a silent abdomen in elderly patients with abdominal scars or evidence of hernias are signals to reconsider the diagnosis of gastroenteritis.

Unusual infections can also mimic a surgical abdomen. Giardiasis is endemic to some areas of the USA. *Yersinia* infections can cause acute ileitis that is not diagnosed until laparotomy. Acute amebiasis not only is a threat to travelers but also is endemic to many areas of the USA. Probably the most common and dangerous of all infections is salmonellosis. Patients treated with antibiotics and those receiving immunosuppressive drugs are at particular risk.

Toxic Lesions of the Bowel

Toxin-producing organisms (eg, staphylococci, *Vibrio cholerae, Campylobacter* sp, and *Clostridium perfringens*) can cause severe enteritis or colitis. From the surgeon's viewpoint, the most important disease is pseudomembranous enterocolitis (see under GASTROINTESTINAL AND INTRA-ABDOMINAL INFECTIONS in Ch. 76).

Malabsorption

Nutritional deficiencies following gastrectomy result from diminished absorption of iron, calcium, fat, and protein and are related to the extent of gastrectomy and the type of anastomosis. Total gastrectomy does not necessarily lead to inanition, but specific nutritional deficiencies (eg, loss of intrinsic factor) must be treated. **Following enterectomy,** depending on the extent of resection, absorption of all nutrients is diminished. Total enterectomy (unless total parenteral nutrition is used) is incompatible with life. **Right colectomy** temporarily diminishes absorption of water and some electrolytes. **Total proctocolectomy** produces no chronic malabsorption after a period of adjustment.

The underlying disease is important. **Gastrinomas** produce the **Zollinger-Ellison syndrome,** originally described as excessive acid secretion causing diarrhea, peptic ulcers, and pancreatic tumor. Further experience has expanded our knowledge of this neuroendocrine neoplasm (see under DISORDERS OF THE PANCREAS, below). Malabsorption of fat may be an early sign of **pancreatic cancer.** Unexplained diarrhea should suggest other **neuroendocrine tumors of the pancreas or the gut,** such as somatostatinomas or vipomas. **Crohn's disease** can cause malabsorption owing to inflamed mucosa or to bowel shortened by resection. Fistulas from the stomach or gastrocolic and proximal enterocolic fistulas, most commonly due to peptic ulcer disease and colonic cancer, respectively, can produce malabsorption.

Symptoms common to most of these syndromes are diarrhea and inanition. Varying degrees of gas, abdominal distention, nausea, and cramps generally also occur.

Celiac disease (nontropical sprue) is a gluten-induced enteropathy characterized by atrophy of intestinal villi. Cramps, diarrhea, and abdominal distention may mimic intestinal obstruction. A barium study of the upper GI tract shows flocculation and scattered areas of distention of the small intestine. Small-bowel biopsy is diagnostic, showing a flattened mucosa. Treatment is a gluten-free diet. Although gluten typically is found in wheat and rye, it is also present in barley and oats and in many prepared foods. Acute symptomatic episodes are managed by nasogastric intubation and IV alimentation. In chronic cases, **lymphoma** or **carcinoma** of the small intestine may develop and must be considered in elderly patients.

Lactase deficiency is manifested by abdominal distention, gas, bloating, nausea, and diarrhea after ingestion of lactose-containing dairy products. Varying degrees of lactase deficiency occur in nearly all geriatric patients.

Motility Disorders

Intestinal motility is influenced by a variety of agents. Laxatives and antidiarrheal drugs, poisons, and food additives (eg, monosodium glutamate and sodium sulfite) are common examples. Ingestion of mushrooms and shellfish can lead to severe diarrhea.

Scleroderma is a well-recognized cause of diminished intestinal motility. In the small bowel, it usually involves the duodenum, leading to megaduodenum. Surgical procedures that bypass the duodenum may provide relief, but other segments of the bowel may become involved. Scleroderma of the colon is manifested by severe constipation, with episodes of fecal blockage that usually can be relieved by laxatives. Diagnosis is aided by barium enema, which often shows short, broad-based diverticula scattered throughout the colon.

Chagas's disease, which is common in Brazil and other tropical areas of South America, is due to infection with *Trypanosoma cruzi.* It leads to megaesophagus, megacolon, and megaduodenum. Colectomy may be required for extreme distention of the colon and unremitting constipation.

Uncommon motility disorders include amyloidosis, mesenteric lipomatosis, desmoid tumors of the mesentery, and Whipple's disease. **Amyloid infiltration of the mesentery** produces symptoms of intestinal obstruction, but laparotomy usually shows such wide infiltration that no curative procedure is possible. **Mesenteric lipomatosis** also produces symptoms of intestinal obstruction; if the disease is not too extensive, a bypass of the mesenteric mass may be possible, but excision is usually impossible. **Desmoid tumors of the mesentery** usually are nonresectable. Improvement after administration of vitamin C has been reported. **Whipple's disease** (intestinal lipodystrophy) occurs in adult males and usually is associated with arthritis as well as diarrhea and malabsorption of fats. It is caused by a bacillary infection, and diagnosis should be confirmed by peroral intestinal biopsy prior to operation.

Neuroendocrine tumors of the gut are a diagnostic challenge because they can produce a wide variety of symptoms. The primary tumor may be located near the intestine or in the pancreas, liver, or elsewhere. About $^2/_3$ are functioning tumors producing several peptides and amines, some of which may cause colic and diarrhea. Malignant carcinoid, insulinoma, gastrinoma, vipoma, glucagonoma, somatostatinoma, adrenal cortical adenomas, and multiple endocrine adenopathy are among the lesions that have been identified. In general, these tumors are rare in older people but must be considered when no other cause can be found for persistent diarrhea.

Functional disturbances of the jejunum and ileum may account for motility disorders. Unfortunately, many patients complain of varying degrees of nonspecific constipation or diarrhea, combined with abdominal distention and flatulence. In nearly all cases, intestinal transit is normal. Patients with permanent ileostomies do not report these symptoms; therefore, it appears that most of these functional complaints arise from the colon rather than the small intestine.

Neoplasms of the small intestine are discussed in Ch. 52.

DISEASES OF THE APPENDIX

Appendicitis

The classic initial symptom of appendicitis is epigastric pain. This is followed by nausea and, later, localization of pain and tenderness in the right lower quadrant. Low-grade fever and leukocytosis are also present. However, in older patients, pain more often *begins* in the right lower quadrant and may not be severe until perforation occurs. Because the blood supply to the appendix is generally less adequate in older than in younger patients, the course of the disease can be fulminant. In some instances, symptoms and signs may be minimal, and chronic infection occurs, marked by low-grade fever and poorly defined localization of abdominal signs.

The treatment is appendectomy. Antibiotics should be given prior to operation and continued for at least 48 h thereafter. If perforation has already occurred and peritonitis is spreading, the value of drainage is controversial. Simple drainage is recommended for a localized abscess and should be followed by appendectomy in a few weeks. In nearly all other cases, however, the appendix can and should be removed at the time of the initial operation.

Appendicitis in the elderly patient occasionally occurs in association with carcinoma of the colon. Low-grade obstruction can lead to appendiceal distention that mimics true appendicitis. If the patient who has had a simple appendectomy fails to recover promptly, the colon should be investigated by endoscopy or barium enema.

Tumors of the Appendix

The most common tumor of the appendix is a **carcinoid**. It is found in approximately one in 1000 resected appendixes and is cured by appendectomy. Rarely, carcinoids are malignant; these are typically > 2 cm in diameter or show evidence of lymphatic or lymph node involvement. If any of these features are present, a right colectomy should be performed.

Primary adenocarcinoma of the appendix is rare, despite the fact that the appendix is lined with colonic mucosa. When present, it may block the lumen, thereby leading to acute appendicitis and perforation.

Mucoceles are manifested by distention of the appendix because of the intraluminal accumulation of mucus. Outlet obstruction is a necessary feature. The symptoms suggest early appendicitis. A mucocele may be demonstrated by CT scan. Although usually benign and curable by appendectomy, some are associated with low-grade adenocarcinoma; if these mucoceles perforate, a form of carcinomatosis known as **pseudomyxoma peritonei** results. Patients with this indolent type of tumor present with increased abdominal girth and a "doughylike" abdomen. They can survive for several years, but repeated accumulation of intraperitoneal mucus or intestinal obstruction occur. Palliative surgical procedures often prolong life and make the patient more comfortable.

DISORDERS OF THE COLORECTUM

The most common colorectal disorders requiring surgery in the geriatric population are cancer, diverticular disease, volvulus, and angiodysplasia. Ulcerative colitis is an uncommon but serious problem. The surgical management of these diseases is discussed below.

COLON CANCER

Benign and malignant neoplasms of the colon and rectum are discussed in detail in Ch. 52.

Cancer of the colon and upper rectum (see Ch. 52) preferably is treated by segmental resection and reanastomosis performed in a single operation. Multiple tumors may necessitate subtotal colectomy. However, because low ileorectal anastomoses may lead to severe diarrhea in older patients, an adequate amount of large bowel should be left whenever possible. Wide excision of the mesentery and regional lymph nodes is preferably performed concurrently. The distal line of resection preferably should be 5 cm beyond the tumor.

Cancer of the mid- and low rectum is more problematic in the elderly because the operation most likely to produce cure—abdominoperineal resection with permanent colostomy—may seem incompatible with a satisfactory life-style to some patients. Fortunately, use of a stapling device permits lower anastomosis than possible with hand-sutured technics.

The anal sphincter can be preserved in only about 5% of low rectal cancers and can be treated with other procedures (eg, coloanal anastomosis after low resection, local excision, electrocoagulation, and intracavitary radiation therapy).

Local excision is satisfactory for polypoid tumors that are not fixed and not > 2 cm in diameter; in 1 series, recurrence was noted in only 8% of cases. However, if the tumor is larger or attached to the underlying muscularis, the recurrence rate rises (about 23% in this study). Papillon's method of **intracavitary radiation,** in which approximately 15,000 rad are delivered to the tumor through a special scope, was successful in his hands with small, polypoid, freely movable neoplasms. In our experience, the larger, fixed tumors are usual; attempts to extend Papillon's method to these less-responsive cancers end in recurrence. **Electrocoagulation** also may be effective for small lesions, but according to one study, when it was used for cancers > 4 cm in diameter, results were poor.

The follow-up of patients after resection of a colorectal cancer is not standardized. Nevertheless, one should make certain that the bowel contains no further cancer or polyps. Patients should be examined every 6 mo with rigid sigmoidoscopy, guaiac stool tests, and carcinoembryonic antigen **(CEA)** determinations. A colonoscopy should be done every 3 yr; if not, a barium enema is indicated. Anastomotic recurrences are most common after low rectal anastomoses, and can be detected by rigid sigmoidoscopy.

A combination of radiation therapy and surgical resection is helpful in many patients. Preoperative radiation permits many fixed and otherwise inoperable tumors to be resected. For the usual cancer of the rectum, postoperative radiation reduces the local recurrence rate in B_2 and C lesions but has not increased the length of survival. Intraoperative radiation, although still investigational, appears to have a favorable influence, particularly in reducing local recurrence.

Chemotherapy has not been proved to be of value, except in some cases of colorectal cancer that have metastasized to the liver. Only 1 study has suggested that it has lowered the recurrence rate when used with surgery and radiation. This finding must be contrasted with the apparently valuable role of chemotherapy in the treatment of perianal cancer.

Immunotherapy has not played any significant role in the treatment of colorectal cancer.

Recurrent cancer: The best marker for recurrent colorectal cancer is serum CEA determination. It is especially valuable postoperatively, when a rise above preoperative baseline levels usually indicates recurrence. Other recurrent cancers, particularly those of the rectum, may not produce an elevated CEA. Some patients can be cured by a second operation for recurrence diagnosed by a rising CEA.

Palliative procedures: In many cases, only palliative procedures are possible, either at the time of initial surgery or later for recurrent disease. A colostomy may help relieve unremitting tenesmus. Radiation therapy can ease the pain of recurrent rectal cancer. Laser therapy has been used to debulk inoperable rectal tumors and prevent obstruction.

Prognosis

The crude 5-yr survival rate for cancer of the colorectum is approximately 50 to 55% in most major centers. When deaths due to other causes are excluded, the adjusted 5-yr survival rate is 90% for Class A disease, about 60 to 70% for Class B, 40% for Class C, and < 20% for Class D. Local recurrence has been reduced significantly by radiation therapy, although life expectancy has not increased beyond that of controls treated by surgery alone.

DIVERTICULAR DISEASE
(See Ch. 48)

VOLVULUS

This arises from *a twist of the colon on its mesentery that is sufficient to produce intestinal obstruction.* An unusually long, mobile mesentery in the affected segment or lack of fixation is necessary for the twist to occur. Unless the obstruction is relieved, it tends to progress proximally and distally because of gas formation within the occluded segment. As a result, the mesenteric vasculature supplying the involved segment is also occluded, and gangrene and perforation can follow.

Volvulus is common in the elderly and is most prevalent in inactive females with restricted mental capabilities living in nursing homes. The combination of an unusually large and long colon with inadequate bowel hygiene is a contributing factor.

Sigmoid volvulus: Volvulus occurs most commonly in the sigmoid. Obstipation, cramps, and marked abdominal distention are the usual complaints. Abdominal x-ray shows a large, distended colon. Distention may be limited to the sigmoid loop but occasionally extends above the liver. A barium enema shows the typical "bird-beak" deformity at the level of the twist.

It usually is possible to pass a long rectal tube through a sigmoido-scope (or colonoscope) and past the obstruction; this can produce explo-sive deflation. If deflation is incomplete or there are indications of gan-grene, immediate laparotomy is necessary. The colonoscope is useful in determining the presence or absence of gangrene.

If deflation occurs, resection of the involved segment of the colon is done electively during the same hospitalization, unless there are overrid-ng reasons to defer surgery. If surgery is *not* performed, the probability of recurrence is very high.

Cecal volvulus: The cecum is also a likely site for volvulus. Diagnosis is made on the basis of abdominal cramps, nausea, vomiting, distention, and obstipation. Abdominal x-ray shows a large bubble of gas, either in the midabdomen or in the left upper quadrant. Barium enema demon-strates the typical bird-beak deformity in the ascending colon and no re-flux into the ileum. *Gangrene supervenes rapidly, so immediate surgery is essential.* If there is no evidence of gangrene, the cecum can be anchored by a cecostomy tube after the twist is reduced. The alternative for low-risk patients is immediate resection and reanastomosis. When gangrene is present in a high-risk patient, resection with the formation of ileal and colonic fistulas is necessary. Intestinal continuity is then reestab-lished at a later date.

ULCERATIVE COLITIS
(See also Ch. 48)

This disease is treated primarily by gastroenterologists. The major complications necessitating surgery include failure to respond to medical therapy, hemorrhage, toxic megacolon, perforation, and late-developing cancer. Ulcerative colitis often pursues a more virulent course in pa-tients > 60 yr of age; with late onset, the mortality in severe cases is > 20%.

Medical therapy in severe cases nearly always includes the use of corti-costeroids. However, these agents increase the risk of spontaneous per-foration, which may be painless and diagnosed only by the presence of subdiaphragmatic gas on an upright abdominal x-ray.

Surgical therapy usually involves either a subtotal colectomy or a total proctocolectomy; in either case, a permanent ileostomy is required. The greatest cause of mortality is protracted delay before surgery is per-formed.

ANGIODYSPLASIA
(See Ch. 48)

ANORECTAL DISORDERS

These disorders occur in the distal 3 cm of rectum, the anal canal, and the area (5 cm in diameter) about the anal verge. Some 50 dermatologic disorders may affect the perianal area; the most common is pruritus ani. Crypts and papillae, which mark the proximal end of the canal, and deep rectal glands may exhibit pathologic changes (eg, inflammation). Rectal continence is discussed in Ch. 48 and neoplasms are discussed in Ch. 52.

PRURITUS ANI

Intense chronic itching in the anal region. Pruritus ani is a very common symptom with multiple causes. Many persons, in their zeal for cleanliness, excoriate and damage the delicate perianal skin. Harsh soaps, excessive wiping with toilet paper, application of sensitizing perfumes or deodorizers, and nylon underwear and tight, warm clothing that promote sweating are the most common exogenous causes. Fungal diseases (eg, epidermophytosis) and parasitism (eg, with pinworms) are examples of infections and infestations, respectively, that cause pruritus ani. Pruritus may accompany local manifestations of more widespread diseases (eg, psoriasis). Psychological problems may also contribute to perianal itching.

Some topical drugs used to treat anal diseases (eg, anesthetic compounds such as lidocaine and benzocaine) may produce contact dermatitis.

Some oral antibiotics can cause an overgrowth of intestinal *Candida* by suppressing the normal bowel flora, resulting in pruritus from perianal candidiasis.

On physical examination, the perianal area may appear essentially normal, but usually, there are excoriations from involuntary scratching during sleep. In advanced cases, there may be secondary bacterial infection.

Treatment

Prior to the introduction of topical corticosteroids, treatment was often unsatisfactory. However, even with corticosteroids, etiologic factors should be sought. Systemic diseases should be identified and fungal infections treated with topical application of antifungal powders available over the counter. Nylon underwear and deodorizers must be avoided. After defecation, the perianal area must be cleaned gently with moist cotton and little wiping. In mild cases due to simple irritation, such cleansing followed by application of petroleum jelly can be very effective. Oral antibiotics should be discontinued if possible.

The most effective local therapy is hydrocortisone cream; several preparations containing 0.5 or 1% hydrocortisone are available. Ordinarily, the cream is applied only at night, when itching occurs. Severe cases may require application several times a day. The cream is discontinued as soon as itching is controlled. Although recurrence is common, retreatment in the same fashion is successful.

Surgical procedures are rarely indicated. Injection of 95% alcohol has been effective but may lead to local necrosis. Excision of skin tags and biopsy of refractory lesions to rule out malignant disease are indicated in refractory cases. Hemorrhoidectomy is not helpful.

HEMORRHOIDS

Abnormally large or symptomatic conglomerates of blood vessels, supporting tissues, and overlying mucous membrane or anorectal skin. They include several types. **Internal hemorrhoids** *arise above the anorectal (dentate) line.* **External hemorrhoids** *arise below that line and form so-called* **piles. Combined hemorrhoids** *include both types.* A **thrombosed external hemorrhoid** *is a localized clot that either forms in the vein of a hemorrhoid or arises from a ruptured hemorrhoidal blood vessel.* **Skin tags** *representing irregular remnants of external hemorrhoids, interfere with proper hygiene.* **Prolapsed internal hemorrhoids** *extend down into the anal canal or through the anus.*

Internal hemorrhoids arise because the vena cava and iliac veins have no valves; erect posture, heavy lifting, and straining all increase distention of the veins. There are 3 veins in which these hemorrhoids develop; they can be observed anoscopically in the right anterior, right posterior, and left posterior positions.

These hemorrhoids may be entirely asymptomatic in their early stages, but later they tend to bleed. The bleeding may vary in amount but usually is minimal and is noted as bright red blood appearing intermittently on the stool or toilet paper. Rarely, significant bleeding occurs; if the blood is retained above the sphincter, a large amount can be expelled at one time. Continued blood loss, even in small increments, can lead to anemia.

Internal hemorrhoids may lead to the formation of **external** or **combined hemorrhoids,** which exhibit the same symptoms. Pain does not occur with hemorrhoids unless there is prolapse of an internal hemorrhoid or thrombosis of an external hemorrhoid.

Diagnosis of internal hemorrhoids requires proctoscopy; hemorrhoids are soft and cannot be detected reliably by finger. It should be kept in mind that they may be a symptom of a lesion higher in the colorectum. In geriatric patients, rectal bleeding always requires a complete examination, including either proctosigmoidoscopy and barium enema or total colonoscopy. External hemorrhoids can be seen on inspection and nearly always indicate the presence of combined hemorrhoids. They are asymptomatic unless a thrombosis or hematoma forms.

Treatment

Mild hemorrhoidal disease is treated by a soft diet and a bulk producer (eg, psyllium hydrophilic mucilloid). Straining at stool must be avoided, as should heavy lifting.

Hemorrhoidectomy is the most effective treatment for combined hemorrhoids or internal hemorrhoids with major prolapse. With proper technic, relief of symptoms is immediate and the long-term results excellent. The main objection of patients to surgery—fear of postoperative pain—indicates the need for long-lasting local anesthetics at the time of surgery.

Rubber bands can be used in the office to treat internal hemorrhoids that have bled or are mildly prolapsed. The bands are placed under tension about the base of each major hemorrhoid in one or more sessions. The bands must be positioned above the anal canal, or great pain results. Several instruments have been devised that make placement relatively simple. When done correctly, the procedure involves no postoperative pain and long-term results are good.

Sclerotherapy also has good early results, although later there is a tendency for secondary hemorrhoids to develop; a hemorrhoidectomy is more difficult at this time. Quinine urea hydrochloride 5% is a widely used sclerosing solution.

Cryosurgery and **laser therapy** also have been used, but the small amount of tissue removed and delayed healing have made these modalities less popular.

A **thrombosed external hemorrhoid** results in sudden, severe, perianal pain. On inspection, a tense blue subcutaneous mass is observed. Subcutaneous injection of a local anesthetic and evacuation of the clot provide immediate relief. A small section of skin also should be excised to allow adequate drainage in case of further bleeding. If the patient is not seen within 48 h of onset, the clot may be difficult to remove. Some small clots resolve without much discomfort, but large ones, if not evacuated, are slow to improve and are painful for many days. Warm sitz baths and analgesics are helpful.

BOWEL INCONTINENCE
(See Ch. 48)

FISSURES

Longitudinal breaks in the squamous epithelium of the anal canal. They may be superficial or deep; in the latter case, the internal sphincter is exposed. A so-called sentinel pile often forms at the lower end of a chronic fissure. Causes are assumed to be large or hard bowel movements, rough fecal debris, straining at stool, diarrhea, or trauma to the anal canal, either by rough wiping or by foreign bodies (eg, thermometers and enema nozzles).

The major symptom is severe pain, aggravated by defecation and persisting for several minutes afterward. There is relative relief until the next bowel movement. Bleeding is rare in adults.

Diagnosis usually can be made by separating the buttocks; as the patient strains, the fissure can be seen. Characteristically, it is in the posterior midline, but occasionally, it is in the anterior midline. If it is not visible, it can be seen on anoscopy if the patient can tolerate this. In some cases, the examination is so painful and associated with so much spasm of the sphincter that either local or general anesthesia is necessary.

Treatment depends on chronicity. Superficial lesions respond to stool softeners (eg, psyllium hydrophilic mucilloid) and warm sitz baths. Topical agents (not suppositories) may be helpful. Creams or ointments that contain local anesthetics or simple protectants may provide relief; they are applied after bowel movements.

Chronic fissures require surgery. Two procedures have been used. One consists of anal dilation and excision of the fibrotic margins of the ulcer, the sentinel pile, and the accompanying papilla at the upper end of the fissure. The hazard in older patients is that excessive dilation may lead to tearing of the sphincter muscle and permanent incontinence.

The second, and more commonly used, method is internal sphincterotomy. A tight band, which is readily palpable at the lower end of the internal sphincter, is divided. Sectioning of this band relieves pain and allows healing. The division must be done on the lateral side of the anus; if it is done posteriorly, permanent incontinence can result. Incontinence after lateral sphincterotomy is uncommon. The procedure is relatively simple and can be accomplished under local anesthesia. There are 2 variants; in 1, an incision is made over the internal sphincter through the mucous membrane, and the muscle band is cut under direct vision; in the other, a scalpel is inserted from below and the band is cut beneath the intact mucosa.

PERIANAL AND ISCHIORECTAL ABSCESSES

Localized collections of pus in cavities due to infections, followed by the disintegration of tissues. Perianal abscesses, the more common, are located close to the anus and are relatively superficial. Ischiorectal abscesses are deep and located at a higher level.

Perianal abscesses usually begin from inflammation of glands located between the sphincters at the dentate line or from inflammation in the crypts at the same level. Pus tends to track both into the lower rectum just above the anal canal and externally, forming a tender swelling that usually is posterior to the midline of the anus but may be anywhere within 1 to several centimeters from the anal verge. **Ischiorectal abscesses** are more difficult to diagnose, usually are larger, and are accompanied by marked systemic symptoms (eg, severe pain and fever). They usually arise from a break in continuity between the extraperitoneal rectum and the fatty tissue in the fossa; however, the source of infection may lie within the peritoneal cavity. Diverticulitis is the most likely cause in older patients.

The cardinal symptom is pain, which, in itself, warrants drainage. If surgery is delayed, signs of sepsis (eg, chills and fever), in addition to local swelling, induration, and tenderness, follow. Spontaneous rupture may occur if the abscess is superficial but should not be expected or awaited. Antibiotics are given but cannot replace drainage. Both aerobic and anaerobic organisms similar to those found in feces can be cultured from the pus. Delayed drainage may lead to life-endangering clostridial infections.

Since nearly all abscesses originate from a break in the continuity of the rectal mucous membrane, a persistent fistula is common after simple incision and drainage. Consequently, a fistula should be sought at the time of the original operation. However, if one is not readily found, it is better to await further developments than to damage the anorectal mucosa and sphincter.

ANAL FISTULA
(Fistula in Ano)

A sinus tract between the rectum and the skin. Fistulas form for several reasons. The most common follow inflammation in rectal crypts or glands, progressing to perirectal abscesses that track internally into the rectum and externally to the skin. Other diseases (eg, Crohn's disease, tuberculosis, and lymphogranuloma) may involve the rectum and lead to fistulas. Intraperitoneal lesions (eg, diverticulitis or Crohn's disease of the small intestine or colon) may cause fistulas that track into the perineum. Trauma, including iatrogenic injuries, childbirth, and cancer can produce fistulas that track into the vagina. Because of these numerous possibilities, microscopic examination of excised tissue is imperative.

Usually, an anal fistula opens near the anus. If the external opening is adjacent to the posterior half of the anus, the tract nearly always runs into the rectum exactly in the posterior midline. On the other hand, if the external opening is adjacent to the anterior half of the anus, the tract runs in a radial direction into the rectum. During initial examination, it may be possible to probe the entire tract, but usually it is difficult to determine the site of the internal opening until the time of surgery.

Most fistulas connect with the rectum just above the anal canal, so that exposing the tract sacrifices very little of the sphincter; this simple procedure is curative. However, if the internal opening is high, the use of a seton is advised to avoid potential damage to the sphincter and resultant incontinence. The seton (either a silk suture or a rubber band) is passed through the tract into the rectum and tied. It gradually cuts through the tissues and leads to fibrosis and fixation, thus avoiding incontinence.

PROLAPSE AND PROCIDENTIA

Protrusion of a portion of the rectum through the anus. **Mucosal prolapse** involves only the mucosa; all other layers of the rectum remain in place. **Complete prolapse** denotes protrusion of all layers. In the most severe form, called **procidentia,** several inches of rectum may pass through the anus, and the pouch of Douglas descends to the level of the anal canal, which remains in place.

Prolapse is common in elderly persons. Women are affected more often than men. The underlying defect is a long and lax sigmoidorectal mesentery; therefore, the rectum is not fixed in the pelvis in its normal position. Unless surgical repair is performed early, continued dilation of the anal sphincters leads to incontinence; the weakened muscular ring often remains incompetent despite later attempts at repair.

Symptoms include protrusion of either mucous membrane or several inches of rectum. Manual reduction is possible initially, but later, protrusion occurs whenever the patient stands, causing pain and discharge of mucus and blood from the inflamed mucosa. Physical examination should include visualization and palpation of the protrusion when the patient is standing or squatting or immediately after a bowel movement, to determine the degree of prolapse. **Mucosal prolapse** is treated surgically by excision of the redundant tissue, similar to standard hemorrhoidectomy.

When prolapse is complete, conservative therapy—avoidance of straining at stool, lifting, and excessive standing; manual reduction whenever necessary—gives temporary help. Attempts can be made to maintain the normal anatomy by strapping the buttocks. Ultimately, surgery is necessary and should not be delayed.

Numerous operations have been devised, but surgeons do not agree on which procedure is optimal. Of the various technics, the best in a good low-risk patient is a transabdominal resection of the redundant colon and rectum together with the corresponding mesentery. After a low anastomosis, the rectum is anchored in the pelvis in its normal position. Resection of excess bowel and a coloanal anastomosis are also possible through a perineal approach, which is less taxing on the patient. Another technic is to anchor the rectum by means of a plastic sling, which also requires an abdominal approach; however, this method makes subsequent sigmoidoscopy or colonoscopy difficult or impossible. The Thiersch procedure, in which a wire loop is passed about the upper end of the anal canal and tightened appropriately, is the simplest operation but has been abandoned. The problems include intestinal obstruction if the wire is tied too tightly, and recurrence due to breakage of the wire.

Postoperative fecal incontinence is common after repair, particularly if it existed beforehand. Procedures in which the sphincters are tightened have been helpful in some cases.

CANCER
(See also Ch. 52)

Cancer may develop in the perianal skin, the anal canal, or the lower rectum. Typically, these are squamous cell tumors except in the rectum, where adenocarcinoma predominates. However, some skin lesions are basal cell carcinoma, and some neoplasms in the low rectum are of squamous cell origin. The term **cloacogenic cancer** refers to the diverse group of epidermoid anal cancers that at times show basal cell or transitional cell histology. Treatment includes radiation therapy (3000 rads) and chemotherapy (5-FU and mitomycin C); surgical resection is reserved for large (> 6 cm) or recurrent tumors. This method of treatment appears to be the most satisfactory.

GALLBLADDER AND BILIARY TREE

Diseases of the gallbladder and biliary tree account for approximately $\frac{1}{3}$ of abdominal operations performed in patients > 70 yr of age. Gallstones, cholecystitis, and carcinoma of the gallbladder are the most important diseases encountered. Neoplasms of the gallbladder and biliary tree are discussed in Ch. 52.

GALLSTONES

The presence of calculi in the gallbladder, (cholelithiasis) is extremely common. It has been estimated that 25% of persons > 50 yr of age will develop gallstones, the indication for nearly all 475,000 cholecystectomies done yearly in the USA (1 in every 500 individuals). The incidence of stones rises with age, and they are present at autopsy in about $\frac{1}{3}$ of individuals > 70 yr old.

Diagnosis

The symptoms of gallbladder disease are primarily those of biliary colic. **Colic,** or steady pain, usually is felt in the right subcostal area, but often radiates to the right scapula or the right shoulder and, in some instances, is similar to angina. At times, the pain may be felt anywhere in the abdomen. Vomiting may occur but is not repetitive. There usually is slight tenderness in the right upper quadrant. Epigastric distention, gas, and vague dyspepsia occur in so many persons that these findings cannot be considered specific for gallbladder disease.

Acute cholecystitis, a complication of cholelithiasis, is characterized by increased local tenderness, fever, and leukocytosis. The gallbladder frequently is palpable. **Migration of a stone into the common duct** can lead to jaundice, chills and fever, and gallstone pancreatitis. **Pancreatitis** is accompanied by more diffuse epigastric tenderness and elevated serum amylase levels.

The best objective evidence is furnished by ultrasound **(US)** examination. When stones are present in the gallbladder, they are visualized in > 95% of cases, and if there is common duct obstruction, the intrahepatic ducts are distended. However, the distal common duct cannot be seen well by US, and CT scan is better for the diagnosis of pancreatic lesions. Transhepatic cholangiography **(THC)** and endoscopic retrograde cholangiopancreatography **(ERCP)** are valuable when common duct involvement is suspected.

Treatment

Current surgical options include cholecystectomy as the first choice, unless the patient decides to live with the stones. Other methods, eg, stone dissolution by chenodeoxycholic acid or destruction by lithotripsy, are successful in some cases but may require continued medication; long-term results of lithotripsy are not yet available. Cholecystectomy combined with common duct exploration is the preferred operation for common duct stones. Endoscopic papillotomy and basket removal of an obstructing stone from the common duct may be advisable in very ill patients or if the gallbladder already has been removed.

However, complications demand consideration of modification of treatment. If the gallbladder is acutely inflamed, **antibiotics** are given for a longer period; surgery should be performed within 2 or 3 days of the onset of acute cholecystitis. Diabetic patients should be brought under control and surgery performed with little delay because the danger of perforation is high. In some instances, the pathologic changes at the base of the gallbladder are so great that the surgeon should perform a cholecystostomy, leaving the elective cholecystectomy for later. The common duct should be explored if the patient has had chills and fever suggestive of cholangitis, if there are small stones in the gallbladder, if the patient is jaundiced, or if there is evidence of pancreatitis.

Many people have asymptomatic gallstones, and the indication for prophylactic surgery is controversial. Surgeons are inclined to advise cholecystectomy for several reasons: The mortality associated with elective operations is about $1/10$ that of emergency procedures, severe complications (common duct stones and pancreatitis) are avoided, and cancer of the gallbladder is prevented. Cholecystectomy performed electively in patients who travel extensively precludes the possible need for an emergency operation far from home.

One study has shown that asymptomatic gallstones lead to biliary colic in $1/3$ of patients within 2 yr. The mortality from elective cholecystectomy in patients < 70 yr old is < 1%. Cancer of the gallbladder is associated with gallstones in 75% of cases and is an incidental finding in about 1 of every 100 cholecystectomies. These are strong arguments for cholecystectomy in patients < 70 yr old who are otherwise healthy. However, above that age the mortality associated with elective cholecystectomy has been estimated at 5%, and many other considerations are important. Thus, surgery for asymptomatic gallstones in older patients rarely is advised.

If an initial attack of biliary colic occurs, a second episode is probable within 2 yr in $2/3$ of patients. The argument for cholecystectomy therefore becomes more compelling. However, one should try to confirm the diagnosis and rule out symptoms from other diseases (eg, coronary insufficiency), especially in elderly patients. In equivocal cases, it is best to await at least 1 more attack before advising surgery. Currently, it is usual for patients to have had several attacks before surgery is advised.

Specific Syndromes

Acute cholangitis: This usually is due to a stone impacted in the ampulla of Vater but may be secondary to cancer of the pancreas. Other, rare, causes include ascending infection after sphincterotomy of Oddi's sphincter or infection secondary to stricture from a previous choledochoduodenostomy or choledochojejunostomy. In the Far East, Oriental cholangitis is due either to ascending infection from the intestinal tract or to parasites.

Treatment varies, depending on the condition of the patient. Patients in septic shock on admission must be treated vigorously with antibiotics prior to surgery. We prefer gentamicin 1 to 1.5 mg/kg IV q 8 h and clindamycin 600 mg IV q 6 h, although, in the future, third generation cephalosporins may replace this preference. Fluid balance must be restored. Emergency operations that precede stabilization are associated with a high mortality.

Alternatively, **endoscopic sphincterotomy** has been valuable in treating Oriental cholangitis and also has been used widely in the USA and in Europe for stones impacted in the distal common duct. A skilled endoscopist is essential because of the hazards of perforation, bleeding, and infection.

Gallstone pancreatitis: Patients with this disease present as do those with acute cholecystitis, except that the pain is more likely to be epigastric and is associated with elevated serum amylase levels and often with increased bilirubin and alkaline phosphatase. Initial treatment is conservative, with the patient taking nothing by mouth and receiving IV alimentation. Pain typically subsides rapidly, and cholecystectomy is performed 5 to 7 days after admission.

Acalculous cholecystitis: This condition tends to occur in patients in intensive care units or in those who have poor oral intake (eg, because of total IV alimentation). Symptoms are minimal. Unexplained fever and vague abdominal distress warrant US examination of the gallbladder. This may show edema of the gallbladder wall and increasing distention on successive examinations. Either cholecystectomy or cholecystostomy is the usual procedure. Percutaneous catheter drainage of the gallbladder has been used, but the frequency of concomitant gangrene makes this procedure somewhat questionable.

Retained stones in the common duct: These are common, particularly if multiple hepatic duct stones were found at the initial exploration. The surgeon must prepare for this possibility in questionable cases by leaving a large T-tube (No. 14 French) to drain the common duct. The radiologist can extract the stones at a later date. As mentioned above, endoscopic removal also is feasible.

Fistulas: These form between the gallbladder and the intestine, allowing gallstones to migrate and cause intestinal obstruction. Patients usually present with signs of distal small-bowel obstruction and often with tenderness over the gallbladder. Abdominal x-ray may show the stone and usually demonstrates gas in the biliary tree. The proper surgical procedure is removal of the stones (if one is faceted, others are present) and cholecystectomy. The latter may be deferred if the patient is very ill.

Iatrogenic stricture of the common duct: A major complication of cholecystectomy is damage to the common bile duct. Usually, the problem is manifested very early by protracted biliary drainage; diagnosis is made by fistulogram. Repair is by a Roux-en-Y anastomosis of the upper duct to the jejunum. A stricture may form at the anastomosis and cause symptoms many years later. Intermittent attacks of pain, fever, and jaundice suggest the diagnosis, which then can be confirmed by transhepatic cholangiography. Operative repair is necessary. Balloon dilation through a transhepatic catheter has been attempted by radiologists, but the stricture usually is too tight to yield a good result.

Polyps of the gallbladder: These usually are small and filiform. They have no malignant potential. Many defects shown on ultrasound simulate polyps but actually are small stones.

Jaundice: (See also NEOPLASMS OF EXTRAHEPATIC BILE DUCTS in Ch. 52.) The differential diagnosis of jaundice is extensive, and many diagnostic methods are available. The physician's first task is to determine whether jaundice is obstructive. The history often is helpful, and the physical examination can give important information. A symmetrically enlarged liver in an alcoholic usually is due to cirrhosis, and in a temperate, elderly person, to metastatic cancer involving the liver. A palpable gallbladder in jaundiced patients usually signifies cancer of the pancreas. Obstructive jaundice is manifested clinically by bile in the urine and acholic stools; in jaundice due to hepatitis, the stools are brown and there is little or no bile in the urine. Serum bilirubin and alkaline phosphatase values document the degree of jaundice, while measurements of such enzymes as AST (SGOT) and LDH confirm the presence or absence of intrinsic liver disease.

When more sophisticated tests are needed, noninvasive procedures should precede. Ultrasonography is valuable in determining the presence or absence of gallstones and the size of the intrahepatic and common bile ducts. If necessary, endoscopy follows, providing direct visualization of the lumen of the stomach and duodenum. ERCP usually can be done safely and, if required, transhepatic cholangiography **(THC)** can follow. If cancer of the pancreas is suspected, fine-needle percutaneous biopsy is positive in nearly 80% of cases.

Both ERCP and THC carry definite hazards of perforation, infection, and hemorrhage. Furthermore, in many instances, it is impossible to establish the differential diagnosis without exploratory laparotomy. The value of radioisotope scans using dyes (HIDA, etc) that are excreted with the bile is somewhat controversial. If the patient has low-grade jaundice and the dye passes through the common duct into the duodenum, obstructive jaundice is unlikely. In our opinion, such scans do not reliably detect acute cholecystitis, although some radiologists believe that inability to visualize the gallbladder after giving the dye is a presumptive sign of a blocked cystic duct, and if associated with local tenderness, of acute cholecystitis.

DISORDERS OF THE LIVER

In the geriatric population, the most common hepatic lesion demanding surgical attention is metastatic cancer. (Cirrhosis and its associated complications are more frequent in younger age groups.) Hepatic surgery is not well tolerated in older patients, so heroic measures that carry a high mortality but possibly could enable long-term survival are not attempted frequently. Hepatic neoplasms are discussed in Ch. 52.

Cysts

These may be congenital or acquired. **Congenital cysts** often are multiple and associated with polycystic disease of the kidney and pancreas. Usually, they are of no significance and if found at operation, can merely be unroofed and left in place. Very rarely, a cyst enlarges during periodic follow-up because it is a cystadenocarcinoma; excision is necessary.

Hydatid cysts, the single important acquired type, are common in many parts of the world. Since they develop slowly, symptoms (eg, epigastric pain, liver enlargement, jaundice, and anaphylactic reactions) may not be noted for many years. These cysts may be huge and are diagnosed by CT scan or US. Aspiration must be *avoided.* Treatment is excision of the entire cyst; care must be taken to avoid spilling daughter cysts or scoleces into the abdomen.

Abscesses

Pyogenic and amebic **abscesses** must be differentiated, since drainage is necessary for the former, and drug therapy (eg, metronidazole), for the latter. **Pyogenic abscesses** arise from the biliary tree in approximately 40% of cases; because of the widespread use of antibiotics, pylephlebitis and secondary abscesses arising from appendicitis are rare. Diverticulitis and sepsis following hemorrhoidal banding are other known causes. Aerobic and anaerobic gram-negative bacteria predominate. Symptoms include upper abdominal pain, chills and fever, and in many cases, right upper quadrant tenderness and mild jaundice.

Diagnosis of hepatic abscess is usually made by CT scan, although both US and radionuclide scan may also be helpful. In nearly half the cases, there are multiple abscesses. Aspiration is helpful to establish the etiology.

Treatment of pyogenic abscess is vigorous antibiotic therapy and drainage (at times, using a percutaneous catheter). The cause should be identified and, if possible, also treated. For example, cholangitis is a frequent finding and requires transperitoneal exploration of the biliary tree, cholecystectomy, and T-tube drainage of the common duct.

Amebic abscesses nearly always respond to metronidazole. Percutaneous aspiration may be required for diagnosis in a few cases. Rupture of the abscess into the peritoneal cavity requires surgery. A few surgeons recommend much greater use of drainage than is customary in the USA today.

DISORDERS OF THE PANCREAS

In older patients, the major disorders of the pancreas are injuries from blunt trauma, gallstone pancreatitis, and cancer.

TRAUMATIC INJURIES

No specific problems exist regarding the diagnosis and treatment of penetrating wounds. However, blunt trauma causes problems, because the diagnosis of pancreatic injury is often difficult and the treatment controversial.

Diagnosis: The most common cause of blunt trauma is a steering-wheel injury. At first, the patient may be asymptomatic, but within a few hours epigastric pain and tenderness supervene. Hyperamylasemia is noted in > 90% of cases. CT scans identify most transections of the gland. Since retroperitoneal rupture of the duodenum often accompanies pancreatic injuries, a diatrizoate meglumine swallow is desirable prior to operation. ERCP also is advisable to identify or rule out injury of the pancreatic duct. Other tests (eg, US and peritoneal lavage) have not proved helpful.

Treatment: Operation is indicated for all suspected pancreatic injuries. The procedure depends on the pathologic changes. Contusions without evidence of ductal or duodenal injury, or minor disruptions, are drained. If the gland has been completely divided or there is disruption of the duct, the portion of the gland distal to the injury is resected. Serious injuries involving the head of the pancreas *and* the duodenum may require pancreatoduodenectomy, or temporary defunctioning of the duodenum as a passage for gastric secretions by closing the pylorus with a temporary suture and emptying the stomach by a gastroenterostomy.

Postoperative complications include abscesses, pancreatic or duodenal fistulas, persistent pancreatitis, hemorrhage, and pseudocyst formation.

PANCREATITIS

Acute Pancreatitis

The major causes are alcohol, gallstones, and postoperative inflammation. The incidence varies with the circumstances and age of the patient. In metropolitan areas, patients tend to be younger, and alcoholism is the most common etiology. In rural areas and in geriatric patients, gallstones predominate. A negative prognostic sign is age > 55 yr.

Diagnosis is based on the sudden onset of severe epigastric pain that may radiate to the back or later involve the whole abdomen. Vomiting and epigastric tenderness follow. In severe cases, shock, mild jaundice, and respiratory distress may then develop. Serum amylase levels are elevated early on in 95% of cases but may fall thereafter. Serum calcium levels also may fall. Leukocytosis is noted and, if there is bleeding, Hct is lowered. Hyperglycemia and hypocalcemia are common in severe cases.

Abdominal x-ray often shows a sentinel loop of gas-filled jejunum in the left upper quadrant. US is particularly valuable in the detection of gallstones but cannot be depended upon in evaluation of the pancreas. For this purpose, CT scan is by far the best method; serial examinations should be performed if the patient fails to improve rapidly.

Other diseases must be excluded. **Perforated peptic ulcer** may be excluded by an upper GI series using a diatrizoate meglumine swallow rather than barium, but **strangulating intestinal obstruction** or **ischemic bowel disease** may be more difficult to diagnose. At times, laparotomy is necessary. **Gallstone pancreatitis** must also be excluded, since patients with this disease require surgery a few days later, if they follow the usual course, in which the severe pain subsides rapidly. There are no chemical tests that can determine the cause of pancreatitis reliably, but CT scan shows a comparatively normal gland in gallstone pancreatitis compared with severe alcoholic pancreatitis. **Vascular disease** (mesenteric thrombosis or embolism) can lead rapidly to gangrene of the bowel; it mimics acute pancreatitis with pain and leaking toxins.

Treatment is supportive. Nasogastric suction, IV alimentation, and fluid replacement are essential. Antibiotics are not used in the early stages. In Europe, there has been much interest in immediate total pancreatectomy, but this procedure is not used in the USA. Early operation is recommended for gallstone pancreatitis. ERCP and endoscopic papillotomy are not used by most surgeons because of the risk of exacerbating the pancreatitis.

Following supportive therapy, the course varies greatly. Many patients, including nearly all those with gallstone pancreatitis, improve rapidly. Those whose condition worsens require ongoing reevaluations with CT scan and surgical treatment of the many serious complications that can follow.

Chronic Pancreatitis

Cases of acute pancreatitis that continue to smolder, or that subside entirely and then recur, are included here. The most severe form is pancreatolithiasis; patients have such severe persistent pain that many become addicted to narcotic analgesics. Loss of weight, diarrhea due to loss of enzymes, and diabetes due to fibrosis of the islets of Langerhans are late complications. A few patients have hyperparathyroidism as well. Appropriate studies include liver function tests—enzymes (AST, SGOT and LDH), alkaline phosphatase, and serum bilirubin—amylase, glucose, calcium, and phosphates.

Several tests have been used to establish the pain as pancreatic. The Nardi test involves subcutaneous injection of morphine and neostigmine; the development of typical pain, together with elevation of serum amylase and lipase concentrations, suggests obstruction at Oddi's sphincter. US observation of dilation of the duct of Wirsung after subcutaneous injection of secretin also suggests sphincter abnormality. There is no consensus concerning the value of these tests. When ERCP shows a large, uniformly dilated duct, obstruction of the ampulla is probable and anastomosis of a Roux-en-Y loop of jejunum to the pancreas (pancreaticojejunostomy) usually is followed by good results.

Treatment: In addition to pancreatojejunostomy, various extirpative procedures may be required. These include distal pancreatectomy when the disease is in the tail of the gland, Whipple's procedure when only the head is involved, or total pancreatectomy in extreme cases of pancreatolithiasis. Splanchnic nerve section for relief of pain has had only sporadic success. In all cases, the patient must abstain from alcohol.

ENDOCRINE TUMORS OF THE PANCREAS

These are not common in the elderly. Generally, they are diagnosed by clinical symptoms and often by specific radioimmunoassays. Localization of the tumor can be aided by CT scan, portal venous sampling, and intraoperative US. (The more common exocrine tumors of the pancreas are discussed in Ch. 52.)

Five important types of endocrine tumors of the pancreas have been described:

1. Insulinomas may be single or multiple. They produce insulin and are identified by episodes of hypoglycemia, which may progress to coma in severe cases. Insulinomas rarely are malignant. Removal of all tumor tissue results in complete cure.

2. Gastrinomas produce the Zollinger-Ellison syndrome, an extremely virulent ulcer diathesis with excessive gastric secretion and diarrhea. They tend to occur near the ampulla of Vater outside the pancreas and are malignant in about 90% of cases. If there are no metastases, complete excision of the tumor is curative. In the presence of metastases, various therapeutic modalities have been used, including large doses of H_2-receptor blockers and gastric surgery to reduce acid secretion. Currently, total gastrectomy is again winning favor.

3. Glucagonomas secrete glucagon and have a high malignant potential. They lead to mild diabetes and a severe dermatitis that involves portions of the lower $1/2$ of the body. Although complete removal may not be possible, the tumor is resected insofar as possible. Streptozocin is very helpful for the treatment of residual disease.

4. Vipomas produce *v*asoactive *i*ntestinal *p*olypeptide, pancreatic polypeptide, and perhaps other hormones. The disease also is known as the **WDHA syndrome,** describing the primary characteristics of severe *w*atery *d*iarrhea, *h*ypokalemia, and *a*chlorhydria. Half of the tumors are malignant. As much tumor as possible should be resected. Residual tumor also is treated with streptozocin.

5. Somatostatinomas are rare tumors that secrete somatostatin. Clinical findings include diabetes, steatorrhea, and achlorhydria.

Cysts of several types occur in the pancreas. **Congenital cysts** can be found in some cases of polycystic disease. The gland may contain many small cysts from which cystadenocarcinoma can develop. Excision or resection of a portion of the pancreas may be necessary. However, these are rare.

Pseudocysts are formed by extravasation of pancreatic secretions into the lesser peritoneal sac. Characteristically, they follow trauma. The patient complains of left upper quadrant pain and tenderness. A palpable mass may be present. Diagnosis may be made by the CT scan, or if the cyst is large, by displacement of the stomach or other viscera shown on an upper GI series. In the early stages, there is only a weak wall about the collection of fluid; generally, surgical intervention is deferred. If an operation is necessary, drainage is all that can be done. Later, as the surrounding wall thickens, or matures, the pseudocyst can be drained internally by anastomosis to the stomach or intestine.

Cysts frequently form in the pancreas or pseudocysts develop in adjacent tissue of patients with alcoholic pancreatitis. Many of these cysts resolve spontaneously, as shown by serial CT scans. If there is no resolution after 6 wk, surgical intervention is indicated. Depending on its location, the cyst is anastomosed to the stomach, the jejunum, or the duodenum.

DISORDERS OF THE SPLEEN

Surgery is limited in the treatment of splenic disorders. Operative measures include splenectomy, repair of injuries by methods other than splenectomy, and drainage of abscesses.

The main indications for **splenectomy** are trauma (either blunt, penetrating, or iatrogenic), disease of adjacent organs (eg, stomach, pancreas, or colon), idiopathic thrombocytopenic purpura, and advanced splenomegaly. Rare indications in the elderly include splenectomy as a requirement of splenorenal shunt for portal hypertension, hypersplenism, and splenic artery aneurysms, or as a staging procedure for Hodgkin's disease.

Trauma

Blunt and penetrating trauma of the spleen frequently requires splenectomy. Furthermore, iatrogenic damage commonly results from vagotomy or operations involving the stomach, tail of the pancreas, or the colon.

The surgeon must decide whether injury is severe enough to warrant splenectomy or whether simple suturing or hemostasis is possible. Although the matter is controversial, seveal facts are clear. Splenectomy is better tolerated by older than younger patients, with a much lower incidence of later fatal sepsis. Continued bleeding is tolerated more poorly by older than younger patients. For these reasons, unless hemostasis is absolute in an elderly patient, splenectomy should be performed.

Idiopathic Thrombocytopenic Purpura (ITP)

In a recent series of > 200 splenectomies for this disease, 12% of patients were > 70 yr of age. ITP usually is treated with corticosteroids, but response to them, or to splenectomy, insofar as correction of the thrombocytopenia, is poorer in older than in younger patients. In this series, splenectomy alone cured only about ½ the older patients; the others required continued corticosteroid therapy.

Massive Splenomegaly

A huge spleen is subject to repeated episodes of minor thromboses, which add to the pain and discomfort of the mass and the pressure on adjacent organs. This can occur, for example, with splenomegaly due to lymphocytic or myelogenous leukemia. In these diseases, splenectomy usually is contraindicated because of high postoperative mortality; patients rarely live for more than a few months after such an operation. However, splenectomy now is urged in some centers for pain relief.

Gaucher's disease is due to the accumulation of glucocerebrosides in the spleen. As the spleen enlarges, hypersplenism (see below) may follow. Some of the largest spleens excised have been removed for Gaucher's disease. After splenectomy, the typical lipid-laden macrophages continue to accumulate in the liver and bone marrow.

Splenectomy for Disease of Adjacent Organs

Surgical treatment of gastric cancer often includes splenectomy because of the frequency of splenic lymph node metastases. Other reasons for splenectomy include cancer of the splenic flexure of the colon, which also may invade the spleen; large cysts of the distal pancreas; and splenic artery aneurysms.

Hypersplenism

Enlargement of the spleen associated with any combination of anemia, leukopenia, or thrombocytopenia. Many diseases, eg, bacterial infections, malaria, kala-azar, and Gaucher's disease, may be associated with hypersplenism. In the USA, portal hypertension and the various lymphomas are the most important.

Abscesses

These may form in the spleen secondary to sepsis. Formerly, diagnosis was difficult and could be established only by splenectomy. Currently, CT scan is helpful in diagnosis. Many abscesses can be drained by radiologists using percutaneous catheters guided by CT scan.

§3. ORGAN SYSTEMS: GENITOURINARY DISORDERS

Contents for HEMATOLOGIC DISORDERS begin on page 643.

---

54.   RENAL SYSTEM

John W. Rowe

A substantial reduction in renal function accompanies normal aging. Function of the senescent kidney, however, ordinarily is sufficient to remove wastes and adequately regulate volume and composition of ECF. Nevertheless, changes in renal function reduce the older individual's capacity to respond to a variety of physiologic and pathologic stresses, with important clinical implications.

EFFECT OF AGING ON RENAL FUNCTION

Renal Anatomy

In the absence of hypertension or marked vascular disease, the senescent kidney maintains its relatively smooth contour. However, advancing age is associated with progressive loss of renal mass, and kidney weight decreases from a normal 250 to 270 gm in young adulthood to 180 to 200 gm in the 8th decade. The loss of renal mass is primarily cortical, with relative sparing of the renal medulla. The total number of identifiable glomeruli decreases with age, roughly in accordance with the decline in renal weight. Aging is associated with a loss of lobulation of the glomerular tuft, thus decreasing the surface area available for filtration. On the other hand, dextran clearance studies indicate no change in glomerular permeability with age.

Several mild microscopic changes occur in the renal tubule with age. Of particular interest is the appearance of diverticula in the distal nephron, reaching a frequency of 3 per tubule by age 90 yr. These diverticula may evolve as the simple retention cysts commonly seen in the elderly.

Histologic studies indicate that normal aging is associated with variable sclerotic changes in the walls of the larger renal vessels. These changes do not encroach on the lumen and are augmented in hypertension. Smaller vessels appear to be spared; only 15% of senescent kidneys from nonhypertensive individuals display arteriolar changes.

X-ray studies in normotensive individuals > 70 yr of age demonstrate an increasing prevalence of abnormalities similar to those seen in younger hypertensives, including abnormal tapering of interlobar arteries, abnormal arcuate arteries, and increased tortuosity of intralobular arteries.

Combined microangiographic and histologic studies have identified 2 distinctive age-related patterns of change in arteriolar-glomerular units. The first pattern consists of hyalinization and collapse of the glomerular tuft and is associated with obliteration of the lumen of the preglomerular arteriole and a resultant loss in blood flow. This type of change is seen primarily in the cortical area. The second pattern, seen primarily in the juxtamedullary area, is characterized by the development of anatomic continuity between the afferent and efferent arterioles during glomerular sclerosis. The endpoint is shunting of blood flow from afferent to efferent arterioles and loss of the glomerulus. Blood flow is maintained to the arteriolae rectae vera, the primary vascular supply of the medulla, which do not decrease in number with age.

Renal Physiology

Renal blood flow progressively decreases from 1200 mL/min in young adulthood to 600 mL/min by age 80 yr. The primary underlying factor is the decreased renovascular bed. However, the reduction in flow is not simply a reflection of decreased renal mass, since flow per gram of tissue falls progressively after the 4th decade. Studies with vasoactive agents indicate that the age-related decline in renal blood flow is due to fixed anatomic changes rather than to reversible vasospasm. There is a highly significant decrease with advancing age in the cortical component of blood flow, with preservation of medullary flow, a finding consistent with histologic studies showing selective loss of cortical vasculature. These vascular changes probably account for the patchy cortical defects commonly seen on renal scans in healthy elderly adults.

Glomerular filtration rate: The major clinically relevant functional defect arising from these histologic and physiologic changes is a progressive decline in the GFR after maturity. **Creatinine clearance** is stable until the middle of the 4th decade, when a linear decrease of about 8 mL/min/1.73 m^2/decade begins.

Longitudinal studies indicate substantial variability in the effect of age on creatinine clearance, with as many as $\frac{1}{3}$ of individuals showing *no* decline in GFR with age. This variability suggests that factors other than aging per se may be responsible for the apparent effect of age on renal function. This view is supported by the finding that increases in BP still within the normotensive range are associated with accelerated, age-related loss of renal function.

The argument that entire nephrons drop out with advancing age is supported by the striking parallel decline with age in GFR and several proximal tubular functions, including maximal excretion of para-amino-hippurate and iodopyracet and maximal absorption of glucose. Additional observations regarding glucose absorption indicate that the renal threshold for glycosuria, which relates inversely to the degree of "splay" in reabsorptive capacity of individual nephrons, increases with age. Thus, in a young diabetic patient, glucose generally spills into the urine at a lower blood glucose level than in an elderly diabetic.

Adjustment of Drug Doses

Although muscle mass, from which creatinine is derived, decreases with age at approximately the same rate as GFR, the decline in GFR is *not* reflected by a concurrent elevation of serum creatinine. Thus, serum creatinine level does not accurately reflect GFR in the elderly. The average healthy 80-yr-old man has a creatinine clearance 32 mL/min less than that of his 30-yr-old counterpart with the same serum creatinine value. Depression of GFR so severe that serum creatinine rises above 1.5 mg/dL is rarely due to normal aging and therefore indicates the presence of renal disease.

In clinical practice, the doses of many drugs excreted primarily by the kidneys are routinely adjusted to compensate for alteration in renal function. Digoxin preparations and aminoglycoside antibiotics are examples. However, these adjustments are usually based on serum creatinine values, with the resultant predictable *overdose* in elderly patients. Ideally, dose adjustments should be based on creatinine clearance, which does not absolutely require 24-h urine collection but can be estimated on a timed urine collection of 8-h duration (eg, overnight). When only data on serum creatinine are available, the influence of age must be considered. This can be accomplished by use of the following formula:

$$\text{Creatinine clearance (mL/min)} = \frac{(140 - \text{age [yr]}) (\text{body wt [kg]})}{(72) (\text{serum creatinine [mg/dL]})}$$

The value is 15% less in women.

RENIN-ANGIOTENSIN-ALDOSTERONE SYSTEM

Basal renin, whether estimated by plasma renin concentration or renin activity, is diminished by 30 to 50% in the elderly despite normal levels of renin substrate. This basal difference between young and old individuals is magnified by maneuvers that augment renin secretion, eg, salt restriction, diuretic administration, and upright posture.

The lowered renin levels are associated with 30 to 50% reductions in plasma concentrations of aldosterone, as well as significant reductions in the secretion and clearance rates of aldosterone. Studies showing that plasma aldosterone and cortisol responses after ACTH stimulation are not impaired with advancing age demonstrate that aldosterone deficiency in the elderly is a function of the coexisting renin deficiency and not secondary to intrinsic adrenal changes.

The impact of normal aging on plasma renin must be considered when assigning hypertensive patients to specific pathophysiologic groups based on renin levels. A hypertensive geriatric patient, or occasionally a patient with modestly elevated systolic BP as normally seen in advancing age, may be categorized as having low-renin hypertension, when actually the renin level is normal for the patient's age.

POTASSIUM BALANCE

Hyperkalemia

The age-related decreases in renin and aldosterone mentioned above contribute to the increased risk for hyperkalemia in the elderly in a variety of clinical settings. Through its action on the distal renal tubule, aldosterone increases Na reabsorption and facilitates the excretion of K. Aldosterone is 1 of the major protective mechanisms in the prevention of hyperkalemia during periods of K challenge. Since GFR (another major determinant of K excretion) is also impaired in older patients, serious elevations of plasma K are likely to develop, especially in the presence of GI bleeding (a major source of K) or when K salts are given IV.

This tendency toward hyperkalemia is enhanced by any clinical setting associated with acidosis, since the senescent kidney is sluggish in its response to acid loading, resulting in prolonged depression of serum pH and concomitant K elevation. Potent antagonists of renal K excretion (eg, spironolactone or triamterene), as well as most nonsteroidal anti-inflammatory drugs (NSAIDs), β-adrenergic blockers, and angiotensin converting enzyme (ACE) inhibitors, which also inhibit K elimination, should be administered *with caution* in the elderly, and the concomitant administration of these agents and K should be *avoided*.

The initial management of hyperkalemia includes discontinuance of K-sparing drugs and any sources of dietary K, as well as prompt optimization of renal function in patients with volume depletion or heart failure. Severe hyperkalemia, manifested by abnormalities in the ECG, including symmetrically peaked T waves and widened QRS complexes, requires prompt treatment with IV Ca salts (calcium chloride or calcium gluconate), which directly antagonize the effect of hyperkalemia on the myocardium and often normalize the ECG. Also indicated are $NaHCO_3$, glucose, and insulin.

Because such emergency treatment is of only temporary benefit in controlling elevated serum K and has no effect on total-body K, efforts toward total-body K depletion should be initiated simultaneously. These include the oral or rectal administration of Na-K exchange resin (sodium polystyrene sulfonate) and IV administration of potent diuretics such as furosemide or ethacrynic acid.

Hypokalemia (see page 642)

RENAL DISEASES

NEPHROTIC SYNDROME

A condition characterized by generalized edema, heavy proteinuria, hypoalbuminemia, and susceptibility to intercurrent infections.

Nephrologists have traditionally taught that age plays an important role in the etiology of nephrotic syndromes (ie, that the likelihood of lipoid nephrosis decreases and that of amyloidosis increases with advancing age). Several reports that include clinical and biopsy data on a large number of elderly nephrotics now indicate that, in general, age has *no* impact on the frequency of any histologic glomerular change. The most common cause of nephrosis in old age is **membranous glomerulonephritis,** and **minimal-change disease** and **amyloidosis** are seen with equal frequency in young and old patients. Clearly, renal biopsy remains a critically important procedure in the evaluation of an elderly patient with nephrotic syndrome.

Age has no influence on the generally excellent response to corticosteroids and immunosuppressants in patients with minimal-change disease. In addition, some elderly patients with membranous disease respond to steroid or cyclophosphamide therapy. In many cases, cyclophosphamide may be the treatment of choice to avoid the steroid-associated exacerbation of common preexisting conditions (eg, glucose intolerance, hypertension, osteoporosis, and cataracts).

ACUTE GLOMERULONEPHRITIS

A disease characterized pathologically by diffuse inflammation in the glomeruli.

Acute glomerulonephritis is receiving increasing recognition as a disease with a clearly age-related presentation and prognosis. In children and young adults, acute glomeronephritis is frequently associated with recent streptococcal infection and, less commonly, with a wide variety of other conditions. Clinical features include hematuria, heavy proteinuria, edema, hypertension, and in many cases, the development of pulmonary congestion. The prognosis is generally good in poststreptococcal disease, with a variable outcome in nonpoststreptococcal cases.

In elderly patients, acute glomerulonephritis is manifestly different. The clinical features are nonspecific, with nausea, malaise, arthralgias, and a striking predilection for pulmonary infiltrates initially, and are believed to represent worsening of a preexisting illness, especially heart failure. Proteinuria is generally moderate. Hypertension or edema, although unusual, indicates a poststreptococcal case and favorable prognosis; otherwise, the prognosis is poor, with crescentic glomerulonephritis associated with focal, segmental, necrotizing, and fibrosing glomerulitis the most frequent histologic finding. The value of treatment with corticosteroids, immunosuppressive agents, anticoagulants, and plasmapheresis remains controversial.

RENAL EMBOLI

Occlusive arterial disease is an important cause of both acute and chronic renal failure in the elderly. Renal arterial emboli occur in any clinical setting associated with peripheral embolization (eg, acute MI, chronic atrial fibrillation, SBE, and aortic surgery or aortography). **The manifestations of renal emboli** in the elderly may vary from an essentially silent event to a full-blown syndrome of severe flank pain and tenderness, hematuria, hypertension, spiking fevers, marked reduction in renal function, and elevation of serum lactic dehydrogenase. Small emboli are very difficult to detect, since renal scans may show focal perfusion defects in many apparently normal elderly patients. Major emboli may be suggested by findings of differential contrast excretion on urography and confirmed by renal scanning and aortography. Surgery is generally not indicated, and anticoagulant therapy may be of major benefit. In many cases in which renal function is discernibly impaired, improvement may occur over a period of several days to weeks.

Renal cholesterol embolization is a specific geriatric syndrome that may occur spontaneously or in association with aortic surgery or angiography in patients with diffuse atherosclerosis. Definitive diagnosis may be difficult, since visualization of cholesterol crystals on renal biopsy is required; a presumptive diagnosis is frequently masked by other possible causes of reduced renal function (eg, hypotension or administration of angiographic contrast material). The clinical course varies, with most patients going on to progressive renal failure. However, some develop only moderate impairment and may regain renal function over time. No specific treatment is available.

RENAL ARTERY THROMBOSIS

Thrombotic occlusive renal artery disease frequently complicates severe aortic and renal arterial atherosclerosis, especially when it occurs with decreased renal blood flow caused by heart failure (**HF**) or volume depletion. Symptoms of renal arterial occlusion may be remarkably absent. In cases in which renal function previously was good, the only manifestation of unilateral thrombosis may be an increase in BUN and creatinine levels and perhaps a modest increase in BP. In patients with preexisting renal impairment and azotemia, renal artery occlusion may precipitate HF, marked hypertension, and the emergence of the uremic syndrome.

Diagnosis: The application of currently available diagnostic tests for detection of renovascular hypertension is determined by the patient's age. The number of false-positive results with either a stimulated plasma renin or saralasin infusion test decreases markedly with age. Similarly, the older the patient, the more likely that a high stimulated renin or positive saralasin infusion result indicates significant renovascular hypertension. Thus, either test is useful in identifying elderly patients for further study, eg, timed IV urography, renal vein renin determinations, and ultimately, angiography.

The patient should be evaluated for a coexisting abdominal aortic aneurysm, which may lead to renal artery occlusion by extension of atheromata or dissection. In angiography, the least amount of contrast material possible should be used to minimize the likelihood of a nephrotoxic reaction; such a reaction, while generally limited to several days of oliguria and mild azotemia, may take the form of severe acute oliguric renal failure.

When technically feasible, surgical revascularization should be considered. Substantial return of renal function can be obtained after prompt revascularization, and in some cases recovery occurs even if surgery is delayed until several months after the vascular occlusion.

ACUTE RENAL FAILURE (ARF)

The clinical conditions associated with rapid, steadily increasing azotemia, with or without oliguria (< 500 mL daily).

Age influences renal disease either by altering the prevalence of specific diseases or by affecting the presentation, course, and response to treatment of conditions seen in both early and late adult life. ARF is seen more frequently in older patients simply because the common inciting events (including hypotension associated with marked volume depletion, major surgery, sepsis, major angiographic procedures, and the injudicious use of nephrotoxic antibiotics) are more common in multi-impaired elderly patients, who are often at increased risk because of pre-existing moderate renal insufficiency.

The management of ARF in the elderly is complex and demanding. The aging kidney retains the capacity to recover from acute ischemic or toxic insults over the course of several weeks. Although typical **acute tubular necrosis** (2 to 10 days of oliguria followed by a diuretic phase preceding recovery of function) is seen in the elderly, **nonoliguric ARF** is being recognized with increasing frequency. In these cases, renal function, reflected by BUN and creatinine levels, is impaired for several days after a brief hypotensive episode associated with surgery, sepsis, overmedication, or volume depletion or after the administration of nephrotoxic radiographic contrast agents. After this brief period of azotemia, renal function gradually returns to its previous level.

Despite the transient loss of renal function, oliguria is not a prominent component of the clinical picture. Since the clinical hallmark of renal failure is generally thought to be a dramatic reduction in urine output, cases of nonoliguric ARF may go unrecognized. This may result in an inadvertent accumulation of drugs excreted predominantly via renal mechanisms during the period of impaired renal function.

The management of elderly patients with full-blown ARF complicated by oliguria is guided by the same general principles used in younger patients. *Most important is the exclusion of urinary obstruction as a cause of the renal failure,* particularly in men with prostatic hypertrophy or carcinoma and in women with gynecologic malignancy.

Treatment

Volume overload precipitating acute pulmonary edema, hypertensive crisis, hyperkalemia, and infection are the major causes of death during ARF.

Either **hemodialysis** or **peritoneal dialysis** is effective, and the complication rate seems to result more from concurrent cardiovascular disease than from age. Dialysis often simplifies management substantially; thus, it is more prudent to initiate dialysis early in a patient with ARF than to wait for an emergency. The immediate indications for emergency dialysis include pulmonary edema unresponsive to diuretics, hyperkalemia, uremic pericarditis, seizures, and uncontrolled bleeding due to uremia.

Femoral vein catheterization for dialysis is a major advance in the management of elderly patients with ARF. These catheters are easily placed, may be left in situ for several days to a week with a very low incidence of infection or thrombosis, and circumvent the need for implantation of A-V shunts for dialysis.

Consideration of **water and sodium balance** is also necessary. The usual patient with ARF loses about 1 lb of body mass/day because of catabolism. Attempts to keep body weight constant result in gradual expansion of ECF volume and a consequent increase in BP with a risk of precipitating cardiac failure. Similarly, overzealous fluid restriction impairs the patient's general condition and CNS function and may delay the recovery of renal function. In general, the administration of approximately 600 mL fluid/day, in addition to insensible losses, provides adequate fluid balance.

K balance is crucial; hyperkalemia must be avoided if possible and treated promptly if present. **Acidosis** progresses with the duration and degree of renal failure, and sodium bicarbonate should be administered to maintain circulating HCO_3^- levels in the range of 15 to 20 mEq/L. Because administration of sodium bicarbonate may expand ECF volume, patients should be observed for evidence of heart failure.

Infection is a common and often lethal complication of ARF. Urinary infection secondary to bladder catheterization is particularly common. Little is gained from placing a urinary catheter in an oliguric patient in whom volume status and BUN, creatinine, and K levels are better guides to treatment than the urinary output. Infection of IV lines is also common; these should be monitored scrupulously and discontinued as soon as possible.

Additional routine measures include the administration of oral phosphate-binding agents to minimize the elevation of serum P associated with ARF and the provision of a limited-protein diet to blunt the rise in BUN. Particular attention should be paid to the alteration in dose interval of drugs excreted via the kidney and recognition of the enhanced sensitivity of elderly uremic patients to psychotropic drugs (eg, hypnotics and major tranquilizers).

CHRONIC RENAL FAILURE (CRF)

The clinical condition resulting from a multitude of pathologic processes that lead to derangement and insufficiency of renal excretory and regulatory function.

Many forms of CRF are seen more commonly late in life, because renal disease is secondary to other age-dependent illnesses, eg, prostatic hypertrophy or cancer leading to hydronephrosis, renovascular hypertension or renal failure secondary to atherosclerosis, multiple myeloma, drug-related causes of renal insufficiency, and perhaps most common, prerenal azotemia from heart failure or volume depletion.

Diagnosis

While general principles of management of renal failure are similar in young and old adults, the geriatric patient with chronic renal insufficiency requires several special considerations. One factor that often delays recognition of CRF in the elderly is its presentation as decompensation of a previously impaired organ system before the emergence of specific symptoms of uremia. Examples include worsening of preexisting heart failure due to inability to excrete Na and water, GI bleeding in the presence of previous GI malignancy or ulcer, and mental confusion in a borderline demented patient who becomes increasingly azotemic.

Once the presence of CRF is established, the definitive cause should be identified. Generally, renal failure in the elderly is due to chronic glomerulonephritis, hypertensive and atherosclerotic vascular disease, diabetes, or in some cases, late-presenting polycystic kidney disease. The most important diagnostic consideration is strict exclusion of potentially reversible causes, such as urinary tract obstruction, particularly in men with symptoms of prostatism; renal arterial occlusion that may be reparable; hypercalcemia; and the administration of nephrotoxic agents.

Treatment

If no reversible cause is identified, the patient should be followed closely so the rate of renal function loss can be accurately assessed. In consideration of the renal failure, appropriate adjustments should be made in the doses and dosing schedules of all drugs, especially digoxin. Hypertension should be controlled. As serum phosphate concentration rises, phosphate-binding antacids should be given with meals to suppress PTH. As serum phosphate falls in response to treatment, serum Ca generally rises toward the normal range. Hypocalcemia that persists after phosphate levels return to normal should be treated with preparations of vitamin D or its congeners (vitamin D_1 tablets 50,000 u. bid or tid; dihydrotachysterol 0.2 to 0.4 mg bid; 1,25-dihydroxyvitamin D_3 0.25 to 0.5 μg bid) to increase intestinal Ca absorption.

Anemia associated with CRF often requires more aggressive management in elderly patients because of coexisting cardiac disease. RBC indexes are not a reliable estimate of iron deficiency in uremia. Iron deficiency should be excluded by evaluation of serum iron and ferritin, and oral or parenteral iron supplements should be administered, if indicated. Non-iron deficiency anemia associated with CRF has been managed with monthly injections of androgens (eg, nandrolone decanoate 200 mg IM). Preparations of erythropoietins developed through genetic engineering are now available and promise to be effective in controlling anemia of CRF.

Dietary management of elderly patients with CRF is often *overdone,* compounding the nutritional impact of the disease. Protein and salt restriction is often needed in young individuals to suppress the volume expansion and BUN elevations, but many elderly patients normally ingest only 60 to 70 gm of protein and 4 to 5 gm of salt daily; thus, strict limitation of these nutrients is often unnecessary. Similarly, hyperkalemia should be avoided and dietary K intake controlled, but the reductions required in the elderly are often moderate. The best approach to these modifications is individual alteration of the diet to meet the needs of the patient.

Pruritus is a major problem in elderly uremic patients, especially in the presence of coexisting xerosis. In addition to skin moisturizers, ultraviolet treatments are effective and safe. Administration of antipruritic agents (eg, antihistamines and ataractics) is rarely helpful, since they act primarily by causing sedation and may produce adverse nervous system effects.

Dialysis: Chronic maintenance dialysis (generally, hemodialysis but occasionally chronic ambulatory peritoneal dialysis) remains the mainstay of treatment in elderly uremic patients. They often do very well on dialysis, with the frequency of complications seemingly related to the coexisting extrarenal diseases more than to age itself. Psychologically, elderly patients often are better able to adapt to chronic dialysis than are their younger counterparts. Once it is clear that a patient will need dialysis in the near future, an A-V fistula should be created to provide access for hemodialysis, since such fistulas often mature slowly in older individuals. Currently, renal transplantation is generally *not* considered in individuals > 60 yr of age.

---

55. DISORDERS OF THE LOWER GENITOURINARY TRACT: BLADDER, PROSTATE, AND TESTICLES

John H. Wasson and *Reginald C. Bruskewitz*

Symptoms of GU tract dysfunction are common in the elderly. Many older persons experience nocturia and frequency, caused by large urine volumes resulting from insufficient urinary concentrating ability as well as age-related changes in neuromuscular coordination of the bladder (described in Ch. 10). However, aging alone is an *insufficient* explanation for GU tract dysfunction unless the conditions listed in TABLE 55–1 have been considered.

DRUG-RELATED URINARY SYMPTOMS

Nocturia is reported in 2/3 of women and men > 65 yr of age who are not taking drugs; for those who take drugs or have more than 3 chronic diseases, the incidence is > 80%. Since > 20% of elderly persons complain of having trouble sleeping "often" or "always," a goal of therapy is to minimize the influence of nocturia on sleep.

Many older patients suffer from losses in bladder distensibility and renal concentrating ability. Therefore, if chronic diuretic therapy is required for hypertension or congestive heart failure **(CHF)**, 2 options should be considered: (1) For hypertension control, a very-low-dose diuretic (12.5 or 25 mg hydrochlorothiazide) in the morning is sufficient. (2) For treatment of CHF, a loop diuretic followed by 1 h of recumbency in the morning often obviates the need for a bid dose. Excessive fluid intake or the use of "natural" diuretics (alcohol and caffeine) before bedtime should be eliminated whenever nocturia is a significant problem.

Relaxation of the internal urinary sphincter, which is innervated in part by α-adrenergic fibers, is important in men with bladder outlet obstruction. Excessive sympathetic (α-adrenergic) nervous system activity from sympathomimetics (eg, cold pills) can imbalance the micturition reflex to the detriment of the patient.

The cholinergic system is needed for detrusor contraction. Thus, anticholinergics, psychotropics, antidepressants, antihistamines, and certain antiarrhythmics should be avoided when possible to prevent weakening the contraction.

The drugs listed in TABLE 55–2 have 2 properties in common: (1) They may weaken the detrusor, inhibit internal sphincter relaxation, or both. (2) They are often effective in older patients at a reduced dose (particularly antidepressants and psychotropics) or they may be unnecessary (particularly antiarrhythmics, antihistamines, or anticholinergics).

URINARY TRACT INFECTION/PROSTATITIS

The diagnosis and treatment of UTI are described in Ch. 56. When urinary symptom exacerbation coincides with prostatic pyuria and bacteriuria, a trial of antibiotics is indicated. Chronic infection suggests significant urinary retention, calculi, or chronic bacterial prostatitis in men. Although reduction of retained urine and removal of stones increase the effectiveness of antibiotic therapy, chronic asymptomatic bacteriuria in the elderly often does not require any therapy.

TABLE 55–1. SYMPTOMS AND CAUSES OF GENITOURINARY TRACT DYSFUNCTION IN MEN

Symptom Group	Common Causes	Less Common Causes
Lower GU tract irritative symptoms Dysuria: Painful urination Frequency: Urinating more than 6 times/day Urgency: Inability to delay urination once the sensation to void is felt Nocturia: Interrupting sleep in order to urinate	**If dysuria present:** Cystitis, prostatitis **If dysuria absent:** Diuretic therapy; heart failure; outlet obstruction from prostatic hypertrophy or urethral stricture; detrusor instability; alcohol, coffee, or excessive fluids before bedtime	Cancer of bladder or prostate, prostatism Cancer of bladder or prostate, neurogenic bladder, uncontrolled diabetes, renal insufficiency, hypercalcemia, extrinsic bladder compression
Lower GU tract obstructive symptoms Hesitancy, intermittency, postvoiding dribbling, retention, and decrease in force and caliber of the urinary stream	Diuretic therapy, prostatic hypertrophy, urethral stricture	Bladder stone, prostatic cancer
Scrotal mass	Epididymitis, varicocele, hydrocele, bowel from hernia	Cancer (lymphoma, spermatocytic seminoma, and seminoma)
Hematuria: Blood, gross or microscopic (> 5 RBC/HPF)	Cystitis, bladder cancer, prostatic hypertrophy, or unknown	Prostatitis, renal disease (cancer or glomerulonephritis), bladder stone, prostatic cancer

TABLE 55–2. DRUGS AFFECTING BLADDER FUNCTION

Classification	Most Problematic	Preferred Alternatives
Anticholinergics	All cause potential problems*	
Psychotropics	Phenothiazines and haloperidol in high doses	Consider short t$_{1/2}$ benzodiazepines
Antidepressants**	Amitriptyline	Desipramine
	Imipramine	Trazodone
Antiarrhythmics/ antianginals	Ca channel blocking agents	β-Blockers Quinidine* Procainamide*
	Disopyramide*	
Antihistamines	All types, particularly when combined with sympathomimetic*	

* Discontinue whenever possible.
** Desipramine is not very sedative; trazodone is somewhat sedative. The more sedative the antidepressant, the more pronounced the anticholinergic effect. Lower dosages may be therapeutic in older persons, eg, desipramine 75 mg daily and trazodone 100 to 150 mg daily.

URETHRAL STRICTURE

Persistent hesitancy and decreased force of stream suggest a diagnosis of urethral stricture. Common antecedents include urethral trauma following catheterization, endoscopy, or prostatic surgery. Rarely, a history of gonococcal urethritis may be obtained.

Direct visualization confirms the diagnosis, excludes cancer of the urethra, and avoids the creation of false channels by blind passage of a urethral sound. Repeated dilatation or direct vision urethrotomy is usually effective therapy.

BENIGN PROSTATIC HYPERTROPHY (BPH)

As men age, the normal golf-ball–sized prostate increases its fibromuscular stroma and encroaches on the urethra. The bladder compensates for the increased resistance by thickening its wall with hypertrophic muscle bundles that, when visualized cystoscopically, appear as trabeculation. Irritation may accompany obstructive symptoms because of noncompliance in the thickened bladder wall or the development of unstable bladder contractions.

TABLE 55–3 lists a scoring system for symptoms of BPH. In an un-referred medical clinic, about 20% of men > 60 yr of age may be moderately symptomatic (with a total score of 10 or more); in a urologist's office, > 50% may be this symptomatic. However, neither BPH nor symptoms of prostatism per se are indications for surgical treatment. Therefore, other factors must be considered.

Unequivocal Factors Favoring Surgical Treatment of BPH

A man with moderate symptoms should at least have renal function tests and a urinalysis. More than 5 RBC/high-power field **(HPF)** in uninfected urine requires cystoscopy to rule out bladder cancer. Abnormal renal function should prompt ultrasonic evaluation of the ureters and postvoiding bladder for signs of obstruction. The presence of hydronephrosis or a large postvoiding residual (> 350 mL) usually requires surgical intervention. Recurrent, severe UTI in the presence of a large postvoiding residual, or the presence of large bladder calculi in a patient with trabeculation and visual prostatic obstruction, is also an indication for surgical treatment.

TABLE 55–3. SYMPTOM SCORING SYSTEM FOR BENIGN PROSTATIC HYPERTROPHY (BPH)

Score	0	1	2	3	4
Stream	Normal	Variable	—	Weak	Dribbling
Voiding	No strain	—	Abdominal strain or Crede's method	—	—
Hesitancy	No	—	—	Yes	—
Intermittency	No	—	—	Yes	—
Bladder emptying	Don't know or complete	Variable	Incomplete	Single retention	Repeated retention
Incontinence	No	—	Yes (including terminal dribbling)	—	—
Urge	None	Mild	Moderate	Severe (incontinence)	—
Nocturia (times per night)	0–1	2	3–4	> 4	—
Diuria	< q 3 h	< q 2 h and up to q 3 h	< q 1 h and up to q 2 h	Once or more q h	—

Factors That May Favor Surgical Treatment of BPH

In the absence of a controlled trial showing the results of surgical treatment compared to observation, many factors have been proposed as indications for surgery: severity of symptoms, previous urinary retention requiring catheterization, low urine flow rate, increased residual bladder volume, or infection. Ultimately, the patient must decide whether the benefits of the intervention outweigh the cost and risk.

Surgery virtually eliminates the small but unpredictable risk of subsequent acute retention and usually reduces obstructive symptoms. Irritative symptoms are less likely to be improved. Surgery is associated with a 0.3 to 1.4% risk of death, a 1% chance of severe incontinence, a 3% chance of stricture, and a 2 to 7% requirement for repeat surgery within 5 yr. Postoperative bleeding and infection are common (occurring in 15 to 20% of cases) but usually mild. The relationship of transurethral resection of the prostate (TURP) to postoperative impotence is controversial (see Ch. 58).

Surgical Treatment Options in BPH

Surgery may be performed under general, spinal, or local anesthesia in an inpatient or outpatient setting. Operations include open prostatectomy, TURP, and transurethral incisions. Since the length of surgery adds significantly to the risk, very ill older patients may benefit from incisions or the removal of small amounts of tissue by TURP. Open prostatectomy, although associated with more short-term complications than TURP, is less likely to require subsequent repeat surgery. In contrast to the radical procedures used for cancer of the prostate, open prostatectomy seldom causes impotence.

Medical Options in BPH

The natural history of untreated prostatism is unclear, but the disorder is not necessarily relentlessly progressive. Nonsurgical treatment of BPH includes patient relaxation during urination, minimization of fluid intake at bedtime, and avoidance of unnecessary diuretics, anticholinergics, and antiarrhythmic agents (see TABLE 55–2). Irritative symptoms *may* be helped by α-adrenergic blocking agents; prazosin 0.5 to 3 mg tid is probably the safest. Numerous endocrine agents have been used experimentally to shrink the prostate, but evidence of their safety and effectiveness has not been documented in long-term controlled trials.

BLADDER CANCER

This neoplasia represents a spectrum of pathologic processes with different tendencies for invasion, spread, and multicentric evolution. Exposure to dyes and cigarettes are particularly important risk factors. Among persons $\geq$ 40 yr of age, the incidence of bladder cancer is 20:100,000; the incidence in men is twice that in women. In general, the depth of tumor penetration and histologic grade correspond best with metastatic potential.

Over 70% of bladder cancers are discovered as superficial tumors. However, unpredictability of spread and recurrence makes treatment of even superficial tumors difficult. Usually, solitary papillary superficial tumors recur least often; multiple superficial tumors, the most often. Although removal of the bladder would seem to be the simplest way to eliminate the risk for metastatic spread, cystectomy is fraught with significant morbid risks for local disease, infection, dehydration, and acidosis. Thus, surgical or laser excision, partial cystectomy, intravesical chemotherapy or bacillus Calmette-Guérin **(BCG)** therapy, and repeated cystoscopic surveillance remain the most common therapies for disease limited to the bladder.

The diagnosis of bladder cancer must be considered in any older patient complaining of gross hematuria and in whom UTI is not the cause. A urinalysis revealing > 5 RBC/high-power field or a positive test for Hb should also prompt cystoscopic evaluation. About 10% of older patients with hematuria have bladder cancer. Other common identifiable causes include urethral inflammation, BPH, and bladder stone. Since renal cell or ureteral cancers occasionally cause hematuria that is missed by cystoscopy alone, renal ultrasound, CT scan, or IV pyelogram is reasonable in the older patient whose hematuria is inadequately explained by cystoscopic findings. The sensitivity and specificity of urine cytology make it inadequate by itself for testing for bladder, ureteral, or renal cancer.

PROSTATIC CANCER

Although > 50% of men > 70 yr of age have histologic evidence of prostatic cancer, only about ⅓ of the cancers become clinically manifest in the patient's lifetime. Nevertheless, prostatic cancer is the second most common cause of cancer death in men > 75 yr of age. Cancer of the prostate is usually anatomically staged as shown in TABLE 55–4, although clinical staging systems have also been proposed. Unfortunately, approximately ½ of prostatic cancers are advanced beyond stages A and B at the time of discovery.

Symptoms, Signs, and Diagnosis

Most patients are asymptomatic or have symptoms compatible with BPH. Few present with acute retention, hematuria, or symptoms related to distant metastases (pain, weight loss, or lymphedema). An annual digital rectal examination is probably justified to screen early for this disease. A firm nodule or induration of the gland should prompt patient referral to a urologist for prostate core biopsy or prostate aspiration. However, screening by digital rectal examination has not resulted in more cures, nor has transrectal ultrasonic screening of the prostate proved more useful than digital rectal examination. Although prostatic acid phosphatase determinations are elevated in 50 to 70% of patients with nodal spread and in 85 to 90% of those with metastatic bone disease, this determination is not sensitive enough to use as a screening test for detecting early disease.

TABLE 55–4. STAGING OF PROSTATIC CANCER

Stage		Positive Nodes (%)	Approximate Actuarial Survival (5 yr) (%)
A_1:	Incidentally found during TURP in about 10% of prostatic fragments	0–5	
A_2:	Incidental but aggressive	25	85
B_1:	Clinically palpable but limited (< 1.5 cm)	5–20*	
B_2:	Seemingly localized within capsule (> 1.5 cm)	15–45*	75
C:	Invasive locally	40–80*	66
D:	Metastatic	> 80*	30

* Depends on tumor grade.

Treatment

A large percentage of men with prostatic cancer will not die from it. Since treatment causes morbidity, the advantages must be weighed against the risks—particularly in older patients whose life expectancy is limited by other diseases or advanced age.

During the past decade, external beam and implant radiation therapy became more popular for Stage B and C disease, even though radiation therapy may cause incontinence (0 to 12%), stricture (0 to 16%), or proctitis. Since recent studies suggest that 40 to 60% of irradiated patients will have metastatic disease and 30 to 85% will have residual cancer in prostate biopsy specimens, the value of radiation therapy for prostate cancer is being reappraised. A nerve-sparing radical prostatectomy is considered the treatment of choice for true Stage B disease.

Treatment for symptomatic, advanced disease (Stage C or D) with diethylstilbestrol (1 to 3 mg/day), gonadotropin-releasing hormone analogs, antiandrogens, and chemotherapeutic agents usually affords the patient temporary relief. Orchiectomy mitigates the risks of antiandrogen therapy but may not be acceptable to the patient.

SCROTAL MASSES

The large, neglected **scrotal hernia** is difficult to correct surgically. However, for the physiologically healthy elderly patient who has neither advanced chronic obstructive pulmonary disease nor prostatism, either primary surgical repair or secondary repair using autogenous fascia or a plastic mesh may be successful.

Hydroceles, which transilluminate, and **varicoceles,** which feel like "a bag of worms," occasionally present de novo in the elderly; testicular and renal cancer, respectively, should be ruled out. When the size of the hydrocele prompts the patient to request treatment, aspiration or surgical excision may be offered. However, aspiration is seldom permanently effective. Varicoceles are treated by ligation or embolectomy of the spermatic vein.

Epididymo-orchitis usually is a temporary sequela of UTI, prostatectomy, cystoscopy, or indwelling catheterization. Treatment of this painful condition consists of bed rest, scrotal support, and an antibiotic that is effective against both gram-negative bacteria and *Chlamydia.*

Painless testicular masses should always be considered **neoplastic.** At a minimum, ultrasonic evaluation is indicated.

Lymphoma is the most common testicular malignancy in the elderly. Unfortunately, even patients whose disease seems to be limited to the testicle may have systemic disease. Therefore, after orchiectomy establishes the diagnosis, further evaluation (CT scan, bone marrow biopsy, chest x-ray) is usually necessary for staging and decisions regarding radiation or chemotherapy. Of the germ cell tumors, **spermatocytic seminomas** occur most frequently in the elderly and carry a favorable prognosis. Orchiectomy is the only treatment required. Other germ cell tumors, including other seminomas, are usually aggressive and metastasize early.

---

56. URINARY TRACT INFECTION (UTI)

S. Ragnar Norrby

UTIs characterized by **significant bacteriuria** are classified according to the following clinical criteria:

1. **Localization,** as **cystitis** and **pyelonephritis.**

2. **Tendency to recur,** as **recurrent** and **sporadic infections** (a term preferred over "acute," because recurrent infections often produce acute symptoms). There is no universally accepted definition of recurrent infection; one proposal is to call an infection recurrent *if the patient has had more than one episode in a 6 mo period or more than 2 episodes in a year.* Recurrent infections are subclassified into **relapses** and **reinfections.** A relapse is caused by the same bacterial strain as the previous infection, ie, therapy failed to eradicate the bacteria or the patient developed a new infection with the same strain. A reinfection is caused by a bacterial strain different from the one that caused the previous infection.

3. **Symptomatology,** as **symptomatic** and **asymptomatic** bacteriuria.

4. **Complicating factors,** as **complicated** and **uncomplicated** infections (see below).

Epidemiology

The incidence of symptomatic bacterial UTIs in elderly persons has been estimated to be as high as 10% per year. Since many of these infections are recurrent, the actual number of infected patients is < 10% of the population. A majority of cases occur in premenopausal women. In the elderly, however, UTIs are more common in men because of the increasing frequency of bladder outlet obstruction from benign prostatic hyperplasia. The reduced incidence in elderly women may result from decreasing sexual activity which is associated with introduction of bacteria into the bladder. Severe UTIs, particularly septicemia originating from the urinary tract, become more common with advancing age, in part because of more frequent bladder catheterization and instrumentation. Recurrent and complicated infections are also more common because of the higher frequency of predisposing anatomic and pathophysiologic factors.

Etiology

UTIs are caused by *aerobic* bacteria. Anaerobes are isolated only from patients with rectovesical fistulas or other abnormal communications between the urinary tract and bowel allowing direct access of the anaerobic fecal flora to the urine. Bacteriologic findings vary according to previous antibiotic therapy, type of infection (complicated or uncomplicated, sporadic or recurrent), and whether bacteriuria is community- or hospital-acquired.

Escherichia coli is the most common pathogen isolated. It accounts for up to 90% of bacteriuria in elderly female outpatients with uncomplicated sporadic cystitis. This percentage decreases to about 40% in patients with indwelling bladder catheters, complicated infections, or hospital-acquired infections.

Klebsiella spp, especially *K. pneumoniae,* are the second most common gram-negative, aerobic pathogens isolated. *Proteus mirabilis, P. vulgaris, P. inconstans,* and *Morganella morganii* are more common in men than in women, because these species tend to dominate the normal aerobic preputial flora. They are also commonly isolated from the urine of patients with calculi, since they grow best in an alkaline milieu, and from patients with urogenital tumors. *Proteus* spp, *M. morganii,* and *Providencia* spp are commonly isolated from patients who are chronically catheterized. *Serratia, Enterobacter, Citrobacter, Acinetobacter,* and *Pseudomonas* spp are seen in patients with **hospital-acquired UTIs.**

In patients with **recurrent infections,** gram-negative bacteria other than *E. coli* and gram-positive bacteria tend to predominate. Of the latter, enterococci are commonly isolated, since many antibiotics used to treat bacteriuria are inactive against these organisms, resulting in enterococcal **superinfection.** With increasing age and in males, *Staphylococcus saprophyticus* becomes rare, and in patients > 60 yr of age it is normally not found.

Pathogenesis

Host factors: In aging women, *atrophic vaginal mucosa* may predispose to bacteriuria, since the vault is often heavily colonized with gram-negative aerobes. However, bacteriuria can occur without obvious cause in women, although traditionally this is considered due to their short urethras, which allow bacteria to be transported easily to the bladder. In aging men, such transport cannot occur unless facilitating factors are present, particularly those causing *turbulent urine flow,* (eg, benign hyperplasia, carcinoma of the prostate, urethral stricture.)

Bacteria proliferate in stagnant bladder urine, and clinically significant bacteriuria becomes established. This is facilitated in patients with postvoiding **residual urine,** possibly associated with a neurologic disorder, bladder outlet obstruction, or urethral stricture. Establishment and maintenance of bacteriuria is also facilitated by **foreign bodies,** most commonly, indwelling bladder catheters. In catheterized patients, significant bacteriuria is established within 14 days unless a closed and aseptically handled system is employed, in which case significant bacteriuria may be delayed for an additional, variable period of time. Bladder calculi can also result in sustained bacteriuria. Development of bacteriuria is facilitated by poorly controlled **diabetes mellitus,** with increased urine glucose providing the substrate for bacterial growth.

In elderly patients with pyelonephritis, bacteria invade the renal parenchyma, usually via the renal pelvis. This is facilitated by **reflux of urine** from the bladder during micturition, by **ureteral or pelvic calculi,** by congenital or acquired **pelvic deformity,** or by **renal parenchymal disease.** Hematogenous spread to the renal parenchyma, although infrequent, may occur in debilitated, septic patients.

Bacterial virulence factors: In most patients, the organism causing bacteriuria is the dominant aerobic fecal isolate. Bacterial species differ in their tendency to colonize urine. The most important bacterial virulence factor seems to be adherence of potential pathogens to epithelial cells lining the urethra and ureter. The bacterial antigen responsible for attachment is located in the pili (fimbriae) of *E. coli* and *Proteus* spp. The receptor is a glycosphingolipid that is present on the surface of uroepithelial cells and also on erythrocytes. Individuals with the rare blood group P lack this glycosphingolipid and are less prone to develop bacteriuria. Attachment of bacteria to epithelial cells seems to be particularly important for development of pyelonephritis. Other important virulence factors are bacterial antigens (eg, the polysaccharide capsule and the O, H, and K antigens of Enterobacteriaceae).

Bacteriologic Diagnosis of UTIs

Bacteriologic diagnosis is usually based on the concept of **significant bacteriuria,** defined as *> 10⁵ colony forming units (CFU)/mL of a midstream urine sample obtained after at least 4 h of bladder incubation.* This figure is based on a statistical analysis of 2 groups, one with and one without bacterial colonization of bladder urine obtained from a catheterized specimen. Depending upon the method of collection, patients without significant bacteriuria in the bladder may yield > 10^5 CFU/mL, and patients with significant bacteriuria in the bladder may have as few as 100 CFU/mL. If there are doubts about the clinical significance of bacteriuria, urine may be obtained by suprapubic **bladder puncture** (which is preferred over bladder catheterization). *Any number* of bacteria is then significant.

For culture, urine samples preferably should be obtained after at least a few hours of bladder incubation. This is not necessary in patients with residual urine or in patients with indwelling bladder catheters.

Rapid tests can provide a semiquantitative determination of significant bacteriuria. The best is the **nitrite test,** in which the conversion of nitrate to nitrite by bacteria in the urine is demonstrated by color change on a dipstick. This test has a high degree of sensitivity and specificity but will not demonstrate bacteriuria caused by *Pseudomonas* spp, staphylococci, or enterococci, which lack the capability to metabolize nitrate. Another rapid diagnostic method for detection of bacteriuria is the **hypoglycosuria test,** based on the demonstration of lack of glucose in urine caused by bacterial consumption. (Uninfected urine normally contains small amounts of glucose.) The test is inferior to the nitrite test because diabetes mellitus and intake of carbohydrate-rich foods give false-positive results and because the test results often are difficult to interpret.

Quantitative urine cultures can be performed by bacteriologic laboratories; the urine must be kept refrigerated if actual culture and incubation are delayed. The physician is provided with both species identification and antibiotic susceptibility. In outpatient clinics, a **dip-slide culture** may be used. With this method, an agar-covered slide is dipped in urine and incubated in a simple device or even left at room temperature overnight. Reliable quantification of the number of bacteria in the sample and differentiation between gram-negative and gram-positive organisms are obtained. A positive dip-slide can later be sent to a bacteriology laboratory for formal species identification and antibiotic susceptibility determination.

CYSTITIS

An *infection localized to the bladder wall,* cystitis is the most common clinical manifestation of bacteriuria. The urethra is often involved **(cystourethritis).** Symptoms are caused by inflammation of the urethral and bladder mucosa following invasion of bacteria.

Symptoms and Signs

The onset is acute, with **urgency, dysuria** (burning sensation during micturition), and **frequency** (pollakiuria). The patient often feels the urge to void 3 to 4 times/h, although little urine is excreted and is frequently foul-smelling. **Gross hematuria** is common, especially in young women with infections caused by *S. saprophyticus.* **Fever** is uncommon but has been reported in patients with their first episode of cystitis. Physical examination reveals *few positive findings;* there may be suprapubic tenderness on palpation.

Diagnosis

The diagnosis is based on the history and the results of urinalysis, rapid tests for demonstration of bacteriuria, and urine culture. **Urine microscopy** shows a large number of polymorphonuclear leukocytes. Erythrocytes may be present, but casts should *not* be seen. Bacteria may be seen (even in normal urine) and infrequently rods can be differentiated from cocci. Bacteriuria cannot be quantified by light microscopy. **Proteinuria** is common, and is the result of the large cellular content (*not* renal disease).

The differential diagnosis is often difficult. **Urethritis** without bacteriuria may cause the same symptoms as cystitis. In patients with pyuria but no growth on routine bacterial culture, **tuberculosis of the urinary tract** should be considered and centrifuged urine should be stained for acid-fast bacilli (Ziehl-Neelsen method) and cultured for mycobacteria. The most important differential diagnostic consideration is between cystitis and **pyelonephritis.** WBC casts seen in the urine on microscopic examination strongly support a diagnosis of pyelonephritis.

Prognosis

Uncomplicated cystitis resolves without sequelae if adequately treated. Recurrence is seen in about 10% of cases, based on follow-up urine cultures obtained 3 to 5 wk after completion of treatment. Most recurrences are reinfections, and relapses are seen in < 3% of properly treated patients. Recurrent infections are often asymptomatic. In patients with complicated cystitis (eg, those with residual urine), the frequency of recurrence is much higher (ie, > 25%). Such patients are also at greater risk for ascending infection and development of pyelonephritis.

Treatment

Cystitis should be treated with renally excreted antibacterial agents active against the most frequently isolated pathogens, especially *E. coli* but preferably also enterococci. Coverage in the antibacterial spectrum of *S. saprophyticus* is not necessary in elderly patients. Since most cases of cystitis are uncomplicated, one should choose an antimicrobial that causes a minimum of adverse reactions and, certainly, none that are life-threatening.

Patients with community-acquired infections can be treated with an oral cephalosporin (cefaclor, cefadroxil, cephalexin, cephradine), norfloxacin, ciprofloxacin, ofloxacin, amdinocillin pivoxil, or trimethoprim. Modern, fluorinated quinolones (eg, norfloxacin, ciprofloxacin, or ofloxacin) are preferred over older, nonfluorinated quinolones (eg, nalidixic acid, cinoxacin, and pipemidic acid) because of their wider antibacterial spectrum and the lower incidence of emerging resistance.

In patients with recurrent or complicated infections, a fluorinated quinolone or trimethoprim is recommended before the cephalosporins and amdinocillin pivoxil, since the first drugs are active also against enterococci. When renal function is markedly reduced, dosage should be decreased accordingly, either by lowering the dose at each administration or by prolonging the interdose interval. Because of a high frequency of adverse reactions, especially in the elderly, combinations of trimethoprim and sulfonamides, pure sulfonamides, and nitrofurantoin are *not* recommended for treatment of uncomplicated cystitis.

The **duration of treatment of uncomplicated cystitis** varies. Single-dose therapy, using 2 or 3 times the normal single dose, has been extensively evaluated. In most studies, such single-dose therapy has been almost as effective as treatment for 7 or 10 days. However, patients with a missed diagnosis of pyelonephritis who are given single-dose treatment for cystitis will experience an exacerbation of symptoms within 48 h. The best-documented duration of treatment is 7 to 10 days, although several studies have indicated that 3 days may suffice. Weighing the increased risk of adverse reactions associated with prolonged treatment against the generally benign nature of this infection, a recommendation that treatment of uncomplicated cystitis not exceed 7 days seems justified.

Prophylactic treatment in patients with complicated cystitis should be considered. Drugs recommended for prophylactic use are nitrofurantoin 50 mg bid or one 100-mg dose at night, or trimethoprim one 100-mg dose at night. With nitrofurantoin, the risk of pulmonary hypersensitivity reactions should be kept in mind, and patients receiving long-term treatment with trimethoprim may require supplementation with folinic acid. When possible, the cause of recurrent cystitis should be sought, identified, and treated. Prophylactic therapy should *not* be used in patients with indwelling bladder catheters.

PYELONEPHRITIS
(Infectious Tubulointerstitial Nephritis)

Infection involving the renal parenchyma and the renal pelvis.

Isolated pyelitis or infectious nephritis is extremely uncommon. **Chronic pyelonephritis** with renal scarring may develop in patients who had childhood renal infections or who have renal tubular necrosis caused by overconsumption of phenacetin derivatives. Chronic pyelonephritis is more common in older patients, mainly because phenacetin derivatives are no longer used.

Symptoms and Signs

Eight to 10% of patients with symptomatic UTIs have pyelonephritis. Patients with pyelonephritis may present with an initial history of cystitis. Typical symptoms of renal infection are **fever, chills,** and **back pains,** which may be unilateral or bilateral. Sudden clinical deterioration may indicate dissemination of bacteria from a renal focus, causing **septicemia.** Urine microscopy shows **pyuria** and often **WBC casts.** ESR will increase but is often initially normal. C-reactive protein **(CRP)** is increased in all patients and is a useful though nonspecific test. Most patients have leukocytosis with an absolute increase in polymorphonuclear leukocytes. Serum creatinine and BUN are elevated in most patients.

Diagnosis

Bacteriuria is demonstrated as it is in cystitis (see above). The bacteriologic tests should always include species identification and antibiotic susceptibility testing in patients with pyelonephritis. In most cases, the clinical features and microscopic findings in urine will provide the diagnosis. **Blood cultures** should be obtained in patients with a deteriorating clinical condition. **IVU** or **ultrasonography** should be performed if renal pelvic or ureteral obstruction due to a calculus is suspected. These procedures are not necessary in patients who have had a normal IVU within the past 3 yr.

Demonstration by immunofluorescence of antibody-coated bacteria in the urine is a test that has been used quite extensively to differentiate pyelonephritis from cystitis. This test has weaknesses, however (ie, low sensitivity [if a positive reaction requires that > 5% of all bacteria be antibody coated] and low specificity [if < 5% of the bacteria is required to be antibody-coated]).

Apart from cystitis, several differential diagnoses should be considered in elderly patients with suspected pyeloneophritis. **Renal pelvic or ureteral stones** may produce similar patterns of pain but do not normally cause fever. **Acute appendicitis** may simulate right-sided pyelonephritis. **Cholangitis** and **cholecystitis** are also important differential considerations in patients with right-sided symptoms. Patients with **lower lobe pneumonia** may have back pain similar to that in pyelonephritis.

Prognosis

The prognosis is good for an adequately treated patient with pyelonephritis. Renal function will return to normal about 3 wk after treatment, unless the patient has had previous renal damage, in which case a permanent reduction in renal function may result. This is a particular risk in older patients who had recurrent episodes of pyelonephritis with renal scarring during childhood. Previous episodes of pyelonephritis that occurred only during adulthood do not normally worsen the prognosis. Patients who develop septicemia have a poor prognosis (see UROSEPSIS, below). To avoid asymptomatic recurrences following treatment of pyelonephritis, all patients should be reevaluated at 1 wk and at 3 to 6 wk after treatment with renal function tests and urine cultures; an IVU can be done if one was not performed during the past 3 yr.

Treatment

Antibiotic treatment should be started as soon as urine cultures and, if necessary, blood cultures are obtained. Many older patients with uncomplicated pyelonephritis can be treated on an outpatient basis, although hospitalization is often necessary. Antibiotics chosen should cover all important gram-negative uropathogens. Duration of therapy should be at least 10 and preferably 14 to 21 days. Patients receiving initial treatment with parenteral antibiotics can continue treatment with oral drugs when improvement occurs. High antibiotic concentrations should be achieved not only in the urine but also in the blood and the renal parenchyma.

Suitable antibiotics for initial **oral treatment** (and for follow-up after initial treatment with parentaral antibiotics) include cephalosporins (cefaclor, cefadroxil, cephradine, cephalexin), ciprofloxacin, norfloxacin, ofloxacin, amdinocillin pivoxil plus pivampicillin (as combination or together), and combinations of trimethoprim and sulfamethoxazole or sulfadiazine.

Patients requiring a **parenteral antibiotic** can be given a cephalosporin or an aminoglycoside, pending results of culture and sensitivity tests. In patients with community-acquired infections who have not received previous antibiotic treatment, a second-generation cephalosporin (eg, cefamandole or cefuroxime) will cover most pathogens; in patients with hospital-acquired infections, a third-generation cephalosporin (eg, cefotaxime, ceftazidime, ceftriaxone) or an aminoglycoside is preferred. Intravenous trimethoprim/sulfamethoxazole is an alternative in the latter.

Dose reductions are often necessary in elderly patients because of the combined effects of aging and pyelonephritis on renal function. If aminoglycosides are used, serum concentrations *must* be monitored at regular intervals (ie, at least twice weekly) to avoid nephrotoxic or ototoxic reactions. Because of the risk of toxicity and serious adverse reactions associated with trimethoprim/sulfonamide combinations, these agents should *not* be used as first-line drugs for this indication. Amoxicillin or ampicillin *alone* is not recommended, since 15% or more of all urinary isolates of *E. coli* and even higher percentages of other gram-negative urinary pathogens are resistant to these antibiotics.

UROSEPSIS

Septicemia originating from the urinary tract. It is very common in the elderly, often occurring 24 to 72 h after a urinary tract procedure, especially after initial insertion or change of a bladder catheter or after cystoscopy, during which bacteria in the urine enter the blood through traumatized urethral mucosa.

Symptoms and Signs

The patient usually has a recent history of catheterization or cystoscopy. Onset is acute with **fever, chills,** and often signs of **septic shock,** although patients who develop septic shock may be afebrile on admission. Renal function is often seriously impaired, and anuria is common.

Diagnosis

The diagnosis is based on the history and the physical findings. Bacteriologic confirmation is obtained from blood and urine cultures. Granulocytosis is usually found, along with increased ESR and CRP. Electrolyte imbalance and elevated serum creatinine and BUN levels are common. Important differential diagnoses are **hypovolemic shock** and **cardiogenic shock.**

Prognosis

The prognosis for geriatric patients with urosepsis is poor; 23 to 30% of those with positive blood cultures die of their infection. In patients who defervesce, the prognosis is good but recurrence should be prevented.

Treatment

Treatment should eliminate bacteria from blood and urine and reverse symptoms of septic shock if present. Antibiotics should always be administered intravenously. The duration of IV treatment and oral follow-up is the same as in pyelonephritis (see above). First-line antibiotics are second- and third-generation cephalosporins and aminoglycosides. Although the initial dose should always be maximal, subsequent doses usually need to be reduced substantially because of markedly decreased renal function.

ASYMPTOMATIC BACTERIURIA

Bacteriuria in a patient who had no symptoms of UTI during the week preceding the time the urine sample was obtained. It is a common finding in the elderly, especially women.

Symptoms and Signs

By definition, a patient with asymptomatic bacteriuria has no symptoms. The patient may complain of foul-smelling urine and difficulty in maintaining normal genital hygiene, but laboratory values are usually normal. Rising serum creatinine or BUN levels indicate underlying urinary tract pathology.

Diagnosis

The diagnosis is based on demonstration of *significant bacteriuria in 2 or more consecutive samples.* Only about 70% of asymptomatic patients with high colony counts in a single urine sample have true bacteriuria; with 2 positive samples, the specificity of the test is about 97%.

Prognosis

Mortality is significantly higher in elderly men with asymptomatic bacteriuria than in elderly women. The reason for this difference has not been determined but may relate to the presence of more malignant diseases in men with asymptomatic bacteriuria.

Treatment

In women, asymptomatic bacteriuria should not be treated, unless other conditions are present that may increase the risk of symptomatic invasive disease. In untreated asymptomatic bacteriuria, the organisms (especially *E. coli*) lose their virulence and become extremely susceptible to the bactericidal effect of normal human plasma. The presence of large amounts of bacteria in the urine may therefore protect against symptomatic bacteriuria caused by more virulent strains. However, besides becoming less virulent, *the bacteria in a patient with asymptomatic bacteriuria become more susceptible to antibiotics.* Thus, asymptomatic bacteriuria can be eradicated with penicillin V, leaving the patient at a higher risk of acquiring a symptomatic urinary tract infection.

In men, asymptomatic bacteriuria should be investigated to exclude complicating factors such as residual urine, calculi or tumors. While the diagnosis is being determined and causative factors eliminated, treatment with the antibiotics indicated by sensitivity testing of identified bacteria should be considered.

Asymptomatic bacteriuria in elderly persons with chronic bladder catheterization is claimed to be associated with increased mortality. This increase is probably due to other diseases or general frailty, leading to a need for chronic catheterization. However, as pointed out above, urosepsis is frequent in patients who are catheterized for prolonged periods, involving catheter changes at regular intervals.

Thus, to prevent increased mortality in the elderly from long-term use of bladder catheters and urosepsis associated with catheter removal or insertion, catheter use must be minimized. *Catheters should be used only when medically indicated* and not in patients with urinary incontinence. Whenever possible, the condition leading to a need for catheterization should be corrected. Bacteriuria should be treated with antibiotics only when a patient shows symptoms of a urinary tract infection. If such rules are followed, the risk of nosocomial spread of multiresistant urinary pathogens is reduced and problems in the choice of antibiotics are minimized.

---

57. FEMALE GENITOURINARY DISORDERS
(See also Chs. 8 and 72)

Edward J. McGuire, John O. L. DeLancey, and *Thomas Elkins*

PELVIC DISORDERS ASSOCIATED WITH ESTROGEN DEFICIENCY

Atrophic changes occur in the GU system and other estrogen-dependent tissues after menopause. Diagnosis of menopause is established by the cessation of menstruation and a characteristic constellation of symptoms and signs. If doubt exists as to its occurrence, an elevated serum FSH level confirms the diagnosis.

Vaginal atrophy is accompanied by a watery discharge, an increased susceptibility to local bacterial infection, and occasional burning vaginal pain. **Dyspareunia** is usually not a problem if intercourse continues at regular intervals, but periods of abstinence can be accompanied by further atrophy and stenosis, causing subsequent sexual activity to be painful.

The treatment of GU menopausal symptoms is hormonal replacement. Estrogen can be given orally, vaginally, parenterally, or transcutaneously. Vaginal application of estrogen is particularly effective in treating atrophic vaginitis. Although therapeutic systemic levels are reached with vaginal administration, this should not be considered an alternative treatment in patients with contraindications to oral estrogen. (See Ch. 72 for a detailed discussion of the menopause and estrogen replacement therapy.)

URINARY INCONTINENCE
(See also Ch. 10)

Poor closure of the proximal urethral sphincter, or that part of the urethra from the vesical outlet to the pelvic floor, is responsible for approximately 46% of cases of incontinence in elderly women. Incontinence in the remainder is thought to be a result of uninhibited detrusor contractility.

Symptoms, Signs, and Diagnosis

Urgency and urge incontinence, characterized by the *sudden need to void and urination before reaching the toilet,* indicate an unstable bladder or a bladder that can contract autonomously. This may be due to a primary bladder disorder, or it may be related to urethral sphincter inefficiency. The latter is associated with a history of urinary leakage with effort, coughing, or sneezing. If a history of such stress incontinence can be elicited, leakage is likely to occur during stress testing (see below). Stress incontinence in the elderly is associated less frequently with disorders of urethral support and more frequently with poor urethral closing pressures; thus, the physical findings associated with surgically remedial stress incontinence in younger women, including prolapse of the urethrovesical junction, are *not* often present.

Hyperreflexia of the bladder is manifested by urgency and wetting that occur frequently at small bladder volumes (eg, 1 time/1 to 1½ h). This kind of bladder hyperactivity is often associated with a neurologic abnormality, eg, stroke or Parkinson's disease. The bladder contraction typically is provoked easily, simply by bladder filling on a cystometrogram.

Intermittent sudden urinary incontinence, which occurs less frequently and at normal as well as large bladder volumes (eg, 1 to 3 times/day) is probably more common than true bladder hyperreflexia. This kind of incontinence appears to result from lack of supraspinal inhibition, which may have a sensory basis. In these patients a detrusor contraction is difficult to provoke during testing by a cystometrogram; thus, patient history is more useful in diagnosis than is urologic evaluation.

A simple stress test can be performed while the patient (with a full bladder) stands over a towel placed on the floor. The patient is asked to cough vigorously several times and, if leakage occurs, stress incontinence is present. The examiner must then determine whether the leakage is associated with loss of urethral support or with poor urethral function. With the patient in the lithotomy position, the examiner determines the location of the urethra and bladder beneath the anterior vaginal wall by gentle palpation. The patient is then asked to cough and strain, and the urethra and bladder base is palpated for motion and posterior rotational descent while intra-abdominal pressure is increased. Leakage from the urethral orifice can also be observed, but the upright stress test is much more accurate in this regard.

If a urethra that has been shown to leak can also be shown to move into the potential space of the vagina, incontinence associated with loss of urethral support is present. If the urethra does not move but remains fixed in its normal retropubic position, leakage due to poor urethral function is likely to be present. The peak age for onset of stress incontinence related to loss of urethral support is 35 to 50 yr. A later onset of stress incontinence suggests poor urethral function.

Treatment

If stress testing is negative for leakage, incontinence can be assumed to be the result of **uninhibited detrusor contractility** (urge incontinence). If there is little or no residual urine (< 30 mL), empiric therapy can be started (see Ch. 10).

Incontinence associated with residual urine should not be treated empirically with anticholinergic agents. This condition may be related to a poor-quality detrusor contraction, cystocele formation, or urethral obstruction. Referral to a urologist or a gynecologist is warranted in this situation, since relatively sophisticated urodynamic evaluation is often required before effective treatment can be initiated (see Ch. 10).

Indwelling catheters should be avoided if possible, since incontinence around the catheter, stone formation, and bladder fibrosis, as well as UTI (including pyelonephritis), often result from such treatment.

Stress incontinence associated with an atrophic vaginal epithelium and little or no urethral hypermobility usually responds to imipramine hydrochloride 10 mg orally tid and intravaginal administration of conjugated estrogens, 1/4 applicator at night or every other night. (See Ch. 72 for a full discussion of estrogen treatment.) Urgency associated with demonstrable stress incontinence usually responds to this treatment as well. **Patients with urethral hypermobility and prolapse of the anterior vaginal wall** may improve with estrogens, tricyclic antidepressants, and a vaginal tampon (which provides support to the vesical urethral junction during periods of vigorous physical activity), but most require definitive surgical repair (see Ch. 10).

DISORDERS OF THE PELVIC-FLOOR SUPPORTING SYSTEM AND GENITOURINARY PROLAPSE

Generally, the patient is aware of a mass at the introitus or a constant feeling of heaviness or pressure within the pelvis. These symptoms may be due to a rectocele, an enterocele, a cystocele, uterine prolapse, or total vaginal vault prolapse, which occurs after hysterectomy and is essentially an eversion of the entire vagina.

Rectocele formation between the levator ani muscles may be associated with difficult passage of stools and may require manual reduction of the prolapsed anterior rectal wall through the vagina. **Enterocele** formation occurs in the cul-de-sac between the uterosacral ligaments and is associated with pelvic pressure and a bulge through the vagina often present at the introitus. Diagnosis is usually made by a bimanual pelvic examination but can be aided by having the patient stand, so the enterocele space can be felt to bulge during the Valsalva maneuver.

A cystocele is recognized as a bulge of the anterior vaginal wall and may be associated with incomplete bladder emptying, UTI and, occasionally, overflow urinary incontinence.

Uterine prolapse is caused by laxity of the supporting uterosacral or posterior ligaments, the cardinal or the lateral ligaments, and the round or anterior ligaments of the pelvis. Uterine prolapse may be classified as 1st degree when the cervix descends to the level of the ischial spines, 2nd degree when the cervix descends to the introitus, and 3rd degree when the cervix descends below the introitus. This classification is related to the degree of difficulty during repair. In patients who have had a hysterectomy, **total vaginal vault prolapse** may occur, although this is uncommon. It presents as a bulge from the introitus, which occasionally may be painful or associated with vaginal mucosal ulceration.

Treatment

The treatment of the various types of pelvic-floor relaxation may be medical or surgical. Medical management involves use of a pessary, which can be cumbersome for many, but is ideal for some elderly patients in whom surgery is contraindicated. Whether done vaginally or abdominally, surgical modalities vary markedly. In general, the earlier surgical treatment is undertaken, the easier and more effective the repair.

CARUNCLE

Erythematous urethral mucosa, protruding from the external urethral orifice, which may bleed or be associated with dysuria. The prolapsed tissue is palpably soft and pliable, as opposed to a neoplastic process, which is palpably firm and nontender.

Treatment: Symptomatic caruncles can be removed under local anesthesia. Asymptomatic caruncles generally require no treatment.

URINARY TRACT INFECTIONS

Recurrent UTIs in elderly women are relatively common. Uncomplicated UTIs are associated with urgency, frequency, dysuria, and, occasionally, lower abdominal or back pain. Fever, hematuria, and flank or costovertebral angle tenderness all are signs of complicated infection and should prompt complete urologic evaluation.

Urologic examination is usually unremarkable, although evidence of residual urine, a cystocele, urinary incontinence, or urethral obstruction (which is rare) should be sought. Baseline laboratory evaluation (CBC, urinalysis, and urine culture) is required, and BUN and serum creatinine determinations are helpful. (For a detailed discussion of UTIs, including treatment, see Ch. 56.)

HEMATURIA

The visible presence of blood in the urine usually prompts a visit to the family physician, who should immediately refer the patient to a urologist. The diagnostic yield of full urologic investigation in elderly women with hematuria is relatively low, but the conditions found can be serious and include transitional cell carcinoma, stone formation, and renal neoplasia. Full evaluation thus cannot be omitted and should include IV pyelography, renal ultrasonography, urinary cytology, and cystourethroscopy. The radiographic studies can be obtained prior to referral to the urologist.

GENITAL MALIGNANCIES

CARCINOMA OF THE VULVA

Carcinoma of the vulva is the fourth most common gynecologic malignancy and has its peak incidence between the ages of 70 and 80 yr. The lesions may be erythematous and flat, condylomatous, or ulcerated; most are symptomatic, causing pruritus, discharge, or local discomfort. Patients with presumed inflammatory lesions that do not respond promptly to topical therapy should be referred for biopsy without delay.

Premalignant vulvar lesions may be confused with cancer of the vulva, especially in the elderly. **Vulvar dystrophy** has been classified into 3 types: atrophic, hypertrophic, and mixed. A similar condition is **lichen sclerosus et atrophicus**. There is some malignant potential, but it is small. Patients with vulvar lesions should be referred to a gynecologist for evaluation. Before initiating therapy, the gynecologist will investigate the lesion by staining the area with toluidine blue and acetic acid, followed by biopsy if indicated by uptake of stain.

Treatment

Treatment is primarily surgical. Vulvar carcinomas, which are mainly intraepithelial, are managed by wide local excision. Radical vulvectomy, although less common, may occasionally be required. In some instances, topical medical therapy with cytotoxic agents has also been found useful, particularly in patients in whom even minor surgical procedures are contraindicated. Prognosis is generally good if the lesions are treated promptly.

CARCINOMA OF THE VAGINA

This is a relatively rare malignancy, usually squamous cell in character. Early symptoms include vaginal bleeding or profuse vaginal discharge. Treatment consists of a combination of surgery, radiation, and topical chemotherapeutic agents. Prognosis is relatively poor.

CARCINOMA OF THE CERVIX

The peak incidence of this disease occurs in the 5th and 6th decades, but 2 to 3% of women will develop cervical carcinoma by the age of 80 yr. The disease is common in elderly women. Several papilloma virus types have been associated with the development of this disease. While 90% of cervical carcinomas are squamous cell tumors, the incidence of adenocarcinoma of the cervix appears to be increasing. The most common symptom is postcoital bleeding in younger women, although many patients are asymptomatic. Symptoms depend on the stage of the tumor.

Cervical carcinoma is diagnosed most commonly by the use of routine Papanicolaou **(Pap)** smears and colposcopic-directed biopsies, along with endocervical curettage. In elderly patients, the cervical transformation zone, where most early cancers originate, may not be visible on colposcopy, and cervical conization is often required for diagnosis. Patients with suspicious Pap smears should be referred for gynecologic evaluation. Elderly women should have routine Pap smears yearly.

Treatment of cervical carcinoma involves both surgery and radiation.

CARCINOMA OF THE OVARY

While ovarian carcinoma constitutes only 5% of malignant disease in women, it is the leading cause of death in women with gynecologic malignancies. Most malignant tumors of the ovary are either serous or mucinous in character, although there are many other varieties. The early symptoms are nonspecific, often nothing more than vague GI discomfort. Patients often present with large pelvic masses. Any palpable ovary found on pelvic examination in a postmenopausal patient should be considered suspicious for ovarian carcinoma, prompting referral to a gynecologist. Treatment is both medical and surgical and sometimes involves radiotherapy. Survival is poor.

CARCINOMA OF THE ENDOMETRIUM

This disease is the most common gynecologic malignancy in the USA, surpassing cervical carcinoma. There are little data about the incidence in elderly women, although it is surely reduced in relation to endometrial involution. Risk factors include obesity and associated conditions, nulliparity, and conditions that predispose to unopposed exogenous estrogens (ie, no periodic progesterone). Estrogen replacement therapy, when combined with progestin therapy at least 12 to 14 days/mo, results in rates of endometrial hyperplasia and carcinoma comparable to those found in women receiving no estrogen replacement. Early symptoms include irregular or heavy postmenopausal bleeding. Diagnosis is made by endometrial biopsy.

Treatment

Treatment is primarily surgical—hysterectomy and associated lymph node sampling. However, radiation therapy or chemotherapy or both are also required in advanced tumor grades or stages. Although the incidence of endometrial carcinoma appears to be increasing, early diagnosis and treatment of this condition have made the prognosis generally better than that of other GU malignancies.

FISTULAS

GU and enterourinary fistulas may occur in the elderly in fairly well-defined circumstances.

Vesicovaginal fistulas may follow hysterectomy for benign conditions or other surgical procedures. Patients present with either continuous or intermittent urinary incontinence and generally with some vulvar and vaginal excoriation and erythema. Vesicovaginal fistulas may occur in the elderly $\geq$ 20 yr following radiation therapy for pelvic malignancy; these patients present with total urinary incontinence.

Diagnosis is established by a number of methods, including cystography (a cystogram with fluid containing a colored dye), cystoscopy, vaginal examination, and vaginography. None of these is sufficiently precise to rule out a fistula if the results are negative. When the cause of involuntary urine loss is a **ureterovaginal fistula,** which occurs after hysterectomy or other surgical procedures, the diagnosis is more accurate and is made either by IV or retrograde pyelography.

Urethral-vaginal fistulas are relatively rare, but typically follow vaginal operative procedures for stress incontinence or urethral diverticula. The history varies with the location and extent of the fistulous tract. Fistulas located above the midurethra may be associated with continuous incontinence. If the bladder outlet is closed by a well-functioning sphincter and fistula lies below the sphincter, postvoiding incontinence resulting from urine pooled in the vagina during voiding is the most common symptom. Fistulous connections distal to the external sphincter are generally asymptomatic, although they also may be associated with postvoiding incontinence.

Diagnosis is made by endoscopy and/or urethrography, performed with a cumbersome technic involving a double-balloon catheter to occlude both the internal and external urethral orifices. Most such fistulas are not found on the first attempt. **Treatment** is surgical, involving closure of the fistula and interposition of some vascularized tissue (eg, a labial fat graft).

Enterovesical fistulas in the elderly are most frequently associated with colonic diverticulitis or, less commonly, with a colonic malignancy. Symptoms include lower abdominal pain, pneumaturia, cystitis, and hematuria. Diagnosis is often difficult. Diagnostic methods include barium enema, sigmoidoscopy, cystography, and oral ingestion of charcoal with subsequent examination of the urine for charcoal particles.

Colovesical fistulas should be sought promptly in the presence of repeated UTIs or UTIs that fail to respond to continuous suppressive antimicrobial therapy. Such fistulas may intermittently seal; failure to find a fistulous tract on the first attempt does not rule it out.

Treatment of colovesical fistulas associated with diverticulitis depends on the extent and nature of the inflammatory process. In some cases, resection of the involved segment of sigmoid colon with immediate reanastomosis and closure of the opening in the bladder can be performed. In other cases, the safest method is to perform a proximal diverting colostomy and allow the inflammatory process to subside before definitive surgical repair and resection of the involved segment of colon are undertaken. Fistulas associated with malignancy usually require excision with proximal diversion.

---

58. SEXUALITY

Robert N. Butler and *Myrna Lewis*

Sexual desire, capability, and satisfaction are important to many elderly persons. However, others have low sexual interest or inhibited sexual desire for a variety of reasons (eg, low intrinsic drive dating back to youth, poor marital relationship, or the death of a spouse or companion). Physicians should be able to handle sexual issues with dignity and skill, despite the apparently common discomfort inherent in discussion of the subject. This discomfort can be traced to negative stereotypes, personal anxieties, objections to the expression of sexuality by the elderly, or simply ignorance.

A sexual history, with emphasis on current sexual function, should be part of the general medical evaluation of an older person. When a problem exists, evaluation of drugs being taken, psychologic testing, referral for sex therapy, and even surgery may be necessary. Much of the expense may be covered by Medicare or private health insurance, but assuming the cost of professional sex therapy (including that for couples) may be a problem for many older people. Medicare allows only $250/yr for outpatient psychotherapy that is administered by a physician. However, Medicare will pay for treatment of sexual dysfunction if the diagnosis can be included in the category of "psychophysiologic genitourinary disorder." Few private insurance programs cover sex therapy.

AGING AND NORMAL CHANGES IN SEXUALITY

Sexual change in old age is a process of gradual slowing; more time is needed to become sexually aroused and to reach sexual climax. This should not be considered an impairment, since it may permit a better response synchronization between the sexes, compared to that in earlier years when men responded more quickly than women.

Special Concerns of Men

In addition to gradual slowing, older men may notice reduced preejaculatory fluid and less forcefulness at ejaculation. In the absence of chronic illness or alcoholism, testosterone levels decline gradually, and some very old men still have levels identical to those in younger men; there is no physiologic male climacteric. Further, since fertility is not associated with potency, men may remain fertile until the end of life. (See also Ch. 73.)

Impotence (erectile dysfunction): A common concern of older men is their ability to maintain sexual potency and performance. Any sign of impotence is distressing and is usually (although inaccurately) attributed to aging. However, impotence may occur from time to time at any age for a variety of reasons (eg, stress, fatigue, tension, guilt, depression, illness, excessive drinking, and anxiety over performance). Psychologic and organic factors are often intermixed. Recent studies suggest that organic causes are a major factor in $\geq$ 50% of persistent male sexual dysfunction.

Drug side effects are perhaps the major cause of impotence. Major physical conditions causing the approximately 5 million cases of impotence are (in descending order) diabetes mellitus, vascular insufficiency, radical surgery, trauma, hypogonadism and other endocrine disorders, multiple sclerosis, and Peyronie's disease. The diagnostic process begins with a history and physical examination. Depression, anxiety, and stress must also be evaluated. Sleep studies that measure nocturnal penile tumescence **(NPT)** help distinguish psychogenic from organic impotence. In most cases of psychogenic impotence, sexual capacity returns spontaneously. Reassurance reduces anxiety and speeds recovery.

Patients with chronic organic impotence and, in rare instances, those with psychologic impotence that is unresponsive to psychotherapy may benefit from permanent penile prostheses or implants. A prosthesis enhances a patient's self-esteem and may improve his partner's pleasure, but it neither produces a sexual climax nor increases sexual desire in the man. The most commonly used device is the ESKA Jonas Silicon-Silver™ implant, a semirigid rod with a central core of braided silver wire. This implant is inserted in each corpus cavernosum, creating a permanent erection. Similar devices include the Small-Carrion semirigid rod prosthesis with a silicone sponge interior and the Flexi-rod® II, a hinged modification of the Small-Carrion device that allows the penis to be bent downward more easily when not in use. An inflatable (Scott—AMS 700 CX™) prosthesis is also available. Contraindications to surgical implants include untreated depression (acute and chronic), psychosis, severe personality disorder, and severe marital problems.

Penile revascularization is still experimental. Even more experimental is the use of papaverine injections to improve penile blood flow. Yohimbine, an α_2-adrenergic blocker also under investigation for the improvement of potency, shows some promise.

Special Concerns of Women

Older women usually can continue their earlier patterns of sexual functioning until the end of life or until serious illness intervenes. They tend to be less concerned about sexual "performance" but more worried about loss of youthful appearance than their male counterparts. Some women enjoy sex more without the fear of pregnancy. The frequency of intercourse for heterosexual women is often more related to the age, health, and sexual function of their partners than to their own sexual capacity or interest. Their partners are usually older and less vigorous than they.

Menopause: For women, most sexual changes are associated with menopause, when estrogen production slows. Although some menopausal women show very few symptoms of estrogen deficiency, the majority have significant symptoms; however, $< \frac{1}{3}$ of these women seek treatment. The effects of menopause on sexuality may include vaginal dryness leading to irritation or pain, a change in vaginal shape (shortening and narrowing), less acidic vaginal secretion with greater possibility of vaginal infections, cystitis due to thinning of vaginal walls with less protection for bladder and urethra, reduction in clitoral size, stress incontinence, and increase in facial hair.

Of the approximately 40 million postmenopausal women in the USA, 4 million take estrogen. Estrogen replacement therapy **(ERT)** has long been used for menopausal symptoms and is especially effective in controlling hot flushes and vaginal dryness. In the late 1970s, however, a higher rate of endometrial cancer was found to be associated with estrogen use, and many women discontinued ERT. Recently, ERT has regained favor for the relief of menopausal symptoms but at a lower dosage and often in combination with a progestin. However, many women are still skeptical and often experience "estrogen anxiety," a new psychologic issue of midlife sexuality.

Specific therapy for menopause is discussed in Ch. 72. Women should be helped to understand and practice self-management of menopausal symptoms. For example, aerobic exercise, relaxation technics, meditation, massage, and yoga may reduce stress, fatigue, and depression. Wearing cotton underwear can help prevent infections by allowing moisture to evaporate from the vaginal area. Girdles, panty hose, and tight slacks should not be worn by women who are susceptible to vaginal infection. Use of water-based vaginal lubricants, eg, K-Y Jelly®, can help prevent or control vaginal dryness and irritation during intercourse.

EFFECTS OF COMMON MEDICAL PROBLEMS

Heart disease: People with angina or heart failure **(HF)** and those who have undergone coronary bypass surgery or have had MI may avoid sex because of an assumed risk to life, but studies indicate that cardiac death following or during sexual activity is rare. Under most circumstances, there are few reasons to abstain from sex after MI and many to continue (eg, an opportunity for mild exercise and release of physical and emotional tension).

Depression and anxiety are common up to 1 yr after MI, and the avoidance of sexual activity may reinforce post-MI depression. Antidepressants may further reduce sexual libido and capacity. A physician's support and encouragement can greatly help patients overcome their fears. An 8- to 14-wk waiting period after MI is generally recommended before resumption of sexual intercourse, depending on the patient's interest, general fitness, and conditioning.

When HF is effectively managed medically, the physical exercise and emotional release associated with sexual activity may contribute to patients' improvement. After an episode of HF, a 2- to 3-wk recovery period is usually advised before resuming sex.

Coronary bypass surgery can produce prolonged sexual problems if the patient is not closely monitored. Physical symptoms, side effects of medical treatment, or fear of sudden death from physical exertion cause many patients to experience sexual dysfunction even before they become candidates for coronary bypass surgery. Patients should be advised about the level of sexual activity they can undertake after surgery without danger of straining the surgical repair. The sternum usually requires 3 mo to heal completely.

Exercise programs to improve cardiac function (eg, increasingly strenuous walking) can reassure patients who are afraid to resume sexual activity. Because of their previous chest pain, some patients become psychologically dependent on nitroglycerin before sexual activity, even though surgery may have eliminated the need for medication. A mild antianxiety agent used briefly may help the patient over this hurdle. Self-stimulation or mutual masturbation may be a less strenuous alternative to intercourse and usually can be started earlier in the recovery period.

β-Blockers can decrease sexual desire and cause impotence, whereas Ca channel blockers have fewer sexual side effects. Patients with arrhythmias may need the reassurance of a treadmill test to overcome anxiety about engaging in sexual activity. When certain antiarrhythmic drugs and β-blockers cannot be avoided, patients may benefit from encouragement to explore forms of intimacy and physical pleasure that are less strenuous.

Hypertension: Men or women with mild to moderate hypertension need not restrict sexual activity, although patients with marked hypertension may require some modification. In men with untreated hypertension, the incidence of impotence is reported to be about 15%; the effects of hypertension on female sexuality have not been as well studied. Selection of antihypertensive drugs should focus on those that do not impair sexual response (see EFFECTS OF DRUGS, below).

Stroke: Sexual activity has not been shown to cause stroke or to increase neurologic deficit following stroke. Unless a stroke causes severe brain damage, sexual desire is usually unimpaired; performance is more likely to be affected. Some male stroke patients experience impotence; others do not. The side of the body that is unaffected by stroke should be emphasized in lovemaking. If a female stroke patient's partner becomes impotent because he fears injuring her, reassurance may be needed.

Diabetes: Sexual problems are common in patients with diabetes. Impotence occurs 2 to 5 times more often in diabetic men than in the general population, even though sexual desire remains unchanged. Good diabetes control may reestablish potency. However, if the diabetic is already well controlled, the impotence is likely to be irreversible. Concurrent endocrine problems may reduce potency (eg, an associated thyroid condition). Diabetes appears to have less of an effect on sexuality in women than in men, although the reasons are unclear.

Arthritis: Osteoarthritis (OA) and rheumatoid arthritis (RA) may interfere with sexual desire or performance, but drugs commonly used to treat arthritis do not. A program of exercise, rest, and warm baths is especially useful in reducing arthritic discomfort and in facilitating sexual performance. Experimentation with new sexual positions that do not aggravate pain in involved joints is often helpful; during sexual activity, the side-by-side position may be preferred by both partners, especially when the patient has many tender areas and pain trigger points. Since OA tends to be less severe in the morning and RA less severe in the afternoon and evening, sexual activity can be planned for times of the day when pain and stiffness have diminished. Some patients report that regular sexual activity produces some relief from the pain of RA for 4 to 8 h. Some researchers have speculated that this may be due to hormone production, release of endorphins, or the physical activity involved.

Chronic prostatitis: Congestive prostatitis has been associated with unusually frequent sex as well as with abstinence, excessive preliminary sexual arousal, and an incomplete orgasm. With chronic or recurrent prostatitis, sexual desire may be diminished because of pain. Mild prostatitis may cause some perineal pain after ejaculation.

Therapy for chronic or recurrent prostatitis includes antibiotics, warm sitz baths, and periodic gentle prostatic massage. The practice of Kegel's exercises, which involve contractions of the muscles of the pelvic floor, may also help.

Recurrent cystitis and urethritis: Some women experience recurrent episodes of cystitis and urethritis following intercourse. Although usually due to the mechanical introduction of bacteria into the urethra during thrusting, the cause may be unclear. A urologic or gynecologic evaluation is indicated to determine the cause, as is a discussion of therapeutic and preventive options.

Peyronie's disease: Intercourse is painful for about 50% of men with Peyronie's disease, and in a few cases, when the penis is angled too greatly, penetration becomes impossible. However, in about 90% of cases tumescence is preserved, even though there may be some pain. Psychotherapy can help the patient adjust to the structural and functional changes in the penis. Results of medical and surgical intervention have not been positive overall, but symptoms sometimes disappear spontaneously after several years.

Chronic renal disease: Men with chronic renal failure are often sterile and may have reduced levels of serum testosterone, although the reason is unknown. Such patients may be treatable if the problems are not strictly organic. Treatment of associated, underlying anxiety and depression and marital counseling can be helpful. Kidney transplants often restore sexual capacity in impotent dialysis patients.

Parkinson's disease: Parkinsonism is commonly associated with depression, which may lead to impotence in men and lack of sexual desire in both men and women. Advanced organic involvement may result in impotence. Some men treated with levodopa (L-dopa) show an increase in sex drive and performance, probably because of greater mobility and an increased sense of well-being. There is little evidence that levodopa acts as an aphrodisiac, and it should not be prescribed as such.

Chronic emphysema and bronchitis: Shortness of breath associated with chronic emphysema and bronchitis hinders physical activity, including sex. Solutions include resting at intervals, finding the least taxing ways to have sexual contact, and using O_2 for shortness of breath during sexual activity.

EFFECTS OF SEXUALLY TRANSMITTED DISEASES

The incidence of sexually transmitted diseases is low in the elderly population. Nevertheless, older persons who are sexually active, and particularly those who have multiple sexual partners, are at risk, as are those who are rape victims.

Older individuals may also acquire human immunodeficiency virus **(HIV)** infection if they belong to a high-risk group (eg, homosexuals and, prior to March 1985, hemophiliacs). The most likely route of infection is through blood transfusions. Elderly IV drug abusers or elderly sexual partners of such persons are rare; thus, HIV infection via this route is less likely.

EFFECTS OF SURGERY

Rate of recovery and return to sexual activity after surgery varies. Thorough explanation of procedures, together with practical advice and emotional support before and after surgery, can enhance recovery and the return to previous levels of sexual activity.

Hysterectomy: Hysterectomy without oophorectomy does not usually cause sexual impairment. However, women who are highly sensitive to cervical and uterine sensations during orgasm are aware of the loss. Although oophorectomy decreases testosterone and other androgen levels, the sexual effects have not been well studied. Emotional reactions, eg, feelings of depression, after hysterectomy are common and can last from 2 to 10 days, although some women report them for 6 mo or longer. Symptoms are rarely sufficiently severe or long-lasting to require psychotherapy. Abstinence from sexual activity for 6 to 8 wk after hysterectomy is usually advised.

Mastectomy: For many women, deep psychologic effects following a mastectomy result from a sense of sexual mutilation. Women may temporarily lose their sexual desire because of embarrassment, inability to accept the loss of the breast, or fear that they have become less attractive to their sexual partners. Periodic depression, with sexual consequences, is common and should be expected during the first year or 2 postmastectomy.

Rehabilitation programs, such as the Reach to Recovery program of the American Cancer Society, help women and their spouses deal with the physical, psychologic, and cosmetic concerns of breast surgery. Couples should share feelings openly and support each other emotionally.

Prostatectomy: Potency is rarely affected by the most common form of prostatectomy, transurethral resection of the prostate **(TURP).** Healing usually takes up to 6 wk, after which sexual activity can be resumed. Retrograde ejaculation is common. However, erection and sexual pleasure are usually not diminished. Most men return to their presurgery sexual functioning; about 10% have some loss of ability to achieve an erection.

The most frequent cause of impotence following TURP is psychologic. Men often assume incorrectly that sexual impairment is inevitable because of the physical proximity of the prostate to the penis. Adequate information from physicians helps alleviate fears. Suprapubic or retropubic surgery is performed when the gland is very large. Perineal surgery, performed when the prostate is substantially enlarged and the patient's physical condition is poor, usually results in impotence.

Orchiectomy: The psychologic impact of this procedure can be devastating. Emotional preparation before and counseling after surgery are essential. Physiologic impotence does occur, but some men are able to have normal erections. Replacement testosterone may be contraindicated in prostatic cancer. When testosterone can be given soon after orchiectomy, potency may be maintained.

Colostomy and ileostomy: Patients who were sexually active before surgery usually continue to be so afterward, although the adjustment can be complex. Couples should be given medical guidance and offered psychologic counseling. Some 250 United Ostomy clubs throughout the USA provide information and help.

Rectal cancer surgery: Removal of the rectum and anus with a permanent colostomy may result in total impotence in men. The proximity of male genital organs to the lower rectum leaves essential nerve fibers vulnerable to damage. Women who undergo this procedure, however, usually maintain capacity for sexual arousal and orgasm, since essential nerves are farther from the surgical site.

EFFECTS OF DRUGS

Many drugs adversely affect sexuality. Some interfere with the autonomic nervous system, which is involved in normal sexual response. Others affect mood and alertness or change the production or action of sex hormones. Assessing the effects of drugs on sexuality is more difficult in women than in men, since potency problems in men are more obvious. However, drugs that affect men may also affect women. Further studies of drug effects in women are warranted.

Patients who develop sexual problems and suspect that their medications are the cause may be tempted to discontinue the drugs or decrease the dosages without informing their physician. It is best to discuss this possibility openly with patients and encourage them to report any side effects.

Tranquilizers, antidepressants, and antihypertensives: Neuroleptics, such as thioridazine and other phenothiazines, may inhibit erection or ejaculation, even though the capacity for erection remains. So-called mild tranquilizers can depress the sexual responses of women and men, and commonly used antidepressants have been reported to inhibit sexual desire.

Antihypertensive drugs are the most common pharmacologic cause of impaired erection. Methyldopa reduces blood flow to the pelvic area, therefore inhibiting erection. The effects of other drugs are listed in TABLES 58–1 and 58–2.

Alcohol: The excessive use of alcohol is a frequent yet seldom-considered factor in sexual problems; although it may increase desire, alcohol decreases performance. Up to 80% of men who drink heavily may experience serious sexual side effects, including impotence, sterility, and loss of sexual desire. Desire in women may also be affected. Fortunately,

TABLE 58-1. POSSIBLE DRUG EFFECTS ON FEMALE SEXUALITY

Increased libido:
androgens; chlordiazepoxide (antianxiety effect); mazindol

Decreased libido:
(See list of drug effects on male sexuality. Some of these *may* have potential for reducing libido in the female. The literature is sparse on this subject.)

Impaired arousal and orgasm:
anticholinergics; clonidine; methyldopa; monoamine oxidase inhibitors (MAOIs); tricyclic antidepressants (TADs)

Breast enlargement:
penicillamine; TADs

Galactorrhea (spontaneous flow of milk):
amphetamines; chlorpromazine; cimetidine; haloperidol; heroin; methyldopa; metoclopramide; phenothiazines; reserpine; sulpiride; TADs

Virilization (acne, hirsutism, lowering of voice, enlargement of clitoris):
anabolic drugs; androgens; haloperidol

(Adapted from J. W. Long: "Many common medications can affect sexual expression," in *Generations,* Vol. 6, pp. 32–34, 1981. Reprinted with permission from *Generations,* Journal of the American Society on Aging, 833 Market Street, Suite 512, San Francisco, California 94103. Copyright 1981 WGS, ASA.)

TABLE 58-2. POSSIBLE DRUG EFFECTS ON MALE SEXUALITY

Increased libido:
androgens (replacement therapy in deficiency states); baclofen; (antianxiety effect); diazepam chlordiazepoxide (antianxiety effect); haloperidol; levodopa (may be an indirect effect due to improved sense of well-being)

Decreased libido:
antihistamines; barbiturates; chlordiazepoxide (sedative effect); chlorpromazine 10–20% of users; cimetidine; clofibrate; clonidine 10–20% of users; diazepam (sedative effect); disulfiram; estrogens (therapy for prostatic cancer); fenfluramine; heroin; licorice; medroxyprogesterone; methyldopa 10–15% of users; perhexilene; prazosin 15% of users; propranolol rarely; reserpine; spironolactone; tricyclic antidepressants (TADs)

Impaired erection (impotence):
anticholinergics; antihistamines; baclofen; barbiturates (when abused); chlordiazepoxide (in high dosage); chlorpromazine; cimetidine; clofibrate; clonidine 10–20% of users; cocaine; diazepam (in high dosage); digitalis and its glycosides; disopyramide; disulfiram (uncertain); estrogens (therapy for prostatic cancer); ethacrynic acid 5% of users; ethionamide; fenfluramine; furosemide 5% of users; guanethidine; haloperidol 10–20% of users; heroin; hydroxyprogesterone (therapy for prostatic cancer); licorice; lithium; marijuana; mesoridazine; methantheline; methyldopa 10–15% of users; monoamine oxidase inhibitors (MAOIs) 10–15% of users; perhexilene; prazosin infrequently; propranolol infrequently; reserpine; spironolactone; thiazide diuretics 5% of users; thioridazine; TADs

(Continued)

TABLE 58-2. POSSIBLE DRUG EFFECTS ON MALE SEXUALITY
(Cont'd)

Impaired ejaculation:
anticholinergics; barbiturates (when abused); chlorpromazine; clonidine; estrogens (therapy for prostatic cancer); guanethidine; heroin; mesoridazine; methyldopa; MAOIs; phenoxybenzamine; phentolamine; reserpine; thiazide diuretics; thioridazine; TADs

Decreased plasma testosterone:
adrenocorticotropic hormone (ACTH); barbiturates; digoxin; haloperidol (increased testosterone with low dosage, decreased testosterone with high dosage); lithium; marijuana; medroxyprogesterone; MAOIs; spironolactone

Impaired spermatogenesis (reduced fertility):
adrenocorticosteroids (eg, prednisone); androgens (moderate to high dosage, extended use); antimalarials; aspirin (abusive, chronic use); chlorambucil; cimetidine; colchicine; co-trimoxazole; cyclophosphamide; estrogens (therapy for prostatic cancer); marijuana; medroxyprogesterone; methotrexate; MAOIs; niridazole; nitrofurantoin; spironolactone; sulfasalazine; testosterone (moderate to high dosage, extended use); vitamin C (in doses of ≥ 1 gm)

Testicular disorders:
Swelling: TADs. *Inflammation:* oxyphenbutazone. *Atrophy:* androgens (moderate to high dosage, extended use); chlorpromazine; spironolactone

Penile disorders:
Priapism: cocaine; heparin; phenothiazines. *Peyronie's disease:* metoprolol

Gynecomastia (excessive development of the male breast):
androgens (partial conversion to estrogen); carmustine; busulfan; chlormadinone; chlorpromazine; chlortetracycline; cimetidine; clonidine (infrequently); diethylstilbestrol (DES); digitalis and its glycosides; estrogens (therapy for prostatic cancer); ethionamide; griseofulvin; haloperidol; heroin; isoniazid; marijuana; methyldopa; phenelzine; reserpine; spironolactone; thioridazine; TADs; vincristine

Feminization (loss of libido, impotence, gynecomastia, testicular atrophy):
conjugated estrogens

(Adapted from J. W. Long: "Many common medications can affect sexual expression," in *Generations*, Vol. 6, pp. 32–34, 1981. Reprinted with permission from *Generations*, Journal of the American Society on Aging, 833 Market Street, Suite 512, San Francisco, California 94103. Copyright 1981 WGS, ASA.)

many of the effects of moderate to heavy drinking are reversible if the drinking is stopped in time. Since tolerance for alcohol decreases with age, smaller and smaller amounts may produce negative effects. People who choose to drink regularly should limit themselves to a maximum of 1.5 oz of hard liquor, 6 oz of wine, or 16 oz of beer in any 24-h period. Drinking should be avoided for several hours before sexual activity or at least limited to 1 drink.

SOCIAL, EMOTIONAL, AND PSYCHOLOGIC ISSUES

Sexuality in old age is associated more with intimacy than just with the act of sex. Sexuality is frequently described in terms that include the opportunity to express passion, affection, admiration, and loyalty; the affirmation that one's body is functioning well; the maintenance of a strong sense of identity; a means of self-assertion; a protection from anxiety; a renewal of a sense of romance; a general affirmation of life, especially the expression of joy; and a continuing opportunity to search for new growth and experience.

However, not all older persons have such positive attitudes. Some, even though they may be physically and mentally healthy, have internalized the negative cultural stereotype of the "typical" older person as a desexualized invalid. They may refuse to discuss the issue of sexuality or to accept help when problems are obvious. The inability to come to terms with aging may lead such persons to envy the young and to feel hostility and bitterness toward them, to show prejudice against other older people and refuse to associate with them, to reject their partner who is also aging, and to make frantic attempts to appear young.

Feelings of sexual guilt and shame may also surface. Some individuals > 60 yr of age, brought up in a climate of Victorian-like prudery, were probably misinformed about issues of sexuality and made to feel guilty about their desires. In many cases, the guilt and shame have become ingrained and inhibit all aspects of sexual expression. Reassurance and information from their physician may help these persons achieve a more positive self-image.

Special Issues in the Later Years

Common emotional reactions (eg, boredom, fear, fatigue, and grief) and problems with a mate influence the sexual behavior of persons of all ages. In addition, elderly persons are likely to experience negative effects of retirement, illness or incapacitation of the partner, and uncomplimentary patterns of personality change (typically, women become more self-assertive and men more nurturant as they grow older).

Older women also face several special problems. In a heterosexual relationship, the man usually becomes incapacitated first, leaving the woman to act as care giver. This change in the relationship can lead to bilateral feelings of frustration, martyrdom, and resentment. Rehabilitation after surgery or illness must include consideration of sexual and emotional issues for patient and partner.

With increasing age, women outnumber men. Over 50% of older women are widows, 7% were never married, and 2% are divorced. Thus, about 60% of older women are without a spouse, in contrast to about 20% of older men. Women living alone constitute a subclass that is more likely to be poor and to have a series of complex and interacting physical and psychosocial problems.

An estimated 10% of older individuals are homosexual. Long-term relationships are common, although many in this generation of elderly homosexuals have not publicly revealed their sexual preference. Their relationships and physical problems with sexuality are not markedly different from those of heterosexuals and require the same thoughtful diagnosis and treatment.

HYPOKALEMIA

A serum K level < 3.8 mEq/L; the condition is considered severe at levels < 3.3 mEq/L. The most common cause of hypokalemia in the elderly is diuretic therapy, which accounts for about 20% of cases in this age group, with women and patients with edematous conditions being more susceptible. The second most common cause is diarrhea from disease or chronic laxative abuse. Other causes are vomiting, renal tubular acidosis secondary to dysproteinemic states, urinary K losses associated with glycosuria and ketonuria, and malnutrition, particularly starvation. In diabetic acidosis, K shifts from the intracellular to the extracellular compartment and may mask losses in the urine. The deficiency becomes evident when acidosis is corrected and fluid is replaced. Secondary hyperaldosteronism (eg, in heart failure, cirrhosis, renal artery stenosis) can also cause hypokalemia in the elderly. Renal losses of K can be induced by gentamicin, amphotericin B, carbenicillin, and massive doses of penicillin. Insulin and β agonists such as terbutaline and metaproterenol can lower K levels substantially without depleting total body stores by shifting K into cells, as can B_{12} therapy for severe pernicious anemia.

Symptoms, Signs, Laboratory Findings, and Diagnosis

Confusion, disorientation, fatigue, weakness, apathy, and anorexia often signal hypokalemia. Muscle cramps and even paralysis result from severe K depletion. Most dangerous are ventricular arrhythmias in patients receiving digitalis.

Metabolic alkalosis usually accompanies low K levels unless the cause is diarrhea or renal tubular acidosis, in which case metabolic acidosis is present. The kidneys may lose their ability to concentrate urine; this is reversed when K is replaced. Characteristic ECG changes include ST segment depression, U waves, flattened T waves, ectopic beats, and tachyarrhythmias. Severe K depletion can disrupt A-V conduction.

Treatment

A K-rich diet or correction of the underlying cause may suffice. Magnesium depletion may have to be corrected before hypokalemia responds to treatment. Use of a K-sparing diuretic or a diuretic/ACE inhibitor combination may mitigate diuretic-induced hypokalemia, but such therapy should be avoided if renal insufficiency is present. When supplementation is required, 10% KCl 20 to 80 mEq/day in excess of losses is given orally in divided doses for several days. For metabolic acidosis, K gluconate or a mixture of K acetate, citrate, and bicarbonate is more suitable. Controlled-release K preparations may cause GI ulceration and bleeding and should be used cautiously.

KCl may be given IV when K depletion is severe or the patient is unable to tolerate oral administration. In acidemia, serum K may be high despite K depletion; K replacement should be delayed until the K level falls. K administration should not exceed a concentration of 40 mEq/L or a rate of 10 to 20 mEq/h unless the situation is critical; concentrations up to 60 mEq/L and rates up to 40 mEq/h may then be used, along with frequent ECG and serum K monitoring.

§3. ORGAN SYSTEMS: HEMATOLOGIC DISORDERS

---

59. NORMAL AGING AND PATTERNS OF HEMATOLOGIC DISEASE

Michael L. Freedman and *Nancy T. Weintraub*

Normal Changes of Aging

Before blood diseases in the elderly can be considered, normal change must be defined. The percentage of the marrow space occupied by hematopoietic tissue varies throughout life, declining progressively from birth until about age 30, when it levels off; after about age 70, it again progressively declines. Whether this second decline is due to a real reduction in the blood-forming elements or to a relative reduction caused by an increase in bone marrow fat is not known.

There is evidence of the following age-related changes in marrow function: (1) Marrow from older individuals can be maintained by serial transplantation in tissue culture just as long as marrow from younger individuals, but the number of stem cells in the marrow decreases significantly with increasing age. (2) Incorporation of iron in marrow culture from older individuals is comparable to that from younger individuals but increases to a lesser degree when stimulated by the addition of erythropoietin. (3) Intact older animals are unable to respond to bleeding or hypoxia with increased erythropoiesis as efficiently as younger animals, but whether the defect lies with the hemopoietic elements or with age-related changes in the marrow environment is unclear. (4) Although iron uptake from the gut is normal in the elderly, ineffective erythropoiesis results in an impaired incorporation of iron into RBCs.

These age-related changes in marrow function are not secondary to nutritional deficiencies, since both total body and bone marrow iron increase with age, and both folate and vitamin B_{12} levels in healthy elderly subjects remain in the normal range.

Age-related changes in the peripheral blood include the following: (1) Average values of Hb and Hct decrease slightly with increasing age but remain within the normal adult range. (2) Mean corpuscular volume **(MCV)** increases slightly with advancing age, but RBC morphology does not change significantly. (3) RBC content of 2,3-diphosphoglycerate (DPG) decreases with increasing age. (4) RBC osmotic fragility increases with increasing age, but the normal circulating RBC life span is not reduced.

Factors that have been measured and do not change with age include RBC survival, total blood volume, RBC volume, and platelet morphology. However, conflicting evidence has been reported concerning other factors: Lymphocyte and granulocyte counts have been reported to be either normal or slightly decreased; platelet counts have been reported to be either normal or slightly elevated; and platelet function in healthy elderly subjects has been found to be normal, decreased, or increased.

Patterns of Disease

Elderly individuals are subject to the same blood disorders as are younger individuals, but only those that are especially common or primarily affect older people are discussed here. Certain age-related adjustments are also required for therapy of some disorders. Procedures and illnesses that are unchanged in the elderly include blood transfusion, granulocytopenias, thrombocytopenias, and clotting disorders. For a discussion of these, the reader is referred to the 15th edition of THE MERCK MANUAL.

---

60. ANEMIAS

Michael L. Freedman and *Nancy T. Weintraub*

Decreases of RBC or Hb content because of blood loss, impaired production, or RBC destruction.

Anemia is common in elderly people, with its incidence ranging to $> \frac{1}{3}$ of outpatients. Anemia is never normal, and when older patients with significant anemia (ie, Hb $<$ 12 gm/dL, Hct $<$ 36%) are evaluated, an underlying disease is often discovered. Because anemia is a symptom, not a diagnosis, its presence indicates the need for an attempt to discover the cause.

Symptoms and Signs

While generally these are similar to those seen in younger people, certain clinical features may be more common in the elderly because of a higher incidence of other, possibly unrelated underlying diseases. Fatigue, shortness of breath, worsening angina, and peripheral edema are more common when there is preexisting atherosclerotic heart disease and/or heart failure. Mental status changes, including confusion, depression, agitation, and apathy, may occur even in previously unimpaired individuals. Dizziness is also common. Pallor may be less noticeable but often can be seen in the mucosa of the oral cavity and in the conjunctiva.

CLASSIFICATION OF ANEMIAS

The most diagnostically useful way to classify anemias is probably by mean corpuscular volume **(MCV)** (see TABLE 60–1). However, there is overlap among categories; anemias of mixed etiologies present atypically.

MICROCYTIC ANEMIA

Anemia in which the MCV is < 80 fL.

IRON-DEFICIENCY ANEMIA

Chronic anemia characterized by small, pale RBCs and depletion of iron stores.

This is the most common microcytic anemia in the elderly, accounting for almost 60% of all anemias in people > 65 yr of age. Iron deficiency is never a normal finding in older individuals. The body has no mechanism for eliminating excessive iron; consequently, total body and bone marrow iron stores increase with advancing age. **Dietary iron deficiency** in adults is virtually unknown in the USA, and **iron malabsorption** occurs only after total gastrectomy or with severe, generalized malabsorption. If these conditions do not exist, iron deficiency implies **blood loss,** most commonly from the GI or genitourinary tract, and investigation of these systems is mandatory. Possible causes include carcinoma, ulcer, atrophic gastritis, gastritis from drug ingestion, postmenopausal vaginal bleeding, and bleeding hemorrhoids. Recurrent hemoptysis may also be responsible.

Pathophysiology

Iron deficiency affects many tissues, most notably the GI tract. Atrophy of the tongue and buccal mucosa and angular stomatitis may occur. Abnormalities of the gastric mucosa are frequent; superficial gastritis is accompanied by a reduction in HCl secretion, which may progress to atrophic gastritis and achlorhydria. In people > 30 yr of age, achlorhydria is not reversible with iron therapy. Inability to secrete intrinsic factor may also occur, resulting in a coexistent B_{12} deficiency (see below).

TABLE 60-1. ANEMIA CLASSIFIED BY USUAL MEAN CORPUSCULAR VOLUME (MCV)

Microcytic (MCV < 80 fL)
 Iron deficiency (can be normocytic)
 Sideroblastic anemia (can be normocytic)
 Thalassemia minor
 Chronic disease (usually normocytic)

Normocytic (MCV 80–100 fL)
 Iron deficiency (usually microcytic)
 Chronic disease (can be microcytic)
 Endocrine disorders
 Sideroblastic anemia (can be microcytic)
 "Unexplained" anemia
 Hemolytic anemia (can be macrocytic)
 Aplastic anemia
 Chronic liver disease (can be macrocytic)
 Bone marrow replacement by metastases
 Multiple myeloma
 Myeloid metaplasia
 Leukemia

Macrocytic (MCV > 100 fL)
 Chronic liver disease (can be normocytic)
 Vitamin B_{12} deficiency
 Folate deficiency
 Hemolytic anemia (can be normocytic)

fL = femtoliter.

Iron deficiency may also cause nervous system dysfunction; fatigue, irritability, and decreased cognitive function have been reported with iron deficiency in younger people, but whether they occur in the elderly is not known.

Diagnosis

The diagnosis is based on the following features: The peripheral blood smear is populated with microcytic hypochromic cells, and the MCV, the mean corpuscular Hb **(MCH),** and the mean corpuscular Hb concentration **(MCHC)** are all reduced. In early iron deficiency, however, these values may still be normal. Chronic bleeding frequently results in an elevated platelet count, but the reticulocyte count is not increased. Measurement of **serum iron** and **transferrin** level (total iron-binding capacity, or **TIBC**) can assist in the diagnosis of iron deficiency if the serum iron is reduced and the TIBC is increased, resulting in a transferrin saturation (serum iron/TIBC) < 16%. However, this ratio is frequently not useful, because the serum iron and TIBC decrease with advanced age. Both serum iron and TIBC are decreased in chronic disease states, and the ratio has been shown to decrease in the evening, even in nonanemic young adults.

Serum ferritin accurately reflects bone marrow iron stores, and a low value indicates reduced marrow iron. However, serum ferritin can be falsely elevated by infection, inflammation, liver disease, and states of increased RBC turnover (eg, ineffective erythropoiesis and hemolysis). In ambiguous cases, the combination of a somewhat decreased serum ferritin and an increased TIBC may help clarify the diagnosis of iron deficiency.

If a conclusive diagnosis still cannot be made, a bone marrow aspirate stained for iron may be performed. In iron deficiency, iron will either be absent or present in only trace amounts. Another option is to give a 1-mo trial of oral iron in the form of ferrous salts (see Treatment, below). If the anemia is due to iron deficiency, both Hb and Hct will increase. If no increase occurs, either the patient is not iron deficient, blood loss is exceeding new blood formation, or an inflammatory or malignant process is contributing to the anemia.

Treatment

This involves both finding and eliminating the source of bleeding and correcting the iron deficiency. Oral iron therapy is inexpensive, safe, and convenient. Approximately 150 to 200 mg iron/day is needed, making dietary replacement impossible. **Only ferrous iron salts should be used,** and enteric-coated or sustained-release preparations should be *avoided,* since they are not well absorbed. The simplest oral preparation is ferrous sulfate 300 mg, which contains 60 mg iron/tablet. One tablet tid, 1 h before meals, supplies 180 mg iron. To prevent constipation and gastric irritation, therapy may begin with 1 tablet/day and the dose gradually increased over 1 to 2 wk. Liquid preparations are available for patients unable to swallow tablets. Response to treatment is monitored serially by Hb, Hct, and ferritin levels. Usually ≥ 6 mo of treatment is needed to replenish iron stores after bleeding has stopped.

In the rare patient who has severe malabsorption, who cannot tolerate oral iron, whose iron stores need rapid replenishing, or whose bleeding is continuing, parenteral iron may be used. **Parenteral iron** is available as iron-dextran and may be given IV or by deep IM injection. The maximal recommended dosage is 2 mL/day, which delivers 100 mg. IV infusion should be given at a rate of ≤ 1 mL/min. *This therapy has been associated with anaphylactic shock, and a test dose of 0.5 mL should be given before treatment begins.* Other side effects include pain at the injection site, fever, and arthralgias. The most expensive and potentially hazardous way to replete iron, of course, is by **transfusion.** Each milliliter of transfused RBCs delivers 1 mg iron.

OTHER MICROCYTIC ANEMIAS

With the exception of **thalassemia minor,** anemias caused by abnormal Hbs are not usually first diagnosed in old age. Thalassemia minor occurs in individuals who are heterozygous for genes that produce very little or no α or β Hb chain. These conditions produce either microcytosis without anemia or a mild, microcytic anemia with hypochromia, target cells, anisocytosis, poikilocytosis, polychromatophilia, and basophilic stippling of RBCs on the peripheral smear. There is no reticulocytosis; serum iron, TIBC, and serum ferritin are all normal. Hb electrophoresis may reveal an increase in the minor Hbs, particularly fetal Hb **(HbF),** or HbA_2 in β-thalassemia; it may be normal in α-thalassemia. No treatment is required for these conditions, and iron therapy is *contraindicated,* since it may produce iron overload.

Anemia of chronic disease may be microcytic but is more commonly normocytic. **Sideroblastic anemia** may also be either microcytic or normocytic and is discussed under MYELODYSPLASTIC SYNDROMES in Ch. 61.

NORMOCYTIC ANEMIA

Anemia in which the MCV is 80 to 100 fL.

ANEMIA OF CHRONIC DISEASE

The most common normocytic anemia in the elderly occurs secondary to other chronic diseases, accounting for up to 10% of the anemias in this population. Following are some of the causes:

Chronic infection or inflammation commonly produces anemia, usually after 4 to 8 wk of illness. The anemia is usually mild, normochromic, and normocytic but may be slightly microcytic. This anemia probably results from a combination of slightly decreased erythropoietin production, decreased RBC survival, and a block in the delivery of iron from the reticuloendothelial system to the bone marrow. The reticulocyte count is low, serum iron and TIBC are normal or reduced, and serum ferritin is normal or increased. Treatment is addressed to the underlying disorder.

Renal insufficiency produces a normochromic, normocytic anemia resulting from decreased erythropoiesis and decreased RBC survival. Serum iron stores are comparable to those described for anemia due to infection or inflammation. Unless the renal disease can be reversed, the only treatment is transfusion when the anemia becomes severe, although the experimental administration of exogenous erythropoietin to small numbers of younger dialysis patients has corrected their anemias.

Chronic liver disease produces a normochromic, normocytic or a normochromic, macrocytic anemia resulting from decreased RBC production and survival. Large quantities of alcohol are directly toxic to the bone marrow as well as the liver. Unless liver disease is complicated by bleeding, TIBC is decreased and serum iron is increased, resulting in an increased transferrin saturation. Serum ferritin in also increased and often reflects total body iron overload.

Endocrine disorders that commonly produce anemia are pituitary insufficiency, adrenal insufficiency, and hypothyroidism. In all 3 disorders, anemia is normocytic and normochromic. Hypothyroidism, however, is sometimes complicated by iron deficiency, producing microcytosis and hypochromia, or by associated megaloblastic anemia (see VITAMIN B$_{12}$ DEFICIENCY and FOLATE DEFICIENCY, below), in which case the cells will be macrocytic and normochromic. Unless a specific deficiency of iron, vitamin B$_{12}$, or folate is identified, treatment is addressed to the underlying disorder.

"UNEXPLAINED" ANEMIA

A mild normochromic, normocytic anemia, with Hb usually between 11 and 12 gm/dL, has been reported in people > 70 yr of age and cannot be accounted for by any underlying disease or deficiency. The bone marrow does not contain ringed sideroblasts. This unexplained anemia accounts for > 30% of the anemias in this age group. It is associated with low neutrophil, lymphocyte, and platelet counts and with increased RBC 2,3-diphosphoglycerate (2,3-DPG) levels, implying that this condition is not merely a normal, age-related variant. Its significance is unknown, but it is probably a myelodysplastic syndrome (see Ch. 61).

HEMOLYTIC ANEMIA

Acquired hemolytic anemia (ie, *hemolysis not due to a congenital abnormality of the RBC*) is a normochromic, normocytic anemia that may occur at any age, but the incidence of this disorder increases with advancing age. Increased peripheral destruction of RBCs results in increased production of immature RBCs by the bone marrow; this produces an increased reticulocyte count and polychromatophilia on the peripheral blood smear. Since reticulocytes are larger than mature RBCs, the RBC indexes may become macrocytic if the reticulocytosis is brisk enough. RBC destruction results in increased unconjugated bilirubin, AST (SGOT), and LDH in the serum, decreased serum haptoglobin, and increased urine urobilinogen. If hemolysis is intravascular, urine hemosiderin is increased as well. The direct antiglobulin (Coombs') test is used to detect antibody or complement on the RBC and can also identify the antigen to which the antibody is reacting.

Causes of acquired hemolytic anemia: Idiopathic autoimmune hemolysis may be a result of warm-reactive antibodies of the IgG class; cold agglutinins that are usually of the IgM class but that may be of the IgG class as well; or a nonagglutinating, cold-activated hemolysin of the IgG class. Idiopathic cold-agglutinin disease is primarily a disease of old age.

Immune hemolysis may also be secondary to a variety of other illnesses. Approximately 30% of secondary immune hemolytic anemias are caused by lymphoproliferative diseases (see Ch. 61), including chronic lymphocytic leukemia, non-Hodgkin's lymphoma, Hodgkin's disease,

and multiple myeloma. Agnogenic myeloid metaplasia (see MYELOPRO-
LIFERATIVE DISORDERS in Ch. 61), SLE, viral infections, *Mycoplasma
pneumoniae* infection, syphilis, and various nonhematologic malignancies
are also associated with immune hemolytic anemia.

Drug reaction is another major cause of hemolytic anemia. The elderly
are prone to develop this problem simply because they generally take
more drugs than younger individuals. Several types of drug-induced hemolysis have been described (see TABLE 60–2). Methyldopa causes auto-
antibody formation, with antibodies directed against normal RBC antigens, in 10 to 40% of people taking the drug. These antibodies attach to
the RBC, resulting in a positive direct Coombs' test against IgG; however, < 1% actually develop hemolysis. Discontinuance of the drug
usually results in a correction of the anemia, but autoantibodies may
persist for months to years. Other drugs that rarely produce autoimmune hemolysis include ibuprofen, L-dopa, and procainamide.

A second type of drug-induced, immune hemolytic anemia results
when the drug binds to the surface of the RBC, acting as a hapten. Antibodies, usually IgG, are produced against the drug-RBC complex. The
direct Coombs' test is positive, and if the offending drug is added to
test RBCs, the indirect Coombs' test is also positive. The drugs most
commonly associated with this problem are the cephalosporins and penicillin. The anemia clears when the drug is discontinued.

A third type of drug-induced, immune hemolytic anemia occurs when
a drug, either alone or bound to plasma protein, stimulates the production of antibodies to the drug. Drug-antibody immune complexes form
in the circulation and bind briefly to the RBC. Hemolysis occurs be-

TABLE 60–2. SELECTED DRUGS CAUSING HEMOLYTIC ANEMIA

Autoimmune	**Immune complex** (continued)
Procainamide	Hydrochlorothiazide
Methyldopa	Ibuprofen
Ibuprofen	Insulin
L-dopa	Isoniazid
Hapten type	Methadone
Cephalosporins	Nalidixic acid
Penicillins	Phenacetin
Tetracyclines	Procainamide
Tolbutamide	Quinidine
Immune complex	Quinine
Acetaminophen	Rifampin
Aminosalicylic acid	Streptomycin
Antihistamines	Sulfonamides
Chlorpropamide	Tetracyclines
Chlorpromazine	Triamterene
Erythromycin	Tolbutamide
Hydralazine	

cause the complex activates complement on the RBC surface. The Coombs' test is positive for complement but not for IgG. The sulfonamides, quinidine, quinine, and insulin, as well as many other drugs, can produce this phenomenon. Hemolysis ceases when the drug is withdrawn.

Treatment

Idiopathic autoimmune hemolysis secondary to warm-reactive antibodies of the IgG class responds to steroid therapy approximately 75% of the time. **Prednisone** 60 mg/day in divided doses is the initial treatment, although occasionally 100 mg/day is needed. A rise in Hb and Hct and a drop in the reticulocyte count usually occur in the first 3 to 14 days, but response may be delayed up to 8 wk. Once remission occurs, steroids may be tapered by 5 mg/wk, but relapse requires increasing the dose by 15 to 20 mg, followed by a more gradual tapering. Some patients continue to require a small daily dose or alternate-day therapy for long periods of time.

If there is no response to 60 mg/day of prednisone after 4 to 8 wk, higher doses may be tried or the weak androgen **danazol** may be added at a dosage of 200 mg bid to qid. If this fails, the next step is usually **splenectomy,** which results in long-term remission in 50 to 75% of cases. In patients who either do not respond to the above measures or who are poor surgical candidates, the **immunosuppressive agents** cyclophosphamide (150 mg/day) or azathioprine (200 mg/day) may be useful.

Most patients with warm-antibody autoimmune hemolysis do not require **transfusion,** but for those experiencing severe symptoms from anemia, transfusion can be considered. Compatibility testing of the blood is problematic, and the autoantibodies will reduce the survival of the transfused RBCs. **Plasmapheresis** is usually not successful, since IgG has a large volume of distribution in the body.

Idiopathic cold-agglutinin disease due to IgM is treated by avoidance of exposure to the cold. **Steroids** and **splenectomy** usually are *not* helpful, although they have been used with some success in small numbers of patients with disease due to either low-titer IgM or to IgG. **Plasmapheresis** may lead to temporary improvement, since the IgM is confined to the intravascular space. Disease caused by cold-activated IgG hemolysin is also treated by avoidance of exposure to the cold. In both of these diseases, **transfusion** should be performed with warmed, washed RBCs.

Immune hemolytic anemia secondary to other diseases usually improves only with treatment of the underlying illness. If this is not possible, treatment may be tried as described above, but success is less likely than in idiopathic disease.

Treatment of **drug-induced hemolytic anemia** usually consists of simply discontinuing the responsible drug. In rare instances, methyldopa-induced autoimmune hemolysis continues long enough to require a course of steroids, as described above.

APLASTIC ANEMIA

Normochromic, normocytic anemia due to decreased bone marrow production of either RBCs alone (pure RBC aplasia) or of all cell lines. In this disorder, the reticulocyte count is low; serum iron, vitamin B_{12}, and folate are normal; and the bone marrow is hypoplastic. If thrombocytopenia occurs, bleeding may become a problem.

Idiopathic aplastic anemia is usually a disease of adolescents and young adults. **Secondary aplastic anemia** can be caused by chemicals, radiation, or drugs, especially antibiotics, gold, and anticonvulsants (see TABLE 60–3). Again, because the elderly are frequently exposed to a large number of drugs, they are especially susceptible to this illness. Thymoma and chronic lymphocytic leukemia are sometimes associated with pure RBC aplasia. Aplastic anemia is not very common; its overall mortality is > 50%.

TABLE 60–3. SELECTED DRUGS ASSOCIATED WITH APLASTIC ANEMIA

Acetazolamide	Gold
Antibiotics	Nonsteroidal anti-inflammatory agents
Anticonvulsants	Oral hypoglycemics
Antihistamines	Phenothiazines
Chloramphenicol	Quinidine
Chlorothiazide	Sulfonamides

All potentially offending drugs must be discontinued. Androgens may be given, but they are rarely successful. Bone marrow transplantation, the only effective therapy in younger adults, is not an option in older patients, who cannot tolerate transplant-related complications. Ongoing supportive treatment with transfusions is therefore required. Pure RBC aplasia may respond to prednisone or cyclophosphamide, and if it is associated with thymoma, resection of the tumor may be helpful.

MALIGNANCY

Replacement of the normal marrow by tumor is a cause of normochromic, normocytic anemia. Serum iron, vitamin B_{12}, and folate values are normal or elevated, and the ESR is usually elevated. Tumor may be metastatic from other sites or a primary disease of the hematopoietic tissue.

MACROCYTIC ANEMIA

Anemia in which the MCV is > 100 fL.

MCV increases slightly with increasing age but not enough to produce significant macrocytosis. Relatively few disorders routinely produce macrocytic anemia. Anemia secondary to chronic liver disease and hemolytic anemia may be macrocytic. The other 2 disorders that produce macrocytosis are the megaloblastic anemias due to either vitamin B_{12} or folate deficiency.

VITAMIN B_{12} DEFICIENCY

This deficiency accounts for up to 9% of anemias in elderly populations. Vitamin B_{12} is stored in the liver in large quantities; thus, after a lesion preventing B_{12} absorption occurs, clinical evidence of B_{12} deficiency may not be apparent for many years. For this reason, patients who are B_{12} deficient may present with profound anemias that are very well tolerated, with no volume depletion or orthostatic hypotension. In fact, transfusion may place these patients at risk for development of heart failure.

Symptoms of B_{12} deficiency may be no more specific than fatigue due to profound anemia. Characteristically, however, patients develop glossitis, with a smooth, red tongue; mild jaundice; and neurologic changes. The latter changes develop in long-standing deficiency and include paresthesias, abnormal position and vibration sensation, gait ataxia due to degeneration of the posterolateral columns of the spinal cord, and various psychiatric disorders. These neurologic changes do not always improve when the deficiency is treated.

Laboratory abnormalities associated with vitamin B_{12} deficiency include macrocytosis and hypersegmented polymorphonuclear leukocytes on peripheral smear, and increased serum bilirubin and LDH levels resulting from ineffective erythropoiesis. The platelet count may be reduced, and serum B_{12} level is low, often < 100 pg/mL. Approximately 30% of patients with B_{12} deficiency have elevated serum folate levels. Examination of the bone marrow shows characteristic megaloblastic changes.

Low serum B_{12} levels have been documented in some older individuals without anemia or characteristic changes on peripheral smear and with normal Schilling tests (see below). Treatment with B_{12} in this group has not been beneficial, although this is still under investigation. Serum B_{12} levels may also be decreased by iron and folate deficiency, even when stores of B_{12} are normal.

The most common cause of B_{12} deficiency is **pernicious anemia (PA),** in which a lack of intrinsic factor prevents B_{12} absorption. In this autoimmune disease, antibodies are produced against parietal cells, in which intrinsic factor is synthesized. It is most common in people > 60 yr of age and is often associated with other autoimmune disorders. **Other causes of B_{12} deficiency** include gastrectomy, intestinal disease, and intestinal bacterial overgrowth. These causes may be identified by the **Schilling test,** which measures the absorption of radiolabeled B_{12} with and without the addition of administered intrinsic factor.

If the patient has PA, the absorption of B_{12} is abnormal but will be corrected by adding intrinsic factor. If absorption is not corrected by intrinsic factor, the patient should be treated for a few weeks with a broad-spectrum antibiotic and the test then repeated. If absorption becomes normal, the problem was bacterial overgrowth. If the patient has PA and has been B_{12} deficient for some time, B_{12} malabsorption may be due to malfunction of the small intestine as a result of the B_{12} deficiency. To test for this possibility, the Schilling test should be repeated after a few months of B_{12} supplementation.

Treatment of B_{12} deficiency requires lifetime parenteral B_{12} administration. Although 100 μg IM daily for the first 5 days is sufficient for initial treatment, it is usually more convenient to give 1000 μg daily for the first week, then weekly for 4 wk or until the Hct is normal, and then monthly for life. The response to treatment is usually a brisk reticulocytosis within 1 wk. While the anemia should be corrected within 1 mo, abnormalities in the peripheral smear may persist for a year. Because hypokalemia and hypophosphatemia may occur early in therapy, serum phosphate and K should be monitored and supplements given, if necessary. Transfusion may produce volume overload; if it is necessary, it should be done slowly and the patient should be monitored.

When B_{12} deficiency has been misdiagnosed as folate deficiency, consequent treatment with folate alone may improve the hematologic disorder, but it will not affect the neurologic changes associated with B_{12} deficiency and, therefore, must be avoided.

FOLATE DEFICIENCY

Deficiency of folic acid produces changes in the peripheral blood smear and the bone marrow that are indistinguishable from those due to B_{12} deficiency. The incidence of folate deficiency in the elderly is controversial, partly because of varying definitions of the lower limits of normal and differences in radioimmunoassay and microbiologic methods used for measuring both RBC and serum folate. Serum folate levels fluctuate rapidly and do not necessarily reflect body stores; RBC folate levels are more stable and, therefore, clinically reliable.

Normal body stores of folate can be depleted in < 6 mo. Rapid folate deficiency can be caused by malabsorption, poor nutrition, alcoholism, and states of increased folate utilization such as hemolytic anemia and neoplasia. Drugs, eg, anticonvulsants, trimethoprim, triamterene, and nitrofurantoin, also cause folate deficiency. Nevertheless, anemia due purely to folate deficiency does not seem to be common in the elderly.

Although according to traditional teaching, folate deficiency alone does not produce neurologic abnormalities, there is evidence that pure folate deficiency may result in nervous system changes that are virtually indistinguishable from those produced by B_{12} deficiency. However, this problem does not seem to be common. Diagnosis of anemia due to folate deficiency depends upon the presence of macrocytic RBCs and hypersegmented neutrophils in the peripheral smear, a normal serum B_{12} level, and a low serum folate level (< 2 ng/mL) or RBC folate level (< 100 ng/mL). Bone marrow is histologically indistinguishable from that seen in B_{12} deficiency.

Treatment of folate deficiency consists of folic acid 1 mg/day orally. A parenteral form is available for patients with severe malabsorption. Treatment with folate alone in a patient with megaloblastic anemia secondary to B_{12} deficiency may correct the anemia but will not reverse neurologic damage.

61. MALIGNANCIES AND MYELOPROLIFERATIVE DISEASES

Michael L. Freedman and *Nancy T. Weintraub*

ACUTE LEUKEMIAS

Accumulation of neoplastic, immature lymphoid or myeloid cells in the bone marrow and peripheral blood, tissue invasion by these cells, and associated bone marrow failure. Untreated, the median survival is 4-6 mo.

Classification

Acute leukemias are categorized as **acute lymphocytic leukemia** or **acute nonlymphocytic leukemia,** according to the cellular morphology in peripheral blood and bone marrow smears, histochemical staining, and immunologic markers. The French-American-British Cooperative Group **(FAB)** classification (see TABLE 61–1) is the most widely used system to facilitate clinical studies and allows for some degree of prognostication. Histochemical and immunologic patterns of the various leukemias are shown in TABLE 61–2.

Etiology

The etiology is unknown in most cases of acute leukemia. Radiation exposure has been implicated as the cause of some cases. Data on atomic bomb survivors from Hiroshima and Nagasaki show a 10 to 20% increase in the incidence of acute nonlymphocytic leukemia. Likewise, studies of diagnostic radiologists and patients who received radiation therapy for ankylosing spondylitis in the earlier part of this century revealed a two-and-one-half- and fourteen-fold increased risk, respectively, of developing acute nonlymphocytic leukemia. High-level benzene exposure in the work place has been strongly implicated as increasing the risk of developing this type of acute leukemia. It is well established that long-term, low-dose therapy with virtually any chemotherapeutic alkylating agent can cause acute leukemia, mostly the acute nonlymphocytic type.

The combination of chemotherapeutic drugs and radiation increases the risk of developing leukemia. Chronic bone marrow disorders (eg, the myelodysplastic syndromes, polycythemia vera, and aplastic anemia) are sometimes followed by a rapidly progressive leukemic phase. Viruses have long been suspected to be the cause of some acute leukemias. Mo-

TABLE 61–1. FRENCH-AMERICAN-BRITISH COOPERATIVE GROUP CLASSIFICATION OF ACUTE LEUKEMIAS AND MYELODYSPLASTIC SYNDROMES

Acute lymphoblastic leukemia

M1: Undifferentiated myelocytic
M2: Myelocytic
M3: Promyelocytic
M4: Myelomonocytic
M5: Monoblastic
  M5 a: Monoblastic
  M5 b: Monocytic
M6: Erythroleukemic
Other: Megakaryoblastic, basophilic, eosinophilic

Acute lymphocytic leukemia

L1: Common childhood type (null or non-B, non-T; pre-B; T cell)
L2: Heterogeneous type (null or non-B, non-T; pre-B; T cell)
L3: Burkitt's type (B cell)

Myelodysplastic syndromes

Refractory anemia
Refractory anemia with ringed sideroblasts (> 15% ringed forms in the marrow)
Refractory anemia with excess blasts (5 to 20% blasts in the marrow, < 5% circulating blasts)
Chronic myelomonocytic leukemia (monocytosis, ≥ 5% circulating blasts)

lecular genetic studies have demonstrated that oncogenes, the cellular homologs of retroviral transforming genes, appear to have a role in the induction and maintenance of the malignant state. Cytogenetic and molecular biologic technics have shown that specific oncogenes are involved in nonrandom chromosome translocations or are found on deleted or reduplicated chromosomes.

Incidence

Acute leukemia is primarily a disease of the elderly. While improvements in the treatment and survival of patients with leukemia have been significant, the most dramatic results have been in the young. Leukemia has an incidence of about 15/100,000 across all age groups. However, the incidence begins to rise at age 40, and by age 80 is approximately 160/100,000. Eighty percent of adults with acute leukemia have the acute nonlymphocytic type, whereas 80% of children with acute leukemia have the lymphocytic type. Nevertheless, the incidence of acute lymphocytic leukemia is 4 times higher in the elderly than in children.

Pathophysiology

Primitive WBCs (eg, lymphoblasts, myeloblasts) accumulate rapidly in the bone marrow and invade many tissues, including the liver, spleen,

TABLE 61–2. HISTOCHEMISTRY AND SURFACE ANTIGENS IN THE ACUTE LEUKEMIAS

	Histochemistry		
	Acute Lymphocytic Leukemia (ALL)	Acute Nonlymphocytic Leukemia (M1-3)	Acute Monoblastic Leukemia (M4, 5)
Peroxidase	0	+ +	0
Esterase			
Chloroacetate	0	+ +	0
Naphthyl butyrate	0	0	0 to + +
Periodic acid-Schiff (PAS) stain	+	0	0
Lysozyme	0	+	+ +
Terminal transferase (Tdt)	+	0	0

	*Surface Antigens**							
	Ia	CALLA	B1	CLG	SLG	E-rosette	My or Mo	Leu 1 or 9
Acute undifferentiated leukemia	+	−	−	−	−	−	−	−
Common ALL (non-B, non-T)	+	+	+/−	−	−	−	−	−
Pre-B ALL	+	+	+	+	−	−	−	−
B cell ALL	+	+	+	−	+	−	−	−
T cell ALL	−	−	−	−	−	+	−	+
Acute nonlymphocytic leukemia	+	−	−	−	−	−	+	−

* Ia = HLA-DR; CALLA = common ALL Antigen; B1 = B-cell–specific surface antigen; CLG = cytoplasmic immunoglobulin; SLG = surface immunoglobulin; E-rosette = the ability to form rosettes with sheep erythrocytes; My or Mo = myeloid or monocyte surface antigens; Leu 1 or Leu 9 = T-cell–specific antigens.

lymph nodes, and CNS. Normal bone marrow and normal leukocytes are replaced by these blasts, resulting in severe anemia, thrombocytopenia with marked bleeding, and great susceptibility to infection.

Symptoms and Signs

Acute leukemia frequently presents as an apparent infection with an acute onset and high fever. The associated thrombocytopenia usually is manifested by petechiae and ecchymoses as well as by bleeding from the nose, mouth, and GI and GU tracts. Often, the liver, spleen, and lymph nodes are enlarged but not always. In the elderly, the disease can present insidiously with progressive weakness, pallor, a change in sense of well-being, and delirium.

Laboratory Findings and Diagnosis

The total peripheral WBC count may be low, normal, or elevated. Blast forms are usually seen in the peripheral blood smear, but a bone marrow aspiration should be performed to confirm the diagnosis. The bone marrow shows excessive blast cells, with decreased or absent normal erythrocytic, granulocytic, and megakaryocytic cells. Histochemical stains and surface antigen markers help identify the type of acute leukemia.

Prognosis

The average untreated patient dies within 4 to 6 mo of clinical onset. Some die within days of onset. Infection, bleeding, advanced age, high blast counts, and chromosomal abnormalities all have been proposed as poor prognostic indicators, while the presence of Auer rods (in acute myelocytic leukemia) and the development of hepatitis have been reported to be advantageous prognostically. Efforts have been made to define morphologic and in vitro growth characteristics as prognosticators; however, data regarding all prognostic signs are contradictory.

Advanced age (defined in most series as > 50 or 60 yr) has typically been considered a bad sign. Much of the problem in treating the elderly seems to be their inability to tolerate the prolonged pancytopenia that accompanies aggressive induction chemotherapy regimens. The elderly also have more complex karyotypic abnormalities than younger patients, and they have more underlying primary marrow disorders (eg, polycythemia vera, myelodysplasia). The presence of a prior hematologic marrow disorder or a leukemia secondary to prior alkylating agent therapy seems to be a poor prognostic sign.

Treatment

Acute lymphocytic leukemia: Older patients have a poor long-term survival rate compared with children, who have an excellent prognosis. The older patient is usually considered high risk and often has 1 or more of the following: a WBC > 20,000/μL, mediastinal mass, L2/L3 morphology, T cell or B cell leukemia, and meningitis. Therapy usually consists of a combination of drugs, including vincristine, prednisone, an anthracycline, and L-asparaginase (which is tolerated poorly by older persons). Most older people relapse within the first year of treatment. Currently, there is no accepted standard therapy.

In acute nonlymphocytic leukemia, a complete remission must first be obtained. The induction phase is the most critical time because the patient is often infected and bleeding and has a large tumor burden with little normal hematopoiesis. A complete remission is defined as the reduction of leukemic blasts to an undetectable level (in practice, < 5%

marrow blasts). Many induction regimens are being studied; the standard combination is cytarabine, 100 to 200 mg/m²/day as a continuous IV infusion for 5 to 7 days and daunorubicin 45 mg/m²/day IV for the first 3 days. With the use of fresh, frozen platelets, packed RBCs, and antibiotics, the current complete remission rate in people > 60 yr of age ranges from 40 to 76%. The median survival is 1 to 2 yr. The value of maintenance and consolidation chemotherapeutic regimens is under study.

Infections are the major cause of morbidity and mortality in the acute leukemias. They result from the severe leukopenia and destruction of normal cutaneous and mucosal barriers. Approximately 500 to 1000 polymorphonuclear leukocytes/μL are necessary for protection against infection. In many patients, endogenous bowel flora is the source of infection, but the pharynx, lungs, perirectal area, and skin are also common sources. The GU tract and meninges are rare sites. Since the source of infection is internal, isolation is of limited value. Viruses, protozoa, and anaerobic bacteria are uncommon pathogens early in therapy.

Fungal infections usually occur after 7 to 14 days of antibiotic therapy in the neutropenic patient. The initial choice of antibiotics depends on the predominant organisms causing infection in a given hospital. An aminoglycoside plus a semisynthetic penicillin or a cephalosporin is usually the drug combination of choice, since the most common organisms in most hospitals are *Pseudomonas* and *Escherichia coli.* Trimethoprim-sulfamethoxazole has been suggested as prophylaxis, particularly in patients who have had frequent admissions with fever and neutropenia.

Metabolic problems are common during induction therapy. Hyperuricemia should be treated prophylactically with allopurinol 300 mg/day. There is often natriuresis and hyponatremia from increased osmolar clearance due to electrolytes, water, and urea released from dead blasts. Hypokalemia can occur from natriuresis, SIADH, physiologic hypervasopressinemia, and/or proximal renal tubular dysfunction. A renal tubular acidosis-like syndrome, with hypokalemia, aminoaciduria, and hyperphosphaturia, occurs but is probably not related to lysozyme. Metabolic alkalosis, metabolic acidosis, hypocalcemia, and hyperphosphatemia are also common complications. Oliguric renal failure will occur due to uric acid nephropathy unless the patient is vigorously hydrated, treated with allopurinol, and has the urine alkalinized.

Aggregates of blasts and thrombi may occlude small blood vessels throughout the body, particularly in the brain and lungs. Therapy revolves around hydration and rapid reduction of the blast count by prompt initiation of chemotherapy. Leukophoresis and cranial irradiation may be temporizing measures.

The CNS is the most common site of extramedullary relapse in acute leukemia. The need for prophylactic meningeal therapy with cranial irradiation and intrathecal methotrexate or cytarabine has not been formally addressed in the elderly. Therefore, these methods currently must be used with extreme caution, if at all. Spinal cord compression, when it occurs, is usually responsive to local radiation. The acute T cell lymphocytic leukemias are most likely to cause either CNS or gonadal invasion. However, the role of prophylactic testicular irradiation in the elderly is currently unclear.

Disseminated intravascular coagulation is an uncommon complication mainly seen in M3 (promyelocytic leukemia). Disseminated intravascular coagulation **(DIC)** is a bleeding disorder due to an underlying illness where the clotting factors and platelets are consumed due to intravascular coagulation. The patient presents either with massive sudden bleeding (acute DIC) or, more usually, with slow bleeding (chronic DIC). In general, it is self-limited and is most problematic during the rapid cell lysis of induction chemotherapy. The use of prophylactic heparin continues to be controversial.

Bone marrow transplantation is rarely used in patients > 35 yr of age and not at all in elderly patients.

MYELODYSPLASTIC SYNDROMES

A heterogeneous group of disorders in which the hematopoietic precursors are abundant but morphologically abnormal. Hematopoiesis is ineffective and mature peripheral blood cells are not produced in normal numbers. The syndromes are vague, with refractory anemia often progressing to a refractory dysmyelopoietic anemia.

Classification

The syndromes are classified according to morphologic criteria. Involvement of the red cell line only with no ringed sideroblasts is **refractory anemia.** If there are > 15% ringed sideroblasts, the diagnosis is **refractory anemia with ringed sideroblasts.** Excessive blasts in the marrow but not in the peripheral blood constitutes **refractory anemia with excess blasts (RAEB).** RAEB accompanied by peripheral blood monocytosis (> $1000/\mu L$) is called **chronic myelomonocytic leukemia.** When $\geq 5\%$ of peripheral blood cells are blasts, the diagnosis is **RAEB in transformation.** Involvement of all 3 cell lines is known as **refractory dysmyelopoietic anemia** or **myelodysplastic syndrome.** These terms have generally replaced the term "preleukemia," since only about 10 to 30% of patients with a myelodysplastic syndrome develop an acute leukemia.

Etiology

The cause in most patients is unknown, but treatment with prolonged courses of alkylating agents is associated with an increased risk of myelodysplastic syndrome and acute nonlymphocytic leukemia. Long courses of melphalan for multiple myeloma or ovarian carcinoma or of chlorambucil or mechlorethamine plus radiation therapy for Hodgkin's disease result in a 2 to 7% incidence of acute nonlymphocytic leukemia in those exposed. Anemia or pancytopenia associated with changes in the bone marrow and peripheral blood identical to myelodysplastic syndrome develops 2 to 10 yr following therapy. The acute nonlymphocytic leukemia that may result is invariably fatal. This long-term complication of successful chemotherapy may become more prevalent as more patients with cancer survive. Chemotherapeutic drugs that are not alkylating agents (eg, methotrexate or hydroxyurea) do not seem to produce this potential complication.

Other possible etiologic factors include RNA viruses, somatic mutations, radiation, and environmental toxins. Aging seems critical, and this has been interpreted as being related to the "multihit" theory of carcinogenesis.

Incidence and Demographics

Actual incidence of these syndromes is not known, but they are fairly common in elderly people. Ineffective erythropoiesis increases with age, and in some studies, up to 20% of people > 65 yr had an unexplained refractory anemia. The syndromes are more common in men and are rare in persons < 40 yr of age. A history of exposure to radiation or chemical leukemogens is common.

Pathophysiology

These syndromes are thought to arise from an as yet undefined cytopathologic alteration of the pluripotential hematopoietic stem cell pool, evolving from the clonal expansion of a single stem cell (or a very small number of such cells). The major specific pathophysiologic consequence is ineffective hematopoiesis, through defective maturation of marrow precursor cells. Proliferation of progenitor and early precursor cells is usually normal or enhanced (giving a hypercellular marrow), but circulating mature cells are deficient. The cells also have a slightly shorter life span, which contributes to the cytopenias.

There are rare familial instances of such myelodysplastic syndromes. A protracted myelodysplastic syndrome lasting for 1 to 20 yr occurs in about 5 to 10% of all cases of acute nonlymphocytic leukemia.

Symptoms and Signs

The patient generally seeks medical care for symptoms of anemia, thrombocytopenia, or leukopenia, eg, fatigue, decrease in exercise tolerance, purpura, fever, or infections. The male:female ratio is 2:1, and the patient is usually elderly. Hepatomegaly is present in about 5% of patients, splenomegaly in about 10%, and pallor in about 50%. Often the patient complains of arthralgias. Because the cytopenias develop slowly, many patients are asymptomatic and the diagnosis is made incidentally, or the anemia is falsely attributed to "aging." Most patients have increased iron stores, and many display clinical hemochromatosis, with diabetes, cirrhosis, infiltrative heart disease, and pituitary dysfunction.

Laboratory Findings and Diagnosis

The hallmark of the syndromes is anemia with reticulocytopenia. The RBC morphology is usually abnormal. A dimorphic population of

RBCs is usually present; some cells are microcytic and hypochromic, and others are normochromic and normocytic or macrocytic. Basophilic stippling, target cells, schistocytes, siderocytes, and nucleated RBCs are often seen.

Leukopenia is moderate, in the range of 1000 to 4000 WBC/μL, with neutropenia more pronounced than lymphopenia. The neutrophils are frequently sparsely granulated; neutrophil alkaline phosphatase may be low, and the acquired (pseudo) Pelger-Huët nuclear anomaly (hypolobulation of the nuclei of the mature neutrophil) may be present. The granulocytes often have abnormal function, which further impairs resistance to infection. Since monocytosis is present in 30% of patients, serum and urinary lysozyme levels may be elevated. Immature myeloid cells may be seen in the peripheral smear.

Thrombocytopenia is common, although occasionally, patients have thrombocytosis. The platelets may have functional defects.

The bone marrow is diagnostic of the myelodysplastic syndromes. Erythroblasts may have double or fragmented nuclei or intranuclear bridging, and budding, ringed sideroblasts (excessive iron in mitochondria) may be prominent. These are usually found primarily in patients with abnormalities in the RBC precursors. With mainly erythroid dysplasia, the ratio of myeloid to erythroid precursors (M:E ratio) is between 1:1 and 1:10 (normal 3:1). Reticuloendothelial iron is increased, and the serum iron and ferritin levels are elevated. Dyserythropoiesis results in moderate elevation of serum LDH and indirect bilirubin. Iron turnover studies reveal the ineffective erythropoiesis; the iron turnover rate is increased but incorporation of iron into circulating erythrocytes is decreased. Iron stores are increased in most patients.

Marrow myeloid cells may show immature to mature neutrophils, may have the acquired Pelger-Huët nuclear anomaly, and are often sparsely granulated. Eosinophils and basophils may also be dysplastic. In patients with mainly myeloid dysplasia, the M:E ratio is between 3:1 and 10 to 20:1. Megakaryocytes may be immature and dysplastic as well.

Prognosis

Prognosis is *very variable,* with survival of a few months to 10 to 15 yr. The median survival is about 3 yr. Approximately 10 to 30% of patients will die from acute blastic transformation (acute nonlymphocytic leukemia), but we are unable to predict which ones. Patients with primarily erythroid dysplasia are at lower risk than those with mainly myeloid dysplasia.

Treatment

Transfusion of blood products is the mainstay of treatment but should be limited. Transfusion of packed RBCs entails the risk of iron overload; alloimmunization to red cell, white cell, and platelet antigens; and transmission of various infections. Washed RBCs may slow the development of alloimmunization. Platelets should be transfused only if bleeding is present or surgery is necessary. Granulocyte transfusions should be given only to neutropenic patients with documented gram-negative infections unresponsive to antibiotics alone.

Occasionally, patients with ringed sideroblasts respond to pharmacologic doses of oral **pyridoxine** 100 to 300 mg/day. The response is only partial, and abnormal RBC morphology usually persists. **Androgens** and **corticosteroids** have benefited a small number of patients. Continuous IV or s.c. use of **deferoxamine** given by portable pumps should be considered when the total number of transfused units of RBCs approaches 100.

Chemotherapy as early treatment of myelodysplasia with excessive blasts has not increased survival. Low-dose cytarabine to induce differentiation of blasts is controversial. When the patient's condition converts to acute nonlymphocytic leukemia, the remission rate is even lower than in those patients with nonlymphocytic leukemia who did not previously have myelodysplasia. Patients with this secondary form of nonlymphocytic leukemia have prolonged marrow aplasia after chemotherapy. One approach in the elderly has involved supportive care with blood products and an attempt to keep the WBC count < 50,000/μL with oral hydroxyurea (10 to 100 mg/kg/day).

CHRONIC LEUKEMIA

A neoplastic accumulation of mature lymphoid or myeloid elements of the blood that usually progresses more slowly than an acute leukemic process. If the neoplastic cells are of the lymphoid type, the disease is called **chronic lymphocytic leukemia.** If myeloid cells are involved, it is called **chronic myeloid (myelocytic, myelogenous) leukemia.**

Classification

Since chronic lymphocytic leukemia is primarily a disease of the elderly, while chronic myeloid leukemia usually occurs in people in their 30s and 40s, this discussion will be limited to the former. **Chronic lymphocytic leukemia** in > 95% of cases involves the neoplastic proliferation of B cells.

Etiology

Ionizing radiation plays no part in the etiology of chronic lymphocytic leukemia, although it does in chronic myeloid leukemia. Rather, a genetic component seems to be involved, since the illness is more common in certain families. Some of these families have immunologic abnormalities. Chronic viral infections (eg, Epstein-Barr virus) have been suggested as possible causes.

Incidence and Demographics

Chronic lymphocytic leukemia is the most common type in Western society, accounting for 25 to 40% of all leukemias. Ninety percent of all patients are > 50 yr of age, with the majority > 60 yr of age. Men are affected twice as often as women.

Pathophysiology

Monoclonal lymphocytes accumulate in the peripheral blood, bone marrow, lymphoid tissues, and sometimes other organs. The cells appear morphologically mature, but the presence of receptors for mouse erythrocytes, ALA-DR antigens, and small amounts of surface immunoglobulin suggests some degree of immaturity. Trisomy 12 has been described in about 25% of cases. Infiltration of the bone marrow may eventually result in pancytopenia. Deficiency of normal B cells often leads to bacterial infection. Transformation to a diffuse, large-cell lymphoma (Richter's syndrome) or to acute prolymphocytic leukemia may occur as a terminal event.

Symptoms and Signs

The presentation is highly variable. Over 25% of patients have asymptomatic disease discovered on routine physical examination or blood count. The most common initial symptoms are fatigue, malaise, and decreased exercise tolerance. In many elderly people, an exacerbation of coronary artery or cerebrovascular disease may be the initial manifestation.

Some patients note enlarged lymph nodes or complain of abdominal pain or early satiety due to splenomegaly. Lymphadenopathy is commonly found in the cervical, axillary, and supraclavicular areas, while inguinal adenopathy is rare. Splenomegaly is found in 50% of patients at presentation. Hepatomegaly may develop as the disease progresses. Lymphocytic infiltration can occur in any organ. Jaundice usually suggests hemolysis, although biliary obstruction due to periportal lymph node enlargement can occur. At late stages, ecchymoses and petechiae may result from thrombocytopenia.

Fever is usually secondary to infection, but in late stages of the disease, progression to acute prolymphocytic leukemia or aggressive lymphoma should be considered. Clinically significant hyperviscosity is rare, occurring only when the WBC is $\geq$ 800,000/μL.

Laboratory Findings and Diagnosis

The diagnosis of chronic lymphocytic leukemia requires the demonstration of sustained lymphocytosis and bone marrow lymphocyte infiltration in the absence of other causes. The absolute lymphocyte count is generally > 15,000/μL. The cells are mature in appearance. These lymphocytes tend to smudge upon preparation of the blood smear.

In **B-cell chronic lymphocytic leukemia,** both T cells and B cells are increased in absolute numbers, but B cells are preferentially increased, making up 40 to 90% of all lymphocytes. They are of monoclonal origin and express the surface immunoglobulins of one light-chain class. The usual surface immunoglobulin is IgM, but less commonly, it is IgD. In B-cell chronic lymphocytic leukemia, the ratio of helper to suppressor T cells is reversed because of an increased number of suppressor cells. This may account for the development of pure RBC aplasia described in a few patients.

Approximately 1% of patients have lymphocytes that form rosettes with sheep RBCs, and their disease is classified as **T cell chronic lymphocytic leukemia**. In **T cell chronic lymphocytic leukemia** both helper (T4) and suppressor (T8) forms are seen. The lymphocytes often inhibit cytoplasmic azurophilic granules. Massive splenomegaly, marked neutropenia, skin infiltration, modest bone marrow infiltration, and a rapid clinical course leading to death are seen in < ¹/₂ of these patients. There is a high concurrence with rheumatoid arthritis; however, most cases have an indolent course.

RBC morphology is usually normal. Anemia is found in 10 to 20% of patients and is most often normochromic and normocytic. The anemia may be due to marrow replacement, hypersplenism, or suppressor mechanisms. The Coombs' test reveals IgG coating of RBCs in about 20% of cases; however, an autoimmune hemolytic anemia is seen only 8% of the time. Thrombocytopenia, which is found in 10 to 20% of cases, may be due to marrow replacement, hypersplenism, or antiplatelet antibodies. Bone marrow morphology shows interstitial or nodular infiltration in early disease and diffuse infiltration in the advanced stages.

In about 5% of cases, the same immunoglobulin found on the cell surface is found in the serum as a monoclonal protein. Hypogammaglobulinemia or agammaglobulinemia is found in 50 to 75% of all patients.

Prognosis

Clinical staging is determined on the basis of examination and CBC (TABLE 61–3). Patients in Stage A have < 3 sites involved while those in Stage B have 3 or more sites involved, including cervical, axillary, supraclavicular, and inguinal lymph nodes, liver, and spleen. Generally, disease progresses in a stepwise pattern from less severe to more severe illness. Patients in Stage C with anemia (Hb < 10 gm/dL) or thrombocytopenia (< 100,000/μL) usually survive < 2 yr.

TABLE 61–3. INTERNATIONAL WORKSHOP STAGING OF CHRONIC LYMPHOCYTIC LEUKEMIA

Stage	Definition
A	No anemia or thrombocytopenia and < 3 areas of lymphoid enlargement Median survival > 7 yr
B	No anemia or thrombocytopenia with ≥ involved areas Median survival < 5 yr
C	Anemia (Hb < 10 gm/dL) and/or thrombocytopenia (< 100,000/μL), regardless of the number of areas of lymphoid enlargement Median survival < 2 yr

Other poor prognostic signs include diffuse replacement of bone marrow, presence of trisomy 12 plus other abnormal chromosomes, and IgM surface immunoglobulin rather than IgD. Although life expectancy in chronic lymphocytic leukemia is often prolonged, the 5-yr survival is only about 50%.

Treatment

Stage A patients usually do not require treatment and this approach is usually extended to **Stage B patients,** since the complications of chemotherapy (eg, infection, development of acute nonlymphocytic leukemia) may be more deleterious than the chronic lymphocytic leukemia.

In Stage C, chlorambucil is the therapeutic agent most often used. It induces responses in 50 to 80% of patients and complete remission rates in 10 to 20%. **Chlorambucil** may be given at a daily dosage of 0.08 to 0.2 mg/kg orally, or for 1 day every 4 wk at 0.4 to 0.8 mg/kg orally in 3 divided doses. **Prednisone** 0.8 mg/kg/day is often used concomitantly and may improve the response rate. Steroids alone are used only in patients with autoimmune hemolytic anemia or thrombocytopenia. **Radiation therapy** is used to reduce local bulky disease, vital organ compromise, or painful bone lesions.

The most common **complications** of chronic lymphocytic leukemia are bacterial infections, especially of the lungs and urinary tract. Gram-positive coccal, gram-negative rod, *Listeria,* fungal, and *Pneumocystis carinii* infections all may occur. Patients with chronic lymphocytic leukemia have at least a four-fold greater risk of developing a carcinoma.

When transformation to either an acute prolymphocytic leukemia or to an aggressive lymphoma occurs, response to chemotherapy or radiation is generally poor.

MULTIPLE MYELOMA

A neoplastic disorder resulting from the proliferation and accumulation of immature plasma cells in the bone marrow. Its major manifestations, which ultimately lead to death, result from the direct effect of these cells, the characteristic proteins they produce, and their secondary effects on other organ systems.

Classification

Neoplastic plasma cells almost always synthesize abnormal amounts of monoclonal immunoglobulin (IgG, IgA, IgD, or IgE) or κ or λ light chains. Therefore, they are usually classified according to their immunoglobulin class. Rarely, there are cases with no detectable production of immunoglobulin.

Etiology

An increased occurrence of myeloma in first-degree relatives, together with the higher frequency of the 4c complex of HLA antigens in myeloma patients and the increased incidence in blacks, suggests that genetic factors play a role. Risk of developing myeloma seems to increase after high radiation exposure, as shown in Hiroshima and Nagasaki atom bomb survivors. Other possibilities include chronic antigenic stimulation due to, for example, cholecystitis, osteomyelitis, repeated allergen injections, rheumatoid arthritis, hereditary spherocytosis, or Gaucher's disease. Asbestos exposure and viral illnesses have also been suggested as possible etiologic factors.

Since myeloma is so age related, 1 potential influence might be the decrease in the T-lymphoid arm of the immune system. As T cells decrease, B cell clones may proliferate excessively. Then, because of such monoclonal expansion, spontaneous or externally induced genetic alteration of such a clone may occur, allowing it to proliferate and produce its immunoglobulin. Since it would remain under some control of the immune system, it would be a **benign monoclonal gammopathy.** A second external oncogenic event could then result in uncontrolled proliferation of these cells (ie, multiple myeloma).

Incidence and Demographics

The annual incidence is approximately 3/100,000 persons. The disease is more common in blacks than in whites. The sex incidence is equal. Multiple myeloma usually occurs in people > 50 yr of age, and the incidence increases progressively with age.

Pathophysiology

The consequences of abnormal plasma cell growth are plasma cell tumors, osteolysis, hematopoietic suppression, hypogammaglobulinemia, paraproteinuria, and renal disease.

Plasma cell tumors usually develop in areas of hematopoietically active bone marrow. They are commonly seen in virtually any bone but rarely in extraskeletal sites. Even plasmacytomas that seem solitary usually become widespread eventually.

Osteolytic lesions, which are very common, are thought to result from the release of osteoclast-activating factor from the neoplastic plasma cell. This stimulates osteoclasts to resorb bone.

Marrow function is impaired in direct proportion to the number of plasma cells in the bone marrow. Anemia is most common, but neutropenia and thrombocytopenia also occur.

In multiple myeloma, the single clone of abnormal plasma cells produces an excess of a single type of immunoglobulin or a portion of the immunoglobulin molecule. Concomitantly, the other normal classes of immunoglobulins are suppressed, resulting in an **actual or functional hypogammaglobulinemia.** In > 50% of patients, the monoclonal protein is an IgG; in 20%, an IgA; and in 12%, an IgM (macroglobulinemia). IgD is found in about 2% of cases, and IgE is rare. About 10% of patients produce only light chains, and < 1% produce only heavy chains. Rarely, patients produce ≥ 2 monoclonal proteins, and about 1% have no monoclonal protein in serum or urine.

Renal disease occurs in about ½ of patients with multiple myeloma. UTIs, glomerular deposits of amyloid, Ca or uric acid calculi, and plasma cell infiltration of the kidney may occur. However, the major cause of renal failure is the tubular damage associated with the excretion of light chains. All light-chain proteins are not nephrotoxic, and some patients may excrete large amounts of light chains for years without developing renal failure. Patients who excrete λ light chains are at greater risk than those who excrete κ light chains.

Symptoms and Signs

Multiple myeloma is usually progressive. It is estimated that the abnormal plasma cells double in 3 to 10 mo. In rare cases, however, the preclinical stage may last for years.

The most frequent symptom of multiple myeloma is **bone pain,** which occurs in about 70% of patients. Pain often occurs in the lower back or ribs and gradually increases in intensity. Sudden onset may mean that a vertebra has collapsed or that there has been a spontaneous pathologic fracture of an involved area (eg, the shaft of a long bone, the pelvis, a rib, or a clavicle).

Systemic symptoms and signs include pallor, weakness, fatigue, dyspnea on exertion, and palpitations, all resulting from the anemia that occurs in about 70% of patients at the time of diagnosis. **Signs of thrombocytopenia** (eg, ecchymoses, purpura, epistaxis, or excessive bleeding from trauma) are common. **Infection** also occurs frequently because of neutropenia and immunoglobulin deficiency, and the patient may present with pneumonia, pyoderma, pyelonephritis. **Cold sensitivity** and **urticaria** may result from cryoglobulinemia. Patients rarely present with **nephrotic syndrome.**

Hypercalcemia is common in patients with destructive bone lesions and may result in anorexia, nausea, vomiting, polyuria, polydipsia, constipation, and dehydration. Particularly in the elderly, drowsiness, confusion, and coma may result from hypercalcemia.

Renal disease may be acute or chronic. The acute disease is usually associated with azotemia, hypercalcemia, hypotension, dehydration, and infections treated with nephrotoxic antibiotics. Dehydration is frequently produced by fluid deprivation or IV use of hypertonic contrast media during a diagnostic procedure. In patients with multiple myeloma, procedures such as IV or retrograde pyelograms or open bone biopsies should *not* be performed unless urine flow is ample and hypercalcemia and hyperuricemia have been corrected.

Hyperviscosity syndrome occurs about 50% of the time when the monoclonal immunoglobulin is IgM (macroglobulinemia). It is uncommon in multiple myeloma with other immunoglobulin classes. Purpura, ecchymoses, epistaxis, GI bleeding, blurred vision associated with venous congestion, intraocular hemorrhages and exudates, and ischemic neurologic symptoms are common.

Neurologic symptoms and signs include mental confusion from hypercalcemia, spinal cord and nerve root compression, myelomatous meningitis, carpal tunnel syndrome (due to deposition of amyloid), and sensorimotor polyneuropathy not due to amyloid or infiltration with plasma cells. Rarer CNS symptoms include intracerebral plasmacytomas, herpes zoster, and multifocal leukoencephalopathy.

Laboratory Findings and Diagnosis

The order in which tests are performed depends on the mode of presentation. If a monoclonal protein is found on serum electrophoresis, the skeleton should be x-rayed and a bone marrow aspiration performed. The absence of both lytic bone lesions and plasma cell infiltration makes a diagnosis of **benign monoclonal gammopathy** likely. Confirming findings for this diagnosis include absence of significant (< 60 mg/24 h) amounts of a single type of light chain (ie, Bence Jones protein) in the urine and a serum monoclonal gammopathy < 2 gm/dL.

The presence of > 10% mature and immature plasma cells in the bone marrow, osteolytic bone lesions, and serum monoclonal protein is diagnostic of **multiple myeloma**. The excretion of light chain > 60 mg/24 h and a monoclonal serum protein > 2 gm/dL is highly suggestive of multiple myeloma. If bone marrow plasmacytosis is not demonstrated in this setting, repeated bone marrow aspirations and a search for an extraskeletal plasma cell tumor should be undertaken. Idiopathic monoclonal components occur with other cancers.

Prognosis

Only time will determine if a diagnosis of **benign monoclonal gammopathy** is really early multiple myeloma. Over 20 yr, about $\frac{1}{3}$ of patients initially diagnosed as having benign monoclonal gammopathy will progress to overt multiple myeloma. There is no evidence that not treating these patients is harmful.

Once a diagnosis of **multiple myeloma** is made, the patient may be classified as a good or a poor treatment risk. **Good-risk** patients have an Hb ≥ 9.0 gm/dL, serum creatinine < 2 mg/dL, and Ca ≤ 12 mg/dL after hydration. **Poor-risk** patients fail to meet these criteria. The good-risk group, with therapy, has a median survival of 42 mo, and the poor-risk group, only 21 mo. Both groups respond equally well to initial therapy.

In some good-risk elderly people, the disease progresses slowly. If the patient is asymptomatic or only mildly symptomatic, the course of the illness can be followed over time to determine the pace of the disease. Occasionally, elderly patients with advanced-stage myeloma do well. In general, if the elderly patient is feeling well, one should wait until the pace of the disease is determined before beginning treatment.

Treatment

Since multiple myeloma is a neoplastic disorder, the mainstay of treatment is chemotherapy. Radiation is useful for localized tumor burden and is widely used to relieve back pain from osteolytic lesions. However, if extensive demineralization of bone is causing the back pain, this is usually not relieved by radiation, and chemotherapy should be begun promptly.

All patients should be encouraged to stay active to prevent further demineralization of bone. Lumbar corsets and braces may help relieve pain and prevent further damage. Large osteolytic lesions should be irradiated before fractures occur. Actual fracture through a lytic lesion requires an intramedullary pin and radiation.

Patients must drink 2 to 3 L fluid/day to maintain increased urine output for excretion of light chains, Ca, uric acid, and other metabolites. All infections must be treated promptly. Hyperuricemia should be treated with allopurinol 300 mg/day. Hypercalcemia is usually treated with either calcitonin 100 to 200 u. s.c. q 12 h or prednisone 40 to 100 mg/day, or both, until the serum Ca returns to normal (usually 1 to 5 days). Plicamycin (mithramycin) 25 μg/kg IV over 1 to 2 h may be used if the above does not work. Oral therapy with 2 gm sodium or potassium phosphate daily may also be useful in some patients with moderate hypercalcemia. IV hydration with saline or saline plus furosemide may also be used on a temporary basis.

Many chemotherapeutic regimens are used for multiple myeloma. In the elderly with decreased bone marrow reserve, the 2 most common regimens are high-dose, intermittent melphalan with prednisone and low-dose, continuous melphalan. In the high-dose intermittent schedule, the dosage of melphalan is 0.25 mg/kg/day orally for 4 days, and the dosage of prednisone is 2 mg/kg/day, also for 4 days. The treatment schedule is repeated every 4 to 6 wk, depending on the degree of bone marrow suppression. In the continuous regimen, the patient is generally first given 8 to 10 mg/day melphalan for about 1 wk (loading dose). The dosage is then reduced to 2 mg/day but must be adjusted frequently, depending on the sensitivity of the bone marrow. In the very elderly, the loading dose is usually reduced to 4 mg/day for 1 wk.

Hyperviscosity may be treated effectively in the short term by plasmaphoresis.

LYMPHOMAS

Primary malignancies of the lymph nodes, including Hodgkin's disease and non-Hodgkin's lymphoma. Lymphomas are distinct entities characterized by different patterns of spread, clinical behavior, and cells of origin. Hodgkin's disease usually has a predictable pattern of spread to contiguous lymph node areas, while non-Hodgkin's lymphoma is usually widespread at diagnosis. The latter is more likely to have extranodal involvement. Both can be divided into subsets based on the histologic appearance of the lymph nodes.

Classification

Fundamental to the diagnosis of Hodgkin's disease is the histologic finding in the lymph node of the giant **Reed-Sternberg cell,** usually with twin nuclei and nucleoli that give it the appearance of "owl's eyes." The Reed-Sternberg cell is probably the malignant cell, and the surrounding cells probably represent tissue reaction.

Histologically, Hodgkin's disease is subdivided into 4 major types: (1) **lymphocyte predominant:** mainly mature lymphocytes with few Reed-Sternberg cells; (2) **mixed cellularity:** a cellular response of mature lymphoid cells, plasma cells, eosinophils, and Reed-Sternberg cells; (3) **lymphocyte depleted:** a paucity of lymphoid cells with a majority of histiocytes, fibrotic reaction, and Reed-Sternberg cells; and (4) **nodular sclerosis:** effacement of lymphoid structure by nodular aggregates of mature lymphoid cells and "lacunar" variants of Reed-Sternberg cells separated by bands of birefringent collagen. Before the introduction of potentially curative treatment, lymphocyte-predominant and nodular sclerosis types carried a better prognosis.

Systemic clinical staging is extremely important in the management of Hodgkin's disease. The currently accepted clinical stages are listed in TABLE 61–4.

The non-Hodgkin's lymphomas are a heterogeneous group of lymphoid malignancies that have some common but many different features. The classification of non-Hodgkin's lymphomas is controversial and has undergone many revisions. Currently, there are 2 complementary approaches to categorizing these illnesses: classic description of lymph node architecture and histology and the use of immunologic markers. TABLE 61–5 shows the histologic classification of Rappaport and the Interna-

TABLE 61–4. CLINICAL STAGING OF HODGKIN'S DISEASE*

Stage	Definition
I	Disease limited to 1 anatomic region
II	Disease in ≥ 2 anatomic regions on the same side of the diaphragm
III	Disease on both sides of the diaphragm but limited to lymph nodes, spleen, and/or Waldeyer's tonsillar ring
III$_1$	Involvement limited to spleen, splenic nodes, and celiac and/or portal nodes, plus disease above the diaphragm
III$_2$	Involvement of para-aortic, pelvic, and disk nodes
IV	Extranodal disease that is not directly contiguous to a nodal area, ie, bone marrow, lung, pleura, liver, plus disease above the diaphragm

* All stages are subclassified as A if there are no systemic symptoms or B if there are any of the following: unexplained fever, night sweats, loss of 10% or more of body weight.

TABLE 61–5. HISTOLOGIC CLASSIFICATION OF THE NON-HODGKIN'S LYMPHOMAS

Working Formulation	Rappaport Classification
Low grade	
Small lymphocytic	Well-differentiated lymphocytic lymphoma
Follicular small cleaved lymphocytic	Nodular poorly differentiated lymphocytic lymphoma
Mixed follicular small, cleaved cell	Nodular mixed lymphoma
Large Cell	
Intermediate	
Follicular, predominantly large cell	Nodular histiocytic lymphoma
Diffuse small cleaved cell	Diffuse poorly differentiated lymphocytic lymphoma
Diffuse large cells (cleaved or uncleaved)	Diffuse histiocytic lymphoma
High grade	

Diffuse large cell immunoblasts
  B cell
  T Cell
  Polymorphous
  Epithelial cell component
	Diffuse histiocytic lymphoma

Lymphoblastic
  Convoluted
  Nonconvoluted
	Lymphoblastic lymphoma

Small noncleaved
  Burkitt's
  Non-Burkitt's
	Diffuse undifferentiated lymphoma

tional Panel Working Formulation based on the type of lymphocyte seen.

Clinical staging is similar to that of Hodgkin's disease (TABLE 61–4). Unfortunately, > 90% of patients have stage III or IV disease at the time of diagnosis.

Etiology

The etiology of Hodgkin's disease remains unknown. However, sero-epidemiologic studies suggest that the Epstein-Barr virus may be involved in this disease. Patients with immunodeficiencies and autoimmune disease are at increased risk, suggesting that the immune system plays a role.

The etiology of most non-Hodgkin's lymphoma is also unknown. However, immunosuppressed patients (eg, renal transplant recipients) or those with excessive function of the immune system, as in Sjögren's syndrome, are at greater risk. A virus is involved in at least some cases. African Burkitt's lymphoma is associated with Epstein-Barr virus infection, and an aggressive T cell leukemia/lymphoma is associated with human T-lymphotrophic virus Type I **(HTLV-I)** infection in Japan and the Caribbean. Similarly, patients with human immunodeficiency virus **(HIV)** infection often develop aggressive non-Hodgkin's lymphoma.

Incidence and Demographics

The incidence of Hodgkin's disease is 2/100,000 persons/yr in the USA. There is a bimodal age distribution: an initial peak between ages 15 and 35 yr and a subsequent peak between ages 50 and 80 yr. At age 25, the incidence is approximately 5/100,000 persons/yr, and at age 75, it is 7/100,000. The incidence rate is slightly greater in men. There appears to be an association between Hodgkin's disease and higher socioeconomic levels. Geographic, occupational (woodworkers), and family clusters of Hodgkin's disease have been noted. The incidence of Hodgkin's and non-Hodgkin's lymphoma is increased in persons with immune deficiencies, autoimmune disease, or who are taking hydantoin drugs such as phenytoin.

The age-adjusted incidence of non-Hodgkin's lymphoma ranges from 2.6 to 5.8/100,000 persons/yr. The progressive increase in incidence with age is similar to that of acute leukemia. At age 80, the incidence is approximately 40/100,000 persons/yr. The incidence of non-Hodgkin's lymphoma is increased in patients with aberrations of the immune system. Some cases seem to be associated with viral infections (see below).

Pathophysiology

Normal lymphoid tissue is replaced by the malignant lymphoma, resulting in immunodeficiency and infections. The bone marrow may be replaced, resulting in pancytopenia and subsequent bleeding and infection. Tumor bulk may obstruct or invade vital organs, ultimately causing death.

Symptoms and Signs

Patients with **Hodgkin's disease** usually have enlarged lymph nodes in the neck upon presentation. Although any nodal group can be involved, the central or axial lymph nodes are most commonly affected. The patient may be asymptomatic or exhibit the "B" symptoms of fever, night sweats, weight loss > 10% of normal body weight, and pruritus, which are often associated with extensive disease. Patients may also present with advanced disease, consisting of diffuse adenopathy and involvement of the spleen, liver, bone marrow, or lung.

The non-Hodgkin's lymphomas appear to be multicentric in origin and widespread early in the course of the disease. A leukemic phase, detectable in the peripheral blood, may occur. Most patients initially seek medical care because of cervical or inguinal lymph node enlargement. However, the skin, GI tract, bone, liver, and CNS make up 10 to 20%

of the primary sites of lymphoma at presentation. Occasionally, spleno-megaly, bone marrow failure, autoimmune hemolytic anemia, and auto-immune thrombocytopenia are presenting features. Systemic "B" symp-toms are not as common as in Hodgkin's disease. Waldeyer's tonsillar ring involvement has a high association with GI lesions. Hypercalcemia is prominent in HTLV-I–related non-Hodgkin's lymphoma, but is rare in the others. Hypogammaglobulinemia may occur, but occasionally, pa-tients have a monoclonal serum M component.

Laboratory Findings and Diagnosis

The diagnosis is made by biopsy and the histologic picture of malig-nant lymphoma.

Clinical staging in Hodgkin's disease is extremely important in deter-mining treatment. Systemic staging includes (1) complete physical exam-ination, with particular attention to all lymph node areas; (2) routine chemistry profile and CBC; (3) CT scans of the abdomen, pelvis, and, in some cases, the chest; (4) lymphangiography via the pedal lymphatics to outline the femoral, inguinal, pelvic, and para-aortic nodes; and (5) in cases in which the clinical stage may change the treatment modality, laparotomy including splenectomy, liver biopsies, and biopsies of grossly suspicious lymph nodes as needed. A bone marrow biopsy is also re-quired if the findings will affect treatment. Clinical and pathologic stages change in up to 30% of patients after laparotomy. In the elderly, Hodgkin's disease is more likely to present as advanced disease (Stage III or IV). Some authorities believe that patients > 40 yr of age, par-ticularly those with mixed cellularity or lymphocyte depletion histolo-gies, may not benefit from laparotomy.

In non-Hodgkin's lymphoma, systemic staging is rarely required. After a complete physical examination, CBC, chemistry profile, bone marrow aspirate, lymph node biopsy, chest x-ray, and abdominal CT scan, about 90% of patients are found to have advanced-stage disease. Staging laparotomy is usually not required. Other studies (eg, serum protein electrophoresis, skeletal x-rays, and IV urography) are sometimes useful.

Prognosis

In Hodgkin's disease, with treatment, almost 70% of patients are long-term survivors, regardless of histology. Success depends upon staging, identifying the spread pattern of disease and the next potential site of involvement, and expert use of radiation and chemotherapy. Elderly per-sons in advanced stages do not do as well as younger people, since they are unable to tolerate maximal radiation and chemotherapy doses.

In non-Hodgkin's lymphoma, the prognosis is related to factors intrinsic to the disease and the patient's age. Indicators of a good prognosis are nodular histology, limited stage, and young age. Marrow involvement is a sign of poor prognosis in the unfavorable histologies but not in the fa-vorable or intermediate histologies. Other poor-prognosis signs are bulky abdominal disease, Hb < 12 gm/dL and serum LDH > 250 u./L.

Treatment

In Hodgkin's disease, the primary therapeutic intervention is treatment of known disease and the next potential site of involvement. In general, limited area radiation therapy is recommended for Stages I and II and chemotherapy with or without radiation is recommended for Stages III and IV. The current recommendations are shown in TABLE 61–6. However, the regeneration of bone marrow after irradiation or chemotherapy is markedly diminished in patients > 40 yr of age, and the GI side effects are much more severe. Thus, consideration should be given to limiting the usual field of radiation in elderly patients with early-stage disease. Similarly, administration of optimal chemotherapy may be impossible in older patients, even though the benefit of aggressive treatment outweighs the risk.

The survival rate of patients given palliative rather than aggressive therapy is dramatically lower. Many elderly patients can tolerate only 30 to 50% of the optimal doses of chemotherapy. The most frequently used regimens in the elderly are MOPP and British MOPP, each of which comprises 4 drugs (shown in TABLE 61–7). The duration of chemotherapy is 6 to 12 mo or at least 2 mo following attainment of a complete remission. The incidence of a second malignancy (usually acute leukemia or non-Hodgkin's lymphoma) increases in patients with Hodgkin's disease who are receiving or have received chemotherapy, especially when combined with total nodal irradiation.

In non-Hodgkin's lymphoma, the prognosis varies markedly according to the pathologic classification. Very few cases are Stage I and, therefore,

TABLE 61–6. TREATMENT OF PATIENTS WITH HODGKIN'S DISEASE

Stage	Therapy	Disease-Free Survival (%)
IA, IIA, and II₁A	Mantle and para-aortic irradiation*	90
IIIA	Total nodal irradiation	50
	Chemotherapy and extended field irradiation**	85
IB and IIB	Similar to IA and IIA	80–90
IIIA and IIIB	Chemotherapy and involved field irradiation**	80–85
IVA and IVB	Chemotherapy with or without irradiation of bulk disease	25–40

* If the mediastinal mass is > 1/3 the diameter of the chest, combined modality therapy consisting of chemotherapy and mantle irradiation is preferable to radiation alone.

** Some groups reserve chemotherapy for Stage IV disease and use irradiation as sole therapy for Stages I to III. The overall disease-free intervals are similar.

TABLE 61-7. CHEMOTHERAPY FOR HODGKIN'S DISEASE*

Regimen	Dosage
MOPP	
Nitrogen mustard	6 mg/m^2 on days 1 and 8 IV
Vincristine	1.5 mg/m^2 on days 1 and 8 IV
Prednisone	40 mg/m^2/day on days 1 to 14 po (cycles 1 and 4 only)
Procarbazine	100 mg/m^2/day on days 1 to 14 po
British MOPP (ChIVPP)	
Chlorambucil	6 mg/m^2/day on days 1 to 14 po
Vinblastine	6 mg/m^2 on days 1 and 8 IV
Prednisone	40 mg/m^2/day on days 1 to 14 po
Procarbazine	100 mg/m^2/day on days 1 to 14 po

* Each regimen is given every 28 days.

curative radiation is rarely possible. However, a true Stage I should be treated with radiation therapy. Most patients have advanced disease at diagnosis and require chemotherapy. Chemotherapeutic "cures" in non-Hodgkin's lymphoma occur paradoxically only in patients with "intermediate-" and "unfavorable-prognosis" histologies. In contrast, aggressive therapy does not seem to prolong survival in the "favorable-prognosis" lymphomas, even though they are extremely sensitive to chemotherapy. For these reasons, therapy should be minimal in favorable-prognosis disease and aggressive in unfavorable-prognosis disease.

Favorable-prognosis histology of non-Hodgkin's lymphoma: In cases appearing to be Stage I or Stage II, regional radiation is used, if any therapy is given. However, most patients relapse because they were not truly in an early stage. In others the disease is so indolent that recurrence does not occur for 5 to 10 yr. Chemotherapy is rarely indicated in Stage I or Stage II; often, no therapy is needed. Particularly in the elderly, close follow-up without treatment until problems develop is a practical approach.

In Stages III and IV, the disease is still very indolent. Most patients respond to chemotherapy, but the relapse rate is 10 to 20%/yr. Even though 80 to 90% of patients with favorable-prognosis histology will achieve a complete remission, at the 10-yr mark, only 10 to 20% will be without disease. Consequently, it is wise to avoid both the serious systemic toxicity inherent in aggressive combination chemotherapy and the potential risk for acute nonlymphocytic leukemia associated with chronic low-dose alkylating agents. Most oncologists use single alkylating agents (eg, chlorambucil at a dosage of 0.4 to 0.8 mg/kg in 3 divided doses for 1 day every 28 days). So-called pulse therapy has less myelotoxicity and, perhaps, less leukomogenic potential. Some physicians use relatively mild combination chemotherapy regimens (see TABLE 61-8).

TABLE 61-8. CHEMOTHERAPEUTIC REGIMENS FOR NON-HODGKIN'S LYMPHOMA*

Regimen	Dosage
CVP or COP	
Cyclophosphamide	750 mg/m^2 on day 1 IV
Vincristine	1.4 mg/m^2 on day 1 IV**
Prednisone	60 mg/m^2/day on days 1 to 5 po
C-MOPP	
Cyclophosphamide	650 mg/m^2 on days 1 and 8 IV
Vincristine	1.4 mg/m^2 on days 1 and 8 IV**
Prednisone	40 mg/m^2/day on days 1 to 14 po
Procarbazine	100 mg/m^2/day on days 1 to 14 po

* Cycles are repeated every 21-28 days.
** Maximum dose 2 mg.

Intermediate and unfavorable-prognosis histologies of non-Hodgkin's lymphoma: These aggressive non-Hodgkin's lymphomas are rapidly growing tumors with a short natural history. Thus, the patients are generally treated with combination chemotherapy. Doxorubicin is not well tolerated in the elderly, nor is methotrexate, because of its renal complications. TABLE 61-8 shows 2 chemotherapeutic regimens that have relatively low toxicity in the elderly.

MYELOPROLIFERATIVE DISEASES

A group of disorders arising from a monoclonal proliferation of the hematopoietic pluripotential precursor cell. In this respect, the diseases may be considered malignancies. Nevertheless, in most of these diseases, the pluripotential precursors retain the ability to differentiate and mature into functional cells, and the disorders are usually clinically benign and chronic.

Classification

The myeloproliferative diseases may be classified by their degree of cell maturation, ranging from benign to dysplastic to malignant (TABLE 61-9). The hyperplastic syndromes are polycythemia and essential thrombocythemia. Myeloid metaplasia is the dysplastic phase, and acute myelosclerosis, paroxysmal nocturnal hemoglobinuria **(PNH)**, aplastic anemia, and acute leukemia are the malignant phases. This classification allows for overlap in the syndromes and the transition from more benign to more malignant phases. These disorders also have variable amounts of fibrosis. Fibroblastic proliferation in myeloproliferative disease is of polyclonal origin and is a reactive phenomenon.

The most **benign proliferative states are characterized by** panmyelosis of the central skeletal marrow with intact maturation of RBCs, WBCs, and platelets **(polycythemia vera** and **essential thrombocythemia). The dysplastic syndromes are characterized by** a reversion to a fetal distribution of the hematopoietic organ involving centrifugal expansion of the bone marrow from the axial skeleton to the long bones and the reactivation of the extramedullary hematopoiesis in the spleen and liver **(myeloid metaplasia).** This occurs in **agnogenic myeloid metaplasia, polycy-**

TABLE 61-9. MYELOPROLIFERATIVE DISEASE CLASSIFIED BY DEGREE OF MATURATION

	Hyperplastic	Dysplastic	Malignant
Typical syndrome	Polycythemia vera, essential throm-bocythemia	Myeloid metaplasia (agnogenic, post-polycythemic)	Acute leukemia, paroxysmal nocturnal hemoglobinuria, aplastic anemia, acute myelosclerosis
Axial marrow			
Cellularity	Panhyperplasia	Panhyperplasia or hypocellularity	Infiltrated by primitive cells
Maturation	Intact	Mild to moderate impairment	Abnormal or absent
Architecture	Normal or slight increase in reticulin	Patchy or extensive fibrosis	Infiltrated by primitive cells
Peripheral marrow	Uninvolved or slightly expanded	Moderate to marked expansion	Infiltrated by primitive cells
Extramedullary hematopoiesis	Slight or moderate splenomegaly	Marked splenomegaly, moderate hepatomegaly	Infiltrated by primitive cells
Circulating mature hemocytic cells	Increased	Variably increased or decreased	Absent or decreased
Complications	Thrombosis, hemorrhage	Thrombosis, hemorrhage, splenic infarction, hypersplenism, hydremia	Hemorrhage, infection, anemia

themia vera with myeloid metaplasia, and postpolycythemia myeloid metaplasia. Further malignant deterioration in myeloproliferative disease is characterized by ineffective erythropoiesis and a decrease in peripheral blood counts. Normal maturation is overtaken by the production of abnormal cells. During this phase, the hematopoietic picture may deteriorate into aplastic anemia, a myelodysplastic syndrome, or paroxysmal nocturnal hemoglobinuria. Final malignant deterioration is seen as acute nonlymphocytic leukemia or lymphocytic leukemia.

Etiology

The etiology of these illnesses is unknown. Rare cases with a familial history or a history of exposure to mutagens or bone marrow toxins (eg, benzene, radiation) suggest that a chromosomal abnormality may be involved.

Incidence and Demographics

Accurate information on the incidence of myeloproliferative disorders is not available. These disorders are found during the middle and later years of life; they are rare in the young. Men are affected slightly more frequently than women. An increased incidence among Ashkenazic Jews has been suggested, but this is questionable.

Pathophysiology

Uncontrolled production of mature RBCs is the predominant proliferative feature of polycythemia vera. The increased blood volume and circulating RBC mass lead to thrombosis and bleeding. Thrombosis may be arterial (coronary, cerebral, peripheral vascular) or venous (peripheral, hepatic, or portal). Small-vessel insufficiency produces cyanosis, erythromelalgia, or even frank gangrene of the fingers and toes. Mild hemorrhagic tendencies (eg, epistaxis, bruising, gingival bleeding) are common, while severe GI, GU, or pulmonary bleeding occurs in about 10% of patients. The major causes of mortality in untreated patients are attributable to thrombosis and hemorrhage.

In essential thrombocythemia, hemorrhage and microvascular occlusions also occur. However, the occurrence of hemorrhagic phenomena generally correlates poorly with the increase in platelet count or the presence of in vitro platelet function abnormalities. The combination of erythrocytosis and thrombocytosis seems to predispose to large-vessel thrombosis. Thrombocythemia in the absence of an elevated RBC mass does not lead to large-vessel thrombosis. However, microvascular occlusion and bleeding occur frequently.

In myeloid metaplasia, the degree of splenic involvement by extramedullary hematopoiesis is independent of the degree of marrow fibrosis. This dissociation invalidates the concept that myeloid metaplasia compensates for diminished bone marrow function. The presence in the peripheral blood of increased numbers of granulocytic stem cells that show fetal characteristics suggests that myeloid metaplasia arises from a homing of these cells to a favorable environment in the spleen and liver.

When myeloid metaplasia occurs de novo it is referred to as **agnogenic myeloid metaplasia.**

In 12% of patients with polycythemia vera, the presentation of this disease evolves about 10 yr postdiagnosis to a picture that is indistinguishable from myeloid metaplasia. This may occur more frequently after radioactive phosphate (^{32}P) treatment. Myeloid metaplasia may also occur early in the course of polycythemia vera. It is far less common to see myeloid metaplasia in the course of essential thrombocythemia.

Patients with polycythemia and agnogenic myeloid metaplasia are at greater risk of developing **acute leukemia.** The leukemia may be acute lymphocytic, acute nonlymphocytic, or biphenotypic and is characteristically resistant to chemotherapy. Transformation to acute leukemia is an expression of myelodysplasia that occurs in both treated and untreated patients, although it is more common in those who have received alkylating agents and radiation therapy.

Symptoms and Signs

The clinical effects of the abnormal hyperplasia or dysplasia are shown in TABLE 61-10. **In polycythemia,** the disease is often discovered in an asymptomatic individual whose Hct is elevated. About $^1/_3$ to $^1/_2$ of patients exhibit plethora, headache, dizziness, visual disturbances, inability to concentrate, and paresthesias. Many patients have hypertension or increased cardiac output and vascular stasis. Signs of large- or small-vessel thrombosis occur in about $^1/_3$ to $^1/_2$ of untreated patients. Major hemorrhage occurs in about 10% of patients. Splenomegaly is present in about 75% at the time of diagnosis. Other symptoms include pruritus, peptic ulcer, and bowel hypermotility from the increase in WBCs. Hyperuricemia and hypermetabolic symptoms also occur.

In essential thrombocythemia, diagnosis is often made in asymptomatic subjects. Patients with complaints have either hemorrhage or microvascular occlusions and thus, may be easily bruised and may have epistaxis, GI or GU bleeding, or postoperative hemorrhage. Microvascular occlusion produces digital cyanosis, erythema, and burning, as well as headache, paresthesias, TIAs, and visual disturbances.

In myeloid metaplasia, about 30% of patients are asymptomatic at the time of diagnosis. The illness is usually detected by the finding of splenomegaly on physical examination. Hepatomegaly may follow splenic enlargement. Complaints in symptomatic patients relate to anemia in 60% (weakness, fatigue, angina, heart failure), splenomegaly in 25% (pressure or pain in the abdomen, postprandial discomfort, and early satiety), and hemorrhage in 20% (patient is easily bruised or has epistaxis, bleeding gums, GI bleeding, CNS hemorrhage from a single vessel, or disseminated intravascular coagulation). Symptomatic splenomegaly may lead to weight loss and malnutrition. Splenic infarction is common and may range from asymptomatic to resemblance of an acute abdomen.

TABLE 61-10. EFFECTS OF ABNORMAL PROLIFERATION ON THE PATHOPHYSIOLOGY OF MYELOPROLIFERATIVE DISEASE

Cell Type	Hyperplastic Phase	Dysplastic Phase

Erythrocyte	Polycythemia vera
	  Hyperviscosity and
	    hypervolemia
	
	  Circulatory overload
	  Thrombosis and
	    hemorrhage
		Anemia
		  Cardiovascular compromise
		  Transfusion requirement
		  Iron overload, hepatitis

Megakaryocyte	Thrombocythemia
	  Thrombosis
	Thrombocytopathy
	  Thrombosis and hemor-
	    rhage
	Release of platelet-derived
	  growth factor
	  ? Fibrosis
		Thrombocytopenia
		  Hemorrhage
		Thrombocytopathy
		  Hemorrhage
		
		Release of platelet-derived
		  growth factor
		  ? Fibrosis

Leukocyte	Basophilia
	  Histamine release
	  Pruritus, ulcer,
	    hyperacidity, bowel
	    hypermotility
	  ? Fibrosis
		Neutrophil function defects
		  Infection
		Leukemic transformation

Pluripotential stem
  cell and progress
	Increased nucleoprotein
	  turnover: hyperuricemia,
	  gout, tophi, uric acid
	  stones, nephropathy
	Hypocholesterolemia
	  ? effect on atherosclerosis
	  ? effect on cell membranes
	Hypermetabolism: fatigue,
	  asthenia, weight loss, fever,
	  diaphoresis
		Myeloid metaplasia
		  Splenomegaly
		  Splenic infarction
		  Hydremia, anemia
		  Hypersplenism,
		    anemia and cytopenia

Malignant myelosclerosis is an acute, rapidly fatal illness with pancytopenia due to a fibrotic bone marrow with circulating myeloblasts; splenomegaly is usually absent. The patient is febrile without necessarily having an infection. Bone pain, arthritis, and generalized wasting are prominent. The symptoms and signs of acute leukemia and aplastic anemia are described above.

Laboratory Findings and Diagnosis

Polycythemia vera must be differentiated from other diseases causing secondary erythrocytosis and from blood volume abnormalities. First, direct measurement must be made of the RBC mass and blood volume. When an increased RBC mass is demonstrated with a normal Sa_{O_2} and an enlarged spleen, the diagnosis of polycythemia is confirmed. If splenomegaly is absent (as it is in 25% of patients at presentation), the presence of 2 other features of pluripotential cell involvement confirms the diagnosis; these include an elevated neutrophil count (50 to 80%), thrombocytosis (35 to 50%), increased neutrophil alkaline phosphatase activity (80%), and an increase in vitamin B_{12} binding proteins (67%).

The bone marrow shows panmyelosis with erythroid hyperplasia and increased megakaryocytes. Increased reticulin is present in 20% of patients, but fibrosis is rare. Cultured bone marrow produces erythroid colonies in the absence of added erythropoietin and a marked increase in the number of erythroid colonies with the addition of erythropoietin. Other laboratory findings include hyperuricemia, hypocholesterolemia, and an elevated blood histamine level.

In essential thrombocythemia, the diagnosis is essentially one of exclusion. The diagnosis may be made if the platelet count is > 1 million/μL and there is no cause of secondary thrombocytosis; the RBC mass is normal; iron is present in the bone marrow and there is no bleeding; collagen fibrosis is absent from the bone marrow biopsy; and the Philadelphia chromosome is absent. Qualitative platelet defects are often found.

In myeloid metaplasia, anemia is the most consistent abnormality. The peripheral smear characteristically shows teardrop and elliptical RBCs and a leukoerythroblastic picture. The WBC count ranges from leukopenia to leukocytosis. Peripheral WBCs are immature, with prominent metamyelocytes and myelocytes and < 5% promyelocytes or blasts. Circulating normoblasts are usually seen. The platelet count ranges from thrombocytopenia to thrombocytosis. The platelets are large, and megakaryocyte fragments are seen. The combination of a leukoerythroblastic peripheral blood picture and splenic enlargement is very suggestive of myeloid metaplasia.

The bone marrow aspirate is often hypocellular or a "dry tap." Bone marrow biopsy has a variable presentation, including hypercellularity, panmyelosis without fibrosis, patchy areas of hypercellularity and fibrosis, or panmyelosis with dense fibrosis, with or without osteosclerosis. Megakaryocytes remain in the bone marrow even after the other hematopoietic elements have disappeared. There is no consistent association between the degree of marrow fibrosis and myeloid metaplasia.

Prognosis

The median survival of patients with **polycythemia vera** who are treated is approximately 10 to 15 yr. In **primary thrombocythemia,** the median survival for untreated patients is only about 5 yr. **Myeloid metaplasia** patients have a 60% decrease in 5-yr survival as compared with controls matched for age and sex. The **acute leukemias** and **myelosclerosis** are usually fatal within months.

Treatment

In polycythemia, the restoration of a normal blood volume and Hct markedly reduces the incidence of complications. At diagnosis, the patient should undergo a series of phlebotomies of 250 to 500 mL every 2nd or 3rd day. If hydration is maintained, the patient's plasma need not be readministered. Patients with cardiovascular disease and people > 75 yr of age usually should be phlebotomized only 250 to 350 mL each time. Once the Hct is reduced to < 42%, phlebotomy should be repeated as required for maintenance at the desired level. Phlebotomy inevitably results in iron deficiency, which limits erythropoiesis and, therefore, the phlebotomy requirement, to less than 8 u./yr. If the Hct is electronically derived, one should keep in mind that the electronic cell counter underestimates Hct by up to 7% when microcytosis is present. Iron should *not* be given to correct the iron deficiency, since it will stimulate erythropoiesis.

Occasionally, a patient will not tolerate phlebotomies, or erythropoiesis is so active that the frequency of phlebotomy is unacceptable. In such patients, myelosuppression, either with chemotherapy or radiation, must be used. However, in patients treated with ^{32}P or chlorambucil, there is a danger of inducing leukemia or a second malignancy. The peak incidence of leukemia approaches 30% 8 yr later, compared with < 1% in patients treated with phlebotomy alone. Currently, when myelosuppression is necessary, hydroxyurea in oral doses of 0.5 to 3.0 gm/day is used, since mutagenicity has not yet been demonstrated with this agent.

In essential thrombocythemia, myelosuppression is indicated in patients > 60 yr of age who have marked thrombocythemia (platelet counts consistently > 1 million/μL, or who have a lower thrombocythemia with a past history of thrombosis or hemorrhage or a coexisting condition that increases the risk for these complications. Myelosuppression is usually achieved with hydroxyurea in the same manner as in polycythemia vera. The platelet count is usually reduced to levels of 500,000 to 800,000/μL. If surgery is necessary, the platelet count should be reduced to < 500,000/μL. Postoperative bleeding should be managed with transfusion of normal platelets, regardless of the platelet count. If the patient with thrombocythemia is bleeding or has active thrombosis, the platelet count should be reduced rapidly with plateletpheresis and hydroxyurea.

In the asymptomatic phase of myeloid metaplasia, no therapy is necessary unless the patient has thrombocythemia and is being prepared for surgery. Splenomegaly is usually responsible for the major complications of myeloid metaplasia, and usually responds to myelosuppression. Hydroxyurea 1 gm/day orally usually reduces the size of the spleen without decreasing marrow function. Anemia is not a contraindication to the use of myelosuppression, since transfusion may be given.

Myelosuppressive therapy cannot, however, be used in the setting of significant neutropenia and thrombocytopenia due to hypoplasia or fibrosis of the bone marrow. Splenic irradiation has been tried, but even localized therapy is myelosuppressive. *Therefore, splenic irradiation must be used rarely and with extreme caution.* Splenectomy is the therapy of choice, but significant mortality and morbidity are associated with this procedure in elderly patients with myeloid metaplasia. Indications for splenectomy include painful splenomegaly, repeated splenic infarction, a short-lived response to hydroxyurea or splenic irradiation, significant thrombocytopenia or neutropenia with bone marrow failure, refractory hemolytic anemia, and portal hypertension. Early splenectomy (at the point significant pancytopenia is present) in the elderly has been advocated before cardiovascular complications occur. However, splenectomy is **contraindicated** if disseminated intravascular coagulation is found on laboratory testing (12% of patients have this without clinical bleeding). Thrombocythemia should be treated with hydroxyurea prior to splenectomy.

Surgery is palliative therapy and usually should not be performed if there is a high serum alkaline phosphatase, anemia with a spleen estimated to be > 3 kg, or anemia with a spleen estimated to be < 1 kg. Measurement of RBC production, survival, and splenic sequestration are not predictive of the effect of splenectomy on the anemia. The anemia should be evaluated to ascertain that deficiencies (eg, iron, folate, B_{12}) are not present. Hemolysis may respond to the use of corticosteroids and should be evaluated by radiochromium (^{51}Cr) RBC survival time. If ineffective erythropoiesis is present (shown by ferrokinetics), pyridoxine and androgens may be tried.

The malignant phases of myeloproliferative disorders are notoriously resistant to therapy. However, treatment is similar to that described for other malignancies.

In all of the myeloproliferative disorders, hyperuricemia is treated with allopurinol 300 mg/day orally. Hydration should be maintained, and hypertonic solutions for diagnostic purposes should be avoided as much as possible. Symptoms of histamine release (pruritus after baths) may be relieved by the potent antihistamine-antiserotonin agent cyproheptadine 4 mg orally. Other antihistaminics are usually not effective. Symptoms of GI hyperacidity may be controlled with H_2-receptor blockers or antacids.

§3.   ORGAN SYSTEMS: MUSCULOSKELETAL DISORDERS

Contents for METABOLIC AND ENDOCRINE DISORDERS begin
on page 773.

---

62. JOINT AND SOFT TISSUE DISORDERS

Walter H. Ettinger

GENERAL PRINCIPLES

Musculoskeletal disease is the leading cause of functional impairment
in the older patient. Being rarely fatal and not curable, these disabling
problems are chronic. However, musculoskeletal disease is not an inevitable consequence of aging and thus should be regarded as a specific
disease process and not just the result of "getting old."

The diagnosis of musculoskeletal disease relies on historical information, physical examination, and judicious use of laboratory tests. However, the clinician must keep in mind that evidence of disease (eg, osteoarthritis [OA]) is commonly found on x-ray or when examining elderly
patients; yet, most patients with such evidence are asymptomatic. The
clinician must not be misled into attributing all complaints to diseases
that are common in the aging patient simply because evidence of such
diseases is found on examination.

History and Physical Examination

The primary complaint of the patient with musculoskeletal disease is
pain, the characteristics of which help narrow the differential diagnosis.
Most important are the location of the pain (regional or diffuse), its
pattern (articular or nonarticular), its time course (when it occurs), and
its association with other symptoms of the inflammatory process (ie,
swelling, warmth, and stiffness). For a differential diagnosis of musculoskeletal disease in the elderly, see TABLE 62–1.

TABLE 62–1. DIFFERENTIAL DIAGNOSIS OF MUSCULOSKELETAL
DISEASE, USING LOCATION AND QUALITY OF PAIN

Generalized pain

Articular
  Noninflammatory
    Osteoarthritis (distal and proximal interphalangeal joints, 1st carpometacarpal
      joints, knees, hips, toes)
  Inflammatory
    Rheumatoid arthritis (proximal interphalangeal and metacarpophalangeal
      joints, wrists, shoulders, elbows, knees, ankles, feet)
    Systemic lupus erythematosus
    Polyarticular gout
    Calcium pyrophosphate dihydrate (CPPD) crystal disease
    Arthritis of malignancy

Nonarticular
  Noninflammatory
    Fibromyalgia
    Metastatic carcinoma
    Multiple myeloma
  Inflammatory
    Polymyalgia rheumatica

Localized pain

Articular
  Noninflammatory
    Fracture
    Osteoarthritis
    Aseptic necrosis
    Internal derangement
  Inflammatory
    Septic arthritis
    Microcrystalline disease (gout, CPPD)
    Bursitis/tendonitis
      Knee (anserine, prepatellar)
      Shoulder (subdeltoid, bicipital)
      Elbow (olecranon)

Nonarticular
  Noninflammatory
    Carpal tunnel syndrome
    Nerve root compression
    Fracture
    Reflex sympathetic dystrophy
    Neuroarthropathy
  Inflammatory
    Soft tissue infection

The clinician must focus on the symptomatic area, while proceeding to examine the entire musculoskeletal system. An evaluation of asymptomatic joints is especially important, because painless swelling or loss of motion in several joints may indicate a systemic or generalized inflammatory process not elicited by the history. Specific aspects of the examination include the presence of tenderness, deformity, swelling, and loss of motion.

A **performance-oriented examination** should include evaluation of the back and all extremities. The clinician should test grip strength and ability to hold objects (eg, eating utensils or writing instruments) as well as the capacity to raise the arms over the head. The back should be examined to assess the ability to bend at the waist, to touch the feet, and to pick up objects on the floor. Examination of the lower extremities focuses on mobility, testing the patient's ability to rise from a chair, to maintain balance, to initiate and maintain gait, to turn, and to return to the sitting position. Additionally, evaluation of the ability to climb stairs and to walk for 5 min (to measure endurance) is important.

Laboratory Tests

Laboratory testing has 3 potential pitfalls: (1) there are no definitive diagnostic tests for most musculoskeletal diseases; (2) many tests that are diagnostic have high sensitivity for disease but lack specificity; and (3) the normal values for certain laboratory tests may change with age, and certain tests (eg, those for autoantibodies) may be positive in older individuals but not indicative of disease (see Ch. 102). Thus *one should not use laboratory tests to screen for rheumatic disease but only when a specific test is indicated to diagnose a disease with a high pretest probability.*

Treatment

In treating the elderly patient, one must separate the direct consequences of musculoskeletal disease from its effects on function. A helpful tool for this is a conceptual framework, such as that of the World Health Organization's International Classification of Impairments, Disabilities, and Handicaps. The terms of this typology are defined as follows: (1) **Impairment:** Any loss or abnormality of psychologic, physiologic, or anatomic structure within an organ system of the body, either temporary or permanent. Examples relevant to musculoskeletal disease include loss of a limb, loss of range of motion, or pain on motion. (2) **Disability:** Inability to perform an activity in the manner or within the range considered normal for the individual. Thus a disability almost always entails lost performance of compound or integrated tasks (eg, walking or combing one's hair). (3) **Handicap:** Limited fulfillment of an individual's role, depending on age, sex, and other social and cultural factors. A handicap, therefore, is a social effect or disadvantage resulting from an impairment or disability (eg, loss of employment or of social interaction). Using this classification, one can determine which disabilities or handicaps are most important to the individual, rather than focusing on impairments that are often irrelevant to function.

Three principles govern treatment of musculoskeletal disease in the elderly: (1) Therapy should be aimed specifically at restoring function and improving quality of life. (2) The patient should be actively involved in decision making, and his preferences should guide the specific goals of therapy. (3) A multifaceted approach to therapy should be used, including treatment of pain, physical or occupational therapy, psychologic support, and environmental manipulation.

The goals of therapy need to be well defined and realistic. For example, a patient may be physically able to undergo rehabilitation after total joint replacement, but lack of social supports or a care giver may prevent his benefiting from such restorative care, therefore resulting in treatment failure.

OSTEOARTHRITIS (OA)

Incidence, Etiology, and Pathogenesis

OA is the most common form of joint disease. It has been estimated that ⅓ of individuals > 35 yr of age have some radiographic evidence of OA, with the prevalence increasing well into the 8th decade. Although a majority of these persons, particularly the younger ones, have mild and relatively asymptomatic disease, OA is 1 of the leading causes of disability in persons > 65 yr of age.

OA is probably not 1 disease but several, all having similar clinical and pathologic features. Thus the typical changes, which include both cartilage deterioration and bony remodeling, occur in a number of diarthrodial joints but may have different etiologies in each. Several factors have been implicated. Aging alone does not cause OA, although cellular or matrix alterations in cartilage that occur with aging probably predispose older persons to OA. Other presumed factors include obesity, trauma, endocrine diseases (eg, diabetes mellitus), and primary disorders of the joint (eg, inflammatory arthritis).

Symptoms and Signs

Because the etiology and pathogenesis are not known, OA is classified according to clinical criteria as primary and secondary (see TABLE 62–2). The disease is called **primary OA** when there is no known predisposing cause. Primary OA can be further divided into distinct subsets on the basis of clinical features. It is not known whether degenerative disk disease or diffuse skeletal hyperostosis represents the same pathologic process as OA of the diarthrodial joints. **Secondary OA** results from a clearly defined underlying condition (eg, trauma, metabolic disease, or inflammatory arthritis) that contributes to its etiology.

Primary OA is characterized by a slow progression of joint pain that is intermittent, then becomes constant, and may be accompanied by limitation of movement and joint deformity. Pain is relieved by rest and exacerbated by movement; it is not associated with inflammatory symptoms. There is a specific pattern of joint involvement that includes the distal and proximal interphalangeal joints, first carpal-metacarpal joint, cervical and lumbar spine, hips, knees, and toes. The metacarpophalan-

TABLE 62–2. CLASSIFICATION OF OSTEOARTHRITIS

Primary
    Peripheral joints (single or multiple)
    Spine
        Diffuse idiopathic skeletal hyperostosis
        Degenerative disk disease
    Subsets
        Erosive inflammatory osteoarthritis
        Generalized osteoarthritis

Secondary
    Trauma (acute, chronic)
    Inflammatory arthritis
    Systemic metabolic disease
    Endocrine disorders
    Microcrystalline disease
    Neuropathic disorders
    Bone dysplasias
    Miscellaneous (avascular necrosis, hypermobility syndrome, etc.)

geal joints, wrists, elbows, shoulders, and ankles are spared in primary OA.

Diagnosis

The diagnosis is made using the clinical findings and the presence of osteoarthritic changes on x-ray. Characteristic x-ray features include the presence of osteophytes, subchondral sclerosis and cysts, and asymmetric loss of joint space (implying degeneration of cartilage). Other laboratory data are not helpful. The ESR and WBC count are normal, and autoantibodies are absent. Examination of synovial fluid from affected joints shows only a mild leukocytosis (< 2000 cells/μL) and no other diagnostic features.

Prognosis and Treatment

When deciding on a therapeutic regimen, the clinician must recognize that several factors may increase morbidity in the older individual (eg, the physiologic changes of aging; the presence of other chronic diseases; and psychologic, environmental, or iatrogenic problems) (see TABLE 62–3). Thus, one must decide if the treatment of OA alone will improve functioning or if treatment of other problems will also be needed. Additionally, the presence of other diseases (eg, renal disease, peptic ulcer, and hypertension) may make treatment of OA more dangerous and difficult.

Comprehensive management involves a balance of psychotherapeutic, physical, pharmaceutical, and surgical measures (see TABLE 62–4). Specific goals of therapy must take into account the functional deficits and the patient's preferences for treatment. The patient should be taught the

TABLE 62-3. CONDITIONS THAT CAUSE COMORBIDITY IN OSTEOARTHRITIS

Physiologic changes associated with aging
Neurologic
  Motor system: Loss of muscle mass and strength; diminished balance reflexes
  Sensory system: Diminished proprioceptive and vibratory input; slowed
    reaction time
Cardiovascular
  Blunted baroreflexes
  Decrease in aerobic capacity

Chronic diseases
Musculoskeletal
  Fractures
  Primary muscle disease
  Painful foot conditions
Neurologic
  Stroke
  Parkinson's disease
  Degenerative dementias
Cardiovascular
  Heart failure
  Atherosclerotic vascular disease
Pulmonary
  Chronic obstructive pulmonary disease
Other
  Blindness
  Severe systemic illness

Psychologic factors
Depression
Fear of injury
Lack of motivation

Environmental and iatrogenic factors
Forced immobility
Physical obstructions
Lack of social support
Drug side effects

nature of the disease and told what can be realistically expected from treatment. Unrealistic expectations can lead to frustration and depression, as well as misunderstanding between the patient and the physician. (See also MANAGEMENT OF OSTEOARTHRITIS in Ch. 66.)

Pain relief is the cornerstone of therapy. Nonpharmacologic strategies include rest when symptoms are at their worst, adjustment of activities to avoid repetitive movements that aggravate symptoms, and weight loss. The most commonly used agents are aspirin and the nonsteroidal anti-inflammatory drugs **(NSAIDs)** (see TABLE 62-5). There is no evidence that 1 NSAID is more efficacious than another in OA. However,

TABLE 62–4. THERAPY FOR OSTEOARTHRITIS

Psychologic support and patient education
Physical therapy
    Range-of-motion exercises
    Strengthening exercises
    Endurance (aerobic) exercises
    Weight loss
Pharmacologic therapy
    Anti-inflammatory agents (aspirin, NSAIDs)
    Intra-articular steroids
    Other non-narcotic analgesics
Surgery
    Arthroscopy
    Total joint arthroplasty

TABLE 62–5. NONSTEROIDAL ANTI-INFLAMMATORY DRUGS

Drug	Dosage
Piroxicam	10–20 mg once/day
Sulindac	150–200 mg bid
Naproxen	250–500 mg bid
Diflunisal	500 mg bid
Diclofenac	50–75 mg bid or tid
Ibuprofen	400–800 mg tid or qid
Fenoprofen	600–800 mg tid or qid
Tolmetin Na	300–400 mg tid or qid
Meclofenamate Na	50–100 mg tid or qid
Indomethacin	25–50 mg tid or qid
Ketoprofen	50–75 mg tid or qid
Aspirin	600–1200 mg tid or qid
Nonacetylated salicylates	3–4 gm/day

individual response to these drugs varies greatly, and several may be tried before relief is obtained. Except for salicylates, which are less expensive, all NSAIDs cost roughly the same at equivalent therapeutic doses.

The dosage schedule for NSAIDs varies from 1 to 4 times/day, and the major side effects of the different agents are similar (see TABLE 62–6). Each drug differs, however, in its propensity for side effects in individual patients. Consequently, the choice of drug should depend partially on the individual's tolerance or potential for developing a toxic reaction. The most common side effect is GI upset, which often occurs without evidence of ulceration or bleeding and may necessitate discontinuance of the drug.

TABLE 62–6. MAJOR SIDE EFFECTS OF NONSTEROIDAL
ANTI-INFLAMMATORY DRUGS

GI
Dyspepsia, anorexia
Gastric and intestinal ulceration
Upper GI bleeding

Nephrotoxicity
Acute renal failure
Interstitial nephritis
Na, water retention
Papillary necrosis
Hyperkalemia

CNS
Headache
Tinnitus
Cognitive dysfunction

Hepatitis

Hypersensitivity reactions
Hives
Anaphylaxis

GI bleeding occurs with all of the agents but may be less of a problem with enteric-coated aspirin, naproxen, sulindac, or ibuprofen. Unfortunately, there is no correlation between ulceration, bleeding, and subjective symptoms; thus, bleeding can occur without warning. Taking these medications with food may help minimize GI symptoms, and the concomitant use of cytoprotective agents is promising in decreasing the incidence of ulceration. In addition, NSAIDs rank second to aminoglycosides as a cause of drug-induced acute renal failure. Therefore, they should be used with caution in the elderly, particularly in patients who have underlying renal disease, heart failure, volume depletion, or liver disease. Preliminary evidence suggests that sulindac may cause less renal toxicity than other NSAIDs, since its active form is not found in the kidney. Other important toxic effects in the elderly are cognitive dysfunction and personality changes. The mechanism of CNS toxicity is unknown, but one should question patients and family about these symptoms.

Other analgesics may be used occasionally. Acetaminophen is not as effective as NSAIDs, but it may be helpful when the latter are not tolerated. In general, systemic corticosteroids and narcotic analgesics should be *avoided*. There is, however, an indication for intra-articular corticosteroids: the presence of a large, painful joint effusion unresponsive to other modalities. The most efficacious steroid preparations are those that are least soluble, and it is recommended that a formulation of triamcinalone be used.

Total joint arthroplasty is highly effective in the management of OA, and age alone should not be a contraindication to its performance. (See also MANAGEMENT OF OSTEOARTHRITIS in Ch. 66.) However, the decision to operate is complex; the goals to be achieved and the needs and capabilities of the patient must first be clearly defined.

RHEUMATOID ARTHRITIS (RA)

Incidence, Etiology, and Pathogenesis

The incidence of RA, unlike OA, declines after age 65. However, since RA is a chronic illness, its prevalence is increased in older populations. The etiology is unknown; however, RA is characterized by intense inflammation of the synovium of the diarthroidal joints. Synovial tissue becomes hyperplastic and infiltrated with lymphocytes and plasma cells. A variety of inflammatory mediators, including interleukin 1, prostaglandins, and immunoglobulins, are found in the synovial fluid.

Symptoms and Signs

Most older patients with RA experience the disease as an ongoing process that began in youth or middle age. While the inflammation is inactive in some, they nevertheless may exhibit joint deformities and degenerative changes.

When RA develops de novo in an older individual, the onset may be insidious or acute. In most patients, the arthritis is accompanied by mild or moderate constitutional symptoms. Usually, RA occurs primarily in the small joints of the hands (proximal interphalangeal, metacarpophalangeal), feet (metatarsal-phalangeal, interphalangeal), and the wrist, later involving the larger joints (eg, elbows, shoulders, knees). When the onset is precipitous, occurring over several days, patients often experience malaise, anorexia, weight loss, and depression. Fever and night sweats occasionally have been reported. Eventually, RA becomes a symmetric, additive disease of the joints, as in younger patients.

Laboratory Findings

Several abnormal test results are found in patients with RA; however, most are common to a variety of inflammatory diseases. Abnormal findings include a normochromic, normocytic anemia; mild leukocytosis; and thrombocytosis. The ESR is elevated in approximately 80% of cases, and positive rheumatoid factor (RF) is present in about 70%. RF in high titer ($\geq$ 1:320) is virtually diagnostic of the disease; in contrast, low titers of RF are seen with other diseases and in up to 25% of older patients without evidence of any disease. X-rays of involved joints usually show only soft tissue swelling until later in the course of the disease. Characteristic late features include periarticular osteoporosis, joint space narrowing, and marginal erosions.

Diagnosis

The diagnosis is based on a clinical judgment and requires that a patient exhibit symmetric inflammatory arthritis involving the appropriate joints and morning stiffness lasting $\geq$ 1 h. Other diseases (eg, polymyalgia rheumatica, SLE, and the arthritis of malignancy) must be excluded.

Treatment

In general, the long-term prognosis for RA is poor; most patients become progressively disabled despite appropriate treatment, and mortality is increased by a higher rate of serious infections and perhaps cardiovascular disease. Nevertheless, many patients do respond to treatment. Therapy should begin with aspirin or another NSAID, as outlined in the discussion of OA, above. Additionally, physical and occupational therapy are essential, along with exercise and assistive devices and, possibly, physical modalities for pain relief (eg, locally applied heat or cold). While rest should be encouraged during periods of severe disease exacerbation, *irreversible immobility may result if an older patient is placed on prolonged bed rest.* Other chronic diseases, as well as the loss of aerobic capacity and muscle strength associated with aging, lower the threshold at which functional ability is so severely compromised that it cannot be restored.

If a patient does not respond favorably to drug treatment and physical measures within 6 to 12 wk, second-line therapy should be initiated. Many patients with active inflammation of the joints respond to systemic corticosteroids (eg, a 1-mo regimen of prednisone, starting at a dosage of 25 mg/day, tapering to 5 to 10 mg/day). Unfortunately, since discontinuance of corticosteroids is difficult, the long-term effects (osteoporosis, cataracts, poor wound healing, hyperglycemia, hypertension, and increased risk of infection) must be balanced against the therapeutic benefits. Intra-articular steroids may be helpful in treating a single acutely inflamed rheumatoid joint.

Longer-acting remissive agents in RA include the following:

Hydroxychloroquine: This antimalarial can be used in dosages of 6.5 mg/kg/day or 400 mg/day to treat RA that is not responding adequately to NSAIDs. Hydroxychloroquine can cause severe and sometimes irreversible adverse effects, particularly loss of visual acuity. However, vision can be spared if it is monitored at 6-mo intervals by an ophthalmologist and the drug is discontinued at the first signs of retinal toxicity.

Gold therapy: Gold can be highly effective in mild-to-moderate RA. Gold sodium thiomalate and aurothioglucose are injectable; auranofin, the oral preparation, appears to be less toxic but is perhaps less efficacious than the injectable forms. Injectable gold is administered in a test dose of 10 mg, followed by a therapeutic dose of 25 to 50 mg weekly for up to 20 wk. If the patient responds, treatment intervals are lengthened to q 2 wk, then q 3 wk, then monthly. Monthly therapy should be continued for a prolonged period to prevent a recurrence. The usual dosage of auranofin is 3 mg bid or 6 mg/day. Dosage may be increased to 3 mg tid after 6 mo if no therapeutic response occurs.

The most common side effects of gold therapy are skin rash, oral lesions, proteinuria, and falling peripheral blood counts. *Proteinuria, leukopenia, or thrombocytopenia necessitates permanent discontinuance of the drug.* Pruritus often precedes stomatitis and a diffuse rash, which may cause exfoliation. *When pruritus or a minor rash occurs, gold should be discontinued.* If the rash resolves, the drug may be restarted at a lower dose. Oral gold causes less mucocutaneous and renal toxicity but more diarrhea and GI reactions.

Penicillamine: The dosage of penicillamine is 125 to 250 mg/day, increasing at 2- to 3-mo intervals by 125- to 250-mg increments to a total of 750 mg/day. Penicillamine should be taken between meals, because food decreases its absorption. Adverse effects include rash, proteinuria, dysgeusia, and thrombocytopenia, and patients taking this medication *must be closely monitored.* Other, more severe side effects (eg, pemphigus, myasthenia gravis, a lupus-like syndrome, and severe bone marrow suppression) have also been reported.

Methotrexate: The dosage of methotrexate is 7.5 mg/wk taken in 3 doses of 2.5 mg; this may be increased to 15 mg/wk. The drug can also be given once weekly, beginning with a 5-mg dose, which is increased gradually. Patients receiving methotrexate require careful monitoring because of the risks of hepatic toxicity, interstitial pneumonitis, bone marrow suppression, and GI ulceration and bleeding. The drug should not be given to patients with renal insufficiency. Aspirin may increase the toxicity of methotrexate by slowing the rate of excretion.

The cytotoxic drugs azathioprine and cyclophosphamide also have been used to treat patients with refractory RA.

SYSTEMIC LUPUS ERYTHEMATOSUS (SLE)

Etiology and Incidence

The etiology of SLE is unknown, but its pathogenesis involves the formation of autoantibodies and immune complexes, resulting in damage to several organs. The incidence of SLE declines in old age, but in large series, patients > 50 yr of age account for approximately 12% of cases. Furthermore, the female:male ratio declines to approximately 3:1 in older populations. In contrast to idiopathic SLE, the prevalence of **drug-induced SLE** increases with age, probably because of the greater use of predisposing drugs (eg, procainamide, hydralazine, and anticonvulsants).

Diagnosis

The diagnosis of SLE is no different in the elderly than in younger persons and includes the usual constellation of symptoms and the presence of antinuclear antibodies **(ANA).** Typical clinical features include rash, asymmetric migratory arthritis, photosensitivity, pleurisy, pericarditis, and pneumonitis. It has been suggested that CNS manifestations, hematologic manifestations, and renal disease are unusual in older patients.

Clinical manifestations of drug-induced lupus are similar to those of idiopathic SLE, although CNS and renal manifestations are uncommon.

Laboratory Tests

The ANA test is positive in 95% of patients with idiopathic SLE and in 100% with drug-induced SLE. Fifty percent of patients taking procainamide have a positive ANA test, and approximately 10% develop an SLE-like syndrome. A multitude of other autoantibodies are present in patients with SLE but are not usually helpful in diagnosis. Serum complement levels may be depressed, particularly in patients with renal disease. The urinalysis may show proteinuria and/or cells and casts on microscopic examination; and CBC may show any or all of the following: thrombocytopenia, leukopenia, and anemia.

Treatment

This depends on the specific manifestations of SLE. Patients with mild disease, presenting primarily as arthritis or skin rash, may respond to a nonsteroidal anti-inflammatory drug **(NSAID)**. Corticosteroids in high dosage are indicated when CNS, renal, or severe hematologic manifestations are present. They are also usually indicated if the patient has fever, weight loss, or severe pleurisy or pericarditis.

In drug-induced SLE, discontinuance of the inciting agent and treatment with an anti-inflammatory drug may be sufficient. However, some patients may require as much as 40 mg/day of prednisone for several weeks, particularly if there is severe pericarditis.

BURSITIS

Etiology

The causes of bursitis are varied and include acute and chronic trauma, crystal deposition disease, and infection. Occasionally, bursae are involved in systemic inflammatory diseases such as RA.

Symptoms, Signs, and Diagnosis

Subdeltoid (subacromial) bursitis: Shoulder pain is a frequent problem in older adults, and bursitis is an important and common cause of nonarticular shoulder pain. The subdeltoid bursa is located between the deltoid muscle and the joint capsule, extending under the acromion and coracoacromial ligament. Bursitis is often accompanied by simultaneous inflammation of the supraspinatus tendon, and the 2 entities may be indistinguishable. Inflammation of the subdeltoid bursa results in painful shoulder movement, particularly *abduction* and *extension*. Pain mainly over the anterior aspect of the shoulder that is aggravated by forearm supination against resistance is more likely to reflect bicipital tendonitis.

Patients with subdeltoid bursitis tend to awaken at night when turning on the affected shoulder. The pain often radiates down the arm in the C-5 dermatome. **Physical examination** indicates tenderness over the lateral aspect of the shoulder and the subacromial space. The pain can be elicited if the arm is abducted and then actively moved toward the body against resistance. Patients report pain on moving the arm downward through the arc of abduction at approximately 90°.

Trochanteric bursitis: The trochanteric bursa lies between the gluteus maximus and the tendon of the gluteus medius. The usual symptom of inflammation is a dull, aching pain or a burning, tingling sensation over the lateral part of the hip. The pain may also be referred to the L-2 dermatome. Pain is worse with activity and after sitting with the affected leg crossed over the other. Sleep disturbance and inability to lie on the affected side are common. **Physical examination** reveals localized tenderness over the bony prominence of the greater trochanter. External rotation with abduction of the hip is often painful, although the range of motion is normal.

Anserine bursitis: The anserine bursa is located about 4 cm below the medial aspect of the knee joint. It lies under the pes anserinus (the insertion tendons of the sartorius, gracilis, and semitendinous muscles). The patient with anserine bursitis complains of knee pain that is worse at night. A pillow between the knees is needed in bed. Physical examination may elicit point tenderness over the bursa and, occasionally, mild-to-moderate swelling.

Olecranon bursitis: The olecranon bursa lies between the skin and the olecranon process. The usual presentation of this bursitis is swelling and tenderness over the most proximal part of the ulna. On careful physical examination, the elbow joint exhibits painless full range of motion.

Treatment

Most important in the treatment of bursitis is determination of the etiology. When the history and physical examination do not yield an obvious degenerative or traumatic etiology, aspiration and examination of the bursal fluid are indicated to determine whether crystal deposits or infection is present. A bursal fluid WBC count of $\geq 2000/\mu L$ suggests an inflammatory process. The fluid should be examined microscopically for crystals and a Gram stain performed to exclude infection.

If infection is present, the most common organisms are those that colonize the skin: *Staphylococcus aureus* and Group A streptococci. Antibiotic therapy should be instituted against these gram-positive organisms. If the patient is not having systemic symptoms such as high fever, antibiotics may be given orally. An infected bursa should not be drained but repeatedly aspirated. If microcrystalline disease and infection have been excluded, the most successful treatment is fluid aspiration and injection of the bursal sac with a mixture of corticosteroids and local analgesics. Use of aspirin or other NSAIDs is also effective.

The patient should be encouraged to move the affected area, particularly the shoulder. Severe, long-term limitation of motion and frozen shoulder can occur if range-of-motion exercises are neglected.

GOUT

Incidence and Pathogenesis

Primary gout is most often a mid-life disease of men. Gout in women most often occurs after menopause. Gout correlates with hyperuricemia; the upper limit of normal serum urate levels is usually 7 mg/dL in men and 6 mg/dL in women. Hyperuricemia represents an imbalance between endogenous production of uric acid and renal urate excretion. Primary hyperuricemia is characterized in most patients by a defect in renal handling of uric acid, as are most cases of secondary hyperuricemia.

Symptoms, Signs, and Diagnosis

The onset of gout is marked by an acute inflammatory arthritis that may follow trauma, illness, or operation. The metatarsophalangeal joint of the great toe is the typical site of the acute attack **(podagra).** Other joints may be involved, either as a monoarthritis or in a polyarticular pattern including the ankle, knee, wrist, elbow, small joints of the hands or feet, and bursae (especially the olecranon bursae).

Fever (up to 39 C [102.2 F]) is often present. Tenderness is usually so exquisite that the patient cannot move the affected joint or tolerate the weight of bedclothes. The inflammatory process often extends beyond the joint, suggesting cellulitis in some cases. Untreated, the acute attack resolves in a few days to weeks. A history of recurrent acute episodes of arthritis, especially involving the great toe, should always suggest the possibility of gout.

Chronic gouty arthritis may cause morning stiffness and aching in joints, mimicking RA and other chronic polyarticular arthritides. It occurs primarily in patients who have tophaceous gout. Such patients often have x-ray evidence of urate deposition in soft tissue or bone adjacent to the joints. The deposition of Na urate in soft tissue increases with the severity of hyperuricemia. These deposits, called tophi, are commonly found in bursae, the articular cartilage, and bone. Tophi may be confused with rheumatoid nodules when they occur in the olecranon bursae or over the extensor surface of the forearm.

About 10 to 20% of patients develop urate stones. Hyperuricemia may be exacerbated by drugs commonly taken by elderly patients (eg, thiazide diuretics and salicylates, even in small doses).

Laboratory Findings

Acute gouty arthritis may be accompanied by leukocytosis and elevation of the ESR. Elevated serum uric acid supports the diagnosis but is not specific. The definitive test is demonstration of urate crystals in the synovial fluid of an affected joint. Synovial fluid should be analyzed particularly when the differentiation of gout from infection is difficult. In acute gout, the synovial fluid shows typical inflammatory changes, with leukocytosis in the 5000 to 50,000/μL range. In 90% of cases, urate crystals can be seen free in the fluid or engulfed by phagocytes. When viewed with a polarizing microscope, they are negatively birefringent.

Treatment

Acute attack: An effective and simple way to manage acute gouty arthritis is with a nonsteroidal anti-inflammatory drug **(NSAID)** at the usual dose (see TABLE 62–5). Relief is seen within 24 h, and symptoms usually resolve within 3 days. Alternatively, colchicine can be given either IV or orally. IV colchicine 1 to 2 mg diluted with 0.9% NaCl and injected over 20 min is highly effective in ameliorating acute symptoms. Oral colchicine at 0.5 mg bid to qid for 2 to 3 days may be necessary to provide complete relief. Also effective acutely, oral colchicine may be given at a dosage of 0.5 mg q 2 h until a favorable response is obtained or GI toxicity supervenes. However, since almost all patients must take colchicine until GI toxicity occurs, this treatment has lost favor in recent years.

Another effective measure in treating acute gout of the large joints is the withdrawal of synovial fluid and injection of deposteroids at a dose of 40 mg (triamcinolone). This is especially effective in patients who are unable to take oral medications or who cannot tolerate NSAIDs or colchicine.

Uricosuric drugs and allopurinol should be *avoided* during the acute attack. The incidence of recurrent acute gouty arthritis may be lowered by chronic administration of colchicine 0.5 mg bid.

Measures to lower serum uric acid may be indicated for the following: (1) presence of tophi, (2) recurrent gouty arthritis uncontrolled by chronic colchicine administration, (3) renal insufficiency, and (4) presence of renal urate stones. One uricosuric drug is **probenicid,** which should be administered initially at 500 mg q 12 h. This may be increased up to 3 gm daily to reduce the serum uric acid level to 6 mg/dL. An alternative to probenicid is **sulfinpyrazone.** This relatively short-acting drug must be given q 6 h in divided doses ranging from 300 to 1000 mg/day.

Allopurinol, a highly effective uricosuric agent, blocks the metabolic pathway of uric acid production, specifically inhibiting xanthine oxidase. Since allopurinol does not produce its effect through the kidney and actually reduces the renal urate load, it is indicated in patients with renal calculi. The initial dosage of 100 mg bid may be increased gradually to 600 mg daily to achieve the desired effect. In severe tophaceous gout, allopurinol may be used with other uricosuric agents.

CALCIUM PYROPHOSPHATE DIHYDRATE (CPPD) CRYSTAL DISEASE

(Pseudogout)

Incidence and Pathogenesis

CPPD crystal disease is a microcrystalline arthritis associated with calcification of hyaline and fibrous cartilage **(chondrocalcinosis).** CPPD crystal disease, which is rare before the 5th decade, is more common with advancing age. The mechanism of cartilage calcification is poorly understood; however, the association of chondrocalcinosis and arthritis with an array of diseases suggests that multiple factors play a role. Certain conditions predispose to CPPD crystal disease, including hyperparathyroidism, acromegaly, and hypothyroidism.

Symptoms and Signs

CPPD crystal disease was originally called **pseudogout** to emphasize the acute, episodic, goutlike attacks of synovial inflammation. However, unlike gout, acute CPPD crystal disease usually occurs in large joints, especially the knee. There may also be involvement of the shoulder, hip, wrist, and elbow. In addition, CPPD crystal disease may cause a chronic, asymmetric, inflammatory polyarthritis, which in some cases mimics RA.

Laboratory Findings

Hematologic findings are nonspecific. There is no abnormality in serum Ca levels unless hyperparathyroidism is present. Hyperuricemia may be present and may play a role in pathogenesis. Chondrocalcinosis of the fibrocartilagenous menisci of the knees, the radial and ulnar joints, the symphysis pubis, and the articular disk of the sternoclavicular joint is frequently seen on x-ray. The synovial fluid in acute CPPD crystal disease is typical of an inflammatory process, with a WBC count of 2000 to $50,000/\mu L$. Intracellular and extracellular crystals of CPPD can be identified on careful examination in 90% of effusions. CPPD crystals are generally rhomboid and, as opposed to urate crystals, are positively birefringent under polarized light.

Diagnosis

This is made by a clinical history of recurrent, episodic acute attacks and the demonstration of CPPD crystals in synovial fluid. Careful search for crystals by polarized light microscopy may be necessary, particularly in patients with polyarticular chronic disease. The diagnosis is supported by x-ray demonstration of chondrocalcinosis of cartilage.

Treatment

As in gout, nonsteroidal anti-inflammatory drugs **(NSAIDs)** are an effective way to treat an acute attack. Similarly, intra-articular corticosteroids may be useful when a large joint is involved. The use of colchicine is controversial, but there is some evidence that it may be efficacious.

SEPTIC ARTHRITIS

Etiology and Pathogenesis

A disproportionate number of cases of septic arthritis occur in patients > 65 yr of age. Bacterial infection arises by direct inoculation or as a result of bacteremia from either a known or an unknown source. In most cases, infections occur in joints with preexisting disease, usually OA or RA. Patients who are immunocompromised as a result of corticosteroid therapy, malignancy, or diabetes, are also more likely to develop septic arthritis.

Symptoms, Signs, and Diagnosis

The disease usually presents as an acute febrile illness associated with either monarticular or polyarticular arthritis. Large joints are primarily affected, most commonly the knee, hip, shoulder, and elbow. Notably, many patients may not look toxemic, particularly elderly persons, who may have low-grade or no fever and whose peripheral leukocytosis may be < 14,000/μL. Diagnosis may be particularly difficult in debilitated or demented patients who cannot accurately describe local symptoms. In febrile patients who cannot give a good history, all of the diarthrodial joints *must be* carefully examined.

Infection is diagnosed by **aspiration of the joint and analysis of synovial fluid.** WBC counts > 50,000/μL indicate infection unless crystals are also seen. Infected fluid can contain < 50,000 WBC/μL, although polymorphonuclear leukocytes predominate in most instances. The glucose level of synovial fluid is also low in most cases, and a difference of 40 mg/dL between serum and synovial fluid glucose is highly suggestive of infection. **Gram stain and culture** demonstrate the infecting organism in up to 50% of cases. **Blood cultures** should be obtained, because the organism often will grow in blood but not in synovial fluid. In general, if all appropriate sites are cultured, a specific organism can be identified in > 80% of episodes of septic arthritis.

Other biochemical tests of synovial fluid include lactate level, bacterial antigen detection, and nitroblue tetrazolium reduction. The most common organism is *Staphylococcus aureus,* as in younger patients; however, gram-negative bacteria are implicated in a significant proportion of cases in older patients.

Treatment

Treatment is urgently required to avoid the destruction of cartilage and permanent joint damage. Joint fluid should be aspirated repeatedly and as completely as possible. If there is no substantial reduction in fever and the signs of arthritis in 48 to 72 h, surgical drainage of the joint is required. Septic arthritis responds to appropriate systemic antibiotic therapy if the organism is sensitive and the dosage is adequate. Intra-articular antibiotics are not necessary.

63. GIANT CELL (TEMPORAL) ARTERITIS AND POLYMYALGIA RHEUMATICA (PMR)

William J. MacLennan

Giant cell arteritis, also called **temporal arteritis,** is a *chronic inflammatory process involving the extracranial arteries.* The latter nomenclature is not ideal because it may direct attention away from more vital cranial blood vessels, which may also be affected. It also does not cover the minority of patients in whom blood vessels not originating from the aortic arch are involved. **Polymyalgia rheumatica (PMR)** is characterized by pain and stiffness in the muscles of the limb girdles and by its response to therapeutic corticosteroids. Since it has few pathologic features, its pathophysiology remains undefined. Rarer forms have little arterial or muscle involvement, and patients may present with cachexia, fever, or anemia.

Epidemiology and Etiology

Although giant cell arteritis and PMR may occur as separate entities, ½ of patients with giant cell arteritis have clinical features of PMR, and ¼ of patients with PMR have clinical or pathologic features of giant cell arteritis. In view of this overlap, most epidemiologic surveys have grouped the 2 conditions together as 1 disorder.

The complex is twice as common in women as in men and shows a striking increase in incidence with age: it is at least 10 times as common in patients > 80 yr of age as in those aged 50 to 59 yr (FIG. 63–1). Hospital surveys report a wide variation in incidence; the number of cases per 100,000 people per year in Tennessee was 1.6; in Scotland, 4.2; in Minnesota, 11.7; and in Sweden, 18.3. The low incidence in Tennessee is partly due to the large black population in that state (the disorder is 6 times less common in blacks than in whites). The higher figures for Minnesota and Sweden may result from the large number of people of Scandinavian descent in both locales. However, hospital surveys may seriously underestimate the rate of occurrence; a recent survey in a British general practice revealed an annual incidence of 4/1000 in patients > 60 yr of age, a figure 20 times higher than that recorded in Swedish hospitals.

Genetic factors appear to be important; several family clusters have been identified. Two centers have reported an increased prevalence in subjects with the HLA-DR4 genotype, which is consistent with the low incidence in blacks, in whom the DR4 genotype is much less common than in whites.

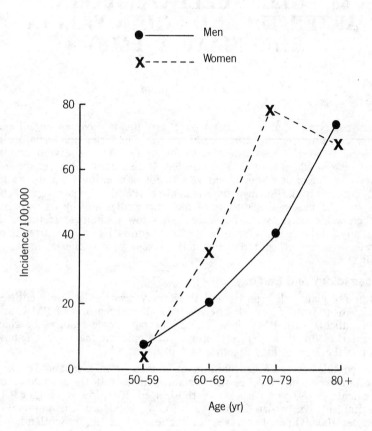

FIG. 63-1. **Incidence of giant cell arteritis and PMR per 100,000 inhabitants ≥ 50 yr of age in Sweden.** (Based on data from B.E. Bengtsson and B.A. Malmvall: "The Epidemiology of giant cell arteritis including temporal arteritis and polymyalgia rheumatica," in *Arthritis and Rheumatism* Journal, Vol. 24, pp. 899-904, copyright 1981.)

Pathology

In giant cell arteritis, the characteristic histologic picture is round cell infiltration of the arterial media. Histiocytes, lymphocytes, and monocytes are numerous, but the presence of typical multinucleated Langhans' giant cells is more useful diagnostically. A large proportion of the lymphocytes are helper/inducer T cells. This, combined with the rarity of immunoglobulin deposits around elastin fibers, suggests that the arterial lesion results from cell-mediated rather than humoral immunity.

The inflammatory process, usually circumferential, involves short segments of the artery. This results in smooth, often dilated, segments of normal artery tapering to a smooth, symmetric stenosis or occlusion of an affected segment. The accessibility of the superficial temporal artery has given the impression that this vessel is most frequently associated with the disease, but autopsy studies have shown that the vertebral, ophthalmic, and posterior ciliary arteries are often concurrently involved. Internal and external carotid and central retinal artery damage is less common, while the intracerebral vessels are hardly ever affected.

Occasionally, aortic arch involvement may lead to simple or aneurysmal dilatation, sometimes complicated by distortion of the aortic valve ring or coronary ostia stenosis. Coronary arteritis is rare.

Smaller arteries in a variety of sites may also be involved. In the lungs, arteritis produces patchy granulomatous infiltration and necrosis, usually centered around a diseased blood vessel. Similar granulomatous lesions are common in the liver and have also been reported in the pancreas, spleen, uterus, and breast. The kidneys may be affected by patchy vasculitis, and a membranous glomerulopathy has occasionally been identified.

PMR is not associated with any histologic abnormalities in skeletal muscle. However, synovitis characterized by round cell infiltration and synovial proliferation is common, although the changes are much less severe than those found in rheumatoid arthritis. Usually, the hips and shoulders are involved, but the knees and sternoclavicular joints may also be affected.

Symptoms and Signs

In giant cell arteritis, the typical presenting feature is a continuous, throbbing temporal headache. Involvement of other branches of the external carotid artery may cause ischemia of the masseter muscles, tongue, and pharynx, resulting in pain at these sites in response to chewing, talking, or swallowing; the pain is relieved by rest. Stenosis of the ophthalmic artery and its branches leads to transient loss of vision (amaurosis fugax), visual field defects, visual blurring and hallucinations, and ocular or orbital pain and may produce sudden blindness. Orbital muscle ischemia may cause diplopia.

Physical examination may reveal characteristic tender, red, swollen, and nodular temporal arteries with diminished pulsations in $2/3$ of patients with the disease. Less common abnormalities include reduced or absent pulsations over other head and neck arteries and, in severe cases, focal necrosis of the scalp, tongue, or face. Ophthalmic artery involvement generally causes a central scotoma or total blindness. Patchy, peripheral visual field defects are less common. Ophthalmic artery blockage initially results in a pale, swollen optic disk surrounded by pericapillary hemorrhage, which progresses to a pale, atrophic disk. Patchy areas of retinal infarction are less common. Patients with orbital muscle damage present with varying degrees of ophthalmoplegia or ptosis.

In PMR, the most common symptoms are bilateral pain and stiffness of the shoulders and thighs, often severe and leading to immobility and other functional losses. Duration of symptoms for < 2 wk and morning stiffness that lasts for > 1 h usually suggest PMR. **Physical examination** elicits tenderness over the affected muscles and painful limitation of hip and shoulder movements.

Both giant cell arteritis and PMR are often associated with depression, weight loss, and fever, in addition to their characteristic features. Weight loss or fever sometimes is the only finding, leading to a fruitless search for malignancy or infection. Thus, the concept of a **malignant,** or **febrile,** form of giant cell arteritis has evolved.

Complications

Vision: *Any delay in starting treatment with corticosteroids may result in permanent unilateral or bilateral blindness.* Thus, every case is treated as a matter of urgency. In 1 survey, 12% of patients with giant cell arteritis suffered eye complications: 5% had transient visual impairment or diplopia, and another 7% had permanent visual impairment. Before routine use of corticosteroids, between 30 and 60% of patients developed visual complications.

Aorta and related vessels: The aortic arch or one or more of its major branches is involved in about 1 out of 8 cases of giant cell arteritis. Subclavian or vertebral artery involvement may lead to brainstem ischemia, which can result in coma and decerebrate rigidity. However, patchy neurologic damage (eg, ataxia, nystagmus, or paralysis of upward gaze) is more usual. Common or internal carotid artery damage may cause either a transient ischemic attack or a full-blown hemiparesis; involvement of both carotid arteries may produce bilateral neurologic signs. Cerebrovascular damage is a relatively uncommon complication of giant cell arteritis and PMR, especially in the absence of other clinical features. Thus, temporal artery biopsy should not be routinely performed in stroke patients.

Unilateral stenosis of a subclavian, axillary, or brachial artery may cause upper limb claudication associated with absent pulse and zero BP on the affected side. The diagnosis should be suspected when these features are present in association with an elevated ESR.

Aortitis may cause associated dilatation and incompetence of the aortic valve. Aortic arch aneurysms also may develop, and cases of dissection have been reported.

Angina pectoris may result from coincidental coronary atheromata or occasionally from obstruction of the coronary ostia by aortitis. Arteritis directly involves the coronary arteries only rarely.

Proof that the aortic arch or its main tributaries are affected by giant cell arteritis requires contrast angiography. The characteristic changes are (1) long segments of smooth luminal stenosis alternating with segments of normal or dilated lumen, (2) smooth tapering of the lumen between normal and affected segments, and (3) absence of ulceration or irregular plaques within the lumen.

Arthritis: Approximately 15% of patients with either giant cell arteritis or PMR have clinical evidence of arthritis affecting the knees or sternoclavicular joints. The usual features are pain, tenderness, swelling, redness, and limitation of motion; evidence of effusion may be found in the knees. The rheumatoid factor test is invariably negative, and radiologic evidence of joint erosion is uncommon. More than 15% of such patients have hip and shoulder joint involvement, which is usually indistinguishable clinically from the tenderness and limited movement associated with PMR.

Respiratory symptoms: One in 10 patients with giant cell arteritis has cough, sore throat, or hoarseness. However, these are rarely the presenting features. The disease may also produce radiologic changes, ranging from vague patches suggestive of infection to large solid lesions easily mistaken for "cannonball" metastases. Pleural effusion occasionally follows pleural involvement.

Renal damage: About 10% of patients with giant cell arteritis have asymptomatic, microscopic hematuria; a few cases of chronic renal failure and nephrotic syndrome have also been reported.

Liver disease: One third of patients with PMR in 1 series had an increased antimitochondrial antibody titer. This finding, combined with the fact that $\frac{1}{2}$ of PMR patients have an increased serum alkaline phosphatase concentration, raises the possibility of a link with primary biliary cirrhosis. However, clinical manifestations of liver involvement are rare.

Other complications: Giant cell arteritis can affect almost any organ (eg, it can mimic breast carcinoma by producing a hard mass attached to surrounding tissue, with axillary adenopathy). Uterine involvement, producing blood and pus in a vaginal smear, has also been reported. Polyneuropathies and mononeuropathies have been encountered. However, all these clinical curiosities are rarely encountered in everyday clinical practice.

Laboratory Findings

The most useful laboratory test is the **ESR.** In both giant cell arteritis and PMR, it is usually > 40 mm/h and often > 100 mm/h. Although the ESR is very sensitive, it occasionally falls within normal values.

C-reactive protein **(CRP)** levels are also usually elevated. While no more specific than the ESR, CRP levels fall more rapidly in remission, and may be of value as a more sensitive monitor of treatment.

Antibody titers (eg, rheumatoid and antinuclear factors) are normal; if they are elevated, the initial diagnosis should be reevaluated. Other biochemical tests are of no value in establishing the primary diagnosis.

Patients often have a normochromic, normocytic anemia, which is of diagnostic value when associated with other clinical features of the condition. If anemia occurs as an isolated finding, diagnostic confusion may result; the disease is identified as the **anemic** form of giant cell arteritis only by a process of exclusion.

Temporal artery biopsy is the most specific test for giant cell arteritis. Three to 5 cm of artery should be excised; a shorter section may miss the segmental area of pathology. The presence of round cell and Langhans' giant cell infiltration of the media confirms the diagnosis, but if the biopsy is negative, there is a 5 to 10% chance that the diagnosis has been missed. Therefore, in exceptional circumstances, a biopsy of the contralateral artery may be justified. Biopsy rarely causes scalp necrosis, but the risk increases considerably if both arteries are removed.

While temporal artery biopsy should be performed in all patients with clinical features of giant cell arteritis, its role in those with symptoms of PMR is controversial. A reasonable approach is to reserve the procedure for patients who fail to respond to corticosteroid therapy.

Differential Diagnosis

The clinical features of giant cell arteritis and PMR are well defined, and even when they overlap, the diagnosis should be straightforward on the basis of the symptoms, signs, ESR, and biopsy as described above. Diagnostic problems arise only in the minority of cases in which evidence of temporal arterial involvement is absent.

In the rare situation in which clinical evidence of temporal arteritis is minimal and radiologic evidence shows extensive pulmonary involvement, **Wegener's granulomatosis** must be ruled out. Evidence of severe upper respiratory involvement (eg, rhinorrhea or epistaxis) and deteriorating renal function favors the latter diagnosis. Although round cell and giant cell infiltration of arteries is found in Wegener's granulomatosis, the temporal arteries are rarely affected.

Although **periarteritis nodosa** can involve almost any system, it usually causes fever, abdominal pain, hypertension, edema, and a polyneuropathy. Albuminuria and hematuria are also prominent. Renal biopsy should clarify the diagnosis.

Takayasu's disease, a rare form of arteritis, causes stenosis and occlusion of the major aortic branches, thus mimicking an atypical presentation of giant cell arteritis. However, because this disease affects primarily young women, it presents few diagnostic problems.

Although approximately 15% of patients with giant cell arteritis have synovitis, only the large and sternoclavicular joints are involved, making the distribution totally different from that found in **rheumatoid arthritis.** Titers of rheumatoid factor are not increased. However, rheumatoid arthritis may mask concurrent PMR, causing a potentially reversible condition to go untreated.

Other causes of polymyalgia: TABLE 63–1 lists other causes of polymyalgia in the elderly. Most of these conditions are rare or rarely present with polymyalgia. An exception is that pelvic girdle pain and tenderness are often the first manifestations of osteomalacia. Also, carcinomatosis in advanced age can present as polymyalgia.

TABLE 63–1. OTHER CAUSES OF POLYMYALGIA

Connective tissue disorders
Dermatomyositis
Periarteritis nodosa
Neoplastic disorders
Carcinoma
Multiple myeloma
Waldenström's macroglobulinemia
Others
Sarcoidosis
Subacute bacterial endocarditis
Osteomalacia

Prognosis

Both giant cell arteritis and PMR are self-limited disorders, resolving within 5 yr of onset. In the interim, without treatment, they may cause considerable discomfort and permanent incapacity. Although death may result from cerebrovascular disease or a ruptured aortic aneurysm, such events are rare, and the life expectancy of most patients is unaffected.

Treatment

Treatment with corticosteroids produces a dramatic response. Symptoms usually remit within the 1st wk of therapy, and even more serious problems (eg, blindness, angina, or upper-limb claudication) may remit if steroid therapy is started soon enough.

The starting dosage should be the equivalent of 40 to 60 mg oral prednisone daily. Efficacy should be monitored by serial determination of ESR; as ESR decreases, the dosage can be progressively reduced to between 5 and 10 mg daily. The temptation to give a lower initial dose of steroids should be resisted, because of the associated risk of a high incidence of complications.

If vision has recently deteriorated or disappeared, a larger dosage of corticosteroids may be effective (eg, 120 mg prednisone orally for 3 days). If this is ineffective, a massive IV infusion of 1000 mg prednisolone bid for 5 days may be indicated. The possible benefit of such treatment has to be balanced with the risk of serious complications (eg, GI hemorrhage, psychosis, and cardiac failure).

Maintenance therapy should be continued for at least 1 yr, then gradual withdrawal should be attempted. During this period, the patient should be carefully monitored for an elevated ESR or a recurrence of symptoms. This happens in $\geq$ $^2/_3$ of patients, and after 2 yr, $>$ $^1/_3$ remain on therapy. Even after 3 yr, $^1/_4$ require continued treatment.

One way to avoid serious side effects of long-term corticosteroid therapy is to treat patients concurrently with an immunosuppressant (eg, azathioprine 100 to 150 mg daily). This reduces the required dose of corticosteroid, and the drugs appear to be well tolerated. However, this approach should be further investigated before it can be generally advocated.

---

64. METABOLIC BONE DISEASE
(See also Chs. 8 and 71)

Robert A. Zorowitz, Marjorie Luckey, and *Diane E. Meier*

Loss of skeletal mass is a universal accompaniment to aging, regardless of race, sex, or habitus. The skeleton is not simply an inanimate scaffold that supports the body, but a living, metabolically active organ. Thus, the structural integrity of the skeleton depends upon the metabolic processes of its composite bony tissue.

The adult skeleton consists of 2 distinct types of bone, cortical and trabecular. **Cortical (compact, or lamellar) bone** forms the outer shell of long bones and the major portion of the cortex of other bones. It accounts for 75% of the total bone mass, comprising approximately 75% of the femoral neck and 95% of the midforearm. **Trabecular (spongy, or cancellous) bone** is formed by a network of intersecting plates (trabeculae), which in turn form the supporting infrastructure of bone. With its greater surface area, trabecular bone is more metabolically active and thus more sensitive to changes in the biochemical milieu. Vertebrae are composed of $>$ 66% trabecular bone, while the distal forearm is only 25 to 30% trabecular bone. The femoral intertrochanteric region is approximately 50% trabecular and 50% cortical bone.

At the cellular level, specialized osteocytes affect the constant modeling and remodeling of bone. Osteoclasts resorb existing bone while new bone is formed by osteoblasts in a tightly coupled process that is responsive to metabolic influences as well as to external agents and stresses. The postpubertal adult experiences a 10 to 15% turnover of the skeleton annually that, until the age of 25 to 30 yr, results in a **net increase in bone density.**

Although resorption and formation of bone continue after age 30 yr, the rate of resorption subsequently exceeds that of formation, resulting in gradual **net bone loss** with age. In women, acceleration of bone loss between 50 and 60 yr of age corresponds to the hormonal alterations of menopause. Cortical bone density is lost at a rate of approximately 3 to 5%/decade in women, increasing to 10 to 20%/decade in the perimenopausal and immediate postmenopausal periods. In men, cortical bone loss occurs at a rate of about 3 to 5%/decade. Loss of trabecular bone in the axial skeleton may start earlier and progress at a greater rate. *Extensive* bone loss increases the risk of fractures.

Factors Affecting Bone Homeostasis

Bone metabolism is influenced by age, activity, dietary minerals, vitamin D, parathyroid hormone, sex hormones, thyroid metabolism, glucocorticoids, and growth hormone, among other factors (see also Ch. 71). However, the complex interactions of these factors are poorly understood. Recent information indicates that Ca intake, sex steroids, and exercise play important roles in normal skeletal aging.

Ca intake is thought to influence the bone loss of aging, although whether its effect is greater on the achievement of peak bone mass or on the moderation of subsequent bone loss is unclear. Ca intake tends to decrease routinely in the elderly and even more so in those with lactose intolerance. In addition, aging decreases GI absorption of Ca, as does inadequate dietary intake of vitamin D, decreased exposure to sunlight, and impaired GI absorption of vitamin D. Moreover, an age-related decline in 1,25-dihydroxyvitamin D production may further contribute to the inability to increase absorption of Ca sufficiently to compensate for reduced intake. Thus, an older person on a Ca-poor diet is more apt to be in negative Ca balance than a younger person on a similar diet.

Exercise is important in achieving and maintaining maximal bone density. Bone density is greater in those parts of the skeleton that are directly stressed by activities. Weight-bearing exercise especially appears to decrease age-related bone loss. However, in women, strenuous exercise (eg, marathons, long-distance runs, and ballet) leading to excessive weight loss and secondary amenorrhea is associated with reduced bone density and increased fracture risk. This suggests that estrogen sufficiency may be more important than exercise in maintaining optimal bone density.

Estrogen deficiency from any cause is associated with accelerated bone loss. Until estrogen receptors were recently identified in bone, estrogen deficiency was thought to indirectly affect postmenopausal and age-associated osteopenia via decreased osteoblast function, increased sensitivity of osteoclasts to the effects of parathyroid hormone, decreased calcitonin secretion, and reduced synthesis of 1,25-dihydroxyvitamin D resulting in decreased GI Ca absorption. Whatever the mechanism, the therapeutic use of estrogen significantly retards bone resorption and decreases fracture risk.

Androgenic hormones slow age-associated osteopenia, although evidence is not as strong as it is for estrogen. Osteoporosis occurs in men with hypogonadism (eg, Klinefelter's syndrome), and a slow decline in gonadal function may be partly responsible for the linear decreases in bone density observed in normal aging men.

OSTEOPOROSIS

A metabolic bone disorder characterized by a gradual decline in absolute bone mass with preservation of the skeletal mineralization process. Declining bone density leads to increased susceptibility to fractures, which may result from seemingly insignificant movements and accidents. The most common fractures occur in the vertebral bodies, the distal radius, and the proximal femur. These and other fractures are discussed in Ch. 8. A major public health problem, osteoporosis affects more than 20 million Americans. The direct and indirect costs of osteoporosis are upward of $6.1 billion annually in the USA.

Etiology

There are 2 types of **primary osteoporosis,** the disorder present in most individuals with metabolic bone disease (see TABLE 64–1). **Type I osteoporosis,** or **postmenopausal osteoporosis,** occurs between the ages of 51 and 75 yr, affecting 6 times as many women as men, and is largely

TABLE 64–1. PRIMARY OSTEOPOROSIS

	Type I	*Type II*
Age (yr)	51–75	70+
Woman:man ratio	6:1	2:1
Type of bone loss	Primarily trabecular	Trabecular and cortical
Rate of bone loss	Accelerated/short duration	Not accelerated/long duration
Fracture sites	Vertebrae (crush) and distal radius	Vertebrae (multiple wedge) and hip
Laboratory values		
Serum Ca	Normal	Normal
Serum phosphate	Normal	Normal
Alkaline phosphatase	Normal (increased with fracture)	Normal (increased with fracture)
Urine Ca	Increased	Normal
PTH function	Decreased	Increased
Metabolism of 25(OH)D to 1,25(OH)$_2$D	Secondary decrease	Primary decrease
Ca absorption	Decreased	Decreased

(Adapted from information appearing in *The New England Journal of Medicine.* B. L. Riggs and L. J. Melton III: "Involutional osteoporosis," Vol. 306, pp. 446-450, 1986. Used with permission of *The New England Journal of Medicine.*)

responsible for their increased risk of osteoporotic fractures. Because it affects mainly trabecular bone, Type I is largely responsible for vertebral crush fractures and Colles' fractures.

In contrast, **Type II osteoporosis** is a protracted slow phase of age-related bone loss. It occurs mainly in individuals > 70 yr. of age, affecting twice as many women as men. It is also known as **involutional** or **senile osteoporosis** and is associated with gradual age-related bone loss. Because density decreases in both trabecular and cortical bone, Type II results in femoral as well as vertebral fractures. While postmenopausal endocrinologic changes are probably responsible for Type I osteoporosis, changes in vitamin D synthesis associated with aging are thought to lead to Type II. In women, Type I and Type II may be present simultaneously, resulting in a biphasic pattern of bone loss.

Accelerated bone loss is also caused by glucocorticoid excess, male hypogonadism, hyperparathyroidism, hyperthyroidism, malignancy, immobilization, hepatic insufficiency, gastrectomy, rheumatoid arthritis, acromegaly, chronic pulmonary disease, chronic renal failure, and heparin therapy. Collectively, these secondary causes account for < 5% of all cases of osteoporosis (see TABLE 64–2). However, in young women and in men of all ages with metabolic bone disease, the percentage due to secondary causes is much higher.

TABLE 64–2. CAUSES OF SECONDARY OSTEOPOROSIS

Endocrinopathies

Hypercortisolism	Hypogonadism
Hyperthyroidism	Hyperprolactinemia
Hyperparathyroidism	

Drugs

Corticosteroids	Alcohol
L-Thyroxine	Aluminum-containing
Barbiturates	antacids
Phenytoin	Tobacco
Heparin	Isoniazid
Methotrexate	

Other conditions

Immobilization	Rheumatoid arthritis
Diabetes mellitus	Osteomalacia
Chronic renal failure	Systemic
Hepatic disease	mastocytosis
Scurvy	Osteogenesis
Malabsorption syndrome	imperfecta
Chronic obstructive lung disease	Sarcoidosis

Endogenous or exogenous glucocorticoid excess is a leading cause of premature osteoporosis. Corticosteroids inhibit osteoblastic function, stimulate bone resorption, increase parathyroid hormone secretion, inhibit intestinal Ca absorption, and cause decreased end-organ response to vitamin D.

Risk Factors

As shown in TABLE 64–3, the major risk factors associated with osteoporosis are aging, female sex, white or Oriental race, early menopause (before 45 yr of age) or oophorectomy, positive family history, thin body habitus, lifelong low Ca intake, and sedentary life-style. Other risk factors include nulliparity, alcohol abuse, cigarette smoking, and a history of drugs or illnesses that predispose to increased bone loss (eg, corticosteroid use, thyrotoxicosis).

Sex: Women have a lower peak bone mass at skeletal maturity and a greatly accelerated phase of bone loss for several years following the menopause. By the 6th decade, their absolute bone density is significantly lower than that in men.

Race: Osteoporosis is more prevalent in whites and Orientals than in blacks, probably because blacks have a greater peak bone mass at skeletal maturity and possibly because of differences in nutrition, exercise, and body weight. A family history of osteoporotic fractures is also thought to be a major risk factor and studies of twins suggest that there is a significant genetic component to attainment of peak bone mass and subsequent bone loss.

Body weight: Low body weight increases the risk for osteoporosis through unidentified mechanisms, which are thought to include decreased availability of biologically active estrogen in thin postmeno-

TABLE 64–3. RISK FACTORS FOR PRIMARY OSTEOPOROSIS

Age
Female sex
Amenorrhea (premature menopause, oophorectomy, secondary amenorrhea)
Family history
Race (white or Oriental)
Low lifelong Ca intake (including lactose intolerance)
Thin body habitus
Sedentary life-style or immobilization
Smoking
Alcoholism
Protein-calorie malnutrition
Gastrectomy

pausal women and lower peak bone mass in thin young women. Obesity may be protective because higher estrogen levels in obese persons of both sexes and their increased skeletal weight bearing may stimulate bone formation.

Symptoms and Signs

Osteoporosis is asymptomatic until fractures occur. The event that precipitates a fracture may be as innocuous as turning over in bed, although falls and lifting are more common causes. In some instances, no precipitating event is recalled. In contrast, osteomalacia often causes diffuse bony tenderness and pain, even in the absence of radiographically evident fractures.

Symptoms and signs of specific fractures are discussed in Ch. 8.

Diagnosis

Since no characteristic symptoms, signs, or laboratory abnormalities are associated with primary osteoporosis, diagnosis requires the exclusion of other causes of metabolic bone disease; ie, osteomalacia, malignancy, and osteoporosis due to other underlying diseases. Usually, history, physical examination, and a few laboratory studies will rule out other causes.

Diagnosis of specific fractures is discussed in Ch. 8.

History and physical examination: The patient with a fracture or radiographic evidence of osteopenia should be questioned about the hallmarks of metabolic bone disease (eg, fractures, loss of height, bone pain, and muscle weakness) and specifically about drugs and disorders associated with vitamin D deficiency and osteomalacia (see below). One should also look for symptoms and signs of alcohol abuse, malabsorption, hypercortisolism, endocrinopathy, malignancy, and other diseases known to lead to secondary osteoporosis (see TABLE 64–2), particularly in men and premenopausal women.

Laboratory evaluation: A history suggesting metabolic bone disease must be followed with appropriate laboratory testing. If the history is negative for causes of secondary osteoporosis, a few tests will usually exclude underlying disorders: CBC with differential, routine serum chemistries, thyroid function tests, serum protein electrophoresis, and serum 25-hydroxyvitamin D concentration. If osteomalacia cannot be excluded with certainty, an iliac crest bone biopsy with double tetracycline-labeled histomorphometric analysis of undecalcified bone may be required.

In an osteopenic patient, any abnormality of the blood count or protein electrophoresis raises the possibility of a malignancy involving bone marrow. In primary osteoporosis, electrolyte, BUN, and creatinine levels are normal unless concomitant renal disease is present. Serum and urine Ca levels are generally within the normal range, although immobility due to a recent fracture may increase urinary Ca excretion. An increased urine or serum Ca level should prompt a thorough investigation into the causes of Ca elevation, which can include malignancy and hyperparathyroidism; low serum Ca or phosphate levels suggest malabsorption and/or osteomalacia.

Serum phosphate and alkaline phosphatase values are also normal, although the latter may be elevated in the presence of a recent fracture. Serum concentrations of vitamin D, 25-hydroxyvitamin D, and 1,25-dihydroxyvitamin D are also normal in primary osteoporosis but may be low because of age-related changes in vitamin D metabolism. However, in elderly shut-ins, malnourished patients, and others at risk for vitamin D deficiency, osteomalacia and osteoporosis may occur concomitantly.

Radiologic findings are insufficient for the differential diagnosis of metabolic bone disease. Radiolucence is the hallmark of osteopenia on conventional x-rays, but it cannot be detected reliably until at least 30% of bone is lost. Nevertheless, incidental skeletal osteopenia on chest x-ray is the most frequent clue to the presence of osteoporosis in asymptomatic postmenopausal women. Generally, the vertical trabeculae of vertebrae and vertebral end-plates appear more prominent because of loss of horizontal trabeculae. In more advanced disease, these end-plates become concave as the intervertebral disks balloon ("codfishing"). Schmorl's nodes are formed when the nucleus pulposus breaks through the weakened end-plate and herniates into the osteopenic vertebral body. Although biconcavity of vertebral end-plates and fractures are common in all metabolic bone diseases, Schmorl's nodes are more common in primary osteoporosis and are rarely seen in osteomalacia.

Compression of the vertebrae results in a wedge fracture if there is predominantly anterior compression and in a crush fracture if the entire body collapses. These compression fractures usually occur in the lower thoracic and upper lumbar vertebrae, although all vertebrae may be affected in severe disease. In long bones, cortical thinning and expansion of the medullary space may be seen. Occasionally, other causes of metabolic bone disease may be suggested by x-ray findings, eg, the lytic lesions of multiple myeloma, the arthropathy of rheumatoid arthritis, and the pseudofractures of osteomalacia.

Prophylaxis

With the success of estrogen replacement therapy in retarding bone loss and reducing the incidence of osteoporotic fractures, it is advisable to evaluate the perimenopausal patient for subsequent risk factors (see TABLE 64–3). Although there is no single, reliable predictor for future fractures, a thorough evaluation of risk factors may help determine the need for preventive therapy.

Bone-density measurement (TABLE 64–4) may help determine the need for estrogen replacement in the patient who is at risk for osteoporosis but who has relative contraindications to or is reluctant to assume the risks of such therapy. It is also useful in patients with minimal vertebral deformities or x-ray evidence of osteopenia to diagnose osteoporosis. Because of problems with precision, serial measurements should be used only to monitor patients receiving therapy expected to cause large changes in bone density, eg, glucocorticoids or fluoride therapy.

The most widely available technic for measuring bone density is **single-photon absorptiometry (SPA)** of the mid- or distal radius. The procedure is inexpensive, exposes the patient to little radiation, and is reasonably accurate, but it does not reflect bone density in the vertebrae or femurs, the most common and disabling sites of osteoporotic fractures. More important, a normal value does not exclude the presence of significant concurrent osteoporosis or fracture. Therefore, SPA is not recommended as a screening tool for osteoporosis in the general population. Furthermore, because annual bone loss in many patients may be less than the

TABLE 64–4. NONINVASIVE TECHNICS OF MEASURING BONE DENSITY

Technic	SPA	DPA	Quantitative CT
Site	Mid-distal radius	Lumbar vertebrae	Lumbar vertebrae
Cortical: trabecular ratio	95:5–75:25	30:70*	5:95†
Accuracy	4%	5–7%	12–30%‡
Precision	1–3%	2–5%	3–15%‡
Radiation	5 mrem	5–30 mrem	200–300 mrem
	Helpful only if abnormal; may be normal despite advanced spinal osteoporosis; does not measure sites most vulnerable to fracture	Most accurate in young and middle-aged subjects; false elevation when degenerative joint disease or compression fractures present; 8–10 studies required over 2–3 yr to accurately determine rate of bone loss	Avoids sclerotic areas; more accurate in elderly; precision error unacceptably high in most nonresearch settings; high radiation precludes frequent serial measurements

SPA = single-photon absorptiometry; DPA = dual photon absorptiometry; CT = computed tomography; mrem = millirem.
* DPA measures entire vetebral body.
† Quantitative CT measures center of vertebral body.
‡ Varies, depending on methodology and center.

reproducibility of the technic, it may be difficult to distinguish actual bone loss from machine variation with serial measurements. The cost of SPA increases with serial measurements as well.

Dual-photon absorptiometry (DPA) overcomes some of the limitations of SPA by directly measuring vertebral and femoral bone density. It is more expensive than SPA, is not widely available, and also results in some overlap in bone density values between individuals with vertebral fractures and age-matched normals. Serial measurements to assess vertebral bone loss require 6 to 7 studies over 2 to 3 yrs to overcome technic reproducibility problems, greatly increasing the cost.

Computed tomography (CT) may yield relatively accurate measurements of trabecular bone density but requires higher radiation exposure than other technics and is more expensive. At present, DPA or CT may aid in the decision to prescribe estrogen replacement therapy, but the technics are not helpful in the differential diagnosis of metabolic bone disease, and their role in the management of established osteoporosis is not yet defined.

Treatment

Agents effective in the prevention of osteoporosis are also useful in the treatment of established primary disease.

Exercise: A regimen of moderate weight-bearing exercise, eg, walking for 45 to 60 min 3 to 5 times/wk, is safe and reasonable. Other forms of exercise must be determined on an individual basis.

Calcium: The average dietary intake of Ca in American women is approximately 400 mg/day, < 50% of the recommended daily allowance. Supplementation is recommended to maintain Ca balance and prevent bone loss. Adequate Ca intake from childhood through the 3rd decade is particularly important; supplements may be required for those who avoid milk products. However, *in postmenopausal women,* while Ca decreases the rate of cortical bone loss, it has not been shown to affect the rate of trabecular bone loss or to reduce the fracture rate.

Despite the uncertain therapeutic benefits of Ca supplementation after skeletal maturity has been achieved, 1000 mg/day of elemental Ca is recommended for premenopausal women and 1500 mg/day for postmenopausal women, except in patients with a history of renal stones or hypercalciuria. Three glasses of milk/day provides approximately 900 mg of elemental Ca, but tablets may be easier to take and are recommended for the elderly, many of whom suffer from lactose intolerance of varying severity.

Calcium carbonate, the most widely available Ca supplement, is 40% elemental Ca by weight. However, it may cause constipation, rebound hyperacidity, abdominal bloating, and other GI side effects. Calcium citrate, which is 22% elemental Ca by weight, is better absorbed, particularly in elderly persons with achlorhydria, and has fewer GI side effects. Serum and urine Ca levels should be monitored before and after initiation of Ca supplementation in patients with renal impairment or with a personal or family history of kidney stones.

Vitamin D has not definitively been shown to be effective in the treatment of osteoporosis, and *pharmacologic doses* of vitamin D present the risk of hypervitaminosis D, which is associated with hypercalcemia, hypercalciuria, acute renal failure, and increased resorption of bone. However, a daily dose of 400 IU vitamin D, the quantity found in most commercially available multivitamin tablets, is safe and adequate for most patients in preventing vitamin D deficiency. If actual deficiency and osteomalacia are suspected (because of low sunlight exposure, avoidance of fortified dairy products, gastrectomy, small-bowel resection, malabsorption syndrome, hepatic disease, renal failure, antiseizure medications), serum concentrations of 25-hydroxy- and, in patients with renal disease, 1,25-dihydroxyvitamin D should be measured. Diagnostic bone histomorphometry and supplementation with appropriate formulations of vitamin D should be considered as well (see OSTEOMALACIA, below, and TABLE 64–5).

Estrogen replacement is the only therapy currently available that prevents the accelerated bone loss associated with menopause or other causes of ovarian failure. To achieve maximal effect, estrogen therapy is best started within 4 to 6 yr of menopause. After this interval, significant and irreversible bone loss will have already occurred. Nevertheless, some studies suggest that estrogen may slow bone loss and decrease the fracture rate even when given well after the immediate postmenopausal period. Upon discontinuance of estrogen, rapid bone loss begins anew. Therefore, estrogen therapy must theoretically be continued indefinitely. See Ch. 72 for details of postmenospausal hormone replacement.

Calcitonin: Salmon calcitonin has recently been approved for treatment of postmenopausal osteoporosis. Although studies have demonstrated that calcitonin can increase total body Ca, they have not shown that calcitonin can retard or reverse loss of bone density or reduce the rate of osteoporotic fractures. Calcitonin must be given parenterally and is expensive. Therefore, it cannot be routinely recommended.

Fluoride: Although not yet approved by the FDA for treatment of osteoporosis, fluoride is known to stimulate osteoblastic activity and increase new bone formation. When given without supplemental Ca, fluoride causes osteomalacia and secondary hyperparathyroidism. An estimated 40% of patients receiving fluoride therapy experience adverse effects, including synovitis with ankle and knee pain, a painful plantar fascial syndrome (both probably secondary to microfractures of the lower extremity because of rapid bone turnover), dyspepsia, recurrent vomiting, peptic ulcers, and iron deficiency anemia resulting from GI blood loss. Because of its high frequency of side effects, fluoride is not routinely recommended for treatment of osteoporosis. Usual doses are 40 to 60 mg/day given with 1200 mg elemental Ca.

Other treatment modalities: Other drugs, such as parathyroid hormone, diphosphonates, oral phosphate, and androgens have not yet been proved to reduce the rate of osteoporotic fractures, although studies are ongoing.

Table 64–5. OSTEOMALACIA

Etiology	Treatment
Dietary deficiency of vitamin D	Vitamin D_3 or D_2 2000–4000 IU daily × 2–3 mo then 200–400 IU daily
Malabsorption syndrome	Treat underlying cause Vitamin D 50,000 IU twice weekly Elemental Ca 1000–3000 mg daily
Hepatic disease	Calcifediol 50–100 μg daily* and Elemental Ca 1000–3000 mg daily
Hypophosphatemia	Phosphate 1000–3000 mg daily in divided doses and Vitamin D 25,000–100,000 IU daily or Calcitriol 0.25–1.0 μg daily
Renal tubular acidosis	Treat underlying disorder (alkalinization) and Vitamin D 50,000–100,000 IU weekly* Vitamin D may be discontinued when alkalinization is achieved
Renal failure	Calcitriol 0.5–1.0 μg daily or Dihydrotachysterol 0.25–0.5 mg daily and Elemental Ca 1000–3000 mg daily Phosphate binders and low-phosphate diet
Anticonvulsants	Routine therapy not recommended; serum vitamin D metabolites should be measured after the patient has been receiving anticonvulsant therapy for several years and replaced if deficient

* Urine and serum Ca should be monitored closely to prevent the complications of hypervitaminosis D, which include hypercalcemia, hypercalciuria, and renal failure.

Treatment of male osteoporosis depends on whether a secondary cause is identified; eg, in men with hypogonadism, androgenic hormones should be replaced, although it is not known whether this will reverse bone loss. Otherwise, Ca supplementation, exercise, a multivitamin preparation, and possibly calcitonin therapy, as described above, may be recommended.

Treatment of drug-induced osteoporosis: All regimens of chronic corticosteroid therapy will lead to osteoporosis. All efforts should be directed toward treating the underlying illness and reducing or discontinuing steroids as soon as possible. Exercise, Ca supplementation, vitamin D, and estrogen replacement may be considered.

Although anticonvulsants (eg, phenytoin and phenobarbital) are known to contribute to loss of bone density by decreasing serum concentrations of the metabolites of vitamin D, routine supplementation of this vitamin is not recommended. After several years of anticonvulsant therapy, serum concentrations of vitamin D should be determined and replacement therapy prescribed as necessary to prevent osteomalacia.

PAGET'S DISEASE OF BONE
(Osteitis Deformans)

A chronic, localized, metabolic bone disorder characterized by an early osteolytic process initiated by proliferating osteoclasts and a later osteoblastic phase resulting in abnormal histology and gross deformity of skeletal structures.

Etiology and Incidence

The etiology of Paget's disease is unknown. With electron microscopy, abnormal inclusions resembling the nucleocapsids of viruses in the Paramyxoviridae family have been observed in osteoclasts, suggesting a slow viral etiology, but many hypotheses are being explored.

It is a common disease, occurring equally in men and women, and is more prevalent in English-speaking countries, but generally rare in China, Japan, India, and the Scandinavian countries. In areas of prevalence, radiologic evidence of Paget's disease is reported in 3% of the population > 40 yr of age, increasing to 10% in those > 80 yr of age.

Pathophysiology

The disease is characterized by multiple localized sites of involvement, leaving most of the skeleton unaffected. The early phase is heralded by an osteolytic process that is initiated by the proliferation of multinucleated and often very large osteoclasts. Enlarged osteoblasts line the bony trabeculae previously resorbed by the osteoclastic phase, initiating exuberant, though disordered, bone formation. The marrow may be filled with connective tissue, blood vessels, and fibroblasts that have displaced hematopoietic tissue. The resultant disordered bone may thus be extraordinarily vascular. A single bone may exhibit evidence of osteolytic, osteoblastic, or "burnt-out" Paget's disease. The osteoblastic phase may occur simultaneously with the osteolytic phase in adjacent bone.

Symptoms and Signs

Paget's disease is asymptomatic in > 75% of those affected and is often detected by an abnormal x-ray or an incidentally elevated serum alkaline phosphatase level. In symptomatic patients, the disease is characterized by deformities in the skull, long bones, and clavicles, pathologic fractures, bone pain, and hypervascularity. Gross enlargement of cranial structures can result in headaches, hearing loss, vertigo, and tinnitus. With bony impingement on the structures at the base of the skull, slurred speech, incontinence, diplopia, and deranged swallowing can occur. Long-bone deformities, eg, bowing of the tibia or femur, and acetabular deformation may occur. When lumbar and thoracic vertebrae are involved, spinal nerve entrapment may follow.

Pain is usually described as vague rather than severe and may be difficult to distinguish from that of concomitant degenerative joint disease of the hips, knees, and lower back. However, pathologic fractures are characteristic of Paget's disease. Vertebral wedge and crush fractures may be heralded by back pain. Tibial and femoral fractures may occur after significant bowing, but generally heal without delay.

The hypervascularity of pagetic bone may be perceived as warmth of the overlying skin. When > 30% of the skeleton is involved or when severe skull involvement is present, high-output heart failure (HF) can result. With concomitant heart disease, less extensive bony involvement may compromise cardiac function sufficiently to cause HF.

Angioid streaks, or defects in Bruch's membrane of the retina, may occur in 10 to 15% of patients but rarely impair vision. Neoplasms occasionally develop from pagetic bone. Osteosarcoma is reported to develop in < 1% of cases and may be heralded by a rapid enlargement of bone, increased bone mass, or an elevation in the serum alkaline phosphatase level. Giant cell tumors are also reported to develop in some patients.

Diagnosis

In a patient with suggestive symptoms and signs, the diagnosis is confirmed by characteristic x-ray findings, bone scan, and elevated serum alkaline phosphatase and urinary hydroxyproline levels. Neither of the latter laboratory values correlates with the extent of involvement, although they may be used to follow disease activity. The serum Ca level is generally normal but may be elevated if the patient is immobilized or if a malignancy is present. In the absence of immobilization, an elevated serum Ca level should be thoroughly investigated. Hypercalciuria, on the other hand, is a common finding and is most likely a result of bone resorption. Immobilization exaggerates hypercalciuria. Hyperuricemia and gout are reported to occur more frequently in patients with Paget's disease.

In the early, or osteolytic, phase of Paget's disease, a localized osteolytic lesion, particularly in the skull or on either end of long bones, may be readily detectable on x-ray. When this lesion is seen in the skull, it is referred to as **osteoporosis circumscripta cranii**. In the extremities, the lesion generally progresses at the rate of about 1 cm/yr in a sharply delineated V shape. In the vertebrae, sclerotic margins may form a "picture frame."

The radiologic findings of osteoblastic activity may not appear until years after the onset of the osteolytic phase but may be the first clue to the diagnosis of Paget's disease. In the skull, a "honeycomb" pattern may be evident, with the appearance of patchy new bone filling in the underlying areas of osteoporosis circumscripta cranii. With increased bone formation and a thickened calvarium, a "cotton-wool" appearance may be evident. In the extremities, x-rays reveal long bones with thickened irregular trabeculation. Thickening of the iliopectineal line in the pelvis is known as the "brim sign."

Bone scan is very sensitive but not specific in identifying Paget's disease, often indicating pagetic bone in otherwise asymptomatic individuals.

Treatment

No treatment is required for the asymptomatic patient with minimal bony involvement. As bone becomes more extensively involved, however, treatment may be initiated to prevent fractures and other complications. Treatment is indicated in patients with skeletal pain or deformity, neurologic or cardiac symptoms, and in candidates for orthopedic surgery, generally about 3 to 4 mo prior to surgery.

Etidronate disodium inhibits osteoclast activity, decreasing bone turnover but does not heal osteolytic lesions. It improves skeletal, cardiac, and neurologic manifestations and reduces serum alkaline phosphatase and urinary hydroxyproline levels. It reduces pain and increases mobility in most patients. When the drug is given in doses of 5 to 20 mg/kg/day, a biochemical plateau may be reached in 3 to 6 mo. Remission may be sustained despite discontinuance of the drug at this point. Generally, treatment for 6 mo at a time with drug-free intervals of 3 to 6 mo constitutes effective therapy. With larger doses, decreased osteoblastic activity predominates, thereby reducing bone formation and leading to a mineralization defect and osteomalacia. Therefore, it is *not* the preferred drug in patients being prepared for orthopedic surgery.

Salmon calcitonin is as effective as etidronate disodium; usually, 80% of patients respond. Unlike etidronate disodium, salmon calcitonin can heal osteolytic lesions, thus making it the preferred drug for patients anticipating orthopedic surgery. Its greatest drawback is that serum antidrug antibodies may form, inducing resistance to the drug. The dosage is 50 to 100 Medical Research Council (**MRC**) u./day or every other day, given s.c. or IM; some patients require more. Side effects, which include nausea, flushing, and polyuria, rarely require that the drug be discontinued.

In patients resistant to salmon calcitonin, **human calcitonin** appears to be effective, although resistance to it has also been noted after prolonged use. The recommended starting dose is 0.5 mg/day s.c. Dosage may be titrated to 0.25 mg daily or 0.5 mg 2 or 3 times/wk, but in patients with extensive osteolytic lesions, doses of up to 0.5 mg bid may be necessary. Both forms are expensive; human calcitonin costs approximately twice as much as salmon calcitonin. Generally, the serum alkaline phosphatase level falls to about $\frac{1}{2}$ of the pretreatment level within several weeks of therapy, and subsequently maintains a plateau. Therapy may be discontinued within 6 to 12 mo and restarted when a relapse is evident.

Plicamycin (mithramycin), not yet approved by the FDA for the treatment of Paget's disease, is a potent inhibitor of osteoclastic function. It is generally given IV and may result in renal, bone marrow, and hepatic toxicity. It may occasionally be used if other regimens fail.

Surgical treatment of pagetic bone may be necessary. Occipital craniectomy may relieve basilar and nerve compression. Osteotomy may be required for extensive involvement in the tibia, and total hip replacement may be necessitated by severe degenerative joint disease.

OSTEOMALACIA

An osteopenic bone disorder caused by a failure of normal mineralization of bone matrix, which results in a decreased mineralized bone:unmineralized matrix ratio. Total bone mass may be normal or increased. It differs from osteoporosis, which is characterized by preservation of the mineralized bone:unmineralized matrix ratio and an absolute decrease in total bone mass.

Pathophysiology

The most common causes of osteomalacia are vitamin D deficiency, abnormal metabolism of vitamin D, and hypophosphatemia. Vitamin D is obtained from the diet (D_2 and D_3) and from biosynthesis following exposure to sunlight (D_3). Its metabolite 1,25-dihydroxyvitamin D enhances GI absorption of Ca and phosphate, and 1,25-dihydroxyvitamin D and 24,25-dihydroxyvitamin D may have direct effects on the bone mineralization process. Vitamin D deficiency may result from dietary restriction of foods (eg, dairy products, fish, and fortified flour), malabsorption of vitamin D, or insufficient exposure to ultraviolet radiation, eg, as occurs in shut-ins, residents in northern climates, and those who wear clothing that allows minimal skin exposure.

Dietary vitamin D, including cholecalciferol (D_3) and ergocalciferol (D_2), is absorbed in the upper small bowel via fat-dependent absorption. Derangements in upper intestinal function or fat malabsorption can result in vitamin D deficiency. Such derangements include the sequelae of surgical procedures such as gastrectomy and intestinal resection, sprue, pancreatic insufficiency, biliary obstruction, or bile salt depletion that accompanies ileal disease or the chronic use of bile-salt–binding resins.

Once absorbed, vitamin D_2 or D_3 is hydroxylated in the liver to 25-hydroxyvitamin D and subsequently in the kidneys to 1,25-dihydroxyvitamin D, the active metabolite. Interference with the metabolism of vitamin D may contribute to the development of osteomalacia. Liver disease, particularly cirrhosis of any etiology, may interfere with hepatic 25-hydroxylation of vitamin D. In renal failure, the deficiency of renal 1-α-hydroxylase activity is the primary cause of osteomalacia, because it produces a deficiency of 1,25-dihydroxyvitamin D.

Increased vitamin D excretion or catabolism may also lead to osteomalacia. Drugs that increase the hepatic degradation of 25-hydroxyvitamin D, particularly phenytoin and phenobarbital, are known to predispose individuals to osteomalacia. In the nephrotic syndrome, there may be an increase in vitamin D clearance and excretion that results in vitamin D deficiency.

Phosphorus is essential for the mineralization process. Hypophosphatemia may result from GI or renal loss of phosphate that is independent of parathyroid or vitamin D metabolism. Malabsorption and subsequent GI wasting of phosphates may be compounded by vitamin D deficiency and hyperparathyroidism and may also be exacerbated by phosphate-binding antacids. Renal wasting of phosphorus is a prominent feature of proximal renal tubular disorders that are associated with normal GFRs. These disorders range from defects that are limited to increased phosphate clearance with a minimum of concomitant abnormalities to more widespread defects involving phosphorus, glucose, amino acids, uric acid, and K. The latter defects are typical of Fanconi's syndrome. In renal tubular acidosis, the acidotic state itself may also contribute to the development of osteomalacia. Osteomalacia and hypophosphatemia with high renal phosphate clearance are also known to occur in a variety of benign and malignant mesenchymal tumors, such as giant cell tumors, hemangiomas, and fibromas, as well as in patients with prostatic carcinoma.

Symptoms and Signs

Bone pain, the hallmark of osteomalacia, may be generalized or localized to the vertebrae, hips, pelvis, ribs, or lower extremities. The pain may be aggravated by movement, and bony tenderness is common. Although deformity is unusual in adults, leg bowing, gibbus deformity, and protrusio acetabuli occasionally develop in severely affected individuals. Pathologic fractures may occur, and when osteomalacia is manifested as vertebral wedge and crush fractures, it may be difficult to distinguish from osteoporosis. The two disorders may in fact exist simultaneously. Muscle weakness is common in osteomalacia but usually absent in osteoporosis.

Diagnosis

Serum alkaline phosphatase levels are usually elevated. Urinary and/or serum Ca levels are generally low in patients with vitamin D deficiency, although serum Ca values may be normal early in the disease. Since vitamin D deficiency can result in secondary hyperparathyroidism, urine concentrations of cAMP and hydroxyproline may increase. If vitamin D deficiency is suspected, levels of 25-hydroxyvitamin D should be measured directly. Serum concentrations of 25-hydroxyvitamin D are usually low, while serum concentrations of 1,25-dihydroxyvitamin D are usually normal, unless renal failure is a contributing cause of the osteomalacia. In hypophosphatemic osteomalacia, serum phosphate levels are low, but serum and urinary concentrations of Ca are generally normal.

Radiologic findings are nonspecific in osteomalacia and difficult to distinguish from those of osteoporosis. Vertebral biconcavity, ballooning of intervertebral disks, and vertebral compression fractures occur in both disorders. Occasionally, thin longitudinal bands of radiolucency may be seen in the pubic rami, ribs, long bones, and scapulae; nonhealing is due to deranged mineralization of the bone. These are known as pseudofractures, Looser's zones, or Milkman's syndrome fractures, and may show increased uptake on bone scan.

If the diagnosis is in doubt, a bone biopsy must be performed. Because the histopathologic findings are similar to those of hyperparathyroidism, hyperthyroidism, and Paget's disease of bone, histomorphometric technics using double-tetracycline labeling are necessary to demonstrate the mineralization defect characteristic of osteomalacia. Although increased amounts of osteoid are seen in all metabolic bone disorders, the distance between the tetracycline bands is reduced or absent in osteomalacia but normal or increased in other conditions.

Treatment

Treatment must be directed at both the underlying cause of the disorder and the consequent derangement in bone mineralization (see TABLE 64–5).

For osteomalacia caused by dietary deficiency of vitamin D, 2000 to 4000 IU/day of vitamin D over 2 to 3 mo may be necessary to restore positive Ca balance and normal bone mineralization. Thereafter, 400 IU/day, the quantity present in most multivitamin preparations, is generally sufficient to prevent subsequent vitamin D deficiency.

For osteomalacia due to malabsorption syndrome, the underlying GI disorder must be treated. In some patients, a relatively selective malabsorption of vitamin D may occur without overt steatorrhea or other obvious manifestations of malabsorption. To overcome the malabsorption defect, relatively large doses of either vitamin D_2 or D_3 are required, usually at 50,000 IU 2 times/wk. The goal is to normalize 25-hydroxyvitamin D (calcifediol) levels in serum, so larger doses may occasionally be necessary. Parenteral therapy is rarely required. Because calcifediol is more polar than its parent compound, it may be more rapidly absorbed, thus facilitating a more reliable clinical response. In patients with severe hepatic disease, the use of calcifediol effectively bypasses the defective biochemical pathway and is the indicated treatment. Calcifediol, in doses of 50 to 100 μg daily or on alternate days, may be used with 1 to 3 gm elemental Ca supplement daily.

Similar principles govern the treatment of **osteomalacia that occurs with increased catabolism or excretion.** Appropriate supplements of vitamin D must be administered to overcome the increased requirements and to normalize serum calcifediol levels. With any vitamin D regimen, improved Ca absorption may lead to vitamin D intoxication. Therefore, careful monitoring of urine and serum levels of Ca and vitamin D is recommended.

Renal osteodystrophy of chronic renal failure is due to abnormalities of acid/base balance, vitamin D metabolism, and parathyroid function. Osteomalacia is a major component of renal osteodystrophy, and is due primarily to a deficiency in 1,25-hydroxyvitamin D. However, hyperparathyroidism, acidosis, and aluminum toxicity may also contribute to the bone disease. This disorder is generally treated with 1,25-dihydroxyvitamin D_3 (calcitriol) 0.5 to 1.0 µg/day or dihydrotachysterol 0.25 to 0.5 mg/day. Elemental Ca 1 to 3 gm/day is added. Finally, phosphate binders and a phosphate-restricted diet are necessary to prevent the hyperphosphatemia of chronic renal failure.

Osteomalacia secondary to hypophosphatemia, such as that seen in X-linked hypophosphatemia or with renal or GI phosphate loss, must be treated with phosphate supplements. Diarrhea is a prominent adverse effect of phosphate supplementation, so it may be advisable to increase the dose of a buffered phosphate solution gradually to 1 to 3 gm/day on a 4 to 6 times/day dosage schedule. Caution must be exercised since rapid phosphate repletion may result in hypocalcemia secondary to accelerated bone remineralization. Therefore, vitamin D supplementation in doses of 25,000 to 100,000 IU or calcitriol 0.25 to 1.0 µg/day is added to this regimen. The metabolic bone disease seen in Fanconi's syndrome is related to the hypophosphatemia that is secondary to the underlying metabolic acidosis. With correction of the acidosis, the metabolic bone disease will be ameliorated.

Patients receiving phenobarbital or phenytoin do not require routine administration of vitamin D. However, after a patient has been receiving anticonvulsant therapy for several years, it is reasonable to obtain serum vitamin D levels and to prescribe vitamin D supplements, as necessary.

---

65. MUSCULAR DISORDERS

Richard T. Moxley

APPROACH TO THE PATIENT WITH PRIMARILY MUSCULAR SYMPTOMS

Healthy elderly persons and younger adults display similar functional ability; eg, climbing stairs, arising from a squat, walking along a straight line, hopping on either foot, and all typical activities of daily living **(ADLs).**

Difficulty and unsteadiness in walking, with occasional falls, and stiffness with leg pains, especially at night, are frequently reported by elderly patients and are often related to degenerative joint disease **(DJD),** rheumatoid arthritis **(RA),** or polymyalgia rheumatica. Significant DJD limits a patient's mobility by producing structural spinal changes and joint symptoms in the limbs and occasionally by damaging the spinal cord, nerve roots, and peripheral nerves.

Cardiovascular, respiratory, endocrine, other systemic illnesses, or anxiety, with fatigue and lack of motivation for ADLs, often limits exercise performance in the elderly, frequently without intrinsic muscle weakness.

CNS disorders can produce abnormalities in gait and lower extremity muscle strength that might be confused with diseases of peripheral nerves or muscle fibers. Papilledema, unilateral weakness or sensory loss, and gait disturbance with the head turned or in flexion suggest a cause within the CNS. Central and peripheral nervous system disorders may present with motor symptoms that are often symmetric and limited to the lower extremities (see TABLE 65–1). Certain features of the clinical history are important in localizing the abnormality (see TABLE 65–2).

Patients with **descending motor pathway dysfunction** (eg, midline subdural hematoma or midline posterior fossa mass) frequently have much greater weakness on functional testing than on direct muscle strength testing. In contrast, patients with **peripheral nerve and muscle damage**

TABLE 65–1. CONDITIONS CAUSING PRIMARILY MUSCULAR SYMPTOMS IN ELDERLY PATIENTS

I.   Lesions affecting the descending motor pathways
A. Intracranial lesions
   1. Midline subdural hematoma
   2. Subfrontal or interhemispheral neoplasm
   3. Communicating hydrocephalus
   4. Midline mass lesion in posterior fossa (such as metastatic tumor in cerebellum)
   5. Degenerative diseases of the central nervous system

B. Spinal cord lesions
   1. Compression of spinal cord secondary to: osteoarthritis and/or disk disease, vertebral collapse (osteopenia vs. neoplasm), epidural metastasis, epidural abscess
   2. Anterior horn cell disease due to amyotrophic lateral sclerosis or post-polio syndrome
   3. Post radiation therapy myelopathy
   4. Lyme disease

II. Lesions affecting the motor nerve roots
A. Comprehensive or infiltrative lesions
   1. Spinal stenosis
   2. Infiltration of roots by lymphoma or carcinoma
   3. Paget's disease

B. Inflammatory lesions
   1. Acute inflammatory polyneuritis
   2. Chronic inflammatory demyelinating polyneuropathy

(Continued)

TABLE 65–1. CONDITIONS CAUSING PRIMARILY MUSCULAR
SYMPTOMS IN ELDERLY PATIENTS *(Cont'd)*

III. Lesions of peripheral nerve motor fibers
  A. Inflammatory or infectious lesions
    1. Acute inflammatory polyneuritis
    2. Chronic inflammatory demyelinating polyneuropathy (idiopathic vs.
       associated with plasma cell disorder producing paraprotein)
    3. Diphtheria
 	
  B. Endocrine disease or lesions due to toxins
    1. Thyroid disease
    2. Heavy metal toxicity (lead, mercury)

IV. Lesions affecting neuromuscular transmission
  A. Autoimmune or neoplasm associated defect
    1. Myasthenia gravis (MG)
    2. MG with thymoma
    3. Lambert-Eaton myasthenic syndrome (LEMS)
 	
  B. Toxin or drug-induced transmission disorders
    1. Botulism
    2. Aminoglycoside toxicity, β-blockers, lithium
    3. Drug-induced myasthenia gravis (such as penicillamine)

V. Abnormality in the muscle fiber
  A. Inflammatory or infectious disorders
    1. Dermatomyositis (with or without associated neoplasm)
    2. Polymyositis (large number of potential causes)
    3. Inclusion body myositis
 	
  B. Endocrine, electrolyte, or drug induced
    1. Thyroid disease
    2. Vitamin D deficiency with osteomalacia
    3. Phosphate, or magnesium
    4. Steroids, penicillamine, chloroquine, emetine, clofibrate
 	
  C. Muscular dystrophies (onset late in life is uncommon)
    1. Myotonic dystrophy
    2. Oculopharyngeal dystrophy
    3. Scapuloperoneal dystrophy

usually have similar weakness on functional and direct muscle testing. Persons with **cerebellar or cerebellar outflow pathway disease** may show no evidence of functional or direct muscle weakness but demonstrate gait disturbances, most apparent when performing tandem gait on tiptoe forward and backward.

Patients with **pathologic fatigue** from a neuromuscular transmission defect (eg, myasthenia gravis) complain of varying ability to perform activ-

TABLE 65-2. PRESENTING CLINICAL FEATURES IN SELECTED CAUSES OF MUSCULAR SYMPTOMS IN THE ELDERLY

Site of Involvement	Frontal Lobes (interhemispheric or subfrontal)	Mid Portion of Cerebellum	Cervical Spinal Cord	Anterior Horn Cell	Peripheral Nerve	Neuromuscular Function	Skeletal Muscle Fibers
Example	Chronic subdural hematoma above and between both frontal lobes	Metastasis	Chronic spinal cord compression due to C5 and C6 osteoarthritis	Amyotrophic lateral sclerosis	Chronic inflammatory demyelinating polyneuropathy	Myasthenia gravis (MG)	Polymyositis
Distribution of Weakness	Symmetric leg weakness	Gait disturbance; often no true weakness	Symmetric or slightly asymmetric weakness in hands and legs	Asymmetric or bulbar	Symmetric, distal $\geq$ proximal	Extraocular, bulbar, proximal limb muscles	Symmetric, proximal limb and bulbar muscles
Muscular Atrophy	None	None	Intrinsic hand muscles	Marked, develops early	Mild to moderate	None	Slight
Sensory Involvement	None	None	Pain and occasional decrease in pin and touch in C6-C7 nerve root distribution	None	Distal dysesthesias and loss of vibration greater than pin and touch	None	Aching

Characteristic Features	Headache, personality change, drowsiness	Unsteady gait, headache	Limited motion of neck, pain with movement, occasional worsening of leg weakness with head flexion or extension	Fasciculations, cramps, tremor	Muscle aches, trouble using stairs, tripping	Weakness fluctuates, diurnal variation	Slowly progressive weakness over weeks to months
Tendon Reflexes	Normal to slightly increased in legs; variable plantar extensor responses	Often decreased; plantar extensor responses variable	Decreased in arms and increased in legs; plantar extensor responses	Variable	Decreased	Normal	Parallel strength
Useful Diagnostic Tests	MRI or CT scan of head; Clotting profile	MRI or CT scan of head with emphasis on posterior fossa	MRI scan of posterior fossa, cervical and upper thoracic spine; X-rays of cervical spine (flexion and extension views)	Electromyography (EMG); Nerve conduction	Nerve conduction; EMG; Nerve biopsy; CSF analysis	Tensilon®* test; Repetitive nerve stimulation; CT scan of chest (thymus); Acetylcholine receptor antibody levels	CK; Sedimentation rate; EMG; Muscle biopsy

* Edrophonium chloride

ities; eg, chewing, keeping eyes open, speaking, and smiling. Pathologic fatigue is characterized by drooping of the eyelids while fixating on a target such as a pen or a flashlight or when repeating movements such as elevating the arms above the head or rising from a chair.

Muscle aches and cramps commonly suggest a peripheral nerve disorder and less commonly may result from a primary muscle fiber disturbance. Before searching for further signs of peripheral nerve dysfunction, one should look for evidence of sensory disturbance, vascular or soft tissue abnormality, or exposure to neurotoxic drugs or toxins. Intense pain, most prominent in the morning in proximal muscles, may indicate polymyalgia rheumatica (see Ch. 63). Pain in specific muscle regions may indicate fibromyalgia. Pain largely restricted to muscle groups and tissue around joints may indicate diffuse arthritic disease with limitation in muscle function. "Non-neurologic" causes for muscular symptoms are much more common in the elderly than nervous system or muscle diseases.

In the absence of significant joint or soft tissue disease, **muscle weakness** is suggested by a patient's inability to walk on his heels and toes, rise from a squat or a chair without using his arms, or step onto the seat of a chair. A normal individual should be able to extend his knee completely against gravity. Any tendency for the knee to remain slightly flexed suggests quadriceps femoris weakness, which is often associated with stumbles and falls. The patient should be able to raise his outstretched arms above his head easily and to blanch his knuckles with a forceful grip. **Focal muscle wasting** indicates derangement in either motor nerve or muscle. Diffuse muscle wasting can occur after as little as 4 to 6 wk of absolute bed rest, usually with remarkable preservation of muscle strength despite the small muscle mass.

Tendon reflexes: In patients with weakness due to CNS disease, tendon reflexes are typically increased with plantar extensor responses. Loss of reflexes with only mild weakness is typical for disease of the peripheral nerve or nerve root, although occasionally cerebellar lesions will depress tendon reflexes and suggest muscle weakness. Loss of reflexes in patients with primary muscle disease often parallels the degree of weakness. Reflexes are usually maintained in disorders of neuromuscular transmission but are frequently lost or hypoactive in patients with Lambert-Eaton myasthenic syndrome **(LEMS),** *a disorder of neuromuscular transmission* (see below under LAMBERT-EATON MYASTHENIC SYNDROME).

SPECIAL TESTS

Imaging Studies

Computerized tomography (CT) and **magnetic resonance imaging (MRI)** can identify lesions within the brain and spinal cord and occasionally in soft tissues and muscle that were previously undiagnosable; eg, lesions producing symmetric dysfunction in the descending motor pathways, thymoma (in myasthenia gravis), or oat cell carcinoma of the lung (in Lambert-Eaton myasthenic syndrome).

Plain spinal x-ray studies can identify chronic osteoarthritis and sometimes signs of chronic disk herniation, early lumbosacral spinal canal narrowing, covert metastatic disease, and vertebral collapse. A skeletal survey may show multiple myeloma or osteomalacia.

Ultrasound (US), CT, and MRI can quantify muscle atrophy and identify for needle biopsy those muscle groups with accelerated damage. US also has helped identify muscle abscess. **Technetium diphosphonate or pyrophosphate imaging** can demonstrate muscle fiber damage in polymyositis. However, at present, imaging studies of skeletal muscle are not routinely performed.

Identification of immune mechanisms for certain chronic and acute inflammatory demyelinating neuropathies and myasthenia gravis has led to greater use of plasmapheresis.

Serum Enzymes

Creatine kinase **(CK)** concentration in skeletal muscle is $>$ 3 times higher than that within heart and brain, the only other tissues with high CK content. Serum CK concentration (normal $<$ 130 IU/L) is determined by its slow release from skeletal muscle and is significantly elevated by muscle damage. CK elevation is a much more sensitive determinant of muscle damage than elevation of any other serum enzyme. Normal exercise causes CK elevation and, depending on its intensity and the conditioning of the individual, there may be as much as a three- to eight-fold rise in CK following exercise, reaching a maximum after several hours and persisting for 24 to 36 h, partly due to the long plasma $t_{1/2}$ of CK (38 to 118 h). CK levels are thus more meaningful in individuals who have not exercised heavily during the previous 48 h.

Elevated CK levels occur in a variety of diseases affecting the motor unit. Mild CK elevations ($<$ 4 times the upper limit of normal) occur in certain normal individuals with a large muscle mass, in families predisposed to malignant hyperthermia, in normal individuals after minor muscle trauma (along with other local trauma such as intramuscular injections or needle electromyography), and in certain chronic anterior horn cell diseases such as amyotrophic lateral sclerosis and postpolio syndrome. Moderate to marked CK elevations occur in inflammatory myopathies such as polymyositis and dermatomyositis, and after conditions that produce muscle necrosis (eg, hypokalemic myopathy).

There are 3 forms of CK: MM (skeletal muscle), MB (cardiac muscle), and BB (brain). Normal adult skeletal muscle contains about 95% MM and 5% MB. However, regenerating skeletal muscle fibers revert to an embryonic isoenzyme pattern, with MB increasing to between 10 and 50%. CK isoenzyme measurements are therefore not useful in diagnosing specific disorders or in monitoring patients with neuromuscular disorders.

Metabolic and Endocrine Studies

Hypokalemia, hypophosphatemia, hypocalcemia, and hypermagnesemia can produce muscle weakness, which usually develops acutely or over several weeks. Measurement of serum electrolytes and evaluation for acidosis or alkalosis are helpful, particularly if weakness is accompanied by muscle cramps and aching. Chronic hypo- or hyperfusion of the thyroid, adrenal, or parathyroid glands also may produce weakness and should be excluded. ESR, serum and urine immunoelectrophoresis to check for a paraprotein, and blood studies to screen for collagen vascular diseases are also useful.

Assessment of Muscle Mass

Occasionally it is helpful to estimate whole body muscle mass through measurement of 24-h urinary creatinine to determine if treatment is increasing the amount of muscle tissue. Conversion of energy-rich creatine phosphate into creatinine occurs in skeletal muscle. The 24-h urinary excretion of creatinine varies < 10% and correlates directly and reliably with total muscle mass.

Electrodiagnosis

Nerve conduction, repetitive stimulation, and electromyographic investigations are the primary electrodiagnostic procedures used to examine the motor unit (anterior horn cell, motor axon and terminal branches, neuromuscular junctions, and muscle fibers) (see TABLE 65–3).

Nerve conduction studies, using skin electrodes, involve stimulation of the mixed peripheral nerve at various points and recording from distal sites to examine amplitudes of compound muscle and sensory action potentials, and latency differences between points of stimulation.

Maximal conduction velocity (m/sec) can be calculated as:

$$\frac{\text{distance between stimulating electrodes (mm)}}{\text{proximal latency} - \text{distal latency (msec)}}$$

In normal adults, conduction velocities over the distal nerve segment typically range from 45 to 75 m/sec. In chronic demyelinating polyneuropathies, the velocity may be decreased by 40% or more.

Limitations of nerve conduction studies: Only the velocity of the fastest, large, myelinated nerve fibers is accurately measured with standard technics, because the much slower small fibers do not contribute significantly to the amplitude of the compound muscle or sensory action potentials. A modest slowing of motor conduction velocity can occasionally result from decreased limb temperature rather than from peripheral nerve demyelination. This can be important in elderly patients with peripheral vascular disease. In neuropathies that produce aching and cramps (eg, alcoholic, nutritional, uremic, diabetic), the axons that survive often have normal or almost normal conduction velocities, despite significant neuropathy.

TABLE 65–3. OVERVIEW OF THE PATTERN OF ELECTRODIAGNOSTIC FINDINGS IN LESIONS CAUSING MUSCULAR SYMPTOMS

	Lesion in Descending Motor Pathways	Lesion of Lower Motor Neuron	Lesion of Neuromuscular Transmission	Lesion of Skeletal Muscle
Nerve conduction	Normal	Often normal. Abnormal only with demyelination of large nerve fibers	Normal	Normal
Repetitive stimulation	Normal	Normal	Variable; usually abnormal if muscle stimulated is weak	Normal
Electromyography	Reduced firing frequency of motor unit potentials	Signs of acute and/or chronic denervation	Normal or myopathic in very weak muscles	Myopathic or normal

Sensory nerve conduction studies have additional limitations. The compound sensory action potential is much smaller than the compound motor action potential and requires considerable amplification to be recorded (which is not possible in some disease states). Other factors may interfere; eg, accurately locating a peripheral sensory nerve requires experience; chronic ankle swelling in elderly patients often prevents accurate measurement of sural nerve conduction.

Repetitive stimulation testing of neuromuscular transmission: Repetitive maximal nerve stimuli are applied to the peripheral motor nerve, and the amplitude of the compound muscle action potential is recorded. Both high and low rates of nerve stimulation have been described. The most used involves low rates of stimulation, usually 3 Hz given before and after a brief period of maximal isometric exercise. An incremental decrease of the action potential amplitude usually indicates a defect in neuromuscular transmission (eg, in myasthenia gravis). In contrast, Lambert-Eaton myasthenic syndrome **(LEMS)** produces an incremental increase with repetitive stimulation.

Electromyography (EMG) records activity at rest and during mild and strong muscle contraction. In normal muscle there is no spontaneous electrical activity at rest. With voluntary contraction, more motor unit potentials of increasing amplitude are recruited as the strength of contraction increases.

In neurogenic disorders that damage the motor axon, EMG findings depend on the type and duration of the nerve disease. If the damage produces axonal death, spontaneous discharges **("fibrillations"** and **"positive waves")** usually develop in single denervated muscle fibers after 3 wk or more.

Fasciculations are a form of spontaneous activity that often do not indicate axonal death. They typically occur with slowly progressive diseases of the anterior horn cell or nerve roots or in electrolyte disturbances. Many normal individuals develop fasciculations, especially following exercise.

EMG often distinguishes primary muscle disease from nerve disease. Typically, myopathic muscle will show a normal number of motor unit potentials, often with decreased amplitude, during maximum contraction. This is in marked contrast to the reduced number of motor unit potentials with very high amplitude seen in chronic denervation. However, inflammatory myopathies, such as polymyositis and dermatomyositis (important causes of muscle weakness in the elderly), may also produce fibrillations and positive waves identical to those following acute nerve damage.

Muscle Biopsy

Muscle biopsy is useful in distinguishing neurogenic from myopathic disease and in diagnosing certain connective tissue diseases (eg, polyarteritis nodosa and polymyositis), and, although rare in the elderly, the muscular dystrophies, congenital myopathies, and specific metabolic diseases of muscle.

Biopsy is not useful for acute generalized weakness or subacute or chronic neurogenic weakness (eg, myasthenia gravis, acute inflammatory polyneuritis, diabetic polyneuropathy).

Nerve Biopsy

Nerve biopsy is more difficult and traumatic than muscle biopsy, and of limited use. It can distinguish segmental demyelination from axonal degeneration and identify inflammatory neuropathies. In certain uncommon diseases it can establish a specific diagnosis; eg, amyloidosis, sarcoidosis, leprosy, and certain unusual metabolic and hereditary neuropathies. In elderly patients, the indications are very restricted.

DISORDERS AFFECTING NEUROMUSCULAR TRANSMISSION

MYASTHENIA GRAVIS (MG)

Etiology, Pathogenesis, and Incidence

MG is an acquired autoimmune disease, with reduced numbers of acetylcholine receptors at the muscle motor endplate. The receptor deficiency is caused by circulating antireceptor antibodies that damage the receptor through complement fixation and activation, block the binding sites for acetylcholine, and accelerate the turnover rate for the receptor (its internalization and destruction). The role of the thymus gland in MG is not known, but ⅔ of patients have thymic hyperplasia, and 10 to 15% have thymoma.

In cases without thymoma and onset after age 40, men are affected more commonly than women (60:40) and exhibit HLA type HLA-A3, HLA-B7, HLA-DRw2. The acetylcholine receptor antibody titer is usually low. About 50% of patients have a positive antistriational antibody titer, and about 33% have other autoimmune diseases. The early onset forms of MG occur more frequently in women (70:30) with HLA types HLA-A1, HLA-B8, HLA-DRw3; there is more pronounced elevation of antireceptor antibody level, and only 5% have positive antistriational antibody titers.

Symptoms and Signs

Initial symptoms are upper eyelid ptosis, diplopia, or blurred vision (from extraocular muscle involvement) in > 50% of patients; generalized weakness and fatigue in about 10%; and difficulty in swallowing, facial weakness, or slurred nasal speech in about 5%. Symptoms remain limited to the extraocular muscles in about 15% of patients, and become generalized in the remaining 85%, usually within the first yr. Symptoms in 50% of patients reach maximum severity in the first yr and in almost all patients by 5 yr.

Symptoms are typically mild and variable at onset. They may be accompanied by general complaints, eg, difficulty in climbing stairs or arising from a seat. On examination, if repetitive tasks are not checked, there may be no evidence of muscle weakness or other localizing signs. Often patients are misdiagnosed as having depression or some other psychiatric disorder. The patient should be asked to perform several deep knee bends, maintain his arms in an extended posture for 30 sec, and gaze without blinking at a target for 1 min. If any of these tests produce obvious fatigue, a disease of neuromuscular transmission (particularly MG) should be suspected. As noted in TABLE 65–2, symptoms typically fluctuate, being relieved by rest, and are most pronounced at the end of the day.

The **Osserman criteria** are often used: Group 1, ocular symptoms; Group 2a, mild generalized symptoms; Group 2b, moderately severe generalized symptoms; Group 3, acute fulminating symptoms; and Group 4, late severe symptoms.

Myasthenic crisis is characterized by the acute onset of respiratory insufficiency, often with difficulty in swallowing and speaking, and increased weakness in the arms and legs. Infection, trauma, and use of certain medications (aminoglycosides, cardiac drugs, antihistamines, and tranquilizers) can precipitate myasthenic crisis in some patients.

Diagnosis

When MG is suspected, a double-blind IV comparison of edrophonium 5 mg vs. placebo should be undertaken to confirm the diagnosis. The ECG should be monitored, with IV atropine available to reverse any toxicity. Equipment and personnel to perform endotracheal intubation should also be available. Edrophonium (or placebo) should be given initially in a dose of 1 mg, and the patient observed for 15 to 30 sec. If there are no obvious side effects, the remaining 4 mg of edrophonium (or placebo) should be given. After the injection is complete, 2 or 3 specific muscles should be evaluated; eg, a positive test is indicated by improvement in ptosis, ability to maintain the arms in the extended position, range of extraocular muscle movements, and forced vital capacity. A period of 4 to 5 min should be allowed before repeating the test.

Circulating levels of antiacetylcholine receptor antibodies and antistriational muscle antibodies should be measured. Patients with thymoma have elevated titers of both antibody types.

MG should be differentiated from neurasthenia, oculopharyngeal muscular dystrophy, progressive external ophthalmoplegia with diffuse limb muscle weakness, posterior fossa mass lesion, drug-induced myasthenic syndromes, LEMS, and botulism. Nerve conduction studies with repetitive stimulation testing often show a decremental response 1 to 2 min following exercise. A positive repetitive stimulation test often occurs in muscles that are clinically weak. However, a negative test does not rule out the diagnosis of MG. Single-fiber EMG studies are quite sensitive in detecting early failure of neuromuscular transmission but are usually not necessary.

Other laboratory tests include antinuclear antibody titer, rheumatoid factor, antithyroglobulin antibody titer, thyroid function tests, and fasting blood glucose. Standard pulmonary function testing is necessary and may need to be repeated throughout the day, depending on patient status. CT scan or MRI imaging of the chest, in addition to a standard PA and lateral chest x-ray, helps evaluate the size of the thymus. A tuberculin skin test is desirable before initiating steroid treatment.

Treatment

Treatment is best carried out by specialists in neuromuscular centers and must be coordinated with routine care to avoid treatment that may acutely worsen symptoms.

Anticholinesterase drugs, such as **pyridostigmine bromide,** are frequently used as first-line therapy. The initial dose is 30 mg ($\frac{1}{2}$ tablet) given 30 to 60 min before meals. Drug effect usually begins within 30 min and reaches a peak at 2 h, gradually declining over the next 2 to 3 h. Dosing is gradually increased depending on patient response. Dosing intervals should be not < 3 h to avoid an excess of cholinergic side effects; eg, abdominal cramps, nausea, vomiting, diarrhea, meiosis, lacrimation, increased bronchial secretions, sweating, and a slowed heart rate. **Ephedrine** 25 mg bid or tid may have a synergistic effect with pyridostigmine. Agitation and insomnia are side effects of ephedrine, and it may be necessary to omit evening doses. Following surgery or in critically ill patients, anticholinesterase treatment is usually given IM. The IM dose of pyridostigmine bromide is $\frac{1}{30}$ of the oral dose. IV injections, with their high potential for uncontrollable cholinergic side effects, are rarely necessary. Excessive use of anticholinesterase drugs can also increase weakness.

Cholinergic crisis rarely occurs with current management of MG. Steroid treatment and other immunosuppressive therapy are generally used to avoid high doses of anticholinesterase drugs. Cholinergic crisis is characterized by increasing muscle weakness and increasing cholinergic side effects. Cholinergic and myasthenic failure of neuromuscular transmission can coexist in different muscles and in different fibers in the same muscle. Therefore, cholinergic/myasthenic crises should be treated by withholding medications and by intubation and ventilatory support. Usually within a few days of supportive treatment, the patient's responsiveness to anticholinesterase medications will return.

Elderly patients typically experience their most severe myasthenic symptoms in the extraocular and bulbar muscles, which are especially resistant to anticholinesterase treatment, and usually require additional therapy. **Immunosuppressive treatment** is the mainstay of chronic management. The decision to start immunosuppressive therapy should be made by a specialist in neuromuscular disease. **Prednisone** can be initiated on an outpatient basis in low doses of 15 to 20 mg/day, and increased by 5 mg q 3 to 4 days until there is a satisfactory clinical response or the dose reaches 60 mg. About 90% of patients improve with steroid therapy, usually beginning within 2 to 6 wk, reaching a maximum after 6 mo or longer. To avoid the significant increase in side effects that occurs after 2 to 3 mo of steroid treatment, it is advisable to switch gradually to alternate-day therapy by incrementally increasing the dose by 5 mg on 1 day and decreasing the dose by 5 mg on the subsequent day over a period of several weeks until the patient is receiving about 100 mg and 10 mg on alternate days. Further adjustments may be necessary. The patient should be monitored frequently for signs of osteoporosis (including vertebral collapse), cataracts, aseptic necrosis of the femoral head, diabetes, increased risk of infection, peptic ulcer activation, hypertension, and excessive weight gain.

Azathioprine 2 to 3 mg/kg/day in divided doses is often started with, or within the first few weeks of, prednisone therapy. Three to 6 mo are required to achieve the maximum beneficial effects. Side effects of azathioprine (eg, pancytopenia, leukopenia, infection, hepatocellular injury) must be monitored with serial blood tests.

Plasmapheresis is frequently helpful for acute worsening of generalized MG. Several treatments, each of which removes at least 2 L of plasma, are usually required. Plasmapheresis is typically done every other day. The beneficial effects usually last only a few weeks.

Thymectomy is indicated in all patients with thymoma, but in elderly patients without thymoma there is no agreement on the need for thymectomy, even in severe cases. Because of the efficacy of immunosuppressive therapy, the role of thymectomy in long-term treatment is being re-examined.

Patients in, or approaching, myasthenic crisis should have frequent measurements of vital capacity, and when it falls to 1 L, they should be transferred to the ICU for ventilatory support through elective tracheostomy or endotracheal intubation. Any associated infection should be vigorously treated. Many antibiotics (eg, aminoglycosides, tetracycline, polypeptide antibiotics) may worsen neuromuscular transmission and precipitate a crisis. Other medications that can block neuromuscular transmission include adrenergic blockers (β-blockers), membrane stabilizers (quinine, quinidine, procainamide), psychotropic drugs (chlorpromazine, lithium), and certain antiarthritics (penicillamine, chloroquine). Medications are often withheld during the first 48 to 72 h of myasthenic crisis, especially if the patient is receiving anticholinesterase drugs. Plasmapheresis is the treatment of choice for crisis. Oral prednisone 50 to 60 mg/day can be initiated subsequently if the patient has not been receiving regular immunosuppressive treatment. Some centers hospitalize those without symptoms of crisis to give high-dose IV methylprednisolone (2 gm IV q 5 days for 3 treatments) before starting oral prednisone.

LAMBERT-EATON MYASTHENIC SYNDROME
(LEMS)

Etiology and Pathogenesis

LEMS is an autoimmune disorder frequently associated with small cell carcinoma of the lung and with autoimmune diseases (especially in women and younger patients). It is characterized by diminished release of acetylcholine from the motor nerve terminal. Serum from patients with LEMS contains circulating IgG antibody that blocks the voltage-dependent calcium channels in the terminals of normal motor nerve fibers.

LEMS occurs about 5 times more frequently in men than in women. Seventy percent of men and 25% of women have an associated malignancy; > 80% of these are small cell carcinomas of the lung. Malignancy can occur before or up to 2 to 3 yr after the onset of LEMS symptoms and is uncommon under age 40. LEMS may occur with autoimmune disorders; eg, pernicious anemia, hypothyroidism, hyperthyroidism, Sjögren's syndrome, vitiligo, celiac disease, and myasthenia gravis. Subacute cerebellar degeneration has occurred in both neoplastic and non-neoplastic LEMS.

Symptoms and Signs

There is muscle fatigue, primarily in the lower extremity and truncal muscles, with little or no muscle atrophy. In contrast to myasthenia gravis, bulbar and extraocular muscles are often unaffected. Also, repetitive testing of muscle strength in the extremities often produces the paradoxic response of increasing power. The same occurs with tendon reflexes. Patients are initially hypo- to areflexic, especially in the legs. However, forceful contraction of the quadriceps femoris, repeated 5 to 10 times, will restore a normal knee jerk. The increase in muscle power and tendon jerk may result from increased calcium mobilization from repetitive firing of the nerve, with increased local calcium concentration in the myoneural junction leading to increased release of acetylcholine.

About 50% of patients with LEMS have autonomic abnormalities; the most frequent symptom is dryness of the mouth. Impotence, decreased lacrimation and sweating, orthostatic symptoms, and diminished pupillary responses to light also occur.

Diagnosis

Fatigability of lower extremity muscles, sparing of cranial muscles, increased strength with repetitive testing, hyporeflexia, and dysautonomic features, particularly dry mouth, distinguish LEMS from myasthenia gravis and other disorders of neuromuscular transmission. Nerve conduction studies with repetitive nerve stimulation produce a characteristic pattern. At rest, the amplitude of the compound muscle action potential is markedly below normal. Following 15 to 30 sec of maximal isometric exercise, there is a several-fold increase in amplitude. Such a response can also be seen in patients with botulism, hypermagnesemia, hypocalcemia, and as a complication of certain antibiotic treatment, usually aminoglycoside therapy. Clinical signs usually differentiate these other conditions. Standard nerve conduction and EMG investigations are normal in LEMS. Single-fiber EMG studies may be abnormal, but (as in myasthenia gravis) are rarely necessary to establish the diagnosis. Edrophonium IV does not produce significant improvement. Occasionally, chronic or subacute forms of inflammatory polyneuropathy will resemble LEMS clinically, but with slowed motor nerve conduction and an elevation of spinal fluid protein.

Treatment

As in myasthenia gravis, drugs are used to increase acetylcholine availability for neuromuscular transmission and to control immune-mediated disease mechanisms.

Guanidine 10 to 35 mg/kg/day increases acetylcholine release at the motor nerve terminals and usually improves strength and exercise tolerance. Side effects include ataxia, paresthesias, GI disturbances, confusion, dry skin, atrial fibrillation, hypotension, bone marrow depression, and renal damage secondary to tubular necrosis and interstitial nephritis. Frequent monitoring is required. **Aminopyridine compounds** are possibly of value but have many serious adverse effects and are considered experimental.

Immunotherapy is usually combined with guanidine. However, many patients respond to immunotherapy alone. Alternate-day treatment with prednisone is frequently effective. Azathioprine can be started with prednisone to allow the prednisone dosage to be tapered after the initial 3 to 6 mo of therapy, as described above for myasthenia gravis.

Plasmapheresis (5 or 6 exchanges) to remove circulating antibodies is used as initial treatment of LEMS at some centers. It is also used if a patient becomes refractory to guanidine and immunosuppressive drugs.

Any elderly patient requires surveillance for malignancy for at least 2 to 3 yr after diagnosis. Neuromuscular transmission improves in some patients following neoplasm removal. Monitoring for the development of other immune-mediated diseases is also necessary.

INFLAMMATORY OR INFECTIOUS MUSCLE DISORDERS

DERMATOMYOSITIS

Etiology and Pathogenesis

Dermatomyositis is considered an autoimmune connective tissue disease. Lymphocytic muscle infiltration is characteristic. Muscle fibers with greatest involvement are perifascicular, consistent with ischemic damage. Some patients have circulating antinuclear antibodies or immune complexes identified in the skeletal muscle vascular endothelium, suggesting an immune basis for the muscle ischemia.

Natural history data for **late-onset** (after age 40) forms are not available. About 10% are associated with malignancy; breast and lung tumors are the most common, with a disproportionate increase in tumors of ovary, uterus, and bowel. There is no consistent relationship between tumor discovery and onset of dermatomyositis.

Symptoms, Signs, and Diagnosis

Skin rash and muscle weakness are the major clinical signs. The rash resembles that seen in other autoimmune diseases. There is erythema and edema of eyelids, malar areas, anterior chest, extensor surfaces of large joints and knuckles, and periungual skin. The rash may appear days or weeks before the muscle weakens. Only rarely does weakness precede the rash.

Proximal limb muscles are typically weaker than distal muscles. Neck flexors are particularly weakened, detection requiring examination of the supine patient who should normally be able to lift his head to his chest against firm resistance. Muscles supplied by cranial nerves are typically spared, except for those involved with swallowing. Dysphagia occurs in about 50% of patients. Mild facial weakness can occasionally appear, but ptosis and paralysis of the extraocular muscles are not generally seen. Respiratory muscles and the heart are rarely involved. Myalgias and muscle tenderness appear in about 50%. The time from onset to peak of muscle weakness is usually days or weeks, but rarely months.

Diagnosis is confirmed by a characteristic rash, proximal muscle weakness, elevation of blood muscle enzyme levels (especially CK), EMG consistent with muscle inflammation, and histologic evidence of myopathy. ESR is frequently elevated.

The differential diagnosis should consider hypogammaglobulinemia, toxoplasmosis, penicillamine toxicity, hypothyroidism, sarcoidosis, ipecac abuse, and hepatitis.

Treatment

In the acute stages, most patients benefit from bed rest while immunosuppressive therapy is initiated. However, physical therapy, frequent monitoring of muscle power, and regular physical activity are vital in long-term management.

Prednisone 1 to 2 mg/kg/day (60 to 100 mg/day) is usually effective in improving muscle strength and is continued for at least 3 to 4 mo before a gradual switch to an alternate-day dosing schedule (see Treatment of myasthenia gravis, above). Changes in prednisone dosage can usually be made at 4-wk intervals without provoking a flare-up. Individual dosage adjustment is required, but prednisone 80 mg on alternate days is usually effective. Because of steroid side effects (eg, increased risk of vertebral collapse or steroid-induced myopathy in elderly patients [see CORTICOSTEROID MYOPATHY, below]), concomitant use of another immunosuppressive drug may be considered. Azathioprine 2 to 3 mg/kg/day in divided doses is often effective. It requires 3 to 6 mo to achieve maximum effect and is often started 1 or 2 mo after prednisone, allowing lower steroid doses after 4 to 6 mo of high-dose prednisone treatment. Cyclophosphamide and methotrexate have also been used for immunosuppression but are more toxic.

Patients are evaluated monthly for muscle strength, joint range of motion, and serum CK. Muscle strength is the critical item in assessing treatment. Occasionally, a marked CK elevation is an early warning of disease flare-up, but periodic CK fluctuations may occur independently of change in muscle strength.

Elderly patients require frequent monitoring for covert neoplasm. There is no predictable relationship between removal of tumor and resolution of myopathy, but some patients show remarkable recovery.

POLYMYOSITIS

Etiology and Pathogenesis

Polymyositis is considered an autoimmune, connective tissue disease, but it may represent the final product of various disorders that cause slowly progressive myopathy with muscle fiber damage due to cytotoxic lymphocytes. No consistent abnormality in cellular or humoral immune mechanisms occurs. On muscle biopsy, most patients show a strong expression of class 1 major histocompatibility complex gene products, whose presence on target cells is necessary for the cytolytic action of cytotoxic lymphocytes. This supports the theory that polymyositis results from a foreign molecule, a viral infection, or some other illness, all of which sensitize muscle cells.

Prevalence ranges from 6/100,000 to 8/100,000, with a peak incidence between 45 and 65 yr. It is most common in blacks and women.

Symptoms and Signs

Muscle weakness usually occurs in the hips and thighs, causing difficulty in arising from squatting, in kneeling, or in climbing or descending stairs. Aching pain may present in the buttocks or thighs in about 10%, while tenderness on palpation occurs as the initial type of pain in another 20%. Distal muscle weakness occurs in only 25%. Muscle atrophy and loss of tendon reflexes are rare in the early stages.

Dysphagia and weakness of neck extensor muscles in a patient with chronic weakness suggest chronic polymyositis.

Cardiac involvement is relatively common, and ECG abnormalities such as A-V conduction defects and bundle branch block occur in about ⅓ of patients. Cardiac disturbances may result from inflammation and fibrosis of the conducting system, correlating with circulating antibodies to cardiac muscle ribonucleoproteins.

About 5% of patients present with pulmonary complaints. Interstitial lung disease occurs in 5 to 10% of those evaluated radiographically and clinically. The most common symptoms are dyspnea and nonproductive cough. Weakness of pharyngeal muscles, which occurs in about 25% of patients in the early stages, may produce an ineffective cough and lead to aspiration pneumonia.

Dysphagia eventually develops in about $2/3$ of patients and varies in severity. Cricopharyngeal achalasia is a less frequent cause of dysphagia, but should be considered since cricopharyngeal myotomy may relieve dysphagia and eliminate the tendency to aspirate. Delayed gastric emptying and esophageal hypomotility appear in about 50% of patients.

Diagnosis

Diagnostic criteria include:

1. Recognition of the symptoms and signs described above.

2. EMG tests indicating a myopathic pattern, muscle biopsy confirming myopathy, and elevated serum muscle enzymes (especially CK).

3. Often evidence of systemic disease, including arthralgia, fever, elevated ESR, and a polyclonal hypergammaglobulinemia on electrophoresis.

4. No evidence of familial muscular dystrophy, no rash typical for dermatomyositis, no overt endocrine disturbance, and no obvious evidence of a primary biochemical disorder in the muscle biopsy.

The differential diagnosis includes (1) collagen vascular disease (eg, systemic lupus erythematosus, rheumatoid arthritis, periarteritis nodosa, systemic sclerosis, giant cell arteritis, Sjögren's syndrome); (2) infections (eg, toxoplasmosis, Legionnaire's disease, influenza virus, mycoplasma); (3) drugs (eg, penicillamine, steroids, clofibrate, kaliuretics, rifampicin, emetine, colchicine, chloroquine, ipecac, IM pentazocine); (4) systemic neoplasm (eg, thymoma, plasma cell diseases); (5) endocrine disturbances (eg, thyroid, adrenal, parathyroid diseases); (6) metabolic disorders (eg, chronic potassium depletion, hypocalcemia, osteomalacia, chronic renal disease); (7) neuromuscular transmission disease (eg, myasthenia gravis, LEMS); and (8) chronic motor neuropathies (eg, chronic inflammatory demyelinating polyneuropathy). A summary of the typical presenting clinical features and useful diagnostic tests are given in TABLE 65–2.

Treatment and Prognosis

Treatment is identical to that for dermatomyositis (see above). The overall mortality is about 4 times that of the general population. Death usually occurs from pulmonary or cardiac complications. Blacks and women have a less favorable prognosis. About 50% of patients recover with treatment, allowing discontinuation of therapy within 5 yr from onset of symptoms. About 20% will have persistent active disease requiring continued therapy, while the remaining 30% will develop inactive disease with permanent residual muscle weakness.

INCLUSION BODY MYOSITIS (IBM)

Etiology and Pathogenesis

The precise cause is unknown. IBM resembles chronic polymyositis and usually occurs in patients > 50 yr of age, affecting men twice as often as women. Cytoplasmic and intranuclear filamentous inclusions of unknown origin are characteristic. The antigen to mumps virus has been identified in muscle biopsies from some patients, but whether there is a relationship to IBM remains unclear.

Symptoms and Signs

Progressive proximal and distal muscle weakness usually develops, without pain, over weeks to months, occasionally causing greater distal weakness; eg, of wrist extensors. In contrast to polymyositis and dermatomyositis, muscular atrophy develops relatively early. Facial muscles are occasionally involved, but extraocular muscles are always spared. Only rarely are spinal, respiratory, and abdominal muscles affected. Tendon reflexes are normal or increased and become reduced only when there is marked muscular wasting. Dysphagia is rare, and no cardiac involvement has been described. IBM is usually very slowly progressive and patients remain ambulatory for many years after onset of symptoms.

Diagnosis

Chronic progressive muscle weakness, with nuclear inclusion bodies on muscle biopsy, is diagnostic. Muscle biopsy often shows a variety of changes, including those typical for mild acute denervation as well as active myopathy. Inflammatory cells are not always seen, and careful serial sections are necessary to detect the inclusion bodies. EMG demonstrates both neurogenic and myopathic features. Plasma CK levels may be normal, slightly increased, or occasionally markedly elevated. The ESR is usually normal.

Differential diagnosis is the same as for polymyositis (see above). Autoimmune diseases, as well as other disorders, show no consistent association with IBM.

Treatment

Although immunosuppressive therapy does not produce predictable improvement in muscle strength, a 4- to 6-mo course of prednisone 60 to 80 mg/day usually is given. Thirty percent of patients may respond to this therapy or to a subsequent 6-mo trial with azathioprine 2 to 3 mg/kg/day. Patients require regular monitoring for side effects and assessment of muscle strength. Supportive care with bracing for occasional foot drop or severe wrist drop is helpful.

ENDOCRINE-INDUCED MUSCLE DISORDERS

CORTICOSTEROID MYOPATHY (CM)

Etiology and Pathogenesis

Usually, CM occurs during corticosteroid treatment for conditions that also cause muscle weakness; eg, myasthenia gravis or inflammatory myopathies. Corticosteroids alter muscle carbohydrate and protein metabolism and the function of the sarcoplasmic reticulum.

CM is associated with selective atrophy of fast-contracting muscle fibers (Type 2) that are more vulnerable than the more slowly contracting oxidative fibers (Type 1). The atrophy is decreased by exercise. CM can occur with all commonly used corticosteroids, and in conditions associated with elevated ACTH levels (eg, Cushing's disease).

The incidence of muscle weakness in Cushing's disease is between 50 and 80%, while in those receiving chronic steroid therapy it is roughly 2 to 20%. In general, the higher the dose, the more likely and more quickly CM will occur, but prednisone 15 mg/day may cause weakness in some patients. Women are twice as likely as men to develop CM at the same steroid dose. The interval between initiation of treatment and the development of CM is usually > 3 wk. Once CM begins, it tends to develop rapidly even though no weakness was observed with the same dose during the previous weeks or months.

Symptoms and Signs

Muscle weakness usually begins in the hip girdle, especially the quadriceps. Over days to weeks, weakness spreads to the trunk, anterior neck, shoulders, and upper arms. Eventually, all muscles are weakened, but the emphasis remains on proximal muscles. In chronically weakened muscles, clinical evidence of muscle wasting is often apparent. Muscles supplied by cranial nerves other than the neck flexors are spared. Occasionally patients experience mild aching of the thigh muscles, but severe pain does not occur. Tendon reflexes remain unchanged and there are no fasciculations. Patients often complain that they fatigue more rapidly during activities demanding sudden bursts of power.

Diagnosis

Serum CK and other muscle enzyme levels are normal. EMG studies are typically normal, as is nerve conduction. Muscle biopsy often shows striking atrophy of Type 2 fibers.

In a patient with polymyositis or dermatomyositis, weakness that increases shortly after the initiation of corticosteroid treatment is almost always *not* due to CM, and usually requires continuing or increasing corticosteroid dosage. Similarly, in patients with inflammatory myopathy, the weakness is probably not corticosteroid induced if it occurs without other clinical signs of steroid use (eg, puffiness of the face or significant increase in body weight). Laboratory data are frequently not helpful. CK elevation can occasionally be seen in CM. Conversely, normal CK does not rule out a flare-up of inflammatory myopathy. Muscle biopsy readily identifies active inflammation, but a normal biopsy does not rule out an inflammatory flare-up. EMG may show signs of muscle irritability and myopathy in the early stages of polymyositis and dermatomyositis. However, after many weeks of steroid treatment, these signs may not be seen during a flare-up. Some have found 24-h urinary creatine excretion helpful. If the weakness is caused by corticosteroids, decreasing corticosteroid dosage lowers creatine excretion and is associated with clinical improvement. In inflammatory myopathy, decreasing corticosteroid dosage increases creatine excretion, with further worsening of muscle weakness.

Treatment

The treatment of CM is empiric. The only certain principles are to reduce corticosteroid dosage carefully and monitor the patient frequently. Complete recovery usually occurs, often 2 to 3 mo after discontinuing corticosteroid treatment. However, when therapy must be continued at reduced dosage, recovery may be much slower. There are no permanent muscular after-effects of CM.

To decrease the likelihood of CM, many recommend switching to alternate-day corticosteroid administration as soon as feasible (see MYAS-THENIA GRAVIS, above). Exercise provides a relative protective effect. Regular physical activity (supervised by a physician to avoid excessive levels) can be helpful. Dietary intervention and the use of androgens have not proved effective. CM in Cushing's disease and other conditions with neoplasm-induced excess of circulating glucocorticoid responds to treatment of the tumor. Once circulating corticosteroid levels return to normal, muscle strength usually normalizes within 3 mo.

MUSCLE DISORDERS IN HYPERTHYROIDISM

Etiology

Hyperthyroidism can cause a subacute proximal myopathy in elderly patients, without the prominent tachycardia or other obvious systemic signs of hyperthyroidism seen in younger patients. It can also cause myokymia *(continuous quivering or undulating movement of muscle surface and overlying skin),* acute bulbar myopathy, ocular myopathy, and, rarely, hypokalemic period paralysis.

Symptoms and Signs

Weakness of proximal limb muscles with increased muscle fatigue are often initial symptoms. There is usually more weakness of the shoulder girdle and upper arm muscles than of the lower extremities. In the legs, the iliopsoas muscle may be primarily affected. Muscle atrophy develops relatively early and may occasionally be pronounced. Over 15% of patients have prominent muscle twitches, often with increased tendon reflexes, which may mimic amyotrophic lateral sclerosis.

Diagnosis

The diagnosis is confirmed by thyroid function tests. Serum muscle enzyme levels are normal. EMG studies often demonstrate fasciculations and myopathic features in weak muscles. Muscle biopsy is usually normal.

Treatment

The euthyroid state should be restored (see Ch. 69). During the first few weeks of treatment, propranolol 120 to 320 mg/day is often effective in reducing proximal muscle weakness.

Long-term prognosis is good. After maintaining the euthyroid state for several months, muscle bulk and strength typically return to normal.

MUSCLE DISORDERS IN HYPOTHYROIDISM

Etiology and Pathogenesis

Hypothyroidism leads to impaired energy metabolism within the muscle fiber and a decrease in contractile force. There is also a defect in the repair and replacement of myofibular proteins due to reduced protein turnover. Slow muscle contraction and relaxation results from diminished activity of myosin ATPase and impaired uptake of calcium by the sarcoplasmic reticulum. Reduced cardiac output results from β-adrenergic hyposensitivity. The pathophysiology responsible for muscle cramps and muscle fiber enlargement is unknown. Muscle deposition of mucopolysaccharides has been seen inconsistently.

Symptoms and Signs

The primary manifestations are proximal weakness, fatigue, slowing of movements, stiffness, myalgias, cramps, and occasionally enlargement of muscles, especially the anterior compartment muscles of the lower extremity. These symptoms develop over weeks to months. Some patients develop pronounced proximal leg muscle weakness and atrophy. Tendon reflexes are slowed, with marked prolongation of relaxation of the Achilles tendon reflex. Myoedema occurs in about $\frac{1}{3}$ of hypothyroid patients, elicited by direct percussion of muscle. A local mounding (electrically silent contraction) of muscle occurs, lasting for 5 sec or longer. A similar response can be seen in disorders associated with malnutrition.

Complications include increased frequency of carpal and tarsal tunnel syndromes and a distal, symmetric, sensory motor polyneuropathy. Rarely, there is marked fatigability of hip girdle and trunk muscles due to neuromuscular transmission abnormality. Repetitive nerve stimulation mimics LEMS.

Diagnosis

A decreased level of circulating thyroid hormone with elevation of thyroid-stimulating hormone **(TSH)** is diagnostic of hypothyroisism. There is usually a several-fold elevation in muscle enzyme levels, especially

CK, and there may be other laboratory abnormalities typical for hypo-thyroidism; eg, an elevation of serum cholesterol.

Electrodiagnostic studies may show compression neuropathies (see above). EMG findings are variable; there may be no abnormality or a mixture of neurogenic and myopathic features. Occasionally, there is evidence of muscle membrane hyperirritability. Muscle biopsy may be normal or occasionally show a reduction in proportion and size of Type 2 muscle fibers.

Differential diagnosis is the same as for polymyositis, above.

Treatment

The goal of treatment is to restore the euthyroid state by careful, slow replacement with increasing doses of thyroid hormone given over a period of weeks (see Ch. 69). Once the euthyroid state is achieved, TSH elevation disappears and serum CK levels return to normal. Surgery is rarely necessary to reverse median or tibial nerve compression.

The long-term prognosis is good. However, patients with severe muscle wasting may never recover full strength and muscle bulk.

MUSCLE WEAKNESS ASSOCIATED WITH DEFICIENCY OF VITAMIN D
(Osteomalacia)
(See also Ch. 64)

Etiology and Pathogenesis

Osteomalacia results from vitamin D deficiency. The pathophysiology of the myopathy is unknown. 1,25-Dihydroxyvitamin D is probably the active form for all tissues. However, some patients with osteomalacia and myopathy have normal levels of this form while levels of 25-hydroxyvitamin D and 24,25-dihydroxyvitamin D are low.

Symptoms and Signs

Patients typically present with pain in the back, hip girdle, and lower extremities; the primary initial complaint in $1/3$ of these patients is muscle weakness (pelvic muscles and thighs). Muscle wasting is proportionate to weakness. About $1/2$ have a waddling gait and use the Gower maneuver to rise from the supine position. About $1/5$ have a marked limp or are unable to walk. Detailed testing of muscle strength is often complicated because of bone pain, but virtually all patients display weakness of pelvic and thigh muscles regardless of whether weakness was a specific complaint. Tendon reflexes are normal to brisk, and sensation is normal. No cranial nerve abnormalities occur. Bone pain and tenderness are most prominent in the pelvis, femurs, spine, and ribs. Collapse of vertebrae frequently occurs, sometimes with skeletal deformities. Occasionally patients describe total body pain, suggesting a primary psychiatric disorder.

Diagnosis

Osteomalacia is suggested by severe pain, especially in the lower lumbar and hip girdle regions, with muscle weakness. Radiographic abnormalities (eg, pseudofractures, biconcave vertebrae) are found in about 70%, serum calcium and phosphorus levels are reduced in about 40%, and serum alkaline phosphatase activity is elevated in > 80% of patients. There is a marked decrease in urinary Ca excretion. Serum levels of vitamin D and its metabolites are decreased. Bone biopsy is a simple confirmatory procedure. Oral tetracycline prior to bone biopsy can be used to label the front of mineralization (see also Ch. 64).

The usual screening tests for primary muscle disease do not provide a specific pattern in osteomalacia. Serum CK is normal or slightly elevated. EMG may show a myopathic pattern. Nerve conduction studies are normal. Muscle biopsy is normal or has nonspecific changes.

Differential diagnosis includes nutritional deficiency or malabsorption (such as occurs with laxative abuse and chronic anticonvulsant therapy), and myopathy of chronic renal failure resulting from phosphate depletion.

Treatment

Initial treatment requires vitamin D 10,000 IU/day IM. Once bone pain has resolved, vitamin D can be given orally. Long-term prognosis is good in most patients. However, if marked wasting, especially of the quadriceps femoris, has occurred, patients may never regain full muscle strength despite normalization of serum levels of vitamin D and phosphate.

HYPOKALEMIC MYOPATHY
(See also Ch. 4)

Etiology and Pathogenesis

A decrease in serum potassium (eg, through chronic use of diuretics) is the most common cause of electrolyte myopathy in the elderly.

Hypocalcemia and hypomagnesemia can also produce prominent neuromuscular symptoms including tetany, irritability, myoclonus, and tremor, but do not typically cause muscle weakness.

Symptoms and Signs

Muscle weakness usually develops slowly over days to weeks. Usually the legs are primarily affected and, in severe cases, weakness spreads to arms, trunk, neck, and, occasionally, thoracic and diaphragmatic muscles. Ocular and bulbar muscles are spared.

The underlying cause of the hypokalemia determines the pattern of weakness. For example, patients with diabetic acidosis (where serum potassium falls rapidly over hours) may present with respiratory weakness, and the arms may become weak before the legs do. In general, chronic hypokalemic myopathy produces greater weakness of proximal than distal muscles. Tendon reflexes become hypoactive and then vanish. There are no sensory complaints and pain is absent.

In severe cases, muscle fiber necrosis with myoglobinuria, muscle pain, tenderness, and muscle swelling can develop.

Diagnosis

Serum potassium is usually < 3 mEq/L. Serum CK may be normal or elevated. Nerve conduction velocities are normal.

Conditions associated with or possibly caused by hypokalemia include chronic alcoholism with alcoholic myopathy, intestinal potassium wastage, Bartter's syndrome, aldosteronism, and licorice intoxication.

Acute hypokalemic paralysis may occur with diabetic ketoacidosis, renal tubular acidosis, or chronic diarrhea; following treatment with amphotericin B; or in most conditions that produce chronic hypokalemia.

Treatment

Chronic myopathy usually reverses over 1 to 4 wk following potassium replacement. If myoglobinuria and rhabdomyolysis have occurred, treatment should include vigorous hydration and alkalinization of the urine to avoid renal tubular necrosis and renal failure. Depending on the etiology, long-term potassium replacement may be necessary.

MYOPATHY DUE TO MUSCULAR DYSTROPHIES

Primary muscular dystrophy presenting for the first time in elderly patients is extremely rare. Three types are particularly variable and are more likely to present in old age.

MYOTONIC DYSTROPHY

Etiology and Pathogenesis

This is an autosomal dominant disorder carried on chromosome 19. The symptoms usually develop in the 20s and 30s, although some individuals have minimal symptoms throughout life. A severe infantile form also occurs.

Symptoms and Signs

Younger patients usually present with distal weakness, primarily in the dorsiflexors of the foot and long flexors of the fingers. There is weakness and wasting of facial and neck muscles, ptosis, and weakness of extraocular muscles. Bulbar muscle weakness manifested by dysphagia and dysarthria is common. However, older patients have minimal muscle weakness with cardiac conduction defects (A-V block, bundle branch block), posterior capsular cataracts, GI hypomotility, and respiratory insufficiency (a decrease in vital capacity, especially when supine). The respiratory insufficiency is due to weakness of respiratory muscles, primarily the diaphragm. Tendon reflexes are depressed, especially in the legs.

Diagnosis

Diagnosis is established by family history and clinical examination. In minimally symptomatic individuals, EMG studies are often necessary. Muscle biopsy usually demonstrates atrophy of Type 1 fibers and an abundance of subsarcolemmal masses, an increase in the number of fibers with central nuclei, and the frequent appearance of ringed fibers. CK levels are mildly to moderately elevated. Slit-lamp examination may show rosette-shaped, subcapsular cataracts. ECG often shows first- or occasionally second-degree heart block with atrial arrhythmias. Bundle branch block may also be present.

Treatment

There is no specific treatment. The goal of therapy is to manage the complications. Respiratory insufficiency is serious, and frequent monitoring of vital capacity, both upright and supine, is necessary. Cardiac arrhythmias, principally conduction block, are managed by ventricular pacemaker. Typical antiarrhythmic medications such as quinidine and procainamide are contraindicated and may worsen the conduction disturbance. Phenytoin has a beneficial effect on arrhythmias and is often useful in controlling severe myotonia. Usually, the myotonia does not require treatment.

GI hypomotility and complaints suggesting intestinal obstruction are not unusual. Conservative treatment, including nasogastric suction and resting the bowel, is usually effective in reversing symptoms.

Surgery should be undertaken with caution. Patients react with a paradoxic rigidity and stiffness to succinylcholine and other depolarizing muscle relaxants. Therefore, nondepolarizing muscle relaxants are recommended for induction of anesthesia. Since halothane has occasionally been associated with muscle rigidity, nitrous oxide with O_2 is preferred, as is spinal anesthesia to general anesthesia. Pentobarbital and phenobarbital have occasionally led to prolonged ventilatory paralysis requiring ventilator support for 1 to 2 days.

Long-term prognosis depends on severity of muscle weakness and presence of complications.

OCULOPHARYNGEAL MUSCULAR DYSTROPHY

This is an autosomal dominant disorder that usually presents in the 50s or 60s.

Symptoms and Signs

Most patients present with ptosis, almost always bilateral, but occasionally asymmetric. Typically, the patient shows a prominent contraction of the frontalis muscle, with the head tipped back to compensate visually for the ptosis. Dysphagia usually follows extraocular weakness, presenting as an intolerance for solid foods. Palatal mobility is often diminished with impaired gag reflex. Some laryngeal weakness with dysphonia is common. Tendon reflexes may be diminished or occasionally absent. Some patients complain of cramps in the calf muscles despite the absence of significant weakness. Years later, the muscles of the limbs, especially of the proximal hip girdle, may become weakened.

Diagnosis

Diagnosis depends on clinical features and a positive family history. It is often confused with myasthenia gravis. In the absence of family history, additional tests are helpful.

Serum CK is usually normal, but may be mildly or moderately increased. EMG studies of limb muscles may show a myopathic or occasionally a mixed myoneuropathic pattern. Muscle biopsy may show nonspecific features; eg, abnormal variation in fiber size and an increase in the number of internal nuclei. Occasionally, there are small angular fibers that react strongly for oxidative enzymes (usually Type 1 fibers) and fibers containing rimmed vacuoles.

Oculopharyngeal muscular dystrophy may occasionally be confused with **oculocraniosomatic disease.** However, patients with the latter often develop symptoms early in life and have progressive external ophthalmoplegia, ataxia, retinitis pigmentosa, cardiac conduction block, hearing disturbance, and other neurologic disturbances. Those who develop ptosis and mild generalized muscle weakness late in life show muscle biopsy findings quite different from those with oculopharyngeal muscular dystrophy (prominent ragged red fibers representing clusters of abnormal mitochondria).

Treatment

There is no specific treatment. Crutches for the eyelids are often helpful. In patients with advanced ptosis, blepharoplasty with resection of the levator palpebral muscles is useful. Dysphagia resulting in significant nutritional deficiency may require tube feeding or the placement of a gastric feeding tube. Some patients benefit from cricopharyngeal myotomy.

MISCELLANEOUS MUSCULAR DISORDERS

IDIOPATHIC "BENIGN" MUSCLE CRAMPS

Electrolyte disturbances and renal failure predispose patients to cramps. However, idiopathic muscle cramps without significant muscle weakness frequently occur in otherwise healthy middle-aged and elderly patients.

Symptoms and Signs

Muscle cramps may develop at rest or with minor exercise. Typically, they occur at night during sleep and affect the calves or foot musculature, with forceful plantar flexion of the foot or toes. Immediate muscle stretching usually relieves symptoms.

Diagnosis

There is no significant muscle weakness or atrophy. All laboratory studies are normal.

Treatment

Conservative treatment is often effective. Stretching the affected muscles prior to sleep for a period of several minutes is often beneficial. A variety of empiric drug treatments is useful; eg, quinine sulfate 200 to 300 mg at bedtime (bitter taste, tinnitus, flushing, pruritus, and GI disturbances may prevent long-term use). Ca supplements (eg, Ca gluconate 1 to 2 gm bid) are well tolerated. Other agents have been used in combination with Ca and quinine treatment, including diphenhydramine 50 to 100 mg at bedtime and magnesium oxide 100 to 200 mg bid.

Occasionally low doses of diazepam 2.5 to 10 mg at bedtime are effective. Clonazepam 0.5 mg bid may also be tried.

---

66. ORTHOPEDIC PROBLEMS

Thomas A. Einhorn, Michael M. Lewis, and *Michael J. Klein*

The most common orthopedic conditions in the elderly are postmenopausal bone loss **(involutional osteoporosis)** and other metabolic bone diseases, eg, **osteomalacia** and **Paget's disease** (see in Ch. 64); a propensity for **fractures** of the hip, distal radius, proximal humerus, and vertebral bodies (see in Ch. 8); acquired angular deformities of the toes (see in Ch. 67); osteoarthritis (see in Ch. 62 and below); and primary and metastatic bone tumors (see below).

MANAGEMENT OF OSTEOARTHRITIS (OA)
(See also Ch. 62)

A degenerative joint disease occurring mainly in older persons and characterized by degeneration of articular cartilage, changes in the synovial membrane, and hypertrophy of bone at the margins. Pain and stiffness, especially after prolonged activity, accompany the degenerative changes.

The early stages of OA are best managed by conservative measures, including treatment with nonsteroidal anti-inflammatory drugs **(NSAIDs),** physical therapy, or no treatment at all (see OSTEOARTHRITIS in Ch. 62). Surgical intervention is appropriate only after significant disease progression has taken place.

External bracing or surgery is indicated when cartilage degeneration has resulted in joint space collapse, when the pain and inflammation can no longer be controlled by conservative measures, or when angular deformities have occurred. **External bracing** is simply a method for maintaining alignment of the spine and improving posture. By improving posture and restricting the extremes of motion, it may alleviate the patient's symptoms, particularly those associated with thoracic or lumbar spondylitis and arthritic pain. Bracing of the spine is best achieved by using a cloth brace such as a Dacron™ corset that can be fastened by hooks or Velcro™ straps. Polypropylene, polyethylene, and Orthoplast™ braces are too heavy, too hot, and too difficult to be fastened by elderly patients who may have limited manual dexterity.

External bracing is of less value in the management of pain or deformity of the appendicular skeletal joints. When indicated, bracing of the peripheral joints (eg, for deformities of the knee) is best achieved by using a light material such as Neoprene™. In patients with severe degenerative arthritis, however, bracing is not a substitute for reconstructive surgery and should be reserved only for those whose medical condition precludes general or regional anesthesia and major surgical intervention.

Advanced OA of peripheral joints frequently requires surgery to alleviate pain and improve function; eg, joint fusion or resection arthroplasty to obliterate the joint space, osteotomy to rebalance mechanical forces, or total joint replacement arthroplasty to resurface joint articulations.

Fusions are effective in most joints but result in loss of flexibility, which tends to transfer loads to adjacent joints that may themselves be diseased. Furthermore, the postoperative period of immobilization required for fusions to heal can lead to adjacent joint stiffness. **Resection arthroplasty,** while sometimes effective in the management of joint pain, results in significant loss of joint function.

Osteotomy is a suitable operation for osteoarthritis of the hip or knee in young persons, but patients > 65 yr rarely do well after the procedure because prolonged postoperative immobilization leads to joint stiffness and impaired ambulation.

Total joint replacement arthroplasty, introduced in the late 1950s, is a major advance in orthopedic treatment. Refinements in technology and surgical technic have resulted in continued improvement of this procedure. Cemented replacement prostheses for the hip, knee, and shoulder continue to provide good results after 10 to 15 yr and are the treatment of choice for advanced, disabling OA of these joints. Prostheses for other joints (eg, elbow, wrist, finger, toe, and ankle) have been less extensively evaluated. The major shortcoming of arthroplasty is its limited long-term success, which is related to the eventual loosening of the cement that affixes the implant to the bone. Newer prostheses have been designed for use without cement, but these are still considered experimental. Since cemented total joint replacement arthroplasty is more successful in older patients than in younger individuals, noncemented arthroplasty may not be an important treatment option for the elderly (see also Chs. 8 and 23).

METASTATIC BONE NEOPLASMS

Metastatic tumors outnumber primary bone sarcomas by 20:1. This ratio becomes even more disproportionate in the geriatric population, in which primary bone sarcomas are exceedingly rare. The proportion of metastatic tumors becomes larger still if autopsy series are included, because carcinomas that metastasize to bone may not produce the symptoms and signs that lead to an antemortem diagnosis.

Metastasis should be strongly suspected in any individual with localized skeletal symptoms and a history of documented malignant epithelial tumor or in any geriatric patient who has unexplained radiolucent or radiodense bone lesions on x-ray. While senile or postmenopausal osteoporosis is implicated in a large percentage of hip fractures and compression fractures of the spine, metastatic carcinoma should also be considered in the differential diagnosis. If a discrete lesion suggesting metastasis is not seen on conventional x-rays, other radioisotopic procedures (eg, radioactive scans, CT, and MRI) may disclose small bone lesions. Nonspecific elevations of serum alkaline phosphatase may occur as a result of bone turnover due to metastatic disease.

While almost any malignancy may produce bone metastases, > 80% of secondary tumors in bone arise from the lungs, breast, prostate, kidney, or thyroid gland. On the other hand, carcinomas of the large intestine usually do not produce bone metastases, even though such tumors may involve adjacent bone by direct extension. Also, carcinomas usually do not produce metastases distal to the elbows or knees.

Capricious patterns of metastatic bone disease suggest primary carcinomas of the kidney, lung, or sometimes an occult malignant melanoma; cortical metastases strongly suggest a pulmonary origin. In most instances of metastatic carcinoma, multiple foci of tumor are present in the skeleton. Occasionally, malignant epithelial tumors, particularly those originating in the kidney, may give rise to a solitary skeletal metastasis. This phenomenon may have therapeutic significance, since a solitary metastasis is not a contraindication to surgical removal of the primary and secondary tumors, which may effect cure.

When an occult primary tumor metastasizes to bone, its appearance on conventional x-ray may hint at its origin prior to a biopsy. Radiolucent osseous lesions are most likely to be pulmonary, renal, or thyroid in origin. Radiodense lesions are usually prostatic in origin in men and of breast origin in women, although breast carcinomas often give a mixed (radiolucent and radiodense) radiographic picture. Tumors that produce bone metastases less frequently (eg, mucinous adenocarcinomas of the upper GI tract and carcinoid tumors) also appear as radiodense bone lesions.

Nonepithelial malignant tumors (eg, lymphomas) may also spread to the skeleton. Non-Hodgkin's lymphomas almost invariably produce radiolucent lesions that may be mistaken for primary osseous lymphomas if nodal disease is either central or not yet clinically apparent. Hodgkin's disease is uncommon in the elderly. When it occurs, osseous involvement usually produces a radiolucent pattern, but it produces radiodense lesions about 20% of the time. While Hodgkin's disease sometimes appears to be a primary osseous lesion, undiscovered lymphadenopathy is almost invariably present when a bone lesion becomes evident.

Biopsy of bone lesions is necessary for a definitive diagnosis of metastatic carcinoma. While needle biopsy may confirm a diagnosis, particularly when the primary site has already been identified, an open technic is preferable when possible, because it ensures better local control of bleeding as well as representative tissue sampling. If the primary site of a bony metastasis is unknown, the histopathology may provide some clue to its origin by revealing glandular or squamous differentiation. Occasionally, the presence of clear cells may suggest a renal carcinoma, while the presence of typical melanin pigment may suggest a malignant melanoma. More recently, histochemical, immunohistochemical, and even electron microscopic analyses have been used with some success to increase the yield of accurate diagnoses of undiscovered primary tumors. However, the ability of a histopathologist to determine the exact site of origin is sometimes limited.

PRIMARY NEOPLASMS OF BONE

Plasma cell myeloma, the most common nonepithelial malignant tumor in bone, is a neoplasm derived from marrow; the tumor cells have the morphologic and functional characteristics of plasma cells. It occurs frequently in a diffuse form and occasionally in a solitary form. In the diffuse form, multiple lytic lesions without reactive borders may be seen on routine x-ray, but the usual finding is diffuse osteoporosis. Patients usually present with weakness, loss of weight, increased susceptibility to infection, and easy fatigability owing to replacement of normal marrow elements, anemia, and decreased antibody production. Diffuse bone pain and, frequently, back pain from spinal involvement is noted. There may be an associated hypercalcemia and, depending on the degree of marrow involvement, anemia, leukocytopenia, and thrombocytopenia.

While metastatic carcinoma is often suspected in patients with these findings, serum protein electrophoresis usually reveals a monoclonal γ-paraprotein and a depression in circulating levels of normal immunoglobulins. When skeletal lesions are discrete, there is often surprisingly little activity associated with their peripheries on radioisotopic scans; this is not the case with metastatic carcinomas. Because the hematopoietic marrow is diffusely involved, myelomatous areas not visible on routine x-ray may yield diagnostic findings on aspiration biopsy from the iliac crest, sternum, or other easily accessible sites.

The less common **solitary plasmacytoma** usually masquerades as a solitary metastasis, a primary bone sarcoma, or a primary benign tumor. It is rarely accompanied by a paraprotein abnormality, and its diagnosis by biopsy is often unsuspected. While the lesion responds well to local irradiation, most patients with solitary plasmacytoma develop generalized myelomatosis with paraproteinemia between 5 and 20 yr after their initial diagnosis.

Chondrosarcoma is the other major class of malignant primary bone neoplasm that occurs in the middle-aged–to–elderly population. Most chondrosarcomas are indolent, slow-growing tumors, with a propensity for local extension and recurrence but little capacity for distant spread. While low-grade chondrosarcomas may, in fact, have been present in a patient for many years, their very slow doubling times permit a very long latency period during which no signs of malignancy are clinically manifest. Moreover, the fact that these neoplasms are often located deep in the extremities or in the pelvis may allow them to reach considerable size before they are discovered. A slowly enlarging mass or gradually increasing pain where none was present previously usually calls attention to the tumor.

Most chondrosarcomas arise de novo, but a small percentage are secondary to a preexisting benign cartilaginous lesion such as an **osteochondroma** or an **enchondroma**. Clinical enlargement of a preexistent exostosis and pain in a bone with a suspected benign preexisting cartilage tumor are ominous symptoms that should raise the clinical suspicion of malignancy. Patients with multiple hereditary exostoses—and especially those with multiple enchondromata—are statistically more likely to develop secondary chondrosarcomas.

Chondrosarcomas are usually diagnosed on routine x-ray. There is usually an area of radiolucency, containing numerous punctate, comma-shaped, and round radiodensities; these correspond histologically to areas of amorphous matrix calcification and endochondral ossification. If the lesion occurs in a long tubular bone, there may be endosteal scalloping, but often there are areas of both resorption and thickening of the bony cortex.

Prognosis depends upon the histologic grade of the tumor and its degree of local spread; high-grade tumors are likely to produce lung metastases. **Dedifferentiation** is a phenomenon that occurs in a small percentage of otherwise low-grade chondrosarcomas, usually in the elderly. In this process, an otherwise indolent, low-grade chondrosarcoma develops within itself an area of high-grade sarcoma, which may be fibrosarcoma, osteosarcoma, malignant fibrous histiocytoma, or a combination of histologic types. The prognosis in patients with this type of tumor is grave.

Treatment

The treatment of metastatic disease requires a team approach and an analysis of the patient's overall care plan. Depending on the clinical situation and the origin of the metastasis, chemotherapy and radiation may be indicated, particularly with metastatic breast disease, lymphoma, and myeloma. In certain circumstances, surgical treatment plays an important role. For example, in the patient with an impending fracture, especially of a long bone, the presence of vague pain may be the first warning. Often, x-rays show a large destructive lesion without evidence of fracture, but if fracture is imminent, prophylactic surgery should be performed (see Ch. 8).

When a pathologic fracture has occurred, surgery should be considered unless other aspects of the patient's condition contraindicate it. In many instances, internal fixation with the use of methyl methacrylate is helpful in stabilizing the fracture. In other instances, especially in a pathologic fracture of the proximal femur or hip, prosthetic replacement, including total hip replacement, is preferred (see Ch. 8). The goals of surgical treatment, whether by internal fixation or prosthetic replacement, are pain relief, local control of the disease process if feasible, and restoration of maximal patient function.

Full surgical resection of primary sarcomas (eg, osteosarcoma, chondrosarcoma, radiation-induced sarcoma, and sarcoma secondary to Paget's disease) should be attempted if possible. This may be accomplished by a limb-sparing surgical procedure using internal reconstruction. Part or all of a bone can be removed and replaced with an internal prosthesis or allograft custom-designed for the patient. However, a limb may need to be amputated, either because of the location of the lesion or the general status of the patient. In such a case, the patient can be fitted with an external artificial prosthesis as part of a general rehabilitation program (see also Ch. 23).

---

67. FOOT PROBLEMS

Barry S. Collet

Foot problems often cause disability and decreased productivity. These problems range from simple ailments (eg, corns or ingrown nails), to more serious conditions arising from complications of diabetes mellitus and peripheral vascular disease.

Neglect of the feet throughout one's active years results in painful conditions in the later years. Foot disorders begin early in life and are influenced by hereditary factors as well as by shoe styles (ie, the geriatric foot has been molded and shaped by years of activity, physical abuse, and possibly ill-fitting shoes).

EVALUATION OF THE FOOT

The patient's chief concern should be recorded in his own words. The nature of the problem as well as the location, duration, onset, severity, symptoms, and prior treatment should be noted. The patient should indicate which part of the foot is most painful when walking; the physician should determine whether or not the same symptoms can be elicited in the nonambulatory state through palpation and range-of-motion testing. If the patient is unable to communicate this information, an appropriate family member should be questioned. Relevant economic, psychologic, and social factors should be recorded. Self-treatment by the patient, proper or improper, should also be noted, as this is often the precipitating factor in his seeking professional help.

An appropriate review of systems should be conducted, and significant findings should be considered in relation to the patient's presenting concerns. Often, symptoms and signs of systemic disease are first noted in the feet. In reviewing the history, diabetes mellitus, cardiac disease, arthritis, hypertension, and peripheral vascular disease in particular should be noted, along with any current treatment for these conditions. Any history of night cramps should also be noted.

Evaluation of the foot requires a consideration of the patient's lifestyle in relation to the presenting problems. The patient's physical environment and degree of ambulation should be considered in the evaluation and treatment plan. Many geriatric patients may be physically unable to seek appropriate attention for their medical problems. Others may not understand a particular treatment plan or may be reluctant to stray from old and outdated remedies. Still others may have delayed seeking professional help for purely economic reasons.

Many foot problems involve the skin. Hyperkeratotic lesions and excrescences should be noted and recorded according to location and size. The presence of bacterial infection, tinea pedis, dry skin, ulcerations, and verrucae should be recorded. The toenails should be inspected for signs of hypertrophy and mycotic infection, and absence of the nail or changes in the color and continuity of the nail plate, as well as any foot odor, should be noted.

A vascular examination should follow. The feet and legs should be evaluated for trophic changes (eg, loss of hair growth; red, shiny, atrophic skin; and pigmentation changes). The temperature of the feet should be noted and information on claudication elicited if present. The presence or absence of pedal pulses (the dorsalis pedis and posterior tibial) should be noted. Check for varicosities and edema. Doppler and plethysmographic studies should be employed if vascular disease is suspected.

Neurologic evaluation should include motor function testing. The Achilles and superficial plantar reflexes should be elicited, and vibratory sensation should be evaluated, along with sensitivity to pain, temperature, and touch. Muscle-strength testing should be performed and recorded and any areas of discomfort noted.

Orthopedic evaluation: One of the most important procedures in the evaluation of the geriatric foot is simply observing the patient's gait. Very often, this will be the key to determining an effective treatment plan for biomechanical conditions. Postural deformities, physical limitations, and the position of the foot at heel strike and through the gait cycle are ascertained by watching the patient walk.

The human foot comprises 26 bones, which, along with ligaments, tendons, and muscles, provide support and mobility. There are 14 phalanges—3 for each of the lesser toes and 2 for the great toe, or hallux; 5 metatarsals; and 7 tarsal bones. The talus, or ankle bone, supports the fibula laterally and the tibia medially. It provides the fulcrum around which motion occurs. The talus is seated on the calcaneus, or heel bone, which makes direct contact with the ground.

Motion occurs primarily around the subtalar, or talocalcaneal, joint. This motion occurs in 3 planes and includes inversion-eversion, abduction-adduction, and dorsiflexion and plantar flexion. A combination of dorsiflexion, abduction, and eversion is commonly referred to as pronation, while a combination of the opposite movements—plantar flexion, adduction, and inversion—is known as supination. It is important that one ascertain the degree of pronation or supination, especially when corrective devices are contemplated.

Structural deformities of the foot are obvious on inspection. **Hallux valgus (bunion deformity),** is a painful condition involving the 1st metatarsophalangeal joint. X-rays should be taken and the degree of deformity noted. A **bunionette** is a similar condition involving the 5th metatarsophalangeal joint, in which the 5th toe is maintained in a varus position. This, too, can be evaluated on x-ray; such studies should also detect any bone changes (eg, osteoporosis, demineralization, old fractures, and arthritis). Range-of-motion testing should be performed for all joints and appropriately graded. Any limitations of movement or the presence of crepitus should be recorded. Finally, the patient's foot type and shoe style should be noted.

COMMON FOOT PROBLEMS

DERMATOLOGIC FOOT PROBLEMS

Corns and calluses, usually the result of undue friction and pressure around a bony prominence, are common problems, and are often associated with improper or tight foot wear. **The corn,** also known as a **clavus** or **heloma,** is *a concentrated hyperkeratotic lesion, somewhat conical in shape, found most commonly on the dorsal surface of the proximal interphalangeal joint of the lesser toes.* This joint also becomes contracted in the hammer toe syndrome, making it most vulnerable to excessive pressure from shoes and stockings. It may be complicated by a bunion deformity, in which the great toe, as it deviates laterally, causes contraction of the 2nd toe. Digital contractures and changes associated with arthritis may also cause lesions to develop on the distal aspect of the toes. The 5th toe is prone to developing a corn because of rotational deformity. These hard hyperkeratotic lesions can lead to inflammation and infection if not properly treated. A **soft corn,** or **heloma molle,** is usually found interdigitally and is caused by pressure from adjacent toes. The lesion becomes "soft" because of moisture that accumulates in the web space.

Treatment is aimed at local debridement of the lesion followed by aperture or balance padding to redistribute pressure away from the painful area. This may consist of a small $1/8$-in. felt pad with a concentric opening, with the hole placed directly over the lesion. Medicated pads should be avoided because their acid content often destroys tissue, leading to further disability. An emollient skin cream should be used afterward to reduce the amount of keratosis. Orthodigital devices, such as tube-shaped foam pads, polyurethane, and silicone molds, may be fabricated for daily use by the patient, whose ability to bend to apply the device, however, must be considered. Another successful method of conservative therapy is the construction of custom-made, molded orthopedic shoes. These shoes are made from casts of the patient's feet and compensate for any bony abnormalities present at the time of casting.

A **callus,** or **tyloma,** is *a diffuse, circumscribed hyperkeratotic lesion found on the plantar aspect of the foot,* where there is friction and pressure. It may also be related to weight changes and improper shoe modifications. Symptoms may range from generalized burning to severe pinpoint pain. A more circumscribed lesion, similar in appearance to tyloma, is the **intractable plantar keratoma.** These painful lesions are usually found directly under the head of the involved metatarsal. They may result from plantar declination of the bone or may be associated with arthritic changes or trauma. They must be differentiated from viral **warts,** which are similar in appearance. Warts characteristically reveal areas of pinpoint bleeding on debridement.

Treatment of a tyloma consists of debridement of the lesion, followed by application of protective padding such as moleskin, lamb's wool, or polyurethane. The local application of an emollient skin cream, preferably with a urea base, is advised to provide dermal hydration. Adhesive padding should be *avoided* in patients with diabetes mellitus or peripheral vascular impairment. **Warts** may be managed with local paring down of the lesion, followed by the application of an acidic preparation, or they may be excised surgically. Excision on the plantar aspect of the foot should be avoided because of subsequent pain and potential scarring.

Orthotic devices should be used when these lesions result from biomechanical factors. X-ray evaluation, as well as clinical examination, provide insight into the cause of the underlying problem. Orthotic devices can be fabricated from a variety of materials, depending on the patient's tolerance, and can be modified if new lesions develop as a result of the bony changes associated with arthritis and aging. Compliance is usually good with these devices, since they can be transferred from one pair of shoes to another.

Dryness and scaling of the skin often caused by a decrease in sebaceous activity, become more apparent with aging. Pruritus may result, and subsequent scratching may produce open wounds and inflammation. Pruritus is also common with conditions such as **tinea pedis, contact dermatitis,** and **eczema.** Low doses of oral antihistamines, in conjunction with a topical corticosteroid, is advised until the symptoms dissipate. Afterward, the prophylactic use of a urea-based, emollient skin cream is usually sufficient to control the condition. In the case of contact dermatitis, the causative factor, usually a pair of shoes or stockings, should be eliminated.

Tinea pedis, commonly known as **athlete's foot,** is usually caused by *Trichophyton rubrum, T. mentagrophytes,* and *Epidermophyton floccosum.* Since fungi thrive in a warm, moist environment, concomitant hyperhidrosis complicates the condition. The most common presentations of tinea pedis are interdigital and the so-called moccasin pattern of eruption, caused by *T. rubrum.* Vesicular eruption, fissuring, loss of the epidermis, and secondary bacterial infection may occur. The elderly are especially susceptible to such outbreaks because of changes in the distal tissues resulting from peripheral vascular disease and the aging process. These patients often develop cracks and fissures, thus providing a convenient portal of entry for invasive organisms. It should be noted that tinea resembles erythrasma, with which it is often confused. The latter is caused by a gram-positive bacillus and is diagnosed by a coral-red fluorescence when examined under a Wood's light. It is treated with oral erythromycin and topical antifungal preparations.

Diagnosis of tinea pedis may be facilitated through the use of a dermatophyte testing medium, in which a simple color change indicates fungal infection. Traditional methods of diagnosis include microscopic examination with a potassium hydroxide preparation and a fungal culture.

Treatment of tinea infections includes soaking the feet in warm water and Epsom salt, followed by the application of a topical antifungal cream. Topical clotrimazole and miconazole nitrate are effective. When edema and bacterial infection are present, the feet should be elevated, ambulation reduced, and oral antibiotics given in conjunction with frequent clinical observation.

Griseofulvin is an effective oral antifungal agent, but **side effects** (eg, urticaria, skin rashes, nausea and vomiting, headache, and fatigue) may preclude its use in the frail elderly. More severe reactions include paresthesias of the hands and feet, proteinuria, and leukopenia. Griseofulvin acts by means of a "curling factor" and relies on an adequate vasculature, which is often absent in the geriatric patient. Griseofulvin incorporates itself into newly formed epidermal tissue and fungal elements actually curl away from the drug. Routine blood chemistry studies should be performed on patients treated with griseofulvin to ensure that the drug has not reached toxic levels.

Psoriasis commonly affects geriatric patients. The characteristic lesion appears on the foot, with hyperkeratosis and fissuring. The nails exhibit pitting and subungual hyperkeratosis. Local treatment consists of the topical application of a corticosteroid and periodic debridement of the nails.

Hyperhidrosis of the feet, or excessive sweating, may result in a foul odor (bromhidrosis). It may be precipitated and/or aggravated by tinea pedis, poor pedal hygiene, or metabolic disease. Usual treatment is with a 10% formalin solution, along with frequent changing of socks and the routine use of a topical foot powder.

NAIL DISORDERS

The primary function of the nail is to protect the distal phalanges against injury and trauma. Many changes in the nail plate can be attributed to aging and are associated with trauma, systemic disease, and dermatologic conditions.

Onychia is *inflammation of the nail matrix* while **paronychia** is *inflammation of the matrix plus the surrounding and deeper structures.* The most common cause of onychia and paronychia is trauma (eg, a direct injury or pressure from shoes that are new or too short). Skin diseases (eg, **psoriasis** and **eczema**) are commonly responsible for inflammatory reactions around the nail. Patients with **diabetes mellitus** are more prone to developing inflammation around the nail bed because of poor circulation and diminished resistance to infection.

Unguis incarnatus, or **onychocryptosis,** is commonly known as an **ingrown toenail.** In this condition, the lateral nail edge penetrates the periungual tissue causing an inflammatory reaction and, at times, bacterial infection. If the infection is not resolved, painful granulation tissue forms, necessitating surgical intervention. Faulty footwear and improper nail care are the primary causes.

Treatment is directed at removing the ingrown portion of the nail. This may be facilitated by the use of an English anvil pattern nail splitter inserted under the nail plate. Local anesthesia may be necessary, depending on the severity of the condition. After the wound is cleansed, a topical antibiotic agent and a dry, sterile dressing are applied. Warm Epsom salt soaks should be used bid, followed by application of a new dressing. When infection is severe, systemic antibiotics should be used.

Onychomycosis, *a localized fungal infection of the nail or nail bed,* is characterized by degeneration of the nail plate, with changes in growth and appearance. Clinically, the nail may present with degeneration ranging from simple scaling to actual destruction of its entire architecture. The nail becomes brittle, hypertrophic, and granular. Infection usually progresses from one nail to the next. The thickened nail plate often demonstrates subungual keratosis and debris. The causative agents are usually *T. rubrum, T. mentagrophytes,* and *E. floccosum,* although monilial infections may also produce onychomycosis. Positive diagnosis may be made through the appropriate dermatophyte-testing technic discussed above.

Onychomycosis can cause severe disability. Repeated microtrauma of the enlarged nail plate due to shoe pressure can cause discomfort and even injury. Antifungal treatment is rarely effective because of the nail matrix involvement. In addition, the diminished pedal blood supply common in many elderly patients precludes the use of oral antifungal agents. Treatment consists of reduction of the nail plates at regular intervals and patient education. The use of topical antifungal agents around the nail bed to keep the tissue soft may be helpful.

Onychauxis and onychogryphosis are other common nail conditions. Onychauxis is *hypertrophy of the nail plate,* while onychogryphosis is long-standing *hypertrophy characterized by a curved or hooked nail* (also known as a ram's horn nail). Severe pain may arise when pressure, including that from the bed sheets at night, is applied to such nails. Because of the severe hypertrophy, the nail may penetrate the adjacent toe, causing local inflammation and pain. In the patient with diabetes or peripheral vascular disease, pressure necrosis may result, causing ulceration and gangrene. Treatment involves frequent reduction of the nails and education in proper foot care and hygiene.

When nail conditions are severe and responsible for pain and disability, and conservative measures have failed, surgery should be considered. A partial or complete destruction of the nail matrix can be performed simply and effectively under local anesthesia, usually on an outpatient basis.

ORTHOPEDIC AND STRUCTURAL DEFORMITIES

Heel pain, which may be unremitting, especially on weight bearing, is common. Symptoms begin almost immediately upon stepping on the foot and may lessen as walking continues, or the pain may be constant. The pain is usually felt around the plantar aspect of the heel and may radiate distally to the arch. Very often this is due to a gradual age-related atrophy of the fat padding beneath the calcaneus. It also may be due to an excessive amount of activity that causes increased pressure and irritation to the area. The patient's entire outlook and ability to carry out simple daily chores may be affected. The most common cause of heel pain is a **heel spur,** in which pain usually arises from inflammation caused by the constant pulling of the plantar fascia at its origin in the calcaneus. In most cases, an abnormal amount of pronation is present, causing excessive tension on the fascial tissue. There may be pain in the area of the longitudinal arch *without* concomitant heel pain; this is known as **plantar fasciitis.**

Treatment for heel pain depends on the nature and extent of bone pathology, as determined on x-ray. In the case of a heel spur, a shelf of bone may be seen at the base of the calcaneus on a lateral view. Local injections of a corticosteroid coupled with an anesthetic agent should be given weekly until symptoms subside. Typically this would consist of 0.5–1 mL of Celestone® Soluspan® (or other suitable agent) and 1 mL 2% plain lidocaine. The injection should originate at the medial side of the heel, aimed toward the area of greatest pain. Plantar strappings are useful in conjunction with injection therapy, since they relieve tension on the plantar fascia. A low-dye strapping may be used to control pronatory motion at the subtalar joint. It should be applied with the foot mildly inverted, and should be replaced in about 1 wk during follow-up evaluation. The addition of scaphoid padding to the strapping provides further support and is highly recommended. The use of oral nonsteroidal anti-inflammatory drugs, physical therapy such as ultrasound and hydrotherapy, heel cups, and plantar paddings may be effective in reducing discomfort in the heel. When the pain has diminished, a biomechanical examination should be performed and an appropriate orthotic device made to compensate for the pronation, alleviate strain on the plantar fascia, and provide adequate support for the heel.

In Haglund's deformity, or **"pump bump, "** pain in the heel may present posteriorly. The condition seems to arise from pressure on the posterior-superior aspect of the calcaneus, where a bursal sac may develop as a result of irritation from the shoe counter. With bursitis, aspiration may be necessary. Heel lifts raise the heel above the counter, alleviating symptoms. Aperture padding around the bursal sac also relieves pressure. Surgical excision may be necessary if conservative therapy fails.

Hallux valgus deformity, or **bunion,** is a common condition in which a deviation of the first metatarsophalangeal joint **(MPJ)** causes the toe to drift laterally, with an accompanying protuberance of the first metatarsal head medially and exostosis formation. (There may also be a metatarsus primus varus deformity, in which the first metatarsal drifts medially away from the lesser metatarsals.) An adventitious bursa may form at the point of greatest pressure. As the hallux drifts laterally, an overriding second toe may develop, causing a painful dorsal lesion. A hammer toe syndrome may develop, followed by a tyloma (see above) beneath the second metatarsal because of contracture of the second toe.

Treatment should be aimed at providing comfort and relieving pain. While surgical correction is usually the treatment of choice, the life-style and ability of the patient to provide self-care should be strongly considered before surgery is contemplated. Often, a bunion is irritated by shoe pressure, since the deformity occupies more space in the shoe than a normal foot and, therefore, is subjected to greater friction and pressure. Removing the tight shoe will afford some relief; when the deformity is severe, a bunion-last type of shoe or a custom-made, molded shoe should be considered. Acute inflammation in the area of the adventitious bursa is usually relieved by the injection of a corticosteroid combined with an anesthetic agent. A cutout should be made in the shoe at the site of greatest pressure until appropriate footwear can be obtained. Oral nonsteroidal anti-inflammatory drugs **(NSAIDs)** are also effective in treating symptoms.

Osteoarthritis often affects the first metatarsophalangeal joint, producing a **hallux rigidus.** There may be pain and swelling at the joint and a limitation of motion caused by exostosis formation. Diagnosis is made by observing the patient walk and noting a decrease in motion at the interphalangeal joint of the hallux. Palpation of the first metatarsophalangeal joint reveals stiffness and pain with a pronounced limitation of motion. **Treatment** consists of local infiltration of a corticosteroid coupled with an anesthetic agent to alleviate the symptoms. Thereafter, exercising the joint and traction of the toe may be useful in increasing range of motion. If this fails, an appropriate orthotic device should be fabricated with a Morton's extension to cushion motion at the metatarsophalangeal joint in an effort to reduce the pain that occurs during walking.

Metatarsalgia is caused by atrophy of the plantar fat pad that supports the metatarsal heads, which then bear the full force of weight bearing. It is described as a generalized ache or soreness directly below the metatarsal heads. It may be accompanied by a plantar callous and, if untreated, may lead to an anterior metatarsal bursitis or arthritis of the involved metatarsophalangeal joints. Treatment consists of redistributing the pressure away from the metatarsal heads. This can be accomplished through the use of an orthopedic shoe, an orthosis, or other accommodative device that provides cushioning and shock absorption to this area of the foot.

In hammer toe syndrome, *the involved toe is in a fixed, contracted position at the proximal interphalangeal joint.* The toe, being higher in the shoe than normal, is exposed to excessive friction, often resulting in a painful heloma. In severe cases, the lesion may become inflamed and ulcerated, leading to secondary bacterial infection and ambulatory disability. Treatment consists of removal of the irritating shoe and debridement of the lesion. Surgical correction, ranging from a simple tenotomy to an arthroplasty of the digit, should be considered in severe cases.

Morton's neuroma is caused by *entrapment of the interdigital nerves as they pass between the metatarsal heads.* It characteristically occurs in the 3rd interspace, where the metatarsal heads are in closest proximity, and causes severe, disabling pain. The patient complains of sharp pain that may radiate to the toes or legs, necessitating removal of the shoe and foot massage. This is pathognomonic. Nonsurgical treatment consists of local injections of a long-acting corticosteroid proximal to the site of pain. If this does not alleviate the symptoms, surgical excision of the neuroma is advised.

Fractures: The geriatric patient, being especially prone to falls and other injuries, may present with a suspected fracture of the foot. Ice should be applied to the injured area immediately to reduce the inflammatory response, and analgesics should be used for pain management. X-rays should be taken to confirm the diagnosis and ascertain the extent of injury; the dorsoplantar, lateral, and oblique views are helpful. Fractures of the toes may be treated by splinting the injured toe to an adjacent one to ensure immobilization. With a displaced fracture of the toe, local anesthesia is necessary for realignment. More severe fractures, such as those of a metatarsal or tarsal bone, require casting, either plaster, semirigid, or Unna's boot. With all fractures, a reduction in ambulation is essential, and crutches may be necessary. Follow-up x-rays should be taken over the next few months to assess healing.

Special shoes: Proper footwear is important in the management of foot problems. The orthopedic molded shoe is helpful in patients with advanced arthritic conditions and structural deformities. These shoes, commonly referred to as "space shoes," are custom-made to the exact contours of the foot impression casts. The shoes can be made to correct specific problems and should afford maximal comfort while providing ease in ambulation.

PEDAL COMPLICATIONS OF SYSTEMIC DISEASE

Peripheral vascular disease and diabetes mellitus can be responsible for major foot problems, thus, an understanding of the nature and consequences of these diseases is essential in planning long-term goals for the patient. (See Chs. 36 and 70.)

Symptoms of vascular diseases in the lower extremities include exertional pain, edema, changes in skin color, coldness, burning, numbness, loss of hair growth, and ulcerations. With advancing vascular disease, changes in the nails are found, most notably thickening and onychomycosis.

Pain on walking indicates intermittent claudication. Patients exhibit a diagnostic limp if walking is continued after symptoms begin. **Pain on resting** indicates more advanced arterial disease and tissue ischemia. With poor circulation, the ability to combat infection is diminished, and even the slightest cut or bruise may cause ulceration and gangrene.

Diabetics demonstrate many of the same symptoms as individuals with peripheral vascular insufficiency. Diabetes affects primarily the small arteries and nerves in the feet, causing paresthesias, motor weakness, numbness, burning, and cramping. Other clinical findings in elderly diabetics include color and temperature changes, dry skin, scaliness, and edema that may be caused by generalized systemic disease or by localized infection. Nail pathology is similar to that seen with vascular insufficiency.

Diabetics are prone to ulcer formation, especially on the weight-bearing surfaces of the foot. Ulcers often lead to infection, osteomyelitis, and gangrene. Often, the diabetic patient precipitates ulcer formation by use of an acidic OTC corn remedy. The medication incites sloughing of the skin and soft tissue destruction.

When an ulcer is present, one should determine whether it is neurotrophic or vascular. The **neurotrophic ulcer** is usually painless, and the patient may be unaware of its presence. In contrast, the **vascular ulcer** is extremely painful and is more prone to infection because of circulatory impairment.

Treatment of sclerotic conditions consists of warm soaks and the use of thermostatically controlled heating elements, under close supervision, to encourage dilation of the blood vessels. Patients need special care, should be seen regularly for evaluation, and should be helped to understand the importance of their role in health care. Many times, simple problems can be resolved if treated early. Daily self-inspection of the feet is strongly advised, especially for patients with neuropathy and an associated lack of feeling in the involved area.

In the case of an ulcerated lesion, necrotic tissue should be debrided aseptically to enable viable tissue to heal. Drainage should be cultured and appropriate antibiotic therapy initiated. An enzymatic debriding agent such as Elase® or Biozyme-C® should be applied, and the foot should be maintained at rest in a level position. Ambulation should be restricted as much as possible, since walking may cause further trauma and increase the likelihood of infection. The patient should be cautioned against cigarette smoking and exposure to temperature extremes. Tissue perfusion may be enhanced by the use of pentoxifylline, a drug that increases the flexibility of RBCs, thereby decreasing blood viscosity and improving blood flow. Aspirin may also be effective in increasing local circulation to ulcerated areas.

After the ulcer is healed, shoes should be modified to divert pressure from sensitive areas. This may be done with padding or other protective devices or with an inlay or an accommodative orthotic device.

When an ulcer cannot be managed conservatively, bypass surgery may be indicated to increase circulation to the limb, provided circulation is adequate above and below the occluded area. In the diabetic patient with vascular insufficiency and microangiopathy, early consultation with a vascular surgeon is extremely important to ascertain whether or not this type of surgery would be beneficial. Plethysmographic and Doppler studies are indicated to evaluate the extent of the pathology. X-rays should be taken to rule out osteomyelitis. If gangrene is present, amputation is usually necessary.

ARTHRITIC CONDITIONS AND GOUT

The most common condition causing pain in the geriatric foot is some form of arthritis. **Osteoarthritis** often involves the ankle and the first metatarsophalangeal joint. Symptoms increase with ambulation and include pain, stiffness, and weakness at the involved joint. Once the disease is established, characteristic x-ray findings include narrowing of the joint space (caused by loss of articular cartilage), osteophyte formation, and increased density of subchondral bone. Exostosis formation is thought to be primarily biomechanical. Treatment is symptomatic, ranging from nonsteroidal anti-inflammatory drug therapy to surgical intervention if marked loss of joint function has occurred.

Rheumatoid arthritis (RA) may produce progressive stiffening of the joints, leading to deformity and ankylosis. Morning stiffness, pain on motion, and subcutaneous nodules may be present. Laboratory findings often include an increase in the ESR, positive RA latex fixation test, and hypochromic anemia. X-ray evaluation typically demonstrates splaying of the forefoot, claw toes, loss of articular cartilage, and bony erosions.

Conservative therapy of the rheumatoid foot includes patient education and support. Periods of rest from weight bearing are essential, as are necessary shoe modifications to accommodate painful plantar areas. The custom-made orthopedic shoe is particularly helpful. Local injection of a corticosteroid helps alleviate joint pain, as do oral doses of anti-inflammatory drugs and analgesics. Numerous surgical procedures are available and should be contemplated when conservative therapy is of minimal value.

Gout is characterized by the deposit of urate crystals **(tophi)** in the synovial membrane and articular cartilage. Typical punched-out lesions may be seen radiographically and are pathognomonic. Diagnosis may be confirmed by microscopic evaluation of aspirated synovial fluid for urate crystals, with their characteristic strongly negative birefringence.

The inflammatory response, initiated by the urate crystals, often begins in the great toe and is characterized by increasing joint pain, swelling, erythema, and heat. While other areas, such as the instep or ankle, may be involved, the majority of cases of acute gouty arthritis seems to affect the first metatarsophalangeal joint. The condition occurs more often in men than in women. Walking is difficult or impossible, even the bed sheets become an irritant during the acute attack. Treatment of the acute gouty attack usually consists of oral colchicine 0.6 mg q h until symptoms subside or GI discomfort develops. Indomethacin has also been used to treat an acute gouty attack; 100 mg q 6 h for the first 24 h followed by 25 mg qid has proved to be effective. Other NSAIDs are also effective. Paragoric is often used to treat the side effects of colchicine therapy. Analgesics may be used for severe pain.

Prevention of future gouty attacks includes modification of life-style as well as drug therapy. Gradual weight reduction should be initiated if necessary and alcohol in any form should be avoided. Increased fluid intake is advised to enhance the excretion of uric acid. Uricosuric drugs encourage the excretion of uric acid as well. Two such drugs, probenecid and sulfinpyrazone, lower serum uric acid levels and help prevent the formation of tophi. They act by blocking the renal tubular resorption of urate. The recommended dosage for probenecid is 0.5 gm bid or tid; for sulfinpyrazone, it is 100 mg tid. Allopurinol, a xanthine oxidase inhibitor, decreases the formation of uric acid. Given at a dosage of 100 mg bid or tid along with a uricosuric agent, it is an effective means of preventing future attacks of gout.

Symptoms of gout may develop after prolonged use of thiazide diuretics. Alternative antihypertensive therapy should be considered if these episodes occur.

NEUROLOGIC FOOT DISORDERS

Tarsal tunnel syndrome denotes compression of the posterior tibial nerve at the ankle and causes severe pain leading to disability and a reduction in ambulation. Presenting symptoms include burning and discomfort, which may be severe and usually radiate to the toes. Pain increases upon ambulation and is relieved by rest. The condition may be diagnosed by Tinel's sign, in which a tapping of the nerve at the site of compression produces distal tingling.

Treatment consists of local injections of a corticosteroid (eg, dexamethasone or triamcinolone acetonide) in combination with a local anesthetic. Strapping to alleviate pressure to the nerve should be used with injection therapy. When conservative measures are ineffective, surgical decompression of the nerve should be considered.

Trauma of the dorsal cutaneous nerves: Pain to the dorsolateral aspect of the foot is usually attributable to pathologic conditions of the intermediate dorsal cutaneous nerve, while similar symptoms involving the dorsomedial aspect of the foot may be caused by conditions of the medial dorsal cutaneous nerve. The latter nerve is often injured in elderly patients who have undergone bunion surgery because of improper surgical technic or entrapment by fibrosis during healing. Again, treatment consists of local corticosteroid injections in conjunction with accommodative strapping or custom-made shoes. Pressure should be avoided at the site of the nerve injury. When severe fibrosis or entrapment of a nerve is suspected, surgical intervention should be contemplated.

§3. ORGAN SYSTEMS: METABOLIC AND ENDOCRINE DISORDERS

68. INTRODUCTION

David H. Solomon

The endocrine and metabolic control systems of the body offer many of the greatest opportunities for preventing the disabilities associated with aging. Thyroid disease is common, often undiagnosed, and easily treated; early detection prevents unnecessary disability. Diabetes mellitus is extremely common, and normalization of blood glucose levels may minimize the devastating vascular and neurologic complications of that disease. Hyperparathyroidism, like hyper- and hypothyroidism, is a clinical masquerader. Early diagnosis by screening for hypercalcemia leads to proper treatment and consequent prevention of disability.

Perhaps most dramatic is the impact of menopause, a "normal" state of ovarian hormone deficiency that affects 100% of older women, with disabling consequences in many. The picture can be radically changed by estrogen replacement therapy. Hypogonadism in older men has been less thoroughly studied, but clearly, much of male sexual disability can be improved by proper diagnosis and treatment. Furthermore, growing knowledge of the importance of disorders of lipoprotein metabolism (particularly cholesterol) has led to improved prevention and treatment, contributing to a reduction in atherosclerosis and its consequences.

Thus, attention to the endocrine and metabolic systems in older persons is not only warranted but mandatory. With aging, many aspects of the endocrine system change but not in a uniform direction. Some endocrine organs and axes become hypoactive, either from diseases of high prevalence or physiologic down-regulation; some change little or not at all; and a few become hyperactive. These diverse and at times striking changes result variously from alterations in hormonal production and secretion rates, metabolic clearance rates, and tissue responsiveness or sensitivity (based on changes in hormone receptors or postreceptor mechanisms). Thus, analysis of the observed changes may be extremely complex.

Hormone levels in serum reflect the sum of all changes. Average age-related changes in serum concentrations of hormones are summarized in TABLES 68–1, 68–2, and 68–3. Many of the changes are closely interrelated, 1 often serving as a compensatory response for another. For example, pituitary gonadotropins rise as gonadal hormones decline. On the other hand, age-associated increases in serum vasopressin and norepinephrine levels, probably result from primary overproduction of vasopressin by the hypothalamo-neurohypophysial system and compensatory hypersecretion of norepinephrine in response to decreased numbers and responsiveness of β-adrenergic receptors in target tissues.

The metabolic systems of the body are also interrelated. Although some steps are still unclear, changes in carbohydrate and lipoprotein metabolism are highly correlated. Further, carbohydrate metabolism af-

TABLE 68–1. SERUM LEVELS OF VARIOUS HORMONES IN
ADVANCED AGE

High
Norepinephrine
Antidiuretic hormone (vasopressin)
Insulin

Normal
Epinephrine
Cortisol
Thyroxine
Growth hormone
Thyrotropin (TSH)*

Low
Triiodothyronine
Adrenocorticotropic hormone (ACTH)* *
Somatomedin C

* TSH may be high, normal, or slightly low but usually falls within the normal range.
* * ACTH is likely to be slightly lower than in youth but generally falls within the
normal range.

TABLE 68–2. SERUM LEVELS OF STEROIDS AND RELATED
HORMONES IN ELDERLY WOMEN

High
Ovarian testosterone*
Follicle-stimulating hormone
Luteinizing hormone

Normal
Total testosterone

Low
Estrone
Estradiol
Progesterone
Androsterone
Dehydroepiandrosterone
Dehydroepiandrosterone sulfate

* May be normal or high.

fects and is affected by changes in fluid and electrolyte balance, acid-base balance, and total energy balance (ie, weight gain or loss). Protein-calorie nutritional status has pervasive effects on metabolic regulatory systems.

Some important mysteries remain in the area of endocrine-metabolic interactions. For example, estrogenic hormone levels profoundly alter li-

TABLE 68–3. SERUM LEVELS OF STEROIDS AND RELATED
HORMONES IN ELDERLY MEN

High
  Dihydrotestosterone (DHT)*
  Free estrone
  Free estradiol
  Follicle-stimulating hormone
  Luteinizing hormone

Low
  Testosterone
  Free testosterone
  Androsterone
  Androstenedione
  Dehydroepiandrosterone
  Dehydroepiandrosterone sulfate

* DHT is high in men with benign prostatic hypertrophy (BPH) but tends to be normal in elderly men without BPH.

poprotein and cholesterol metabolism and may affect the rate of athero-genesis. This set of interrelationships is under study. Similarly, the effects of male hypogonadism in the elderly are unknown, except for decreased sexual function. Another example is uncertainty regarding the pathogenetic importance of the "normal" impairment in glucose tolerance associated with aging.

69. THE NORMAL AND DISEASED THYROID GLAND

David H. Solomon

The thyroid gland produces thyroxine (T_4) and triiodothyronine (T_3), hormones that are essential for life and health. The gland's function changes with normal aging. More important, the thyroid gland may be affected by 2 major conditions that increase in incidence with age (hypothyroidism and nodule formation) and 1 that remains constant with age (hyperthyroidism).

THYROID FUNCTION IN NORMAL AGING

With advancing age, the thyroid gland undergoes moderate atrophy and develops nonspecific histopathologic abnormalities—fibrosis, increasing numbers of colloid nodules, and some degree of lymphocytic infiltration. Correspondingly, its production of T_4 declines nearly 50%

between young adulthood and advanced old age. However, this decline is generally thought to be a physiologic compensation for a decreased rate of tissue utilization of the hormone rather than a manifestation of primary thyroid failure. The crucial evidence for this conclusion is that serum T_4 levels remain unchanged with advancing age; if thyroid dysfunction were the major cause for decreased hormone production, serum T_4 would fall.

The decrease in utilization rate for T_4 correlates well with age-related decline in lean body mass, suggesting that the primary event is shrinkage with age of metabolically active, protein-rich tissues (muscle, skin, bone, and viscera). This may lead to reduced utilization and catabolism of thyroid hormones and, sequentially, to a subtle rise in thyroid hormone levels, a resultant decrease in thyrotropin **(TSH)** output, a decrease in thyroidal T_3 and T_4 output, and a return of serum T_4 levels to normal. However, when stimulated by increased TSH, the nondiseased, aged thyroid gland can increase its hormone production normally.

Serum levels of assayed thyroid hormones change very little with age. Serum T_4, free T_4 index **(FT$_4$I)** and free T_4 **(FT$_4$)** remain unchanged. Serum T_3, free T_3 index **(FT$_3$I)** and free T_3 **(FT$_3$)** fall slightly with normal aging. In contrast to the case with T_4, the metabolic clearance rate of T_3 falls little or not at all with aging. Thus, with a decreased amount of T_4 being metabolized to T_3 daily and an unchanged clearance of T_3, serum T_3 levels must fall. Combining the results of many studies, the best estimate is a 10 to 15% decrease. Normal ranges for persons $\geq$ 70 yr of age should be adjusted accordingly.

Since acute and chronic illnesses are more common in older persons, a low serum T_3 level or the whole **euthyroid sick syndrome (ESS)** is common. Features and variants of ESS are (1) low serum T_3; (2) high serum reverse T_3; (3) low serum T_4 and FT$_4$I; (4) euthyroid hyperthyroxinemia (high serum T_4, FT$_4$I, and FT$_4$); (5) normal to low FT$_4$ in the most seriously ill; and (6) blunted TSH response to thyrotropin-releasing hormone **(TRH)**.

The average serum TSH rises in population-wide studies, a fact that appears to directly contradict the above explanation for the constancy of serum T_4. However, good evidence suggests that the rise in TSH reflects the high prevalence of Hashimoto's thyroiditis in the older population. In 1 study, for example, the rise in mean serum TSH was completely eliminated by excluding persons with positive titers for antimicrosomal antibody.

THYROID DISEASE IN OLDER PERSONS

The 3 most important conditions of the thyroid are hypothyroidism, hyperthyroidism, and nodules. The incidence of **hypothyroidism** is 2 to 5% in those > 65 yr and rises with age; it is much higher in women than in men at all ages and is always higher in geriatric inpatients (hospital or nursing home) than in community-dwelling older persons. The incidence and prevalence of **hyperthyroidism** remain relatively constant with age, but the etiologic spectrum shifts somewhat from Graves' disease toward multinodular and uninodular toxic goiter. The prevalence of hyperthyroidism averages about 0.4%, and it also is higher in women and inpatients. The prevalence of **thyroid nodules** increases with age. One study showed that by 80 yr, 9% of women and 1.5% of men living in the community had 1 or more palpable thyroid nodules.

HYPOTHYROIDISM

The characteristic effects of thyroid hormone deficiency.

Etiology

The dominant causes of irreversible thyroid failure in adults are chronic autoimmune thyroiditis, iatrogenic hypothyroidism due to irradiation or surgical removal of the gland, and idiopathic hypothyroidism. Infrequent causes are pituitary or hypothalamic lesions with TSH deficiency, iodine-induced hypothyroidism, or ingested antithyroid drugs or natural substances in the diet, eg, goitrin in rutabagas, thiocyanate in cabbage, aminotriazole in cranberries. Transient hypothyroidism may occur after thyroid surgery or treatment with radioactive iodine (^{131}I), or during episodes of subacute thyroiditis. Chronic autoimmune thyroiditis may be divided into its milder form, lymphocytic thyroiditis, or its more full-blown expression, Hashimoto's disease.

The treatment of hyperthyroidism and thyroid cancer account for most cases of iatrogenic hypothyroidism. Irradiation with ^{131}I is the most frequent treatment for Graves' disease or a solitary hyperfunctioning adenoma. Over 50% of patients with Graves' disease who receive therapeutic doses of ^{131}I ultimately develop hypothyroidism. On the other hand, hyperthyroidism associated with nodular goiter rarely leads to hypothyroidism when treated with ^{131}I.

Thyroidectomy is the treatment of choice for some cases of hyperthyroidism (certain Graves' disease patients and most patients with multinodular goiter) and all suspected or confirmed cases of cancer. Hypothyroidism is invariably the outcome of thyroid cancer, because the goal of therapy is complete ablation of the gland; this is usually accomplished by radical subtotal thyroidectomy followed by large doses of ^{131}I.

Idiopathic hypothyroidism in adults is generally thought to be the result of undiagnosed chronic autoimmune thyroiditis. Supporting this theory, antithyroid antibodies are sometimes detected in the serum, even though antibodies tend to disappear in known chronic thyroiditis when the gland reaches an advanced stage of atrophy. Direct cytologic proof of this line of reasoning is lacking, since the biopsy or aspiration of an atrophic, nonpalpable gland is unwarranted.

Pathogenesis and Pathophysiology

Hashimoto's disease is an *autoimmune inflammatory process of the thyroid gland.* Thyroid-directed antibodies of 4 types are found in the serum of patients with the disease, but the mediator of the inflammatory and cytotoxic lesion remains unknown. Inhibitory antibodies that bind to the TSH receptors, displacing TSH from that site, have been identified, and may account for some of the decline in thyroid function. Recently, antimicrosomal antibody was shown to be targeted to thyroid peroxidase as its antigen; this may explain inefficient synthesis of thyroid hormone in this circumstance. As the disorder progresses, destruction of thyroid follicles is seen histologically, along with florid lymphocytic infiltration and eosinophilic changes in the cytoplasm of thyroid epithelial cells. In some cases, fibrosis supervenes and the gland ultimately becomes devoid of thyroid epithelium.

Hypothyroidism after ^{131}I therapy is difficult to predict because its pathogenesis is not fully understood. In Graves' disease, pathologic changes associated with Hashimoto's disease are often seen concurrently, but the presence of lymphocytic infiltration prior to ^{131}I therapy is not a good predictor of the subsequent development of hypothyroidism. Many cases of hypothyroidism appear during the first year after ^{131}I therapy, but new cases continue to appear at a rate of 2 to 5%/yr over the next 15 or 20 yr. This linear relationship to time suggests that irradiation produces a delayed effect, with the length of the delay varying widely. This is compatible with accepted principles of radiation biology. Early hypothyroidism appears to be dose related and attributable to acute radiation thyroiditis, whereas lower doses appear to cause failure of DNA replication, so that thyroid cell replacement ceases and eventually hypothyroidism supervenes.

On the other hand, the presence of Hashimoto's thyroiditis preoperatively predicts a higher incidence of hypothyroidism after subtotal thyroidectomy for Graves' disease. Naturally, the size of the remnant left by the surgeon and the integrity of its blood supply also determine the likelihood of hypothyroidism.

The frequency of serum antithyroid antibodies and of clinical or histologic evidence of Hashimoto's disease rises sharply with advancing age, especially in women. Thus, the likelihood of developing hypothyroidism, either spontaneously or after subtotal thyroidectomy, increases in the elderly. Furthermore, DNA in older people is more susceptible to radiation-induced damage and less well repaired, so hypothyroidism following treatment with ^{131}I also increases with age.

Symptoms and Signs

Hypothyroidism in the elderly is 1 of the great masqueraders. The clinical presentation is usually obscure. Most commonly, the symptoms are attributed by the unsuspecting to aging—fatigue, loss of initiative, depression, myalgia, constipation, and dry skin. Less than $^1/_3$ of elderly patients with hypothyroidism present with the classic complex of symptoms and signs. Most develop nonspecific syndromes common in the frail elderly—mental confusion, anorexia, weight loss, falling, incontinence, and decreased mobility, plus the above. Musculoskeletal symptoms, including arthralgias, are frequent but arthritis is rare. Muscular aches and weakness, often mimicking polymalgia rheumatica or polymyositis, and an elevated CK in hypothyroidism make the differential diagnosis even more difficult.

The findings on physical examination are similarly difficult to interpret. Puffiness around the eyes and the myxedematous facies are difficult to distinguish from normal facial changes associated with aging. Even the most reliable sign, prolonged relaxation time following muscular contraction, may be unavailable because of decreased amplitude or absence of normal reflexes. Noninflammatory effusions may be present in joints and pleural, pericardial, and peritoneal cavities, adding to the diagnostic confusion.

Laboratory Findings

The diagnosis of hypothyroidism is based on precise and reliable radioimmunoassays or immunoradiometric assays of TSH and T_4 serum levels. The serum T_3 level is of little value, since $1/3$ of patients with hypothyroidism have serum T_3 concentrations within the normal range. An elevated serum TSH is extremely sensitive (approximately 0.99) for the diagnosis of hypothyroidism, while a subnormal serum T_4 is highly specific. A subnormal FT_4I (**FT₄I** [serum T_4 multiplied by an index of protein-binding, such as a T_3 resin uptake]) is even more sensitive and specific, because it corrects for abnormalities in the thyroxine-binding proteins. An FT_4I should be obtained in any patient suspected of having hypothyroidism, although a serum TSH > 15 $\mu U/mL$ is probably diagnostic on its own. Once thyroid-hormone binding has been estimated, it remains constant thereafter (unless estrogenic medication is started or discontinued), so the less expensive serum T_4 may be used in all follow-up tests.

Many older patients have moderately elevated serum TSH (from the upper limit of normal, 4 or 5 $\mu U/mL$, to about 15 $\mu U/mL$) but serum T_4 remains within normal range. This condition is often termed "subclinical hypothyroidism." Better descriptors are **compensated hypothyroidism** or **mild hypothyroidism.** The latter term is favored, because if serum T_4 is in the lower $1/3$ of the normal range in the presence of an elevated serum TSH, it is quite likely that T_4 is actually subnormal for the patient.

The concept of compensated hypothyroidism depends on the assumption that the serum T_4 level is normal for that patient and is being kept normal in the presence of thyroid disease by the effect of a moderate excess of TSH. The clinical picture in patients with compensated or mild hypothyroidism is highly variable. Some have mild symptoms that disappear with thyroid hormone replacement, so the term "subclinical" is unsatisfactory. Other patients are truly asymptomatic.

Antimicrosomal antibody assay is occasionally useful in the diagnosis of hypothyroidism, because it confirms the presence or absence of Hashimoto's thyroiditis. Serum cholesterol and CK are elevated in hypothyroidism, but this information is rarely useful diagnostically except in reverse; ie, diagnosing hypothyroidism explains the abnormal cholesterol and CK values.

Similarly, anemia, hyponatremia, hypoglycemia, and hypercapnia all can be explained by hypothyroidism. The anemia is usually mild, with Hb no lower than 9 gm/dL. Typically, it has the characteristics of the anemia of chronic disease but may be mildly macrocytic. Because auto-immune diseases tend to coexist, frank pernicious anemia occurs in perhaps 5% of patients with hypothyroidism. Older persons have more circulating antidiuretic hormone (vasopressin) than younger persons and, accordingly, a greater susceptibility to hyponatremia. Hypothyroidism accentuates this tendency to excessive water retention without proportionate Na retention. Hypoglycemia and hypercapnea, which are manifestations of advanced thyroid deficiency, are frequent findings in myxedema coma.

A key problem in older people is distinguishing hypothyroidism from severe cases of the euthyroid sick syndrome **(ESS)**, or detecting hypothyroidism superimposed upon ESS. Since serum T_3 has little bearing on the diagnosis of hypothyroidism, the low T_3 aspect of ESS should pose little problem. The difficulty arises primarily in the critically ill patient who has the **low T_4 syndrome.** FT_4I, as well as total T_4, is subnormal in ESS, because the circulating inhibitor of protein binding also inhibits the binding of thyroid hormones to the inanimate sites such as resin or charcoal used in the T_3 uptake assay.

Therefore, the keys to the diagnosis of hypothyroidism during ESS are serum TSH and serum FT_4 by equilibrium dialysis. Serum TSH is normal to slightly subnormal in ESS but never elevated. When hypothyroidism is superimposed on ESS, serum TSH rises, although slightly less vigorously than in the person who is not severely ill. Equilibrium dialysis of T_4 shows the full effect of the circulating inhibitor of protein binding; thus, the serum FT_4 is generally normal in ESS (ie, low total T_4 multiplied by high dialyzable fraction of T_4, yielding a normal serum FT_4). A low serum FT_4 in the presence of elevated TSH establishes the diagnosis of primary hypothyroidism in the patient with severe nonthyroid illness, while a low serum FT_4 with subnormal TSH is compatible with ESS alone but would also raise the question of pituitarigenic hypothyroidism.

Diagnosis

The diagnosis of hypothyroidism requires a high index of suspicion and reliable laboratory tests appropriately selected and interpreted (see above). The differential diagnosis includes normal aging, ESS, depression, the various causes of dementia, idiopathic obesity, Cushing's syndrome, myopathies, neuropathies, various arthritides, fibrositis, myositis, Parkinson's disease, various colonic conditions that cause constipation or ileus, pericarditis, heart failure, cirrhosis, renal disease, and various dermal conditions.

The disorder is so frequently present in the elderly, the diagnosis so difficult to make on clinical grounds, and so easy when based on laboratory data that the physician should be quick to order blood tests. A recommended policy is that serum FT₄I and TSH be measured in any person > 65 yr of age who presents for a diagnostic evaluation or a comprehensive geriatric assessment, whether inpatient or outpatient. This policy also applies to any person being admitted to a board-and-care residence or a nursing home.

Thus, this policy calls for extensive diagnostic case finding of an easily treatable condition. Whereas this policy is not controversial, *population-wide screening* in the elderly is. Theoretically, such screening would be analogous to the highly successful screening programs for neonatal hypothyroidism. All studies to date, however, have concluded that the prevalence of undiagnosed hypothyroidism, even though greater in persons > 65 yr of age compared with younger persons, is still too low to make this process cost-effective, since the diagnosis is likely to be made through the patient-care system before great harm is done. In the latter respect, the situation differs from that involving the newborn.

Treatment

The treatment of hypothyroidism is straightforward. The average replacement dose is 0.075 to 0.1 mg/day of sodium-L-thyroxine in patients ≥ 65 yr of age, in contrast to 0.125 to 0.15 mg/day in younger patients.

Unless the patient is in impending or actual myxedema coma, replacement therapy should be conducted cautiously, starting with a dose of 0.0125 to 0.025 mg/day and increasing at intervals of ≥ 2 wk. Each step-up in dosage should be by no more than 0.025 mg/day.

The most serious hazard of this phase of therapy is MI. Patients should be monitored closely for angina, dyspnea, arrhythmias, or unusual weakness, although serious cardiac complications of T₄ therapy are actually quite uncommon. By and large, T₄ therapy in proved hypothyroidism is among the safest and most effective treatments in medicine.

One or 2 mo after reaching a dose of 0.075 mg/day of sodium-L-thyroxine, serum TSH should be measured, always by the new generation of sensitive assays (s-TSH) capable of detecting < 0.1 μU/mL TSH. If s-TSH is still above normal, the dose may be increased to 0.1 mg/day. If s-TSH is below normal (usually cited as < 0.4 μU/mL), the dose should be lowered.

Serum T₃ and T₄ measurements may add reassurance but are usually unnecessary, since continued hypo- and hyperthyroidism can be detected reliably by serum TSH measurements alone. The only major qualification to this statement is that the serum TSH sometimes falls slowly; thus, if TSH is still high 1 to 2 mo after reaching a dosage of 0.1 mg/day of sodium-L-thyroxine in a geriatric patient, the dosage should be left the same for another 2 mo. If TSH is still elevated at that time, the dose should be raised to 0.125 mg/day.

HYPERTHYROIDISM

Hyperthyroidism is *the condition in which the thyroid gland delivers a supranormal amount of its hormones to the blood.* **Thyrotoxicosis,** on the other hand, is *the state of the body when it is exposed to an excess of thyroid hormones from any source.*

Etiology

Thyrotoxicosis is usually caused by hyperthyroidism but occasionally by ingestion of excessive amounts of pharmaceutical thyroid hormone and rarely by an extrathyroidal source, such as an ovarian struma. The causes of hyperthyroidism are Graves' disease, single hyperfunctioning adenoma, multinodular goiter, some forms of subacute and chronic thyroiditis, and rarely, a primary TSH-producing pituitary lesion. Although hyperthyroidism may appear to be uncommon in older persons, in fact, the prevalence changes little with age, when shrinkage of the population at risk (ie, alive) is considered. Graves' disease becomes somewhat less common, while hyperthyroidism associated with multinodular goiter increases in frequency.

Pathogenesis and Pathophysiology

The common denominator in hyperthyroidism is a loss of normal physiologic regulation of the output of thyroid hormones. **In Graves' disease,** an autoimmune disorder leads to the production of an antibody to the TSH receptor on thyroid follicular cells. This antibody has the surprising property of behaving like TSH itself, ie, of activating the adenylate cyclase system, thereby stimulating the thyroid cell.

In hyperthyroidism associated with adenomas (single or multiple), the area of the thyroid gland responsible is autonomous, ie, it produces and secretes too much thyroid hormone even though serum TSH is fully suppressed. The cause of this autonomy is unknown; it is clearly not due to a thyroid-stimulating antibody and is presumably intrinsic to the cells making up certain adenomas.

In subacute thyroiditis, either the granulomatous or lymphocytic type, damaged follicles leak thyroglobulin, T_3, and T_4 into the circulation. In some cases, the resultant level of hormones in the blood is sufficient to cause thyrotoxicosis. In certain cases of **Hashimoto's thyroiditis,** there may be a similar leakage, causing thyrotoxicosis, usually of short duration.

In all of these conditions characterized by excess thyroid hormone release independent of TSH control, the pituitary responds normally to the excess by shutting down its production of TSH. Thus, the hypothalamo-pituitary sector of the axis is normal; the dysregulation occurs in the immune system or in the thyroid gland itself.

A TSH-secreting adenoma of the pituitary rarely is the cause of hyperthyroidism, and even more rare is a **hypothalamic disorder** in which thyrotropin-releasing hormone **(TRH)** is overproduced, leading sequentially to hypersecretion of TSH and thyroid hormones.

Regardless of the cause of thyrotoxicosis, the final common path is the presence of supranormal levels of thyroid hormones in T_3-responsive tissues. Overproduction of both T_3 and T_4 characterizes the various types of hyperthyroidism, T_3 generally to a greater extent that T_4. The ultimate in this trend is so-called T_3 thyrotoxicosis, in which serum T_4 is normal despite clinical evidence of hyperthyroidism. T_3 thyrotoxicosis accounts for about 5% of thyrotoxicosis at all ages.

In hyperthyroidism, extrathyroidal tissues convert the excess of secreted T_4 to an excess of T_3, in addition to the T_3 secreted by the thyroid. Thus, a supraphysiologic concentration of T_3 arrives at target tissues and is transported into the nucleus, where it binds to a receptor. The hormone-receptor complex then binds to the promotor region of T_3-responsive genes, leading to production of enzymes and other proteins that mediate the characteristic actions of T_3. All of this occurs excessively in hyperthyroidism.

The clinical picture differs in the elderly (see below), and a precise explanation for this is not possible. The illness is probably the same (ie, overproduction of thyroid hormones), but age and concomitant disease may change the manifestations by altering the response of various organs and tissues. For example, response to catecholamines is decreased in older persons and animals, possibly because of a decreased number of or affinity for catecholamine receptors. Since catecholamines are synergistic with T_3 in producing many of the typical symptoms and signs of thyrotoxicosis, reduced responsiveness to catecholamines could explain the frequent atypicality. Another possible factor is aging of heart muscle; the aged heart may be more prone to react unfavorably to thyroid hormones.

Symptoms and Signs

Hyperthyroidism in the elderly is even more of a masquerader than hypothyroidism. Older patients exhibit fewer of the classic symptoms of thyrotoxicosis than younger patients; only about 25% of persons $\geq$ 65 yr of age present with the typical complex of symptoms and signs. In 1 recent study of hyperthyroid patients, advanced age was associated with significant decreases in the percent of patients complaining of increased perspiration, heat intolerance, increased appetite, irritability, and thyroid enlargement. Average heart rate and thyroid size also decreased with age.

However, some symptoms and signs were highly sensitive and specific for distinguishing hyperthyroidism from euthyroidism in the 7th and 8th decades of life. While the overall number of typical hyperthyroid symptoms was definitely lower in older patients with hyperthyroidism, thyroid enlargement, weight loss, pulse rate $\geq$ 90, and fatigue had sensitivities > 0.70; an increased number of bowel movements, lid lag, increased appetite, fine tremor, heat intolerance, and increased sweating had specificities $\geq$ 0.98. Weight loss and atrial fibrillation were significantly more common in the 7th and 8th decades.

Common atypical presentations in the elderly may be classified roughly into cardiovascular, GI, neuropsychiatric, or neuromuscular types, although aspects of each may coexist in the same patient. TABLE 69–1 summarizes clinical features of thyrotoxicosis that are likely to be different in older patients. **Cardiovascular features** are atrial arrhythmias, heart failure, and angina; these may dominate the clinical picture to the exclusion of the usual features of thyrotoxicosis. Since cardiac disease is so common in the elderly, the possibility of underlying hyperthyroidism may be unsuspected.

TABLE 69–1. CLINICAL FEATURES OF THYROTOXICOSIS IN THE ELDERLY

Thyroid gland smaller	Less diarrhea
Multinodular goiter	More constipation
Lower incidence of Graves' disease	Less excitability
Less tachycardia	Less hyperkinesis
More arrhythmias	More apathy
More angina	More depression
More heart failure	More arthralgias
Less hyperphagia	More muscular weakness
More anorexia	More hepatomegaly
More weight loss	

The GI picture is that of "failure to thrive." Anorexia, dyspepsia, abdominal distress, rapid weight loss, exhaustion, and bowel disturbances (diarrhea, constipation, or an alternation of both) are the symptoms. GI malignancy is almost always at the top of the differential diagnostic list; hyperthyroidism may not be on it at all.

The neuropsychiatric type is most often a picture of depression. Lahey called this condition "apathetic thyroidism," and it is characterized by apathy, listlessness, anorexia, marked weight loss, weakness, and mental confusion. It may be classified primarily as depression, often meeting the criteria of the *Diagnostic and Statistical Manual of Mental Disorders,* Third Edition, revised **(DSM III-R)** for that diagnosis. Finally, **the neuromuscular type of presentation** is dominated by symptoms and signs of proximal and some distal myopathy with severe weakness and usually some of the wasting features described above.

Laboratory Findings and Diagnosis

The crux of diagnosis in young and old persons is the measurement of serum levels of thyroid hormones and TSH by a sensitive assay method, now referred to as an s-TSH assay. The best single test is the measurement of s-TSH. Its sensitivity and specificity are both ≥ 0.98. A subnormal value strongly suggests the diagnosis of thyrotoxicosis, and an undetectable level (usually $< 0.05 \ \mu U/mL$) is almost pathognomonic. Serum thyroid hormone levels may be measured just to confirm the diagnosis or, in the infrequent case in which the serum s-TSH concentration is normal but clinical suspicion persists, that the patient is not euthyroid.

Many physicians still order measurement of serum T_3 and T_4 (or FT_3I and FT_4I) out of long-established habits, but this is probably wasteful. If ordered, it should be noted again that T_3 is more sensitive than T_4 for the diagnosis of thyrotoxicosis because it tends to rise earlier and more sharply.

All geriatric patients presenting with chronic symptoms should be tested for hyperthyroidism, as is the case with hypothyroidism. Case-finding for both diagnoses is done most cost-effectively with a sensitive TSH assay alone, even though this costs more than an FT_4 assay. However, screening of entire populations of persons over a certain age is not justified, because too few cases are detected.

While laboratory testing is the sine qua non of diagnosis of hyperthyroidism in the elderly, it is by no means a panacea. Patients who are starved or very ill as a result of thyrotoxicosis or concomitant disease invariably show a lower serum T_3 concentration than would be expected from the level of thyroid activity, and it may fall into the normal range. With more serious illness, the T_4 and FT_4I may also decline into the normal range. A still-elevated FT_4 by equilibrium dialysis, an above-normal radioiodine uptake test, or an undetectable serum s-TSH usually provides the correct diagnosis.

More confusion is added by the transient occurrence of **euthyroid hyperthyroxinemia** in some patients with acute systemic illness (eg, pneumonia) and in many patients with acute psychiatric illnesses. This condition can be fairly reliably differentiated from hyperthyroidism by the serum s-TSH, but most reliably by repeating thyroid function tests after 2 wk. By that time, serum FT_4I has generally returned to normal.

In all varieties of the ESS, a single measurement of serum s-TSH has replaced the more tedious and expensive TRH response test, although the latter still may be useful when findings are particularly puzzling. However, advanced age, depression, or ESS may blunt the TRH response test or cause a subnormal s-TSH. The key distinction is that absolute nonresponse to TRH or an undetectable basal s-TSH is extremely rare in these conditions, whereas it is the rule in thyrotoxicosis.

Treatment

The treatment of choice for most elderly patients with hyperthyroidism due to **Graves' disease** or a **single autonomous nodule** is ^{131}I. Age-related risks of surgery and special difficulties in antithyroids drug therapy combine to favor radioiodine. Antithyroid drugs are effective in elderly patients with Graves' disease if compliance is high, but they are slow to work and almost never lead to permanent remission in uninodular toxic goiters.

In **multinodular toxic goiter,** response to ^{131}I therapy is often delayed and incomplete. Many doses of ^{131}I may be required, leaving the patient still hyperthyroid many months after the diagnosis has been made. Thus, surgery may be preferred, at least in low-risk patients.

Administration of antithyroid drugs in older persons is the same as in younger individuals. **Propylthiouracil (PTU)** is started at a dosage of 100 to 150 mg orally q 8 h and continued at that dosage until serum hormone levels reach the normal range. The dosage is then lowered sequentially, with appropriate monitoring of clinical symptoms and signs and of serum hormone levels approximately q 2 mo. If response is inadequate, PTU dosage may be increased to 300 mg q 8 h.

Methimazole is longer acting than PTU and therefore can be given as a single daily dose; the initial dose is 30 to 45 mg/day. This needs to be adjusted upward or downward q 1 or 2 mo, depending on the response. With either methimazole or PTU, if the patient's course is erratic (eg, slipping quickly into hypothyroidism after small increases in dose), the simplest, surest solution is to add a small dose of **sodium-L-thyroxine,** usually 0.05 mg/day.

Giving antithyroid drugs for 2 or 3 mo before administering a therapeutic dose of ^{131}I restores a euthyroid condition rapidly, at least in Graves' disease. It also depletes the thyroid gland of its store of hormone, thereby minimizing the possibility of a post-^{131}I exacerbation of thyrotoxicosis due to dumping of stored hormone into the blood during the acute radiation thyroiditis.

In thyrotoxic patients with atrial fibrillation, cardioversion should not be attempted until the patient is euthyroid. Approximately $^2/_3$ revert spontaneously in the first 4 mo after euthyroidism is reestablished. Psychiatric symptoms in elderly thyrotoxic patients should be treated on a prn basis; they usually clear completely when the patient has become euthyroid.

Propranolol or other **β-adrenoceptor blockers** are useful in the symptomatic management of thyrotoxicosis, unless contraindicated by the presence of heart failure. One of this class of drugs may be given along with an antithyroid drug before treatment with ^{131}I or in preparation for surgery. β-Adrenoceptor blockers do not affect thyroid hormone secretion rates. Their benefit is due to a blunting of the interaction of thyroid hormones with catecholamines. In high doses (eg, propranolol 320 mg/day), the extrathyroidal conversion of T_4 to T_3 is inhibited as well. Dosage must be individualized but 40 mg tid would be typical.

Oragrafin, a now rarely used cholecystographic contrast material, is an extremely potent inhibitor of the enzyme that converts T_4 to T_3 in extrathyroidal tissues (and probably in the thyroid gland as well). Although not approved by the FDA for treatment of thyrotoxicosis, it is extremely effective, lowering the serum T_3 into the normal range within 48 to 72 h. It is quite useful in thyroid storm or pre-storm and in patients with serious complications of thyrotoxicosis, such as heart failure.

THYROID NODULES

Although death due to thyroid cancer is exceedingly rare (1100/yr in the USA, 4/yr/10^6 population, 0.24% of all cancer deaths, and 0.05% of all deaths), the thyroid nodule is a topic of great concern. Most nodules are either altogether benign or, even if interpreted as carcinoma histologically, behave in a benign manner. The 5-yr survival of all patients with thyroid cancers is 93%, compared with average noncancer survival of the age-adjusted population. Nodules tend somewhat more toward malignancy and invasiveness in the elderly, but the majority are papillary or papillofollicular, with an excellent prognosis. Most of the 7% deficit in survival can be accounted for by cases of anaplastic carcinoma and lymphoma, which often present in ways other than the asymptomatic thyroid nodule. While the mortality of patients with thyroid nodules is extremely low, the hypothesis that this is because of an aggressive medical approach to diagnosis and surgical resection cannot be excluded; thus, this practice must continue.

Symptoms, Signs, and Diagnosis

Evaluation of thyroid nodules differs little by patient age group. A nodule may be merely an enlarged lobe, a lobule in a diffuse goiter, or a pyramidal lobe. Nodules may also be regenerating areas after subtotal resection, localized subacute or chronic thyroiditis, cysts, or colloid accumulations with hemorrhage and calcification. Concern for malignancy is lowest if the dominant nodule is not the only one, if both lobes are abnormal to palpation, or if the history describes sudden appearance with pain and tenderness, suggesting hemorrhage into a degenerating colloid adenoma. Radiation-induced cancer has occurred 35 yr after exposure, and it is not known if the latency can be even longer. Thus, a history of radiation to the face, neck or thorax is important, even in the elderly.

Physical examination may be helpful in assessing the significance of a thyroid nodule. Hashimoto's thyroiditis causes the gland to feel very firm with multiple small nodules. Colloid adenomas may be softer than normal, though their consistency is quite variable from patient to patient. Tenderness suggests hemorrhage into a colloid adenoma. Fluctuation suggests cystic changes, but these are more likely due to hemorrhage or necrosis of a colloid adenoma than to a simple, water-clear cyst.

Anaplastic carcinoma often presents with features suggestive of malignancy, including a large, growing thyroid mass, stony hardness, irregularity, immobility, fixation to other tissues, and hoarseness. It poses no diagnostic problem.

Evaluation of a thyroid nodule remains controversial, regardless of patient age. Thyroid function tests are normal except in the relatively uncommon hyperfunctioning nodule. In that case, serum T_4 and T_3 are high and serum s-TSH is subnormal. A **radionuclide scan** should then be done to prove that the nodule is "hot." If thyroid function tests are normal, a radionuclide scan has routinely been done in the past to exclude a functioning lesion, which is almost always benign, and an **ultrasonogram** has been done to identify simple cysts, also usually benign.

However, these expensive procedures have a low diagnostic yield because of their extremely poor specificity for malignancy.

In other words, most "cold" nodules identified by scintigram and solid nodules by sonogram are benign. Thus, **fine-needle aspiration** is now used as the first step in diagnosis; often, it is the only study needed. Elevated serum thyroglobulin is another test of interest, but specificity is low, whereas the finding of microcalcifications on x-ray, representing psammoma bodies, has low sensitivity but high specificity for the diagnosis of papillary adenocarcinoma.

Treatment

In deciding whether to treat nodules surgically, one must consider the higher risk of surgical morbidity in older persons. Cytologic evidence of malignancy or suspicion of malignancy based on the fine-needle aspiration calls for surgery unless concomitant medical conditions absolutely contraindicate it. If one has doubts about the cytologic impression (eg, the cytologist can diagnose a follicular neoplasm but usually cannot tell if it is benign or malignant), a better treatment choice is TSH-suppressive therapy with sodium-L-thyroxine and a repeat fine-needle aspiration in 6 to 12 mo.

If thyroid carcinoma is discovered at surgery, the next step is also controversial. Most physicians recommend a near-total thyroidectomy followed by ^{131}I therapy to ablate the remainder. After this, a total-body scan is performed to search for residual tissue capable of capturing [131]I. If results are positive, a therapeutic dose is administered.

However, there is no evidence that this plan is superior to near-total thyroidectomy alone, since its alleged advantage derives solely from nonrandomized studies with prominent selection bias. At all times, except when preparing for a scan or a therapeutic dose of ^{131}I, the patient should receive doses of sodium-L-thyroxine sufficient to lower serum TSH into the subnormal range but not enough to cause symptoms of hyperthyroidism.

---

70. CARBOHYDRATE METABOLISM AND DIABETES MELLITUS

Mayer B. Davidson

Diabetes mellitus is *a syndrome with interrelated metabolic and vascular components.* The **metabolic syndrome,** secondary to absent or markedly diminished insulin secretion or ineffective insulin action associated with a moderate decrease in insulin secretion, is characterized by hyperglycemia. The **vascular syndrome** consists of abnormalities in both small vessels (microangiopathy) and large vessels (macroangiopathy). Microangiopathy is expressed clinically as diabetic retinopathy and nephropathy. Macroangiopathic changes cause cerebral vascular accidents, MIs, and peripheral vascular disease. These large-vessel sequelae, especially peripheral vascular disease, appear earlier and are more severe in diabetic than in nondiabetic patients.

A variety of **peripheral nervous system abnormalities** also contribute to the clinical picture of diabetes; most are due to metabolic alterations, although a few may be secondary to vascular causes. Neuropathy seems fairly common in the older diabetic population.

Physiology

Glucose is produced by the liver through 2 separate pathways: (1) **Glycogenolysis** is the breakdown of glycogen and provides about 75% of the glucose after an overnight fast. (2) **Gluconeogenesis** is the synthesis of new glucose from noncarbohydrate precursors delivered to the liver. Glycogenolysis decreases considerably as the fasting period lengthens, and gluconeogenesis becomes the predominant pathway.

Glucose production is regulated by insulin, which decreases it; by glucagon, which increases it; and by autoregulation, a process by which the glucose concentration mediates hepatic glucose production independent of external hormonal stimuli. Insulin concentrations fall while glucagon levels rise during fasting.

However, after a meal, the increasing plasma concentration of glucose stimulates pancreatic β cells to release insulin, while glucagon production by the α cells of the islets is suppressed. The newly secreted insulin traverses the liver first, where about 50% is degraded on each passage. The remainder escapes into the general circulation, where its half-life ($t_{1/2}$) is about 5 min. Insulin binds to specific receptors on the cell surfaces of liver, muscle, and fat tissue, where it may exert an effect for several hours following its binding.

The metabolic result of these hormonal changes is that hepatic glucose production is markedly suppressed and the carbohydrate content of the meal is stored in the tissues. About 25% ends up in the liver and the remainder in peripheral tissues—mostly muscle.

In younger subjects without diabetes, plasma glucose levels usually rise 20 to 50 mg/dL immediately after a meal and return to baseline 2 h later. With aging, resistance to insulin gradually increases so that **postprandial plasma glucose (PPG)** concentrations rise about 5 mg/dL more with each decade. **Fasting plasma glucose (FPG)** concentrations change little during aging—1 to 2 mg/dL/decade.

Five mechanisms have been proposed to explain the effect of aging on carbohydrate metabolism: (1) poor diet, (2) physical inactivity, (3) decreased amounts of lean body mass in which to store the ingested carbohydrate, (4) impairment of insulin secretion, and (5) insulin antagonism. Although low carbohydrate intake and physical inactivity contribute to glucose intolerance, these factors do not entirely explain the age-associated deterioration of carbohydrate metabolism. Similarly, although lean body mass definitely diminishes with age, this tissue redistribution cannot explain age-related changes in carbohydrate metabolism. Diminished insulin secretion does not cause the glucose intolerance of aging. Almost all studies in which the insulin response to various stimuli (oral or IV glucose, amino acids, and tolbutamide) has been assessed in aging have shown normal or even increased insulin concentrations in older individuals.

In contrast, insulin antagonism has consistently been shown to be associated with aging, especially in persons $\geq$ 60 yr of age. The mechanism, however, remains unclear. Some studies have documented decreased insulin binding, while others have shown normal results. Decreased insulin binding may be due to down-regulation, in which the internalization of the insulin-receptor complex leaves a diminished number of unoccupied receptors on the cell surface. Studies showing normal or even some with decreased insulin binding also indicate evidence of a postbinding defect to explain the insulin antagonism associated with aging. However, there is little evidence to suggest the site or nature of the defect.

Classification and Pathogenesis

Diabetes mellitus can be divided into 3 general types. Patients with **Type 1, or insulin-dependent diabetes mellitus (IDDM),** are individuals with certain HLA antigens (DR3 and/or DR4) who produce autoantibodies against pancreatic β cells. These antibodies may be present for years before symptoms appear.

Type 1 patients develop ketosis, signifying an almost complete lack of effective insulin. Almost all of these patients have the symptoms and signs of uncontrolled diabetes at the onset of the disease. Without insulin therapy, they usually progress to diabetic coma and die. Although most of these patients are children and young adults (ie, < 30 yr of age), the older term **juvenile-onset diabetes** was not entirely accurate, since some lean adult and elderly patients also have ketosis-prone diabetes. Of the 5% of the total population with documented diabetes, only 10% have Type 1 diabetes mellitus. It has been estimated that about 10% of patients diagnosed after age 40 yr have islet-cell antibodies and eventually require insulin. Even patients in their 70s and 80s can present with diabetic ketoacidosis.

Type 2, or **non-insulin-dependent diabetes (NIDDM)** (older terms were **adult-onset, maturity-onset,** or **ketosis-resistant diabetes**), involves both *relative* insulin deficiency and resistance to insulin action. The combination of normal or high insulin concentrations and hyperglycemia implies the presence of insulin resistance. Both increased insulin levels and decreased insulin action have been documented in the 2 groups of individuals at increased risk; ie, the obese and the elderly. If pancreatic β-cell reserve is sufficient, normal plasma glucose levels are preserved at the expense of hyperinsulinemia. Impaired glucose tolerance appears, although hyperinsulinemia continues. This state may persist indefinitely, but in certain patients (presumed to have increased genetic susceptibility) with progressive β-cell failure, plasma glucose concentrations increase to values consistent with diabetes, and plasma insulin concentrations fall to normal or below.

Type 2 diabetes is distinguished by the absence of ketosis; this signifies the presence of at least some effective insulin. The term "non-insulin-dependent diabetes mellitus" may be confusing, since about 25% of such patients receive insulin. The difference is that *they do not need insulin to sustain life, as Type 1 diabetic patients do.* Obesity and older age are independent risk factors for Type 2 diabetes; 80 to 90% of Type 2 diabetics are obese, and the prevalence is estimated to double for every 20% increase over ideal body weight and for each decade after the 4th, regardless of weight. The prevalence in persons aged 65 to 74 yr is about 20%. An even higher percentage of people beyond the 9th decade may have diabetes mellitus.

The third kind of diabetes mellitus is now termed **other types** (the older term was **secondary diabetes**). This category includes patients with diseases that destroy the pancreas (eg, hemochromatosis, pancreatitis, or cystic fibrosis); those with certain endocrine diseases in which excess hormones interfere with insulin action (eg, growth hormone in acromegaly, cortisol in Cushing's syndrome, or catecholamines in pheochromocytoma); and those taking certain drugs that suppress insulin secretion (eg, phenytoin) or inhibit insulin action (eg, estrogens or glucocorticoids).

Symptoms and Signs

As carbohydrate metabolism deteriorates, postprandial glucose concentrations fail to return to the preprandial level until 3 to 5 h after eating, but no symptoms or signs occur as long as plasma glucose concentrations do not exceed the renal threshold. With a normal GFR, the plasma glucose concentration can reach 160 to 180 mg/dL before glucosuria occurs; it can be even higher in older people or in those with renal disease. When **glucosuria** occurs, urine formed after meals tests positive for glucose while urine formed before meals tests negative. Thus, patients are only intermittently glucosuric and usually are asymptomatic.

As the metabolic abnormality worsens, plasma glucose concentrations often remain above the renal threshold throughout the day. Such patients have persistent glucosuria but most often have no symptoms, except perhaps fatigue.

With further progression, regulation of hepatic glucose production diminishes, resulting in fasting hyperglycemia and plasma glucose levels exceeding the renal threshold for most or all of the 24-h period. This persistent glucosuria usually causes osmotic diuresis. Patients experience **polyuria**, which leads to dehydration and **polydipsia**. Since insulin is increasingly ineffective, the body is unable to use sufficient calories, leading to weight loss, even though patients have increased hunger with **polyphagia**. Such patients may also complain of **blurring of vision**, the result of alterations in the shape of the ocular lens due to osmotic changes induced by hyperglycemia. Patients may also show **increased susceptibility to certain infections**, especially fungal (usually candidiasis) and staphylococcal.

Ketosis and the presence of ketone bodies in the urine indicate that insulin effects are either absent or almost so. Ketone bodies are used for energy to a limited extent only by the peripheral tissues. Since they are weak acids, they are neutralized by the body's buffer systems. The remainder are excreted by the kidneys. When the buffer systems are exceeded, renal excretion soon becomes inadequate to rid the body of excess ketone bodies and they start to accumulate in the blood, causing **anorexia** and, occasionally, nausea. Further accumulation of the acidic ketone bodies depletes body bases, resulting in **ketoacidosis.** If the patient is not treated quickly and appropriately, coma and death follow. While most patients with diabetes never develop ketosis and a few do so over a period of years, most ketosis-prone diabetics probably progress from normal metabolism to ketoacidosis in a matter of weeks; almost all have symptoms and signs of uncontrolled diabetes at the time of diagnosis.

If hyperglycemia is unrecognized in patients who do not develop ketosis, especially in association with another medical stress (eg, urosepsis), **hyperosmolar, nonketotic syndrome (HNKS)** or **coma** may be the first indication of diabetes. In this situation, hyperglycemia becomes so profound and prolonged that the patient develops extreme dehydration, with plasma glucose levels often exceeding 1000 mg/dL, and suffers decreased mentation that may progress to coma. Many patients show focal neurologic signs (including seizures) that resolve when normal metabolism is restored. Since mortality is high, elderly diabetics must be followed closely to prevent this situation.

Diagnosis

The diagnosis of ketosis-resistant diabetes is usually made in asymptomatic patients undergoing screening during a routine physical examination or in conjunction with another medical problem. This is especially true in older persons, partly because of their increased renal threshold for glucose. The elderly may simply complain of vague constitutional symptoms (eg, fatigue or loss of energy). Occasionally, symptoms or signs of **peripheral or autonomic neuropathy** may be the initial manifestation.

Any 1 of 3 criteria is sufficient to diagnose diabetes mellitus: (1) random plasma glucose concentrations $\geq$ 200 mg/dL (whether or not associated with symptoms of uncontrolled diabetes), (2) fasting plasma glucose **(FPG)** concentrations $\geq$ 140 mg/dL, or (3) plasma glucose concentrations $\geq$ 200 mg/dL 2 h after oral glucose (see TABLE 70–1). For whole-blood glucose levels, these values are 10 to 15% lower; ie, 180 and 120 mg/dL, respectively. These abnormal values must be confirmed to avoid misdiagnosis due to laboratory error.

Persons whose plasma glucose levels are between normal (ie, FPG concentrations $<$ 115 mg/dL and 2 h after glucose $<$ 140 mg/dL) and diabetic are designated as having **impaired glucose tolerance** (former terms included **chemical, latent, subclinical, borderline,** or **asymptomatic diabetes**) (see TABLE 70–1). Ten to 30% of the population $>$ 65 yr of

TABLE 70–1. WORLD HEALTH ORGANIZATION CRITERIA FOR
DIABETES MELLITUS AND IMPAIRED GLUCOSE TOLERANCE

	Venous Plasma Glucose Levels (mg/dL)		
	Fasting		2 h*
Diabetes mellitus	≥ 140	or	≥ 200
Impaired glucose tolerance	< 140	and	140 to 199

* After ingesting 75 gm glucose.

age are glucose intolerant. Although these patients do not develop the microvascular complications, they are much more prone to the macrovascular complications of stroke, coronary occlusion, and peripheral vascular disease (especially the latter). If followed over many years, about 50% of these patients will remain glucose intolerant, 30% will return to normal, and only 20% will progress to diabetes mellitus, and then only at the low rate of 1 to 5%/yr.

TREATMENT

There are 4 components of therapy for diabetic patients: diet, exercise, sulfonylurea agents, and insulin. Ketosis-prone patients must be treated with insulin. About 25% of ketosis-resistant patients also take insulin, 50% receive sulfonylurea agents, and the remaining 25% are controlled by diet alone.

Diet

Diet should be balanced and nutritious to maintain ideal body weight, but its application differs, depending on whether the patient is receiving insulin or is obese. Most patients on insulin regimens have less flexibility with the timing and carbohydrate content of their meals than do those not taking insulin. The rate of insulin absorption is mainly dependent on the kind and amount given. Since the times at which insulin starts to become effective and peaks are predictable, patients should follow their prescribed diet and eat (especially carbohydrates) at appropriate times to avoid hypoglycemia. Patients receiving intermediate- or long-acting insulin need a bedtime snack. Some who are receiving intermediate-acting insulin require a midafternoon snack if they take their injection early in the morning and eat dinner late. Since exercise increases the rate of insulin absorption and enhances its effectiveness in tissues, patients should ingest enough calories for anticipated exercise in advance.

For patients not taking insulin, the timing and content of meals are less important, as long as the total number of calories taken in is appropriate. Since 80 to 90% of Type 2 diabetic patients are obese, the low-calorie aspect of the diet is the most important factor.

An appropriate diabetic diet should be ordered and detailed dietary counseling carried out by trained dietitians. Three steps are involved (see TABLE 70–2). **The first step is to determine the patient's ideal body weight.** A simple approach for women is to assign 100 lb for the first 5 ft of height and 5 lb for each additional inch. For men, allow 106 lb for the first 5 ft and 6 lb for each additional inch. If the body frame is small, decrease the calculated ideal body weight by 10%; if the body frame is large, increase the ideal body weight by 10%.

The second step is to estimate the appropriate number of total calories. Fifteen kcal/lb ideal body weight is assigned to patients who need to maintain their weight; 10 kcal/lb ideal body weight is for weight loss; 20 kcal/lb ideal body weight is allowed for those who need to gain weight and those engaged in heavy physical activity. However, the number of total calories should be *lowered by 10% for each decade after the age of 50 yr* because decreased physical activity, lean body mass, and resting metabolic rate are all associated with aging.

The third step is to apportion the calories among carbohydrate, protein, and fat. There are 2 general kinds of carbohydrates: simple and complex. Simple carbohydrates are monosaccharides and disaccharides; eg, sucrose (table sugar), fructose (a constituent of honey), lactose (milk sugar), and glucose (dextrose). If eaten alone, simple carbohydrates are absorbed rapidly. In diabetic patients, this may lead to a rapid rise in plasma glucose concentrations because the normal insulin response is lacking. Limited amounts of simple carbohydrates ingested with meals are less likely to lead to hyperglycemia. Complex carbohydrates are long polymers of glucose found in starches such as rice, potatoes, and vegetables. Although low-carbohydrate diets were popular in the past, evidence shows that high-carbohydrate diets are not detrimental to diabetic control when most of the carbohydrates are complex. Diabetic diets should contain about 55% carbohydrates, with 35 to 45% derived from complex and 10 to 20% from simple carbohydrates.

Most noncarbohydrate calories should come from fat, but diets rich in fat cause high cholesterol levels and should be discouraged. Thus, the fat content of the diet should be low (30% of total calories) and consist of approximately equal amounts of saturated, monounsaturated, and polyunsaturated fat and < 300 mg of cholesterol. The remaining 15% of calories are derived from protein. Recent evidence suggests that high-protein diets may cause the patient to be more susceptible to the eventual development of nephropathy.

To maximize compliance, the diabetic diet should be as close as possible to the patient's usual diet, although patients taking insulin require a bedtime snack. Once the food plan is agreed on, the insulin dose is adjusted to the prescribed diet rather than vice versa. Recent studies sug-

TABLE 70–2. CONSIDERATIONS IN ORDERING DIABETIC DIETS

1. Determine ideal body weight of patient

Women	5 ft, allow 100 lb; for each in. > 5 ft, allow 5 lb	Large frame, add 10%
Men	5 ft, allow 106 lb; for each in. > 5 ft, allow 6 lb	Small frame, subtract 10%

(If the metric system is preferred, change to kilograms by dividing the number of pounds by 2.2.)

2. Determine total caloric intake

To maintain weight	15 kcal/lb or 30 kcal/kg	
To lose weight	10 kcal/lb or 20 kcal/kg	*For each decade over 50 yr of age, decrease by 10%*
To gain weight, in adolescents, or with increased physical activity	20 kcal/lb or 40 kcal/kg	

Round off to the nearest 50 kcal. Although the total number of calories will differ slightly between calculations based on pounds or kilograms, this difference is of little practical importance, since neither prescribing nor following diets is that exact.

3. Calorie composition

Carbohydrate	Approximately 55% of total calories	Complex carbohydrates 35–45% of total Simple sugars 10–20% of total
Protein	Approximately 15% of total calories	
Fat	Approximately 30% of total calories	Saturated, monounsaturated, and polyunsaturated fat should *each* be approximately 10% of total calories Cholesterol < 300 mg/day

gest that eating foods high in fiber or fiber supplements, such as bran or guar, is associated with lower postprandial and perhaps decreased FPG levels. However, the amount of fiber required to accomplish this often leads to bloating, flatulence, abdominal cramping, and occasionally, diarrhea. Although most of these symptoms improve or disappear with time, they are unacceptable to many patients. Therefore, natural foods that are high in fiber should be encouraged, but external sources of fiber are not usually recommended.

In the case of obesity, both patient and physician must have a realistic expectation of the response to hypocaloric diets. On average, the caloric intake on a weight-reduction diet calculated in TABLE 70–2 is about 500 kcal/day less than the caloric expenditure. Since the catabolism of 1 lb of body fat releases 4000 kcal, it would take about 8 days for the patient to lose 1 lb (500 kcal/day × 8 days). This results in a loss of 46 lb/yr. More important, this approach restructures the patient's eating habits, which is critical for long-term success.

Fortunately, the weight loss need not be large before control of diabetes improves. For unknown reasons, insulin sensitivity increases when obese subjects are in negative caloric balance. This can occur within weeks (ie, long before much of the extra weight has been lost). As hyperglycemia lessens, depressed insulin secretion may improve, leading to better control. *The importance and efficacy of weight reduction in obese diabetic patients cannot be too strongly emphasized.*

Lean patients may make their own food choices to maintain ideal body weight. Therefore, except for possible recommendations concerning fat intake, dietary changes should be minimized to enhance compliance. This is especially true in older individuals, whose lifetime eating habits are usually difficult to alter.

Exercise

Regular exercise makes people feel better, has beneficial effects on the cardiovascular system when vigorous and sufficiently prolonged (see Ch. 25), and expends additional calories in obese patients. However, in patients taking insulin, moderate to vigorous exercise can lead to hypoglycemia, primarily because of increased absorption of insulin from the injection site. Patients taking intermediate- or long-acting insulin may have hypoglycemia hours after exercising, unless appropriate dietary interventions are carried out.

A secondary cause of hypoglycemia during physical activity is the increased use of glucose by exercising muscles. On the other hand, if a Type 1 patient has poor control of diabetes prior to exercising, glucose concentrations may rise further, and ketosis may develop or worsen. This is more likely to occur with vigorous exercise and is probably due to increasing concentrations of catecholamines, glucagon, and growth hormone opposing the action of insulin.

Physical training also increases insulin sensitivity (ie, patients respond better to either insulin injection or endogenous insulin). However, for this training effect to occur, exercise must be sufficient to lower the resting heart rate, and it must be sustained, since the increased insulin sensitivity disappears within 1 wk after the training regimen is curtailed.

Exercise rarely leads to significant weight loss without a concomitant decrease in caloric intake. For example, walking 1 mi consumes about 100 kcal, the equivalent of 2 cookies. The same amount of calories is used if the patient runs a mile; it simply takes less time. A list of representative activities and their caloric expenditures is provided in TABLE 70–3. Few obese patients undertake, much less sustain, a vigorous exercise program. Usually, the first step is to encourage them to take regular walks.

Sulfonylurea Agents

All sulfonylureas stimulate insulin secretion directly and potentiate the effect of other insulin secretagogues. They also potentiate the action of insulin in peripheral insulin-sensitive tissues (liver, muscle, and fat). Although this was initially thought to be the result of increased insulin binding, evidence now suggests that these agents act beyond the receptor, within the cell. They may also act directly on insulin-sensitive tissues. Sulfonylureas should be used only in patients with Type 2 diabetes; they are ineffective in Type 1 patients.

The sulfonylureas available in the USA are listed in TABLE 70–4 in the order in which they were introduced. No evidence is available to indicate which drug is best. In making a selection, physicians should weigh 4 criteria: (1) effectiveness, (2) side effects, (3) ease of compliance, and (4) cost. Potency (ie, the amount of drug necessary to achieve the desired results) is clinically irrelevant.

Tolbutamide is the least effective drug, followed by acetohexamide. Chlorpropamide, tolazamide, glyburide, and glipizide are equally effective, but *chlorpropamide should not be used in patients > 65 yr of age because of the risk of both hyponatremia and prolonged hypoglycemia in this age group* (see below). A patient who fails to achieve control with maximal doses of 1 of the 4 most effective agents has about a 10% chance of succeeding with 1 of the other 3.

Side effects are relatively uncommon with sulfonylureas, occurring in < 5% of all patients. Of these, GI and dermatologic reactions are most common. Chlorpropamide can cause the **alcohol flushing syndrome,** which may occur in 10 to 30% of patients. Additionally, chlorpropamide can cause **hyponatremia** via the **syndrome of inappropriate antidiuretic hormone (SIADH) secretion.** This is more likely to occur in older patients and especially in those also receiving thiazide diuretics.

Hypoglycemia can occur with all sulfonylureas, especially in patients who eat irregularly. Although hypoglycemia may last for several days, regardless of the inciting drug, it may last longer with chlorpropamide because of the drug's extensive duration of action. *Because of the extended duration of all sulfonylurea-induced hypoglycemia, patients with changes in mentation must be admitted to the hospital and treated with IV glucose until they are capable of maintaining a normal, or raised, glucose level.* **Reversible intrahepatic cholestasis** leading to obstructive jaun-

TABLE 70–3. CALORIC EXPENDITURE DURING VARIOUS
ACTIVITIES*

Level	Activity	Calories Expended/h*
Light		50–199
	Lying down or sleeping	80
	Sitting	100
	Driving an automobile	120
	Standing	140
	Domestic work	180
Moderate		200–299
	Walking (2½ mph)	210
	Bicycling (5½ mph)	210
	Gardening	220
	Canoeing (2½ mph)	230
	Golf	250
	Lawn mowing (power mower)	250
	Lawn mowing (hand mower)	270
	Bowling	270
Marked		300–399
	Fencing	300
	Rowing (2½ mph)	300
	Swimming (¼ mph)	300
	Walking (3¾ mph)	300
	Badminton	350
	Horseback riding (trotting)	350
	Square dancing	350
	Volleyball	350
	Roller-skating	350
	Table tennis	360
Vigorous		≥ 400
	Ditch digging (hand shovel)	400
	Ice-skating (10 mph)	400
	Chopping wood or sawing	400
	Tennis	420
	Climbing hills (100 ft/h)	480
	Skiing (10 mph)	490
	Squash	600
	Jogging (6 mph)	600
	Handball	600
	Bicycling (13 mph)	660
	Scull rowing (racing)	840
	Running (10 mph)	1000

* The number of calories that would be expended by a 150-lb person is shown. Caloric expenditure will be slightly lower for lighter persons and somewhat higher for those who are heavier.

TABLE 70–4. DOSES AND SELECTED CHARACTERISTICS OF
SULFONYLUREA AGENTS

Agent	Usual Daily Dose Tablet Strength (mg)	Usual Dose Range (mg)	Maximal Dose (mg)	Duration of Action (h)
Tolbutamide	250, 500	500–2000 (divided)	3000	6–12
Chlorpropamide	100, 250	100–500 (single)	750	60
Acetohexamide	250, 500	250–1500 (single or divided)	1500	12–24
Tolazamide	100, 250, 500	100–750 (single or divided)	1000	12–24
Glyburide	1.25, 2.5, 5.0	2.5–15 (single or divided)	20	12–24
Glipizide	5.0, 10.0	5–30 (single or divided)	40	10–24

dice is a rare side effect of sulfonylureas, but it is more common with chlorpropamide. These drugs do *not* have deleterious effects on the cardiovascular system, despite the contention of the University Group Diabetes Program (UGDP) study, which was not borne out by further analysis of their data or by 6 additional studies.

Sulfonylureas are simple to use. General guidelines are shown in FIG. 70–1. About 75% of Type 2 diabetics are asymptomatic and should be treated first with diet alone. If diet fails, a sulfonylurea should be started. The criterion for unsuccessful dietary management is 1- to 2-h postprandial plasma glucose (PPG) levels consistently exceeding 180 mg/dL.

The suggested initial doses of the sulfonylureas are listed in TABLE 70–5. Plasma glucose responses should be monitered every week or 2. The dose should be increased gradually until either the FPG level falls to < 180 mg/dL or the maximal dose is reached with the FPG remaining > 180 mg/dL. In the latter situation, the patient should be switched to a maximal dose of 1 of the other 4 most effective agents. Any response will be evident within several weeks. If the FPG remains > 180 mg/dL, the sulfonylurea should be discontinued and the patient started on an insulin regimen.

If the FPG falls to < 180 mg/dL as the amount of the sulfonylurea is being increased, PPG should be monitored. The dose should continue to be increased until either this value falls to < 150 mg/dL or the maximal dose is reached. As long as the FPG remains < 180 mg/dL (regardless of the PPG), the patient is usually not switched to insulin,

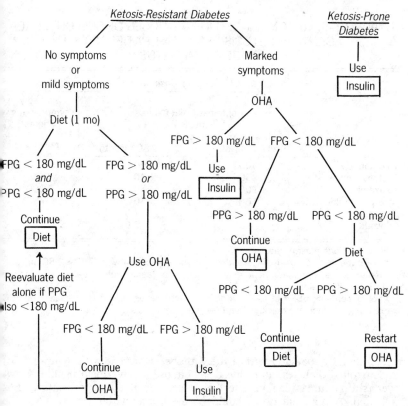

FIG. 70–1. Algorithm for use of sulfonylurea agents. FPG = fasting plasma glucose concentration; PPG = 1- to 2-h postprandial plasma glucose concentration on usual diet; OHA = oral hypoglycemic agents.

since in many cases no better control would be attained (especially in obese patients) and a marked change in life-style is required for successful insulin therapy. Since older patients are more sensitive to sulfonylureas, the dose increments should be smaller than in younger individuals.

The cutoff value of 180 mg/dL, both in the fasting state and 1 to 2 h after eating, is only a guide to aid the clinician in deciding among the various therapies available. If the renal threshold is relatively normal and if chemical measurements of circulating glucose are not available, persistent glucosuria can be substituted for the plasma glucose value of 180 mg/dL. The value of 180 mg/dL should be used only in deciding when to *change* therapy.

TABLE 70-5. RECOMMENDED INITIAL DOSES OF SULFONYLUREA
AGENTS IN KETOSIS-RESISTANT PATIENTS WITH
DIABETES MELLITUS

	Initial Total Daily Dose (mg) for Indicated Group*		
	Asymptomatic diet failures† with FPG		Markedly symptomatic patients‡
	(<180 mg/dL)	(>180 mg/dL)	
Tolbutamide	500	1000	—
Acetohexamide	250	500	—
Tolazamide	100	250	1000
Chlorpropamide	100	250	750
Glyburide	1.25	2.5	20
Glipizide	2.5	5.0	40

FPG = fasting plasma glucose.
* For patients > 65 yr of age, use dose for younger patient with FPG < 180 mg/dL.
† Relatively asymptomatic patients who should be treated with diet alone initially; see text for full discussion.
‡ For patients > 65 yr of age, use dose for younger asymptomatic patient with FPG > 180 mg/dL; increase quickly after 1 wk if no response seen.

Occasionally, patients with Type 2 diabetes present with symptoms of uncontrolled diabetes, and physicians choose to give them insulin. However, sulfonylureas can be effective, especially if an appropriate diet is followed. A maximal dose should be used, and within 1 wk it will be apparent which patients are not responding and should be switched to insulin therapy. If the FPG stabilizes at > 180 mg/dL, insulin should be started. If the FPG falls to < 180 mg/dL but the postprandial value remains at > 180 mg/dL, maximal doses of the sulfonylurea are maintained. If 1- to 2-h PPG levels drop to < 150 mg/dL, the sulfonylurea dose should be gradually reduced to determine whether dietary management alone may be suitable. Such responses, especially when weight loss occurs, are not uncommon.

The issue of **compliance** in sulfonylurea therapy involves only remembering to take the tablets. Tolbutamide is inactivated rapidly in the liver and therefore must be taken at least bid and sometimes tid. A reasonable dosage progression is 250 mg bid, 500 mg bid, 500 mg tid, 1 gm bid, 1 gm tid. Tolazamide, glyburide, and glipizide are also degraded to mostly inactive metabolites in the liver but apparently at a slower rate. The first ½ of a maximal dose of these 3 drugs is usually given before breakfast (ie, tolazamide up to 500 mg, glyburide up to 10 mg, and glipizide up to 20 mg). If greater amounts up to the maximal dose are needed, they are usually taken before dinner.

Acetohexamide is rapidly metabolized by the liver, but the resulting product is 2.5 times as active as the parent compound; thus, the timing of its effect is similar to that of tolazamide, glyburide, and glipizide. The first gram of acetohexamide is taken before breakfast, while the remaining 500 mg is taken before dinner. The relationship between drug and meal ingestion is unimportant except in the case of glipizide, which seems to be slightly more effective if taken at least 30 min before eating.

Although **cost** is an important consideration, it is difficult to generalize, since prices of drugs vary in different locales. A phone call to the patient's pharmacy is the only way to determine the cost of these drugs.

Some additional points should be made about sulfonylurea therapy. First, a few drugs will potentiate the effects of sulfonylureas by displacing them from serum albumin to which they are bound. Most important among these are the sulfonamides; others include chloramphenicol, clofibrate, dicumarol, phenylbutazone, and oxyphenbutazone. Second, use of 2 sulfonylureas together is *inappropriate,* since there is no additive benefit.

Third, available data do not make a strong case for combining insulin and a sulfonylurea. Studies have shown either no benefit or only modest improvement over use of insulin alone. The additional expense involved should be considered, as well as the fact that increased amounts of insulin would have achieved the same, if not better, results.

Fourth, if sulfonylurea therapy fails in obese patients, they should be treated with insulin. Although this may cause them to gain more weight (the evidence is conflicting), a few extra pounds adds little additional health risk compared to the eventually devastating effects of hyperglycemia.

Fifth, plasma glucose concentrations should be lowered to as near normal as possible without subjecting the patient to the risk of frequent or profound hypoglycemia. For instance, if a diabetic patient who takes insulin maintains an FPG concentration between 175 and 200 mg/dL, insulin should be increased to lower this value to < 150 mg/dL. Similarly, if a patient taking 500 mg tolazamide consistently has FPG and/or PPG levels between 150 and 200 mg/dL, the dose should be increased to 750 mg in an attempt to decrease both values to < 150 mg/dL. If such a patient had been taking maximal doses of tolbutamide or acetohexamide, full doses of 1 of the 4 more effective sulfonylurea agents should be substituted, with the choice initially influenced by the age of the patient.

Insulin

Goals of therapy: The effect that control of diabetes has on the complications of the disease is the same, regardless of age. Overwhelming evidence shows that near euglycemia delays, ameliorates, and possibly prevents the development of retinopathy, nephropathy, and neuropathy. However, the closer the attainment of euglycemia, the greater the risk of hypoglycemia. A balance must be struck between the benefits of tight diabetic control and the risks of hypoglycemia. Since many older diabetic patients have coronary artery and cerebrovascular disease, hypoglycemia may be a greater risk for them. Therefore, the balance may need to be shifted toward less strict control in these patients (see below).

The limiting factor for monitoring patients who take insulin is the amount of self-testing they will perform. Many patients are unwilling to consistently perform home blood glucose monitoring qid. A urine test for glucose may be substituted for the blood glucose test before a meal or at bedtime but is not suitable for monitoring when tight control is the objective. However, many patients can be persuaded to perform a combination of blood and urine tests. A first-voided urine sample should be tested, since it reflects a large part of the period of greatest interest. A positive result is considered unsatisfactory (ie, the target plasma glucose level has been exceeded), while a negative result is considered satisfactory (ie, the target level has been met).

The physician should continually encourage patients to increase the frequency of home blood glucose monitoring, to start it if they are relying only on urine testing, or to start urine testing if they are not monitoring themselves at all. Diabetes educators and patient-support groups often can influence patient acceptance of more vigorous attempts to achieve better diabetic control. Frequently, patients need to be persuaded for months to several years before monitoring themselves appropriately.

Glycated (glycosylated, glucosylated) Hb is the product of an irreversible, nonenzymatic reaction between blood glucose and Hb. Because of the 120-day lifespan of the RBC, this value reflects the average glucose concentration to which the cell was exposed over the preceding 2- to 3-mo period. The goal of therapy is to achieve normal values in this test performed q 2 to 3 mo. However, the closer insulin-dependent patients are to normal, the more hypoglycemia they will experience. Therefore, a balance must be struck. In practice, glycated Hb values do not guide day-to-day therapeutic decisions but are used to help decide whether greater efforts are needed to optimize control. Continued elevated glycated Hb values motivate some patients to undergo the discipline of home blood glucose monitoring.

Suggested levels of diabetic control for patients who use a home blood glucose monitoring device are listed in TABLE 70–6. The glucose concentrations correspond to the values represented by the colors on a Chemstrip® comparison chart or the values halfway between 2 colors. (Chemstrip® is a type of home blood glucose monitoring strip that can be read visually as well as by a meter.) Most individuals are able to judge whether the color on the strip is near one of those shown on a chart or is about halfway between 2 values.

Which level of control to select, at least initially, is influenced by (1) the age of the patient, (2) the length of time a Type 1 patient has had

TABLE 70–6. LEVELS OF DIABETIC CONTROL IN ORDER OF INCREASING STRICTNESS

1. Before meal and bedtime snack glucose concentrations of $\leq$ 180 mg/dL

2. Before meal and bedtime snack glucose concentrations of $\leq$ 150 mg/dL

3. Before meal and bedtime snack glucose concentrations of $\leq$ 120 mg/dL

4. 1- to 2-h postmeal glucose concentrations of $\leq$ 210 mg/dL*

5. 1- to 2-h postmeal glucose concentrations of $\leq$ 150 mg/dL

* $\leq$ 200 mg/dL if a glucose meter is used, $\leq$ 210 mg/dL if a visual reading of Chemstrips® is used.

diabetes, (3) the patient's awareness of hypoglycemic symptoms, and (4) clinical evidence of autonomic neuropathy.

Level 1 of diabetic control as shown in TABLE 70–6 is selected for (1) Type 1 patients who have had diabetes for > 5 yr, (2) any patient who has hypoglycemia without concomitant symptoms, (3) any patient with clinical evidence of autonomic neuropathy, and (4) any patient who is taking insulin and is > 65 yr of age. If preprandial values < 180 mg/dL can be achieved without significant hypoglycemia, the target range is carefully advanced to Level 2 for all of these groups except patients > 80 yr of age. Because of their limited life expectancy and the increased danger of hypoglycemia when associated with coronary artery and cerebrovascular disease, these patients are maintained at Level 1 indefinitely.

Because patients between 65 and 80 yr of age have a longer life expectancy, they should be advanced carefully to Level 2 of control. This target level (preprandial values < 150 mg/dL) is the initial goal in all other groups of patients except those who begin insulin therapy in a hospital. Patients with autonomic neuropathy (especially those who have hypoglycemia without premonitory symptoms), as well as those between 65 and 80 yr of age, are maintained at Level 2. All other patients who are able to achieve Level 2 without significant hypoglycemia are carefully advanced to Level 3 (ie, preprandial values < 120 mg/dL). Levels 4 and 5 require measuring blood glucose concentrations postprandially and are attempted (unfortunately) by very few patients.

For insulin-dependent patients to achieve tight control requires relatively constant patterns of eating and exercise and a stable emotional state. A balance must always be achieved between euglycemia and the risk of hypoglycemia. Under the current, relatively crude system of replacing or supplementing endogenous insulin with exogenous insulin, some episodes of hypoglycemia are almost unavoidable if glucose concentrations are to approach normal most of the time. Nevertheless, since tight control has such important benefits, patients should be asked to tolerate occasional (2 to 3 times/wk) mild episodes of hypoglycemia. However, if these episodes occur more frequently, are distressing to the patient, are not quickly aborted, and, most important, are not easily recognized, the insulin dose should be reduced and the patient must settle for the next lower level of control.

The same principles apply to achieving control in patients willing to perform self-testing more sporadically (eg, several times/day, 2 to 4 times/wk). If the data they provide appear to represent relatively consistent values, insulin doses can be adjusted accordingly. However, if the glucose levels vary considerably, hypoglycemia may become a problem if insulin doses are increased and these patients must settle for looser control.

In patients who perform only urine testing, the goal of therapy is no glucosuria in all first-voided urine samples. Initially, preprandial urine samples are tested. Once they become routinely negative for glucose, postprandial urine samples should be tested. In patients with an increased renal threshold for glucose, even negative urine tests may not ensure very good control. Conversely, in the rare patient with a lowered threshold for glucose, negative urine test results may be associated with unacceptable hypoglycemia.

Choice of insulin preparation: The most important criterion for selecting an insulin preparation is its time course of action: specifically, the onset, peak, and duration. These relationships are summarized in TABLE 70–7, but the values given are only approximations. Responses vary widely among different patients and even in the same individual from day to day. In addition, a small number of patients have a delayed response to regular insulin, so that the time course of this short-acting agent is similar to that of Semilente® insulin. Further, regular insulin added to Lente® or Ultralente® insulin in the same syringe has a delayed response in all patients. Apparently, the excess zinc in the lente series of insulins binds the regular insulin and retards its absorption.

Thus, when combinations of short- and intermediate-acting insulins are used, regular insulin should be added to neutral protamine Hagedorn **(NPH)** insulin. On the other hand, if short- and long-acting insulins are used together, regular insulin should be added to Ultralente® insulin. Although absorption of the regular insulin is delayed somewhat, the problem would be even greater with protamine zinc insulin **(PZI)** suspension, where the excess protamine would make very little short-acting insulin available until the regular:PZI ratio exceeds approximately 1:1.

Once the kinds of insulin (short-, intermediate-, or long-acting) have been selected, other variables (ie, concentration, purity, species source, and cost) may be considered. Over 90% of all insulins used are U-100; U-40 is used mostly for children, who usually need lower doses. Since differences in purity are no longer a major consideration, the species source and cost are the major factors on which to base a decision.

TABLE 70-7. APPROXIMATE TIME-ACTIVITY RELATIONSHIPS OF
VARIOUS INSULIN PREPARATIONS

Kind of Insulin	Preparation	Onset of Action (h)	Maximal Action (h)	Total Duration of Action (h)
Short acting	Regular*	0.5–1	2–4†	4–6
	Semilente®	1–2	3–6	8–12
Intermediate acting	NPH‡	3–4	10–16	20–24
	Lente®	3–4	10–16	20–24
Long acting	PZI§	6–8	14–20	> 32
	Ultralente®	6–8	14–20	> 32

* Also called crystalline zinc insulin (CZI).
† In some patients, the action of regular insulin may peak later than indicated here
(between 4 and 8 h) and last considerably longer. Therefore, addition of regular insulin
to intermediate-acting insulin may cause afternoon hypoglycemia in these patients.
‡ Neutral protamine Hagedorn.
§ Protamine zinc insulin.

Beef insulin is more antigenic than **pork** and **human insulin.** However,
titers of IgG antibodies that bind insulin are extremely low with the
current, more pure insulins, and their clinical significance is unknown.
Therefore, the most important consideration is cost, and the local pharmacy can provide this information.

With **human insulin,** there are other important considerations. Although most studies report no differences between the time course of
human and pork insulin, a more rapid onset, an earlier peak, and a
shorter duration of action has been reported for human insulin in some
patients in a few studies. Occasionally, human insulin forms aggregates
appearing as small white precipitates that stick to the vial walls of floc-
culate in the solution when larger. Agitation and higher temperatures
(eg, as occur when an insulin vial is kept in a purse) seem to enhance
this reaction. Therefore, vials of human insulin should be checked when
patients inexplicably lose control.

Sensitivity to exogenous insulin can vary over time, even in the absence of a recognizable cause (eg, infection, weight change, emotional
stress). Therefore, patients need to be monitored and insulin doses need
to be adjusted more frequently (about monthly) than at the interval between office visits (usually 3 to 6 mo). This requires ongoing communication between physician and patient, a family member, or nursing
home personnel. Decisions regarding changes in the insulin dose are
based on the results of blood and/or urine tests and on the degree of
diabetic control desired. Some patients (even those who are elderly) can
be taught to adjust their own insulin doses based on their home glucose
monitoring results.

The more often patients perform home glucose monitoring (or even urine testing), the tighter their control will be. Under ideal circumstances, the physician needs home blood glucose monitoring results 7 times/day and overnight. However, this much monitoring is unrealistic for most patients; glucose values before each meal and the bedtime snack are adequate in most instances.

Insulin regimens: The times in a 24-h period during which each type of insulin is effective and the timing of the tests reflecting that activity are summarized in TABLE 70–8. Five insulin s.c. regimens are summarized in TABLE 70–9. In regimen E, the Ultralente® insulin may be given before supper or the dose may be split (ie, before breakfast and before supper). The fasting test is still used to regulate the amount of Ultralente®, and if 2 doses are given, both are changed concurrently.

Starting insulin in the hospital: For lean patients (< 125% ideal body weight) starting insulin therapy, **using either regimen A or B** in TABLE 70–9, 10 u. of NPH are given in the morning and 4 to 5 u. in the evening. For obese patients (> 125% ideal body weight), the initial doses are 20 and 10 u., respectively. The doses are increased gradually until Level 1 of control (see TABLE 70–6) is reached before breakfast and dinner. At that point, the need for regular insulin is assessed by evaluating

TABLE 70–8. PERIOD DURING WHICH GLUCOSE IS CONTROLLED BY VARIOUS COMPONENTS OF INSULIN REGIMEN AND TIMING OF TESTS REFLECTING THAT ACTIVITY

Insulin	Time Injected	Period of Activity	Test Reflecting Insulin Action
Regular	Before a meal	Between that meal and either the subsequent one or the bedtime snack (if insulin taken before supper)	Both following meal before which insulin is injected and before subsequent meal or bedtime snack (if insulin is taken before supper)
NPH	Before breakfast	Between lunch and supper	Before supper
NPH	Before supper or before bed	Overnight	Before breakfast
Ultralente®	Before breakfast and/or before supper	Overnight	Before breakfast

TABLE 70–9. VARIOUS INSULIN REGIMENS FOR ACHIEVING STRICT
DIABETIC CONTROL*

Regimen	Before Breakfast	Before Lunch	Before Supper	At Bedtime
A	NPH/regular	—	NPH/regular	—
B	NPH/regular	—	Regular	NPH
C	Regular	Regular	NPH/regular	—
D	Regular	Regular	Regular	NPH
E	Ultralente®/regular	Regular	Regular†	—

* Insulin usually injected 30 min before designated meal.
† Either half or the entire Ultralente® dose may be given before supper since the long-acting preparation is thought to provide a basal level of insulin whose activity mostly affects the overnight period.

the before-lunch and before-bedtime-snack glucose values. The initial dose is usually 2 to 4 u. in lean patients and 6 to 8 u. in obese ones. These amounts are gradually increased until Level 1 of control is reached. Because of pressures not to prolong hospital stays, the initial doses of regular insulin can be started with the NPH insulin. However, these are not increased until before-breakfast and before-supper glucose concentrations of < 180 mg/dL have been achieved.

Further increases in intermediate- and short-acting insulin to attain more strict control should be made in the patient's home environment, not in the hospital. Eating, activity, and emotional patterns usually differ in the 2 settings, and *tight control in the hospital can lead to hypoglycemia at home.*

The regimens that use regular insulin before each meal **(C, D, and E** in TABLE 70–9) are begun with 4 to 5 u. for lean patients and 8 to 10 u. for obese patients. The initial dose of NPH and Ultralente® insulin in these regimens is 10 u. for lean patients and 16 u. for obese individuals. All doses are then adjusted according to the appropriate tests as summarized in TABLE 70–8. If insulin therapy is started in the hospital using regimens C, D, or E, final insulin adjustments must be made in the patient's typical daily home environment. If patients are switched from regimen A or B to regimen C, D, or E, the old insulin dose may provide clues to the new one; the initial doses discussed above may not be appropriate.

Changes are made daily, depending on the results of the appropriate tests. Once stable doses are achieved, changes are made less frequently: weekly if the patient performs self-tests often enough (bid to qid) and can be taught algorithms or monthly if the results of the tests have to be reviewed by a physician. In general, if most of the tests before meals or bedtime are higher than the target level, the appropriate part of the insulin dose is raised by about 10% or 4 u., whichever is less. If most of the test results are < 70 mg/dL (or 100 mg/dL in older patients and those who either are unaware of hypoglycemia or have clinical evidence of autonomic neuropathy), the appropriate part of the insulin dose is decreased by about 10% or 4 u., whichever is less.

If unexplained hypoglycemia occurs during the period when 1 of the components of the insulin dose is active (see TABLE 70–8), the glucose value before the subsequent meal must be considered < 70 mg/dL (even though if measured, it is likely to be high because of the action of counterregulatory hormones).

Certain concerns should be kept in mind with the regimens used to achieve tight control. **Regimens A and B** offer the least flexibility in the timing and content of meals; hypoglycemia is most likely to occur if meals are delayed. **In regimens A and C,** the intermediate-acting insulin given before dinner may have peak activity in the middle of the night rather than toward morning; increasing the dosage may lead to hypoglycemia at that time, before the prebreakfast target level of glucose is achieved. Administering the intermediate-acting insulin before bedtime (regimens B or D) should solve this problem.

In regimens C and D, if the period between lunch and dinner is prolonged (usually > 5 to 7 h), the before-dinner blood glucose level may be too high because the effect of the regular insulin given before lunch may have worn off. **In regimen E,** since Ultralente® insulin starts to work 6 to 8 h after injection, hypoglycemia may occur between lunch and dinner, especially if dinner is eaten late, or before breakfast if Ultralente® is given in the evening. This is usually not a problem when the dose of long-acting insulin is low (about 10 u.).

Many patients who rely exclusively on home blood glucose monitoring prefer not to test their urine at all. However, since diabetic ketoacidosis often can occur with blood glucose levels < 300 mg/dL, *physicians must insist on urine testing for ketone bodies in patients with Type 1 diabetes who are sick.*

Besides hypoglycemia, insulin therapy has 5 side effects: (1) a delayed reaction at the site of injection (dermal reaction); (2) an immediate reaction at the site of injection, often spreading as an urticarial rash to other areas (also called systemic or true insulin allergy); (3) clinical insulin resistance; (4) lipoatrophy; and (5) lipohypertrophy.

Local dermal reactions are small, 2- to 3-cm erythematous, pruritic papules that appear several hours after the injection and gradually disappear over the next several days. They seem to be a delayed sensitivity response to impurities in the insulin preparation. They were fairly common at the initiation of insulin therapy with older, less pure preparations and ceased within several months. They can occasionally be seen, however, with the newer pure insulin preparations.

Systemic insulin allergy is uncommon (< 0.1% of insulin-dependent patients). Within 10 to 60 min, a local reaction occurs at the site of injection and often soon spreads into a generalized urticarial pattern. It is more common with intermittent insulin therapy. Insulin and penicillin allergies are similar in their association with occasional angioneurotic edema and/or anaphylactic shock, positive skin tests, mediation by IgE antibodies, and treatment by desensitization.

Clinical insulin resistance is *an insulin requirement of > 200 u./day for several days in the absence of infection or diabetic ketoacidosis.* Except for gross obesity, the most common cause is immune-mediated, due to high titers of IgG (insulin-binding) antibodies. Like systemic insulin allergy, clinical insulin resistance is uncommon (< 0.1% of insulin-dependent patients) and more likely with intermittent insulin therapy. Although most insulin-dependent patients generate low titers of IgG antibodies, the reason for high titers in a few patients is unknown. Fortunately, the situation is self-limiting and insulin responses return to normal, usually within 6 mo.

Lipoatrophy *(loss of subcutaneous fat tissue at sites of insulin injection)* was much more common with older impure preparations, especially in young females. It is thought to be due to an immune response to impurities in the preparations. Lipoatrophy often can be successfully treated by injecting the patient's usual dose of a pure insulin preparation into the area. Within several weeks, the lipogenic effect of insulin starts to restore the local fat deposits. Paradoxically, however, a patient occasionally develops lipoatrophy when starting to take a pure insulin preparation.

Lipohypertrophy, *an accumulation of subcutaneous fat,* occurs with repeated injections at the same site, presumably because of the local lipogenic effect of insulin. Although injections in these areas may be less uncomfortable, insulin absorption may be erratic. Therefore, rotation of injection sites must be encouraged.

HYPEROSMOLAR NONKETOTIC SYNDROME (HNKS)

HNKS is due to a marked deficiency of effective insulin. Although small amounts of circulating insulin can be measured, the presence of large amounts of the "stress" hormones (glucagon, epinephrine, norepinephrine, cortisol, and growth hormone) antagonizes its effects. The ensuing hyperglycemia causes an osmotic diuresis, leading to dehydration and electrolyte depletion. The absence of significant ketosis implies that the production of free fatty acids via lipolysis is not markedly elevated. This is probably because of the restraining effects of the remaining insulin (lipolysis is much more sensitive to insulin than the pathways of carbohydrate metabolism) and to an independent inhibition by the markedly increased plasma osmolality.

Since there is no buildup of ketone bodies and subsequent acidosis, patients do not immediately seek medical attention because they do not have marked symptoms. They are often able to tolerate polyuria and polydipsia for weeks. This leads to severe electrolyte depletion and dehydration until renal plasma flow is impaired, allowing the glucose concentrations to reach extremely high levels. Thus, HNKS is characterized by severe hyperglycemia (> 800 mg/dL) and hyperosmolality (> 350 mOsm/kg) and by profound dehydration in the absence of significant ketosis (usually defined as a nitroprusside reaction of < 2+ in a 1:1 dilution of plasma). Plasma osmolality (P_{osm}) can be estimated from the following formula:

$$P_{osm} \text{ (mOsm/kg)} = 2([Na] + [K]) + \frac{[glucose]}{18} + \frac{BUN}{2.8}$$

where Na and K are given as mEq/L and glucose and BUN concentrations are in mg/dL.

Some important distinctions between the pure syndromes of HNKS and diabetic ketoacidosis (DKA) are presented in TABLE 70-10. Older patients often have a mixed syndrome with very high glucose and osmolality values but a compensated acidosis (ie, with significant ketosis, low

TABLE 70-10. COMPARISON OF SOME SALIENT FEATURES OF HYPEROSMOLAR NONKETOTIC SYNDROME AND DIABETIC KETOACIDOSIS

Feature	Condition	
	HNKS	DKA
Age of patient	Usually > 40 yr	Usually < 40 yr
Duration of symptoms	Usually > 5 days	Usually < 2 days
Glucose*	Usually > 800 mg/dL	Usually < 800 mg/dL
Na*	More likely to be normal or high	More likely to be normal or low
K*	High, normal, or low	High, normal, or low
HCO3*	Normal	Low
Ketone bodies	< 2+ in 1:1 dilution of serum or plasma	At least 4+ in 1:1 dilution of serum or plasma
pH	Normal	Low
Serum osmolality	Usually > 350 mOsm/kg	Usually < 350 mOsm/kg
Cerebral edema	Not clinically evident	Occasionally clinically evident
Prognosis	Approx 30% mortality	< 10% mortality
Subsequent course	Insulin therapy not required in many cases	Insulin therapy required in virtually all cases

* Serum concentration.

TABLE 70-11. FACTORS ASSOCIATED WITH THE ONSET OF
HYPEROSMOLAR NONKETOTIC SYNDROME

Condition	Drug	Miscellaneous
Diabetes mellitus*	Diuretic (potassium	Burns
Infection	depleting)	Hemodialysis
Acute pancreatitis	Diazoxide	Peritoneal dialysis
Pancreatic carcinoma	Phenytoin	Hypothermia
Acromegaly	Propranolol	Heat stroke
Cushing's syndrome	Glucocorticoids	
Thyrotoxicosis	Hypertonic $NaHCO_3$	
Subdural hematoma		
Uremia (with vomiting)		

* Initial manifestation without known precipitating cause.

P_{CO_2} and bicarbonate values, but a normal pH). Conditions associated with HNKS are listed in TABLE 70-11. If HNKS is not the initial presentation of diabetes, it often occurs when the Type 2 patient has another, often severe, illness.

The treatment of HNKS in patients with either the pure form or in those with a compensated acidosis involves fluid, insulin, and K replacement. Adequate fluid replacement is critical for lowering glucose concentrations. Hyperglycemia persists (even with appropriate insulin therapy) with underreplacement of fluid. Initial fluid replacement with 0.45% or 0.9% NaCl solution should be at least 500 to 1000 mL/h for at least the first several hours. However, *since older patients often have limited cardiac reserve, their lungs must be evaluated frequently to avoid overhydration and pulmonary edema* (which, unfortunately, is commonly seen in the treatment of HNKS). Patients with a history of heart disease should be monitored by measuring pulmonary wedge or central venous pressure.

In the absence of indexes of overhydration, the rate of saline repletion depends on the signs of dehydration. Failure of the neck veins to fill *from below* while the patient is completely horizontal (an indirect assessment of central venous pressure), indicates modest dehydration. An orthostatic fall in systolic BP > 20 mm Hg signifies more marked volume depletion. The goal of normal hydration (filling of neck veins to $\frac{1}{2}$ to $\frac{2}{3}$ of the way up to the angle of the jaw), can finally be attained by the oral route once the patient can ingest fluids.

Low-dose insulin administration is effective in HNKS, as it is in DKA. An initial bolus injection does not improve the response and is unnecessary. Doses between 2 and 10 u./h seem equally effective. The usual route of administration is IV, which should be continued until the patient can eat; then intermediate-acting insulin can be given s.c.

Even though there is marked total-body depletion of K (which must eventually be replaced), initial serum K levels may be low, normal, or high. K repletion often must be delayed because of the cardiac response to elevated serum K levels. During treatment, however, serum K invariably decreases, so K repletion is necessary in all patients (assuming urine flow) but may be started at different times.

On ECG, T waves in lead II, V_1, or V_2 reflect serum K and can aid in determining K administration, since there is often a delay of several hours before laboratory results are available. High-peaked T waves reflect hyperkalemia, and low T waves sometimes accompanied by U waves are noted in the presence of hypokalemia. Therefore, initially, patients with high-peaked T waves should not receive K; patients with normal T waves should receive K at a modest rate (about 20 mEq/h); and patients with low T waves with or without U waves should receive higher amounts (about 40 mEq/h). The lead that best shows the T waves should be repeated q 1 or 2 h, and the changing configuration of the T waves dictates the rate of K replacement. Laboratory K values are then used to confirm the decisions based on the T wave patterns.

The prognosis is worse for patients with HNKS than for those with DKA (TABLE 70–10). Although this difference is partially secondary to the delay in diagnosis of HNKS, most fatal outcomes are related to older age and severity of complicating illness that is either present initially or develops during treatment in most patients. Thrombotic complications are not unusual. Thus, death is most often due to these associated conditions rather than to the metabolic derangements per se.

Long-term treatment of patients after recovery from HNKS may not require insulin. In contrast to the Type 1 diabetic patient after recovery from DKA who requires continued insulin therapy, many Type 2 diabetic patients after recovery from HNKS can be treated successfully with sulfonylureas and/or diet alone.

SPECIAL CHALLENGES IN THE ELDERLY

Diabetes care in the elderly can be particularly difficult because of special circumstances associated with aging. Older patients may have trouble preparing meals because of tremors, osteoarthritis, or affective or cognitive disorders. Depression commonly occurs in the elderly. Depression or bereavement may lead to inattention to hygiene, inability to care for oneself, anorexia, and skipping medications. Cognitive impairments can also contribute to these factors, and severely affected individuals may not sense hunger or thirst, the former leading to weight loss, the latter to dehydration and, if uncorrected, the HNKS. Lack of educability and inadequate financial support (both of which are common in the elderly) prevent the patient from understanding what should be done and taking appropriate action.

Taste perception can change, with bitter or salty tastes becoming more predominant. Many older people are either edentulous or have poorly fitting dentures, interfering with chewing. All of these factors make it difficult for older diabetic patients to eat appropriate nutritious meals at regular intervals. This can be particularly dangerous in patients who are taking insulin and somewhat less so in those taking sulfonylureas. There is often a diminished appreciation of raised serum osmolality by thirst in older people, leading to an increased possibility of severe dehydration.

These factors make care of diabetes in the elderly a particular challenge. Since prevalence is so high in this population, the problem is enormous. Such patients should be approached with patience and understanding, and available support systems should be used as much as possible.

71. DISORDERS OF MINERAL METABOLISM

Lawrence G. Raisz

There is an increasing frequency of disorders of mineral metabolism in the aging population. Among these are disorders of Ca metabolism, which include not only diseases of bone, eg, osteoporosis, osteomalacia, and Paget's disease (see Ch. 64), but also disorders of Ca regulation resulting in hypercalcemia or hypocalcemia.

DISORDERS OF CALCIUM METABOLISM

Normally, serum Ca concentration ranges between 8.8 and 10.4 mg/dL (2.2 to 2.6 mM). Approximately 45% of the total blood Ca is bound to serum proteins, 5% is complexed with anions, such as phosphate, bicarbonate, and citrate, and only 50% is ionized. The ionized fraction affects cellular function and is normally maintained over a narrow range of 4.8 to 5.2 mg/dL (1.2 to 1.3 mM). The proportion of ionized to total Ca is affected not only by the amount of protein (particularly albumin) and anion-binding to ionized Ca but also by the pH of the blood; acidosis decreases protein-binding and alkalosis increases it. Moreover, the interaction between ionized Ca and the cell membrane is affected by the pH. Thus, at the same level of ionized Ca, alkalosis can precipitate tetany and acidosis can prevent it. Changes in K and Mg concentrations can also alter the response to Ca.

Although most hospital laboratories still routinely measure only the total serum Ca, measurement of ionized or ultrafilterable Ca is increasingly available. Ionized Ca is a more precise and appropriate parameter, since the value is unaffected by changes in bound Ca. If only total Ca is available, a simultaneous albumin determination should always be obtained. It is possible to have a normal total serum Ca with an abnormally high ionic Ca concentration because the albumin concentration is low.

If ionized Ca cannot be measured, the total Ca value must be corrected to compensate for any deficit in albumin. This can be done by adding 0.8 mg/dL (0.2 mM) total Ca for each 1 gm/dL decrease in albumin below normal (4 gm/dL). Thus, a patient with a total Ca of 10.4 mg/dL and a serum albumin of 2.5 gm/dL would have a deficit of approximately 1.2 mg/dL of protein-bound Ca (0.8 mg/dL × 1.5 gm/dL albumin deficit) and a corrected total serum Ca of 11.6 mg/dL, which is clearly abnormal. Conversely, a low total serum Ca is often simply the result of decreased serum albumin concentration. Since hypoalbuminemia is common in the elderly, particularly in chronically ill or malnourished patients, this correction assumes increasing importance with aging.

In interpreting any abnormality of serum Ca concentration, it is also important to assess acid-base balance, as well as K and Mg levels. Measurement of serum phosphate concentration is important, not only for diagnosis but because changes in phosphate can alter serum Ca (as discussed below).

Ca Regulation

The serum ionized Ca concentration is maintained at a constancy, with variations in an individual generally < 5% at different times of day and under different dietary conditions. This constancy is the result of a complex interaction among 3 major Ca-regulating hormones: **PTH**; 1,25-dihydroxyvitamin D (calcitriol) and calcitonin. In addition, other systemic growth regulators, such as glucocorticoids and thyroid hormones, can affect Ca regulation. Also, there are important local factors that act on bone, such as prostaglandins, interleukins, and growth-stimulating factors. The physiologic roles of these factors are unknown, but they have been implicated as the cause of hypercalcemia in malignancy.

PTH, the most important regulator of serum Ca concentration, is an 84-amino acid, single-chain polypeptide secreted by the parathyroid glands. Although the biologically active portion of the PTH molecule is in the first 30 or so amino acids at the N-terminal, the active circulating form is probably the intact 1-84 molecule. This molecule is cleaved in the liver and kidneys and has a short half-life ($t_{1/2}$). Some of the N-terminal fragments may circulate and have biologic activity, but the amount appears to be small. The C-terminal fragments are biologically inactive but have a longer $t_{1/2}$.

Increasing serum Ca concentration produces a rapid **decrease** in PTH secretion (proportional control). Prolonged increases in serum Ca concentration can result in atrophy of the parathyroid glands. More important, prolonged **hypocalcemia** can result in massive **hyperplasia** (integral control). These integral responses are slow; when the hypocalcemic stimulus is removed, hyperplasia persists and may produce rebound hypercalcemia. This has been termed **tertiary hyperparathyroidism**, and it has been suggested that the glands have become autonomous. However, in most situations, they are simply slow to involute.

PTH increases serum Ca concentration by at least 4 actions: (1) increased resorption from bone; (2) increased distal renal tubular reabsorption of Ca; (3) stimulation of the production of 1,25-dihydroxyvitamin D in the kidney, which results in increased intestinal absorption of Ca; and (4) decreased renal tubular reabsorption of phosphate. The reduction of serum phosphate concentration may enhance the bone resorptive response to PTH and prevent redeposition of the Ca mobilized from bone.

The effects of PTH on bone formation are complex. PTH can inhibit collagen synthesis by osteoblasts, but when given intermittently in low doses, it produces an anabolic effect that has been used to treat osteoporosis. The bone-resorptive effect of PTH is blunted in patients who are deficient in vitamin D or Mg. In the former group, this effect was thought to be due to a requirement for vitamin D as a cofactor in PTH action, but studies suggest that it is due to decreased mineralized bone surfaces. The osteoclasts, which resorb bone and release Ca into the ECF under PTH stimulation, cannot act on unmineralized bone surfaces.

The effects of PTH on the kidney appear to be mediated at least in part by stimulation of adenylate cyclase and increased cAMP concentration. Although PTH also increases cAMP in bone, the precise role of this mediator in bone resorption is not clear. The increase in cAMP occurs in osteoblasts, and these **may be the major target cells for PTH,** with bone resorption produced indirectly by the release of a mediator from osteoblasts. Although osteoclastic bone resorption is usually increased only by increasing the size and number of these cells, rapid changes in their activity have been observed after PTH administration, evidenced by an expansion of the ruffled border, the bone-resorbing apparatus that secretes hydrogen ions and lysosomal enzymes onto the bone surface, removing both mineral and matrix from bone.

With aging, there appears to be an increase in the level of PTH that is required to maintain a normal serum Ca concentration. This is most probably due to decreased PTH-mediated renal synthesis of 1,25-dihydroxyvitamin D as a result of reduced renal mass. There is no evidence that the increased tubular reabsorption of Ca, the decreased tubular reabsorption of phosphate, or the stimulation of bone resorption by PTH is impaired in the elderly. In fact, there is some suggestion that the catabolic effects of PTH on bone are enhanced.

In the parathyroid glands of the elderly, the proportion of mitochondria-rich oxyphil cells is increased, while the capacity to secrete PTH is sustained. The increase in serum immunoreactive PTH concentration with age may be relatively greater for assays that measure the C-terminal inactive metabolite of PTH, which is normally excreted by the kidneys and thus retained as renal function decreases. However, increased PTH with age is also seen with immunoassays that measure the whole molecule or with bioassays.

The second important Ca regulator is 1,25-dihydroxyvitamin D. It is clearly a hormone, since it is synthesized in the body from a readily available precursor, 7-dehydrocholesterol. The concept of vitamin D as a nutrient resulted from the fact that inadequate endogenous production occurred in populations living in northern latitudes and working largely indoors with inadequate sun exposure.

The synthesis and activation of vitamin D is complex. First, 7-dehydrocholesterol is converted to vitamin D in the skin under the influence of ultraviolet radiation; vitamin D is then hydroxylated in the liver to a circulating form, 25-hydroxyvitamin D, which is tightly bound to a vitamin D-binding protein (DBP). Finally, it is converted to the active hormone, 1,25-dihydroxyvitamin D, in the kidneys.

The production of 1,25-dihydroxyvitamin D is stimulated by low and inhibited by high Ca or phosphate concentrations in the blood. The effect of Ca is largely mediated through PTH. The concentration of 1,25-dihydroxyvitamin D in the blood is 16 to 40 pg/mL (40 to 100 pM), and 99% is bound to DBP. 25-Hydroxyvitamin D is present in much higher concentration, 8 to 40 ng/mL (20 to 100 nM) and is even more tightly bound to DBP. The serum also contains another renal oxidation product, 24,25-dihydroxyvitamin D, the precise function of which is not known, although it may simply be an inactivation product.

At physiologic concentrations, the major effect of 1,25-dihydroxyvitamin D is to enhance the intestinal absorption of Ca. These concentrations may also promote the synthesis of Ca-binding and transport proteins in many cells, since vitamin D-dependent proteins and receptors for this hormone are found in most tissues. High concentrations of 1,25-dihydroxyvitamin D have a catabolic effect on bone, stimulating bone resorption and inhibiting formation. These effects are probably important only when there is a marked deficiency of Ca or phosphate intake. Under these circumstances, 1,25-dihydroxyvitamin D levels increase, making more Ca and phosphate available for the needs of soft tissues and for vital bone remodeling (eg, fracture repair). There is recent evidence of an additional loop in Ca regulation, through which 1,25-dihydroxyvitamin D directly inhibits PTH synthesis and secretion. The absence of this feedback may be important in the increased PTH levels seen with aging.

Although 1,25-dihydroxyvitamin D synthesis and response to either PTH or low serum Ca are impaired in older individuals, serum levels are usually within normal limits, except in individuals who have severe renal disease or are vitamin D deficient. Serum 25-hydroxyvitamin D concentrations also tend to decrease with age, probably mainly because of decreased intake or decreased sun exposure. Levels are normal in older persons who receive vitamin D supplements or are exposed to the sun for at least 1/2 h/wk.

Calcitonin was the last of the Ca-regulating hormones to be identified, perhaps because it is the least important in man. Calcitonin is a 32-amino acid peptide, secreted in response to hypercalcemia, which reduces serum Ca concentration by decreasing bone resorption. Calcitonin acts directly on osteoclasts, stimulating cAMP production and causing cell contraction, loss of ruffled borders, and decreased resorptive activity. It is secreted by parafollicular, or C, cells, which in man have migrated to the thyroid gland from the ultimobranchial body.

Calcitonin deficiency occurs after thyroid ablation but is not associated with difficulty in maintaining a normal serum Ca concentration. Conversely, patients with medullary carcinoma of the thyroid, who produce excessive calcitonin, can still maintain normal serum Ca concentration and bone remodeling. The main importance of calcitonin for disorders of Ca regulation and bone metabolism is as a therapeutic agent in hypercalcemia, Paget's disease, and osteoporosis. Unfortunately, its effect on hypercalcemia is short-lived, probably due to a desensitization or "escape," which may represent down-regulation of calcitonin receptors or postreceptor desensitization.

HYPOCALCEMIA

Corrected serum Ca < 8.8 mg/dL (2.2 mM) or ionized Ca < 4.4 mg/dL (1.1 mM).

Etiology and Pathogenesis

TABLE 71-1 lists the causes of hypocalcemia. A decreased total serum Ca concentration is common among chronically ill, elderly patients. However, most such patients have a normal corrected or ionized Ca concentration with a low serum albumin. **Vitamin D and Ca deficiencies** are common causes of hypocalcemia in the elderly. The causes in the remaining patients can be divided into 3 groups: (1) primary hypoparathyroidism due to a loss of parathyroid gland mass or secretory function, (2) a relative decrease in parathyroid function, and (3) parathyroid hormone resistance. These divisions are not absolute, and in many cases hypocalcemia is due to multiple abnormalities.

Primary hypoparathyroidism occurs most often in the elderly following surgical damage to the parathyroid glands. Transient hypoparathyroidism is common following thyroid or parathyroid surgery. It is presumably the result of (1) damage to the parathyroid glands or to their blood supply; (2) prior suppression of normal parathyroid tissue in both hyperparathyroidism and hyperthyroidism; and (3) the so-called hungry-bone syndrome, in which increased bone formation and mineralization results in rapid removal of Ca from the circulation. Permanent hypoparathyroidism is most common after complete thyroidectomy for cancer, but this complication is infrequent in patients operated on by experienced head and neck surgeons.

Idiopathic hypoparathyroidism can be isolated or familial and may be associated with autoimmune failure of multiple endocrine glands. Metabolic or infiltrative damage to the parathyroids can occur in hemochromatosis and malignancy. Antiparathyroid antibodies that inhibit glandular function have been detected in some patients, particularly those with multiple endocrine failure.

TABLE 71-1. CAUSES OF HYPOCALCEMIA

Primary hypoparathyroidism
  Surgical (transient or permanent)
  Idiopathic (autoimmune)
  Mg deficiency (severe)
  Infiltrative (hemochromatosis or malignancy)

Relative hyperparathyroidism
  Inhibition of bone resorption (calcitonin, plicamycin, diphosphonates)
  Hyperphosphatemia
  Pancreatitis

PTH resistance
  Pseudohypoparathyroidism (PHP)

Osteomalacia and rickets
  Vitamin D deficiency
  Vitamin D resistance

False hypocalcemia
  Decreased serum albumin

Severe hypomagnesemia is associated with hypocalcemia and impaired parathyroid secretion. Hormone synthesis is less impaired, and there is a rapid release of PTH after infusion of Mg. However, the serum Ca response is slower. This has been attributed to end-organ resistance, particularly of bone. **Hypermagnesemia** may also inhibit PTH secretion, but this is not a clinically important cause of hypocalcemia. (See below for further discussion of Mg metabolism and hypomagnesemia.)

Relative hypoparathyroidism occurs when the entry of Ca into the ECF is so diminished or its exit so accelerated that an increase in PTH secretion cannot adequately compensate. Inhibitors of bone resorption can produce hypocalcemia, particularly plicamycin and other cytotoxic agents. These drugs may also impair the function of the parathyroid glands themselves. Calcitonin can produce hypocalcemia in patients with high bone turnover (eg, as in Paget's disease), but this is transient.

Phosphate excess is a cause of hypocalcemia in the elderly that can occur from a variety of sources. Rapid cell breakdown in rhabdomyolysis or during chemotherapy for leukemia or lymphoma, retention of phosphate in acute renal failure and shock, and excessive administration of phosphate given IV or by enema can all cause a marked reduction in serum Ca concentration with accompanying tetany. *Phosphate excess is particularly dangerous,* because it not only reduces serum Ca concentration but also results in soft tissue deposition of Ca and phosphate, with damage to the kidneys, blood vessels, and lungs.

In acute pancreatitis hypocalcemia has been attributed to a sequestration of Ca by fatty acid salts in the retroperitoneal space and occasionally in the peritoneal cavity by chylous ascites. True hypocalcemia is rare in patients with osteoblastic metastases and presumably is related to rapid mineralization, which exceeds Ca entry from intestinal absorption or bone resorption. Most patients with low total serum Ca concentration and pancreatitis or osteoblastic metastases have a normal ionized Ca and a low serum albumin concentration.

PTH resistance has been clearly delineated in several syndromes of pseudohypoparathyroidism (PHP). In classic PHP Type 1A, there is a defect in PTH response because of a reduction in the amount of the guanyl nucleotide regulatory protein (G_s), which links the PTH receptor with adenylate cyclase. This is usually associated with other structural abnormalities, such as short metacarpals, short stature, and mental retardation, as part of Albright's hereditary osteodystrophy. These patients do not respond to an injection of PTH with the expected increase in renal cAMP excretion and phosphate clearance. Other patients with PHP do not show a defect in G_s and may have postreceptor abnormalities or a circulating inhibitor of PTH.

Symptoms and Signs

Mild hypocalcemia may be asymptomatic or accompanied by nonspecific CNS symptoms. Chronic hypocalcemia is associated with an increased incidence of cataracts and calcification of the basal ganglia. Associated endocrine syndromes and chronic moniliasis are seen in some patients with multiple endocrine failure. Chronic hypocalcemia may also present with mild diffuse brain disease mimicking depression, dementia, or psychosis.

When hypocalcemia is severe, or when an associated alkalosis increases neuromuscular irritability, tetany develops. Tetany is characterized by paresthesias, particularly around the mouth, and muscle spasms, particularly of the hands, feet, and face. It usually does not occur until the serum Ca is < 7 mg/dL (1.75 mM) or ionized Ca is < 3 mg/dL (0.75 mM) unless there is concurrent alkalosis. Patients who do not have tetany may still have latent neuromuscular irritability, which is demonstrable by provocative tests. Chvostek's sign is a *contraction of the facial muscles elicited by tapping the facial nerve*. It can be present in normal individuals. Trousseau's sign is *carpopedal spasm caused by reduction of the blood supply to the hand* when a tourniquet is applied to the arm above systolic BP for 3 to 5 min. The ECG can be helpful diagnostically, since it shows prolongation of the QT interval in hypocalcemia.

Differential Diagnosis

A low corrected total Ca or ionized Ca concentration cannot be assessed adequately without concomitant measurement of phosphate, Mg, K, bicarbonate, and renal function. When serum Ca is low, serum phosphate concentration is usually high. This occurs even in severe vitamin D deficiency, when phosphate reserves are low, possibly because of a physicochemical effect on exchangeable Ca and phosphate in the skeleton. However, mild hypocalcemia can occur with hypophosphatemia, not only in patients with vitamin D deficiency but also in those who have both Mg and phosphate depletion.

The differential diagnosis is usually easy when hypocalcemia is caused by vitamin D deficiency, pancreatic disease, or renal failure. The distinction between primary and pseudohypoparathyroidism (PHP) can be made by measuring immunoreactive PTH concentration; PTH is high only in PHP. The response to PTH administration is also helpful. Human synthetic amino N-terminal 1-34 PTH (teriparatide acetate) has been used investigationally for this purpose and has just become available for diagnostic use.

Treatment

The immediate treatment of tetany is IV infusion of Ca. This is effective even in patients in whom the major precipitating cause is alkalosis or an abnormality of Mg or K. Usually 10% Ca gluconate is given IV, initially over a few minutes, but subsequently, substantial amounts of Ca gluconate may need to be added to a continuous IV drip. The amount of Ca required may be large if there is a substantial sink in the skeleton. This is seen particularly in patients with primary or secondary hyperparathyroidism. A 10-mL Ca gluconate ampule contains only 90 mg Ca, and the skeleton contains 600 to 1000 gm. If there is a large amount of unmineralized osteoid, several grams of Ca may be needed during repletion. The dose is determined by carefully monitoring serum Ca concentration.

Although any form of tetany will respond to Ca, in hypomagnesemic hypocalcemia the response will be short-lived until Mg is also administered.

The management of hypocalcemia lasting > 1 day has been considerably altered by the availability of 1,25-dihydroxyvitamin D as **calcitriol.** Calcitriol in doses of 0.5 to 2.0 μg/day orally is usually given in divided doses at 12-h intervals because of its relatively short $t_{1/2}$. This treatment, together with oral Ca supplements of 1 to 2 gm/day, can increase serum Ca concentration rapidly in most patients. Hence, it is usually possible to avoid symptomatic hypocalcemia after thyroid or parathyroid surgery by administering calcitriol as soon as the serum Ca concentration begins to fall. **For chronic hypocalcemia in primary hypoparathyroidism and PHP and in renal failure,** calcitriol is also effective.

Although calcitriol is expensive, it has several advantages over other agents. It is rapidly absorbed, does not require further metabolic alteration, and is rapidly cleared. One of the greatest problems in vitamin D therapy is the development of toxicity, ie, severe symptomatic hypercalcemia. Although calcitriol can cause hypercalcemia and hypercalciuria when given in a dose only slightly greater than the physiologic replacement dose, these effects are transient and disappear rapidly when the drug is discontinued. Nevertheless, serum Ca should be monitored in patients receiving calcitriol. There is a greater margin of safety with **vitamin D** itself or with **25-hydroxyvitamin D,** but these agents require further metabolism to become active, and toxicity is more prolonged, particularly when large amounts of vitamin D, given for long periods, accumulate in adipose tissue. **Dihydrotachysterol,** a "pseudo" 1-hydroxylated analog of vitamin D, has been used in renal failure and in vitamin D-resistant syndromes in the past, but calcitriol appears to be more effective and reliable.

In the treatment of primary hypoparathyroidism or PHP, calcitriol can be combined with a Ca supplement of 1 to 2 gm of elemental Ca/day. A **thiazide diuretic** or **chlorthalidone** has been used in some patients to increase phosphate excretion and decrease Ca excretion.

Hypocalcemia due to phosphate excess can be avoided by decreasing phosphate intake or by using aluminum hydroxide gels or large doses of Ca carbonate, which bind phosphate in the intestine and reduce its absorption.

HYPERCALCEMIA

Corrected total serum Ca > 10.4 mg/dL (2.6 mM) or ionized Ca > 5.2 mg/dL (1.3 mM).

Etiology and Pathogenesis

TABLE 71–2 lists the causes of hypercalcemia. In most cases of hypercalcemia, excessive bone resorption is the primary pathogenetic factor, but there is often the additional effect of increased intestinal absorption or renal tubular reabsorption of Ca. In contrast to a low total serum Ca concentration due to hypoalbuminemia, an elevation of serum Ca due to increased protein-bound Ca (with a normal ionized Ca value) is less common and usually drug related (see below). **False hypercalcemia** can occur when there is hemoconcentration due to diuretic therapy or prolonged hemostasis, and also in rare cases of myeloma in which the immunoglobulin is atypical and binds Ca strongly.

Clinically, it is useful to divide hypercalcemia into mild and severe forms. Prolonged, mild elevations of serum Ca concentration are almost always due to primary hyperparathyroidism, but a few may be due to hyperthyroidism, sarcoidosis, or familial benign hypocalciuric hypercalcemia. In contrast, acute, severe symptomatic hypercalcemia is most often caused by malignancy but can also result from any of the other causes, particularly when aggravated by a vicious circle of dehydration, producing increasing serum Ca with further fluid loss and decreased capacity for renal Ca excretion.

Primary hyperparathyroidism is common in the elderly. There is an increased incidence in postmenopausal women, perhaps related to the loss of an opposing effect of estrogen on PTH-stimulated bone resorption. At least 80% of patients with primary hyperparathyroidism have a single parathyroid adenoma. The remainder have multiple adenomas or pluriglandular hyperplasia. Primary hyperplasia is often seen in associa-

TABLE 71-2. CAUSES OF HYPERCALCEMIA

Increased bone resorption
Primary hyperparathyroidism
Persistent secondary (tertiary) hyperparathyroidism
Metastatic malignancy
Hematologic malignancy
Humoral hypercalcemia of malignancy
Immobilization
Hyperthyroidism

Increased intestinal absorption
Vitamin D toxicity
Sarcoidosis and other granulomas
Milk-alkali syndrome

Miscellaneous
Familial benign hypocalciuric hypercalcemia
Addison's disease
Acute renal failure (recovery phase)

False hypercalcemia
Hemoconcentration
Increased Ca-binding proteins or anions

tion with other endocrine neoplasms in 2 multiple endocrine neoplasia **(MEN)** syndromes: Type 1, in which pancreatic, parathyroid, and pituitary tumors are seen, and Type 2, in which hyperparathyroidism is associated with medullary carcinoma of the thyroid and pheochromocytoma.

Secondary hyperparathyroidism generally is due to development of parathyroid hyperplasia by prolonged Ca deficiency, and hence is ordinarily associated with low or normal serum Ca concentration, but patients with marked secondary hyperplasia can develop hypercalcemia under certain circumstances, eg, chronic renal failure in association with phosphate depletion, aluminum intoxication, and following renal transplantation. The last has been termed **"tertiary" hyperparathyroidism,** but the implication that the parathyroid glands are truly autonomous is probably incorrect. Most often the prolonged hypercalcemia is due to the slow regression of the hyperplastic glands. Hypercalcemia can also occur after recovery from acute renal failure associated with rhabdomyolysis, probably due to release of Ca previously deposited with phosphate in soft tissues.

Hypercalcemia of malignancy can occur by several different pathogenetic mechanisms. **Metastatic involvement of bone** with a local increase in resorption is the most common. This is probably not due to direct osteolysis by the tumor but to the local release of resorbing factors either from the tumor cells themselves or from adjacent hematopoietic or bone cells stimulated by the tumor. This syndrome often occurs in carcinoma of the breast.

Hematologic malignancies frequently cause hypercalcemia. In multiple myeloma an osteoclast activating factor **(OAF)** released by the myeloma cells has been implicated. This has been identified as tumor necrosis factor **(TNF)** β. Other lymphomas may produce interleukin-1 or TNF-α, which are also potent OAFs. Some lymphomas produce hypercalcemia by excessive conversion of 25-hydroxyvitamin D to 1,25-dihydroxyvitamin D, which also occurs in sarcoidosis and other granulomas.

In humoral hypercalcemia of malignancy (HHM), a circulating substance produced by a tumor acts on bone and probably also on the kidneys to increase serum Ca concentration. HHM is most commonly seen with squamous cell tumors, renal tumors, and hepatomas. Rarely, the factor is prostaglandin E$_2$; more often, it is a peptide that has a PTH-like action. This HHM factor is chemically distinct from PTH, although there is some amino acid homology. There is also evidence that a transforming growth factor of either the α or β type can be produced by tumors and stimulate bone resorption.

Vitamin D intoxication, milk-alkali syndrome, and sarcoidosis are major causes of hypercalcemia in which intestinal absorption plays an important role. **Massive doses of vitamin D** can produce prolonged hypercalcemia, while the metabolites 25-hydroxyvitamin D and 1,25-dihydroxyvitamin D have a more transient hypercalcemic effect. **Milk-alkali syndrome** is probably the combined result of a defective barrier to intestinal Ca absorption and decreased renal function associated with nephrocalcinosis, so the increased load cannot be excreted. **Sarcoidosis** and other granulomatous diseases (tuberculosis, histoplasmosis, and foreign-body granulomas) produce hypercalcemia by excessive, unregulated synthesis of 1,25-dihydroxyvitamin D.

Other causes of hypercalcemia include **hyperthyroidism,** which directly increases bone resorption but usually causes only a modest increase in serum Ca concentration. **Familial benign hypocalciuric hypercalcemia** is important, because it may be mistaken for primary hyperparathyroidism and result in inappropriate and useless parathyroid surgery. **Immobilization** can produce hypercalcemia in individuals with rapid bone turnover. In the elderly, rapid remodeling is rare except in Paget's disease. Hypercalcemia can occur in **Addison's disease,** probably due to a combination of increased bone resorption and hemoconcentration.

Hypercalcemia due to **increased protein binding** can occur in the early phases of diuretic therapy, particularly with thiazides or amiloride, which not only cause hemoconcentration but **also decrease urinary Ca excretion.** Compensation usually occurs and sustained hypercalcemia that develops while receiving these drugs is usually due to primary hyperparathyroidism.

Symptoms and Signs

Most patients with hyperparathyroidism are discovered by routine measurement of serum Ca and often do not have any characteristic symptoms. However, patients with primary hyperthyroidism may have many different symptoms and signs, some of which can be reversed by surgical extirpation. In the elderly, these clinical features include hypertension, muscular weakness, irritability, mild GI disturbances, renal colic, bone cysts, and decreased bone mass. However, it is common for hypertension and CNS symptoms to persist after surgery.

Hypercalciuria and nephrolithiasis can be asymptomatic. Moderate or severe renal impairment progress after hypercalcemia and hypercalciuria are reversed. When nephrocalcinosis develops, irreversible damage has already occurred. Although symptomatic cystic bone lesions are rare, mild degrees of osteitis fibrosa cystica with subperiosteal bone resorption in the hands and a "salt-and-pepper" appearance of the skull can be observed radiologically. Except for these bone lesions, the symptoms and signs described here are not specific for hyperparathyroidism but can occur with other forms of hypercalcemia.

Severe hypercalcemia, whatever the cause, is associated with progressive dehydration due to direct inhibition of renal tubular reabsorption of Na and water and the associated anorexia, nausea, and vomiting that diminish fluid intake. Occasionally, patients with mild primary hyperparathyroidism develop severe hypercalcemia because of an intercurrent illness that results in dehydration. When the serum Ca concentration exceeds 12 mg/dL (3 mM), mental confusion can occur. As the patient becomes increasingly dehydrated, higher Ca concentrations may be reached, resulting in coma and death. *Hence, Ca concentrations > 16 mg/dL (4 mM) are life-threatening and constitute a medical emergency.*

Laboratory Findings and Diagnosis

In primary hyperparathyroidism, the serum Ca concentration is elevated, and the phosphate concentration is low. Tubular reabsorption of phosphate is decreased and of Ca is increased. Because the filtered load of Ca is also increased, Ca excretion is usually high, although it rarely exceeds 500 mg/24 h. The levels of urine and serum Ca and P in primary hyperparathyroidism can be mimicked exactly in hypercalcemia of malignancy and hence are not useful in differential diagnosis.

A sustained mild elevation of serum Ca over several years is strongly indicative of primary hyperparathyroidism, although it can occur occasionally in sarcoidosis. On the other hand, rapid onset of hypercalcemia, especially with anemia, weight loss, and hypoalbuminemia, suggests malignancy. Serum protein electrophoresis, thyroid function tests, and a chest x-ray should be obtained in all cases. Additional tests for specific malignant disorders should be carried out when appropriate. Because mild hyperchloremic acidosis can occur in hyperparathyroidism, the chloride/phosphate ratio may be used as a diagnostic indicator. Hyperchloremia is useful diagnostically because it is less likely to occur in other forms of hypercalcemia.

In vitamin D toxicity, milk-alkali syndrome, and thyrotoxicosis, serum phosphate is usually normal or elevated. Vitamin D toxicity can be detected by measurement of serum 25-hydroxyvitamin D concentration. The measurement of 1,25-dihydroxyvitamin D, which is elevated in primary hyperparathyroidism, sarcoidosis, and occasionally in hematopoietic malignancies, is not useful.

Measurement of circulating immunoreactive PTH has become increasingly useful in the differential diagnosis of hypercalcemia. Based on currently available assays, most patients with primary hyperparathyroidism have elevated PTH values, while those with malignancy generally have low values, although there is still occasional overlap. Patients with vitamin D intoxication, milk-alkali syndrome, and sarcoidosis have low PTH values.

In the elderly, interpretation of PTH assays is complicated because the levels are normally increased with aging, but the increase is slight. Moreover, older patients often have impaired renal function and hence accumulate the C-terminal fragments of PTH, which are measured in most immunoassays. Thus, the combination of N- and C-terminal assays or an immunoradiometric assay, which detects only intact PTH, may be a better discriminator. Because elderly patients are more likely to have a second disease in combination with primary hyperparathyroidism, such signs of malignancy as hypoalbuminemia, anemia, and weight loss may be present. Coexistent hyperparathyroidism and malignancy are not rare in elderly patients.

Nephrogenous cAMP has been used as a biologic marker of PTH action but is not helpful in differentiating hyperparathyroidism from HHM, which is also associated with increased cAMP excretion.

Localization of a parathyroid adenoma, although not strictly diagnostic, may help to avoid prolonged surgical exploration and permit use of local anesthesia. The thallium-technetium digital subtraction scan is the most useful test for this purpose. However, false-positive results often occur in patients with multinodular goiter, which is common in older patients.

Treatment

The approach to treatment depends on the level of serum Ca, the severity of associated symptoms, the rapidity with which hypercalcemia developed, and the underlying cause. In patients with serum Ca concentrations > 12 mg/dL, especially of recent onset, immediate efforts should be made to reduce Ca levels while diagnostic studies are undertaken.

Since dehydration and impaired renal function are often contributing factors, the first step is rehydration by expanding ECF volume with IV isotonic NaCl solution. However, elderly patients may have difficulty handling large fluid loads, and furosemide may be needed as well. This diuretic increases urinary Ca as well as Na excretion, but should be given only if necessary to prevent or treat fluid overload. Effective reduction of serum Ca with furosemide requires large doses (80 to 100 mg IV q 2 h), which can be dangerous in elderly individuals, resulting in recurrent dehydration or hypotension. Rarely, hemodialysis is used to treat severe hypercalcemia that does not respond to other therapy.

Hypercalcemia can produce K loss, and this may be aggravated by saline loading. Therefore, serum K levels should be monitored and K replaced as necessary. Hypophosphatemia is usually not a problem, but when the serum inorganic P concentration is < 1 mg/dL, it may be appropriate to replace phosphate cautiously by IV administration. *Except under these circumstances, IV phosphate therapy should be avoided,* particularly in the presence of hypercalcemia. IV phosphate therapy should be closely monitored and stopped when serum phosphate levels reach the usual range or if any decrease in renal function occurs. IV phosphate can cause irreversible damage because of tissue deposition of Ca phosphate salts in the kidneys, blood vessels, and lungs. See below for further discussion of hypophosphatemia.

Calcitonin is a useful antihypercalcemic agent. It lowers serum Ca rapidly, although usually not to normal levels. The main disadvantage is that the effects are short-lived. Despite continued administration of calcitonin, "escape" occurs in 48 to 72 h in most patients. **Prednisone** in doses of 20 to 40 mg/day reduces hypercalcemia in patients with vitamin D intoxication and sarcoidosis and in some patients with hypercalcemia of malignancy. The combination of calcitonin and prednisone may produce a greater and more prolonged effect than is obtained with either drug alone. Rarely, patients with prostaglandin-dependent hypercalcemia may respond to nonsteroidal anti-inflammatory drugs (eg, indomethacin). However, these drugs can result in further impairment of renal function, particularly in the presence of dehydration or renal damage, and should probably be avoided.

In either hypercalcemia of metastatic malignancy or humeral hypercalcemia of malignancy, plicamycin is the most widely used drug, given in dosages of 15 to 25 μg/kg IV over several hours. In most patients, it produces a decrease in serum Ca in 24 to 48 h; this decrease usually lasts for several days. Repeat doses can be given, but toxic effects on marrow, liver, and kidney limit its long-term use. **Diphosphonates** are potent inhibitors of bone resorption that have been shown to reduce serum Ca in hypercalcemia due to increased resorption of bone. Etidronate disodium, the form currently available in the USA, is not highly effective except when given IV in large doses (7.5 mg/kg in 250 mL isotonic NaCl given as once-daily infusions for 3 to 6 days). New forms under study in Europe appear to be more effective.

The treatment of **primary hyperparathyroidism** is surgical. Surgical exploration of the neck should be considered as soon as the diagnosis is made, although some patients with mild asymptomatic hypercalcemia due to primary hyperparathyroidism may not be candidates and should be treated conservatively. Age alone is not a contraindication to surgery. In the hands of a skilled head and neck surgeon, the operation is well tolerated even in patients > 80 yr of age and often results in a substantial improvement in health. Although elderly patients can tolerate parathyroid surgery, they often develop "rebound" hypocalcemia after removal of adenoma, probably because of the combination of suppression of the remaining parathyroid glands and the hungry-bone syndrome. Vigorous treatment with 1,25-dihydroxyvitamin D as well as Ca IV and orally should be instituted early to avoid tetany.

If surgery is contraindicated, refused, or delayed, the most important treatment for mild hypercalcemia is avoidance of dehydration. Chronic therapy with oral phosphate has been used, but this often produces diarrhea and may result in further impairment of renal function. Small oral dosages of 1 to 1.5 gm/day of elemental P should be considered in patients who have a low serum phosphate concentration. In postmenopausal women with hyperparathyroidism who generally show low bone mass, presumably due to excessive resorption, treatment with **estrogens** (and progestins to prevent endometrial hyperplasia) decreases serum Ca concentration and urinary Ca and hydroxyproline excretion, suggesting that bone resorption has been decreased.

HYPOPHOSPHATEMIA

Serum P levels show much greater variation than those of serum Ca. The normal range is 2.5 to 4.5 mg/dL of inorganic P (0.8 to 1.5 mM phosphate). While 80% of the body's phosphate is stored in bone as hydroxyapatite, the remaining 20% is largely organic. Nucleic acids, nucleotides, phospholipids, and phosphoproteins are vitally important for energy metabolism, membrane function, and cell regulation. Phosphate depletion can occur as a result of poor intake, impaired intestinal absorption, or excessive renal loss.

Mild hypophosphatemia is common, probably resulting from both decreased intake and impaired intestinal absorption. The age-related increase in parathyroid function might also lower the renal threshold for tubular reabsorption of phosphate. **Severe phosphate depletion,** with *serum levels < 1 to 1.5 mg/dL (0.3 to 0.5 mM),* usually results from more prolonged and severe impairment of dietary intake and absorption. Vomiting, acidosis, and alcoholic ketoacidosis may contribute to hypophosphatemia. Aluminum hydroxide antacids, renal dialysis, and rapid recovery of renal function after acute renal failure or transplantation are other important causes of phosphate loss. Serum phosphate concentrations may also be extremely low, with relatively mild degrees of intracellular phosphate depletion, when there is a rapid shift of extracellular phosphate into the cells. This usually occurs when insulin and glucose are administered together in the treatment of diabetes.

Because IV phosphate can cause hypocalcemia and soft tissue calcification and because many elderly patients have impaired renal function and do not handle phosphate loads well, *it is necessary to be cautious in administering phosphate, even when serum concentrations are extremely low.* Patients who have severe phosphate depletion often have depletion of other ions, particularly K and Mg; it may be difficult to determine which abnormality is causing the symptoms. However, patients with extremely low phosphate concentrations who have evidence of impaired CNS function and muscular weakness should be given IV sodium phosphate or potassium phosphate if there is also K depletion. Serum Ca, inorganic P, K, and Mg concentrations should be monitored. Oral phosphate supplements are usually unnecessary in patients who are eating an adequate diet, but they are useful in hypophosphatemic individuals who also have hypercalcemia, since this may lower serum Ca concentration. Elderly patients have difficulty taking more than 1 to 2 gm/day of P given as oral phosphate, even when administered in divided doses, because of diarrhea.

DISORDERS OF MAGNESIUM METABOLISM

Mg is a cation that is abundant in the body, almost equally distributed between bone and soft tissue. Unlike Ca, serum Mg concentration is not tightly regulated and can vary considerably with diet and with changes in cellular uptake. Normal plasma Mg is between 1.9 and 2.5 mg/dL (0.8 to 1.1 mM or 1.6 to 2.1 mEq/L). About 20 to 30% of serum Mg is bound to plasma proteins, and there may be some competition between Ca and Mg for protein binding.

There is little evidence for primary regulation of serum Mg, but high concentrations can inhibit PTH secretion, presumably acting at the same sites as extracellular Ca. Low Mg concentrations may stimulate PTH secretion transiently; however, when there is a marked Mg depletion with levels < 0.9 mg/dL (0.4 mM), PTH secretion may be impaired and hypocalcemia can develop. Mg in bone is probably largely on the surface of hydroxyapatite crystals and can slow crystal growth. Intracellular Mg is required for a large number of enzyme activities, particularly those involving nucleotide phosphate metabolism, and plays a vital role in DNA, RNA, and protein synthesis. Maintenance of serum Mg concentration depends mainly on dietary intake, but normally there are extremely effective renal and intestinal mechanisms for conservation; with a Mg-deficient diet, both renal and fecal Mg excretion fall rapidly to low levels.

Hypermagnesemia is rare except in renal failure or after parenteral Mg administration. It can cause depression of CNS and cardiac function and may occasionally itself be an indication for dialysis.

HYPOMAGNESEMIA

Serum Mg concentration < 1.9 mg/dL (0.8 mM or 1.6 mEq/L).

Mild to moderate hypomagnesemia is common in elderly patients. It is probably not an accurate reflection of intracellular or bone Mg stores, which can be maintained for long periods after serum concentrations begin to fall. Nevertheless, a decrease in serum Mg is a warning sign that depletion may develop. Renal losses can occur in a variety of conditions, including aldosterone excess, diuretic therapy, and diabetes. A few patients develop marked Mg depletion because of a primary defect in renal tubular reabsorption of Mg. Alcoholism and malabsorption syndromes associated with steatorrhea are frequent causes of Mg depletion. Serum Mg concentrations fall rapidly in some patients after removal of parathyroid adenomas, presumably because of rapid uptake in bone.

The symptoms and signs of Mg depletion are nonspecific. Neuromuscular irritability and muscle weakness are common. Because hypomagnesemia is frequently associated with low serum concentrations of Ca, K, and phosphate, it is difficult to ascribe particular symptoms or signs to Mg depletion. Nevertheless, when hypomagnesemia occurs in these settings, vigorous treatment may result in a more rapid recovery.

Treatment: When possible, Mg depletion should be avoided by maintaining adequate dietary intake. Mild hypomagnesemia can usually be reversed by feeding the patient a Mg-rich diet. If there has been prolonged depletion or if the serum concentration is likely to impair parathyroid function as well as to affect cell function, parenteral magnesium sulfate **(MgSO₄)** can be given; 50% MgSO₄ can be given IM in doses of 2.5 mL. However, since this may result in hypotension, smaller doses should be given to high-risk patients. IV Mg can be given but only as a more dilute solution (MgSO₄ 10% or lower) and at a rate not exceeding 1 mEq/min.

Because Mg salts are powerful laxatives and depletion often occurs in individuals with GI disease, it is difficult to achieve replacement by the oral route. Small amounts of oral magnesium hydroxide can be used, but some patients require IM MgSO₄ at regular intervals to prevent deficiency.

---

72. MENOPAUSE AND OVARIAN HORMONE THERAPY

Brian W. Walsh and *Isaac Schiff*

MENOPAUSE

The permanent cessation of menses.

This results when the dwindling number of ovarian follicles lose their ability to respond to stimulation by gonadotropic hormones and estrogen levels fall. After 1 yr without menses, a woman generally is considered to have passed the menopause. If doubt exists as to its occurrence, an elevated follicle-stimulating hormone **(FSH)** level will confirm the diagnosis, but this is rarely needed.

The average age at which menopause occurs is 51 yr. This is not influenced by prolonged periods of hypothalamic amenorrhea, number of pregnancies, or oral contraceptive use. Although the average age at menopause has not changed since antiquity, increases in life expectancy have meant that US women will spend ¹/₃ of their lifetime after ovarian failure. Thus, management of menopause-related problems will become increasingly important in the coming decades.

VASOMOTOR FLUSHES
(Hot Flashes)

A **hot flash** is *the subjective sensation of intense warmth in the upper body, typically lasting 4 min but ranging from 30 sec to 5 min.* A hot flash may follow a prodrome of palpitations or a sensation of pressure within the head and is frequently accompanied by weakness, faintness, or vertigo.

A **vasomotor flush** is the objective counterpart of this phenomenon, with *a visible ascending flush of the thorax, neck, and face, followed by profuse sweating.* The first observable event is an increase in distal perfusion occurring 1¹/₂ min before the subjective sensation and 6 min before the peak increase in peripheral skin temperature. This increase in peripheral blood flow releases heat, causes a simultaneous fall in core temperature, and is followed 6 min later by a peak in serum luteinizing hormone **(LH)**.

Hot flashes frequently awaken patients from sleep, causing insomnia and fatigue and leading, in turn, to other symptoms (eg, irritability, impaired memory, poor concentration).

Incidence

About ¹/₂ to ³/₄ of all menopausal women complain of hot flashes. Of these, 85% are symptomatic for > 1 yr, and 25 to 50%, for up to 5 yr. Hot flashes lessen in frequency and intensity with advancing age, unlike the other sequelae of menopause, which progress over time.

Etiology

Hot flashes result from acute withdrawal of estrogen, by either natural or surgical menopause or by discontinuance of exogenous estrogen. The ovary does not usually stop functioning at one particular moment— typically, its function waxes and wanes over a number of years. When the estrogen secretion declines, flashes occur, but the flashes stop when the estrogen secretion increases. This rise and fall in estrogen production may occur for many years. Women with Turner's syndrome, who are hypoestrogenic, do not have hot flashes unless exogenous estrogen is withdrawn. Similarly, men with prostatic cancer who discontinue estrogen treatment develop hot flashes. This phenomenon does not require an intact pituitary, since a total hypophysectomy does not prevent its occurrence. Presumably, estrogen influences central neurotransmitters, which regulate the thermoregulatory center in the hypothalamus. Estrogen withdrawal alters central neurotransmitters, producing instability of the thermoregulatory center of the hypothalamus. Adjacent hypothalamic centers controlling LH release are also stimulated, resulting in the associated peaks of serum LH.

Diagnosis

A thorough history and physical examination should be sufficient to diagnose menopause and exclude other conditions (eg, thyrotoxicosis, carcinoid, pheochromocytoma). Menopause may be confirmed, if necessary, by demonstrating an elevated serum FSH. However, a low level of serum estradiol is not diagnostic, since premenopausal women frequently have low levels during menses.

Treatment

Optimal treatment of menopausal symptoms is with hormone replacement. Estrogen and progestogen treatment regimens are discussed fully below.

Clonidine, a centrally acting α-adrenergic agonist/antagonist, is 30 to 40% effective. A proposed mechanism is that it may inhibit the binding of norepinephrine in the hypothalamus; norepinephrine release may be the event that initiates hot flashes. The initial dose of clonidine is 0.1 mg bid; this may be increased to 0.2 mg bid if no adverse effects occur and hot flashes persist. This drug has a high incidence of side effects (eg, postural dizziness), but it is better tolerated by hypertensive patients, who may be the best candidates for this treatment.

OSTEOPOROSIS
(See Chs. 8, 64, and 71)

GENITAL ATROPHY

Atrophy of estrogen-dependent genitourinary tissue.

The tissues of the lower vagina, labia, urethra, and bladder trigone are of common embryonic origin, derived from the urogenital sinus; all are estrogen dependent. Following the loss of estrogen, the vaginal walls become pale (because of diminished vascularity) and thin (perhaps only 3 or 4 cells thick). The epithelial cells contain less glycogen, which prior to menopause had been metabolized by lactobacilli to create an acidic pH, thereby protecting the vagina from bacterial overgrowth. Loss of this protective mechanism leaves the thin, friable tissue vulnerable to ulceration and infection. The vagina also loses its rugae and becomes shorter and inelastic.

The urethra and the trigone undergo atrophic changes similar to those of the vagina. Dysuria, urgency, frequency, and suprapubic pain may occur even in the absence of infection. A proposed mechanism is that the markedly thin urethral mucosa may allow urine to come in close contact with sensory nerves. In addition, the menopausal loss of resistance to urinary flow by thick, well-vascularized urethral mucosa has been hypothesized to contribute to stress incontinence.

Symptoms and Signs

Patients may complain of symptoms secondary to vaginal dryness, such as dyspareunia and vaginismus, leading to diminished libido. These symptoms are less likely if intercourse continues at regular intervals; periods of abstinence are more likely to be associated with stenosis and discomfort with sexual activity. Patients may also present with symptoms secondary to vaginal ulceration and infection, such as vaginal discharge, burning, itching, or bleeding. Atrophic urethritis and trigonitis may present as urinary urgency, frequency, dysuria, and suprapubic pain.

Diagnosis

Atrophic vaginitis may be diagnosed by its typical appearance, but any atypical lesions should be biopsied. If a discharge is present, it should be cultured for pathogens such as *Neisseria gonorrhoeae, Chlamydia, Trichomonas,* and *Gardnerella (Hemophilus vaginalis).* If *Candida* is found, the patient should be screened for diabetes, since the low glycogen content of unestrogenized vaginal epithelial cells ordinarily will not support its growth. Atrophy may be confirmed by a vaginal cell maturation index, using scrapings from the lateral vaginal wall at the level of the cervix. The exfoliated cells may be classified by degree of maturation, with a small proportion of superficial cells indicating a high degree of vaginal atrophy.

Atrophic urethritis/trigonitis is diagnosed by urinary symptoms in the absence of infection and the presence of vaginal atrophy. Urethroscopy reveals a pale, atrophic urethra.

Treatment

Estrogen is the only effective therapy. The dose required is generally less than that needed for hot flashes or osteoporosis; thus, treatment for those conditions is adequate for genital atrophy. If the latter is the only indication for estrogen treatment, daily use for a minimum of 2 to 12 wk is required to reverse the atrophic changes; intermittent therapy, 2 to 3 times/week, should then be prescribed. Usual daily oral doses are as follows: **conjugated equine estrogens (CEEs)** 0.3 or 0.625 mg; estrone 0.3, 0.625, or 1.25 mg; or **micronized estradiol-17β** 1 or 2 mg. **Transdermal estradiol** 50 μg/24 h twice weekly, is also effective. Estrogens such as CEEs 0.625 mg or micronized estradiol-17β 0.1 mg used daily for 2 to 12 wk until atrophy is reversed, then 2 to 3 times/wk prn, may also be administered vaginally. Although these preparations exert a local effect, they are rapidly absorbed systemically. Thus, the addition of a progestational agent is advised for patients with an intact uterus (see ESTROGENS and PROGESTOGENS, below).

If estrogens are contraindicated, water-soluble lubricants may relieve dyspareunia. Improvement of vaginal stenosis has been accomplished by the careful use of graduated vaginal dilators.

ATHEROSCLEROSIS

Oral estrogens raise high-density lipoproteins (**HDLs**) and lower low-density lipoproteins (**LDLs**) in a dose-dependent fashion. This may be clinically significant, since elevations in HDL and decreases in LDL lower cardiovascular risk. The effects of oral estrogens are thought to be due to a direct action on the liver following intestinal absorption, since vaginal and transdermal estrogens do not affect lipoproteins similarly. One exception is s.c. estradiol implants 50 to 100 mg which favorably alter serum lipids, perhaps because of the supraphysiologic levels of estradiol initially released.

Some epidemiologic studies have found a decreased incidence of cardiovascular disease in postmenopausal estrogen users as compared with nonusers; other series have concluded the opposite. Although the former analyses were controlled for numerous cardiovascular risk factors, estrogen users may have been healthier initially and, therefore, thought to be better candidates for hormonal treatment. Since no long-term, prospective, randomized, controlled studies have addressed this issue, the effect of estrogen replacement on cardiovascular disease remains unknown.

OVARIAN HORMONE THERAPY

ESTROGENS

Pharmacology

Synthetic estrogens are chemical derivatives of estradiol and are 100 times as potent, on a per-weight basis, as are natural estrogens in stimulating the production of hepatic proteins. Since the minimal dose for therapeutic effect exceeds the lowest dose that markedly elevates hepatic globulins (5 μg), synthetic estrogens are *not* routinely recommended for postmenopausal use.

Nonsynthetic (natural) estrogens may be administered by oral, vaginal, transdermal, or subcutaneous routes. Orally administered estradiol is rapidly converted in the intestinal mucosa to estrone, which is then presented to the liver, where 30% of an initial dose is conjugated with glucuronide on the first pass. These conjugates undergo rapid renal and biliary excretion. The biliary conjugates are hydrolyzed by the intestinal flora, allowing 80% to be reabsorbed and returned to the liver. Estrogen may then be reconjugated and excreted, or it may enter the systemic circulation.

This enterohepatic circulation contributes to the prolonged effect of orally administered estrogens. Thus, patients with altered gut flora (eg, due to antibiotic therapy) may not sufficiently hydrolyze these conjugates, thereby preventing reabsorption, and may require higher doses for a therapeutic effect. Also, patients chronically maintained on phenytoin have enhanced glucuronidation and therefore excrete estrogens more rapidly; they, too, may require higher doses.

The most common nonsynthetic estrogens used orally are **conjugated equine estrogens (CEEs)** 0.625 mg; **estropipate** (piperazine estrone sulfate) 1.25 mg; and **micronized estradiol-17β** 1 mg. At these doses, the mean peak serum estradiol level ranges from 30 to 40 pg/mL, similar to that of the premenopausal early follicular phase; the estrone level ranges from 150 to 250 pg/mL. These doses are generally effective in relieving menopausal symptoms (eg, hot flashes), as well as in normalizing urinary Ca/creatinine ratios, without producing a clinically significant effect on the liver.

In general, CEEs are twice as potent as estrone preparations. This increased potency is due to their equine estrogens, which have a prolonged action, due in part to storage in, and slow release from, adipose tissue.

Since the concentration of estrogen after oral ingestion is 4 to 5 times higher in the portal than in the general circulation, more estrogen is presented to hepatocytes than to cells of other organs. Thus, the liver is more profoundly affected by oral than by parenteral estrogens. Although many of these actions on the liver may potentially be deleterious (eg, stimulating renin-substrate and coagulation factors), some effects may be beneficial (eg, increasing HDL and decreasing LDL).

In any case, appropriate doses of parenteral estradiol given vaginally or transdermally can result in therapeutic serum estradiol levels, with relief of hot flashes and restoration of urinary Ca/creatinine ratios, with minimal effect on the liver. In addition, estradiol enters the systemic circulation directly, without significant conversion to estrone, so the level of serum estradiol exceeds that of estrone, as occurs physiologically prior to menopause.

Parenteral estrogens may be given by the vaginal, transdermal, or s.c. routes. **Vaginal estrogens** are absorbed and enter the systemic circulation, achieving ¼ the circulatory level of an equal oral dose. However, vaginal estrogens exert a potent local effect: 0.3 mg CEEs given vaginally produces the same degree of epithelial maturation as does 1.25 mg given orally. The continued use of estrogen vaginally leads to increasing blood levels because of enhanced transfer across a healthier, better vascularized epithelium.

Subdermal estradiol pellets 25 mg are effective but have variable life spans of 3 to 6 mo and are difficult to remove. **Transdermal skin patches** applied twice weekly provide constant serum estrogen levels: the 50-μg/24-h patch yields mean serum levels of 60 pg/mL estradiol and 50 pg/mL estrone, which are usually adequate to reduce hot flashes significantly.

Adverse Effects

Estrogens may cause nausea, mastalgia, headache, and mood changes. More serious risks include the following:

Endometrial neoplasia: Unopposed estrogen use (ie, without the addition of a progestin) may induce endometrial hyperplasia and, ultimately, adenocarcinoma. Endometrial carcinoma associated with estrogen use has an excellent prognosis, since it is generally low grade and less apt to have invaded myometrium. The adjusted 5-yr survival rate is 94%, possibly because of earlier diagnosis. Unopposed estrogen use appears to increase the risk of endometrial cancer two- to fourfold, from 1/1000 women/yr to 4/1000 women/yr, and is related to both the dose and the duration (minimum, 1 to 2 yr). Reducing the dose, or treating cyclically, will *not* provide adequate protection.

Concomitant use of progestins is advised in a patient with an intact uterus. Progestins can both prevent and reverse hyperplasia. Their use reduces the incidence of endometrial cancer below that of women not receiving hormonal therapy. The duration of progestin use is important; although administration for 7 days/mo significantly reduces the incidence of hyperplasia, 10 to 13 days offers greater protection.

Ovarian neoplasia: Estrogen replacement may increase the risk of endometrioid cancer of the ovary (which accounts for 10 to 20% of all ovarian malignancies), but this association has *not* been conclusively established. It is not known if progestin use will reduce the risk, if it indeed exists.

Breast neoplasia: The possibility has been raised that estrogen use increases the risk of breast cancer, since (1) breast cancer can be an estrogen-sensitive tumor, (2) estrogens can induce mammary tumors in rodents, and (3) women with prolonged endogenous estrogen exposure (eg, early menarche, late menopause, nulliparity) are at increased risk for breast malignancies. However, many epidemiologic studies have not found an association between estrogen replacement and breast cancer, except for a possible modest increase in risk with long-term use (ie, > 10 yr). Nonetheless, women at particularly high risk for breast cancer may decline estrogen treatment for menopause. High risk for osteoporosis represents a different risk:benefit consideration. It is especially important that women receiving estrogens undergo yearly mammography. (The American Cancer Society advises this for all women ≥ 50 yr of age.)

The assumption that the addition of a progestin may protect the breast, as it does the endometrium, is unsubstantiated. Moreover, this hypothesis is contrary to the facts that the mitotic activity of the breast increases during the luteal phase (peak endometrial mitosis occurs during the follicular phase) and that progesterone induces mammary ductal growth in rodents. Since there is no good evidence that progestins reduce the risk of breast cancer, but they may adversely affect lipoproteins and thus increase cardiovascular mortality, **the use of progestins in women without a uterus is unnecessary and possibly detrimental.**

Gallbladder disease: Estrogen replacement doubles the incidence of gallbladder disease. A proposed mechanism is that estrogens decrease chenodeoxycholate in bile. This, in turn, will stimulate 3-hydroxy-3-methylglutaryl-coenzyme A (HMG CoA) reductase, the rate-limiting enzyme of cholesterol synthesis. Since bile is 75 to 90% saturated with cholesterol, this increase in biliary cholesterol may lead to precipitation and stone formation.

Thromboembolic disease: Oral contraceptives, particularly those with the highest estrogen content, are associated with thromboembolic disease. This effect appears to be dose related; controlled epidemiologic studies of postmenopausal estrogen replacement at physiologic doses have shown no increase in thrombosis. Moreover, a consistent biochemical effect of estrogen replacement on the coagulation and fibrinolytic systems has not been found.

Hypertension: Estrogen replacement may modestly lower BP in some women but may also induce or exacerbate hypertension in others. Oral estrogens may increase the hepatic production of renin substrate or may stimulate the production of an aberrant form. In either case, associated elevation in BP is usually reversible on discontinuance of estrogen. Moreover, estrogen replacement is not associated with an increased risk of stroke.

Glucose tolerance: Although oral contraceptives are associated with impaired carbohydrate metabolism, the lower doses used for estrogen replacement have not been linked to impaired glucose tolerance. Postmenopausal women with diabetes show either no change with estrogen use or an improvement in their disease, evidenced by lower glucose levels or reduced insulin requirements. This response is consistent with the observation that estrogen appears to increase the binding of insulin to its receptor. Moreover, animal models have shown that experimentally induced hyperglycemia improves with estrogen therapy.

Contraindications

Absolute contraindications to postmenopausal estrogen replacement are as follows: (1) known or suspected endometrial or breast cancer, (2) undiagnosed genital bleeding, (3) active liver disease, and (4) active thromboembolic disease or a history of estrogen-related thromboembolic disease.

Relative contraindications include (1) Chronic liver dysfunction: The liver's ability to metabolize estrogen is impaired, leading to excessive levels of estrogen; this may be compensated for by using smaller and/or less-frequent doses. (2) Preexisting uterine leiomyomata or active endometriosis: Estrogen use may prevent the involution of these conditions, which would be expected following the menopause. (3) Poorly controlled hypertension. (4) History of thromboembolic disease. (5) Acute intermittent porphyria: Estrogens are known to precipitate attacks.

PROGESTOGENS

The primary purpose of postmenopausal progestin use is reduction of the risk of endometrial hyperstimulation caused by estrogen replacement. Progestins may also be used for the relief of hot flashes or for prophylaxis of osteoporosis in patients who are not candidates for estrogen replacement.

Available Preparations

Progesterone and its derivatives are well absorbed by the vaginal, rectal, and IM routes. The oral route, although convenient and commonly used, provides a highly variable degree of absorption with as much as a three-fold difference among patients. For this reason, variable clinical effects may be seen in patients given the same dose. Following absorption, oral progestins are presented to the liver in high concentration, where they may greatly affect the hepatic metabolism of serum lipoproteins. These progestins are then rapidly metabolized by the liver to desoxycorticosterone.

Medroxyprogesterone acetate (MPA) 10 mg, the most commonly used progestin in the USA, is effective against hyperplasia and has only minor effects on serum lipids. Patients unable to tolerate this dose may use 5 mg. In most cases, the 5-mg dose offers similar protection against hyperplasia, except in individuals who absorb oral MPA poorly. MPA given IM as its depot formulation is well absorbed but has a highly variable duration of action and is commonly associated with irregular vaginal bleeding. The usual dose is 50 to 150 mg IM every 1 to 3 mo; the 50-mg dose is usually adequate to relieve hot flashes, while the 150-mg dose may be as effective as 0.625 mg CEEs in reducing urinary Ca loss.

Megestrol acetate is also effective in suppressing hot flashes and restoring Ca/creatinine ratios to premenopausal levels. Daily dosages of 40 to 80 mg are required, since this agent has $1/4$ to $1/8$ the potency of MPA on a per-weight basis. Micronized progesterone 200 to 300 mg is also active against hyperplasia and does not significantly alter serum lipids.

19-Nortestosterone derivatives are the progestins used in oral contraceptives; they have partial androgenic properties and an adverse action on serum lipids. **Norethindrone (norethisterone, NET)** was initially used in doses of 2.5 to 5 mg, but recent work has shown that 1 mg (as used in low-dose oral contraceptives) is equally effective against hyperplasia but has much less impact on lipids. **D,L-norgestrel,** known for its more potent androgenic properties, was also used in a 0.5-mg dose, but 0.15 mg appears equally effective. Only the *l* isomer is biologically active, so 0.15 mg *d,l*-norgestrel is equivalent to 0.075 mg levonorgestrel. The effect of this dose on lipids is unknown.

Adverse Effects

Progestins may produce abdominal bloating, mastalgia, headache, mood changes, and acne. Progestins, particularly the 19-nortestosterone derivatives, also affect serum lipids adversely, decreasing HDL and increasing LDL in a dose-dependent manner. Thus, the risk of developing cardiovascular disease may outweigh the benefit of preventing endometrial cancer. Since the protective activity of progestins on the endometrium appears related more to the duration of use (ie, 13 out of 25 days) than to the dose, the minimal effective dose should be used. For

MPA, this is 10 mg, and for NET, 1 mg; both these doses have minimal effects on serum lipids. Since progestins have not been proved to protect against breast cancer and may adversely affect lipoproteins, thus predisposing to cardiovascular disease, these agents are not recommended for women without an intact uterus who are receiving estrogens.

HORMONE REPLACEMENT REGIMENS

Insufficient data are available to indicate that all postmenopausal women must be treated with estrogen replacement. For that reason, the benefits and risks (see above) as they pertain to each individual patient should be reviewed with her in detail. She must ultimately decide whether to receive therapy and give informed consent.

Prior to initiation of hormonal therapy, the patient must be evaluated with a thorough history and physical examination, including BP, breast and pelvic examinations, and Papanicolaou **(Pap)** test. BP should be monitored after 3 to 6 mo, then annually. Mammography should be performed (and repeated annually) to avoid prescribing estrogens to a patient with preexisting subclinical breast cancer.

An endometrial biopsy should be considered if the patient has a history of abnormal vaginal bleeding, is at increased risk for preexisting endometrial hyperplasia, bleeds at any time other than during the drug-free interval, or has heavy bleeding. Biopsy may be accomplished by vabra aspiration or, if adequate tissue cannot be obtained, by fractional D & C. A patient receiving unopposed estrogens for an extended time should have a biopsy prior to the start of therapy and annually thereafter, regardless of the presence or absence of bleeding.

The most commonly used schedule of oral hormone replacement in the USA is cyclic, with conjugated equine estrogens **(CEEs)** 0.625 mg given on days 1 through 25, and medroxyprogesterone acetate **(MPA)** 10 mg given on days 13 through 25, each month. No hormones are given the remainder of the month. On this regimen, many patients demonstrate withdrawal bleeding. The schedule may be modified by substituting another estrogen for CEEs and/or another progestin for MPA.

To avoid withdrawal bleeding, continuous rather than cyclic treatment has been proposed. CEEs 0.625 or 1.25 mg as needed to control symptoms are given continuously with norethindrone **(NET)** 0.35 mg. The dose of NET is serially increased q 2 to 3 mo by 0.35 mg up to a limit of 2.1 mg, until all bleeding is abolished. Ninety-five percent of patients become amenorrheic by 1 yr, but higher doses of NET are required with 1.25 mg CEEs. These higher doses are associated with abdominal bloating and mastalgia, which may cause the patient to discontinue therapy. The effect of this regimen on lipids is unknown. The use of MPA 2.5 to 10 mg has been suggested as a substitute for NET in this schedule.

Treatment of genital atrophy is discussed above.

73. MALE HYPOGONADISM AND IMPOTENCE

Stanley G. Korenman

HYPOGONADISM

The testis is the site of spermatogenesis (in the seminiferous tubules) and androgen production (by the Leydig cells). Although rarely evaluated in elderly men, spermatogenesis is remarkably sustained despite advanced age in the presence of adequate testicular androgen synthesis. In this discussion, **hypogonadism** is defined as *inadequate testicular androgen production.*

Reproductive Physiology of the Aging Male

Androgen production declines with aging. However, the consequences of this reduction for health and well-being have not been determined. As testosterone **(T)** secretion diminishes, its diurnal variation is blunted, resulting in a lower 6 to 8 AM peak. Mean gonadotropin levels slowly rise but **luteinizing hormone (LH)** pulse frequency is reduced, impairing pulsatile testicular response. Binding of testosterone to **sex hormone-binding globulin (SHBG)** reduces the tissue availability of the former. Testosterone binding increases with age, resulting in a substantial decline of unbound, bioavailable testosterone **(BT)** and in a slowing of testosterone metabolism. Low levels of both gonadotropin and testosterone (particulary bioavailable testosterone) suggest hypothalamic-pituitary dysfunction.

Testosterone acts on most body tissues either unchanged (as in muscles), after conversion to dihydrotestosterone **(DHT)** (as in reproductive tissues), or after conversion to estradiol (as in certain brain nuclei).

Sexual potency requires the interaction of libido ("sexual appetite") and erectile capacity. The best evidence suggests that androgens play an important role in libido and influence the frequency of nocturnal erections, but they do not seem to be involved in erections associated with erotic stimuli. (See also Ch. 58.)

Symptoms and Signs

Hypogonadism is suspected on the basis of relatively nonspecific complaints (eg, impotence, decreased libido, or gynecomastia). Patients may also have hot flashes, increased irritability, inability to concentrate, and a depressed mood. Severe and prolonged hypogonadism is marked by loss of body hair and reduced skeletal muscle mass, with loss of masculine habitus. Small, soft testes and a loss of scrotal pigmentation and rugation are important clues. Mild cases of hypogonadism usually have no characteristic findings.

Laboratory Assessment

Assessment of Leydig cell function is commonly made by radioimmunoassay of testosterone and LH. Fasting morning blood samples are obtained daily for 3 days or 3 samples are obtained 20 min apart. The average value is derived, to minimize fluctuation due to pulsatile LH secretion. The normal range of testosterone is 300 to 1000 ng/dL. Normal LH values vary with the laboratory standard used.

Because secretion of testosterone is reduced and binding is increased with age, assessment of BT may be very valuable in the elderly, but the methodology is not widely available. Elevated SHBG (> 13 ng/mL) suggests reduced testosterone tissue availability, even in the presence of normal serum testosterone levels. Dynamic testing of the pituitary-testicular axis through the use of gonadotropin-releasing hormone **(GnRH)** and human chorionic gonadotropin **(HCG)** merely confirms data from the basal tests and is not of great value in diagnosis.

Differential Diagnosis

Although newly diagnosed hypogonadism in the older man occasionally is caused by Klinefelter's syndrome, panhypopituitarism, Cushing's syndrome, Kallmann's syndrome, or mild androgen resistance, it usually results from acquired causes associated with other illnesses. Viral orchitis due to mumps, lymphocytic choriomeningitis, arboviruses, or, rarely, to echovirus, may occur, but the ensuing testicular atrophy may take years to develop. Testicular trauma or exposure to heavy metals should also be considered. Radiation therapy or the combination of radiation and chemotherapy frequently results in seminiferous tubular failure. Insidiously developing hypogonadism may also occur.

Treatment with spironolactone, cyproterone acetate, ketoconazole, and medroxyprogesterone acetate interfere with testosterone biosynthesis and may cause hypogonadism in a small percentage of men. Addiction to marijuana, heroin, or methadone may result in low testosterone levels without LH elevation, suggesting pituitary as well as testicular inhibition.

A large number of drugs impair sexual function without specific impairment of the hypothalamic-pituitary-testicular axis. These include virtually all antihypertensives, as well as phenothiazines and other psychotropic drugs. (See also EFFECTS OF DRUGS in Ch. 58.)

The autoimmune endocrine deficiency syndrome that includes adrenal, thyroid, and ovarian failure and diabetes mellitus occasionally results in testicular failure. However, primary testicular failure is associated with leprosy and myotonic dystrophy. Primary hypogonadism with gynecomastia is common in uremia, even with chronic dialysis. It may improve after renal transplantation.

Hepatic cirrhosis causes hypogonadism and gynecomastia as a result of a markedly increased circulating bioavailable estrogen/androgen ratio, with reduced Leydig cell responsiveness to gonadotropin stimulation. Alcoholic cirrhosis seems to produce a greater degree of testicular failure than that produced by cirrhosis due to hepatitis or hemachromatosis.

Severe stress, as occurs with surgery, MI, stroke, or burns, causes a profound fall of serum testosterone levels, with slow subsequent return to normal. This is probably due to high cortisol levels, which inhibit gonadotropin secretion.

A substantial number of older men have low serum testosterone and BT levels, with elevated or normal levels of gonadotropins, without an identifiable basis for these findings. An explanation gaining acceptance is that these findings reflect a form of hypogonadism that may result from both pituitary and testicular hypofunction.

Treatment

Profound hypogonadism is the chief indication for **androgen therapy.** The principal available forms of androgens are injectable long-acting esters of testosterone and 19-nortestosterone (the enanthate and the cyclopentylpropionate) and oral forms of testosterone derivatives, which have an alkyl group in the 17 position. The oral agents may cause hepatotoxicity with reversible elevation of hepatic enzymes, occasional episodes of cholestatic jaundice, and, rarely, hepatic tumors; their use is rarely justified.

The long-acting esters of testosterone are administered IM in a dosage of 100 to 200 mg every 1 to 3 wk. Testosterone is effective in restoring the muscle strength, hair pattern, sexual function, bone formation, and well-being of hypogonadal men. However, therapy often results in stimulation of erythropoietin sufficient to increase the Hct by several percentage points, sometimes requiring dosage reduction or periodic phlebotomy.

Testosterone enhances the activity of hepatic lipoprotein lipase, resulting in a decrease of high-density lipoprotein (**HDL**) cholesterol; total cholesterol is unaffected. Androgens increase sensitivity to the action of warfarin derivatives. They do not appear to affect benign prostatic hypertrophy, but a clinically significant increase in obstructive symptoms is possible. There is a theoretical risk that testosterone therapy will stimulate tumor aggressiveness in preexisting prostatic carcinoma.

IMPOTENCE

Secondary impotence, *the inability to have an erection with vaginal penetration on more than 50% of attempts following a period of normal erectile function,* is progressively frequent with age. The incidence of secondary impotence is high in men with chronic illnesses, including diabetes mellitus, hypertension, atherosclerotic cardiovascular disease, stroke, neuromuscular disease, and major psychiatric disorders, as well as with hypogonadal states. Secondary impotence has interdependent multifactorial origins, including penile arterial and venous insufficiency, sacral and autonomic neuropathy, hypogonadism, and emotional disorders. (See also Ch. 58.)

Only hypogonadism may be treated successfully with androgens. The mainstays of the treatment of nonendocrine secondary impotence currently include the use of intracorporeal papaverine to dilate the penile arteries, vacuum tumescence devices to induce cavernosal filling and impair venous return, and, as a last resort, penile prosthesis. In the older man, psychotherapy alone is not likely to be successful.

74. LIPOPROTEIN METABOLISM

Charles J. Glueck and *E. Gordon Margolin*

A new era of preventive medicine has dawned in the management of atherosclerosis. Better understanding of lipoprotein metabolism and coronary heart disease **(CHD)** suggests that atherosclerotic disease is controllable in the elderly and that the major risk factors contributing to CHD (hypertension, dyslipoproteinemia, smoking, obesity, and impaired glucose tolerance) can be reduced by dietary changes, weight control, smoking reduction or cessation, and (if needed) drug therapy.

Seven major primary and secondary CHD prevention trials have recently demonstrated that lowering plasma total cholesterol **(TC)** and low-density lipoprotein cholesterol **(LDL-C)** and raising high-density lipoprotein cholesterol **(HDL-C)** by diet alone or with a variety of lipid-modulating drugs (cholestyramine, nicotinic acid, colestipol plus nicotinic acid, gemfibrozil) may be effective in prevention of CHD, in stabilization of the arterial atherosclerotic lesion, and in regression of some arterial atherosclerotic lesions.

LIPIDS AS CORONARY HEART DISEASE RISK FACTORS

Primary Prevention

The Oslo Heart Trial compared subjects who used dietary and smoking-reduction interventions with a nonintervention group; this was, of necessity, not a blind study. The intervention group showed a 47% reduction in CHD events.

The Lipid Research Clinics' Coronary Primary Prevention Trial **(LRC-CPPT)** was a multicenter, randomized, double-blind, 7-yr test of the efficacy of lowering cholesterol in 3806 asymptomatic men with primary hypercholesterolemia. The men, aged 35 to 59 yr at study onset, were initially free of overt CHD. With cholestyramine resin and dietary intervention, their TC and LDL-C levels were reduced by 8 and 11% beyond placebo levels, and HDL-C increased by 3% on the average. A 21% reduction in deaths from CHD was reported, along with a 17% reduction in all CHD endpoints and a 19% reduction in CHD events.

The Helsinki Heart Trial was a multicenter, randomized, double-blind, 5-yr study of the efficacy of simultaneously raising HDL-C and lowering non-HDL cholesterol with gemfibrozil and diet. Studies were carried out in 4081 asymptomatic men 40 to 55 yr of age with non-HDL cholesterol $\geq$ 200 mg/dL. One group of men (n=2051) received 600 mg gemfibrozil bid while another group (n=2030) received placebo. Gemfibrozil increased HDL-C by 11% and reduced TC by 10%, LDL-C by 11%, and triglycerides by 35% from baseline levels.

In the gemfibrozil group, the cumulative rate of cardiac endpoints at 5 yr was 27.3/1000 compared with 41.4/1000 in the placebo group, a reduction of 34% (p < 0.02). The reduction in incidence of CHD in the subjects receiving gemfibrozil became evident in the 2nd yr of the trial and continued throughout. From the 3rd to the 5th yr, the number of CHD endpoints in the gemfibrozil group was about $^1/_3$ to $^1/_2$ the number in the placebo group. On the basis of the Cox proportional hazards model, the reduction in CHD risk could be attributed to both decreased LDL-C and increased HDL-C.

Secondary Prevention

Four major recent secondary prevention studies based on dietary intervention alone (Leiden Heart Study), diet plus nicotinic acid (Coronary Drug Project), cholestyramine plus diet (National Heart, Lung, and Blood Institute [NHLBI] Type II trial), and diet plus colestipol plus nicotinic acid (Cholesterol-Lowering Atherosclerosis Study [CLAS]) all suggest that reductions in LDL-C and/or increases in HDL-C can reduce progression of coronary artery atherosclerosis, and in some cases, induce regression. Of these, CLAS is probably the most important study.

The CLAS was a randomized, placebo-controlled, angiographic trial to evaluate the effects of lowering LDL-C and elevating HDL-C with combined colestipol and niacin in 162 nonsmoking men, aged 40 to 59 yr, who had previous coronary artery bypass surgery. These subjects received 30 gm colestipol plus 3 to 12 gm niacin/day; over 2 yr of treatment, there was a 26% reduction in plasma TC, a 43% reduction in LDL-C, and a concurrent 37% increase in HDL-C. Compared with the placebo group, the drug-treated group had a progressive reduction in average number of coronary artery atherosclerotic lesions per subject (p < 0.03), as well as a reduction in percentage of subjects with new atheromata formation in the native coronary arteries (p < 0.03). In addition, the percentage of drug-treated subjects with new lesions (p < 0.04) or any adverse change in bypass grafts (p < 0.03) was significantly reduced. Atherosclerosis regression, as indicated by perceptible improvement in overall coronary artery status, occurred in 16.2% of the treatment group, compared with 2.4% of the placebo group (p = 0.002).

The CLAS was the first controlled clinical angiographic trial to provide unequivocal evidence that lowering LDL-C, elevating HDL-C, and reducing triglycerides leads to both cessation of progression and regression of human coronary atherosclerotic lesions. Evidence remained strong even when the results were divided to compare treatment effects when plasma TC entry levels were above and below 240 mg/dL. This evidence implies that all cholesterol levels ranging from 185 to 350 mg/dL are relevant to coronary risk and should be reduced through appropriate medical treatment.

Effects of Age

In the LRC-CPPT, which enrolled men at baseline ages of 35 to 59 yr, it was found over a 7-yr follow-up period that for every 1% drop in plasma TC, there was a 2% reduction in CHD events. The latter reduction *was not* affected by age at entry into the study. Reduction of plasma TC and LDL-C by diet alone was greater in older than in younger subjects.

The geriatric population has been included in the sharp decline in cardiovascular mortality during the past 2 decades. This decline may reflect the effects of reduced CHD risk factors (eg, lower plasma cholesterol, increased physical activity, reduced dietary intake of saturated fats and cholesterol, reduced smoking, and better control of hypertension). The 20-yr follow-up of the Framingham study found that the following cardiovascular risk factors were significantly and positively associated with the incidence of CHD: LDL-C elevation, systolic hypertension, electrocardiographic evidence of left ventricular hypertrophy, and diabetes (only in women). In addition, in both men and women, HDL-C was significantly inversely associated with CHD incidence.

Most recently, on the basis of the 32-yr follow-up data from the Framingham study, the atherogenic potential of serum cholesterol has been reexamined. The TC/HDL-C ratio accounts for a significant CHD risk gradient associated with CHD > 50 yr of age. The average serum TC for patients with CHD was 225 mg/dL in men and 248 mg/dL in women; average HDL-C levels for men and women with CHD were 43 and 48 mg/dL, average LDL-C levels were 148 and 164 mg/dL, and TC/HDL-C ratios were 5.6 and 5.0 for men and women, respectively. Triglyceride levels influenced CHD risk at any HDL-C level but only in women. However, in both sexes, CHD risk at any triglyceride level was strongly influenced by the level of HDL-C.

On a population-wide basis, Framingham data indicate that the TC/HDL-C ratio is highly predictive of CHD in the elderly. In 26-yr follow-up Framingham data, the risk of CHD in subjects between the ages of 50 and 90 yr increased with the ratio of TC to HDL-C as follows: At a TC/HDL-C ratio < 3.5, the risk of CHD (age-adjusted rate/1000) was 70 for men and 36 for women; at a ratio of 3.5 to 5.4, the risk was 93 and 86, respectively. At a ratio of 5.5 to 7.4, the risk was 152 for men and 70 for women; at a ratio of 7.5 to 9.4, it was 176 and 171, and at a ratio ≥ 9.5, it was 275 and 281, respectively.

In both the Framingham and LRC-CPPT studies, the levels of plasma TC in men increased until about age 60, then declined; in women, the increase was more gradual and, at approximately age 55 to 60, plasma

TC values exceeded those in men. In both studies, mean levels of HDL-C increased after age 55 in men but declined after age 65 in women. However, even in elderly women, mean HDL-C levels were approximately 10 mg/dL higher than in men. In the Framingham study, the ratio of plasma TC/HDL-C increased up to age 80 in women, while it peaked at age 45 and remained stable in men, albeit at a higher level than in women. Similar findings, particularly for HDL-C, have been reported in the Oslo study and in the Israeli Ischemic Heart Disease Study.

Most mammalian species age without developing atherosclerosis. *CHD is neither natural nor necessary, and its prevention does not mean that it will be replaced by other chronic diseases. It is reasonable to expect that CHD morbidity and mortality can be reduced in older persons.*

There is substantial evidence that blood lipid and lipoprotein cholesterol levels, which are so potently influenced by heredity, diet, and obesity, influence atherogenesis in the elderly. In individuals with primary and familial aggregations of top decile HDL-C levels (familial hyperalphalipoproteinemia), CHD is rare and life expectancy is prolonged. Similarly, in individuals with familial hypobetalipoproteinemia with hereditary depression of LDL-C (bottom decile), CHD is rare and life expectancy is prolonged. Conversely, in **progeria,** a premature aging syndrome, moderate elevation of plasma TC and LDL-C and marked depression of HDL-C have been reported. Moreover, in total lipodystrophy and Cockayne's syndrome, 2 other premature aging syndromes, very low levels of HDL-C are common.

Although in aggregate, epidemiologic studies show a clear-cut relationship between LDL-C, TC, HDL-C, and CHD morbidity and mortality in the elderly, the relationship of these factors to stroke is less clear. Specifically, no positive relationship between serum cholesterol and the occurrence of atherothrombotic brain infarction has yet been demonstrated in the Framingham study.

Postmenopausal Estrogens, Lipids, and CHD

One special consideration in older women is the effect of menopause on lipids, lipoproteins, and the development of atherosclerosis. The life expectancy of USA women is about 78 yr, with approximately ⅓ of these years being postmenopausal. CHD events increase substantially during menopause for women > 50 yr of age. Heart disease accounts for approximately ⅓ of all deaths in 50- to 69-yr-old women.

The lower rates of CHD in premenopausal women compared with those in men may be related to their lower plasma LDL-C and higher HDL-C levels, which result in part from endogenous estrogens. This protection against CHD is lost in women who undergo surgical or early natural menopause. In the Lipid Research Clinics' 1972 to 1976 prevalence study, approximately ⅓ of postmenopausal women received estrogen replacement; this was associated with lower LDL-C and higher HDL-C levels, resulting in a substantial decrease in the LDL-C/HDL-C ratio. Such changes might be expected to reduce CHD risk in women.

In the Lipid Research Clinics' 8-yr longitudinal follow-up study of postmenopausal women, comparing 1677 nonusers of estrogen with 593 users, the relative risk for cardiovascular death in estrogen users was 0.34, a statistically significant reduction. It was hypothesized that this benefit was mediated by higher HDL-C and lower LDL-C levels associated with estrogen use. Similar benefits were reported in a prospective study of estrogen use by nurses, published in 1985, but such observations are not uniform. For example, Framingham participants using estrogen after menopause were reported at $\geq$ 1 examinations to have a > 50% higher risk for cardiovascular morbidity and more than twice the risk for cerebrovascular disease than nonusers. Mortality from all causes and cardiovascular disease did not differ between the 2 groups.

Because of the increased risk of endometrial hyperplasia and cancer from unopposed estrogen, postmenopausal estrogen is often administered in combination with progestins, many of which lower HDL-C and raise LDL-C levels. Almost all epidemiologic studies of postmenopausal estrogen use and CHD were done *before* the current practice of adding progestins evolved. Moreover, a fasting lipid profile should be obtained before initiating estrogen supplementation, since estrogen use is contraindicated in women with familial hypertriglyceridemia because of the increased risk of pancreatitis.

Much of the evidence regarding postmenopausal estrogen use suggests, but not unequivocally, that the resultant alterations in lipids and lipoprotein cholesterol may reduce CHD morbidity and mortality. Controlled clinical trial data are needed to document whether and to what degree postmenopausal estrogen supplementation ameliorates CHD. (See also OVARIAN HORMONE THERAPY in Ch. 72.)

Age-Related Distribution of Lipids and Lipoprotein Cholesterol

In 1988, the National Cholesterol Education Program (NCEP) recommended simplified guidelines not specific to race or sex for identifying elevated cholesterol and LDL-C levels; it also identified a single HDL-C level (< 35 mg/dL) as being associated with increased CHD risk (see TABLE 74-1). According to these guidelines, if TC is < 200 mg/dL, measurement of TC every 5 yr, using a nonfasting blood sample, is recommended, with no further follow-up. If initial TC $\geq$ 240 mg/dL, a repeat fasting TC measurement is advised. If the average of the 2 samples is $\geq$ 240 mg/dL, follow-up lipoprotein analysis after a 12-h fast is recommended.

For persons with an average TC of 200 to 239 mg/dL (on 2 samples), who have no CHD and a CHD risk factor score < 2 (as described below), NCEP guidelines recommend that TC be measured at least annually and that a low-saturated-fat, low-cholesterol diet be followed. For individuals with a TC of 200 to 239 mg/dL *and* CHD *or* a CHD risk factor of $\geq$ 2, lipoprotein analysis (after a 12-h fast) is recommended for follow-up. The CHD risk score is determined by totaling points for the following risk factors, each of which is assigned 1 point: male sex, family history of heart attack in parents or siblings < 55 yr of age, smoking $\geq$ 10 cigarettes/day, high BP, low levels of the protective lipoprotein cholesterol (HDL-C $<$ 35 mg/dL on 2 measurements), diabetes mellitus, definite stroke or peripheral vascular disease, severe obesity ($\geq$ 30% overweight).

TABLE 74–1. RECOMMENDATIONS OF THE NATIONAL CHOLESTEROL EDUCATION PROGRAM FOR CLASSIFICATION, TREATMENT, AND RISK DETERMINATION OF CORONARY HEART DISEASE

Initial Classification and Recommended Follow-up Based on Total Cholesterol

Classification, mg/dL	
< 200	Desirable blood cholesterol
200 to 239	Borderline-high blood cholesterol, borderline-high risk
≥ 240	High blood cholesterol, high risk
Recommended follow-up	
Total cholesterol < 200 mg/dL	Repeat within 5 yr
Total cholesterol 200–239 mg/dL	
Without definite CHD or 2 other CHD risk factors (1 of which can be male sex)	Dietary information and recheck annually
With definite CHD or 2 other CHD risk factors (1 of which can be male sex)	Lipoprotein analysis; further action based on LDL-C level
Total cholesterol ≥ 240 mg/dL	Lipoprotein analysis; further action based on LDL-C level

Classification and Treatment Decisions Based on LDL-Cholesterol

Classification, mg/dL		
< 130	Desirable LDL-C	
130 to 159	Borderline-high-risk LDL-C	
≥ 160	High-risk LDL-C	
	Initiation level, mg/dL	Minimal goal, mg/dL
Dietary treatment		
Without CHD or 2 other risk factors*	≥ 160	< 160†
With CHD or 2 or other risk factors*	≥ 130	< 130‡
Drug treatment§		
Without CHD or 2 other risk factors*	≥ 190	< 160
With CHD or 2 other risk factors*	≥ 160	< 130

(Continued)

CHD = coronary heart disease; LDL-C = low-density lipoprotein cholesterol.
(Please see next page for explanation of footnote symbols.)

TABLE 74–1. RECOMMENDATIONS OF THE NATIONAL
CHOLESTEROL EDUCATION PROGRAM FOR CLASSIFICATION,
TREATMENT, AND RISK DETERMINATION OF CORONARY HEART
DISEASE *(Cont'd)*

Risk Status Based on Presence of CHD Risk Factors Other Than LDL-C

The patient is considered to have a high risk status if he has 1 of the following:
  Definite CHD: the characteristic clinical picture and objective laboratory findings of
    either:
  Definite prior myocardial infarction, or
  Definite myocardial ischemia, such as angina pectoris
  2 other CHD risk factors:
    Male sex* *
    Family history of premature CHD (definite myocardial infarction or sudden death
      before 55 yr of age in a parent or sibling)
    Cigarette smoking (currently smokes > 10 cigarettes/day)
    Hypertension
    Low HDL-C concentration (< 35 mg/dL confirmed by repeated measurement)
    Diabetes mellitus
    History of definite cerebrovascular or occlusive peripheral vascular disease
    Severe obesity (≥ 30% overweight)

CHD = coronary heart disease; LDL-C = low-density lipoprotein cholesterol.

  * Patients have a lower initiation level and goal if they are at high risk because they already have definite CHD, or because they have any 2 of the following risk factors: male sex, family history of premature CHD, cigarette smoking, hypertension, low high-density lipoprotein (HDL)-cholesterol, diabetes mellitus, definite cerebrovascular or peripheral vascular disease, or severe obesity.

  † Roughly equivalent to total cholesterol level of < 240 mg/dL, which can be used as a goal for monitoring dietary treatment.

  ‡ Roughly equivalent to total cholesterol level of <200 mg/dL, which can be used as a goal for monitoring dietary treatment.

  § Drug treatment should usually not be considered until at least 6 months of dietary treatment has been intensively applied, with initiation levels given referring to levels on dietary treatment.

  * * Male sex is considered a risk factor in this scheme because the rates of CHD are 3 to 4 times higher in men than in women in the middle decades of life and roughly 2 times higher in the elderly. Hence, a man with 1 other CHD risk factor is considered to have a high-risk status, whereas a woman is not so considered unless she has 2 other CHD risk factors.

  (From the National Cholesterol Education Program Expert Panel Recommendations, *Archives of Internal Medicine,* Vol. 148, pp. 36-69, 1988. Used with permission.)

Although the NCEP guidelines are very useful for wide scale population screening, they pose a disadvantage to the elderly. Because of the importance of HDL-C to CHD risk, there is a relatively high possibility that elderly persons would be misclassified under these guidelines, by not measuring low HDL-C in those who seem to have desirable TC levels (< 200 mg/dL) or by not obtaining lipoprotein profiles in those whose TC is 200 to 239 mg/dL. Within this frame of reference, it is probably reasonable in screening the elderly to obtain a fasting lipid profile and to use age-sex-race–specific data to characterize CHD risk.

The American Heart Association's **(AHA)** position paper on hyperlipidemia in adults used age- and sex-specific lipid and lipoprotein cholesterol cutpoints from LRC prevalence studies, as summarized in TABLES 74–2 to 74–5. On the basis of the AHA guidelines for healthy American adults, desirable TC and LDL-C levels are below the LRC 25th percentile, while high levels are at or above the LRC 75th percentile.

TABLE 74–2. PLASMA TOTAL CHOLESTEROL (mg/dL)
POPULATION DISTRIBUTION

	White Men					White Women				
	Percentiles					Percentiles				
Age (yr)	10	25	50	75	90	10	25	50	75	90
45–49	171	188	210	235	258	162	182	204	231	256
50–54	168	189	211	237	263	171	188	214	240	267
55–59	172	188	214	236	260	182	201	229	251	278
60–64	170	191	215	237	262	186	207	226	251	282
65–69	174	192	213	250	275	179	212	233	259	282
70+	160	185	214	236	253	181	196	226	249	268

(From *The Lipid Research Clinics Population Studies Data Book, Vol 1: The Prevalence Study.* NIH publication No. 80-1527. Copyright 1980 by National Institutes of Health.)

TABLE 74–3. PLASMA LDL-C (mg/dL) POPULATION DISTRIBUTION

	White Men					White Women				
	Percentiles					Percentiles				
Age (yr)	10	25	50	75	90	10	25	50	75	90
45–49	106	120	141	163	186	89	105	127	150	173
50–54	102	118	143	162	185	94	111	134	160	186
55–59	103	123	145	168	191	97	120	145	168	199
60–64	106	121	143	165	188	105	126	149	168	191
65–69	104	125	146	170	199	99	125	151	184	205
70+	100	119	142	164	182	108	127	147	170	189

(From *The Lipid Research Clinics Population Studies Data Book, Vol. 1: The Prevalence Study.* NIH publication No. 80–1527. Copyright 1980 by National Institutes of Health.)

TABLE 74–4. PLASMA HDL-C (mg/dL) POPULATION DISTRIBUTION

| | White Men | | | | | White Women | | | | |
| | Percentiles | | | | | Percentiles | | | | |
Age (yr)	10	25	50	75	90	10	25	50	75	90
45–49	33	38	45	52	60	41	47	58	68	82
50–54	31	36	44	51	58	41	50	62	73	85
55–59	31	38	46	55	64	41	50	60	73	85
60–64	34	41	49	61	69	44	51	61	75	87
65–69	33	39	49	62	74	38	49	62	73	85
70+	33	40	48	56	70	38	48	60	71	82

(From *The Lipid Research Clinics Population Studies Data Book, Vol. 1: The Prevalence Study.* NIH publication No. 80–1527. Copyright 1980 by National Institutes of Health.)

TABLE 74–5. PLASMA TRIGLYCERIDES (mg/dL) POPULATION DISTRIBUTION

| | White Men | | | | | White Women | | | | |
| | Percentiles | | | | | Percentiles | | | | |
Age (yr)	10	25	50	75	90	10	25	50	75	90
45–49	65	88	119	165	218	55	71	94	139	180
50–54	75	94	128	178	244	58	75	103	144	190
55–59	70	85	117	167	210	65	80	111	163	229
60–64	65	84	111	150	193	66	78	105	143	210
65–69	61	78	108	164	227	64	86	118	158	221
70+	71	87	115	152	202	68	83	110	141	189

(From *The Lipid Research Clinics Population Studies Data Book, Vol. 1: The Prevalence Study.* NIH publication No. 80–1527. Copyright 1980 by National Institutes of Health.)

Particularly in women, the increase in plasma TC with age is due primarily to an increase in LDL-C and much less to the small increase in very low-density lipoprotein cholesterol **(VLDL-C).** There is a small increase in HDL-C in men > 65 yr of age, compared with a decrease in HDL-C in women of that age. The rate at which LDL-C rises accelerates from age 25 to 50, and by age 55, the concentration in women equals (and later exceeds) that in men.

Because LDL-C levels increase with age, and because in women HDL-C levels actually fall with age, the risk for CHD in the elderly gradually increases in the absence of intervention. CHD mortality in men and women $\geq$ 70 yr of age is 2.5 times greater in those with cholesterol concentrations in the upper quartile than in those with concentrations in the lower quartile.

The lipid and lipoprotein cholesterol values in TABLES 74–2 to 74–5 were obtained using the Centers for Disease Control standardized methodology and plasma samples drawn after a 12-h fast. Because many commercial laboratories do not use these standards, they tend to report higher cholesterol levels and are less accurate in measuring TC and HDL-C. Physicians should determine whether the laboratories they use follow a national standardization program, because a difference of 5 mg/dL in HDL-C level has significant consequences in CHD rate.

MANAGEMENT OF HYPERCHOLESTEROLEMIA

*The National Cholesterol Education Program **(NCEP)** Guidelines for 1988 (which are not specific for age, sex, or race) identified a TC level of < 200 mg/dL as desirable, 200 to 239 mg/dL as borderline high, and ≥ 240 mg/dL as high.*

According to these cutpoints, approximately ⅓ of adult Americans have TC levels of ≥ 240 mg/dL, approximately ⅓ have levels of 200 to 239 mg/dL, and ⅓ have levels of < 200 mg/dL. Predating the introduction of these simplified NCEP guidelines, the National Consensus Conference on lowering cholesterol identified for persons < 20, 20 to 39, and ≥ 40 yr old cholesterol levels of 200, 220, and 240 mg/dL, respectively, as representing moderate risk, and 220, 240, and 260 mg/dL, respectively, as high risk. These moderate and high-risk cutpoints correspond roughly to the 75th and 90th percentiles of the population. The National Consensus Conference guidelines and the NCEP guidelines recommend respectively that individuals in the top quartile for plasma TC should be treated, as should those with LDL-C ≥ 160 mg/dL.

Treatment should be primarily dietary in those between the 75th and 90th percentiles, and with diet and medications when necessary in those above the 90th percentile. Familiarity with the following is particularly important: the phenotypic classification of dyslipidemia (TABLE 74–6), the differentiation of primary from secondary causes (TABLE 74–7), the history and major physical findings associated with the dyslipoproteinemias (TABLE 74–8), the systematic approach to the diagnosis and therapy of hypercholesterolemia (TABLE 74–1 and FIG. 74–1), including stepped dietary interventions (TABLES 74–9 and 74–10) and, if necessary, drug therapy (TABLE 74–11).

Screening for Hypercholesterolemia

In the interpretation of cholesterol measurements, no single value should be relied upon to classify a patient clinically. There may be significant day-to-day variations in values; the phenomenon known as regression toward the mean predicts that the second measurement in individuals having a high initial value will often be considerably lower. If a lipid or lipoprotein cholesterol abnormality is found on the first screening test, at least 2 subsequent evaluations should be performed (FIG. 74–1).

TABLE 74–6. PHENOTYPIC CLASSIFICATION OF DYSLIPIDEMIA*

Phenotype	Lipoprotein Abnormality	Typical Lipid Values (mg/dL)	Comments
I	Chylomicrons	TC 150–400 TG 1000–15,000 HDL-C ≤ 35	Typically presents in childhood; risk of pancreatitis; creamy layer over a clear plasma layer after centrifugation
IIA	LDL	TC 250–1000 TG 50–200 LDL-C ≥ 160	Severe premature atherosclerosis; plasma clear or may have increased orange tint
IIB	LDL and VLDL	TC 250–1000 TG 200–400 LDL-C ≥ 160	Severe premature atherosclerosis; plasma cloudy, opalescent
III	IDL and chylomicron remnants	TC 200–800 TG 300–1400 HDL-C ≤ 40	TC and TG often nearly equal; plasma cloudy, opalescent; possible creamy layer on top; very diet sensitive; severe premature atherosclerosis
IV	VLDL	TC 150–350 TG 300–800 HDL-C ≤ 40	TG much higher than TC; plasma cloudy, opalescent; often secondary to other diseases/drugs; premature atherosclerosis
V	VLDL and chylomicrons	TC 200–800 TG 1,000–150,000 HDL-C ≤ 35	Creamy layer over an opalescent or cloudy layer after centrifugation; premature atherosclerosis; abdominal pain, pancreatitis

(Continued)

TABLE 74–6. PHENOTYPIC CLASSIFICATION OF DYSLIPIDEMIA*
(Cont'd)

Phenotype	Lipoprotein Abnormality	Typical Lipid Values (mg/dL)	Comments
Hypoalphalipoproteinemia	HDL	HDL-C ≤ 35 TG < 250 TC < 250	Severe premature atherosclerosis, stroke, peripheral vascular disease
Hyperalphalipo-proteinemia	HDL	HDL-C ≥ 75 TG < 250 TC < 250	Protection against CHD, stroke; increased longevity
Hypobetalipoproteinemia	LDL	LDL-C ≤ 100 TG < 250	Protection against CHD, stroke; increased longevity

TC = total cholesterol; TG = triglycerides; HDL-C = high-density lipoprotein cholesterol; LDL-C = low-density lipoprotein cholesterol; IDL = intermediate-density lipoprotein.

* Phenotype is qualitative; quantitation of the lipoprotein cholesterols and triglycerides is required.

There are 2 major disadvantages to obtaining only TC values for the initial screening test. First, many people with CHD have normal TC and triglyceride levels but an HDL-C ≤ the 10th percentile. They are at *very high risk* for progression of CHD. Second, particularly in the elderly, it is probable that some physicians will misclassify as hypercholesterolemic some persons with a high HDL-C level, not recognizing that this accounts for their high TC and that they are, in fact, at *reduced* risk for CHD.

In the elderly, a better screening test might include TC and HDL-C, both of which can be obtained using nonfasting blood; or most definitively, TC, triglycerides, HDL-C, and calculated LDL-C (if triglycerides are < 400 mg/dL) after a 12-h fast. The TC and, to a lesser degree, the HDL-C measurements are not significantly affected by eating, whereas triglyceride levels are very sensitive to food and can be accurately measured only after a fast.

Cholesterol and lipoprotein cholesterol fractions should *not* be measured in the following situations, since the levels found are usually *not* representative of basal state and could be misleading: (1) when a patient is febrile; (2) during or within 4 wk of an acute MI, stroke, or major surgery (eg, coronary artery bypass or peripheral bypass surgery); (3) immediately following acute excessive alcohol intake; (4) during any ma-

TABLE 74–7. SECONDARY CAUSES OF BLOOD LIPID
ABNORMALITIES

Increased Cholesterol, LDL-C	Increased TG, Low HDL-C
Diseases	
Hypothyroidism*	Poorly controlled diabetes*
Obstructive liver disease†	Alcoholic hepatitis, alcoholism*
Nephrotic syndrome†	Severe metabolic stress (MI, cerebrovascular accident)*
Uremia†	Hypothyroidism*
Orthostatic proteinuria	Obstructive liver disease, acute hepatitis†
Dysproteinemias (myeloma, Waldenström's)‡	Nephrotic syndrome†
Acute intermittent porphyria‡	Uremia (with or without dialysis)*
Anorexia nervosa‡	Dysproteinemias, lupus erythematosus‡
Cushing's syndrome‡	Glycogen storage disease‡
Poorly controlled diabetes*	Idiopathic hypercalcemia‡
	Chlorinated hydrocarbon exposure‡
Diet	
Excess dietary saturated fat, cholesterol*	Alcohol excess* (may elevate both TG and HDL-C)
Drugs	
Corticosteroids*	Corticosteroids*
Androgenic steroids*	Estrogens, oral contraceptives*
Progestins*	Synthetic vitamin A compounds (for acne)*
Thiazide diuretics*	β-Blockers*
	Androgenic steroids (*low* HDL-C)*
	Smoking (*low* HDL-C)*
	Zinc (*low* HDL-C)

* Common.
† Occasional.
‡ Rare.

jor infection (eg, pneumonia, pyelonephritis); (5) when diabetes mellitus
is severely out of control; or (6) during rapid weight loss from severe
hypocaloric intake.

Classification of Dyslipidemia

Phenotypes are a qualitative way of categorizing patients. In the past,
electrophoretic lipoprotein phenotyping (which was qualitative), coupled
with measurement of TC and LDL-C, was used to segregate and differentiate various types of dyslipoproteinemia. More recently, quantitation
of lipoprotein cholesterol and triglyceride levels has supplanted the

older phenotypic system. The parallel and supplementary natures of these 2 classification systems are summarized in TABLE 74–6.

The NCEP guidelines use total serum cholesterol as the initial discriminant, and then move to LDL-C as a major determinant of risk. HDL-C < 35 mg/dL is also identified as a discriminant associated with increased risk.

Most individuals with dyslipidemia fall into 3 major categories, as follows:

1. Hypercholesterolemia with elevations of LDL-C, often with moderate elevations of triglyceride and modest reductions in HDL-C levels. In the older, qualitative phenotypic system, the lipoprotein phenotypes are IIA (triglyceride levels normal) and IIB (triglyceride levels high).

2. Hypertriglyceridemia, with elevations of VLDL-C, usually with low HDL-C and normal or low LDL-C levels.

When triglycerides are markedly elevated (usually > 1000 mg/dL), chylomicrons are usually present in addition to the increased triglycerides and VLDL-C.

3. Hypoalphalipoproteinemia (bottom decile for HDL-C), often with normal TC and LDL-C and normal to modestly elevated triglyceride levels.

After documenting the nature of the dyslipidemia (TABLE 74–6) and evaluating for secondary causes of blood lipid abnormalities (TABLE 74–7), if secondary causes can be ruled out, the dyslipidemia is usually one of the common familial hyperlipidemias (TABLE 74–8).

When familial, the 3 dominantly transmitted dyslipoproteinemias—elevations of LDL-C, elevated VLDL-C and triglycerides, elevated VLDL-C plus triglycerides *with* associated chylomicronemia (types II, IV, and V hyperlipoproteinemia in the older lipoprotein phenotyping system)—are common in free-living, unselected individuals, each type estimated to affect approximately 1/200 to 1/500 persons. Familial hypercholesterolemia or hypoalphalipoproteinemia may not be as prevalent in the elderly as in the general population because of the higher mortality (especially from CHD) in the former, which removes affected subjects from survival cohorts.

Most physicians will probably never see a patient with typical familial chylomicronemia (Type I hyperlipoproteinemia). However, familial chylomicronemia with increased VLDL triglyceride (Type V lipoproteinemia) is more common, although not nearly as common as familial hypercholesterolemia and hypertriglyceridemia (TABLES 74–6 and 74–8).

There are also a significant number of elderly persons with predominant hyperalphalipoproteinemia, ie, HDL-C levels > 75 mg/dL (TABLE 74–6). These individuals, usually with hereditary high HDL-C, are *protected* against CHD and stroke and have increased longevity. Similarly,

TABLE 74–8. CLINICAL HISTORY AND PHYSICAL FINDINGS FOR
FAMILIAL HYPERLIPIDEMIA

Lipoprotein Phenotype/ Lipoprotein Abnormality	Physical Findings	Clinical History and Findings	Mode of Inheritance; Estimated Prevalence
I High TG, primarily chylomicrons	Eruptive xanthomas* Hepatosplenomegaly* Lipemia retinalis*	Recurrent abdominal pain* Pancreatitis*	Recessive; 1/1,000,000 (?)
II High TC, LDL-C, with or without high TG	Periorbital xanthelasma† Tendon xanthomas*‡ Tuberous xanthomas‡§ Arcus juvenilis corneae*	MI, angina*, **, †† Tenosynovitis (achilles, patellar)*	Dominant; 1/200-1/500
III High TC, high TG, high IDL (beta migrating VLDL)	Palmar-planar xanthomas††‡ Tuberous xanthomas††‡ Tendon xanthomas‡§	MI, stroke, peripheral vascular disease, claudication, carotid obstruction*, **, †† Glucose intolerance† Hyperuricemia† Essential hypertension* Obesity*	Recessive; 1/1000 (?)

(Continued)

TG = triglycerides; TC = total cholesterol; LDL-C = low-density lipoprotein cholesterol; IDL = intermediate-density lipoproteins, VLDL = very low-density lipoproteins; HDL-C = high-density lipoprotein cholesterol.

* Common.

† Occasional.

§ When present, these physical findings are almost always diagnostic of familial hyperlipidemia.

‡ Rare.

** Often in subject *and* common in first-degree relatives.

†† Premature cardiovascular disease in subject and, commonly, in first-degree relatives.

there are a significant number of individuals with familial hypobetalipoproteinemia, usually with LDL-C levels < 100 mg/dL and with normal triglyceride levels (TABLE 74–6). These persons are also *protected* against CHD and stroke.

The genes responsible for the eventual clinical expression of Type III hyperlipidemia (TABLES 74–6 and 74–8) appear to be relatively common, but clinical cases are very rare, occurring in only an estimated 1% of those with the appropriate genetic background.

TABLE 74–8. CLINICAL HISTORY AND PHYSICAL FINDINGS FOR
FAMILIAL HYPERLIPIDEMIA (Cont'd)

Lipoprotein Phenotype/ Lipoprotein Abnormality	Physical Findings	Clinical History and Findings	Mode of Inheritance; Estimated Prevalence
IV High TG, VLDL TG, and cholesterol	Periorbital xanthelasma[†]	MI, stroke*, **, †† Glucose intolerance* Hyperuricemia* Obesity* Essential hypertension*	Dominant; 1/200
V High TG, VLDL TG, and chylomicron TG	Eruptive xanthomas[†] Hepatosplenomegaly* Peripheral sensory neuropathy*	MI, stroke*, **, †† Abdominal pain, pancreatitis* Glucose intolerance* Hyperuricemia* Essential hypertension* Obesity*	Dominant; 1/1000 (?)
Hypoalphalipo-proteinemia Low HDL-C with normal TC and TG	None	MI, stroke*, **, †† Hyperuricemia* Glucose intolerance* Essential hypertension* Obesity*	Dominant; 1/200

In familial type III hyperlipidemia, the basic metabolic defect involves an abnormality in apolipoprotein E. Changes in the charge of apolipoprotein E appear to retard the clearance of the E-rich, intermediate-density lipoproteins in the liver by the B-E receptor. However, the apolipoprotein E defect, while apparently *necessary* for the expression of the type III phenotype, is not *sufficient*. There are other, as yet poorly understood, contributing factors that in the presence of this defect, lead to the expression of the dyslipoproteinemia.

Secondary Causes of Dyslipidemia

After finding an abnormal lipid or lipoprotein cholesterol level (and confirming it on at least 1, and preferably 2, follow-up samples), before any therapeutic intervention is initiated, particularly in older persons, it is important to distinguish between primary and/or familial dyslipoproteinemia and that which is secondary to a variety of diseases, diets, and drugs (TABLE 74–7).

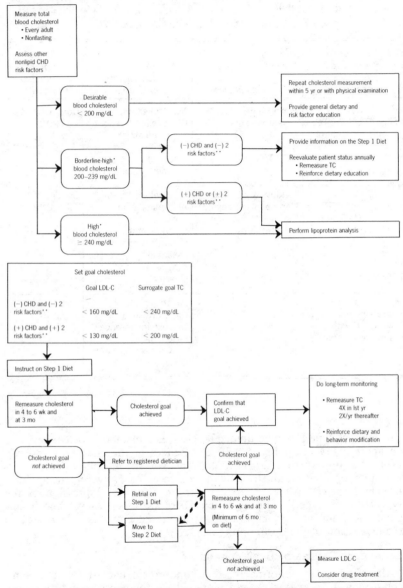

FIG. 74–1. Stepwise National Cholesterol Education Program approach to the diagnosis and therapy of elevated total serum cholesterol and LDL-C. (From the National Cholesterol Education Program Expert Panel Recommendations, *Archives of Internal Medicine*, Vol. 148, pp. 36-69, 1988. Used with permission.)

* Must be confirmed by obtaining repeat blood cholesterol measurements and then using the mean value.

** Male sex; family history of heart attack in parents or siblings before age 55 yr; ≥ 10 cigarettes/day; high BP; low levels of protective lipoprotein cholesterol (HDL-C < 35 mg/dL on 2 measurements); diabetes mellitus; definite stroke or peripheral vascular disease; severe obesity (≥ 30% overweight).

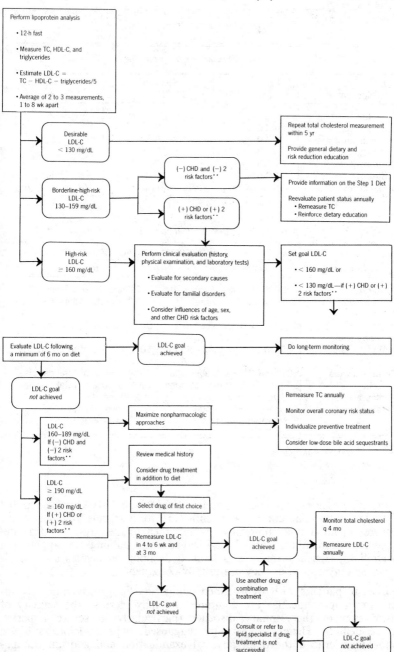

Perform lipoprotein analysis

- 12-h fast
- Measure TC, HDL-C, and triglycerides
- Estimate LDL-C = TC − HDL-C − triglycerides/5
- Average of 2 to 3 measurements, 1 to 8 wk apart

Desirable LDL-C < 130 mg/dL

Repeat total cholesterol measurement within 5 yr

Provide general dietary and risk reduction education

Borderline-high-risk LDL-C 130–159 mg/dL

(−) CHD and (−) 2 risk factors**

(+) CHD or (+) 2 risk factors**

Provide information on the Step 1 Diet

Reevaluate patient status annually
- Remeasure TC
- Reinforce dietary education

High-risk LDL-C ≥ 160 mg/dL

Perform clinical evaluation (history, physical examination, and laboratory tests)
- Evaluate for secondary causes
- Evaluate for familial disorders
- Consider influences of age, sex, and other CHD risk factors

Set goal LDL-C
- < 160 mg/dL or
- < 130 mg/dL—if (+) CHD or (+) 2 risk factors**

Evaluate LDL-C following a minimum of 6 mo on diet

LDL-C goal achieved

Do long-term monitoring

LDL-C goal not achieved

LDL-C 160–189 mg/dL If (−) CHD and (−) 2 risk factors**

Maximize nonpharmacologic approaches

Remeasure TC annually

Monitor overall coronary risk status

Individualize preventive treatment

Consider low-dose bile acid sequestrants

LDL-C ≥ 190 mg/dL or ≥ 160 mg/dL If (+) CHD or (+) 2 risk factors**

Review medical history

Consider drug treatment in addition to diet

Select drug of first choice

Remeasure LDL-C in 4 to 6 wk and at 3 mo

LDL-C goal achieved

Monitor total cholesterol q 4 mo

Remeasure LDL-C annually

LDL-C goal not achieved

Use another drug or combination treatment

Consult or refer to lipid specialist if drug treatment is not successsful

LDL-C goal not achieved

TABLE 74–9. STEPWISE APPROACHES TO DIETARY TREATMENT OF HYPERCHOLESTEROLEMIA

American Heart Association Diet

Nutrient*	Phase I (%)	Phase II (%)	Phase III (%)
Total fat	30	25	20
Saturated	10	8	7
Polyunsaturated	10	8	7
Monounsaturated	10	8	7
Carbohydrate	55	60	65
Protein	15	15	15
Cholesterol	< 300 mg/day	200–250 mg/day	100–150 mg/day

National Cholesterol Education Program Diet

Nutrient	Recommended Intake	
	Step-1 Diet	Step-2 Diet
Total fat	< 30% of total calories	< 30% of total calories
Saturated fatty acids	< 10% of total calories	< 7% of total calories
Polyunsaturated fatty acids	Up to 10% of total calories	Up to 10% of total calories
Monounsaturated fatty acids	10% to 15% of total calories	10% to 15% of total calories
Carbohydrates	50% to 60% of total calories	50% to 60% of total calories
Protein	10% to 20% of total calories	10% to 20% of total calories
Cholesterol	< 300 mg/day	< 200 mg/day
Total calories	To achieve and maintain desirable weight	To achieve and maintain desirable weight

* As % of total calories

In the absence of clinically useful dichotomous markers of familial dyslipoproteinemia, current convention is to first rule out secondary causes of blood lipid abnormalities and then to identify other first degree family members with dyslipidemia, thus enabling the appellation "familial." Hence, primary and familial dyslipoproteinemias are not always synonymous, but they are usually congruent.

Even in patients with well-defined familial dyslipoproteinemia, secondary dyslipoproteinemias are common and may increase the severity of expression of the primary disorder (particularly in severe hypertriglyceridemia). Hence, all newly diagnosed hyperlipidemic subjects should undergo a thorough physical examination and a drug, occupational, family, dietary, and alcohol-intake history. The following laboratory tests should also be performed: urinalysis, T_4, BUN or creatinine, fasting blood sugar, and liver function (TABLE 74–7). The causes of secondary hyperlipidemias should be treated when possible.

If all elderly Americans with TC > 200 mg/dL ($\geq$ 240 mg/dL for NCEP guidelines) are considered as being at moderate or high risk, the most common cause of secondary hypercholesterolemia is probably a diet high in saturated fat or cholesterol or such a diet superimposed on a polygenic tendency for hypercholesterolemia. Diseases and drugs that commonly cause high TC in this age group are listed in TABLE 74–7.

In older persons, the most common secondary causes of hypertriglyceridemia are excessive alcohol intake, exogenous estrogen supplementation, poorly controlled diabetes, uremia, corticosteroid use, and use of β-blockers. Isolated low levels of HDL-C, when plasma triglycerides are normal, may be secondary to smoking, androgenic steroid use, severe restriction of physical activity, or morbid obesity. Treatment of the underlying diseases or elimination of the offending drugs should ameliorate these conditions.

Primary and/or Familial Hyperlipidemia

Any geriatric patient who sustained an MI or stroke prior to age 60 should be assessed for primary and/or familial dyslipoproteinemia (TABLE 74 –8). An important factor in documenting familial dyslipidemia in this age group is that the most common familial dyslipoproteinemias are transmitted as autosomal dominant traits; hence $\frac{1}{2}$ of the offspring (themselves adults) of the geriatric population are similarly affected and should be screened.

Certain characteristic clinical and laboratory findings are useful in identifying subjects with primary and/or familial hyperlipidemia, eg, tendon, tuberous, and palmar-planar **xanthomas.**

Findings of obesity (with or without concurrent essential hypertension), glucose intolerance, and hyperuricemia should alert the physician to the likelihood of a concurrent primary hypertriglyceridemia or hypoalphalipoproteinemia.

Dietary Treatment

According to NCEP guidelines, if a person is identified as requiring lipoprotein analysis, the diagnostic and therapeutic goals shift from focusing on TC to LDL-C, as summarized in Table 74–1. **Treatment for high LDL-C should always be initiated with diet** (FIG. 74–1 and TABLES 74–9 and 74–10). The 3-phase diet approach recommended by the AHA has been simplified by the NCEP into a 2-step diet (TABLE 74–9). The NCEP panel recommends the Step 1 diet for high-risk persons but does not recommend intensive dietary therapy (eg, the Step 2 diet or the AHA Phase III diet) for most elderly patients. According to the panel,

TABLE 74–10. PRACTICAL APPROACH TO A LOW-CHOLESTEROL, LOW-SATURATED FAT DIET

Reduce Intake of:	Choose:	Use Substitutes:
1. **Meats and meat products** Fatty cuts of beef, lamb, pork, spareribs, organ meats, regular cold cuts, sausage, hot dogs	Fish, chicken and turkey (without the skin), lean cuts of beef, lamb, pork, veal	Cold cuts prepared from processed turkey, except those containing organ meats
2. **Dairy products, eggs** Whole milk (4%) fat, evaporated or condensed whole milk, cream, half-and-half, most nondairy creamers, whipped toppings	Skim or 1% fat milk Buttermilk	Polyunsaturate based cream substitutes
Whole milk yogurt, whole milk cottage cheese (4%), all natural cheeses (blue, Roquefort, Camembert, cheddar, Swiss), cream cheese, sour cream, ice cream	Nonfat (0%) or low-fat yogurt; low-fat cottage cheese (1%, 2%); low-fat cheeses (should be labeled no more than 2-6 gm fat/oz)	Sherbet, sorbet, frozen low-fat yogurt made from skim milk and no eggs
Butter Eggs (< 3/wk)	Margarines made from liquid vegetable oils Egg substitutes; egg whites (2 whole egg whites = 1 egg in recipes); cholesterol-free egg substitutes	
3. **Commercial baked goods** Pies, cakes, doughnuts, croissants, pastries, muffins, biscuits, high-fat crackers, high-fat cookies, egg noodles, breads in which eggs are a major ingredient	Homemade bread goods, using unsaturated oils, angel food cake, low-fat cookies, crackers, pretzels Rice, pasta Whole-grain breads and cereals (oatmeal, bran, rye, multigrain)*	Pastries made with polyunsaturated or monounsaturated oils, egg substitutes or egg whites

(Continued)

* Fruits, vegetables, grains, seeds, and nuts contain no cholesterol and most contain no saturated fat.

TABLE 74-10. PRACTICAL APPROACH TO A LOW-CHOLESTEROL, LOW-SATURATED FAT DIET *(Cont'd)*

Reduce Intake of:	Choose:	Use Substitutes:
4. Saturated fats and oils, dressings Chocolate, butter, coconut oil, palm oil, kernel oil, lard, bacon	Unsaturated vegetable oils: corn, olive, rapeseed, safflower, sesame, soybean, sunflower	Cocoa powder, carob
Butter, butter-margarine mixture	Margarine made from liquid oils, as above	Diet margarine made from liquid oils
Dressing made with egg yolk	Mayonnaise, salad dressings made with liquid oils, as above	Low-fat diet dressings made with liquid oils
Coconut	Seeds and nuts*	
5. Vegetables prepared in butter, saturated fats, cream, or in sauces with saturated fat	Fresh, frozen, canned, dried fruits or vegetables*	

sound clinical judgment is required in modifying diet for older individuals classified as high risk, particularly because adequate calorie and protein intake can be a major problem among the elderly.

TABLE 74-10 presents a practical guideline to dietary modification that approximates the goals of the Step 1 diet. The NCEP guidelines recommend that intervention proceed by steps in elderly hypercholesterolemic persons. The Step 1 dietary interventions listed in TABLES 74-9 and 74-10 should be adequate and safe for older adults, including diabetics.

Generally, changes in the steps of dietary therapy should be made slowly and only if the LDL-C reduction is short of targeted levels, since it may take 8 to 12 wk to achieve the full effects of dietary intervention at any 1 step (TABLE 74-9, FIG. 74-1). Reduction of obesity greatly facilitates the reduction of TC and LDL-C in hypercholesterolemic subjects.

In patients with hypertriglyceridemia and low HDL-C who are at increased risk for CHD, the dietary interventions appear to be appropriate: Ongoing Framingham studies have demonstrated that even when HDL-C is considered, for women > 50 yr of age, triglycerides appear to be an independent risk for heart disease, providing further justification for treatment of hypertriglyceridemia in adult women. The objec-

TABLE 74–11. DRUG THERAPY FOR HYPERLIPIDEMIA

Agent	Indications	Usual Dosage	Adverse Effects
Cholestyramine*†‡	High LDL-C Type II	8–24 gm resin (2–4 packets) daily in 3 or 4 divided doses; many patients respond to 8 gm/day	Constipation; other GI symptoms; increased VLDL (and TG); binds other drugs; augments coumadin effect; rarely (reversibly) elevates liver enzymes
Colestipol* (in conjunction with nicotinic acid‡	High LDL-C Type II	10–30 gm resin (2–6 packets or scoops) daily in 3 or 4 divided doses; many patients respond to 10 gm/day	Same as above
Nicotinic acid§ (in conjunction with colestipol)‡	High LDL-C with high TG High TG Type II (especially IIB) Synergistic with resins in Type II Type IV (if others fail) Type V (if others fail)	2–6 gm daily in 3 or 4 divided doses (4–12 500-mg sustained-release capsules); take with meals to minimize flushing	Cutaneous flush and pruritus; GI symptoms, ulcer, gastritis; frequent liver function abnormality; impaired glucose tolerance; hyperuricemia; toxic amblyopia

(Continued)

LDL-C = low-density lipoprotein cholesterol, TG = triglycerides, HDL-C = high-density lipoprotein cholesterol, CHD = coronary heart disease, VLDL = very low-density lipoproteins.

* Always start with small doses, 2 packs or 2 scoops per day; gradually increase dose prn.

† CHD event rate reduction proven by controlled clinical trials.

‡ Cessation of progression of coronary artery atherosclerosis and/or regression of lesions proven by controlled clinical trials.

§ Always start with small dose, 500 mg/day; gradually build dose by 500-mg increments.

** Reduce dose if uremia is present.

TABLE 74–11. DRUG THERAPY FOR HYPERLIPIDEMIA
(Cont'd)

Agent	Indications	Usual Dosage	Adverse Effects
Probucol CHD event rate reduction not proven	High LDL-C Type II (use with resin to achieve added lowering of LDL)	500 mg bid	Minor GI symptoms; lowers HDL as much as or more than LDL; rarely, foul-smelling sweat; prolongs QT interval
Gemfibrozil[†,**]	High TG Low HDL-C High LDL-C with high TG Type IV Type III Type V	600 mg bid; maximum dose 1.5 gm/day	Minor GI symptoms; rash, eosinophilia, etc; ? increased gallstones; rarely, muscle cramps, aches (myositis); myositis more common if patient has uremia or is receiving lovastatin or cyclosporine
Lovastatin CHD event rate reduction not proven	High LDL-C High LDL-C with high TG: Type IIB	20–80 mg/day; at 20–40 mg dose, give in evening; at 60–80 mg, in divided doses, give in AM and PM	Liver function test abnormalities; myalgia (myositis); evaluate for lens opacities (ongoing experience suggests *no* effect on augmentation of cataracts)
Cholestyramine + nicotinic acid	LDL-C > target on single drug	8–24 gm resin + 2–6 gm nicotinic acid	Same as individual drugs
Colestipol + nicotinic acid	LDL-C > target on single drug	10–30 gm resin + 2–6 gm nicotinic acid	Same as individual drugs
Cholestyramine + lovastatin	LDL-C > target on single drug	8–24 gm resin + 20–80 mg lovastatin	Same as individual drugs
Colestipol + lovastatin	LDL-C > target on single drug	10–30 gm resin + 20–80 mg lovastatin	Same as individual drugs

(Continued)

TABLE 74–11. DRUG THERAPY FOR HYPERLIPIDEMIA
(Cont'd)

Agent	Indications	Usual Dosage	Adverse Effects
Probucol + **cholestyramine** *or* **colestipol**	LDL-C > target, HDL-C < target on single drug	1 gm probucol + 8–30 gm resin	Less constipation than on resin alone; less diarrhea than on probucol alone; HDL-C higher than on probucol alone
Resin + **gemfibrozil**	LDL-C at target TG > 250 mg/dL HDL-C < 35 mg/dL	8–30 gm resin + 1200 mg gemfibrozil	Same as individual drugs
Lovastatin + **gemfibrozil**	LDL-C at target TG > 250 mg/dL HDL-C < 35 mg/dL	20–80 mg lovastatin + 1200 mg gemfibrozil	Myositis or ↑ CPK is more common than with the drug alone

tive of dietary treatment in hypertriglyceridemia is to raise HDL-C, but as noted above, treatment that lowers triglycerides alone may be valuable in women > 50 yr. The NCEP panel lists changes in life-style (control of weight, increased physical activity, restriction of alcohol, and in some cases, restriction of dietary fat) as the primary modes of therapy for hypertriglyceridemia.

Dietary interventions are as follows:

1. Weight loss using a low-fat diet, if the patient is overweight. In most overweight patients, including those with primary and familial hypertriglyceridemia, triglyceride levels drop sharply with only modest weight loss. A patient usually does not need to reach ideal body weight or even to effect more than a 5- to 10-kg weight loss to bring triglycerides within normal range.

2. Reduction in alcohol intake to 3 or fewer alcoholic beverages per week. If triglyceride levels are ≥ 500 mg/dL, all alcohol consumption should be discontinued.

3. Reduction in intake of total fat, saturated fat, and cholesterol, following the guidelines of the Phase III and Step 2 diet.

In severely hypertriglyceridemic persons (triglycerides ≥ 1000 mg/dL) with mixed elevations of chylomicron and VLDL triglyceride, or the much rarer primary hyperchylomicronemia (TABLES 74–6 and 74–8), total fat intake should be restricted to 10 to 20% of total calories. This rigid low-fat diet is instituted primarily to prevent pancreatitis, a major outcome of uncontrolled hypertriglyceridemia in such individuals. A secondary benefit may be realized from the sharp reduction of VLDL-C and increases in HDL-C that may further help protect individuals with the chylomicronemia-increased VLDL triglyceride syndrome from severe premature CHD. Weight loss is crucial in obese persons, and all alcohol intake should be discontinued. Estrogen use is proscribed.

For individuals with Type III hyperlipidemia (increased TC, triglycerides, and intermediate-density lipoprotein cholesterol), the *single* most important factor is weight reduction in those who are overweight. Patients should reduce intake not only of total fat, saturated fat, and cholesterol (Steps 1 and 2 as for hypercholesterolemia), but also of dietary sucrose.

For patients with hypoalphalipoproteinemia there is no known consistently effective dietary intervention except weight loss, which may raise HDL-C levels. Supplementation with omega-3–rich fish oils (4 to 12 gm/day) may help raise HDL-C levels. Reduction of smoking is very important in raising HDL-C levels, as is supervised aerobic physical activity, up to five 30-min periods/wk. Increased physical activity in older persons should be undertaken with physician supervision, at least initially. (See also Ch. 25.)

The targets for dietary treatment of hypercholesterolemia should be reduction of TC and LDL-C according to NCEP guidelines (TABLE 74–1) and the reduction of triglycerides to < 500 mg/dL (to avoid pancreatitis). For HDL-C, the goal should be to elevate levels to > 35 mg/dL and preferably to 40 mg/dL. Controlled clinical trial data concerning the cardiovascular effects of such changes in lipids and lipoproteins are available for both TC and LDL-C (LRC-CPPT, Oslo Heart Study, Helsinki Heart Study, NHLBI Type II Study, CLAS) and for HDL-C (Helsinki Heart Study, NHLBI Type II Study, CLAS). Moreover, in CLAS, the benefits of lowering cholesterol have been demonstrated throughout the cholesterol range, as low as TC 185 mg/dL. CLAS suggested that if TC could be lowered < 180 mg/dL and LDL-C < 120 mg/dL, the progression of atherosclerosis could be stabilized or stopped, and regression could be observed. Regression of coronary artery atherosclerosis occurred in 16.2% of the CLAS intervention patients compared with 2.4% of the placebo patients.

Drug Therapy

TABLE 74–11 provides one approach to drug therapy in patients with persistent primary and/or familial hyperlipidemias, including those ≥ 65 yr of age. Drugs should be used when diet fails to produce the targeted changes in lipoprotein cholesterol (FIG. 74–1), with attention to the patient's cardiovascular status, enthusiasm, and desire for therapy, as well as any concurrent illnesses. Recent publications of the Helsinki Heart Study and CLAS emphasize the effectiveness and importance of treating atherosclerosis in all adults, including the elderly. CLAS in particular documents the capability of protecting both native coronary arteries and coronary artery bypass grafts (and probably peripheral bypass grafts) in persons at increased CHD risk; if untreated, these individuals would have a high likelihood (70% or more) of reocclusion in both of the grafts and native coronary arteries, within 10 yr.

Currently, the major emphasis for initial drug use in hypercholesterolemia lies with nonabsorbable bile acid–binding resins. **Cholestyramine and colestipol,** 2 such resins, interrupt the normal enterohepatic circulation of bile acids and indirectly increase the liver's catabolism of LDL-C through increased LDL-receptor synthesis by hepatocytes. A very small bile acid–binding resin dose (8 to 10 gm/day) should be used initially, particularly in the elderly, and the reduction in LDL-C should be titrated against the dose provided (TABLE 74–11). The major side effect is constipation, which can usually be avoided by having the patient ingest dried fruit (eg, prunes, raisins, apricots) or use stool softeners.

Bile acid–binding resins potentiate warfarin effect and should be used cautiously, if at all, with warfarin-like anticoagulants. The resins should *not* be given concurrently with exogenous thyroid hormones, sex steroids, prednisone, or digoxin, all of which may be bound in the intestine by resins. These drugs should be given at least 2 h before the day's first resin dose. Because resins are not systemically absorbed, they have essentially no systemic side effects (aside from rare, mild, reversible changes in liver enzymes) and have been shown to be safe and effective in reducing CHD morbidity and mortality.

CLAS used 30 gm colestipol/day plus 3 to 12 gm niacin. This study demonstrated significant reduction in progression of atherosclerosis in coronary arteries, *and* initiation of regression.

In individuals whose primary defect is high LDL and whose triglyceride levels are < 250 mg/dL, the bile acid–binding resins are effective and safe, as documented by the LRC-CPPT. In individuals with elevated LDL-C and triglycerides ≤ 250 mg/dL, bile acid–binding resin therapy may concurrently raise triglycerides; either nicotinic acid alone as a primary drug or the addition of gemfibrozil to the resins should be contemplated. Alternatively, lovastatin (20 to 80 mg/day) could be used.

Given the frequency of side effects of nicotinic acid, however, our choice in individuals with mixed elevations of LDL-C and triglyceride in whom triglycerides rise to > 300 mg/dL during bile acid–binding resin therapy is to add gemfibrozil 1200 mg/day. The bile acid sequestrants are probably contraindicated as single drug therapy in patients with high LDL-C *and* marked hypertriglyceridemia (triglycerides > 500 mg/dL) and in those with severe hemorrhoids or history of bowel resection or severe constipation. In these patients, lovastatin is the drug of choice.

Nicotinic acid: Use of this agent in the Coronary Drug Project was associated with a reduction in recurring myocardial infarction and hence in CHD morbidity. Moreover, 10 yr after the trial had been formally ended, a reassessment of participants disclosed a significant reduction in all causes of total mortality. Nicotinic acid inhibits secretion of very low-density lipoproteins from the liver, which accounts for its ability to reduce both VLDL-C and LDL-C.

Nicotinic acid should be started at a low dosage, 100 to 250 mg/day. The initial dose should probably be given after the evening meal to minimize flushing during the day. The frequency of administration, as well as the total daily dose, should be very slowly increased (approximately once a week) with titration against the LDL-C reduction. Generally, a first-level therapeutic dosage of 1.5 to 2 gm/day is required to produce targeted reductions of LDL-C. Every 6 to 8 wk, patients receiving nicotinic acid should be monitored with laboratory tests, including liver function tests, blood glucose and uric acid concentration, and stool tests for occult blood. They should also be evaluated to determine whether the targeted LDL reduction has been reached. Although nicotinic acid can be used as a primary drug to lower LDL-C, it is usually added to the resins when they fail to produce satisfactory results.

Nicotinic acid side effects are frequent, bothersome to the patient, and often severe, although flushing and tachycardia may be reduced by taking a small dose of aspirin simultaneously. In addition to the side effects listed in TABLE 74–11, nicotinic acid very rarely produces toxic amblyopia. Close follow-up for side effects is necessary, particularly the measurement of liver function, blood sugar, and uric acid q 6 to 8 wk.

The FDA has recently approved specific competitive inhibitors of the rate-limiting enzyme of cellular cholesterol biosynthesis (HMG CoA reductase), opening up a remarkable new avenue for therapy of persons with primary hypercholesterolemia. The first such drug to be approved is **lovastatin;** other related drugs should be approved in the near future. Lovastatin blocks intracellular cholesterol biosynthesis, forcing the cell to synthesize more LDL receptors, which increases the catabolism of LDL-C.

In clinical trials with 2 yr of follow-up, side effects of lovastatin appear to be relatively rare, with the major biochemical changes including **increases in liver enzymes** (particularly transaminase) and in CPK levels with myositis. The current convention is *not* to discontinue lovastatin unless the liver function test results rise to levels $\geq$ 3 times the upper limit of normal. Approximately 1.9% of patients have developed persistent increases of transaminase levels > 3 times normal requiring discontinuance of therapy. These elevations appear to be entirely reversible. Approximately 0.5% of patients develop **increases in CPK levels with symptomatic myositis.** The myositis is particularly common in individuals receiving lovastatin plus cyclosporine, where **rhabdomyolysis and myoglobinuria** have also been reported. The concurrent use of these 2 drugs should be restricted to special situations where other cholesterol-lowering regimens are ineffective, and patients treated with this drug combination very closely monitored.

Other clinical side effects of lovastatin, which are usually transient, include skin rashes, headaches, fatigue, and constipation. Despite an initial concern that lovastatin might potentially increase the likelihood of cataract formation, subsequent studies have not borne this out. Close follow-up is recommended, with evaluation of liver function tests at least q 4 to 6 wk, along with measurement of CPK, where indicated. Evaluation of the eyes (for cataract formation) by slit lamp examination should be carried out annually.

Patients should generally be started on a regimen of 20 mg lovastatin, given with the evening meal, with the dosage increased to 40 and then 60 mg/day as a single evening dose, or given bid when the level reaches 80 mg/day. Lovastatin alone usually achieves a 25 to 40% reduction of LDL-C, may produce a modest reduction of triglycerides (5 to 20%), and a modest (5 to 10%) increase in HDL-C. If long-term safety can be established, the HMG-CoA reductase inhibitors will probably become the cholesterol-lowering drugs of choice, given their ease of administration and effectiveness in reducing LDL-C concentrations.

Lovastatin can be effectively combined with resins, but it probably should *not be used concurrently with niacin because of increased myositis and hepatoxicity.* Lovastatin plus gemfibrozil is effective in lowering LDL-C, raising HDL-C, and lowering triglycerides; however, *the risk of myositis is increased by the concurrent use of these 2 drugs,* and CPK levels should be monitored routinely (q 6 wk). *Combined use of lovastatin plus gemfibrozil should not be used,* except for special patients in whom neither drug alone (after a thorough trial) is sufficient. Patients treated with this combination should be monitored with exceptional care, particularly if there is also concurrent use of cyclosporine, since risk of myositis and even rhabdomyolysis is high.

Thus, the major drugs for treatment of hypercholesterolemia include the bile acid–binding resins, nicotinic acid, gemfibrozil (if triglycerides are also elevated), and lovastatin.

Probucol, another cholesterol-lowering drug, may be used but is considered a second-choice agent by NCEP guidelines. Probucol therapy usually reduces LDL-C by about 8 to 15% but usually with a concurrent *reduction* in HDL-C up to 25%. Probucol appears to increase the rate of LDL catabolism, probably through nonreceptor-mediated pathways. A recent hypothesis is that in animal models, probucol's antioxidant effect might reduce atherosclerosis by reducing the atherogenic effect of oxidized LDL. No extensive, long-term clinical studies are available to assess the safety of probucol or its effect on CHD risk. As noted by the NCEP, "the role of probucol in the treatment of patients with high LDL-C is uncertain because of concerns about the reductions in HDL-C, but xanthoma regression has also been reported as the HDL-C level decreases."

Probucol is generally well tolerated; diarrhea is the most common side effect. The drug causes prolongation of the QT interval and is probably *contraindicated* in patients with ventricular irritability with an initially prolonged QT interval, or those taking other drugs that prolong the QT interval. The combination of probucol plus resins is effective, with less reduction in HDL-C than with probucol alone and much less constipation than with resins alone.

The drug of choice for treatment of hypertriglyceridemia and hypoalphalipoproteinemia in the elderly is **gemfibrozil**, a fibric acid derivative that increases the hydrolysis of VLDL triglycerides and the syntheses of HDL-C and apolipoprotein Al. When NCEP guidelines were published, the outcome of the Helsinki Heart Trial was just being revealed. Subsequently, this trial demonstrated that gemfibrozil, which produced a 10 to 16% increase in HDL, a 30 to 40% decrease in triglycerides, and an 8 to 10% decrease in LDL, was associated with a 34% reduction in CHD morbidity and mortality. Moreover, long-term safety (> 5 yr) was observed, with no significant differences in side effects between placebo and active drug.

Gemfibrozil is well tolerated by most patients. It rarely causes GI upset and myositis. The latter is particularly common when gemfibrozil is given to patients with poor renal function. Such patients, and especially those also receiving cyclosporine, should be given a reduced dose. Gemfibrozil should be particularly useful in individuals with high-risk LDL-C levels who also have elevated triglycerides (250 to 500 mg/dL) and low HDL-C levels.

New drugs for lowering cholesterol and/or triglyceride levels currently under development include several HMG-CoA–reductase inhibitors whose efficacies are apparently similar to or better than that of lovastatin, and fenofibrate, a fibric acid derivative that has effects on triglycerides and HDL-C similar to those of gemfibrozil.

Recently, **omega-3–rich fish oils** have been used to lower triglyceride levels, usually in dosages > 15 gm/day. These agents are not useful as cholesterol-lowering drugs; they may elevate HDL-C slightly. These fish oils, available over the counter, may increase the hydrolysis of VLDL triglyceride. At much higher dosages (usually > 50 gm/day), they may be associated with thrombocytopenia and increased bleeding time; thus, platelet counts and bleeding time should be followed during therapy at doses > 20 gm/day. At higher doses, they may also interfere with euglycemic control in diabetics. There are very few controlled, long-term clinical study data for showing the lipid-lowering effectiveness or side effects of these agents, although at ≤ 15 gm/day, they appear to be safe in short-term trials.

§3. ORGAN SYSTEMS: INFECTIOUS DISEASE

Contents for NEUROLOGIC DISORDERS begin on page 925.

---

75.   NORMAL CHANGES IN HOST DEFENSE

Bruce E. Hirsch and *Marc E. Weksler*

Infectious diseases occur with greater severity in the elderly, partly because of the effect of age on host defenses. Although older persons may have increased experience with pathogens, the time between primary exposure and rechallenge, as well as immune senescence, diminishes the vigor of their immune responses. In addition, age-related diseases and associated conditions not only increase the susceptibility of older persons to infection but also may depress the immune response. Thus, adequate care of older patients depends on an understanding of the changes in host resistance that occur with age.

CELLS OF THE IMMUNE SYSTEM

The immune system comprises several cell types, which form a network of interacting elements that together generate **humoral immunity (B lymphocytes)**, **cell-mediated immunity (thymus-derived, or T lymphocytes)**, and **nonspecific immunity (monocytes and polymorphonuclear neutrophil leukocytes [PMNs])**. The immune system is an important defense against microbial pathogens. Mononuclear cells (monocytes, macrophages, and Langerhans' and dendritic cells) are the first cells to interact with antigen. They present antigen to T cells in an immunogenic form in association with major histocompatibility complex **(MHC)** Class II molecules on the mononuclear cell surface.

A variety of regulatory and effector T lymphocytes are activated in the immune response. **T helper cells** interact with antigen associated with MHC Class II molecules, while **T suppressor** and **T cytotoxic cells** interact with antigen associated with MHC Class I molecules. These interactions result in the production of soluble mediators. The inflammatory response derives to a considerable extent from the secretion of interleukin-1 **(IL-1)** by macrophages. IL-1 produces fever, increased vascular permeability, and other signs of inflammation. IL-1 facilitates the activation of T cells, which in turn produce the T cell growth factor interleukin-2 **(IL-2)**. IL-2 stimulates the proliferation of (1) additional T lymphocytes and other lymphokines, including γ-interferon, which activate macrophages and B cell growth, and (2) differentiation factors, which promote the expansion of B lymphocyte populations and the production of antibody. T suppressor cells down-regulate the immune response, maintain self-tolerance, and provide a regulatory counterbalance to the action of T helper lymphocytes. Other T cells, large granular lymphocytes, have natural killer activity.

Regulation of the immune system depends on the balance between T helper and T suppressor cells. In old age, there is a decline in function of the essential T cells, causing diminution of cell-mediated immunity, humoral immunity, and self-tolerance. These changes lead to a decline in the response to foreign antigens and the emergence of autoimmune phenomena.

CELL-MEDIATED IMMUNITY AND AGING

Involution of the thymus is a universal accompaniment of aging. In man, the loss of thymic mass begins at 30 yr of age and continues until the age of 50, at which time only 5 to 10% of maximal thymic mass is retained. The thymus contributes in at least 2 ways to immune function: (1) It provides a microenvironment in which T lymphocyte precursors from the bone marrow mature. (2) It produces a family of polypeptide hormones that induce further maturation of T lymphocytes. The serum activity of thymic hormones is maintained until age 30, after which it declines, becoming undetectable by age 60.

Most investigators have found that the total number of T lymphocytes and B lymphocytes in the peripheral blood changes little with age. However, modest changes in T lymphocyte subpopulations occur. T lymphocytes expressing the CD4 determinant increase in number, while T lymphocytes expressing the CD8 determinant decrease. CD4+ T cells are usually associated with helper cell activity, stimulating humoral immunity. CD8+ T cells are associated with suppressor cell activity and down-regulate humoral immunity. The number of immature T cells in the thymus and in the blood also increases, as the thymus loses its capacity to induce differentiation of T cell precursors. A decrease in the germinal centers in lymph nodes and an increase in plasma cells and lymphocytes in bone marrow are also seen.

With aging, a remarkable **loss of functional capacity of cell-mediated immunity** occurs, as evidenced by diminished delayed hypersensitivity reactions to common skin-testing antigens (eg, *Candida,* mumps, and purified protein derivative of tuberculin). Another manifestation of delayed hypersensitivity is the lymphocyte transfer test. In this model of the graft-vs.-host reaction, the functional capacity of lymphocytes injected into the skin is assayed. Lymphocytes from older donors are less capable of inducing a positive reaction than lymphocytes from younger donors.

In vitro studies reveal that T lymphocytes from older persons are less able to proliferate in response to mitogens. Lymphocytes from elderly persons sensitized to *Mycobacterium tuberculosis* and the influenza and varicella-zoster viruses show an impaired proliferative response to these antigens, compared with lymphocytes from sensitized younger persons. This observation is consistent with the increased incidence and severity of these infections in older persons.

Studies in animals reveal functional consequences of the decline in cell-mediated immunity. The graft-vs.-host reactivity of lymphocytes from old animals is impaired. Lymphocytes from old mice are less capable of rejecting tumor implants or skin grafts than are lymphocytes from young mice. The induction of cell-mediated immunity by viral infection is diminished in older mice. Old animals infected with *Listeria monocytogenes* express only $1/1000$ the level of T lymphocyte immunity found in young mice.

Laboratory investigations have focused on the changes in T lymphocytes from older persons. While the total number of T lymphocytes in the peripheral blood does not change with age, only $1/5$ to $1/2$ of these cells respond to mitogen. In addition, the ability of the responding cells to divide sequentially in culture is impaired. Studies of the subcellular locus of the proliferative defect have demonstrated the same number and affinity of mitogen receptors in lymphocytes from older and from younger persons. Furthermore, the generation of a cytoplasmic factor that stimulates DNA synthesis by isolated nuclei is also comparable. However, nuclei isolated from the lymphocytes of older donors show an impaired response to this cytoplasmic factor. *Thus it appears that the roliferative defect is due to the failure of the nucleus to synthesize DNA,* ven though many of the cell surface and cytoplasmic events following ctivation proceed normally in lymphocytes from older persons.

HUMORAL IMMUNITY AND AGING

The total **concentration of immunoglobulin** in serum changes little with ge. Modest changes in the **distribution** of antibody classes have been reported: The concentrations of **IgA** and **IgG** are increased in older persons, while the concentration of **IgM** is decreased.

The **antibody response** to vaccines for influenza, parainfluenza, pneumococcus, and tetanus is diminished in older persons. The class of immunoglobulin produced in response to foreign antigen changes with aging. Of the total antibody formed, relatively more IgM and relatively ess IgG are produced. The maximal antibody response requires a larger lose of foreign antigen and is maintained for a shorter time.

Despite a diminished antibody response to foreign antigens, autoantibodies are more frequently found in the serum of elderly persons. This phenomenon is not associated with an increased incidence of autoimmune lisease but reflects dysregulation of the immune system. One such class of autoantibodies is **autoanti-idiotypes,** which may directly inhibit the antibody response to foreign antigens. Findings of **monoclonal immunoglobulins** not associated with malignant myeloma increase dramatically vith age. Less than 0.1% of persons < 50 yr of age have **benign monoclonal gammopathy.** In contrast, 2% of persons > 70 yr of age and (in study) 19% of those > 95 yr of age have benign monoclonal immunoglobulins in their serum.

The primary cause of the changes in humoral immunity is impaired T lymphocyte function. The changes in B lymphocyte functions appear to be secondary to the decline in T cell function that occurs with age.

NONSPECIFIC IMMUNITY AND INFLAMMATION IN AGING

Inflammation, one of the earliest responses to injury and infection, is characterized by increased local blood flow, increased vascular permeability, and the rapid mobilization of PMNs. This first line of defense is mediated by various substances, including catecholamines, histamine, serotonin, and prostaglandins. The coordination of the clotting, kinin, and complement systems provides for the elaboration of chemotactic factors and opsonins and heralds specific immune responses.

In general, the inflammatory and nonspecific immune defenses are moderately diminished, if at all, by the aging process. Elevations of the serum complement components C3 and properdin have been reported in some healthy elderly persons. Macrophages from old and young mice have shown comparable ability to phagocytize antigen, support T lymphocyte proliferation, and secrete lymphokines. However, PMNs from the elderly have been reported to be impaired in their capacity to migrate and kill *Candida albicans* in vitro.

The elderly are burdened with numerous pathologic conditions, some of which impair host defenses. For example, the hyperglycemia of diabetes mellitus is known to impair the function of PMNs. Vascular disease reduces blood flow and compromises resistance to local infection and wound healing.

The febrile response and leukocytosis—but not the relative increase in immature PMNs and PMN precursors (the "shift to the left")—traditionally were thought to be diminished in older patients. However it now appears that, as with local inflammatory responses, *disease burden and loss of physiologic reserve account for the impaired nonspecific inflammatory responses to infectious disease.* Thus the clinical response to infection is also blunted in younger patients with equally severe multisystem illness. It is the accumulation of diseases, not the passage of years, that impairs nonspecific immunity in some elderly persons.

HOST DEFENSE CHANGES AND INFECTIOUS DISEASES

Depressed Cell-Mediated Immunity

The decline in T cell function in older persons leads to a moderate deficiency of cell-mediated immunity. Approximately $1/4$ of healthy persons can be shown to have a marked decline; $1/2$, a moderate decline; and $1/4$, no decline relative to younger subjects. However, even those with the most compromised functional deficiency are not subject to *Pneumocystis carinii* or *Aspergillus* infections, as often occur in patients with severe cell-mediated immunodeficiency syndromes.

The **age-associated T lymphocyte defects** contribute to reactivation of *Mycobacterium tuberculosis* and varicella-zoster infections. Cell-mediated immunity is a major factor in the host response to these infections. Reactivation in late life may, in part, be due to waning cellular immunity. In the USA, **tuberculosis** is now primarily a disease of the elderly, and reactivation correlates with other diseases or with immunosuppressive therapy, which may accentuate the decline in cell-mediated immunity. Similarly, **reactivation of varicella-zoster virus,** or shingles, is more common in healthy older persons who have declining cellular immunity. Disorders that impair cell-mediated immunity (eg, Hodgkin's disease) also are associated with varicella-zoster reactivation.

General Host Defenses and Frequent Infections

The pattern of infections in a compromised host often reflects the nature of the defect or defects in host defense. The infectious diseases that occur with increased frequency and severity in the elderly include most bacterial infections (eg, pneumonia; UTI; gram-negative bacteremia; intra-abdominal infections, such as cholangitis and diverticulitis; and skin and soft tissue infections) and some viral diseases (eg, influenza).

Numerous factors contribute to the increased frequency and severity of infection in the elderly. The presence of **associated diseases,** rather than an age-dependent decline in immunity, seems to be the major factor. Even certain remedies may lead to **infectious complications**—eg, prosthetic joints and heart valves, pacemakers, and other implanted devices, any of which can be sites of infection. In addition, the elderly are more frequently hospitalized or placed in nursing homes, where the risk of **nosocomial infections** is high. **Socioeconomic factors** contribute to the risk of infection in those who cannot afford appropriate nutrition and housing. Social isolation, death of a spouse, and loss of independence are sources of **psychologic stress** that may also compromise immunologically mediated host resistance.

Respiratory Tract Infection (see also Ch. 39)

Pneumonia and influenza together are the seventh leading cause of death in persons between 65 and 74 yr of age, the fifth leading cause in those between 75 and 84, and the fourth leading cause in those ≥ 85 yr.

Colonization of the oropharynx with coliform bacteria occurs in approximately 6% of healthy elderly individuals vs. 3% of normal younger subjects. This rate increases to 40% in hospitalized patients > 65 yr of age.

Fibronectin, a high molecular weight glycoprotein, binds to bacteria and blocks sites on the microbial cell surface necessary for adhesion to buccal epithelium. A rise in salivary protease activity occurs with illness, destroys fibronectin, and promotes colonization of the oropharynx by coliform bacteria. The elderly often have an **impaired cough reflex** and a decreased ability to clear respiratory tract secretions. **Aspiration** of altered microbial flora may overwhelm the defenses of the lower respiratory tract and lead to pneumonia.

The elderly are also more susceptible to **influenza,** in part perhaps because of an impaired immune response to the virus. Infection with influenza destroys ciliated epithelial cells of the respiratory tract and depresses mucociliary clearance. There is **increased mortality** because of frequent and numerous complications, including secondary bacterial infections (eg, with *Streptococcus pneumoniae* or *Staphylococcus aureus*) and nonseptic problems, usually cardiovascular or respiratory in origin.

Microbes that reach the alveolus activate macrophages and T cells, which then initiate local inflammatory and immune responses. The functional defect in T lymphocytes may contribute to a diminished immune response in the alveolus and, consequently, to the increased severity of pneumonia in older persons. For these reasons, immunization with influenza and pneumococcal vaccines is recommended for persons > 65 yr of age; the quantitative diminution in immune response to these antigens may limit their effectiveness in increasing host resistance to either pathogen.

Urinary Tract Infections (see also Ch. 56)

UTIs are the most common nosocomial infections in the elderly. **Adherence of bacteria** to urogenital epithelial cells is increased in women with frequent UTIs, and **urine loses bacteriostatic properties** in some elderly individuals. Decline in renal function is accompanied by **reduced ability to concentrate and acidify urine**—all of which favors bacterial growth. Age-related prostatism in men and relaxation of pelvic musculature in women lead to incomplete bladder emptying and thus to **urinary stasis.** Elderly patients are frequently subjected to **instrumentation** of the urinary tract, which may introduce bacteria and lead to colonization and subsequent infection.

GI Tract and Intra-abdominal Infections

The GI tract undergoes age-related changes that compromise its resistance to infection. **Achlorhydria** allows colonization of the stomach and upper small intestine by coliform bacteria, thus increasing the risk of gram-negative pneumonia in elderly patients who aspirate gastric contents. Elderly patients are also more susceptible to *Salmonella* infections because of the **higher pH of the upper GI tract** and possibly diminished IgA production. GI diseases common in old age also favor the development of infection. Alteration in gallbladder function leads to **gallstones,** which can cause local obstruction, cholecystitis, and cholangitis. Obstruction and perforation of colonic **diverticula** can lead to life-threatening systemic infection.

Dissemination of Infection

Not only are the elderly more susceptible to infection, but they are also less able to contain infections and more often experience **local spreading** and **bacteremia.** For example, erysipelas, a rapidly spreading Group A β-hemolytic streptococcal infection of the dermis, occurs more often in infants and older persons than in the rest of the population. The skin of older persons is characterized by thinning, loss of Langerhans' cells (skin tissue macrophages), and diminished blood supply in certain areas. Aggressive infections are favored by this decrease in local defense.

The older patient can more often develop gram-negative bacteremia without an obvious primary site of infection, although the urinary tract is a frequent source. The mean age of patients with reported cases of infective endocarditis is increasing, in part because of the increased susceptibility of sclerotic or prosthetic heart valves to infection.

GENERAL PRINCIPLES OF MANAGEMENT

Risk Assessment and Preventive Medicine

Older individuals with associated diseases and degenerative changes are at increased risk for infection. Comprehensive assessment of health status allows the clinician to take steps that prevent or limit the seriousness of infectious diseases.

Adequate nutrition is required for normal wound healing and maximal host resistance. Nutritionally compromised persons given a 3-mo course of nutritive supplements have been reported to show improvement in in vitro immunologic function. Oral administration of 220 mg zinc sulfate/day to a population of institutionalized elderly also has been reported to enhance in vitro lymphocyte function. Detecting frank nutritional deficiency states and providing nutritional supplements may improve host defenses.

Structural abnormalities that increase the potential for infection should be corrected when possible. For example, prostatectomy can improve urine flow and decrease the incidence of UTIs. Tracheostomy or enteral feeding may be considered in individuals with recurrent, life-threatening aspiration pneumonia. Orthopedic procedures that enhance mobility and improve the quality of life can improve host resistance.

Recognition and careful control of **disease states,** such as diabetes mellitus, heart failure, thyroid disease, and occult malignancy, are essential to reduce the risk and severity of infections.

Vaccination

The decline in the immune system that occurs with aging impairs the magnitude of antibody response to vaccines. In 1 study, only 40% of healthy older individuals responded to influenza vaccination compared with 100% of the younger adults. While quantitative antibody responses may decline, vaccination with tetanus toxoid, pneumococcal vaccine, and annual influenza vaccine nevertheless is indicated in many elderly persons. Optimization of dosage schedules and use of immune response enhancers, such as thymic hormones, are currently under investigation.

---

76. EPIDEMIOLOGY AND PATHOGENESIS OF INFECTIOUS DISEASES

Larry M. Bush and *Donald Kaye*

Infectious diseases are the second most frequent cause of death and a major cause of morbidity in the elderly. The frequency of infections is greater and the epidemiology and pathogenesis often quite different in the elderly than in the younger population. These differences are due to anatomic and physiologic changes and socioeconomic influences that occur with aging. Immunologic senescence affects host defenses, causing a decline in both cell-mediated and humoral immunity (see also Ch. 75). Data regarding the effect of age on the inflammatory process are inconclusive; however, polymorphonuclear leukocyte function may be diminished by chronic illnesses. The competence of nonspecific host defenses declines as organ systems undergo progressive degenerative changes.

Other factors, eg, malnutrition, decreased physical activity, and increased drug use, also influence the epidemiology, pathogenesis, and prognosis of infections. As the percentage of elderly persons continues to increase, more people will spend time in acute- and chronic-care facilities and thus be vulnerable to nosocomial infections, as described below.

PNEUMONIA
(See also PNEUMONIA in Ch. 39)

Bacterial pneumonias are the leading cause of death from infections and the 5th most common cause of death overall, accounting for a reported mortality of 184.8/100,000 elderly persons. The yearly incidence varies from 20 to 40/1000 for community-acquired pneumonias to 100 to 250/1000 for pneumonias acquired in chronic-care facilities. At any given time as many as 2.1% of nursing home residents may have lower respiratory tract infections. The hospitalized elderly have a three-fold greater incidence of **nosocomial pneumonia** than do younger patients. Without an underlying high-risk condition, age-related **excess mortality** from lower respiratory tract infections is 9/100,000. This can rise to 217/100,000 with 1 high-risk condition and to 979/100,000 with 2 or more risk factors.

Microorganisms reach the tracheobronchial tree via 4 routes: (1) inhalation; (2) aspiration; (3) direct inoculation from contiguous sites; or (4) hematogenous spread. The first 2 routes are much more frequently involved than the latter 2. Pneumonitis occurs when the normal defense mechanisms of the lungs (eg, the cough reflex, airway patency, mucociliary transport, macrophage-phagocytic activity, and immunoglobulin function and secretion) are overwhelmed or impaired.

Two major factors predisposing to pneumonia are oropharyngeal colonization and silent aspiration. **Colonization of the oropharynx** with various gram-negative bacilli is frequent, especially in patients whose underlying illness requires treatment in an intensive care unit. Predisposing factors include poor oral hygiene; decreased saliva; abnormal swallowing; increased adherence of gram-negative bacilli to mucosal cells; debility from cardiac, respiratory, or neoplastic diseases; reduced ambulation; and frequent exposure to broad-spectrum antibiotics. **Silent aspiration of oropharyngeal secretions,** the most common mechanism of pulmonary infection, is often related to alcoholism, use of sedatives or narcotics, cerebrovascular disease, esophageal disorders, and nasogastric intubation.

COMMUNITY-ACQUIRED PNEUMONIA

Streptococcus pneumoniae (Diplococcus pneumoniae, pneumococcus) causes 40 to 60% of all bacterial pneumonias in the elderly. The attack rate of **pneumococcal pneumonia** is estimated to be 45.6 cases/1000 persons $\geq$ 65 yr old, and mortality is more common in the elderly than in the young.

Gram-negative bacilli, excluding *Hemophilus influenzae,* are isolated from 6 to 37% of patients with community-acquired pneumonia. *Klebsiella pneumoniae* and *Enterobacter aerogenes* are the most common enteric gram-negative isolates. Both typeable and nontypeable strains of *H. influenzae* account for 8 to 20% of pneumonias. These organisms are frequently recovered from the oropharynx of patients with chronic bronchitis, as is *Branhamella catarrhalis,* which can also invade the lower respiratory tract. Estimates of community-acquired pneumonia caused by *Legionella* spp vary, ranging from 2 to 20%. *Staphylococcus aureus* causes 10 to 14% of pneumonias. *S. aureus* pneumonia is often found during viral influenza epidemics, although pneumococcal disease is more common. Anaerobes are estimated to account for 1 to 20% of community-acquired pneumonia; these common oropharyngeal commensals probably play a role in almost *all* aspiration pneumonias. The more common anaerobes include *Fusobacterium nucleatum, Bacteroides melaninogenicus,* peptostreptococci, peptococci, and occasionally *B. fragilis.* Although *Mycoplasma pneumonia* is an unusual cause of pneumonia, it should be considered when infection involves an entire family.

Infection due to influenza A or B virus is particularly important in patients with chronic diseases. Older persons account for at least 50% of all hospitalizations and 75 to 80% of all deaths attributed to influenza. The disease is acquired via inhalation of aerosolized droplets. The majority of affected patients develop bronchitis without other involvement of the lower respiratory tract. When pneumonia does occur, several patterns may be seen. One is **diffuse bilateral primary viral pneumonia,** which is characterized by high fever, dyspnea, and bloody sputum. Mortality is high. **Bacterial superinfection** with *S. pneumoniae, S. aureus, H. influenzae,* or others may complicate the patient's course. Respiratory syncytial virus, adenovirus, and parainfluenza virus are uncommon causes of pneumonia.

Mycobacterium tuberculosis is common in the elderly, with > 25% of newly reported cases occurring in those > 65 yr of age. The elderly now account for the single largest group with active tuberculosis. Although most cases are due to reactivation of latent foci, primary infection may occur. Miliary tuberculosis also affects the elderly (see Ch. 39).

INSTITUTION-ACQUIRED PNEUMONIA

The epidemiology and pathogenesis of pneumonia acquired in acute- or chronic-care facilities may differ from that seen in the community setting. **Nosocomial pneumonia** accounts for approximately 15% of all hospital-acquired infections and is the leading cause of death from such infections in the elderly. The risk is comparable in **nursing homes,** where the number of beds is double that in US hospitals. Underlying illnesses are often more complex in the hospitalized and institutionalized elderly than in community dwellers. The former often receive multiple drugs, including antibiotics. They are also subject to endotracheal intubation, mechanical ventilation, invasive monitoring, intravascular catheterization, nasogastric intubation, and indwelling urinary catheterization, all of which predispose them to direct inoculation, bacterial colonization, and bacteremia.

Isolates from patients with pneumonia generally reflect the prevalent bacterial flora of the institution. Gram-negative aerobic enteric bacilli, excluding *Pseudomonas,* cause 35% of nosocomial pneumonias. *Klebsiella, Enterobacter, Escherichia coli,* and *Proteus* are most commonly isolated. *Serratia, Acinetobacter, Citrobacter,* and *Providencia* spp are common isolates in intensive care units, survive well in fluids, and are easily spread by the hands of the hospital staff. *Pseudomonas aeruginosa,* which can invade the lower respiratory tract via aspiration or bacteremia, causes approximately 12% of nosocomial pneumonias. Overall mortality in patients with gram-negative pneumonia and bacteremia has been reported to be 57 to 76%.

Other organisms associated with nosocomial pneumonia include *S. aureus, S. pneumoniae, Legionella* sp, anaerobic bacteria, influenza virus, and *M. tuberculosis.*

URINARY TRACT INFECTION (UTI)
(See also Ch. 56)

The urinary tract is the most frequent site of bacterial infection in older persons. Urinary tract infections **(UTIs)** increase in prevalence with advancing age. **Asymptomatic bacteriuria** is $> 10^5$ colony-forming units/mL of urine in a person without symptoms of UTI. **Symptomatic infections** (eg, pyelonephritis, cystitis, and prostatitis) are especially important causes of morbidity. In the absence of obstruction, UTI does not lead to decreased renal function. The urinary tract is the most common pathway by which bacteremia ensues, and the resultant mortality is greater in the elderly.

Whereas the female:male ratio of bacteriuria in young adults is approximately 30:1, this ratio in patients > 65 yr progressively decreases to approximately 2 to 3:1. Epidemiologic studies have shown that about 15 to 20% of women and 0 to 3% of men 65 to 70 yr of age have bacteriuria, compared with approximately 20 to 50% of women and 20% of men > 80 yr of age. In general, about 20% of elderly women and 10% of elderly men living at home have bacteriuria. These percentages increase to about 25 and 20%, respectively, in nursing homes and 40 and 30%, respectively, in hospitals. The higher rates of bacteriuria found in these institutions probably are related to greater patient debilitation and attendant fecal incontinence, incomplete bladder emptying, and urethral catheterization.

Bacteria usually invade the urinary tract by the ascending route. Bacteriuria develops following a single urethral catheterization in about 1% of healthy ambulatory subjects. Micturition with complete bladder emptying is an important defense mechanism.

Once bacteria gain access to the bladder, they may multiply and migrate to the kidneys, especially if vesicoureteral reflux is present. The capacity of certain bacteria to adhere to uroepithelial cells has been associated with UTIs. However, studies have shown that increased bacterial adherence to uroepithelial cells is not responsible for the high prevalence of bacteriuria in elderly women, although it may play a role in elderly men. Loss of bactericidal secretions from the prostate also leads to increased bacteriuria in men. Renal defense mechanisms in both sexes include the flow of urine and a systemic antibody response, which does not occur with bladder infection.

Although *E. coli* is the most common infecting organism, bacteriuria in the elderly is more often due to *Proteus, Klebsiella-Enterobacter-Serratia* and *Pseudomonas* spp, or to enterococci than is bacteriuria in younger populations. *E. coli* is also a relatively more common isolate in community-acquired bacteriuria than in institutional cases. The increased occurrence of other gram-negative bacilli in the institutionalized elderly may be related to the frequency of structural abnormalities of the urinary tract, increased urethral catheterization and instrumentation, and repeated courses of antimicrobial therapy in institutionalized patients.

Chronic bacterial prostatitis contributes to the relapse of UTI in elderly men. Prostatitis is most often caused by *E. coli,* but *Klebsiella-Enterobacter, Proteus mirabilis,* and enterococci are also common pathogens. *Staphylococcus epidermidis, S. aureus,* and diphtheroids are less commonly found.

Catheter-associated bacteriuria partly accounts for the high incidence of UTIs (35 to 40% of all nosocomial infections). Intermittent straight catheterization is less likely to cause bacteriuria than an indwelling bladder catheter, particularly if the latter remains in place for an extended time. Fifty percent of patients develop bacteriuria within 24 h and virtually 100% in 3 to 4 days when open drainage systems are used. Closed drainage systems have been shown to prevent infection for up to 10 days in 50% of patients. This effect can be matched by open drainage systems when continuous antimicrobial bladder rinses are used.

MENINGITIS

The incidence of bacterial meningitis in the elderly is 15 cases/100,000/yr. The elderly account for approximately 10% of all cases of meningitis, with > 50% of the fatal cases occurring in those > 60 yr of age. Mortality is high (53 to 79%) owing to patient debilitation and associated illnesses, along with frequent delays in diagnosis and isolation of more problematic infecting organisms.

Although the mechanism of infection is the same in the elderly and the young, **the bacteriology of meningitis** differs somewhat in the elderly. *Streptococcus pneumoniae* predominates (about 55% of cases), generally causing infection through bacteremic pneumonia, otitis media, or skull fracture. *Neisseria meningitidis* is next most common (about 15%); its usual site of entry is the pharynx. Gram-negative aerobic bacilli (8%) cause meningitis through bacteremia from pneumonia, decubitus ulcers, osteomyelitis, or urosepsis or from head trauma or neurosurgery. *Listeria monocytogenes* accounts for 10% of all cases of bacterial meningitis and is associated with a very high mortality. Although infection is often coupled with diseases affecting cellular immunity or with chronic corticosteroid use, the apparently healthy elderly also show increased susceptibility to this organism, which causes infections more frequently during the summer.

S. aureus, another cause of meningitis (about 5%) is isolated more frequently in hospitalized patients, particularly those who have had endocarditis, pneumonia, or neurosurgery. *S. epidermidis* is the most common cause of CSF shunt infections. Organisms less commonly associated with meningitis include *H. influenzae* (as protective serum bactericidal antibody decreases with age), various streptococcal species, and anaerobic organisms. The latter may be associated with head and neck malignancy, upper respiratory tract infections, or neurosurgery.

Viral (aseptic) meningitis is less common in elderly than in younger populations, whereas meningitis from *M. tuberculosis* is seen more often in the elderly. Other pathogens (eg, the fungus *Cryptococcus neoformans*) may be implicated when there is use of immunosuppressive drugs or depressed cell-mediated immunity associated with malignancy.

ENDOCARDITIS

Infective endocarditis has become more prevalent in the elderly in the modern antibiotic era, and more than half of all cases occur in persons > 60 yr of age. Several factors account for this epidemiologic shift: an increase in the number of elderly persons, an increase in prosthetic valve implantation, an increase in the frequency of hospital-acquired bacteremia, a decrease in the number of new cases of rheumatic heart disease, and prolongation of the life span of persons with rheumatic valvular lesions.

The development of infective endocarditis requires 2 events. First is an alteration in the endocardial surface, which then permits the deposition of platelets and fibrin. The resulting thrombus or vegetation most often arises in areas of increased turbulence. Second is transient bacteremia, which allows colonization of the thrombus. Bacterial properties, eg, the increased adherence of certain streptococcal and staphylococcal species, make particular organisms more common etiologic agents than others.

The underlying cardiac lesions that predispose the elderly to endocarditis tend to differ from those in younger patients. In most series, about 40% of elderly patients with endocarditis had either no valvular lesions or undetermined ones. Rheumatic valvular lesions were found in about 30%, calcified valves in 25%, and mitral valve prolapse in about 5%. The increased incidence of atherosclerotic disease in the elderly may also be a factor, since atheromatous deposits can cause turbulence and, hence, thrombus formation. The aortic valve is involved in 20 to 40% of cases.

This percentage, which is higher than that in younger persons, probably reflects the increased prevalence of calcific aortic stenosis in the elderly. Until age 60, rheumatic heart disease is the most common cause of calcific aortic stenosis. A calcified congenital bicuspid valve is the most common cause from age 60 to 75. After age 75, aortic stenosis with calcification, resulting from degeneration of a normal valve, becomes the leading cause. Mitral valve involvement occurs in 25 to 70% of cases of endocarditis, and both aortic and mitral valve involvement are found in approximately 10 to 25% of cases. Infections involving congenital heart defects other than those of the bicuspid valve occur infrequently in the elderly.

The source of bacteremia is unknown in 28 to 63% of cases of endocarditis. The sites of primary infection include the mouth, the GU tract (particularly postinstrumentation), skin and decubitus ulcers, surgical wounds, and IV catheters.

The causative organisms are similar to those in younger patients. *Streptococcus* spp remain the most common, accounting for 25 to 70% of cases. However, *S. viridans* is less prevalent than in the younger population, owing to the greater prevalence of enterococci, which are frequent inhabitants of the GU and lower GI tracts and can account for as many as 25% of all cases of endocarditis in elderly men. Frequent GU tract infections and instrumentation (especially in men with prostate disease) explain the increased frequency of enterococcal bacteremia and endocarditis.

Streptococcus bovis, a nonenterococcal group D streptococcus, can be isolated in up to 25% of cases in persons over 55 yr old. Many such cases of endocarditis are associated with underlying and often asymptomatic malignant or premalignant GI lesions, especially colon carcinoma. Staphylococci account for 20 to 30% of all cases of endocarditis in the elderly. The predominant species, *S. aureus*, is a frequent cause of nosocomial endocarditis, and many cases are only discovered incidentally at autopsy.

S. epidermidis is isolated in < 5% of cases of native valve endocarditis, but as in younger persons, it is the most common single cause of prosthetic valve endocarditis. Gram-negative aerobic bacilli remain a rare cause of endocarditis (only 2 to 3% of cases), often involving a prosthetic valve. *Bacteroides* spp are rare isolates in older patients, as in younger ones. Mixed infections are rare in the geriatric population. Fungal endocarditis occurs in 0 to 5% of cases. It is usually due to *Candida* spp, often affects a prosthetic valve, or is secondary to fungemia from an indwelling intravascular catheter.

Culture-negative endocarditis, *a suggestive clinical syndrome without an isolated organism,* accounts for 10 to 20% of cases. The inability to isolate an organism from blood cultures may be due to prior antibiotic administration, fastidious pathogens, inadequate laboratory technics, and obligate intracellular organisms (ie, *Rickettsia*). Endocarditis is more often missed in the elderly because the diagnosis is not considered.

GASTROINTESTINAL AND INTRA-ABDOMINAL INFECTIONS

INFECTIOUS DIARRHEA

Although the exact incidence of infectious diarrhea in the elderly is unknown, it is higher than in younger adults and has a higher mortality. Anatomic and physiologic changes that occur with aging, chronic illnesses, and increased drug administration make the elderly more susceptible to GI infections. **Gastric acidity,** which aids in the inactivation of ingested bacteria, is generally decreased because of mucosal atrophy, frequent use of H_2-receptor blockers and antacids, or possible previous gastric resection. **Intestinal motility,** another defense mechanism, is also decreased secondary to intrinsic neuronal degeneration, vascular ischemia, diabetes mellitus, or frequent use of anticholinergic drugs or narcotics. As a result, pathogenic organisms and their toxins can remain in the gut for an extended period and may thus overgrow. **Intestinal mucosal immunity** (ie, IgA secretion) is also believed to be decreased, although this has not been proved.

The **causative agents,** similar to those in other age groups, include bacteria, viruses, and parasites. Illness may also occur from ingestion of a *preformed toxin* contained in certain foods. The toxins responsible for such "food poisoning" are produced by *S. aureus* and *Bacillus cereus.* Food poisoning also results from the ingestion of food contaminated with *B. cereus* or *Clostridium perfringens,* which then produce enterotoxin in vivo. Other pathogens (eg, *Shigella, Salmonella,* and *Campylobacter* spp; enteroinvasive *E. coli; Vibrio parahaemolyticus;* and *Yersinia enterocolitica*) may produce disease by direct invasion of the intestinal mucosa.

Gastroenteritis caused by *Salmonella* is found more frequently in patients > 60 yr of age, partially because of reduced gastric acidity. *Salmonella* bacteremia also occurs more often in the elderly than in young adults with *Salmonella* gastroenteritis, and is potentially more harmful to them, since it tends to colonize the endothelial surfaces of atherosclerotic aortic aneurysms.

Some bacteria (eg, *Vibrio cholerae* and toxigenic *E. coli*) cause diarrhea by forming toxins that alter epithelial cell function. Some toxins (eg, those produced by *Clostridium difficile* and *E. coli* serotype 0157;H7) actually destroy epithelial cells. The incidence of *C. difficile* pseudomembranous colitis is largely influenced by the use of antibiotics that selectively allow overgrowth of this organism. Older persons are more susceptible to this problem and have higher mortality rates as well, in part because of the frequency with which they receive antibiotics.

Viruses responsible for infectious diarrhea include the Norwalk virus-like agents and, less commonly, rotavirus. The exact pathogenetic mechanism is unclear. Diarrhea due to Norwalk virus occurs throughout the year, whereas rotavirus infection occurs more often in the cooler months. Both agents have caused epidemic diarrhea in nursing homes and are easily spread by the fecal-oral route.

The parasites causing infectious diarrhea most frequently are *Entamoeba histolytica,* which produces inflammation by direct invasion of colonic mucosa, and *Giardia lamblia,* which involves the small bowel and can cause malabsorption.

BILIARY TRACT INFECTION

Biliary tract disease is the most common reason for abdominal surgery in the elderly. The incidence of cholelithiasis in persons > 60 yr of age approximates 50%. Bactobilia is present in 54 to 72% of those > 70 yr of age who undergo cholecystectomy and may result in abscess formation. Bacterial invasion of the biliary system occurs following impeded bile flow, usually secondary to stones or sludge. The subsequent pathophysiologic events may lead to focal necrosis, empyema, perforation, and gangrene of the gallbladder. Mortality from cholecystitis is about 7%, compared with < 2% in the general population. Acute cholangitis results when the hepatic or common bile duct becomes obstructed, most often from a stone; however, carcinoma, a benign stricture, or a fistula to the GI tract may be responsible.

Organisms commonly isolated from the biliary tract are enteric (eg, *E. coli, Klebsiella-Enterobacter, Proteus* spp, enterococcus, *B. fragilis,* and *C. perfringens*). Infection is caused by mixed aerobic-anaerobic organisms in about 50% of cases.

DIVERTICULITIS

The prevalence of diverticular disease is directly proportional to the age of the population, occurring in about 40% of those > 65 yr of age and in 50% of those > 80 yr of age in Western societies. Most diverticula are located in the sigmoid colon. These can undergo subclinical microperforations as a result of normal circular muscle contraction and intracolonic pressures. Eventually, frank perforation may occur and lead to focal peritonitis, local or disseminated intra-abdominal abscesses, and adhesions with intestinal obstruction. The incidence of diverticulitis increases with the duration of diverticulosis and varies from 10 to 40% after 5 to 20 yr. The organisms involved include the usual colonic flora (eg, aerobic and anaerobic gram-negative bacilli). The role of enterococci, however, is uncertain.

APPENDICITIS

The mortality associated with appendicitis in the elderly may be up to 10 times that in younger individuals because of delayed diagnosis leading to perforation, and the increased prevalence and severity of underlying illnesses. The incidence of acute appendicitis in persons > 65 yr of age is 20/100,000 and accounts for about 1.6/1000 hospital admissions. Anatomic changes in the appendix (eg, thinning of the mucosa, narrowing and obliteration of the lumen, and reduced number of lymphoid follicles) account for the greater severity of appendicitis and the greater risk of perforation. Anaerobes predominate in the infectious complications that follow perforation, with *B. fragilis* being the most common organism. *E. coli* and other enteric gram-negative bacilli also play a role. It is not unusual for periappendiceal abscess, with fever, mass, and weight loss, to be the initial presentation of appendicitis in the elderly.

INTRA-ABDOMINAL ABSCESSES

Intra-abdominal abscesses result from the increased frequency of abdominal surgery, diverticulitis, ulcer perforations, and the complications of appendicitis and cholecystitis. The peak incidence occurs in persons > 50 yr of age, and mortality increases with age, most likely reflecting frequent and severe underlying illnesses and complications.

OSTEOMYELITIS AND SEPTIC ARTHRITIS

Osteomyelitis can be classified into 3 major pathogenetic categories. **Hematogenously induced disease** is bimodal, often causing bone infection in children and showing a second peak in persons > 50 yr of age. Antecedent bacteremia may result from a concurrent UTI but is often untraceable. Although the vertebrae are most often involved, the long bones (eg, femur, tibia, humerus) may also become infected. Vertebral osteomyelitis particularly is more prevalent in older people, with about 60% of documented cases presenting in persons > 50 yr of age.

Generally, only 1 organism is isolated. *S. aureus* is the most common; however, gram-negative aerobic bacilli are also frequently found. In vertebral osteomyelitis, *E. coli* is the second most common isolate and most likely arises from GU tract infection and/or instrumentation.

A contiguous focus of infection is more commonly associated with osteomyelitis in patients > 50 yr of age. Contiguous septic foci usually result from postoperative infections, decubitus ulcers, radiotherapy, or foreign bodies. Infection involves the head of the femur (often secondary to prosthetic hip infections) in about 40% of cases, the tibia in 30%, the mandible in 16%, and the skull in 14%. The bacteria found in these infections are often mixed and frequently include *S. aureus, S. epidermidis,* gram-negative aerobic bacilli, and anaerobic species.

Vascular insufficiency most commonly causes osteomyelitis in patients between the ages of 50 and 70 yr, owing to the greater presence of associated conditions in this population (eg, diabetes mellitus, atherosclerotic cardiovascular disease, vasculitis). The small bones of the feet and toes are most often involved. The infections are commonly mixed and may involve *S. aureus, S. epidermidis,* streptococci, gram-negative aerobic bacilli, and anaerobic organisms.

Septic arthritis is often associated with underlying systemic illnesses, resulting in bacteremia superimposed on chronic joint disease (ie, rheumatoid arthritis, osteoarthritis, and crystal-induced arthritis). Although septic arthritis is usually preceded by bacteremia, organisms may be introduced directly by arthrocentesis. In order of descending frequency, the joints involved are the knees, hips, shoulders, and wrists. *S. aureus* is the most commonly isolated pathogen, and gram-negative aerobic bacilli are more often found in older than younger patients.

TETANUS

People > 60 yr of age account for > 50% of all reported cases of tetanus in the USA, which has a mortality ≥ 75%. Many cases are *not* associated with injury, but occur following surgery or are secondary to skin ulcers (chronic or decubitus). The higher incidence of tetanus in the elderly is attributed to their decreased immune status against the toxin of *Clostridium tetani*. Protective serum antibody levels, defined as 0.01 u./mL, are present in only 40% of men and 30% of women > 60 yr of age. Undetectable or nonprotective antibody levels indicate a lack of previous immunization with tetanus toxoid or an extended time lapse since the last booster injection. Antibody levels fall below the protective range in about 25% of elderly persons who received a booster dose ≥ 8 yr earlier but are easily restored following reimmunization.

HERPES ZOSTER

This disease primarily affects the elderly. The annual incidence is 6.5/1000 persons between 60 and 79 yr of age, and increases to 10/1000 persons 80 or older. The development of herpes zoster requires previous infection with varicella virus. The increased frequency among older persons may partially be explained by a decrease in cellular immune response to varicella-zoster antigen, which is undetectable in up to 30% of previously immune healthy persons > 60 yr of age. However, the majority have detectable antibody levels, which may be why dissemination of zoster is uncommon. Other factors that predispose to a reactivation of varicella virus include immunosuppressive drugs or corticosteroids, malignancy, local irradiation, trauma, and surgery. Herpes zoster recurs in about 6% of cases, usually at the same site as the initial episode.

The distribution of dermatomal zoster infections is 50 to 60% thoracic, 10 to 20% trigeminal, 10 to 20% cervical, 5 to 10% lumbar, and < 5% sacral. Herpes zoster infection is usually self-limited unless the person has an underlying immunologic abnormality. Most morbidity is a result of postherpetic neuralgia, which occurs more frequently (10 to 50% of cases) in the elderly. Other complications include encephalitis, ophthalmic disease, motor neuropathies, Guillain-Barré syndrome, and urinary retention.

77. ANTIMICROBIAL AGENTS

S. Ragnar Norrby

Epidemiology of Infections (See also Chs. 75 and 76)

Infections are more common and often more severe in older than in younger adults. This can be explained largely by an increased frequency of other diseases in the elderly. However, old age per se is a risk factor in some infections. Underlying conditions (eg, cardiovascular diseases, alcoholism) usually can be identified in patients with pneumococcal septicemia who are between ages 1 and 65 yr, while no such risk factors are present in about 25% of neonates and older patients.

The mortality in pneumococcal septicemia varies between < 10% in patients aged 2 to 17 yr and 25% in patients > 65 yr of age. Studies of septicemia caused by gram-negative bacteria or fungi have demonstrated that elderly persons have a higher incidence of these infections and are at higher risk of dying. *Salmonella* infections occur infrequently in the elderly, but when they do, the risk of septicemia and death is considerable. In younger adults, septicemia caused by *Salmonella* sp other than *S. typhi* and *S. paratyphi* is extremely rare and often indicates an underlying malignancy.

The etiology of infections tends to be different in the elderly. Septicemia caused by gram-negative aerobic pathogens increases in frequency, partly because of a higher incidence of urinary tract disorders and more frequent use of urinary catheters, leading to bacteriuria. Further, while gram-positive species dominate the normal aerobic oropharyngeal flora in healthy individuals, illness facilitates attachment of gram-negative organisms to the buccal mucosa. These organisms may be aspirated and cause gram-negative pneumonia.

Frequent hospitalization also affects the etiology of infections in the elderly. In the past, nosocomial infections were caused mainly by gram-negative antibiotic-resistant aerobes (eg, *Pseudomonas* spp, *Acinetobacter* spp, and *Serratia marcescens*). Currently, these infections are often caused by methicillin-resistant strains of *Staphylococcus aureus* or *S. epidermidis,* although variably resistant gram-negative strains are still common.

One explanation for the increased incidence and severity of infections is that the elderly have an impaired immune response; nevertheless, the type and degree of age-related impairment is insufficient to explain their increased susceptibility to infections.

Pharmacokinetics of Antimicrobial Agents

Many drugs, including some antimicrobial agents, are handled differently by the elderly than by the young, healthy male volunteers normally used for determining the pharmacokinetics of new agents. For example, peak plasma concentrations of ciprofloxacin, a new fluorinated 4-quinoline derivative, are about 2 times higher in elderly, sick patients than in young volunteers receiving the same dose. Considering that 4-quinolones seem to have dose-dependent side effects, such differences may be of considerable clinical importance. General aspects of geriatric clinical pharmacology are discussed in Ch. 18; issues specific to antimicrobial agents are discussed below.

Absorption: Aging results in decreased production of gastric acid, prolonged gastric emptying, and decreased small-bowel motility. The effects of these changes on drug absorption have not been thoroughly investigated. Theoretically, the effects could be either positive (ie, increased absorption) or negative. Generally, drug absorption is not altered in the elderly (see Ch. 18).

Distribution: The lean body mass of an elderly person is about 20% lower than that of a younger adult. As a result, water-soluble antimicrobial agents (eg, aminoglycosides, penicillins, cephalosporins, and amphotericin B) reach higher plasma and tissue fluid concentrations. Conversely, fat-soluble antimicrobial agents (eg, chloramphenicol, doxycycline, and ketoconazole) achieve lower plasma and tissue concentrations in older than in younger patients, given the relatively higher percentage of fat in the former.

Protein binding: With few exceptions, antimicrobial agents are bound to albumin in plasma to some extent. The bound portion cannot penetrate to extravascular compartments and thus lacks antibacterial effect. In most cases, protein binding is rapidly reversible, and the drug may be displaced from the albumin by highly bound drugs and substances, such as bilirubin. This may have clinical consequences. The only antibacterials that are highly protein bound and that may displace other drugs and bilirubin are the sulfonamides.

Plasma albumin concentration decreases somewhat with age. While this is probably of little importance, the changes in protein binding that occur from diseases can lead to hyperbilirubinemia or to uremia. In hyperbilirubinemia, bilirubin displaces antimicrobial agents from albumin and the plasma concentration of free drug increases. In uremia, marked hypoalbuminemia gives the same result. More free drug also leads to more rapid elimination.

Elimination: Metabolism and biliary excretion of antimicrobial agents seem to be relatively constant with age. A possible exception is the first-pass metabolism of some drugs (eg, ciprofloxacin), which may decrease with age, leading to increased plasma concentrations. Since aging is associated with reduced kidney function, renally excreted antimicrobial agents may have markedly altered pharmacokinetics. This is especially true if renal excretion is the only mode of elimination. The plasma half-life ($t_{1/2}$) of such drugs is longer in older than in younger adults. The increase is moderate in patients with a creatinine clearance > 30 mL/min. Lower clearances result in a drastic increase in the plasma $t_{1/2}$, with considerable risk of drug accumulation and adverse reactions. As noted in Ch. 18, serum creatinine is not a reliable indicator of kidney function in older patients; therefore, a creatinine clearance value should be estimated with a nomogram or a formula that takes into account age, sex, body weight, and serum creatinine.

Choice of Antimicrobial Agent

The increased risk for certain infections and the high frequency of nosocomial infections in the elderly should be considered in the choice of antimicrobial agent. In patients with symptoms and signs of bacteremia, empiric treatment must be correct, since mortality can be very high. In contrast, the mortality rates for some infections are unaffected by early treatment. The mortality in pneumococcal septicemia did not differ during the first 5 days of hospitalization in a comparison of patients who received no antibiotics with those who received benzylpenicillin. Afterward, however, mortality was close to zero among the treated patients, while almost all of the untreated patients died.

ANTIBIOTICS

AMINOGLYCOSIDES

Aminoglycosides irreversibly inhibit bacterial protein synthesis and are rapidly bactericidal against staphylococci and gram-negative aerobic bacteria, including *Pseudomonas*. The most important aminoglycosides are amikacin, gentamicin, neomycin, netilmicin, and tobramycin. Neomycin is used topically or orally for treatment of hepatic coma or for sterilizing the large bowel before colorectal surgery. Amikacin, gentamicin, netilmicin, and tobramycin differ in resistance to bacterial aminoglycoside-inactivating enzymes; amikacin and netilmicin are most resistant.

Pharmacokinetics: Aminoglycosides are not absorbed from the GI tract. Excretion is renal, exactly as for creatinine, and there is no metabolism. Aminoglycosides are reabsorbed in the renal tubules and accumulate in these cells. Because the drugs have a narrow therapeutic spectrum, antibacterial levels in peripheral compartments are difficult to achieve. In individuals with normal renal function, the half-life ($t_{1/2}$) is about 2 h. It is increased with reduced renal function and is about 4, 9, 18, and 29 h in patients with creatinine clearances of 70, 35, 18, and 9 mL/min, respectively. Thus, dose adjustment proportional to creatinine clearance estimation or measurement is essential.

Side effects and interactions: Aminoglycosides reduce glomerular filtration and may cause tubular necrosis at toxic levels. As a consequence of **nephrotoxicity** the $t_{1/2}$ increases during therapy; if doses are not reduced, accumulation may result, increasing the risk of **ototoxicity.** While nephrotoxicity is reversible in most patients, ototoxicity is often irreversible. It may affect the vestibular or the cochlear branch of the 8th cranial nerve and can be unilateral or bilateral. The risk of ototoxicity increases with age. However, because of reduced renal function, it is also more difficult to avoid overdosing in the elderly. Ototoxicity is related to the aminoglycoside serum levels at the end of a dose period, which should not exceed 2 mg/L of gentamicin, netilmicin, or tobramycin or 10 mg/L of amikacin.

In all patients receiving aminoglycoside therapy, especially the elderly, serum-concentration monitoring is strongly recommended. Samples should be drawn before and 1 h after administration of a new dose. The second sample is drawn to ensure that therapeutic concentrations have been achieved and may not have to be repeated during treatment. Concentration monitoring should begin on the second treatment day and be repeated at least twice weekly during treatment. There are no clinically significant differences among the 4 most important aminoglycosides (amikacin, gentamicin, netilmicin, and tobramycin) relative to risk of nephrotoxicity or ototoxicity or auditory vs. vestibular toxicity in the latter category. Establishment of a causal relationship between an ototoxic reaction and a drug requires a pretreatment audiogram, often difficult and impractical in an older patient with a severe systemic infection.

The risk of nephrotoxicity and ototoxicity is increased in patients receiving cisplatin or methotrexate, in whom aminoglycosides should be avoided.

β-LACTAM ANTIBIOTICS

All β-lactams inhibit the final steps in bacterial cell wall synthesis by binding to penicillin-binding proteins, which are enzymes that catalyze that process. They are bactericidal, although there may be large differences between bacteriostatic and bactericidal concentrations. Resistance to β-lactam antibiotics is due to production of β-lactamases, to alteration of the bacterial cell wall rendering it impermeable to the drugs, or to alterations of the penicillin-binding proteins.

Benzylpenicillin (Penicillin G)

Penicillin G is active against gram-positive bacteria (eg, β-hemolytic and α-hemolytic streptococci and *Streptococcus pneumoniae*). Enterococci are less susceptible. Most strains of staphylococcus are resistant, owing to penicillinase production. Of the gram-negative bacteria, *Neisseria* spp are highly susceptible and *Hemophilus influenzae* is intermediately susceptible. Many gram-negative anaerobes are sensitive, but *Bacteroides* spp are often resistant because of β-lactamase production.

Pharmacokinetics: Penicillin G is acid labile and should be administered parenterally. Excretion is renal with a serum $t_{1/2}$ of approximately 1 h in patients with normal renal function. Doses should be adjusted in patients with severe renal impairment (creatinine clearance < 30 mL/min). About 30% of the dose is metabolized, mainly to penicilloyl-polylysine, which is microbiologically inactive but may cause hypersensitivity reactions.

Indications: Penicillin G is indicated in infections caused by streptococci (eg, endocarditis, erysipelas, and pneumococcal pneumonia or meningitis) or by meningococci. In the treatment of streptococcal endocarditis, penicillin G is combined with an aminoglycoside to obtain synergistic antibacterial activity.

Side effects and interactions: Penicillin G has a high degree of safety. Hypersensitivity reactions occur in about 5% of patients. Nonurticarial rashes predominate and contraindicate continued treatment, but not the later use of penicillin (after 2 mo). In ≤ 1% of patients, IgE-mediated reactions are seen. Most are urticarial. Anaphylactoid reactions are rare, especially in the elderly. All IgE-mediated reactions contraindicate further use of any penicillin. Drug fever and hematologic reactions (neutropenia, thrombocytopenia, or anemia) are seen in patients treated for prolonged periods with high doses (eg, for endocarditis). Such reactions are rapidly reversible if treatment is discontinued. Neurotoxicity may develop if high doses are used in patients with renal failure. Penicillin G interacts with phenylbutazone, which has a probenecid-like effect and increases the antibiotic's $t_{1/2}$.

Phenoxymethyl Penicillin (Pencillin V)

The antibacterial spectrum and activity of penicillin V are identical to those of penicillin G. Penicillin V is acid resistant and is given orally. Absorption is about 50% of the dose and is reduced by food. Kinetics after absorption are the same as for penicillin G. Penicillin V is a first-line antibiotic for oral treatment of infections caused by β-hemolytic streptococci or pneumococci. Hypersensitivity reactions occur at the same frequency as with penicillin G.

Penicillinase-Resistant Penicillins

This group includes cloxacillin, dicloxacillin, floxacillin, methicillin, nafcillin, and oxacillin. Their antibacterial spectrum includes all penicillin G-susceptible organisms plus penicillinase-producing staphylococci. Resistance (methicillin resistance) is relatively uncommon in *S. aureus* but is frequent in *S. epidermidis*.

Pharmacokinetics: Methicillin and nafcillin are not absorbed after oral administration and must be given parenterally. Cloxacillin and oxacillin are absorbed to a lesser degree than dicloxacillin and floxacillin. The protein binding of oxacillin, cloxacillin, floxacillin, and dicloxacillin is > 90%, leading to slow penetration of peripheral compartments. Therapeutic concentrations cannot be achieved in CSF. Excretion is renal, with a $t_{1/2}$ ≤ 1 h; $t_{1/2}$ increases in renal failure, but since the drugs are also metabolized in the liver, it rarely exceeds 4 h.

Indications: These penicillins are used to treat staphylococcal infections. Since their spectrum is similar to that of penicillin G, they are effective in infections caused by either staphylococci or β-hemolytic streptococci (eg, soft tissue infections).

Side effects: These are the same as for penicillin G. All, and especially dicloxacillin, may cause thrombophlebitis when given IV.

Ampicillin, Ampicillin Esters, and Amoxicillin

These penicillins are more active than penicillin G against gram-negative aerobes (eg, *E. coli, Proteus mirabilis,* and *H. influenzae*) and against enterococci. They are hydrolyzed by β-lactamases and, therefore, penicillinase-producing staphylococci are resistant.

Pharmacokinetics: Only 60% of orally administrated ampicillin is absorbed. Ampicillin esters, pivampicillin and bacampicillin, are pro-drugs; during absorption, the esters are split off. The active substance is ampicillin. Amoxicillin is well absorbed. Excretion is renal and the $t_{1/2}$ is approximately 1 h. About 25% of the dose is metabolized.

Indications: Because there is a relatively high frequency of ampicillin- and amoxicillin-resistant strains of *E. coli,* these antibiotics have limited value in UTIs and are mainly indicated for *H. influenzae* or enterococcal infections.

Side effects and interactions: Ampicillin and amoxicillin cause a higher frequency of skin rashes than penicillin. A morbilliform rash is occasionally seen in patients with viral infections 10 to 12 days after the start of ampicillin therapy. Diarrhea is common with oral ampicillin; therefore, an ampicillin ester or amoxicillin should be used. An increased frequency of rashes has been reported in patients given ampicillin in combination with allopurinol.

Antipseudomonal Penicillins

Azlocillin, carbenicillin, mezlocillin, piperacillin, and ticarcillin are β-lactamase–sensitive penicillins whose spectrums, while similar to those of ampicillin, also include gram-negative aerobes, such as *Enterobacter* and *Pseudomonas* spp. The most active are azlocillin and piperacillin. All are poorly absorbed from the GI tract and must be given parenterally. The sodium salt of the indanyl ester of carbenicillin may be used orally. Pharmacokinetics are similar to those of penicillin G. Carbenicillin and ticarcillin are rapidly cleared by the kidneys.

Antipseudomonal penicillins are indicated in patients with severe infections known or believed to be caused by *Pseudomonas.* For infections outside the urinary tract, they should be combined with an aminoglycoside to avoid emergence of resistance. Side effects are similar to those of ampicillin. Bleeding complications have been reported with these penicillins, especially with carbenicillin and ticarcillin, when used in high doses. In most cases, the cause seems to have been platelet dysfunction. With high doses of carbenicillin, patients with severe renal impairment may develop hypernatremia.

Amdinocillin (Mecillinam), Pivmecillinam

The penicillins described above are all aminopenicillins; ie, they have an amino group at the 6 position in the penicillin nucleus. If the amino group is replaced by an amdino group, the antibacterial spectrum changes drastically. Mecillinam is active only against gram-negative aerobic bacteria; it is active against most species except *Pseudomonas* sp.

Pharmacokinetics: Mecillinam is poorly absorbed from the GI tract, but the pivaloyl ester, pivmecillinam, is orally active. It is well absorbed and deesterified to mecillinam during absorption. The pharmacokinetics are otherwise similar to those of ampicillin.

Indications and side effects: Mecillinam and pivmecillinam are used as monotherapy to treat UTIs but can be combined with other β-lactams (eg, ampicillin). Such combinations are frequently synergistic, owing to selective binding by different penicillin-binding proteins. A fixed combination of pivmecillinam and pivampicillin has been licensed in several countries for use in UTIs and lower respiratory tract infections. The side effects are the same as those of penicillin.

First-Generation Oral Cephalosporins

Cephalosporins have been subdivided into generations, on the basis of their spectrum of activity. Oral cephalosporins (eg, cefaclor, cefadroxil, cephradine, and cephalexin) all belong to the first generation and are active against gram-positive aerobes (including penicillinase-producing staphylococci but excluding enterococci) and against *E. coli, Klebsiella* spp, and some *Proteus* spp. Cefaclor alone is active against *H. influenzae*. All are sensitive to hydrolysis by cephalosporinase-type β-lactamases.

Pharmacokinetics: Oral cephalosporins are well absorbed. They are renally excreted, with $t_{1/2}$s of approximately 1 h. Metabolism is minimal.

Indications and side effects: Oral cephalosporins are used for treatment of UTIs and in patients who are allergic to penicillin. Elderly patients requiring suspensions for oral treatment of staphylococcal infections should be given a cephalosporin rather than a penicillinase-resistant penicillin, which has a very bitter taste. Oral cephalosporins are safe, with a frequency of side effects similar to or lower than that of penicillin.

First-Generation Injectable Cephalosporins

This group includes the older cephalosporins: cefazolin, cephradine, cephaloridine, and cephalothin. Their antibacterial spectrum is similar to that of the oral derivatives.

Pharmacokinetics: Cephalothin is metabolized in the liver by deacetylation to about 40% active drug. All of these cephalosporins are eliminated renally, with $t_{1/2}$s between 0.7 (cephalothin) and 2 h (cefazolin). Dosage should be adjusted in patients with renal impairment.

Indications: These antibiotics are indicated mainly in community-acquired infections, especially those due to a gram-positive organism. In many countries, they have been replaced by newer, cephalosporinase-resistant derivatives.

Side effects: *Cephaloridine is nephrotoxic and should not be used.* The others share a high degree of safety. The frequency of hypersensitivity reactions is lower than with penicillin. The risk of cross-reaction between cephalosporins and penicillins has been recognized for many years. However, studies have demonstrated that patients with serologically and clinically verified hypersensitivity to the penicillins do not react when given therapeutic doses of cephalosporins. Despite that, care is recommended in patients with a history of anaphylactic reactions to a penicillin.

Second-Generation Cephalosporins and Cephamycins

The 2 most important second-generation cephalosporins are cefuroxime and cefamandole. Cefuroxime has a high, and cefamandole a moderate, degree of stability to cephalosporinase. The antibacterial spectrum is similar to that of first-generation agents but, because of enhanced β-lactamase stability, includes more strains. Second-generation cephalosporins are also active against *H. influenzae,* but enterococci and methicillin-resistant staphylococci are resistant.

The cephamycins differ from the cephalosporins in that they have a methoxy group at the seventh position in the nucleus. This moiety confers such a high degree of β-lactamase stability that the cephamycins are resistant to the β-lactamase produced by *Bacteroides fragilis.* Two members of this group, cefoxitin and cefotetan, have similar antibacterial spectrums, they cover the same organisms as the second-generation cephalosporins, plus most strains of *B. fragilis,* but show reduced activity against methicillin-sensitive staphylococci.

Pharmacokinetics: These antibiotics are poorly absorbed from the GI tract and must be given parenterally. They are not metabolized, and—with the exception of cefotetan, which is partly eliminated in bile—they are excreted renally and have a $t_{1/2}$ of approximately 1 h. The $t_{1/2}$ of cefotetan is $3 \frac{1}{2}$ h. The dosage should be reduced in patients with renal impairment.

Indications: Second-generation cephalosporins and cephamycins are used to treat community-acquired infections, especially when a mixed gram-positive and -negative etiology is suspected or when the patient is allergic to penicillins. The main role of the cephamycins is as therapeutic or prophylactic agents in mixed infections. The efficacy of cefuroxime in the treatment of bacterial meningitis is well documented.

Side effects and interactions: Cefuroxime and cefoxitin have a high degree of safety. Cefamandole and cefotetan have a 3-methylthiotetrazole side chain, leading to hypoprothrombinemia, especially in the elderly. The hypoprothrombinemia is reversible with administration of vitamin K. As with the penicillins, prolonged treatment with high doses of injectable cephalosporins may cause drug fever or hematologic reactions. Diarrhea may occur; in the elderly especially, it may be caused by the cytotoxin of *Clostridium difficile,* leading to colitis or pseudomembranous colitis. The frequency of hypersensitivity reactions is low, and it is doubtful that there is a cross-allergenicity with the penicillins.

Like other β-lactams, these antibiotics (especially cefoxitin) may induce cephalosporinases in certain species (eg, *Enterobacter* and *Pseudomonas* spp). Combinations with other β-lactams may therefore result in antagonism.

Third-Generation Cephalosporins

This rapidly growing group of antibiotics includes, among others, cefmenoxime, cefoperazone, cefotaxime, ceftazidime, ceftizoxime, ceftriaxone, and moxalactam. They are highly resistant to cephalosporinases. In addition to their activity against organisms covered by the second-generation derivatives, they are active against a majority of strains of *Proteus* spp, *Enterobacter* spp, and *Serratia* spp. Ceftazidime is the only 1 with generally high activity against *Pseudomonas* spp. Moxalactam and cefoperazone have high activity against anaerobes, while ceftazidime is inactive and the others show an intermediary effect. Gram-positive organisms other than enterococci and methicillin-resistant staphylococci are susceptible, although at higher concentrations than needed with the first- or second-generation cephalosporins.

Pharmacokinetics: The pharmacokinetics of these antibiotics differ considerably. Since none is absorbed after oral administration, all must be given parenterally. Cefotaxime is metabolized by deacetylation in the liver to a considerably less active compound. Cefotaxime, ceftizoxime, and moxalactam are excreted only via the kidneys, with serum $t_{1/2}$s of between 1 and 2 h. Cefmenoxime, cefoperazone, and ceftriaxone are also excreted in bile, leading to high fecal concentrations of active drug. Their $t_{1/2}$s vary between 1 ½ h for cefmenoxime and 8 h for ceftriaxone, which can be given once daily. Dosage must be reduced in patients with diminished renal function; this does not apply to drugs excreted in bile, whose elimination increases with declining renal function.

Indications: Third-generation cephalosporins are indicated for nosocomial infections caused by susceptible gram-negative or -positive pathogens (eg, urosepsis and pneumonia). With the exception of ceftazidime, they should not be used when *Pseudomonas* is the verified or suspected pathogen. Cefoperazone and moxalactam may be used in patients with infections caused by mixed aerobic/anaerobic bacteria. The efficacy of cefotaxime and ceftriaxone in meningitis is well documented. Ceftazidime has been used as monotherapy in febrile neutropenic patients.

Side effects and interactions: Biliary-excreted derivatives tend to disturb the normal fecal flora, causing diarrhea. *C. difficile* cytotoxin-induced diarrhea or colitis is relatively common in the elderly. Cefoperazone, ceftizoxime, and moxalactam have a 3-methylthiotetrazole side chain and may cause hypoprothrombinemia, which has been reported mainly in elderly patients. The frequency of other side effects is low.

Monobactams

These are β-lactam antibiotics with a simple nuclear structure. Only 1, aztreonam, is in clinical use. It is active only against gram-negative aerobes. Gram-positive organisms and anaerobes are naturally resistant, since aztreonam has no affinity for their penicillin-binding proteins. Aztreonam is as active as ceftazidime against gram-negative aerobes.

Pharmacokinetics: Aztreonam is not orally absorbed and must be administered parenterally. It is excreted renally, with a $t_{1/2}$ of approximately 2 h. In renal failure, the $t_{1/2}$ is increased. Approximately 30% of the dose is metabolized.

Indications: Aztreonam is indicated in hospital-acquired infections caused by gram-negative aerobes. In lower respiratory tract and skin and soft tissue infections, it should be combined with an antibiotic active against gram-positive organisms to avoid superinfection.

Side effects: The safety of aztreonam is comparable to that of an injectable cephalosporin that is excreted renally and lacks a 3-methylthiotetrazole side chain. No cross-allergenicity with the penicillins has been demonstrated. When aztreonam is used to treat lower respiratory tract and skin and soft tissue infections, superinfection from gram-positive aerobes frequently occurs.

Carbapenems (Thienamycins)

Carbapenems are β-lactams with an exceptionally broad antibacterial spectrum. The first member of the group, imipenem, is active against all bacteria except *Pseudomonas maltophilia, Streptococcus faecium,* JK corynebacteria, methicillin-resistant staphylococci, and about 50% of strains of *Pseudomonas cepacia.* Imipenem is resistant to virtually all β-lactamases and is hydrolyzed only by enzymes containing zinc, which appear mostly in *P. maltophilia.*

Pharmacokinetics: Imipenem has complicated pharmacokinetics. It is not absorbed from the GI tract and is given IV. About 30% of the dose is metabolized in patients with normal renal function. The metabolite and the parent compound are excreted renally. Imipenem given alone is metabolized in the kidneys by an enzyme, dehydropeptidase I, to a microbiologically inactive compound. The degree of metabolism varies between 30 and 65% of the dose. In heavy metabolizers, urine concentrations of active imipenem are low and fall rapidly below inhibitory levels for some bacteria, mainly *Pseudomonas* spp. To avoid this, imipenem is combined at a 1:1 ratio with cilastatin, an inhibitor of dehydropeptidase I, which has no antibacterial effect of its own. Thus combined, imipenem undergoes no renal metabolism, and about 70% of the dose is excreted unchanged in the urine. Imipenem is not excreted via bile, and the $t_{1/2}$ is approximately 1 h. The dose should be adjusted in patients with decreased renal function.

Indications: Imipenem is indicated for infections caused by mixed aerobic/anaerobic flora (eg, intra-abdominal infections) and for empiric treatment of serious hospital-acquired infections (eg, septicemia) pending results of cultures.

Side effects: Imipenem and cilastatin have high degrees of safety. Nausea may develop if large doses are administered rapidly. Seizures have been reported in patients who receive doses that are excessive relative to body weight and renal function. However, neurotoxicity is rare if dosage recommendations are followed. Given alone, imipenem is nephrotoxic in rabbits; when it is combined with cilastatin, the nephrotoxicity is not seen, and nephrotoxicity has been rarely reported in humans.

CHLORAMPHENICOL

Chloramphenicol is a broad-spectrum, bacteriostatic antibiotic active against a wide range of gram-positive and -negative aerobic and anaerobic species. Resistance to chloramphenicol is often plasmid mediated and varies in frequency, depending on the extent of usage. In most Western countries, resistance is rare.

Pharmacokinetics: Chloramphenicol is rapidly and almost completely absorbed from the GI tract and can be administered orally or IV. IM administration should be avoided because of the risk of inactivation at the site of injection. It penetrates well into all peripheral sites, including CSF and brain, and is eliminated by hepatic metabolism. The $t_{1/2}$ is 2 to 3 h.

Indications: Because of its side effects (see below), systemic chloramphenicol is indicated only in life-threatening infections. The main indications are purulent meningitis, brain abscesses, enteric fever, and paratyphoid.

Side effects and interactions: One patient in every 5000 to 100,000 who receive chloramphenicol develops a dose-independent aplastic anemia with pancytopenia; mortality is $> 50\%$. This condition may have an onset in direct relation to treatment but can be seen up to 6 mo afterward. Reversible dose-dependent bone marrow toxicity may develop if large doses (total dose > 25 gm) are used for prolonged periods. The hematologic side effects are not seen when chloramphenicol is used topically (eg, in ophthalmic ointment).

Chloramphenicol interacts with several other drugs. If given with phenytoin, metabolism of the latter will be reduced, possibly resulting in toxic serum levels. This interaction is important, since patients with intracerebral infections often receive both drugs. Chloramphenicol also inhibits the metabolism of tolbutamide, with risk of hypoglycemia, and of dicumarol, with risk of hypoprothrombinemia.

CLINDAMYCIN AND LINCOMYCIN (LINCOSAMIDES)

These antibiotics inhibit bacterial protein synthesis and are active against anaerobes and gram-positive (but not gram-negative) aerobes. The aerobic spectrum includes streptococci (not enterococci) and staphylococci. Most anaerobes, including *B. fragilis* are susceptible. *C. difficile* is resistant. Clindamycin is generally more active than lincomycin; strains may be resistant to lincomycin and susceptible to clindamycin but not vice versa.

Pharmacokinetics: Lincomycin is slowly and incompletely absorbed from the GI tract, whereas clindamycin is well absorbed. Both drugs can be administered IV. They are eliminated by hepatic metabolism and by biliary and renal excretion. The $t_{1/2}$ is approximately 4 h for lincomycin and about 2½ h for clindamycin. Dosage should be reduced in patients with diminished liver or kidney function.

Indications and side effects: With its superior pharmacokinetic properties, clindamycin is the preferred antibiotic. It is indicated for anaerobic and staphylococcal infections. Antibiotic-associated colitis, or pseudomembranous enterocolitis, caused by the cytotoxin of *C. difficile* is reported relatively frequently after treatment with lincomycin or clindamycin. It is more common in elderly than in younger patients.

ETHAMBUTOL

Ethambutol is an antibiotic active only against species of *Mycobacterium,* mainly *M. tuberculosis* and *M. bovis.* Other atypical mycobacteria (eg, *M. avium, M. intracellulare*) are resistant. As with other tuberculostatic agents, resistance is a problem, and the in vitro mutation frequency is high.

Pharmacokinetics: Ethambutol is given orally, and 80% of the dose is absorbed. It penetrates to CSF, where therapeutic concentrations are achieved. It is eliminated via the kidneys and is only moderately metabolized. The $t_{1/2}$ is approximately 4 h. Dosage should be reduced in patients with renal impairment.

Indications and side effects: Ethambutol is used only for treatment of mycobacterial infections and should be combined with other tuberculostatic agents to minimize the risk of resistance. Optic neuritis has been reported with high doses. It is reversible if treatment is stopped but may otherwise be irreversible. Patients receiving the drug should have baseline and monthly visual acuity examinations.

FUSIDIC ACID

Fusidic acid is a bacteriostatic agent that inhibits bacterial protein synthesis. It is active mainly against staphylococci. If it is used alone, resistance commonly develops in vitro. Fusidic acid is given orally or IV. Elimination occurs by hepatic metabolism, and the $t_{1/2}$ is approximately 6 h. Dosage should be reduced in patients with hepatic dysfunction.

Fusidic acid is used mainly to treat staphylococcal infections when the organisms are methicillin resistant. It is often combined with another antibiotic to avoid development of resistance. After oral administration of fusidic acid, side effects are few and reversible. Liver toxicity, nausea, and vomiting have been reported. IV administration commonly causes thrombophlebitis, while hemolysis may result if the drug is infused too rapidly.

ISONIAZID

Isoniazid is a tuberculostatic agent active against only *M. tuberculosis* and *M. bovis.*

Pharmacokinetics: Isoniazid is rapidly absorbed after oral administration and can also be given parenterally. It penetrates well into peripheral compartments, including the CSF, and is metabolized by the liver. The rate of metabolism varies among individuals. Two genetic populations have been identified; rapid metabolizers, in whom the drug has a $t_{1/2}$ of approximately 1 h, and slow metabolizers, in whom the drug has a $t_{1/2}$ of 2½ to 3 h. About 35% of whites and 80% of Asians are rapid metabolizers. Both parent compound and metabolites are excreted renally.

Indications, side effects, and interactions: Isoniazid is used to treat mycobacterial infections and should be combined with another tuberculostatic agent (eg, rifampin and/or ethambutol). Adverse effects are dose dependent. The most common is neuritis. Because of the genetic differences in rate of metabolism, serum-concentration monitoring should be considered. Isoniazid interacts with several other drugs. Antacids reduce its absorption. In slow metabolizers, the metabolism of phenytoin, phenobarbital, and carbamazepine may be inhibited, with subsequent drug accumulation. Isoniazid treatment may lead to vitamin B_6 deficiency; thus, pyridoxine is administered concurrently.

MACROLIDES

The macrolide group of antibiotics includes, among others, erythromycin, spiramycin, and troleandomycin, but only erythromycin is discussed here. Macrolides inhibit bacterial protein synthesis and are bacteriostatic. Erythromycin is active against gram-positive aerobic bacteria (eg, streptococci and staphylococci), gram-negative bacteria (eg, *Campylobacter* spp, *Branhamella catarrhalis, Listeria monocytogenes,* and *Legionella pneumophila*), and some gram-negative anaerobes. It is also active against *Mycoplasma pneumoniae* and *Chlamydia* spp. *Enterobacteriaceae* and *Pseudomonas* spp are resistant. Resistance may develop in staphylococci and is common in *B. fragilis.*

Pharmacokinetics: Erythromycin base is acid labile and cannot be absorbed after oral administration unless it is enterocoated. Erythromycin salts are more acid stable. Although absorption is improved if the drug is taken with food, it does not exceed 55% of the dose. Erythromycin can also be given parenterally. Elimination is by metabolism and biliary excretion. Serum $t_{1/2}$ is approximately 1 h. Renal elimination is negligible. Dosage should be reduced in patients with severe liver dysfunction.

Indications and side effects: In the elderly, erythromycin is used mainly for the treatment of *Mycoplasma, Legionella,* and *Campylobacter* infections. It can also be used instead of penicillin in allergic patients. Oral erythromycin often causes upper GI disturbances, especially if used in high doses. Erythromycin estolate may cause cholestatic hepatitis.

NITROFURANTOIN

Nitrofurantoin is active against gram-negative and -positive urinary tract pathogens. It is well absorbed after oral administration and is not used parenterally. It is excreted unchanged in urine, and its $t_{1/2}$ is short in patients with normal renal function (approximately 20 min). Dosage should be reduced in those with renal impairment.

Nitrofurantoin is used primarily for treatment of or prophylaxis against bacterial cystitis. It is not indicated for renal cortical or perinephric abscesses. Nausea and vomiting may occur. Skin reactions tend to be more common in the elderly. Toxic hepatitis may develop if the drug is used in high doses for a prolonged duration. The most severe adverse effect is interstitial pulmonary infiltrates, which cause dyspnea and may result in pulmonary fibrosis if treatment is not discontinued. Lung reactions have been reported mainly in elderly women and are associated with high doses given for > 10 days. Deaths have occurred, mainly in patients with cardiac decompensation.

NITROIMIDAZOLES

This group of drugs includes metronidazole and tinidazole. Metronidazole was developed for the treatment of protozoal infections (trichomoniasis, giardiasis, and amebiasis) but was found to be bactericidal against obligate anaerobic bacteria (eg, *Clostridium* spp and *B. fragilis*). These drugs are not active against aerobes and microaerophiles, including anaerobic streptococci, which are not obligate anaerobes. Resistance rarely develops.

Pharmacokinetics: These drugs are rapidly and completely absorbed after oral administration and can be used orally, rectally, or parenterally. They penetrate well into peripheral compartments, including the CSF and brain, as well as into abscesses. Renal elimination follows metabolism in the liver. The $t_{1/2}$ is approximately 4 h for metronidazole and 12 h for tinidazole. Dosage should be reduced in patients with hepatic dysfunction or severe renal impairment.

Indications: Nitroimidazoles are used for the treatment of protozoal infections and infections caused by obligate anaerobes. Since anaerobic infections are often mixed, nitroimidazoles should be combined with an antibiotic active against aerobes (eg, an aminoglycoside or a cephalosporin) when used in cases of systemic bacterial infections. An important indication is oral treatment of *C. difficile* cytotoxin-induced, antibiotic-associated colitis.

Side effects and interactions: Nitroimidazoles cause few adverse reactions. Neuritis may develop with overdosage. If taken with alcohol, metronidazole may provoke a disulfiram-like reaction.

Cimetidine reduces plasma clearance of metronidazole by about 30%, leading to risk of overdose. Phenobarbital has been found to induce hepatic enzymes that metabolize metronidazole, leading to reduced levels of active drug. Metronidazole increases the effect of warfarin and hence the risk of bleeding. The effect of disulfiram is increased if it is coadministered with metronidazole. These interactions are also likely to occur with tinidazole.

POLYMYXINS

Polymyxins (polymyxin B, colistin) are bactericidal polypeptide antibiotics that interact with phospholipids in the bacterial cytoplasmic membrane. The derivatives discussed here are active exclusively against gram-negative aerobes, including *Pseudomonas*. Resistance is uncommon among gram-negative aerobic bacilli.

Pharmacokinetics: Polymyxins are available only for parenteral or topical use. They are not metabolized and are excreted renally, with $t_{1/2}$s heavily dependent on renal function (4 h for polymyxin B and 3 h for colistin). Dosage must be reduced even in the presence of slightly decreased renal function.

Indications and side effects: Polymyxins are indicated mainly for the treatment of infections caused by multiresistant strains of *Pseudomonas* spp. Polymyxins may cause neurotoxicity, nephrotoxicity, and hypersensitivity reactions, especially if used in high doses. For these reasons, use should be restricted, especially in elderly persons, who frequently have reduced renal function.

QUINOLONES

Quinolones are synthetic carboxylic acids that inhibit DNA gyrase (topoisomerase II). This enzyme supercoils DNA in the bacterial chromosome and plasmids, giving quinolones a rapid bactericidal effect. The older quinolones are nonfluorinated (eg, nalidixic acid, cinoxacin, and pipemidic acid); the newer derivatives are fluorinated (eg, norfloxacin, ofloxacin, enoxacin, pefloxacin, and ciprofloxacin). Nonfluorinated quinolones are active only against gram-negative aerobes, excluding *Pseudomonas* spp. Fluorinated quinolones have markedly improved antibacterial activity and are also effective against *Pseudomonas* spp and many gram-positive aerobes. Anaerobes are resistant to quinolones. Development of resistance is always chromosomal and occurs more frequently with nonfluorinated than with fluorinated quinolones.

Pharmacokinetics: With the exception of norfloxacin and ciprofloxacin, which are approximately 50% absorbed, the quinolones are well absorbed from the GI tract. All quinolones are available in oral forms; ofloxacin, ciprofloxacin, and pefloxacin are also available in forms for parenteral administration. They are metabolized to varying degrees. Elimination is renal, with $t_{1/2}$s varying between $1\frac{1}{2}$ and 8 h. Dosage should be reduced in the presence of renal impairment.

Indications: The older, nonfluorinated derivatives have no advantages over the fluorinated quinolones. The latter offer an oral alternative to parenteral treatment in patients with infections caused by multiresistant gram-negative aerobes, such as *Pseudomonas aeruginosa*. Norfloxacin is indicated in the treatment of UTIs and in the treatment of and prophylaxis against enteric bacterial infections. It can be used prophylactically in neutropenic patients, thus reducing the incidence of gram-negative septicemia. These indications also apply to ciprofloxacin, which has similar pharmacokinetics and poor GI absorption. Treatment of systemic infections outside the urinary tract is being studied for each of the new fluorinated quinolones.

Side effects and interactions: All quinolones may cause nonspecific neurologic side effects (eg, dizziness, headache, dimmed vision, and paresthesia). These adverse effects are dose dependent, reversible, and infrequent after oral administration of the new derivatives. Nalidixic acid causes phototoxicity in some patients, as do some of the new quinolones. Nausea and vomiting may occur after oral administration. Arthritis has been reported with IV ofloxacin.

Nalidixic acid, which is > 90% bound to plasma protein, has been reported to displace coumarin derivatives from albumin, leading to risk of bleeding. This should not occur with the fluorinated quinolones, which are less bound to albumin. Ciprofloxacin, pefloxacin, and especially enoxacin interact with theophylline, which may result in adverse theophylline reactions. All derivatives seem to interact with antacids, reducing their absorption, but not with the H_2-receptor antagonists.

RIFAMPIN

Rifampin is bactericidal and inhibits RNA synthesis in aerobic bacteria, including mycobacteria. Its spectrum includes many methicillin-resistant staphylococcal strains. Development of in vitro resistance is rapid. Antagonistic antibacterial effects have been found in vitro when rifampin was combined with other antibiotics.

Pharmacokinetics: Rifampin is highly lipid soluble and is rapidly absorbed after oral administration. It can also be given parenterally. Tissue penetration is good. Elimination occurs via liver metabolism and biliary excretion of metabolites. The $t_{1/2}$ is approximately 2 h. Dosage should be reduced in the presence of liver failure.

Indications: Rifampin is used to treat mycobacterial infections in combination with other tuberculostatic agents (eg, isoniazid, with or without ethambutol). It is also used in other bacterial infections, especially those caused by methicillin-resistant staphylococci.

Side effects and interactions: The main adverse effect of rifampin is hepatotoxicity, and liver function should be monitored during therapy. Because of its hepatic metabolism, rifampin may interact with many other drugs. It may even induce enzymes that increase its own metabolism. Enzyme induction has been reported when rifampin is combined with any of the following drugs: digitoxin, cyclosporine, coumarin derivatives, quinidine, theophylline, disopyramide, mexiletine, metoprolol, propranolol, verapamil, sulfasalazine, dapsone, chloramphenicol, glucocorticoids, tolbutamide, chlorpropamide, and diazepam.

SULFONAMIDES AND TRIMETHOPRIM (BACTERIAL FOLATE INHIBITORS)

Most bacteria (excluding enterococci) require para-aminobenzoic acid (PABA) to begin folic acid synthesis. Sulfonamides compete with PABA to induce a bacteriostatic effect. They are active against streptococci other than enterococci (which are naturally resistant) and some aerobic gram-negative bacilli. Trimethoprim and some other antimicrobial agents (eg, pyrimethamine) inhibit dihydrofolic acid reductase, thereby interfering with the synthesis of tetrahydrofolic acid. Trimethoprim is also bacteriostatic and active against gram-positive and -negative aerobes.

When sulfonamides and trimethoprim are combined, they are often synergistic, making the combination bactericidal. The most commonly used combination is trimethoprim and sulfamethoxazole (TMP/SMX) in a 5:1 ratio. This combination is also active against protozoa, especially *Pneumocystis carinii* . Development of resistance to sulfonamides is common; resistance to TMP/SMX also has increased, especially in the Third World.

Pharmacokinetics: The sulfonamides are classified into those with short $t_{1/2}$s ($\leq$ 8 h), those with intermediate $t_{1/2}$s (8 to 16 h), and those with long $t_{1/2}$s (> 16 h). Their absorption varies when they are given orally. Protein binding also varies; the greater the binding, the longer the $t_{1/2}$. Elimination is renal, and the derivatives are metabolized to varying extents. Trimethoprim is well absorbed and is excreted renally, with a $t_{1/2}$ of approximately 10 h following partial liver metabolism. Dosages of all drugs in this group should be reduced in the presence of renal failure.

Indications: Given their side effects (see below), the sulfonamides and TMP/SMX should be used restrictively in the elderly. Trimethoprim has a broader spectrum than the sulfonamides, causes fewer serious side effects, and can be used to treat or prevent UTIs. TMP/SMX is indicated in acute exacerbations of chronic bronchitis and in some serious systemic infections (eg, enteric fever, paratyphoid, and infections caused by *P. carinii*).

Side effects and interactions: Sulfonamides frequently cause skin rashes. In some patients, febrile mucocutaneous syndromes may occur. Such reactions are more common in adolescents and young adults than in the elderly. If these agents are used for > 7 days, toxic hepatitis may develop. With sulfonamides and TMP/SMX, hematologic reactions (neutropenia, thrombocytopenia, pancytopenia) have been reported frequently, especially in older persons who have received high doses for $\geq$ 10 days. *Hematologic reactions may be fatal.* Side effects of trimethoprim alone are normally mild and reversible. If used for prolonged periods, trimethoprim (alone or in TMP/SMX) may cause folic acid deficiency. This can be prevented by administering folinic acid.

Since both sulfonamides and trimethoprim are metabolized in the liver, they may interact with other drugs. Sulfonamides have been reported to displace methotrexate from albumin, leading to enhanced methotrexate activity. Similarly, sulfonamides may increase the activity of other highly protein-bound drugs. Trimethoprim and especially TMP/SMX interact with phenytoin and coumarin derivatives, increasing both their activity and the risk of toxic reactions. If combined with cyclosporine, TMP/SMX may increase the nephrotoxicity of that drug.

TETRACYCLINES

Tetracyclines inhibit protein synthesis in aerobic and anaerobic bacteria, *Rickettsia, Mycoplasma, Chlamydia,* and some protozoa. The various derivatives (eg, tetracycline, chlortetracycline, oxytetracycline, lymecycline, doxycycline, and minocycline) do not differ markedly in antimicrobial spectrum. Resistance is common and often plasmid mediated (ie, transferrable between bacterial cells).

Pharmacokinetics: The main differences among the various tetracyclines concern pharmacokinetics. All are absorbed after oral administration, doxycycline and minocycline more efficiently than the others. Penetration into peripheral compartments is good, especially of doxycycline and minocycline. The different drugs are eliminated by renal metabolism and biliary excretion with $t_{1/2}$s of approximately 10 h for most, 15 h for minocycline, and 18 h for doxycycline. However, renal elimination is low for doxycycline and negligible for minocycline.

Indications: In elderly persons, tetracyclines are used for the treatment of *Mycoplasma* infections and exacerbations of chronic bronchitis. Use in sinusitis is of doubtful value.

Side effects and interactions: In the elderly, the most important side effects are **ecologic** (ie, diarrhea, *Candida* overgrowth, and induction of resistance in the normal flora). Phototoxic reactions may occur. Nephrotoxicity has been reported with older tetracyclines but not with doxycycline and minocycline. Bleeding diathesis may develop from a reduction in vitamin K–producing bacteria in the gut.

Absorption of tetracyclines is reduced if they are coadministered with antacids, because of chelate binding to metal ions. Carbamazepine, phenytoin, and barbiturates induce liver metabolism of the tetracyclines, leading to a reduced $t_{1/2}$. The administration of methoxyflurane may increase the nephrotoxicity of the older tetracyclines.

VANCOMYCIN

Vancomycin is a polypeptide antibiotic active against gram-positive aerobes and anaerobes, including enterococci, methicillin-resistant staphylococci, and *C. difficile.* Resistance to vancomycin has not been reported. The drug is not absorbed after oral administration. When given IV, vancomycin is eliminated renally, with a $t_{1/2}$ of 2 to 4 h. Penetration into CSF is poor. Dosage should be adjusted in patients with renal impairment.

912 Organ Systems: Infectious Disease

Vancomycin is used IV to treat serious gram-positive infections (eg, endocarditis and infections caused by methicillin-resistant staphylococci). It is also used orally to treat *C. difficile*–induced diarrhea and colitis. If administered by rapid IV infusion, vancomycin may cause acute "red-neck syndrome." Allergic reactions, mainly rashes, have been reported in 4 to 5% of patients. Nephrotoxicity and ototoxicity may occur; serum concentrations should be monitored when the drug is used parenterally.

ANTIFUNGAL AGENTS

AMPHOTERICIN B

Amphotericin B is a polyene macrolide that interacts with sterols in the cytoplasmic membrane of many fungal species. It is fungicidal and has a wide spectrum, which includes *Candida* spp, *Aspergillus* spp, *Cryptococcus* spp, *Coccidioides* spp, *Histoplasma* spp, and *Blastomyces* spp. Resistance to amphotericin B is uncommon.

Pharmacokinetics: Amphotericin B is not absorbed after oral administration but is used orally to treat oral and intestinal mycoses. In systemic mycoses, it must be given by IV infusion. It is highly protein bound and is excreted slowly via the kidneys, with a $t_{1/2}$ of 18 to 24 h in patients with normal renal function. Dosage must be adjusted in patients with renal impairment.

Indications and side effects: Amphotericin B is widely used to treat systemic mycoses and is the drug of choice for all infections (except candidiasis) caused by flucytosine-susceptible strains (see below). It frequently causes adverse reactions. Fever, chills, and nausea are common with infusion, and the dose must be increased slowly over several days to mitigate these effects. Concurrent administration of corticosteroids or antiemetics may be necessary. Nephrotoxicity is very common, and renal function must be monitored in all patients.

FLUCYTOSINE

Flucytosine (5-fluorocytosine) is active mainly against *Candida* spp (including *C. glabrata,* previously called *Torulopsis glabrata*). When entering the fungal cell, flucytosine is deaminated to 5-fluorouracil, which disrupts RNA synthesis. Development of resistance is common, especially if the drug is used topically or in systemic doses that are too low.

Pharmacokinetics: Flucytosine is well absorbed after oral administration and can be given both orally and by IV infusion. It penetrates well into peripheral compartments, including CSF. It is not metabolized; elimination is renal, with a $t_{1/2}$ of 2½ to 4 h in patients with normal kidney function. Dosage should be reduced in patients with renal failure. Serum concentrations should be monitored to avoid overdosage, which increases the risk of toxicity, or underdosage, which increases the risk of resistance.

Indications and side effects: Flucytosine is indicated for the treatment of systemic *Candida* infections caused by susceptible strains. It can be combined with low doses of amphotericin B if synergy is likely. Topical use should be avoided because of the risk of resistance. Flucytosine causes few adverse reactions in correct doses. If overdosage occurs (serum concentrations > 100 mg/L), 5-fluorouracil may be found in serum and may cause bone marrow depression.

IMIDAZOLES

The imidazole group of antifungal agents includes, among others, miconazole and ketoconazole. Their fungicidal activity is still under investigation. Susceptible fungi include *Trichophyton* spp, *Epidermophyton* spp, *Candida* spp, *Cryptococcus* spp, *Coccidioides* spp, *Blastomyces* spp, and *Histoplasma* spp. Resistance may occur in all of these species.

Pharmacokinetics: Ketoconazole is available only in oral forms and is moderately well absorbed in patients with normal gastric acidity. Miconazole is poorly absorbed and can be used only IV. Both drugs are eliminated by liver metabolism, with $t_{1/2}$s between 4 and 8 h.

Indications: The role of the imidazoles is still unclear. They are used therapeutically in cases of severe cutaneous mycoses and prophylactically in severely immunocompromised patients. They are also used topically for the treatment of cutaneous mycoses and vaginal candidiasis.

Side effects and interactions: When used topically, the imidazoles cause few adverse reactions. Systemic use may lead to hepatic toxicity, manifested in most cases by elevated liver transaminase. Endocrine disorders (eg, gynecomastia and reduced libido) have been reported with high doses.

The imidazoles interact with a number of other drugs. The absorption of ketoconazole is reduced in patients treated with cimetidine, ranitidine, or antacids. Severe interactions have been described between cyclosporine and ketoconazole; in transplant recipients, the blood levels of cyclosporine increased twentyfold, resulting in nephrotoxicity when the 2 drugs were given together. Metabolic interactions are described with rifampin, isoniazid, and methylprednisolone, resulting in increased metabolism of the first 2 and decreased metabolism of the last. Imidazoles may also induce their own metabolism.

NYSTATIN

Nystatin is a nonabsorbable agent that interferes with sterols in the cytoplasmic membrane of yeast cells, especially *Candida*. It is used topically for the treatment of cutaneous, vaginal, and oral candidiasis and prophylactically in immunocompromised patients.

ANTIVIRAL DRUGS

ACYCLOVIR

Acyclovir acts specifically on herpes simplex virus **(HSV)** and varicella-zoster virus **(VZV)**, both of which use thymidine kinase in DNA synthesis. This enzyme metabolizes acyclovir to acyclovir triphosphate, which then acts as an inhibitor and a substrate of herpes-specific DNA polymerase. Other viruses, including cytomegalovirus and Epstein-Barr virus, do not have a thymidine kinase and are resistant to acyclovir. Development of resistance has been described in HSV but is of little clinical significance.

Pharmacokinetics: Acyclovir, only about 20% absorbed when given orally, is also available for IV use. It penetrates well into peripheral compartments including CSF and the brain. It is not metabolized and is excreted renally, with a $t_{1/2}$ of approximately 3 h. Dosage should be reduced in patients with renal impairment.

Indications: Oral acyclovir is indicated for the treatment of and prophylaxis against cutaneous HSV infections. To be effective, treatment must be started early after the onset of symptoms. IV acyclovir is used to treat severe HSV infections (eg, HSV encephalitis), severe cases of varicella, and disseminated herpes zoster. Higher doses are required in infections caused by VZV, which is less susceptible than HSV.

Side effects: When used orally, acyclovir causes few adverse reactions. IV, it may cause thrombophlebitis; if infusions are given rapidly, marked increases in BUN and serum creatinine may occur.

AMANTADINE AND RIMANTADINE

These synthetic amines inhibit the uncoating of influenza A virus nucleic acid and thus viral replication. Resistance has been reported in some strains. Both drugs, especially amantadine, are well absorbed and are excreted in the urine, with a $t_{1/2}$ of 14 h for amantadine and approximately 30 h for rimantadine. Amantadine is not metabolized, while rimantadine undergoes hepatic metabolism.

These prophylactic agents are indicated in persons who are likely to develop serious symptoms if infected with influenza A—eg, elderly persons with severe cardiac decompensation or lung disorders. Furthermore, they may be used prophylactically in institutional outbreaks of influenza A when vaccination is ineffective or incomplete. Used early in illness, they ameliorate disease and hasten recovery. Rimantadine has few side effects. Amantadine may cause neurotoxicity, especially neuritis. Both drugs have cholinergic effects and may interact with anticholinergic drugs.

78. VACCINES AND IMMUNIZATION

Theodore C. Eickhoff

The principal targets and greatest successes of immunization in the USA have been in pediatric age groups. Less attention has been paid to immunization of adults, particularly the elderly. Recognition of the underutilization or inappropriate utilization of immunizing agents recommended for older adults and of underutilization of recently introduced vaccines has resulted in a renewed interest in adult immunization, with particular emphasis on influenza and pneumococcal vaccines.

For example, an estimated < 20% of the recommended recipient population has actually been immunized with pneumococcal vaccine. Of patients with serious pneumococcal infections who were hospitalized at least once within 5 yr of the illness, ≤ $\frac{1}{3}$ received pneumococcal vaccine. In one survey, > 50% of physicians gave pneumococcal vaccine only to patients with cardiopulmonary disease and not to otherwise healthy elderly patients. Similarly, only about 20% of the population recommended to receive influenza vaccine are actually immunized in any given year.

Serologic surveys carried out in the past 10 yr indicated that > $\frac{1}{2}$ of the group > 60 yr of age did not have protective levels of antitoxin antibodies against either tetanus or diphtheria.

GENERAL PRINCIPLES

Immunization is considered active or passive. **Active immunization** is usually carried out in anticipation of exposure to a disease; the immunizing agents are vaccines or toxoids. Protection depends on an immune response by the vaccinee. **Vaccines** may consist of whole killed bacterial cells, wholly or partially purified bacterial proteins or polysaccharides, inactivated viruses or purified viral proteins, or live attenuated viruses. **Toxoids** consist of bacterial toxins that have been modified to render them nontoxic, although they retain the ability to induce formation of antitoxin antibodies.

Passive immunization, in which no immune response occurs in the subject, is used when exposure to a disease has recently occurred or is anticipated. It is accomplished by administering **immune globulins,** usually of human but sometimes of animal origin. Specific hyperimmune globulin preparations are derived from donor pools preselected for a high level of antibody against a specific disease, eg, tetanus, rabies, hepatitis B, or varicella zoster. Since 1985, all human plasma entering such donor pools has been screened to exclude donors with detectable antibody to human immunodeficiency virus **(HIV).** Furthermore, the purification process excludes HIV in donated plasma.

Vaccines and toxoids may contain other substances in addition to specific immunogens. Awareness of the presence of such adventitious materials is important, since they may cause untoward or allergic reactions. The suspending fluid may contain minute amounts of protein or other components of the biologic system in which the immunogen was produced, eg, egg antigens or antigens derived from the cells in which vaccine viruses were grown. Preservatives, stabilizers, or antibiotics used in viral cell cultures may also be present in minute amounts. Further, adjuvants, usually consisting of aluminum salts, are sometimes added to enhance the immune response. Such adjuvants are believed to be harmless when injected IM but, if given s.c., they may produce granulomatous inflammation or even necrosis.

The use of both active and passive immunization in older persons should be based on risk-benefit considerations. In general, demonstrated hypersensitivity to a component of a vaccine is a *contraindication* to using that vaccine. A very small segment of the population is allergic to eggs, and some commonly used vaccines, including that for influenza, are prepared in eggs. Hypersensitivity to antibiotics used in culture media is another possible but infrequent risk. Penicillin, for example, is not currently used in preparing any vaccine.

The immunologic response to most vaccines decreases quantitatively with advancing age. This is well documented in the case of influenza vaccine; elderly nursing home residents respond with much lower levels of antibody than do young adults. This also occurs with pneumococcal vaccine. However, whether increasing age per se is the major attenuating factor or simply a marker for increased prevalence of underlying disease in an aging population is unknown.

Persons whose immune competence is decreased, either as a result of underlying disease or its treatment, should not be given live attenuated viral vaccines because of the risk of vaccine-induced disease. In general, individuals who have received immune or hyperimmune globulin within the preceding 3 mo should not receive live attenuated virus vaccines, because the passively administered antibody may interfere with the attenuated, subclinical infection that is the desired response to the vaccine.

A number of vaccines may be given together without loss of efficacy. For example, influenza and pneumococcal vaccines may be administered concurrently but at separate sites. TABLES 78–1 and 78–2 list the active and passive immunizing agents recommended for elderly patients and the usual circumstances in which they are recommended.

GENERAL IMMUNIZATIONS

TETANUS AND DIPHTHERIA TOXOIDS

Tetanus and diphtheria toxoids for adult use **(Td)** consist of formalinized toxoids derived from tetanus and diphtheria toxins and are indicated for use in all adults. Persons who have been primarily immunized previously in adult life or as children need only booster doses at 10-yr intervals to maintain adequate immunity. Pediatric immunization schedules generally end with a preschool booster dose of these antigens; therefore, subsequent booster doses might be given at the mid-decade birthday (eg, 15, 25, 35, 45, 55, etc), which is a convenient recall date. Booster doses of Td have few contraindications; the major one is a neurologic or severe hypersensitivity reaction after a previous dose.

The product for use in adults (Td) differs from that used in pediatrics (diphtheria, pertussis, tetanus [**DPT**]). The adult product contains no pertussis component and a reduced dose of diphtheria toxoid component to minimize reactions. Tetanus toxoid alone (**T**) is recommended for persons who have had adverse reactions to the reduced diphtheria component in Td. If there is serious doubt that an individual was primarily immunized with tetanus and diphtheria toxoids, 2 doses of Td IM should be given a month apart, followed by the usual schedule of booster doses at 10-yr intervals.

For trauma management, an additional dose of Td is recommended only in the presence of major, contaminated or severe puncture wounds, and then only if > 5 yr have elapsed since the last dose. Td is preferred to T alone.

INFLUENZA VACCINE

Influenza vaccine consists of inactivated whole influenza viruses or subunit components. Preparation of the split-virus, or subunit, vaccines consists of disruption of the viral membrane with organic solvents and subsequent purification and concentration. Influenza vaccine differs from other products routinely recommended for adults in that its composition is likely to be changed each year. Changes are based on the specific immunologic characteristics of the influenza viruses present at the time and the need to give the vaccine annually because of the relatively short-lived immunity it confers. The late-1980s vaccine is a trivalent product containing the 2 influenza A strains (H1N1 and H3N2) predominant during recent influenza seasons, as well as an influenza B strain.

The vaccine is recommended for annual use in any adults who have high-risk conditions (eg, chronic pulmonary, cardiac, renal, or metabolic diseases) and for those > 65 yr of age. In young adults, influenza vaccines have a protective efficacy against influenza of about 75%. The efficacy declines, even with annual immunization, in adults > 65 yr of age, but the vaccine is still effective in reducing severity of illness, protecting against serious complicating bacterial pneumonia, and reducing mortality rates.

An unanticipated association of swine influenza vaccine with subsequent development of the Guillian-Barré syndrome in vaccine recipients was detected following the swine influenza vaccination program in 1976. The risk of Guillian-Barré syndrome associated with swine influenza

TABLE 78–1. COMMONLY USED ACTIVE IMMUNIZING AGENTS

Agent	Type of Preparation	Dosage Schedule	Comments
For general use			
Tetanus and diphtheria toxoids, for adult use (Td)	Bacterial toxoids	IM q 10 yr; use mid-decade birthday	Also used in wound management and for diphtheria
Influenza virus vaccine, trivalent	Inactivated virus	s.c. annually	Used in persons > 65 yr of age and in those of any age with chronic disease
Pneumococcal polysaccharide vaccine	23-valent, purified capsular polysaccharides	s.c. once	Used in high-risk adults, in those with asplenia, and in all adults > 65 yr of age
For selective use			
Cholera vaccine	Whole killed *Vibrio cholerae*	2 doses IM 4 wk apart; booster doses at 6-mo intervals	Used only in travelers to countries requiring cholera vaccination
Hepatitis B vaccine	Purified HBsAG, produced in yeast	3 doses IM	Used in persons at risk, especially health care workers, homosexual males, IV drug abusers, sexual contacts of HBsAG carriers, persons with prolonged residence in areas in which the disease is highly endemic
Meningococcal vaccine	Purified polysaccharides, serogroups A, C, Y, W-135	s.c. once	Used for outbreak control and in persons at increased risk

Poliomyelitis vaccine	Live attenuated virus (oral polio vaccine)	3 doses po	Used for booster doses in adults, if needed in special circumstances; do not use for primary immunization of adults
	Inactivated virus (inactivated polio vaccine)	3 doses s.c.	Used for primary immunization of adults, if needed
Rabies vaccine	Inactivated virus, grown in human diploid cells	5 doses IM for postexposure prophylaxis	Preexposure prophylaxis in special circumstances (3 doses)
Typhoid vaccine	Whole killed *Salmonella typhosa*	2 doses s.c. 4 wk apart; booster doses at 3-yr intervals	Used only in travelers to areas in which the disease is known to be endemic
Yellow fever vaccine	Attenuated live virus	Single dose s.c. and booster doses at 10-yr intervals	Used only in travelers to areas in which the disease is endemic

TABLE 78–2. AGENTS USED IN PASSIVE IMMUNIZATION

Disease	Agent	Comments
Hepatitis A	Immune globulin (IG), human	For susceptible contacts, outbreak control
Hepatitis B	Hepatitis B immune globulin (HBIG), human	For exposed susceptibles; begin active immunization with hepatitis B vaccine
Rabies	Rabies immune globulin (RIG), human	For post-exposure prophylaxis; begin active immunization with rabies vaccine
Tetanus	Tetanus immune globulin (TIG), human	For management of tetanus-prone wounds
Varicella zoster	Varicella zoster immune globulin (VZIG), human	For use in immunocompromised, exposed susceptibles; may modify but not prevent disease
Botulism	Monovalent E; bivalent A-B; trivalent A-B-E antitoxins, equine	For treatment of botulism

Note: Equine antivenins directed against coral snake, pit viper (including rattlesnake), and black widow spider venins are also available.

immunization at that time was approximately 1 case/100,000 persons vaccinated. Since the swine influenza antigen was removed from influenza vaccines, no such association has been noted.

Influenza outbreaks in the USA are regularly associated with increased mortality, and the impact is most severe in elderly persons, who account for 60 to 80% of all influenza-associated deaths. Approximately 90% of these deaths occur in persons with recognized underlying high-risk conditions, but some deaths also occur in apparently healthy older adults. Thus, annual use of influenza vaccine is strongly recommended in the target populations.

PNEUMOCOCCAL VACCINE

The currently available pneumococcal *(Streptococcus pneumoniae)* vaccine consists of 25 μg each of 23 individual pneumococcal polysaccharides, derived from the 23 pneumococcal capsular types that account for most bacteremic pneumococcal infections in the USA. Indications for this vaccine include splenic dysfunction or anatomic asplenia, chronic diseases associated with increased risk of pneumococcal disease (eg, chronic cardiopulmonary disease), and age > 65 yr. While the indications for pneumococcal vaccine are similar to those for influenza vaccine, pneumococcal vaccine need be given only once rather than annually.

Recommendations for pneumococcal vaccine in the USA have been controversial because of conflicting efficacy data and differing perceptions of the importance of pneumococcus as a cause of pneumonia, bacteremia, and death, particularly in the elderly. The most reasonable conclusion based on studies of efficacy is that the vaccine is effective in preventing pneumococcal bacteremia and death in patients able to mount a satisfactory immunologic response. In high-risk patients and in those compromised by underlying cardiopulmonary disease or malignancy, the vaccine is less effective. Thus, consideration should be given to immunizing older adults at an earlier age (eg, 55 yr) before the age-related increase in frequency of underlying disease occurs and at a time when a brisk immunologic response can be anticipated.

SELECTED IMMUNIZATIONS

POLIOMYELITIS VACCINES

Two types of poliovirus vaccine are currently available in the USA: live oral polio vaccine (**OPV**) and inactivated polio vaccine (**IPV**). OPV is the most widely used but is not recommended for primary immunization of adults. Routine polio vaccination of elderly adults who have not been primarily immunized is no longer necessary, since the risk of poliomyelitis in the USA is exceedingly low. Poliomyelitis vaccines should be considered only for elderly adults who plan international travel, with prolonged exposure in an area in which the disease is endemic. Those who were primarily immunized earlier with either OPV or IPV need only a booster dose of IPV. If primary immunization is necessary, IPV is recommended.

HEPATITIS B VACCINE

The first vaccine against hepatitis B consisted of purified, inactivated hepatitis B surface antigen **(HBsAg),** derived from plasma obtained from chronic HBsAg carriers. The current hepatitis B vaccine, introduced early in 1987, is derived from yeast cells into which the gene coding for the production of HBsAg has been inserted. Such yeast cells have been genetically coded to synthesize large amounts of HBsAg. This product will eventually replace the plasma-derived hepatitis B vaccine.

The vaccine should be administered IM in the deltoid region in 3 doses, the second dose 1 mo after the first, and the third dose 6 mo later. Major target populations for whom the vaccine is recommended include homosexual males, IV drug abusers, certain institutionalized populations, household or sexual contacts of chronic carriers of HBsAg, and health care personnel who have occupational exposure to blood or blood-contaminated body fluids. Under most circumstances, the use of hepatitis B vaccine in elderly adults need be considered only in the instance of international travel, with possible exposure in areas in which the disease is endemic.

RABIES VACCINE

The current preparation is an inactivated vaccine from rabies virus grown in human diploid-cell cultures. This represents a substantial improvement over the vaccines available prior to 1980. The current vaccine has a high degree of efficacy both in preventing rabies after exposure and in providing preexposure prophylaxis against rabies in certain populations.

Following exposure to animals known to be or suspected of harboring rabies virus, five 1-mL doses of rabies vaccine are given IM. The initial dose is given as soon as possible after exposure, with the additional doses given on days 3, 7, 14, and 28 after the initial dose. Postexposure rabies prophylaxis should include the use of human rabies immune globulin **(RIG),** consisting of antirabies globulin concentrated from the plasma of hyperimmunized donors.

RIG should be administered only once, at the time of the first dose of rabies vaccine, to provide passive antirabies antibodies until the vaccine response is established. The recommended dose of 20 IU/kg should be divided approximately in $1/2$, with up to 50% of the dose injected in the area around the wound and the rest administered IM. The recommended dose of rabies globulin results in only very little, if any, attenuation of the host's immunologic response to rabies vaccine.

Preexposure rabies immunization should be considered only in elderly adults at high risk for exposure (eg, veterinarians, animal handlers, persons with occupations or hobbies resulting in unavoidable exposure to potentially rabid animals, and laboratory workers who work with wild rabies virus). For preexposure immunization, 3 injections of the vaccine are required, the second 1 wk after the initial dose and the third 3 or 4 wk later. Booster doses are recommended every 2 yr in persons at continuing risk for exposure. If an individual who has received preexposure immunization is subsequently bitten by an animal known or believed to be rabid, two 1-mL doses of the vaccine should be administered, 1 immediately and the other 3 days later. RIG need not be given to such patients.

Any decision to provide postexposure rabies prophylaxis should take into account the animal species involved, the circumstances of the bite or other exposure, the vaccination status of the exposed person, and the presence of rabies in the region. Local or state public health officials should be consulted if questions arise about the need for rabies prophylaxis. In some jurisdictions, any animal bite is reportable to the responsible governmental agency.

MENINGOCOCCAL VACCINE

Two meningococcal vaccines, directed against *Neisseria meningitidis* of serogroups A, C, Y, and W-135, are available in the USA. These are a bivalent A-C and the quadravalent A, C, Y, and W-135 product. These vaccines consist of purified capsular polysaccharides that induce specific serogroup immunity and have been shown to be highly effective in preventing meningococcal disease caused by these serogroups in approximately 90% of susceptible adults. Only a single dose is required, and the immunity is believed to be long-lived.

The use of meningococcal vaccine in elderly adults need be considered only in the case of international travel to areas in which the disease is known to be highly endemic or epidemic. In local epidemics or household cases, chemoprophylaxis may be used in those intimately exposed.

TYPHOID VACCINE

The administration of typhoid vaccine is no longer recommended routinely in the USA. It should not be administered routinely to victims of natural disasters, such as earthquakes and floods. It should be considered in elderly adults only for international travel to areas in which the disease is known to be endemic.

CHOLERA VACCINE

Cholera vaccine is marginally effective, and immunity lasts for little more than 6 mo. It is recommended only for travelers to countries that require cholera vaccination for entry.

YELLOW FEVER VACCINE

Yellow fever vaccine is recommended only for international travel to areas in which the disease is endemic. Because this vaccine consists of live attenuated virus, it should be used cautiously in elderly adults. I there is underlying immunocompromising disease, a letter from the pa tient's physician outlining the medical contraindications to the vaccine will usually suffice to obtain an entry waiver to areas in which the vac cine is required.

PASSIVE IMMUNIZATION

Immune globulins, of either human or equine origin, that are some times indicated for older adult populations are summarized in TABL 78-2. Immune or hyperimmune globulins derived from humans have a high degree of safety. Immune globulins of equine origin (eg, botulism antitoxin and the several antivenins) must be used with caution and pre ceded by an intradermal test dose to determine if the patient is allergi or hypersensitive to horse serum. Serum sickness is a late, dose-related complication of equine globulin products.

FUTURE TRENDS

A number of additional vaccines are under development and may be licensed for use in the USA within the next 10 yr. New or improved versions of classic vaccines will continue to be introduced, and standard technics will be used to develop bacterial or viral component vaccines or live attenuated viral vaccines. Examples include purified pertussi vaccines and live attenuated varicella vaccine, both currently under in vestigation.

In addition, recombinant DNA technology will be increasingly impor tant in the future; the recently released recombinant yeast-derived hepa titis B vaccine represents the first major example of this trend. The use of such technology may result in the development of vaccines effective against meningococci of serogroup B, respiratory syncytial virus, enteric virus, and cytomegalovirus and against hepatitis types A and non-A non-B, and malaria. An effective vaccine directed against human im munodeficiency virus (HIV) infection will depend heavily on continuing advances in DNA technology.

Few, if any, of these anticipated developments will be appropriate for widespread use in elderly adults. Major emphasis will continue to be placed on more extensive use of diphtheria and tetanus toxoids, influ enza vaccine, and pneumococcal vaccine in this population. Nonetheless future vaccine development appears promising.

§3. ORGAN SYSTEMS: NEUROLOGIC DISORDERS

79. NORMAL AGING AND PATTERNS OF NEUROLOGIC DISEASE

Robert J. Joynt

Neurologic disorders account for > ½ of all disabilities requiring supervision in a nursing home in the elderly. The cost is inestimable, encompassing not only the expense of medical care but the diversion of human resources, including both trained health care personnel and family members acting as care givers.

The emotional burdens are also incalculable. In dementia, for example, all that was endearing to spouses, family, and friends is lost as the patient's mind, capabilities, sensitivities, and humanity disintegrate. Therefore, the appreciation that normally would be shown to the care giver of an elderly mate, parent, or friend is often missing and this may destroy the care giver's incentive to carry on.

Interest in the neurologic disorders of the aged derives in part from the growing number of elderly people in the population, the prevalence of neurologic disorders among them, and their increasing longevity. Another factor is advancing technology. For example, noninvasive and less innocuous means of visualizing the nervous system are providing increased knowledge of disease.

The new modes of therapy can successfully ameliorate many neurologic disorders. Cerebrovascular disease has decreased markedly in the USA, largely because of detection and treatment of hypertension. This therapeutic success has encouraged investigators to seek new understanding of the etiology, pathophysiology, and prevention of strokes. Similarly, the successful treatment of Parkinson's disease has led to increased knowledge in neuropharmacology.

Advances in research technics have been applied extensively to diseases of the nervous system. For example, advances in molecular biology have led to identification of the chromosomal locus for familial Alzheimer's disease.

Neurologic diseases encountered in old age fall into 3 categories. First are the degenerative and cerebrovascular disorders. The term "degenerative disorder" implies ignorance of causation; some diseases (eg, familial Alzheimer's disease) may be classified differently as we learn more about them. Second are disorders that occur at any age but have different implications, manifestations, treatment, and prognosis in the elderly (eg, seizures in the elderly are more likely to be the result of some structural abnormality, such as a brain tumor). Third are diseases of the nervous system that are not characteristic in the elderly (eg, epilepsy, muscular dystrophies, demyelinating disorders, migraine, and others). If such disorders occur, other explanations or disorders are often found.

Aging and the Nervous System

The fact that **cells in the nervous system cannot reproduce** sets them apart from cells in other organ systems. The damaged liver, lung, or bowel, for example, may regenerate in part, but cells lost in the brain disappear after injury.

There is a **decrease in the number of nerve cells** with normal aging. The degree of cell loss varies in different parts of the brain; some areas (eg, brainstem nuclei) are resistant to cell loss, while others (eg, the hippocampus) exhibit a rapid decrease in number of cells. This has been confirmed by studies showing both reduction in brain weight after the 2nd or 3rd decade and an enlargement of the cerebral ventricles with aging.

Other changes include deposition of the aging pigment lipofuscin in nerve cells, deposition of amyloid in blood vessels and cells, and appearance of senile plaques and neurofibrillary tangles. Although the latter are the hallmarks of Alzheimer's disease, they appear in the brains of older people without evidence of dementia.

Other properties of the nervous system mitigate these adverse changes. First, there is **redundancy,** ie, many more nerve cells are present than are needed. The number of cells required for certain functions is not known, so the extent of redundancy is difficult to estimate. As one example, diabetes insipidus (which arises from a lack of ADH) does not appear until < 10 to 15% of the normal number of nerve cells are present in the supraoptic and paraventricular nuclei. Further, normal intelligence has been seen in hydrocephalic patients having only a thin cerebral cortical mantle.

Second, **compensatory mechanisms** are available in the nervous system that may appear only after damage. For example, speech function gradually returning after serious injury to the dominant hemisphere appears to emanate from the nondominant hemisphere.

Finally, **more plasticity at the nerve cell level** probably exists than was previously recognized. Recent studies have shown 2 simultaneous processes: a gradual deterioration and dying off of nerve cells, accounting for the decreased number, and compensatory lengthening and an increasing number of dendrites in the remaining nerve cells. With the increase in the dendritic tree, new connections are possible, to make up for the loss in number of cells. This attempt at regeneration is seen even in Alzheimer's disease.

Both the negative and positive aspects of these changes are affected by exogenous factors that enter into any disease process at any age but are particularly influential in neurologic disorders in the elderly. Older people, particularly those with some degree of brain disease, are especially susceptible to the actions of drugs. Sleeping medications, which may be effective and innocuous for most people, may make an older person confused or delirious. Otherwise healthy older people may experience cognitive or behavioral abnormalities with minor illnesses that decrease O_2 to the brain; eg, pneumonia, heart failure, and anemia.

Neurologic Evaluation

Several complicating factors enter into the neurologic evaluation of the elderly. First, the assumption that deterioration of the nervous system is a **normal** consequence of aging is false. Despite the changes described, most people retain normal cognition and behavior. Second, acceptance of the first assumption leads to the mistaken notion that careful evaluation is not warranted, since there is likely to be no therapy. Third, the high probability that other diseases are present complicates evaluation and therapy. An elderly patient with hemiplegia often develops periarthritis of the shoulder. Depression, which is common in the elderly, confuses the mental status examination and makes the diagnosis of dementia difficult. Fourth, there are few standard tests for evaluating the aged. This is attributable partly to past lack of interest in this population but also to the difficulty of obtaining satisfactory control populations for testing. Simple questions, such as What is the acceptable memory loss for an 80-yr-old? can't be answered. However, large-scale longitudinal studies now in progress may provide better data.

Certain findings on neurologic examination of the elderly may be considered concomitants of aging. The clinician must decide which can be dismissed and which may truly indicate a neurologic lesion. All systems must be systematically tested. Some areas require special attention because of the nature of disease in the elderly and the changes in the nervous system generally associated with aging.

The **pupil** of the eye is often smaller in older people. Also, the pupillary light reflex may be sluggish and the pupillary miotic response to near vision may be diminished. Upward gaze, and, to a lesser extent, downward gaze, is limited in elderly patients. The smooth pursuit movements in tracking a moving finger may be diminished and appear more jerky and irregular. **Bell's phenomenon** (reflex upward movement of the eyes on closure) is occasionally absent in elderly patients. It is tested by first having patients close their eyes tightly and then forcing the lids open to see the eye.

In checking the **motor system,** the physician must remember that elderly people, particularly women, often appear weak on routine testing; ie, it is easy to overcome sustained contraction of the extremities. If the weakness appears to be symmetric and is not accompanied by any complaints, it is most likely normal. Tone, usually detected by flexion and extension movements at the elbow, may be increased to a slight extent; this is not unusual. Greatly increased tone is, however, an early sign of parkinsonism.

The muscle stretch reflexes usually show no changes with aging except for the Achilles tendon jerk, which is often diminished or absent. This is likely the result of loss of elasticity of the tendon rather than neurologic deficit.

Muscle atrophy, or at least the loss of muscle bulk, particularly in the small muscles in the hand, may be seen in the elderly. Again, unless accompanied by loss of function, it is of little significance.

The **sensory examination** is usually within normal limits except for the ability to perceive vibration. This is commonly absent below the knees in the elderly and is usually not accompanied by loss of proprioception, as tested by perception of joint position. Loss of vibratory sensation has been attributed to small-vessel changes in the posterior column of the spinal cord. However, joint position sense, which presumably uses a similar pathway, is preserved.

Signs elicited at the neurologic examination must be considered in light of the patient's age, history, and other findings. Any finding that is symmetric and is unaccompanied by other neurologic signs or complaints, should be recorded but viewed as a variant of aging. Findings that appear to be abnormal may be reevaluated at intervals to note changes, development of asymmetry, or new complaints.

80. MENTAL STATUS EXAMINATION (MSE)

Marshal F. Folstein and *Susan E. Folstein*

That part of the medical examination that assesses the appearance, speech, mood, perceptions, beliefs, fears, and cognitive state of patients.

The purpose of the mental status examination **(MSE)** is to determine the patient's mental capacity at the time of the evaluation. It is thus distinguished from other aspects of the traditional medical history that would address only distressing mental experiences or behaviors that occurred in the past. The medical history and the manner in which it is elicited can give clues to the patient's current mental status, but a separate evaluation is needed to determine and document it.

Cognitive impairment and other psychiatric symptoms are relatively common in the elderly. Often, the psychiatric, neurologic, or metabolic diseases responsible for these clinical findings are curable or treatable. In addition, assessment of the mental status of elderly patients is needed to establish their legal competence to make a will, or to give informed consent for procedures, or to manage their own care.

The MSE and its quantitated derivatives (eg, the General Health Questionnaire **[GHQ]** for emotional disorders and the Mini Mental State **[MMS]** examination for cognitive impairment) can be used for case finding, diagnosis, and assessment of treatment. The MSE alone does not provide a diagnosis; that requires a history, physical examination, and laboratory tests as well.

Clinical Assessment

The MSE is begun by explaining the necessity for the evaluation and by requesting the patient's permission and cooperation. For example, the physician says, "As a routine part of the examination, I would like to ask you some questions about how you feel and how you think. Is it all right to ask you about your thinking?"

The MSE is conducted supportively, but direct questions are asked to elicit specific insights into the patient's current psychiatric state. For example, the patient may be asked, "Do you hear voices?" Ambiguous or uncertain responses are followed by further questioning to determine whether the patient is reporting an experience that meets the definition of the phenomenon. For example, the physician may ask, "Are the voices you hear as clear as mine is now?" The cognitive examination must be conducted empathetically to avoid emotional responses to failure (catastrophic reactions), which in themselves can worsen cognitive performance.

The MSE is divided conventionally into the following sections:

Appearance: The patient's dress and grooming are assessed for signs of self-neglect or inability to dress, perhaps because of apraxia. Also noted are the patient's level of activity, which may reveal agitation or motor slowing; gait disturbances; presence of a hearing aid or glasses; and signs of lethargy, such as may occur in delirium or confusional states.

Speech: The physician notes whether the patient speaks rapidly, as in mania, or slowly, as in depression or dementia; whether his speech is clear or slurred, as in dysarthria secondary to stroke or parkinsonism; and whether he has trouble naming objects or uses jargon, as occurs in aphasia due to stroke or Alzheimer's disease.

Mood: The physician should ask, "How are your spirits?" or "How is your mood?" and note whether the patient feels depressed, hopeless, worthless, or guilty or, alternatively, unduly cheerful, optimistic, or overconfident. Mood-associated disturbances of appetite or sleep are determined at this point. A sense of dread or impending doom, as seen in panic or anxiety attacks, should be noted. In the elderly, a lack of feeling, apathy, or a nonspecific irritability can be prominent.

Suicidal thoughts and intentions must be assessed in depressed patients, since suicide rates are high, particularly in elderly men with physical impairment. The physician asks, "Have you thought of harming yourself or doing away with yourself?" If the patient admits to suicidal thinking, an inquiry is made into specific plans. Psychiatric referral and hospitalization are indicated for such patients.

Emotional disorders can be detected through brief quantitated screening tools such as the GHQ, a self-rated questionnaire derived from the Cornell Medical Index. The GHQ is designed to detect emotional disturbances of all sorts and has been extensively tested in general practitioners' offices in outpatient settings, and in field surveys involving large numbers of older individuals. A score of $\geq$ 5 on the 30-item version indicates an emotional disturbance.

Delusions are *false, fixed, idiosyncratic, and ego-preoccupying ideas*. The physician may ask, "Is anyone harassing you or trying to harm you?" He also should assess the patient's possibly false feeling of poverty or suspicion that someone is stealing from him or poisoning his food. Delusions occurring in late-life schizophrenia or paraphrenia should be distinguished from overvalued ideas (which may appear as a preoccupation or hobby that overrides all other activities and concern) or from culturally determined beliefs (eg, religious or superstitious ideas that, while not deeply held, are part of the patient's cultural identity). Delusions should also be distinguished from obsessions or hypochondriacal preoccupations, which are not idiosyncratic and appear to arise from an obsessive personality.

Obsessions or compulsions: Obsessions are *recurrent unwanted ideas* that the patient tries unsuccessfully to resist. Compulsions are *recurrent unwanted behaviors* (eg, hand washing) that also defy resistance. The physician may ask, "Are there thoughts that keep coming back that you can't get out of your mind?"

Hallucinations are *false visual, auditory, olfactory, or tactile perceptions.* The physician asks questions such as, Do you see visions of people? Is there any buzzing or ringing in your ears? Are there voices around you? Are they as clear as my voice? Do you smell anything unusual? Do you feel things crawling on your skin? Hallucinations are prominent in delirium, dementia, and schizophrenia, and may occur in late-life depression and even occasionally during grieving.

Phobias are *irrational fears of particular places, things, or situations; the fear is severe enough to cause the person to avoid the provocation.* For example, the patient may stay at home because he fears going out or may avoid high buildings because he fears elevators. The appearance of phobias, obsessions, or compulsions in the elderly can be the first sign of a severe depression.

Cognition is *the capacity to think in order to know the world.* Cognition is related to intelligence; it depends on alertness and is hampered by drowsiness, stupor, or coma. Assessment of cognition involves testing **attention, memory,** and **language functions.** Cognition is best tested using a quantitative procedure. This ensures a systematic, standardized comparative assessment and the clear documentation of change due to illness or treatment.

Quantitative Assessment

The clinical MSE can be supplemented with reliable quantitative procedures that are useful for case finding and patient follow-up or, in some instances, for buttressing one's clinical impression of impairment. Extensive batteries of neuropsychologic tests are part of the psychologist's armamentarium. Briefer quantitated measures are available, however, for use at the bedside by physicians, nurses, social workers, or technicians.

Among these, the Mini Mental State **(MMS)** examination (FIG. 80–1) is a useful screening tool for cognitive disorders. The MMS has been found valid in field studies and hospital settings. In one study of community-dwellers > 65 yr of age, 95% achieved a score of ≥ 24 out of

30 on this test. Scores < 24 are associated with delirium or dementia and can also reflect severe depression. The sensitivity and specificity are adequate for the detection of dementia in a community or hospital population.

However, many patients with no diagnosable disorders have low scores. Although reasons for this are not understood, such *low scores do not necessarily indicate a medical diagnosis.* In general, individuals with little education score lower than those with more education. Race and sex do not appear to influence scores if the level of education is controlled.

Mini Mental State Inpatient Consultation Form

Maximum Score	Score	
		Orientation
5	( )	What is the (year) (season) (date) (day) (month)?
5	( )	Where are we: (state) (county) (town) (hospital) (floor)?
		Registration
3	( )	Name 3 objects: 1 second to say each. Then ask the patient all 3 after you have said them.
		Give 1 point for each correct answer. Then repeat them until he learns all 3. Count trials and record.
		Trials
		Attention and calculation
5	( )	Serial 7s. 1 point for each correct answer. Stop after 5 answers. Alternatively, spell "world" backwards.
		Recall
3	( )	Ask for 3 objects repeated above. Give 1 point for each correct answer.
		Language
9	( )	Name a pencil and watch (2 points)
		Repeat the following "No ifs, and, or buts." (1 point)
		Follow a 3-stage command: "Take a paper in your right hand, fold it in half, and put it on the floor." (3 points)
		Read and obey the following: "Close your eyes." (1 point)
		Write a sentence. (1 point)
		Copy design. (1 point)

Total Score

ASSESS level of consciousness along a continuum.　Alert　Drowsy　Stupor　Coma

FIG. 80–1. **Mini Mental State Examination form.** (Reprinted with permission from *Journal of Psychiatric Research,* Vol. 12, M. F. Folstein, S. E. Folstein, P. McHugh, "Mini-mental state: A practical method for grading the cognitive state of patients for the clinician," copyright 1975, Pergamon Press PLC.)

81. SENILE DEMENTIA OF THE ALZHEIMER TYPE (SDAT)
(Alzheimer's Disease; Primary Degenerative Dementia)

Robert N. Butler

A progressive neuropsychiatric disease of aging found in middle-aged and, particularly, in older adults affecting brain matter and characterized by the inexorable loss of cognitive function as well as affective and behavioral disturbances. It is a major public health issue. Long-term care costs now exceed $40 billion/yr.

Incidence

Two million Americans have SDAT. It accounts for > 50% of the dementias in the elderly. About 60% of people in long-term care facilities have SDAT, and 20% of patients with Parkinson's disease develop this dementia. Multi-infarct dementia and SDAT coexist in about 15% of cases. SDAT is the fourth or fifth leading cause of death in Americans > 65 yr of age. It is seen more commonly in women (perhaps because women live longer than men, but female gender may be a risk factor). SDAT increases in incidence with advancing age; eg, < 1% of individuals < 65 yr of age are affected, but 20% of those > 80 yr have some measure of dementia. Chances of developing SDAT after age 85 may be reduced.

Etiology and Pathology

SDAT appears to result from a degenerative process characterized by loss of cells from the cerebral cortex, hippocampus, and subcortical structures, including selective cell loss in the nucleus basalis of Meynert, as well as the presence of neuritic or senile plaques (nerve cells surrounding an amyloid core) and neurofibrillary tangles (comprising paired helical filaments). Although neuritic plaques and neurofibrillary tangles occur in the normal aging process, they are much fewer in number. There are specific protein abnormalities and a marked reduction in choline acetyltransferase, decreasing the availability of acetylcholine. Somatostatin, corticotropin releasing factor (CRF), and other neurotransmitters are also significantly reduced. Thus, in SDAT there is a multiple neurotransmitter deficiency. A reduction in cerebral glucose utilization also occurs in some areas of the brain (parietal association and temporal cortices in early-stage SDAT, prefrontal cortex in severe-stage SDAT), as determined by positron emission tomography (PET). However, whether this reduction precedes or follows cell death is not known. Loss of cells in the locus ceruleus and nuclei raphes dorsalis also occurs. The microvasculature may be affected, as seen in angiophilic angiopathy.

The etiology of Alzheimer's disease appears to be familial (ie, genetic) in approximately 50% of cases and "sporadic" in 50%. A marker pointing to the locus of a gene involved in SDAT has been found on chromosome 21. This genetic finding supports the epidemiologic observation of an autosomal dominant genetic disease with low but variable late-life penetrance. Retrospective epidemiologic studies of the genetic aspects of SDAT are difficult, since family members may not have lived long enough for the disease to be expressed. As more is understood about the factors that regulate genetic expression, it may be possible to postpone or prevent the disease's occurrence.

Infectious agents and environmental contaminants, including slow viruses and metals (eg, aluminum), have been suspected etiologic factors. The roles of these factors have not been substantiated as yet; however, such environmental factors are the focus of active investigation. Normal aging has been associated with decrements in some neurotransmitters as well as with some of the neuropathologic findings in SDAT. Therefore, the question has arisen, is the disease due to an acceleration of normal aging changes?

A majority of patients with Down's syndrome who live long enough to develop the additional brain disorder of SDAT (usually after age 40) exhibit the same neuritic plaques and neurofibrillary tangles.

Symptoms and Signs

The first reported case of SDAT was in a presenile 51-yr-old man. SDAT and the originally described Alzheimer's presenile dementia have similar neuropathologic and clinical features, although the presenile form progresses more rapidly.

SDAT can be subdivided according to clinical stage, *but there is great variability and the progression of stages often is not as orderly as the following description implies.*

The early stage of SDAT is characterized by recent memory loss, inability to learn and retain new information, language problems, lability of mood, and possibly, changes in personality. Patients may have progressive difficulty performing activities of daily living (eg, balancing their checkbook, finding their way around, or remembering where they put things). They may be unable to think in the abstract or to use proper judgment. Irritability, hostility, and agitation may occur as responses to loss of control and memory. Other patients may present with an isolated aphasia or with visuospatial difficulties. The early stage may not, however, compromise sociability. Patients may be alert, making it difficult for the practitioner to uncover problems with cognition. However, families may report strange behavior (eg, the patient's getting lost on the way to the store or forgetting who a recent dinner guest was). This may be accompanied by the onset of emotional lability.

The intermediate stage of SDAT finds the patient completely unable to learn and recall new information. Patients frequently get lost, often to the point of being unable to find their own bedroom or bathroom. Although they remain ambulatory, they are at significant risk for falls or accidents secondary to confusion. Memory of remote events is affected but not totally lost. The patient may require assistance with activities of daily living (eg, bathing, eating, dressing, toileting). Behavioral disorganization occurs in the form of wandering, agitation, hostility, uncooperativeness, or physical aggressiveness. At this stage, the patient has lost all sense of time and place, since normal environmental and social cues are ineffectively utilized. Neuroleptic agents or antianxiety drugs may be required to stabilize the patient.

The severe, or terminal, stage of SDAT finds the patient unable to walk, totally incontinent, and unable to perform any activity of daily living. Patients may be unable to swallow and may require nasogastric feeding. They are at risk for pneumonia, malnutrition, and pressure necrosis of the skin. They are totally dependent on their family care giver, or a long-term care facility. Eventually, they become mute. Recent and remote memory is completely lost. The patient cannot relate any symptoms to the physician. In addition, since there may be no febrile or leukocytic response to infection, the clinician must rely on experience and acumen whenever the patient looks ill.

The progress of the disease is gradual, not rapid or fulminating; there is a steady decline, although some patients' symptoms seem to plateau for a time. No motor or other focal neurologic features occur until very late in the disease. **The end stage of SDAT** is coma and death.

Complications

Complications fall into 3 categories: behavioral, psychiatric, and metabolic. **Behavioral complications** include hostility, agitation, wandering, and uncooperativeness. Depression, anxiety, and paranoid reactions are common **psychiatric complications.** In addition, perhaps 80% of family members or care givers develop depression over time. **Metabolic problems** (eg, dehydration, infection, and drug toxicity) may also occur, adding to cognitive impairment and making management of the patient more difficult. **Other complications** include falls, "sundowning" (confusion after dark) (see "Sundowning" in Dementing Illnesses in Ch. 12), and incontinence. These complications are risk factors for premature institutionalization of the elderly patient and should be treated, since many can be controlled or reversed.

Diagnosis

The diagnosis of SDAT remains clinical. Definitive diagnosis can be made only from brain tissue obtained at biopsy, which is not ordinarily performed. Therefore, the diagnosis is usually made on the basis of history, physical examination, tests, and the exclusion of a variety of other causes of similar mental manifestations.

Clinicians need to be able to differentiate SDAT from depression and delirium, as well as from other psychiatric syndromes with which it can be confused (see also Chs. 9 and 82). Diagnosis may be further complicated by the fact that depression and delirium may coexist with dementia. Major depression is a mood disorder characterized by persistent diminished interest and pleasure in daily activities, insomnia or hypersomnia, psychomotor agitation or retardation, fatigue, feelings of worthlessness, decreased ability to concentrate, thoughts of death, and weight loss or gain. Delirium causes disorganized thinking (eg, rambling, irrelevant, or incoherent speech); reduced ability to maintain or shift attention; decreased level of consciousness; sensory misperceptions; disturbances of the sleep-wake cycle and level of psychomotor activity; disorientation concerning time, place, or person; and memory impairment. The onset of delirium is rapid and the duration is brief. In dementia, however, the essential feature is impairment of short- and long-term memory and of abstract thinking and judgment as well as other disturbances of higher cortical function or personality change.

In the earliest stage of the disease, the clinician should differentiate the cognitive deficit from benign senescent forgetfulness (eg, the patient's problem is simply the slow speed at which he can learn and recall new information; when he is given extra time for such tasks, his intellectual performance is adequate). Since many such individuals are concerned about having early SDAT, they should be reassured that a decrease in learning speed and recall is part of the aging process.

A diagnosis of SDAT should be made only when all other reversible and irreversible causes of dementia have been ruled out. Clinical confirmation of the diagnosis rests in the progressive nature of the cognitive impairment (ie, no improvement is seen in SDAT). A report from the National Institute of Neurological and Communicative Disorders and Stroke **(NINCDS)** and the Alzheimer's Disease and Related Disorders Association **(ADRDA)** lists the following criteria for the probable clinical diagnosis of SDAT, although it points out that these criteria are tentative and subject to change: (1) dementia established by clinical examination and documentation by the Mini Mental State Examination, Blessed Dementia Scale, or some similar examination and confirmed by neuropsychologic tests; (2) deficits in $\geq$ 2 areas of cognition; (3) progressive worsening of memory and other cognitive functions; (4) no disturbance of consciousness; (5) onset between ages 40 and 90 yr, most often after age 65; and (6) absence of systemic disorders or brain diseases that could account for the progressive deficits in memory and cognition.

According to this report, clinical criteria for probable Alzheimer's disease plus histopathologic evidence obtained from brain biopsy (or at autopsy) make up the criteria for the definitive diagnosis of Alzheimer's disease.

The **differential diagnosis** includes multi-infarct or vascular dementia; the dementia subgroup associated with Parkinson's disease; Creutzfeldt-Jakob disease; cerebral vasculitis; end-stage multiple sclerosis; progressive multifocal leukoencephalopathy; metabolic, endocrine, and nutritional dementias (including hypo- and hyperthyroidism); adverse and long-term drug reactions; dementia associated with alcoholism; and dementia pugilistica.

Prior to the imposition of stricter diagnostic criteria, SDAT was misdiagnosed up to 50% of the time. Since depression, the most common psychiatric problem of the aged, closely mimics early-stage SDAT and co-exists in about 20% of SDAT cases, depression should be considered a distinct possibility in patients who present with cognitive impairment. (See Chs. 9 and 82 for information on other illnesses, some of which are treatable, that share features of SDAT.)

The basic evaluation should include a CBC, electrolyte panel, SMA-12 (Sequential Multiple Analyzer tests), thyroid function tests, folate and vitamin B_{12} levels, VDRL test, urinalysis, ECG, and chest x-ray. Scales, such as the Hachinski, are available to help rule out multi-infarct dementia (see Ch. 82). CT is required to rule out tumors, infarcts, subdural hematoma, and normal pressure hydrocephalus. It should be performed when the history suggests a mass, when there are focal neurologic signs, or when there is dementia of brief duration. MRI is more sensitive than CT for detection of small infarcts, mass lesions, and so on. PET remains primarily a research technic.

Prognosis

No predictable stages or patterns can be discerned in the course of SDAT, but cognitive decline is inevitable. Survival ranges from 2 to 20 yr, with an average of 7 yr.

Treatment

SDAT is not curable. Nevertheless, treatment is essential, since the patient's ability for self-care and adaptation depends on CNS function. Each patient's level of impairment progresses differently, and most interventions are directed at complicating factors that can quickly emerge, resulting in failure of self-care, medical problems, and poor nutrition. The physician must treat medical problems, maintain the patient's nutrition, and monitor drug use.

Many drugs can have an adverse effect on the CNS, causing increased confusion and lethargy. Drug-drug interactions can also produce unwanted side effects. Since the anticholinergic activity of antidepressants and antihistamines can worsen the symptoms of Alzheimer's disease, these drugs must be avoided or prescribed judiciously. For example, tricyclic antidepressants are not as useful as trazodone, which has less anticholinergic activity.

Obtaining clarification of the patient's wishes prior to his incapacitation is important. Financial and legal arrangements, such as durable power of attorney, should be arranged in the early stage of the illness (see also Chs. 97, 99, and 100).

In the early stage, cueing and scheduling may help keep the patient functional. Drugs are generally unnecessary, since behavioral disorganization occurs later. Remote memory deficits are less prominent, but word-finding difficulty may occur.

Management includes simplification, definition, and familiarization of the patient's environment, while avoiding isolation and understimulation. Other treatment includes orientation therapy (eg, familiarization with digital clocks and calendars), exercise to reduce restlessness, occupational and music therapy, analysis of the environment for safety and security (including signal systems to monitor wandering), group therapy (reminiscence and socialization), and family counseling services.

The physician must emphasize the importance of drawing on team members (social worker, nutritionist, nurse, home health aide, and others) to assist both patient and care giver. They can provide counseling and support to family members and patients, who frequently deny the severity or existence of cognitive deficits. The physician should help the family understand the progressive nature of the disease but should also emphasize that many of the complicating factors can be controlled. The stress of caring for an SDAT patient may adversely affect the physical and emotional health of family members, resulting in compromised care.

The Alzheimer's Association and its support groups have been instrumental in the treatment of SDAT. Day-care centers have been established that provide respite for family care givers and increased socialization for patients. The presence of paranoia, depression, and agitation may, however, require psychoactive medications, making day care more difficult. To avoid tardive dyskinesia and extrapyramidal symptoms, shorter-acting benzodiazepines should be the first choice in treating agitation and sundowning. However, butyrophenones or phenothiazines may be required for persistent agitation.

Severely ill patients may be cared for in nursing homes, particularly those that have special units for Alzheimer's patients. Currently, there are no adequate government-supported programs or affordable private insurance coverage for long-term institutional or noninstitutional (home) care.

---

82. ORGANIC BRAIN DISORDERS
(See also Chs. 9, 80, and 81)

Trey Sunderland

Syndromes that affect proper cognitive, physical, or behavioral functions and are associated with an acute or chronic CNS disorder.

An estimated 4 to 5 million Americans (about 2% of all ages) suffer from some form of organic brain syndrome. Of this group, approximately 50% have Alzheimer's disease **(AD)**, leaving more than 2 million patients with other conditions, categorized as follows: **(1) delirium and confusional states, (2) amnestic syndromes,** and **(3) non-Alzheimer dementias.**

Although many organic brain syndromes are chronic and irreversible, others are not. This makes careful evaluation and differential diagnosis extremely important. Since there is no reliable laboratory test to establish a definitive diagnosis, the history and physical examination are usually the cornerstones of any evaluation. Routine laboratory tests are useful in excluding other causes of reversible brain disorders. Because the clinical condition in a patient with a brain syndrome can fluctuate and be influenced by other medical problems, it is important to differentiate among the various causes as rapidly as possible to maximize therapeutic options and avoid potential iatrogenic problems.

DELIRIUM

Clinical states characterized by fluctuating disturbances in cognition, mood, attention, arousal, and self-awareness, which can arise acutely or be superimposed on chronic intellectual impairments.

Etiology

The causes of acute delirium or confusional states can be categorized into 3 main groups: **(1) metabolic, (2) structural,** and **(3) infectious.** In each case, the normal physiology of consciousness in the cerebral hemispheres or the arousal mechanisms of the reticular activating system in the brain stem is impaired, leading to a variable clinical picture, described below. Although a large number of individual disease processes can result in these changes, they share many clinical characteristics.

Metabolic: The confusion and transient delirium associated with the **postictal state** is one of the more common and reversible deliria seen in clinical practice. A similar presentation can be observed **postconcussion** without concurrent evidence of intracranial bleeding. **Anoxia** and **transient ischemia** may also present acutely with delirium, as may **hypoglycemia** in a patient with poorly managed diabetes.

Perhaps the most common cause of acute delirium and confusional states is **iatrogenic toxicity** from potent drugs with CNS activity. **Tricyclic antidepressants** and **antiparkinsonian agents** are particularly likely to cause toxic confusional states in the elderly, who may have increased sensitivity to the potent central anticholinergic effects. The widely prescribed **sedatives of the benzodiazepine class** are also frequently responsible for iatrogenic delirium or confusion. Because of reduced metabolism and decreased excretion of these drugs in the elderly, effects are longer lasting and potentially deleterious after weeks or even days of use. **Alcohol and other CNS depressants** can contribute to chronic confusion or even delirium, particularly when used in combination with the aforementioned agents.

Accidental or purposeful **self-induced intoxication** is another major cause of delirium, especially in patients who are mildly impaired at baseline or suffer from chronic depression. Metabolic imbalances associated with **nutritional deficiencies** or **chronic organ failure** (eg, liver, kidney) may also lead to confusional states chronically and to delirium when the underlying condition precipitates **acute electrolyte disturbances** (eg, hyper- or hypokalemia, metabolic acidosis, etc). **Chronic endocrine abnormalities** (eg, hypo- or hyperthyroid and hypercalcemia due to hyperparathyroidism) can present clinically with delirium as well.

Structural: Most structural lesions can be detected with CT scan and MRI. Acutely, these lesions include **vascular occlusion and cerebral infarction, subarachnoid hemorrhage,** and **cerebral hemorrhage.** Usually developing more chronically, **primary** or **metastatic brain tumors, subdural hematomas,** or **brain abscesses** can also lead to delirium or confusional states. Because the therapeutic approaches to each of these causes can differ, speedy and careful differentiation is imperative.

Infectious: Delirium caused by **acute meningitis** or **encephalitis** can often be diagnosed clinically because of the association with a concomitant febrile episode and systemic infection. However, if treatment is to be successful, antibiotic therapy and supportive measures must be instituted before the causative agent has been identified, pending culture results. Slower-developing **embolic abscesses** or **opportunistic infections** are more difficult to diagnose clinically and in some cases even require brain biopsies for proper evaluation. Because patients displaying cognitive deficits at baseline are usually more susceptible to the added confusion associated with central or systemic infections, particular vigilance with older impaired individuals is advised.

Symptoms and Signs

The clinical picture is extremely varied and often changes rapidly. The most prominent manifestation is a clouding of consciousness, with an attendant disorientation to time, place, or person. The syndrome may occur at any age but is more common in elderly persons, particularly those with baseline cognitive impairment. Changes in personality and affect are prevalent, with symptoms of giddiness, irritability, inappropriate behavior, fearfulness, excessive energy, and even frankly psychotic features such as hallucinations or paranoia. Contradictory emotions are often displayed in the same individual within a short time span. Disordered speech is frequently noted, with prominent slurring, rapidity, neologisms, aphasic errors, or chaotic patterns.

Confusion regarding day-to-day events and daily routine, as well as individual roles, is common, and normal patterns of sleeping and eating are usually grossly distorted. Physical restlessness is often seen in the form of pacing, but apathy can also be a manifestation of delirium. In fact, the severity and progression of each of these symptoms may vary widely from patient to patient and within each patient at different times. Family members and friends usually report that the recent changes in behavior are alarming and "out of character" for the patient. The time course for these changes is rarely more than hours or days, and they almost always precipitate a medical emergency.

Confusional states (see Ch. 9), which are milder cases of this cascade of symptoms, develop more slowly and persist for weeks or even months before being detected. The symptoms of confusional states may resemble those of delirium, but they are usually less obvious and less likely to require an emergency consultation.

Diagnosis

A rapid medical evaluation of patients with **delirium** or **confusional states** is imperative because the underlying condition often changes acutely and is sometimes reversible. In the absence of a known cause, a thorough evaluation should include a detailed history (including information from as many relatives or care givers as possible), physical examination, and mental status examination. Laboratory testing should include an SMA-12, CBC with differential, Venereal Disease Research Laboratory **(VDRL)** test, urinalysis with culture, blood cultures, thyroid function tests, and a toxicology screen. Further evaluation with a chest x-ray, CT scan of the brain, EEG, and a CSF examination is indicated if the cause has not yet been determined. Etiologic diagnosis is based on the causes described above.

Prognosis and Treatment

When the underlying cause is identified quickly and managed properly, many symptoms are reversible, particularly in cases due to infections, iatrogenic causes, drug withdrawal, or electrolyte imbalances. In addition to specific treatment of individual causes, several general principles can help in management.

First, adequate fluids and nutrition should be administered under supervision, since the patient frequently has neither the desire nor the physical capacity to maintain a balanced intake. Nutrition should include multivitamins, especially thiamine for the patient in alcohol withdrawal. Second, the environment should be as quiet and calm as possible, preferably with low lighting (ie, avoiding total darkness). Staff and family members should offer reassurance as well as reinforce orientation and explain current proceedings at every opportunity. Third, additional drugs should be avoided unless relevant to the reversal of the underlying condition. However, because agitation can exacerbate delirium, it must sometimes be treated symptomatically, particularly when the physical agitation threatens the well-being of the patient, a care giver, or members of the staff.

Low doses of haloperidol (as little as 0.25 mg) can help in managing the confused geriatric patient, although larger doses (2 to 5 mg) are often needed. Individually titrated doses of benzodiazepines (eg, diazepam) can also be useful to control agitation. These drugs must be administered in the context of care by the physician or nurse. The continuing presence of familiar physicians and nurses often helps alleviate this problem.

AMNESTIC SYNDROMES

A seemingly contradictory state in which a patient can perform some complex tasks learned previously but cannot remember other simple tasks or learn new material, despite repeated trials.

Etiology

Amnestic syndromes can be associated with bilateral cerebral infarctions, severe head trauma involving bilateral brain lesions, chronic or acute brain anoxia, nutritional deficiencies, encephalitis, large subdural hematomas, bilateral brain tumors, postoperative brain lesions, subarachnoid hemorrhage, status epilepticus, and certain medications.

Perhaps the best known of the amnestic syndromes is **Korsakoff's psychosis.** This severe impairment of recent memory is often associated with chronic alcoholism, leading to protracted thiamine deficiency and pathologic involvement of the mamillary bodies as well as other areas of the cerebral cortex.

Transient global amnesia (TGA) is probably associated with ischemic episodes in an otherwise intellectually intact person who generally returns to normal baseline functioning within minutes to hours after the start of the attack. This amnesia is to be differentiated from that following a **seizure** in which the EEG may reveal an underlying abnormality after or between episodes.

Another clinically important entity is that of **psychogenic amnesia** associated with acute psychologic stress (eg, posttraumatic stress disorder) or a more chronic process (eg, **depression**) in which memory functions are commonly impaired to the point that diagnostic confusion, especially in the elderly, may arise (ie, **pseudodementia**). Retrograde amnesia also is frequently reported by depressed patients after they have received a course of **ECT,** even after they have recovered fully from their depressed state. More commonly, mild amnesia is reported with the short- and long-acting benzodiazepines as well as with agents having anticholinergic activity (eg, scopolamine, atropine, or benztropine).

Symptoms and Signs

Amnestic syndromes can involve memory for past events **(retrograde amnesia)** or current events **(anterograde amnesia).** The forgetfulness associated with amnesia is far greater than the "benign senile forgetfulness" often found with normal aging and frequently interferes with the activities of daily living. Cases of memory loss associated with discrete brain injury have demonstrated that areas of the limbic system are central to memory formation and retrieval, but other brain areas also play important roles. Combinations of injuries to the cerebral hemispheres, hippocampus, amygdala, thalamus, hypothalamus, or other subcortical regions can lead to any of a series of memory disturbances, including amnesia.

Patients may attempt to camouflage their memory deficits by replacing lost circumstances with imaginary ones, often formulated on the spur of the moment and replaced with yet another explanation at the next examination. This **confabulation** can be misleading to the clinician when accurate details are not immediately available, and many casual observers are deceived by the attempted cover-up. Because this symptom requires the use of continued language and social skills, it is seen far more often in patients with amnesias than in those with progressive dementias, in which other cognitive functions are also lost or at least more impaired.

Other symptoms associated with amnesia may include emotional changes ranging from apathy in some patients to mild euphoria and intrusiveness in others. Patients often do not have insight into either their memory losses or their personality changes and may in fact deny them when they are pointed out. These emotional symptoms and the memory difficulties may present acutely or may develop slowly over time, depending on the underlying cause.

Diagnosis

Because an amnesia can present acutely and herald further neurologic and intellectual damage, a rapid but thorough evaluation is indicated. The memory deficit is generally more discrete than in delirium or confusional states, and there is usually no clouding of consciousness or marked impairment of attention. In addition, the amnesias commonly lack the pervasive impairments of other intellectual activities seen in the progressive dementias. Cognitive function may, in fact, remain intact except for the memory deficit.

In the absence of an acute medical emergency, which would usually be discovered by routine examination and the laboratory evaluations previously outlined (see under DELIRIUM, above), the amnesia patient should undergo neuropsychologic tests to pinpoint the focal nature of the amnesia and to distinguish the condition from a dementia syndrome. Knowledge of the patient's history or consultation with staff or visitors concerning a current experience can help determine whether the patient is confabulating.

Prognosis and Treatment

Not all amnesias are permanent. In TGA, the memory problems can last for 6 to 36 h, then fully resolve without residual damage other than memory loss for the period of time encompassing the TGA. The progressive amnesia associated with chronic alcoholism can sometimes be slowed or even partially reversed if alcohol is discontinued permanently and the concomitant nutritional deficiencies corrected. On the other hand, amnesias associated with bilateral brain lesions or severe subarachnoid hemorrhages are rarely reversible.

As with delirium and confusional states, the treatment of amnesia depends on the underlying cause; eg, in TIAs, correction of the associated hypertension or atherosclerotic difficulties may help prevent future episodes. Although not always as immediately responsive to treatment, some amnesias resolve slowly over months and years if the underlying problem is corrected.

NON-ALZHEIMER DEMENTIAS

A deterioration of intellectual function and other cognitive skills, leading to a reduction in the previously normal performance of activities of daily living.

Symptoms and Signs

Although new memory retention decreases with increasing age, other cognitive functions normally remain relatively intact. Dementia, therefore, represents a marked change from the age-dependent normal level of functioning. The non-Alzheimer dementias can present similarly to Alzheimer's disease (see Ch. 81). Specifically, impairment may be seen in areas of higher function, including speech (aphasia), motor activity (apraxia), interpretation of sensory input (agnosia), judgment, short-term memory, and attention span. In addition, behavioral manifestations of agitation, anxiety, depression, apathy, irritability, or superficial euphoria often occur.

Personal habits or interests can be altered dramatically or dropped entirely without obvious explanation. In contrast to the cognitive and behavioral changes of Alzheimer's dementia, these changes can occur suddenly and are not necessarily progressive. Associated gait abnormalities, seizures, incontinence, muscle abnormalities, or other medical symptoms may also be part of the non-Alzheimer dementia syndrome and can occur early in the course of the illness.

Diagnosis

There is no clinically available pathognomonic marker for dementia; *dementia is a clinical diagnosis.* The diagnosis implies that a marked change in mental or intellectual capacities has already taken place and that the condition is relatively stable. Although patients with non-Alzheimer dementia can worsen over time, the condition is usually not as volatile as delirium and should not be confused clinically with a clouding of consciousness, which is characteristic of delirium.

The general assessment must include many of the tests previously listed for the evaluation of delirium and confusional states (see above) to exclude the possible reversible causes of dementia; ie, diagnostic tests should be thought of as *tools of exclusion.* For example, whereas a brain CT scan showing cortical atrophy is consistent with a diagnosis of dementia, it does not establish the diagnosis. Rather, such a report should be viewed as probably excluding at least a large tumor or cerebrovascular accident as the cause of the patient's dementia. The underlying cause usually remains unknown; only autopsy or brain biopsy findings provide a definitive neuropathologic diagnosis.

Special attention must be paid to the possibility of a psychiatric condition. **Pseudodementia,** a common manifestation of depression (especially in the geriatric population), may be difficult to differentiate from dementia. **Depression associated with dementia** can make this differentiation even more difficult. Neuropsychologic test batteries may help in distinguishing the various dementias but are not unequivocal. Sometimes, only the clinical course and response to antidepressants confirm these conditions.

The causes of non-Alzheimer dementia, like those of delirium (see above), can be categorized into 3 main areas: (1) metabolic, (2) structural or intrinsic, and (3) infectious.

Metabolic: Some of the metabolic causes of acute delirium can result in chronic dementia if not corrected, eg, **chronic anoxia,** such as that associated with severe chronic obstructive pulmonary disease. The more profound acute anoxias accompanying **cardiac arrest, anesthesia accidents,** or **carbon monoxide poisoning** can also result in permanent anoxic brain damage and dementia, occasionally with accompanying myoclonus.

Conditions resulting from nutritional and vitamin deficiencies, eg, **pernicious anemia** or **pellagra,** can cause a chronic memory disorder. Failure of other organ systems, including the liver and kidneys, is frequently associated with intellectual impairments and dementia-like syndromes. Full-blown **hepatic** or **uremic encephalopathy** usually presents as a change in consciousness, as well as asterixis or myoclonus, but subclinical variations of these conditions can be present with dementia symptoms alone. The hypercalcemia associated with **hyperparathyroidism** can also cause decreased intellectual performance. **Hypoglycemia,** if sufficiently severe and frequent, can lead to a progressive dementia, especially in a diabetic who has brittle disease and a history of poorly controlled serum glucose.

Structural or intrinsic: This is by far the largest category of non-Alzheimer dementias. The most common diagnosis is probably **multi-infarct dementia (MID)** or the dementia associated with cerebrovascular disease. The symptoms are identical in some cases to those of Alzheimer's disease and the 2 are often difficult to distinguish. An associated history of heart disease, previous strokes, focal neurologic signs, hypertension, or an intermittent course of clinical progression can be helpful differentiating points, but even with careful evaluation, there may be considerable diagnostic confusion. Laboratory evaluations, including CT scan and MRI, also support the diagnosis of MID, but there is currently no foolproof diagnostic method. Even at autopsy, definitive diagnosis is impossible in some cases because of the neuropathologic overlap between MID and Alzheimer's disease.

Binswanger's dementia or **subcortical arteriosclerotic encephalopathy (SAE)** involves multiple infarcts in hemispheric white matter associated with severe hypertension and systemic vascular disease. Clinically, the dementia is similar to MID, although there may be more focal neurologic symptoms associated with acute strokes and more rapid clinical deterioration.

Dementia is present in > 25% of patients with **Parkinson's disease (PD);** some estimates of the incidence are as high as 80%. In addition, at autopsy, PD patients may show some of the same neuropathologic brain findings seen in AD patients, and the 2 groups share numerous biochemical changes. The diagnosis is futher confusing because AD patients also frequently demonstrate progressive symptoms of parkinsonism. Clinically, the diagnosis is often based on the time and course of symptoms, specifically, whether the motor signs were present before or after the cognitive decline. Also, tremor is uncommon in the extrapyramidal syndrome of AD.

Huntington's chorea can also present with symptoms of dementia, but the clinical picture is usually clarified by the obvious family history and the motor abnormalities characteristic of the disease process.

Pick's disease is a less common form of dementia, involving the frontal and temporal regions of the cortex. Patients with this disease have prominent apathy as well as memory disturbances; they may show increased carelessness, poor personal hygiene, and decreased attention span. Clinically, this condition is often confused with Alzheimer's disease. While the symptom presentation and CT scan findings of Pick's disease can be quite distinctive, absolute diagnostic differentiation is possible only at autopsy. The **Klüver-Bucy syndrome** can be seen early in the course of Pick's disease, with emotional blunting, altered sexual activity, hyperorality, and visual agnosias.

Frontal lobe syndromes can be due to intrinsic pathology, such as with Pick's disease, but they may also be associated with **primary or metastatic tumors, previous surgical manipulation,** or **irradiation** to these areas of the brain, which results in residual intellectual damage. Dementia can sometimes be the presenting clinical symptom of primary or metastatic neoplasms. **Repeated head trauma** (eg, that received by professional fighters, or **dementia pugilistica**) can also lead to a frontal lobe dementia syndrome, but again the history is of great value in the differential diagnosis.

Normal-pressure hydrocephalus (NPH) can cause a progressive dementia with an insidious onset. The clinical triad of gait disturbance, incontinence, and dementia, along with a brain CT scan showing enlarged ventricles without cortical atrophy, can help differentiate this illness, but the clinical presentation is variable. NPH is more common in men than in women and may be associated with previous attacks of meningitis or head injury.

Progressive multifocal leukoencephalopathy (PML) may be present in patients with other concurrent debilitating diseases (eg, tuberculosis, lymphoma, sarcoidosis) or with disorders involving compromised immunologic functioning. The dementia is usually accompanied by numerous other systemic and CNS symptoms, including hemiparesis, ataxia, blindness, and behavioral alterations. The dementia associated with **progressive supranuclear palsy** is commonly preceded by other neurologic symptoms, eg, pseudobulbar palsy, dystonic axial rigidity, supranuclear ophthalmoplegia, and dysarthria.

Infectious: The most publicized infectious cause of dementia is probably **Creutzfeldt-Jakob disease (CJD),** in which memory deficits, electroencephalographic changes, and myoclonus are prominent. The onset of illness is generally in the fifth or sixth decade, and the duration of illness is usually less than a year. The infectious agent is a so-called slow virus, which has been successfully transmitted in laboratory settings to lower animals and results in a characteristic spongiform encephalopathy quite different from that of AD. Patients with CJD may resemble those with frontal lobe syndromes; they are often apathetic, are personally unkempt, and display psychomotor retardation. They can also develop motor symptoms, incontinence, and seizures later in the course of the disease. The typical course is much more rapid than that of AD and usually lasts from 6 to 24 mo.

Gerstmann-Straussler's syndrome is another dementia with known transmissibility to animals, which typically presents as ataxia, followed later by the onset of cognitive decline.

General paresis was once a more common cause of dementia occurring as a late sequela of syphilis. It is currently much less common in Western societies but is still prevalent in developing countries. In addition to intellectual decline, there are associated tremors and pupillary changes. Serologic examination of the CSF should be positive for syphilis.

Patients with **acquired immune deficiency syndrome (AIDS)** can also develop dementia. This dementia, clinically similar to progressive multifocal encephalopathy, is usually caused by the virus itself or by a variety of opportunistic infections including fungal, bacterial, other viral, or protozoal agents, which can be identified at autopsy.

Prognosis and Treatment

Dementia is usually considered an irreversible condition that is progressive and incurable. Although this is often true, certain conditions are treatable or at least partially reversible, and many palliative measures can be instituted in any dementia patient. If the dementing process is acute, as with some of the metabolic, intrinsic, or infectious causes, treatment of the underlying conditions can arrest progression of the dementia and, in some cases, allow partial recovery over time.

Even when the dementia is chronic and a return of intellectual function is not possible, simple supportive measures (eg, frequent orientation reinforcement, limited expectations, a bright and cheerful environment, a minimum of new stimulation, and regular low-stress activities) can be of great help. If daily routines can be simplified and the expectations of the care givers reduced without the patient sensing a total loss of self-control or personal dignity, the patient may actually show some improvement.

Functioning can be further improved by the elimination or strict limitation of drugs or nonessential medications with CNS activity. On the other hand, some patients may develop clinical depression and can be helped by the addition of antidepressants. However, the lowest possible effective dose should be used, since dementia patients appear to be particularly sensitive to the anticholinergic effects of such drugs and may react with increased confusion.

Once the acute medical evaluation is completed and a course of treatment is established, most responsibility falls on the shoulders of the family, especially with chronic dementias. The stresses on the family are tremendous. Although curative medical intervention is rarely available to the patient, the clinician can still be of great help to the families. By recognizing the early symptoms of "care giver burnout" and guiding the families through the myriad of social agencies and nursing institutions often required, the clinician can remain sensitive to the needs of the family support system, thereby enhancing overall care for the patient.

83.   CEREBROVASCULAR DISEASE

(Stroke; Cerebrovascular Accident [CVA])

Louis R. Caplan

Magnitude of the Problem

In 1984, 500,000 Americans had a stroke, more than 155,000 died of a stroke, and there were more than 2 million stroke survivors. A majority of the stroke deaths occured in individuals $\geq$ 65 yr of age. TABLE 83–1 shows the stroke death rates/100,000 population for whites and blacks in the USA in 1983. The rates dramatically increase after age 65. In nearly all age groups, men have more strokes and more of them die of stroke than women.

More impressive than the mortality rates are the qualitative aspects of life after stroke. Many patients are impaired in their ability to walk, see, and feel. In some cases, they cannot speak or otherwise communicate, read, recall, or think as well as they could before their stroke. Daily functions in the work place, home, and community may be affected.

TABLE 83–1. STROKE DEATH RATES PER 100,000 POPULATION BY AGE, SEX, AND RACE IN THE USA, 1983

Race and Sex	Age (yr)					
	35–44	45–54	55–64	65–74	75–84	> 84
White	5.6	18.0	49.1	167.6	643.5	1950.9
Men	5.5	19.1	56.5	197.1	714.8	1862.9
Women	5.6	16.9	42.6	144.6	602.0	1986.5
Black	22.0	64.0	143.0	341.5	807.4	1570.7
Men	24.3	74.1	163.8	388.0	844.1	1479.4
Women	20.1	55.7	126.0	308.4	786.7	1603.1

Classification

Stroke is *a heterogeneous category of illness that describes brain injury, usually sudden, caused by vascular disease.* The 2 major categories are **brain hemorrhage** and **brain ischemia.** Brain hemorrhage can be subdivided into **subarachnoid hemorrhage (SAH),** *bleeding into the spaces and spinal fluid around the brain,* and **intracerebral hemorrhage (ICH),** *bleeding directly into the brain.*

These different patterns of hemorrhage have different causes, symptoms, signs, outcomes, and treatments. In ICH, bleeding injures tissue by local pressure effects, and the blood interrupts important brain pathways. SAH suddenly increases the pressure within the cranium, impairs the drainage of spinal fluid, and irritates the arteries at the base of the brain. Each type of hemorrhage accounts for about 10% of all strokes but a much higher percentage of stroke deaths.

Ischemia, *injury to brain tissue caused by an inadequate supply of blood and nutrients,* accounts for about 80% of strokes. **Ischemic stroke** is also a heterogenous category that can be subclassified into (1) diseases of the large arteries (carotid and vertebral) in the neck and within the cranium; (2) diseases of the small penetrating arteries deep within the brain; (3) embolism arising from the heart or great vessels; and (4) general circulatory failure caused by shock, poor cardiac output, or hypotension. These different subgroups of ischemia have varied causes, symptoms and signs, prognoses, and treatments.

SAH is less common after age 60, probably because of the reduced frequency of arteriovenous **(A-V)** malformations and saccular aneurysms that remain life threatening by that age. Penetrating artery occlusive disease, cerebral hemorrhage, and cerebral embolism increase in frequency during old age, probably because of increased prevalence of hypertension, the effects of age on the cerebral vessels, and cardiac disease and arrhythmias (eg, atrial fibrillation).

General Principles of Evaluation

Since the middle of the 20th century, most texts have emphasized the temporal features of stroke. The terms **transient ischemic attacks (TIAs), stroke in progress, reversible ischemic neurologic deficit (RIND),** and **completed stroke** describe only the time course of ischemia and not the cause. However, as in any other human disease, the physician should concentrate on the cause of the stroke or the temporary episode in the individual patient.

The physician should ask the following questions, generally in the order suggested: Using the classification of hemorrhage and ischemia noted above, what is the type and subtype of stroke present? How severe is the brain damage? Is there still tissue at risk that could soon suffer further damage? Can and should the patient be treated other than just in a supportive way? Are there limitations to acceptable and potentially effective treatments in this patient? What is the nature and severity of the patient's disability? What are the available personal, family, medical, social, economic, and community resources that could help the patient cope with and adapt to any resultant disability?

Extent of brain damage is determined by the severity of neurologic abnormalities and the findings in brain-imaging studies. To assess the tissue still at risk for further damage, the physician must know the cause as well as the vessels and arterial territory involved. For example, 1 patient with a sudden hemiparesis has a tiny infarct in the internal capsule that represents the total supply of a single penetrating lenticulostriate artery that has been blocked by hyaline material because of hypertension. Another patient has weakness of 1 arm due to occlusion of the contralateral internal carotid artery in the neck. The patient with unilateral paralysis caused by penetrating artery disease has little immediate risk of worsening, but in the future, that patient will be at risk for further penetrating artery occlusions unless the cause of the disease—hypertension—is recognized and effectively treated.

The patient with carotid artery occlusive disease is at immediate risk of serious worsening. A patient with an infarct at the periphery of a cerebral hemisphere, caused by an embolus from a clot within a left ventricular aneurysm, is in imminent danger of brain damage from further embolization to other cerebral arteries.

Prophylaxis

Prevention of stroke is clearly preferred to treatment after stroke, yet preventive measures are often overlooked. While introducing treatment for a given stroke, the physician should begin to institute general health practices to prevent additional strokes and progressive vascular disease. These principles are applicable to all geriatric patients and include control of hypertension; treatment of cardiac disorders, coronary artery disease, heart failure, and arrhythmias; treatment of hematologic problems (eg, anemia, polycythemia, and bleeding diathesis); measurement of blood lipids and treatment of hyperlipidemia; forceful admonition to stop smoking, to avoid recreational drugs, and to use alcohol only in moderation; encouragement of regular exercise; and avoidance of overeating, undereating, and exhaustion. A positive psychologic outlook is also critical; the physician must take time to listen and understand the patient's situation.

All prospective studies show dramatically increased stroke risk in patients who have had one or more TIAs. Prospective studies of patients with stenosis of the internal carotid artery in the neck, detected by noninvasive technics, show a low rate of stroke ($< 2\%$) without preceding TIAs. Detection of TIAs is essential; their presence should trigger a search for their cause, to prevent stroke.

Most patients are not knowledgeable about nervous system anatomy and physiology and do not know about the afferent and efferent connections of the brain, limbs, and senses. They attribute numbness and weakness of the limbs and dimness of vision to the symptomatic body parts and not to the CNS. The patients must be asked specific questions, eg, Have you had temporary prickling or loss of feeling in your arms or legs? Have you had a temporary limp or other walking problem? Have you ever had a "shade" or "curtain" come over one of your eyes? Recent headaches can be an indication of occlusive disease and should be diagnostically pursued.

Patients who have had TIAs should *not* simply be given an aspirin a day (or whatever the most recently touted panacea may be) but instead should be assessed for the specific cause. A TIA is not a homogeneous entity but is a *symptom* of heterogeneous vascular, cardiac, and hematologic problems. No one treatment has proved or will prove effective for all, and delay in diagnosis can be disastrous if the patient has a disabling stroke.

General Principles of Treatment

In some patients, the stroke is so severe that it results in an extremely poor quality of life; in others, no available treatment is likely to help. Patients with stroke may also have other serious diseases (eg, cancer, incapacitating heart or lung disease, or dementia) that affect treatment decisions. Nevertheless, all stroke patients deserve humane supportive care (eg, hydration, avoidance of decubitus ulcers, and maintenance of parenteral nutrition).

Clearly, aggressive treatment may not be warranted in everyone. In some patients, certain treatments are contraindicated (eg, anticoagulants in patients with severe hypertension or GI bleeding), but other therapeutic interventions may be applicable. Age alone is never an absolute contraindication for treatment. Many treatments (eg, anticoagulants and vascular and brain surgery) have higher risk and complication rates in the elderly, but older patients are also more easily disabled than are younger patients, and their daily routines may be destroyed by handicaps that could have been more readily overcome in their youth.

Retraining and adaption to neurologic handicaps depend on the nature of the underlying anatomic abnormality, ie, what part of the brain is injured, and not on the cause of the injury. Visual field defects, aphasia, spatial disorientation, paralysis, and gait ataxia all require very different rehabilitation and adjustment strategies. Recovery depends as much, if not more, on the personal and socioeconomic circumstances of the stroke victim as on the injury itself.

Are good medical and rehabilitation facilities available? Stroke is a complex disease. If expertise and technology to care for the stroke patient are not available locally, treatable patients should be transferred to a center with special stroke capabilities. Similarly, rehabilitation is best performed in specialized units.

The prior capability and physical as well as psychologic health of the patient are important predictors of subsequent ability to cope and work toward recovery. If there is no one at home to help the patient, recovery is extremely difficult. Social and economic factors are also influential. A patient who lives on the first floor; owns and can drive a car or has access to a driver; has nearby convenient shopping, recreational, and medical facilities; and has the economic resources to afford needed equipment and personnel is much more likely to return to an active, useful life than someone without these resources. Acute depression following stroke, a common complication, or a history of chronic or recurrent depression also can be a barrier to recovery.

HEMORRHAGIC STROKE

Cerebrovascular disorders caused by bleeding into brain tissue or meningeal spaces.

SUBARACHNOID HEMORRHAGE (SAH)

Sudden bleeding into the subarachnoid space.

The most common causes of SAH are cerebral aneurysms, arteriovenous **(A-V)** malformations, bleeding diatheses, head trauma, and amyloid angiopathy. A-V malformations rarely present first in the later years of life without earlier symptoms of bleeding or epilepsy. Aneurysms do occur in the elderly, but they are slightly more common in younger populations. The most common bleeding disorder leading to SAH in the elderly is iatrogenic, due to prescribing warfarin and other anticoagulants.

Head trauma is common in the elderly because of their increased tendency to fall. The patient is often confused or amnesic after the fall and cannot provide a clear account of the event. Head injury is often not diagnosed: the physician incorrectly attributes the blood found in CSF at lumbar puncture to a spontaneous SAH that caused the fall and confusion rather than evaluating the fall and injury as the initial event. Such trauma victims are often needlessly subjected to angiography in search of aneurysms.

Amyloid angiopathy is a degenerative hyalinization of the arteries in the brain and subarachnoid spaces that can cause SAH and intracerebral hemorrhages. Bleeding episodes in patients with amyloid angiopathy are often recurrent and multiple, and the patient may be demented because of frequently coexisting Alzheimer-like changes in the cortex.

Symptoms, Signs, and Diagnosis

Headache is an invariable symptom in patients with SAH. Head pain often begins suddenly, usually while the patient is physically active, and becomes severe almost immediately. The pain is usually diffuse but at times is most severe at the back of the head and neck and may radiate down the back in a sciatic pattern. Nausea and vomiting are common. Usually such patients must interrupt their activity, and they often become restless, agitated, and confused.

Unlike persons with intracerebral hemorrhage or ischemic stroke, patients with SAH are generally not paralyzed and most often do not have important focal neurologic signs. The headache, vomiting, and confusion are all caused by a sudden increase in intracranial pressure.

Blood is usually released quickly into the subarachnoid space at arterial pressure and widely disperses around the brain and spinal cord.

On examination, the most important abnormality is usually alteration of level of consciousness—restlessness, delirium, sleepiness, stupor, or coma. Stiff neck, difficulty concentrating, and impairment of immediate past memory and extensor plantar reflexes are also common. Focal neurologic signs (eg, hemiparesis, hemisensory loss, hemianopia) are usually absent because most SAH patients do not have focal collections of blood within the brain. Focal signs can develop later because of vasoconstriction and delayed ischemia.

The most important diagnostic tests are CT, lumbar puncture, and cerebral angiography. CT within the first 24 to 48 h of bleeding is likely to show blood as hyperdensity within the cisterns, between the cerebral gyri, and in the ventricles on unenhanced scans. However, small SAHs or those occurring days before may not be visible. CT can also show small contusions, subdural hematomas, and skull fractures, and sometimes an aneurysm can be visualized on an enhanced scan. Restlessness and agitation compromise the patient's ability to cooperate for a high-quality cranial CT.

All patients with symptomatic SAH have grossly visible blood-stained CSF under increased pressure when lumbar puncture is performed within a few days of SAH. If the patient with severe unexplained headache requires hospitalization, performance of a CT scan before lumbar puncture is usually preferred. If the patient has no focal neurologic signs and can walk normally, a spinal tap can be safely performed without CT to exclude an SAH or meningitis. Angiography is the only available procedure by which an aneurysm and its feeding vessels can be visualized. When the diagnosis of SAH is definite, angiography usually should be delayed until the patient is relatively fit for surgery.

The most common complications of SAH are cardiac arrhythmias, hydrocephalus, delayed vasoconstriction (so-called spasm), and rebleeding. Blood can induce vasoconstriction of cerebral arteries beginning $\geq$ 48 h after the SAH; vasoconstriction can continue for $\geq$ 1 wk. Vasoconstriction can also follow surgical manipulation of the vessels, especially if blood is released into the subarachnoid space during or after surgery. Large hemorrhages, or those in which there are thick focal collections of blood, are particularly likely to be complicated by spasm and delayed cerebral ischemia.

Headache, decreased alertness, and focal neurologic signs (eg, hemiparesis) are the most common findings in patients with spasm. The major differential diagnostic consideration is rebleeding. In patients with vasospasm, CT shows no new bleeding and may reveal a hypodense area of cerebral infarction. Rebleeding is manifested by suddenly increased headache, decreased alertness, and new blood on CT or lumbar puncture. Angiography not only defines the aneurysm but shows general or focal vasoconstriction.

Treatment

Treatment of SAH depends on the specific cause. In SAH due to an aneurysm or A-V malformation, the aim is to clip or coat the involved vessels before the next episode of bleeding. Mortality increases greatly with each bleed. When SAH is due to the use of warfarin, hypoprothrombinemia must be quickly reversed with vitamin K. Patients with SAH due to head trauma should be quickly evaluated and managed neurosurgically if indicated.

All SAH patients should be monitored in a quiet room. Dehydration should be avoided, since it can lead to decreased cerebral blood flow. Severe hypertension should be controlled, but one must remember that the increased systemic BP may be precipitated by the sudden increase in intracranial pressure. Increased intracranial pressure causes an increase in venous pressure in the brain and dural venous sinuses; the systemic BP must exceed this elevated venous pressure if the brain is to be perfused. Corticosteroids in doses equivalent to 60 to 100 mg prednisone/day help control increased intracranial pressure and brain swelling.

INTRACEREBRAL HEMORRHAGE (ICH)

Bleeding into the brain usually arises from small arteries or arterioles. The most common cause is hypertension. The coexistence of degenerative changes due to aging and hypertension leads to an increased susceptibility to ICH in the elderly. Bleeding diatheses, especially warfarin-induced hypoprothrombinemia, are especially treacherous causes of ICH because the bleeding is more gradual and progressive and more often results in death than other causes.

Amyloid angiopathy is a common cause of ICH, accounting for up to 20% of hematomas in patients > 70 yr of age. Special stains are needed to detect the congophilic changes in the blood vessels of surgical or postmortem specimens. Aneurysms and A-V malformations are unusual causes of ICH. Bleeding occasionally occurs into a previously unsuspected brain tumor, especially if it is metastatic.

Symptoms, Signs, and Diagnosis

When blood is released into the brain, the earliest symptoms result from the loss of the functions subserved by that brain region. Bleeding into the left putamen and internal capsule causes paralysis of the right limbs; hemorrhage in the right occipital lobe causes a left visual field defect; and cerebellar hemorrhage causes deficits of coordination. The hemorrhage may expand within minutes, or at most a few hours, and lead to a progressive increase in focal neurologic symptoms and signs. The expanding hematoma acts like a solid mass, increasing intracranial contents and pressure and causing headache, vomiting, and decreased alertness. If the hemorrhage remains small, symptoms of increased intracranial pressure do not occur. Nearly 50% of patients with small-to-moderate ICHs do not have headache and remain alert. This is especially true in the elderly, because previous atrophy provides ample space to accommodate the extra contents.

On examination, signs of focal abnormality of brain function are apparent. The most common locations for hypertensive ICH are listed in TABLE 83–2, along with the most important accompanying neurologic signs. Putamenal hemorrhages account for approximately 35% of cases of hypertensive ICH; lobar hematomas, approximately 25%; and thalamic hemorrhages, approximately 20%. Caudate, pontine, and cerebellar locations each account for about 7% of cases.

Warfarin-induced hemorrhages tend to occur in the lobes of the cerebrum and the cerebellum, begin more insidiously, and progress more gradually. Amyloid angiopathy hemorrhages are almost always lobar and do not usually involve the other common sites for hypertensive hemorrhage (putamen, caudate, thalamus, pons, cerebellum). Traumatic hematomas are usually multiple and located on the surface of the brain,

TABLE 83–2. NEUROLOGIC SIGNS IN PATIENTS WITH HYPERTENSIVE INTRACEREBRAL HEMORRHAGE AT COMMON LOCATIONS

Putamen	Contralateral hemiparesis, hemisensory loss, and at times hemianopia; conjugate deviation of eyes to side of hemorrhage; normal pupil size and reaction
	Left putamen—aphasia; right putamen—left visual neglect
Thalamus	Contralateral hemisensory loss with slight hemiparesis or hemiataxia; eyes deviated down or down and in; reduced vertical gaze; small, poorly reactive pupils
Caudate nucleus	Contralateral slight transient hemiparesis; restlessness and confusion; occasionally, ipsilateral Horner's syndrome
Lobar	Frontal lobe—decreased spontaneity; contralateral Babinski's sign
	Parietal lobe—contralateral hemisensory loss and hemineglect; left parietal reading/writing deficits and aphasia
	Temporal lobe—agitation and upper quadrantanopia contralaterally; left temporal—Wernicke's fluent aphasia
	Occipital lobe—contralateral hemianopia
Pons	Quadraparesis; reduced alertness; absent horizontal gaze; small reactive pupils; some pontine hemorrhages affect the tegmentum or base unilaterally causing a hemiparesis and crossed cranial nerve signs
Cerebellum	Gait ataxia; vomiting; sometimes conjugate gaze paresis or 6th nerve palsy to the side of the hemorrhage

especially the orbital frontal lobes and the tips of the temporal lobes, sites that are in close contact with rough bony ridges at the base of the skull.

Diagnosis of ICH has been revolutionized by CT. Hematomas appear as white, hyperdense, well-circumscribed lesions. CT can give accurate information about the hematoma location and size, drainage into the ventricles or onto the surface, and shifts of intracranial contents. CT can also show an unsuspected tumor or vascular malformation adjacent to the hematoma. When the patient is anemic, the hematoma may appear hypodense or have a fluid level.

MRI can also readily show hemorrhages and can better reveal the extent and dissection of the hemorrhage in the coronal and sagittal planes. Separation of hemorrhage and ischemia is less obvious on MRI than on CT and requires an analysis of the differences in T-1 and T-2 weighted images. Old hemosiderin is also detected by MRI.

Treatment

Treatment of ICH depends on cause, location, and amount of bleeding. Large hemorrhages are usually fatal before treatment can be initiated. Small hemorrhages are self-contained and have self-limited clinical courses requiring little treatment except prophylactic measures (eg, control of hypertension to prevent a recurrent ICH). Moderate-sized (2 to 4 cm) hematomas are the most important to treat, especially if the patient's condition is worsening.

Progression is usually manifested by a decrease in alertness and consciousness and an increase in focal neurologic signs. For example, on admission, a patient with a right putamenal hemorrhage has left hemiparesis and conjugate deviation of the eyes to the right. The left plantar response is extensor, and the pupils are normal. If the hematoma expands or the region surrounding the hematoma becomes edematous, the right plantar response may become extensor, the eyes may fail to move in either horizontal direction, the right pupil may become dilated and fixed, and stupor may develop. Without aggressive treatment, such patients, who worsen while under medical observation, have a high fatality rate. Surgical drainage of an expanding hematoma can be lifesaving, decompressing the brain and decreasing intracranial pressure; however, because surgical drainage substitutes a cavity for the hematoma, it does not diminish the extent of the paralysis or other focal abnormalities.

Surgical decompression is most feasible for cerebellar hemorrhages and lobar hematomas near the brain surface. An excellent example is the case of a vigorous hypertensive man of 82 who presented with headache, left hemianopia, and decreased alertness. CT showed a right temporal lobe hemorrhage about 4 cm at its greatest diameter. He gradually became stuporous and developed bilateral extensor plantar reflexes. His physicians struggled with the decision of whether or not to drain the hematoma surgically, fearful that he might survive severely disabled and become a permanent burden to his family and society. Because of his previous vigor and a supportive family with ample resources and optimism, neurosurgical drainage was performed. He was left with only a nondisabling visual field defect and lived another 10 yr, surviving to dance at his granddaughter's wedding.

Thalamic and pontine hematomas are not accessible surgically. Hypertension should be controlled but BP should not be reduced to normal levels, which could compromise cerebral perfusion. Corticosteroids and osmotic agents, such as mannitol and glycerol, may help control increased intracranial pressure (see TABLE 83–3).

TABLE 83–3. TREATMENT OF INCREASED INTRACRANIAL PRESSURE

Medical
Intubation and mechanical hyperventilation
Dexamethasone 4 mg q 6 h IM
Mannitol 0.5–1 gm/kg q 4 h IV
Glycerol 1–1.5 oz po q 6 h
Furosemide 40 mg (4 mg/min) IV

Surgical
Drainage of hematoma or large infarct
Ventricular drainage or shunt
Excision of bleeding A-V malformation or tumor
Repair of aneurysm

ISCHEMIC STROKE

Cerebrovascular disorder caused by insufficient cerebral circulation.

Except for systemic hypotension, which usually begins abruptly, the characteristics of ischemic stroke are TIAs and a fluctuating, stepwise, or progressive clinical course. Ischemia is caused by an impediment to blood flow, almost always in the form of a narrowed or occluded artery leading to a local brain region. Arterial occlusion sets in motion a chain of events, some tending to increase the ischemia and worsen the neurologic deficit, and others (ie, compensatory body reactions) acting to limit the ischemia and reduce the deficit (see TABLE 83–4). During the first week after ischemia begins, a thrombus gradually adheres to the arterial wall and becomes organized, diminishing the early tendency of the loosely attached clot to embolize or distally propagate. Also, time is needed for collateral circulation to become established and stabilized.

During this relatively unstable period of a few days to 2 wk after occlusion, any decrease in cerebral perfusion should be avoided. BP should not be lowered unless it is ≥ 170/110 mm Hg. Cardiac output should be maximized. Hypovolemia, a frequent problem in the stroke patient who may eat and drink suboptimally, should be avoided. Since the simple act of sitting up or standing may worsen the ischemia early in its

TABLE 83–4. INSTABILITY AFTER A VASCULAR OCCLUSION

Factors promoting deficit
  Reduced regional cerebral blood flow in territory supplied by occluded artery
  Local stagnant flow and activation of clotting factors enlarge the clot
  Clot propagates distally
  Loosely adherent clot embolizes, blocking distal arteries

Factors limiting deficit
  Reduced pressure and tissue acidosis stimulate opening of collaterals
  Collateral arteries dramatically increase flow in the supply area of occluded artery
  Fibrinolytic systems are activated
  Emboli pass

course, patients should be watched carefully when they first sit or stand; they should also be observed for postural hypotension or increases in symptoms or signs related to posture. Patients whose signs fluctuate or worsen usually should be maintained in the supine position to maximize cerebral blood flow until the instability passes. Other factors in the management of ischemia include the location and severity of the occlusive vascular lesion, the status of the blood and its constituents, and the degree and reversibility of any damage to the target organ, the brain.

ATHEROSTENOSIS OF THE LARGE EXTRACRANIAL AND INTRACRANIAL ARTERIES

Atherosclerosis is a generalized process. In whites, atherosclerosis in the cerebrovascular bed is most common at the origins of the internal carotid artery **(ICA)** and the vertebral artery **(VA)** in the neck and at the intracranial basilar artery **(BA).** The large intracranial arteries (anterior, middle, and posterior cerebral arteries **[ACA, MCA, PCA]**) and their superficial convexal artery branches are affected much less often.

Atherosclerosis of the extracranial ICA and VA is twice as common in white men as in white women and correlates highly with coronary and peripheral vascular occlusive disease and hyperlipidemia. A history of angina pectoris, prior MI, or leg claudication makes a diagnosis of extracranial atherostenosis quite likely in a patient with a TIA.

In blacks and in individuals of Japanese and Chinese descent, antherostenosis of the neck arteries is less common but the major intracranial arteries are more predisposed to stenosis than in whites. In these populations, intracranial artery stenosis does not correlate epidemiologically with coronary or peripheral vascular disease or hyperlipidemia, occurs at a younger age than extracranial disease, and does not have a strong male preponderance. Diabetics are prone to intracranial disease, and populations with a high prevalence of intracranial disease also have a high incidence of hypertension.

Symptoms and Signs

The most common presenting symptom is ≥ 1 TIAs. These attacks are often brief and may recur for weeks or months if untreated. Some present as a sudden onset stroke, probably caused by embolization of intraarterial clot or plaque material arising from regions of extracranial atherostenosis, and traveling distally to block intracranial recipient arteries. Headache is also common and is probably caused by dilatation of collateral arterial channels. Specific symptoms and signs relate to the anatomy of the involved artery and the area it supplies.

Internal carotid artery (ICA) in the neck: The first branch of the ICA is the ophthalmic artery, which arises intracranially and supplies the optic nerve, retina, and iris. Transient decreases in flow in the ICA cause attacks of transient monocular blindness, or amaurosis fugax, on the side of the ICA lesion. These attacks are usually described as a shade falling or a curtain moving across the eye from the side. Transient monocular blindness spells are usually brief, lasting 30 sec to a few minutes. Some attacks are precipitated by the patient's suddenly standing or bending or by exposure to bright natural light.

Patients with carotid artery disease often have attacks of hemispheric ischemia characterized by weakness or numbness of the contralateral limbs or the opposite part of the face. The hand and arm are more often involved than the face or leg. The attacks vary; the hand may be involved in 1 spell, the leg in another, and the arm and leg in a third. Aphasia is common when the left ICA is involved.

When spells of transient monocular blindness and attacks of numbness or weakness of the opposite limbs occur in the same patient, the physician can be confident about the diagnosis of ICA disease within the neck or within the carotid siphon before the ophthalmic artery branch. Plaque disease and stenosis are most severe at the origin of the ICA from the common carotid artery. TABLE 83–5 lists some of the signs found in patients with atherostenosis of the ICA.

Subclavian artery: Atherostenosis usually affects the subclavian arteries proximal to the origins of the vertebral artery branches. The left side is stenosed more often than the right. The most frequent symptoms involve the ischemic arm, which often aches, is cool, and becomes fatigued easily on exercise. The radial pulse on the ischemic side is usually weak or delayed and the BP is lower than in the opposite arm. A bruit is at times audible in the supraclavicular fossa. TIAs, which are much more common than stroke, are characterized by temporary dizziness, blurred vision, diplopia, or staggering and at times are provoked by exercising the ischemic arm. These patients usually do well, unless the arm is used vigorously in sports (eg, golf), and treatment is usually not indicated.

Vertebral artery (VA) in the neck: TIAs usually are characterized by evanescent dizziness or vertigo, diplopia, or blurred vision. The clinical findings are identical to those in subclavian disease, except that the arm

TABLE 83–5. PHYSICAL SIGNS IPSILATERAL TO THE VASCULAR LESION IN PATIENTS WITH INTERNAL CAROTID ARTERY ATHEROSTENOSIS

Neck
Bruit best heard with stethoscope bell—long, focal, high-pitched

Face
Increased pulsation in facial, preauricular, and superficial temporal arteries (STA) when CCA is normal and ECA acts as collateral vessel. Decreased pulsations in facial, preauricular, and STA when CCA or ICA and ECA are stenosed
Increased ABC pulses: A—angular near medial corner of eye; B—brow laterally; C—cheek
Coolness in supraorbital region
Reversal of blood flow in frontal artery

Eyes
Iris	Red speckling (rubeosis iridis)
	Fixed, dilated, or irregular pupil
	Horner's syndrome
Retina	White retinal infarcts
	Hollenhorst plaques—bright refringent cholesterol crystals usually at bifurcations of retinal arteries
	Decreased caliber of retinal arteries
	Asymmetric hypertensive retinopathy—less on side of stenosis
	Central venous retinopathy—engorged veins, microaneurysms, small-dot hemorrhages, sometimes papilledema

CCA = common carotid arteries; ECA = external carotid arteries; ICA = internal carotid arteries.

is not ischemic and pulses and BPs in the upper limbs are equal. Sometimes occlusion of the VA in the neck presents as a sudden posterior circulation stroke with ischemia caused by blockage of the intracranial VA, the PCA, or its branches, resulting from embolic material originating in the proximal VA. A similar situation is commonly found in thrombosis of ICA origin. The most frequent site of VA atherostenosis is the origin and first few centimeters of the vessel. The distal portion of the VA in the neck is vulnerable to tearing or dissection during neck trauma, sudden movement, or manipulation.

Intracranial carotid artery and MCA and ACA branches: When stenosis affects the intracranial carotid artery proximal to the ophthalmic artery branch, the syndrome is similar to that of ICA origin, but there is no neck bruit and noninvasive studies of the ICA are normal. Stenosis of the intracranial carotid artery beyond the ophthalmic artery origin is accompanied by spells of hemispheric ischemia, but transient monocular blindness does not occur. Also, the signs and noninvasive evidence of decreased ophthalmic artery flow are absent.

MCA disease usually is most severe in the proximal segment of the MCA or its upper trunk branch. ACA disease is less common than MCA disease, but the former usually affects the proximal portions of the artery. The TIA/stroke ratio is much lower in disease of these intracranial arteries than it is in disease of the ICA and VA in the neck.

MCA disease usually causes weakness and numbness of the contralateral limbs, trunk, and especially the face. When the left MCA is affected, aphasia is usually present; visual-spatial dysfunction and neglect of the left side of space occur with right MCA disease. ACA disease causes weakness and numbness of the contralateral lower extremity. At times, lack of spontaneity, disinterest, and incontinence occur. In the intracranial ICA siphon and MCA and ACA disease, stroke is more common than TIA. The stroke is caused primarily by hemodynamic insufficiency, with poor perfusion of the affected vascular territories and is often gradually progressive.

Intracranial VA: Occlusion or severe stenosis of the intracranial VA blocks flow through the posterior-inferior cerebellar artery **(PICA)** branch, causing ischemia of the lateral medulla and cerebellum. The most common symptoms and signs of lateral medullary ischemia are listed in TABLE 83–6. Cerebellar ischemia is manifested by staggering gait, ataxia, sensations of dysequilibrium, and nausea. Large cerebellar infarcts can cause posterior fossa pressure and coma from compression of the brainstem; this potentially fatal complication is treated by surgical decompression of the lesion and removal of infarcted tissue.

Basilar artery (BA): The most frequent symptoms and signs of BA atherostenosis are listed in TABLE 83–7. BA occlusion is potentially fatal unless collateral circulation is quickly established. The BA supplies the pons; the region most vulnerable to ischemia is the base of the pons, which the long motor tracts pass through. Ischemia causes bilateral weakness of the trunk and limbs with exaggerated reflexes and extensor plantar signs. Sometimes premonitory spells of dizziness and diplopia occur, especially when the occlusive lesion begins in the VA and spreads to the BA.

Posterior cerebral arteries (PCAs): The cardinal symptoms and signs of atherostenosis of PCAs relate to the visual fields. Patients may have transient attacks of hemianopia or scotomata. The hemianopia often develops suddenly. Loss of memory, alexia, and an agitated delirium also occur when the lesion is large and includes the temporal lobe territory of the PCA.

Laboratory Findings and Diagnosis

CT and MRI can be useful in delineating the affected vascular territory when an infarct is present. Negative studies give hope that the ischemia is reversible, whereas a large infarct carries a poor prognosis for good recovery. The distribution of infarction yields clues as to the likely vascular lesion. Carotid occlusion often causes infarction near the border zones between the ACA and the MCA, between the MCA and the

TABLE 83–6. SYMPTOMS AND SIGNS OF LATERAL MEDULLARY ISCHEMIA

Symptoms	Signs
Ipsilateral	
Jabbing pain in eye or face	Decreased pain and temperature sense along trigeminal distribution
Lid droop; decreased facial sweating	Horner's syndrome
Dizziness and feelings of motion	Nystagmus
Hoarseness and dysphagia	Decreased movement of ipsilateral palate, pharynx, and vocal cord
Incoordination of arm and leg	Incoordination, tremor, and rebound of arm and leg
Contralateral	
Difficulty telling temperature over arms and legs	Decreased pain and temperature sense over limbs and trunk
General	
Walking imbalance	Gait ataxia
Difficulty sitting or standing	Falls to side when sitting or standing Tachycardia Labile BP

PCA, or in the deep white matter. A small zone of infarction in the central part of the MCA territory suggests a small pial territory embolic infarct arising from the heart or the ICA. CT and MRI also can show zones of edema and shifts of intracranial contents.

Sometimes occlusions are caused by hematologic abnormalities, either alone or superimposed upon a stenotic lumen. Polycythemia and thrombocytosis are major causes of vascular occlusion. A hypercoagulable state can complicate cancer, systemic illness, and pregnancy. A CBC, prothrombin time test, and platelet count should be performed routinely in every patient with TIA or stroke.

A host of **new noninvasive technics** allow imaging of the VAs and carotid arteries in the neck, as well as measurement of pressure and flow in the neck and intracranial arteries. TABLE 83–8 lists common noninvasive tests that give information about the location and severity of stenosis of the ICA in the neck. In general, there are 2 types of tests: those that give direct information about the ICA origin from ultrasonography and spectral analysis of bruits and those that analyze pressure and flow in the ICA tributaries in and around the orbit and cranium. When performed by an experienced technologist, transcranial Doppler ultrasonog-

TABLE 83–7. SYMPTOMS AND SIGNS IN BASILAR ARTERY
ATHEROSTENOSIS

Symptoms
  Diplopia
  Dysphagia
  Dizziness
  Dysarthria
  Bilateral leg or leg and arm weakness
  Crossed weakness—one side of face, opposite side of body and limbs
  Ataxia
  Bilateral numbness
  Deafness or tinnitus
  Occipital headache

Signs
  Palsies of extraocular movement (III, IV, VI)
  Internuclear ophthalmoplegia
  Nystagmus—horizontal or vertical
  Bilateral bulbar weakness (face, lips, palate, pharynx, tongue)
  Crossed 6th or 7th nerve paralysis and hemiparesis
  Decreased hearing
  Pseudobulbar palsy
  Quadraparesis
  Bilateral extensor plantar reflexes
  Gait ataxia
  Limb ataxia
  Stupor
  Locked-in syndrome
  Bilateral decreased position sense in limbs

raphy also allows measurement of pressure in the intracranial MCAs, VAs, and BA.

Angiography remains the definitive test for imaging the extracranial and intracranial arteries and veins. The use of a computer to generate images allows rapid real-time subtraction of images with contrast from those without, to obtain high-resolution pictures with the use of small amounts of contrast material. This procedure, called digital subtraction angiography, can be performed via either the venous or the arterial route on an outpatient basis in many institutions. Although angiography has definite risks, they can be minimized by using the least amount of dye and the smallest number of injections needed for accurate diagnosis. The experience of the angiographer and the information supplied by the responsible clinician are vital to these decisions.

Two commonly cited rules, when applied literally, have led to problems in the past. These are (1) that angiography is warranted only if surgery is planned or considered, and (2) that visualization of all 4 major arteries and the aortic arch is needed for diagnosis. Angiography is needed when the diagnosis is unclear despite clinical, imaging, and

TABLE 83–8. NONINVASIVE TESTS OF INTERNAL CAROTID ARTERY ATHEROSTENOSIS

Indirect　Yield information about flow and pressure in tributary vessels
Ophthalmodynamometry
Oculoplethysmography
Radionuclide angiography
Thermography
Directional Doppler ultrasonography of orbit
Transcranial Doppler ultrasonography
Direct　Yield direct information about carotid bifurcation
Spectral analysis of bruits
B-mode ultrasonography (echo) of neck in real time
Continuous wave and pulsed Doppler ultrasonography

noninvasive tests. *Treatment based on accurate diagnosis is more rational than empiric guesswork.* Some medical treatments, eg, use of anticoagulants, are potentially risky, especially when unwarranted. One should begin angiography by injecting the artery most likely to harbor the lesion. When sufficient information is obtained to dictate treatment, angiography can be discontinued.

Treatment

Treatment depends on the location and severity of the occlusive lesion. There are 5 principal, specific treatment alternatives: surgical endarterectomy, warfarin, aspirin or other platelet antiaggregates, heparin, or surgical bypass of an occlusive lesion. General treatment considerations have been discussed at the beginning of this chapter. In choosing among these alternatives, the following guidelines are suggested:

1. If the vascular occlusive lesion is seriously stenotic (ie, there is < 2 mm residual lumen), the lesion is surgically accessible, and the patient has not already had a severe stroke in the territory of supply, endarterectomy is the procedure of choice.

2. When the vascular lesion is severely stenotic and the lesion is inaccessible (eg, ICA siphon or MCA), or the patient is not a surgical candidate or refuses surgery, warfarin should be used. The prothrombin time should be kept at approximately 1.5 times the control value. Warfarin is most effective in preventing "red clots" composed of erythrocytes and thrombin that might be expected to form in regions of very reduced flow (eg, very stenotic arteries, veins, or dilated cardiac chambers).

3. If the vascular lesion is not stenotic, aspirin is prescribed. The optimal dose is still undetermined; 1.2 gm/day in divided doses has been effective in trials, but theoretically as little as 100 mg/day might work as well, if not better. Aspirin and other platelet antiaggregates would be

expected to prevent "white clots" composed of fibrin-platelet clumps that form in fast-moving streams on irregular surfaces (eg, craggy plaques in nonstenosed arteries).

4. Heparin is prescribed for short-duration (2- to 3-wk) treatment in patients with complete occlusion of large arteries to prevent propagation and embolization of clot until the loosely adherent thrombus becomes organized on the vascular wall and collateral circulation is well established. Heparin may also be used when the neurologic signs are fluctuating, the occluding lesion is undefined, and more definitive information is not yet available. Heparin should be given in a continuous IV infusion, avoiding bolus injection (especially in the elderly), and keeping the activated partial thromboplastin time **(APTT)** 1.5 to 2 times the control value.

5. The indications for extracranial-intracranial bypass surgery are currently unknown. A controlled randomized international study showed conclusively that the procedure is no better than medical therapy for most patients with an inaccessible occlusive vascular lesion in the anterior circulation. Bypass might be considered for isolated, well-studied patients refractory to medical treatment.

PENETRATING ARTERY DISEASE

The small arteries that penetrate into deeper brain structures (eg, the basal gray nuclei, internal capsule, thalamus, and pons) are especially susceptible to degenerative changes caused by hypertension (see FIG. 83–1). Medical hypertrophy, fibrinoid changes, and lipohyalinosis gradually narrow the lumens of these arteries, impeding blood flow. Patients with fibrinoid degeneration and lipohyalinosis of penetrating arteries are invariably hypertensive or have a history of hypertension.

When a penetrating artery becomes occluded and flow is sufficiently diminished, a small, deep infarct, usually called a lacuna, results. The lesions are < 2 cm at their greatest diameter and affect only deeper structures. At times, microatheromata or microdissections occlude the origins of the penetrating arteries, causing infarcts in identical distributions. Plaques within arteries, blocking or extending into the orifices of penetrating arteries, and microatheromata are more common in diabetics. Small, deep infarcts are relatively more common in the posterior circulation and increase in frequency with age. There seems to be no definite race or sex predilection for lacunar infarcts.

Symptoms and Signs

Because the lesions are small and deep, symptoms related to vasodilation or increased intracranial pressure, eg, headache, vomiting, and decreased alertness, do not occur. The clinical syndrome develops during a short period—usually < 1 wk. TIAs may occur but are less frequent than in patients with large-artery atherostenosis. When present, TIAs are characteristic and brief, usually lasting no longer than a few days. Symptoms of brain dysfunction relate to the ischemic region. The most common patterns are unilateral weakness of the face, arm, and leg and unilateral paresthesias of the face, trunk, and limbs.

On examination, abnormalities are limited to dysfunction of deep structures. When lacunae are located deep in the cerebral hemisphere, hemianopia, visual field loss or neglect, and abnormalities of cognitive func-

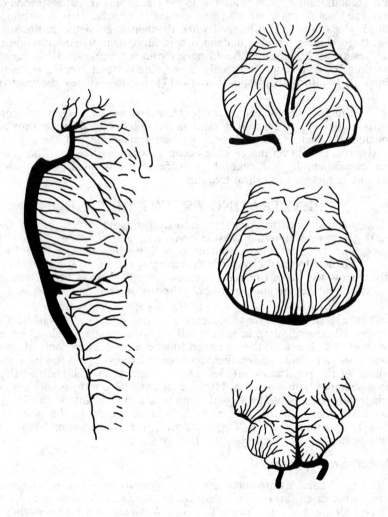

FIG. 83–1. **Penetrating arteries to brainstem.** (From *Human Neuroanatomy* by M. B. Carpenter. © 1976, the Williams & Wilkins Co., Baltimore. Used with permission of Williams & Wilkins Co. and the author.)

tion or behavior should not accompany the weakness or numbness. When the brainstem is involved, the signs are seldom if ever limited to dysfunction of tegmental structures (cranial nerve nuclei and eye movements). The most common lacunar syndromes are listed in TABLE 83–9; pure motor hemiparesis and pure sensory stroke are by far the most common.

Laboratory Findings

In patients with lacunae, CT and MRI show either normal findings or small, deep infarcts. When these imaging technics show superficial infarcts that could account for the symptoms, the diagnosis of lacunar infarction is excluded. EEG usually shows normal findings or minor symmetric abnormalities. Angiography is usually not indicated in patients with typical lacunar infarcts. Hypertension, the cause of lacunae, often leads to coexistent atherostenosis of larger arteries; thus, in patients with typical lacunae, vascular narrowing is often found during noninvasive tests or angiography.

Diagnosis

Diagnosis depends on a combination of epidemiologic features, symptoms and signs, and laboratory findings. In a typical example, the pa-

TABLE 83–9. LACUNAR SYNDROMES

Pure motor hemiparesis: Unilateral weakness of face, arm, and leg, usually with exaggerated reflexes and Babinski's sign; dysarthria may be present but dysphasia and other cognitive and behavioral abnormalities are absent

Pure sensory stroke: Unilateral paresthesias, dysesthesias, or numbness of face, arm, leg, and trunk; no accompanying weakness, ataxia, hemianopia, or cognitive or behavioral abnormalities

Sensory-motor stroke: Unilateral numbness and weakness of face and limbs without cognitive, visual, or behavioral abnormalities

Dysarthria–clumsy hand syndrome: Slurred speech; facial and tongue weakness with ipsilateral clumsiness of the hand; increased reflexes and Babinski's sign may be present

Ataxic hemiparesis: Unilateral combined ataxia and weakness with exaggerated reflexes in arm and/or leg and Babinski's sign

Pure dysarthria: Dysarthria, sometimes with dysphagia without other findings

Hemi-Parkinson or hemidystonia: Unilateral abnormal posture, tone, and movement

Sensory stroke limited to the face: Like pure sensory stroke, but limited to the face

Hemiataxia: Unilateral incoordination, often with abnormal gait

tient has a history of hypertension, rapidly evolving clinical symptoms and signs typical of one of the lacunar syndromes (TABLE 83–9), and CT or MRI evidence of lacuna or no relevant lesion. When this combination of findings is present, no further testing is needed to establish the diagnosis. The diagnosis of lacunar infarction ordinarily should not be made in patients with no history of hypertension or diabetes; more often than not, in such cases, it would be incorrect. When the clinical evaluation and/or imaging features are atypical, further testing, including angiography, may be necessary.

Treatment

Treatment consists of control of hypertension after the acute period of vulnerability to ischemia has passed. For the first 1 to, at most, 3 wk, changes in position, BP, blood volume, and blood flow can increase the ischemic deficit. Deep penetrating arteries are end vessels, and any decrease in flow though adjacent arteries can enlarge the infarct. Only when BP is in the so-called malignant range (> 200/120 mm Hg) should it be immediately lowered. Diabetes should also be controlled. A high Hct causes increased blood viscosity and contributes to susceptibility to lacunar infarction as well as to large artery occlusion. Phlebotomy and cessation of smoking are important in patients with a Hct > 45%.

CEREBRAL EMBOLIZATION

Cerebral emboli are being recognized with increasing frequency. Emboli can arise from the aortic arch or from plaques or dissections in the proximal portions of the large extracranial and intracranial arteries, in which case the epidemiology and clinical findings will be the same as those discussed under ATHEROSTENOSIS OF THE LARGE EXTRACRANIAL AND INTRACRANIAL ARTERIES, above.

The heart is also frequently a source of emboli, especially in the elderly. The advent of newer cardiac diagnostic tests and brain imaging has led to identification of more cases of cerebral embolization than in the past. The most common potential cardiac sources of cerebral embolization are listed in TABLE 83–10. Most important are all varieties of valvular disease, myocardial ischemia, and atrial fibrillation. The incidence of atrial fibrillation increases with age. Some have estimated that as many as 5% of individuals > 70 yr of age have atrial fibrillation.

Symptoms and Signs

Neurologic symptoms usually begin abruptly, often while the patient is awake and active. Most often the deficit is maximal at or near onset, because the sudden blockage of a distal artery does not allow time for adequate collateralization. Emboli do pass distally, and when this occurs, the deficit may worsen or improve. Stepwise worsening is usually limited to 48 h. When angiography is performed later than 2 days after the onset of symptoms, emboli are usually no longer visible in the intracranial arteries. In the anterior circulation, emboli most often reach MCA and ACA branches, while in the posterior circulation, long cir-

TABLE 83–10. COMMON CARDIAC SOURCES OF CEREBRAL EMBOLIZATION

Valvular disease
Rheumatic valvulitis
Prosthetic heart valves
Calcific aortic stenosis
Mitral annulus calcification
Nonbacterial thrombotic (marasmic) endocarditis
Bacterial and fungal endocarditis

Myocardial ischemia
Acute infarction
Ventricular aneurysms
Akinetic zones
Mural thrombi

Arrhythmias
Atrial fibrillation
Sick sinus syndrome

Lesions within cardiac chambers
Myocarditis
Cardiomyopathy
Sarcoidosis
Amyloidosis

cumferential cerebellar arteries and branches of the PCAs are most often terminal sites. When the embolus causes a large infarct, headache and decreased alertness commonly occur. Neurologic signs are identical to those discussed under ATHEROSTENOSIS OF THE LARGE EXTRACRANIAL AND INTRACRANIAL ARTERIES, above.

Laboratory Findings and Diagnosis

Brain imaging technics, **CT** and **MRI,** usually reveal superficial, slice-of-pie–shaped infarcts in the cerebral hemisphere or cerebellum in the territories of the ACA, MCA, PCA, and cerebellar arteries. There may be multiple, scattered infarcts, some unexpected, in different vascular territories. **Noninvasive tests** (see TABLE 83–8) can reveal embolic sources within the proximal extracranial arteries. **Angiography** can show abrupt distal cutoff of intracranial branch arteries without underlying local atherostenosis, filling defects in the form of thromboemboli, and proximal regions of atherostenosis.

ECG can document myocardial ischemia, chamber hypertrophy, and arrhythmias. **Echocardiography** is especially useful, demonstrating valvular disease, regions of locally decreased contractility, tumors such as myxomas, and chamber enlargement. Paradoxic embolism can be studied by the introduction of saline IV and use of Doppler ultrasound to detect the passage of bubbles through septal defects during echocardiography. **Holter monitoring** can detect intermittent arrhythmias. **Radionuclide cardiac scans** can corroborate regions of ischemic damage and abnormal function.

Treatment

Treatment depends on the nature of the embolic source. Treatment of proximal atherostenotic embolic sources has already been discussed in the section on atherostenosis, above. Specific medical treatment may be available for the cardiac abnormality (eg, antiarrhythmic agents or coronary vasodilators for ischemia). Some cardiac lesions require surgical correction.

Anticoagulants are usually indicated during the period of vulnerability to further emboli. In some patients (eg, those with recent MI or reversible arrhythmia), this risk is acute, while in others (eg, those with intractable atrial fibrillation), it is lifelong. One may start therapy with heparin in a constant infusion, controlled to keep the activated partial thromboplastin time **(APTT)** at 1.5 to 2 times the control value, and gradually change to warfarin for long-term use, keeping the prothrombin time at about 1.5 times control. Intracranial bleeding has been described above, especially in elderly patients with large infarcts, hypertension, and excessive anticoagulation.

Anticoagulants should not be used if the infarct is large; hypertension is a contraindication to anticoagulation, unless BP can be reduced but not to an extent that will increase the neurologic deficit. Conservative doses of anticoagulants should be given, with monitoring of the APTT and prothrombin time and observation for early signs of systemic bleeding.

Anticoagulation therapy should be continued while the patient is still at risk for further emboli. In patients with artificial valves who develop new emboli while taking warfarin, the addition of dipyridamole in dosages of 400 mg/day may be helpful. The risk/benefit ratio of prophylactic anticoagulation in patients with potential cardiac embolic sources, such as atrial fibrillation, is currently under study.

SYSTEMIC HYPOPERFUSION

Cerebral ischemia can be caused by circulatory failure or inability of the heart to pump adequate amounts of blood and nutrients to the brain. Acute MI, cardiac arrest, and life-threatening ventricular arrhythmias are the most common causes. Less often, pulmonary embolization, acute GI or systemic bleeding, or shock is responsible. Most often, the patient is pale, sweating, and hypotensive when first examined. When poor cerebral perfusion has been severe or prolonged, the patient is usually comatose.

Symptoms, Signs, and Diagnosis

The onset of neurologic dysfunction is usually abrupt and follows systemic symptoms related to the underlying disorder. The most prominent findings are decreased alertness and symmetric depression of hemispheric functions. When ischemia is severe, the brainstem may not function normally and brainstem reflexes may be absent (pupillary, corneal, doll's eyes, pharyngeal). When the motor system is involved, there is bilateral weakness or decorticate or decerebrate rigidity. In some patients, the arms are most severely affected, with relative sparing of the face and legs, a distribution described as "a man in a barrel." Loss of brainstem reflexes for > 24 h carries a poor prognosis, as does persistent coma. When stupor lightens, patients may show deficits in visual function and memory. CT is usually normal during the acute period in all but the most severely affected, but EEG usually shows severe bilateral slowing.

Treatment is directed at the underlying cardiac or systemic process.

CHRONIC CEREBROVASCULAR LESIONS
("Multi-Infarct Dementia")

Although many lay people refer to senile intellectual loss as being caused by "hardening of the arteries," there is absolutely no evidence that cerebrovascular disease plays any etiologic role in Alzheimer's disease, the most common cause of dementia in the elderly. Control zones for basic functions needed for daily life (eg, moving, feeling, seeing, eating, speaking, and excreting waste) are strategically placed in the middle of the main arterial supply areas.

Other functions (eg, the ability to calculate, plan, discipline, and read) are more dependent on "associative cortical areas," which are generally located between zones of arterial supply. These higher functions are readily affected by intoxicants, metabolic disorders, and degenerations, while cerebrovascular disease tends to interrupt basic functions more than higher cognitive functions. Vascular disease "bites the soma and licks the mind," whereas degenerative and toxic-metabolic diseases waste the intellect while sparing somatic functions until late in their course. However, patients with cerebrovascular disease do become demented when brain damage is severe. Comparing the brain to a pie, when enough nibbles or slices are removed, the pie is decimated.

Most patients with chronic vascular dementia have (1) high stroke risk factors (eg, hypertension, diabetes, coronary and peripheral vascular occlusive disease, cardiac disease, and hyperlipidemia); (2) a history of TIAs or sudden-onset neurologic deficits (strokes); and (3) abnormal, often asymmetric neurologic signs (eg, weakness, sensory loss, exaggerated reflexes, Babinski's signs, visual field defects, pseudobulbar palsy, and incontinence).

There are 3 major subcategories of vascular dementia: large-artery thromboembolism, état lacunaire (the lacunar state), and subcortical arteriosclerotic encephalopathy **(SAE, Binswanger's disease). In large-**

artery thromboembolism, cerebral damage is due to multiple large-vessel occlusions or cardiogenic emboli. CT should show multiple areas of damage to superficial cerebral arterial territories. **État lacunaire** is due to decimation of the deep cerebral and brainstem structures by multiple lacunae, which give the brain a Swiss-cheese–like appearance at necropsy or on CT. There is a reduction in the volume of the white matter, with resulting ventricular enlargement. Patients have a plethora of pyramidal and extrapyramidal signs and pseudobulbar palsy. They look stiff, exhibit parkinsonian signs, and walk slowly.

SAE describes damage to broad areas of the cerebral and cerebellar white matter and basal gray matter, resulting from hypertension and partial occlusions of many deep-penetrating arteries. CT and MRI show periventricular and white matter abnormalities, which include hypodensities and periventricular lucencies without zones of cortical infarction.

Treatment of vascular dementia depends entirely on control of risk factors and specific therapy aimed at the cause of the individual stroke. L-dopa and its analogs may help control some of the parkinsonian symptoms.

STROKE COMPLICATIONS

At times, the complications of stroke are more devastating than the stroke itself. A patient's relatives often say that their parent or grandparent was doing well until "complications set in." Stroke seems to activate the body's clotting system, leading to the development of venous thromboembolism and MI during the acute period or during convalescence from the stroke. At times, it is difficult to know whether the myocardial or cerebral ischemia came first.

Elderly patients respond to aggressive diagnostic tests, invasive medical and surgical therapies, and prolonged bed rest by losing a great deal of their former spirit and vigor. Pneumonia, limb contractures, pressure sores, and depression are particularly common and must be prevented or at least treated when they appear. Antidepressants may help.

The following strategies may be helpful in preventing and treating stroke complications: (1) Prescribe tight stockings or inflated hose and frequent active and passive leg motion. (2) Turn patients in bed frequently, with special attention to pressure sites. (3) Maintain adequate fluid intake and nutrition. (4) Administer small doses of heparin (5000 u.) s.c. q 8 to 12 h (so-called miniheparin) to prevent thromboembolism, when not contraindicated. (5) Encourage early ambulation (as soon as the patient's signs become stable), always with close monitoring by nurses and doctors. (6) Pay attention to pulmonary hygiene. Cessation of smoking, encouragement of deep breathing, and use of respiratory therapists are important. (7) Watch closely for infectious complications, especially pneumonia, urinary tract infections, and skin infections; treat early. (8) Avoid overdistention of the urinary bladder preferably without use of an indwelling catheter.

(9) Begin rehabilitation strategies early during the acute hospitalization. This includes active and passive exercises, full range-of-motion movement, and teaching patients about the nature of their functional disabilities. (10) Emphasize risk factor control early: cessation of smoking, weight loss, control of dietary factors, etc. (11) Maintain positive outlook; all members of the health care team should emphasize regaining a good, active life. Do not emphasize returning to previous, normal functions, since that may not be possible, but many patients can lead an active life despite residual handicaps. Many well-meaning patients concentrate so much on returning their arm or hand function to normal that they lose sight of the fact they can regain nearly all other premorbid activities despite the loss of hand dexterity.

(12) Prepare the family early and continuously for the patient's return home. Family members should be educated regarding the patient's needs and changes in the home that may be necessary. When returning the patient home is not feasible, early search for a suitable alternative is important. (13) Continue the preventive measures and treatments begun at the acute-care hospital when the patient is transferred to a rehabilitation facility. Stroke clubs and contact with other individuals who have overcome similar stroke handicaps are often valuable to the patient.

---

84. MOVEMENT DISORDERS

Melvin D. Yahr and *Stuart W. H. Pang*

Diseases of the basal ganglia, or **extrapyramidal diseases,** are a frequent cause of motor disability in the elderly. They comprise a complex group of clinical disorders characterized primarily by abnormal involuntary movements (dyskinesias), alterations in muscle tone, and disturbances in bodily posture. The major clinical states are parkinsonism, chorea, athetosis, dystonia, and hemiballismus.

These terms not only denote particular disease entities but in a descriptive sense refer to constellations of symptoms that may occur in a variety of disorders, some intrinsic to the CNS, others of a generalized nature that involve the basal ganglia or their connections. The disorders are distinguishable by the degree, form, and combination of the triad of symptoms noted above and are recognizable as disease entities by the age at and mode of onset, the identification of particular etiologic and genetic factors, and the rate and manner at which symptoms progress.

Although much is known about the clinical aspects of extrapyramidal disorders, information concerning their fundamental anatomic, physiologic, and pathogenetic bases is deficient. However, a growing body of information regarding biochemical alterations in the basal ganglia has provided considerable understanding of the mechanisms by which symptoms occur and has suggested a rational approach to their treatment.

The most prominent biochemical feature of the basal ganglia is a high content of putative neurotransmitter agents, notably acetylcholine **(ACh)**, dopamine **(DA)**, and γ-aminobutyric acid **(GABA)**. The substrates and enzyme systems for their production and degradation are found within the cellular components of the basal ganglia. In some instances, these neurotransmitter agents are produced within the segment in which their action is based; in others, cellular elements in 1 area are responsible for their production but they are transported via connecting axons to another area where their action occurs. Experimental evidence is available indicating that DA, for example, is produced in the pars compacta of the substantia nigra and is transported via a neuronal tract, the nigral-striatal pathway, to the caudate nucleus and putamen.

Normal function in the basal ganglia appears to depend on an exquisite balance between these various neurotransmitter agents (ie, they may be viewed neurophysiologically as being either **inhibitory** [DA and GABA] or **excitatory** [ACh]). Disturbances in their homeostasis result in symptoms that are generally attributed to this area of the brain. In general, DA deficiency allows for cholinergic hyperactivity and can be correlated with the akinetic rigid disorders, such as parkinsonism. DA hyperactivity, cholinergic hypoactivity, or both result in the hyperkinetic phenomena encountered in Huntington's chorea. To a considerable extent, current approaches to the treatment of basal ganglia disorders rely on the use of agents capable of reestablishing neurotransmitter balance.

PARKINSONIAN SYNDROME

The major clinical manifestations of this syndrome are tremor, muscular rigidity, akinesia, and loss of postural reflexes. It is 1 of the most frequently encountered disorders of the basal ganglia and is a prominent cause of disability in those > 50 yr of age. Its prevalence has been placed at close to 1 million patients in the USA, with the addition of 50,000 new cases each year. The incidence increases with age, peaking at about 75 yr. While it is < 1% below 50 yr of age, it may exceed 2% thereafter. The estimated overall lifetime risk is 2.5% among Caucasians. *As a symptom complex,* its occurrence has been noted in a number of disease processes, either as the sole manifestation or in association with other symptoms. However, in most cases, no definable cause has been found; since the latter cases seem to have many features in common, particularly in regard to evolution, they have been designated as primary parkinsonism.

The cases in which definable processes are found are best classified as **secondary or symptomatic parkinsonism.** This separation into clinical groups cannot be construed as indicative of a difference in pathophysiology or even pathogenetic mechanisms for the production of symptoms, since all cases of parkinsonism may have a common origin. From the standpoint of what is currently known about its biochemical basis, a deficiency of striatal DA is common to all types of parkinsonism. In some cases of parkinsonism, regardless of cause, cell loss is consistently found in the substantia nigra in association with other changes diffusely distributed in the corpus striatum and cortex.

No specific laboratory tests exist to aid in establishing the diagnosis of parkinsonism. Routine examination of blood, spinal fluid, and urine yields normal results. The disturbance in cerebral DA metabolism may result in a decrease in CSF homovanillic acid **(HVA)**; however, it has limited reliability in confirming the diagnosis. The EEG is usually normal, although diffuse slowing may be present and sleep recordings may be abnormal. CT scans and MRI scans of the head show no abnormalities in primary parkinsonism but are helpful in some of the secondary forms and in eliminating disorders with symptoms that mimic these conditions. Such scans should be performed routinely as a screening procedure and as a baseline for future reference.

PRIMARY PARKINSONISM
(Parkinson's Disease, Paralysis Agitans)

Most cases of parkinsonism fall into this category. The disease most frequently appears between the ages of 50 and 79 yr, but the incidence declines above the 8th decade of life. A rarely encountered juvenile form has been described in persons < 30 yr of age. The disease affects both sexes and all races. There is no evidence to indicate a hereditary factor, although a familial incidence is claimed by some authorities.

Symptoms and Signs

The disease begins insidiously; any of its cardinal manifestations may appear alone or in combination. **Tremor,** usually in 1 or sometimes in both hands, involving the fingers in a pillrolling motion, is the most common initial symptom. **The tremor is present at rest,** accentuated by sustension, but decreased during active movements and eliminated by sleep. It is rhythmic, alternately affecting flexor and extensor muscles, and may involve upper and lower limbs, mouth, or head. This is often followed by stiffness of the limbs, generalized slowing of movements, and inability to carry out normal and routine daily functions with ease.

Muscular rigidity is readily evident on passive movement of a joint and manifested by a series of interrupted jerks **(cogwheel phenomenon)** rather than a smooth-flowing, easy motion. **Bradykinesia** is the tendency to slowness in the initiation of movement and sudden unexpected arrest of volitional movement while carrying out purposeful acts. The parkinsonian patient appears disinclined to move, and in the middle of performing a routine function suddenly becomes "frozen" and unable to follow through the sequence of motion necessary to complete the action. This is especially evident in writing or feeding and can be striking when, in attempting to walk, the patient finds that his feet are suddenly "frozen to the ground." Rapid alternating movements of the extremities are slowed. As the disease progresses, the face becomes "masklike," with failure to express emotional feeling and with diminished eye blinking but ready induction of blepharospasm when the frontalis muscle is tapped **(Meyerson's sign).**

The body becomes stooped, the gait becomes shuffling, there is a loss of arm swing, and the patient is unable to readily gain and maintain an erect posture. **Postural abnormalities** are evident in the erect and sitting positions. The patient has a tendency to let the head fall forward on the trunk, and the body tends to fall forward or backward unless supported when the patient is seated on a stool. When pushed from in front **(propulsion)** or from behind **(retropulsion)** in the erect position, the patient falls, and no attempt is made to stop the fall either by a step or by movements of the arms. **Deformities of the trunk, hands, and feet** tend to occur. Kyphotic deformity of the spine, causing a stooped posture, is a hallmark. Ulnar deviation of the hands, flexion contractures of the fingers, or an equinovarus posture of the feet can be found.

Speech becomes slow and monotonous. The patient tends to drool. The skin takes on an oily quality, and there is a tendency to seborrheic dermatitis. Mood abnormalities, usually in the form of depression and anxiety, are frequent. In some instances, they may be the heralding symptoms of the disorder, while in others they are a reaction to the slowing of motor activity. Although intellectual impairment does occur, controversy exists as to whether it is intrinsically part of the disease or related to associated dysfunction in this age group.

Although paralysis agitans is invariably progressive, the rate at which symptoms develop and disability ensues is extremely variable. In some instances, the disease is rapidly progressive and patients become disabled within 5 yr of onset. More often, a slower, more protracted course of evolution of symptoms occurs and patients remain functional for extended periods of time. **Treatment** follows discussion of secondary parkinsonism, below.

SECONDARY OR SYMPTOMATIC PARKINSONISM

The parkinsonian syndrome occurs in numerous situations as the predominant clinical manifestation. Those most commonly encountered are listed in TABLE 84–1.

The parkinsonian syndrome is occasionally seen during the acute phase of several types of **viral encephalitis,** although permanent extrapyramidal residua are rare. The exception is the parkinsonian syndrome that developed following the epidemic of encephalitis lethargica from 1915 to 1926; sporadic cases still occur occasionally.

Cerebral atherosclerosis with multi-infarcts of the cerebrum produces a parkinsonism-like state. Lack of initiation of movement and gait disturbances occur with cerebral arteriosclerosis and are more properly classified as **"pseudoparkinsonism."** They rarely respond to therapeutic measures effective for Parkinson's disease. Parkinsonism has been reported following **poisoning with carbon monoxide. Chronic manganese intoxication,** seen in several industrial situations, produces a parkinsonian syndrome accompanied by dystonia and mental changes.

Parkinsonism may appear as a **side effect of drugs that deplete or block the action of cerebral monoamines.** Most commonly, it appears as

TABLE 84-1. CAUSES OF SECONDARY PARKINSONISM

Infections
  Postviral encephalitis
Arteriosclerosis of cerebral vessels
Drugs
  Neuroleptics
  Reserpine
  Metoclopramide
  Methyldopa
Toxins
  Carbon monoxide
  Manganese
  Meperidine analog (MPTP)
Metabolic disorders
  Parathyroid dysfunction
  Anoxia
Tumors
Head trauma
Degenerative disorders
  Parkinson's dementia complex (Guam)
  Striatonigral degeneration
  Progressive supranuclear palsy
  Olivopontocerebellar atrophies
  Parkinsonism with autonomic dystrophy (Shy-Drager syndrome, multisystem atrophy)

a side effect of various neuroleptic drugs, such as the phenothiazines and butyrophenones. Occasionally, antihypertensive agents (eg, reserpine and methyldopa) are the cause. The use of metoclopramide for gastric dysfunction may induce parkinsonism. In some instances, these reactions are dose dependent; in others, they are related to individual susceptibility. Once the drugs are withdrawn, the symptoms usually disappear within a few days, although occasionally they persist for months. In some persons, permanent remnants of parkinsonian symptoms have been found years after the elimination of the drugs. Recently a meperidine analog, MPTP (1-methyl-4-phenyl-1,2,5,6-tetrahydropyridine), used IV by drug abusers, has induced an irreversible parkinsonian state.

Hypoparathyroidism is associated with calcification of the basal ganglia, which may produce parkinsonism as well as chorea and athetosis. CT scan may demonstrate small calcific deposits in the basal ganglia. **Brain tumors** in the region of the basal ganglia may present with hemiparkinsonism. Frontal lobe tumors also occasionally produce gait and movement abnormalities that may mimic parkinsonism. Other disorders that may be confused with parkinsonism include **myxedema, normal pressure hydrocephalus, hepatic encephalopathy,** and **depression.**

A parkinsonian syndrome may be present to varying degrees in several so-called **degenerative diseases of unknown cause** that involve multiple areas of the CNS (eg, progressive supranuclear palsy [PSP], olivopontocerebellar atrophy, and the Shy-Drager syndrome).

In PSP (Steele-Richardson-Olszewski syndrome), the major abnormalities are parkinsonian symptoms, subcortical dementia, pseudobulbar signs, and vertical-gaze palsies. About 4% of parkinsonian patients actually have the clinical manifestation of PSP. Onset is usually during or after the 6th decade, but PSP can present during the 40s. Men are more commonly affected, and there is no ethnic or racial predilection. The course of the disease is usually rapid, with marked incapacity occurring within 2 to 3 yr and death within 10 yr, generally due to intercurrent infection.

Pathologic examination shows degenerative changes in the brainstem, diencephalon, and cerebellar nuclear masses. Other findings include nerve cell loss, neurofibrillary tangles, granulovacuolar degeneration, gliosis, and occasionally, perivascular cuffing. The pathogenesis of this disease is unknown. Evidence for a transmissible etiology is lacking, and there are no reports of familial cases of PSP.

The clinical manifestations of PSP include progressive impairment of voluntary gaze of supranuclear origin, with vertical-gaze palsy (downward more than upward) being most prominent. Other ophthalmologic symptoms include blurring of vision, diplopia, photophobia, burning eyes, tearing, and retraction of the upper lids leading to a staring, astonished-like appearance. Other findings are unsteadiness of gait with falling, dysarthria, dysphagia, rigidity, bradykinesia, and tonic contraction of facial muscles with hypomimia and hyperactive neck extension. Tremor is not prominent. Depression or dementia of the subcortical type is common later in the course of PSP; disturbances of sleep (insomnia or hyposomnia), agitation, irritability, apathy or slowed thinking, and pseudobulbar affect are also seen.

CT scan and MRI may show mild to moderate atrophy of the midbrain, cerebellum, and occasionally, the cerebral hemispheres. Routine laboratory studies are normal, except for an occasional increase in CSF protein. The EEG often shows nonspecific abnormalities early in the course of the disease, but after progression, bifrontal nonrhythmic bursts of delta activity may be seen. No fully effective treatment is available. Although dopaminergic agents can control the parkinsonian symptoms, they have no effect on the ocular motor difficulty and tend to accentuate the behavioral abnormalities.

Shy-Drager syndrome is *a multisystem degenerative disease with involvement of the central (preganglionic) autonomic, cerebellar, basal ganglia, pyramidal, and spinal motor neurons.* The mean age of onset is 55 yr (range, 37 to 75 yr). A male predominance is noted, with a 2 or 3:1 ratio. There is no genetic predisposition, and familial incidence has been reported in only 1 case. About 11% of patients with orthostatic hypotension have this syndrome. The disease is progressive, and patients die 7 to 10 yr after the onset of neurologic symptoms. Cardiac arrhythmia, aspiration, sleep apnea, and pulmonary emboli are common causes of death.

The major manifestation is autonomic insufficiency with wide swings in BP but no changes in pulse rate. Patients complain of dizziness, syncope, or light-headedness on standing; postexertional weakness; unsteadiness of gait; or dimming of vision. Impaired temperature control, reduced sweating, sphincter disturbance with incontinence of urine or stool, diarrhea, constipation, nocturnal diuresis, sexual impotence, iris atrophy, impaired eye movements, Horner's syndrome, anisocoria, nystagmus, and abnormal convergence also may be found.

Central neuron degeneration is manifested by parkinsonian features, intention tremor, ataxia, dysarthria, and in some cases, corticobulbar and corticospinal tract signs. Evidence of anterior horn cell degeneration with wasting and fasciculation of distal muscles can be seen. Intellectual and emotional function is preserved until late in the course of the disease. Laboratory studies are usually normal, with some nonspecific EEG abnormalities reported. The EMG may show involvement of anterior horn cells.

Nonpharmacologic treatment of the autonomic dysfunction includes avoidance of extreme heat, alcohol, large meals, getting up rapidly, and excessive straining. In addition, compressive clothing and stockings, increased salt and fluid intake, and sleeping in a reverse Trendelenberg position may ameliorate some of the orthostatic symptoms. Fludrocortisone, starting at dosages of 0.1 mg daily, can be used to expand the plasma volume. Additional drugs for the orthostatic hypotension include indomethacin, midodrine, propranolol, and pindolol.

In olivopontocerebellar atrophy (OPCA), cerebellar incoordination is an additional finding. The incidence is 5/100,000, with an estimate that it represents 5 to 6% of all parkinsonism. It is a heterogeneous group of disorders, with sporadic dominant and recessive inherited forms. A deficiency in the enzyme glutamate dehydrogenase has been associated with the recessive form.

The disease usually begins in adult life with progressive cerebellar signs (ataxia, nystagmus, scanning speech, oscillatory tremor of the trunk and head, and impairment of equilibrium). Bulbar dysfunction, with dysarthria, dysphagia, and facial and oculomotor palsies, may occur with parkinsonian features. Some patients have a peripheral neuropathy, with loss of knee and ankle jerks. A mild dementia, retinal degeneration, and impairment of sphincter function may also be present.

The disease is predominantly localized in the pons, medulla, and cerebellum, with marked atrophy grossly, which can be seen on CT scan or MRI. Severe loss of cells in the pontine nuclei and olives, as well as demyelination in the middle cerebellar peduncle and cerebellar hemisphere, is seen histologically. Involvement of the striatum is seen in cases with extrapyramidal features, and the disease is more widespread. The disease is progressive and disabling; no specific therapy is available.

Treatment

Currently, no curative therapy is available for most cases of parkinsonism. Only in the exceptional case of secondary parkinsonism, resulting from drugs or occurring with a specific disease, can treatment of the causative factor result in eradication of symptoms. All other cases require lifelong treatment with pharmacologic agents whose actions are palliative and directed toward symptom control. In this regard, hard and fast rules applied indiscriminately to all patients give less than optimal results. *Treatment programs should be personalized,* using as a guide the type and severity of symptoms, the degree of functional impairment, the existence of associated disease processes, and the expected benefits and risks of available therapeutic agents. This applies especially to the elderly, who may have reduced tolerance for dopaminergic and anticholinergic agents, the mainstays of parkinsonism therapy.

Patients with symptoms of recent onset, primarily tremorgenic, and with mild functional impairment, are best treated with agents whose pharmacologic action is central inhibition of cholinergic activity. **Diphenhydramine,** an antihistamine with such action, in a dosage of 25 mg tid is well tolerated and may suffice. If that is ineffective, **amantadine** 100 mg bid may be useful. More effective is **trihexyphenidyl** 2 mg 3 to 5 times/day. However, elderly persons are prone to the side effects of the latter agent, including confusion, urinary retention, and visual impairment; it must be administered with caution and usually below the optimal dosage.

Patients with fully established parkinsonian symptoms that impair motor function should be treated with agents capable of replenishing or activating striatal dopaminergic effects. The best way to accomplish this is to use **levodopa combined with carbidopa.** The combination tablets contain a fixed ratio of carbidopa 10 or 25 mg to levodopa 100 or 250 mg. Treatment should begin with a low dosage, ½ tablet of the 25:100 combination 2 or 3 times/day, and gradually increase to a total daily dosage of 100:400 or 125:500 mg. In most patients, this will alleviate, although not completely eradicate, symptoms. However, for older patients, these levels should be maintained, rather than risk subjecting them to distressing side effects at higher dosage (eg, confusional states, involuntary movements, GI distress, and hypotension). Striatal dopaminergic activity can also be stimulated by DA receptor agonists. **Bromocriptine** is the only agent of this type currently available. A cautious induction period, beginning with 1.25 mg/day and gradually increasing to 2.5 mg tid or qid, can be effective. The selective monoamine oxidase-β inhibitor **(MAO β1)** L-Deprenyl is available in many countries but not currently in the USA. It prevents the oxidative metabolism of dopamine, hence making it more readily and continuously available. Administered 5 mg bid concomitantly with levodopa/carbidopa, it can produce a more salutary therapeutic response than the latter combination alone.

In addition to the pharmacologic treatment, supportive care of the patient with physical, occupational, and speech therapy is important to slow the progressive disability and social withdrawal often seen in these patients.

TREMOR

ESSENTIAL TREMOR
(Familial Tremor; Senile Tremor)

A monosymptomatic, usually benign, condition that involves the hands, head, or face, or all 3. **Essential tremor** *refers to sporadically occurring cases,* while **familial tremor** *refers to cases with an associated positive family history.* Essential tremor may occur in several successive generations and members of the same family, but the genetic pattern of inheritance has not been determined. Its transmission as an autosomal dominant trait has been suggested. It is commonly seen in patients with torsion dystonia and in males with sex chromosome abnormalities. No specific pathologic lesion has been reported in the nervous system of people with this condition. Rarely, it is a prodrome of primary parkinsonism and may be an abortive form.

The age at onset is variable, but in most cases, is before 25 yr; it tends to persist throughout life. The overall incidence of essential tremor is about 5.5/1000.

Essential tremor usually begins asymmetrically, more often in the dominant hand, and tends to remain asymmetric, with tremor frequency, amplitude, and movement not in phase. The tremor is initially distal, becoming more proximal later in its course. The tremor is not present at rest, occurs with suspension of the limbs (postural), and is more rapid than that encountered in parkinsonism. It is accentuated by emotional factors and fatigue, may be worsened by volitional movements, and is usually suppressed by alcohol. Some progression in intensity and spread to other bodily parts usually occur over the years and may result in significant physical and social disability. Involvement of the head, with either vertical or horizontal movement accompanying hand tremor or as an isolated phenomenon, can be seen. In addition, speech distortion with a quivering voice may be a prominent symptom.

No specific effective therapy is available for controlling essential tremor, although β-adrenergic blocking agents (eg, propranolol in dosages up to 250 mg/day divided equally into 3 or 4 doses) are occasionally effective. The anticonvulsant primidone in a dosage of 50 to 100 mg qid has been helpful to some. Sedatives (eg, phenobarbital 15 mg tid or diazepam 10 mg tid) may reduce the intensity of the tremor. Anxiety and hyperthyroid tremors are similar in appearance and may be mistaken for essential tremor. *Essential tremor must be differentiated from parkinsonism.* The distinguishing characteristics are earlier age at onset; lack of severe progression, akinesia, rigidity, or postural abnormalities; and a strong family history of tremor.

Senile tremor *refers to cases in which the tremor begins in old age*, with the highest prevalence in the 7th decade and seen in men and women equally. This disorder is more prevalent in whites than in blacks.

Senile tremor most often involves the upper limbs and head. At first, it occurs only with voluntary movements, but later, it becomes more constant and even occurs while the limbs are at rest. There is no associated weakness or alteration in muscle tone. The cause is unknown; however, since senile tremor has both cerebellar and extrapyramidal features (in that it occurs both at rest and with movement), the assumption is that some critical pathway linking these systems has undergone degeneration.

No effective treatment is available, although mild benefit may be derived from sedatives or from diphenhydramine 25 mg tid. Most patients accept this condition as another of the many changes that come with advancing years.

CEREBELLAR TREMOR

Elderly patients with cerebellar disease may have both a postural and a characteristic kinetic tremor, which is readily demonstrated on finger-nose or heel-shin testing. The tremor results from lesions of the lateral cerebellar nucleus dentatus or its projections. The tremor frequency is 3 to 5 Hz. It is generated proximally and may wax and wane in amplitude and have a coarse side-to-side component. It tends to increase with prolonged posture of the limbs but is not evident during sleep or with complete relaxation. The tremor differs from cerebellar ataxia in that the latter is irregular, uncoordinated, and nonpatterned and consists of decomposition of movements.

Titubation refers to *a rocking forward and back movement with a rotating or side-to-side component* that can be seen with midline cerebellar disease (of the vermis cerebelli). There is no effective treatment for cerebellar tremor.

NEUROPATHIC TREMOR

Although rare, tremor may be seen as a manifestation of peripheral neuropathy due to porphyria, diabetes, alcohol, uremia, amyloidosis, vincristine, or relapsing polyneuropathy. The mechanism of this tremor is unclear, with some suggestion that it results from an imbalance in the sensory input to the motor neuron pool. However, it may be an enhancement of physiologic tremor by weakened muscle or impaired stretch reflexes. This tremor is not responsive to propranolol therapy.

OTHER TREMORS

Tremor may be seen in **alcohol withdrawal,** in which it is rapid and coarse and involves the entire body. It is characteristically abolished or diminished by a drink of alcohol. A permanent tremor of different quality (more generalized and akin to tremulousness) may be seen in **chronic**

alcoholism. The pathophysiology is unknown. **Narcotic withdrawal** in the elderly, although uncommon, may be manifested by a fine tremor of the facial muscles and fingers.

Drugs may also induce tremor, especially in the geriatric population, in whom drug tolerance is reduced and polypharmacy common. These drugs include theophylline, tricyclic antidepressants, terbutaline, metaproterenol, valproic acid, lithium, and some neuroleptics. In addition, caffeine may induce tremor. **Heavy-metal poisoning** with mercury, arsenic, or bismuth, or poisoning with methyl bromide can cause tremor.

Metabolic encephalopathy due to liver failure, uremia, or respiratory acidosis may cause **asterixis,** which is characterized by irregular flapping movements of the outstretched hands. Electromyographic data indicate that the loss of sustained muscle contraction is a result of intermittent loss of tone in the outstretched muscle.

The tremor of hyperthyroidism is fine, regular, and rapid; it is usually confined to the outstretched hands and fingers. **Hysteric tremor** in the elderly is unusual but can be distinguished by its irregularity, variability from time to time, and tendency to diminish when the patient is distracted.

These tremors can be treated by attending to the underlying etiology.

THE CHOREAS

Disease entities that, although wholly unrelated etiologically, are manifested primarily by choreiform movements. In some, close relationships to infectious processes have been found, whereas in others, familial tendencies suggest a strong genetic component. In the light of newer concepts of inheritance, a common pathogenesis may exist for all.

Considerable controversy exists as to the exact anatomic site from which these movements derive. Pathologic changes have been found in various components of the basal ganglia, many of which influence the motor system via the globus pallidus. It is postulated that choreiform movements result from a loss of inhibition of the pallidum because of impaired afferent connections. Chorea is induced by biochemical agents that enhance dopaminergic activity at the striatal level when supersensitivity to this neurotransmitter exists. This most commonly occurs when the small-cell components of the caudate nucleus and putamen are involved.

Choreic movements may be noted in any part of the body (eg, limbs, face, hands, tongue, or trunk). At first, they may appear to be a part of the natural pattern of coordinated movements, but soon they are noted to be completely random, jerking, aimless, and purposeless. They occur at rest, are accentuated by an attempt at volitional movement, and disappear during sleep. They may be very mild and only minimally affect normal function, or they may be so forceful and frequent as to be totally disabling. Facial grimacing and difficulty in speaking, chewing, and swallowing occur when the muscles subserving these functions are involved. Interruption of voluntary movements by involuntary ones leads to incoordination. Frequently, objects drop from the hands, walking is awkward and ungainly, and a general appearance of incoordination is present.

Other prominent features found in almost all patients include pronation of the forearm when the upper limbs are raised or extended; inability to sustain muscle contraction when the examiner grasps the patient's hand or when the patient protrudes the tongue so that it darts rapidly in and out of the mouth; and abnormal posturing of hands, in which the wrists are noted to be sharply flexed and the fingers hyperextended at the metacarpophalangeal joints.

There are no specific laboratory tests for chorea. The CSF is normal. The EEG may or may not show diffuse abnormalities that correlate with the severity of the disease. Unless associated diseases are present, blood count, ESR, and blood chemistry studies are normal. CT and MRI of the head may be helpful in identifying the underlying nature of the disease.

Considered a symptom complex rather than a specific disease entity, choreiform movements are seen as initial manifestations of various conditions. **The classification of chorea** into separate entities is currently somewhat arbitrary and is based on age at onset, association with identifiable diseases or familial tendency, and association with other neurologic abnormalities. The major disorders in which chorea occurs in the elderly are listed in TABLE 84–2. Few distinctive features of the movements indicate the underlying cause. Therefore, each patient must be thoroughly evaluated with a view to uncovering the associated disease. The conditions more frequently encountered in the geriatric population are detailed below.

ACUTE CHOREA

Choreic movements, either localized to a body segment or generalized, may occur in association with systemic disease or may be induced by pharmacologic or toxic agents. There are no characteristic features of the choreic state nor any fixed time course that might be helpful in diagnosis. Early recognition and institution of appropriate therapy for the basic disease usually eliminates the choreic movements, but in some instances, they persist and require symptomatic treatment.

SLE is a common cause of acute chorea, especially in middle-aged women. Chorea may occur as the initial manifestation during the course of the illness. Frequently, it is associated with other CNS manifestations, such as seizure phenomena or behavioral disturbances. **Autoimmune disorders; blood dyscrasias, such as polycythemia; and endocrine disorders, such as parathyroid or thyroid dysfunction,** must be considered when chorea is a prominent clinical manifestation.

Iatrogenic chorea induced by drugs is most frequently seen in epileptics taking anticonvulsants, in psychiatric patients using neuroleptics, and in

TABLE 84–2. CONDITIONS ASSOCIATED WITH CHOREA

CNS infections
  Encephalitis lethargica (von Economo's disease)
  Meningoencephalitis secondary to virus
  Parenchymatous neurosyphilis
Autoimmune disorders
  Systemic lupus erythematosus (SLE)
  Henoch-Schönlein purpura
  Rheumatoid arthritis
  Periarteritis nodosa
  Serum sickness reaction to tetanus antitoxin
  Lyme disease
Metabolic disorders
  Thyrotoxicosis
  Hypo- and hyperparathyroidism
  Hypocalcemia
Drug intoxications
  Atropine poisoning and other anticholinergic intoxications
  Anticonvulsants
  Amphetamines
  Levodopa
  Lithium
  Phenothiazine and related neuroleptic drugs
  Isoniazid
Genetic disorders
  Huntington's chorea
  Acute intermittent porphyria
  Wilson's disease
  Acanthocytosis
  Olivopontocerebellar atrophy, dominant form
Miscellaneous disorders
  Pick's and Alzheimer's disease
  Senile chorea
  Benign familial chorea
  Polycythemia
  Beriberi
  Cerebrovascular disease
    Arteriosclerotic vascular disease
    Meningovascular syphilis
  Brain tumor, primary or metastatic
  Trauma, subdural hematoma

parkinsonian patients being treated with levodopa. In most instances, withdrawing the offending drug eliminates the choreic movements within a few days. Occasionally, choreic movements persist for extended periods of time, particularly with the use of neuroleptics. Since their induction and persistence may be related to dosage and duration of administration of the drug, early recognition and discontinuance of the offending drug is of primary importance.

HUNTINGTON'S CHOREA
(Chronic Progressive Chorea; Hereditary Chorea)

A progressive degenerative disease of the basal ganglia and cerebral cortex beginning in adult life and characterized by choreiform movements and mental deterioration.

Inheritance is based on a single dominant autosomal gene localized to chromosome 4. Approximately 50% of the offspring are affected. The disease is relatively rare, with a prevalence of 4 to 8/100,000, but its incidence may be high in places where affected families have resided for many generations.

Pathophysiology

Widespread degenerative changes, with cell loss and reactive gliosis, are found, primarily in the cerebral cortex and caudate nucleus. Glutamic acid decarboxylase activity and choline acetyltransferase activity are reduced in the basal ganglia of patients with Huntington's chorea, resulting in a deficiency of γ-aminobutyric acid **(GABA)**, an inhibitory transmitter substance in the brain, as well as depressed function of the excitatory transmitter acetylcholine **(ACh)**. Disruption of the homeostatic relationship of these neurotransmitters may underlie the choreic manifestations of this disorder.

Symptoms and Signs

The clinical manifestations consist of choreic movements, emotional disturbance, and intellectual deterioration, all of which vary in degree, rate of appearance, and progression. The disease usually appears, somewhat insidiously between the ages of 35 and 50 yr, with any of the symptoms listed but usually with abnormal movements.

The movements are similar to those of acute chorea but usually more jerky and less lightning-like. They involve primarily the trunk and shoulder girdle and the lower limbs more often than the upper. This pattern of involvement tends to produce a dancing sort of gait, which is a prominent feature of the disease. Rarely, a parkinsonism-like rigidity rather than involuntary movements is the major manifestation. Mental deterioration is progressive, with impairment of memory and intellectual capacity and inattention to personal hygiene. Emotional disturbances include heightened irritability, bouts of depression, and fits of violent behavior.

Diagnosis

With the typical triad of choreiform movements, dementia in adult life, and documentation of similar symptoms in family members, the diagnosis is readily evident. However, families tend to deny the existence of mental disease, and it is sometimes difficult to obtain corroborative data.

Few laboratory tests are helpful. The EEG usually shows nonspecific abnormalities. Caudate atrophy may be demonstrable on CT scan or

MRI in association with generalized cerebral atrophy, but this may not occur until late in the disease process. PET scan may show decreased uptake in the caudate region well before any loss of caudate tissue appears on CT scan. Decreased CSF GABA levels, reflecting the reduced synthesis of this neurotransmitter, have been reported but not confirmed.

Differentiation from senile chorea may be a problem. The latter, which presents late in life, involves few, if any, mental changes; lacks a familial history; and is usually benign. Because of the dementia and the similarity in age at onset, distinguishing this chorea from other diseases (eg, the presenile psychoses—Alzheimer's and Pick's disease) may offer some diagnostic difficulty, especially when choreiform movements are inconspicuous. CT scan of the brain may help to establish the correct diagnosis. There is a tendency to overdiagnose hereditary chorea, applying this diagnosis to diverse neurologic disorders, such as cerebellar degenerations and familial tremors. *The dire prognostic implications of Huntington's chorea require strict adherence to the diagnostic criteria.*

Treatment

There is no effective therapy. Theoretically, drugs that are capable of elevating GABA levels or enhancing the brain's cholinergic activity should be helpful. Some (eg, phenelzine sulfate and deanol) have been tried with inconsistent therapeutic effects. Levodopa worsens chorea in affected individuals and may induce chorea in those at risk for the condition. This may be a useful provocative test for early identification of affected individuals before onset of the disease. In view of the psychologic trauma imposed, ethical issues regarding the desirability of such a test have been raised.

Huntington's chorea is relentlessly progressive, leading to total incapacity and, inevitably, death, usually within 15 yr of onset. In the early stages, the patient can be managed at home with supervision and phenothiazines, haloperidol, or reserpine to reduce the intensity of the movements and control the behavior to some extent. As the disease advances, confinement to a psychiatric facility becomes necessary.

SENILE CHOREA

Choreiform movements encountered as an isolated symptom in persons > 60 yr of age. This occurs infrequently and, usually, the movements are mild and may involve the limbs, unilaterally or bilaterally. Involuntary complex movements of the face, mouth, and tongue may occur alone or in association with limb movements. There is no associated mental disturbance or family history of Huntington's chorea. Symptoms often come on abruptly; are usually unilateral; and show little if any progression. This has suggested an underlying vascular lesion, which may be found only in exceptional cases.

The pathologic findings are similar to those of Huntington's chorea insofar as involvement of the caudate nucleus is concerned, but the cerebral cortex is spared. Some consider these cases to be a variant of Huntington's chorea, but senile chorea probably has several causes. Since the symptoms are mild and the course benign, therapeutic considerations are unimportant.

TORSION DYSTONIAS

A group of movement disorders characterized by intense, irregular, sustained torsion spasms of the musculature, resulting in marked abnormalities of bodily posture. The dystonic movements may be (1) focal, involving 1 body site, eg, foot or hand; (2) segmental, involving > 1 site, eg, shoulder, or pelvic girdle, or both; and (3) generalized, involving the limbs and trunk simultaneously. The pathophysiology and underlying morbid anatomy are unknown.

Based on genetic, clinical, and presumed causative factors, 3 forms can be recognized: (1) inherited (autosomal recessive, autosomal dominant, X-linked recessive); (2) idiopathic; and (3) symptomatic. The inherited and idiopathic forms are often considered primary dystonia, in contrast to the symptomatic form, which is considered secondary. In the primary dystonias, no neurologic abnormalities are found except for the dystonic movements and postures.

PRIMARY DYSTONIA

Spasmodic Torticollis

Dyskinetic movements are limited to neck muscles, so that abnormal posture of the head results in the distinguishing characteristic of this symptom complex. Involuntary activity involves the sternocleidomastoid, trapezius, and scalene muscles in sustained contractions that result in slow, twisting, turning movements of the head **(torticollis)** or, less often, forward flexion **(anterocollis)** or forceful extension **(retrocollis).**

In most cases, there is bilateral involvement, and the resultant postural deformity is maintained for varying lengths of time. The muscles of the neck appear tense, and the continual muscular activity may lead to some degree of hypertrophy, especially evident in the sternocleidomastoid muscles. Similar activity may spread to facial and brachial musculature. The amount of active motion or static postural deformity is extremely variable. A brief tremor may be present with the spasm. Cervical arthropathy is a common sequela of prolonged spasm.

Spasmodic torticollis is variably described as a psychogenic disorder, a limited form of dystonia musculorum deformans, or a compensatory postural defect in persons with congenital ocular muscle imbalance or defects of the cervical spine or musculature. Hyperthyroidism is present in a few patients. In some instances, the torticollis is part of a wide spectrum of extrapyramidal disorders that follow encephalitis lethargica. Currently, there is no information regarding either its pathophysiology or its pathology.

The disorder can occur at any age but most frequently appears during the 3rd to 6th decades of life. The course varies, being transitory and remitting after a few months in some patients and relentlessly progressive, leading to incapacity, in others. Some patients reach a static phase in which movements cease or are minimal, and a minor postural deformity of the head persists.

The evaluation of this condition includes a search for ocular and vertebral signs, major psychiatric disturbances, and other associated neurologic conditions. Definable conditions account for only a small percentage of cases. In most patients, no underlying cause is found.

Cranial Dystonias

Blepharospasm, oromandibular dystonia, and laryngeal and pharyngeal dystonia all are cranial dystonias. They all occur in adult life, usually in the 5th or 6th decade; their cause is unknown; and they are resistant to most therapeutic measures. Each is characterized by intermittent spasms of selected groups of muscles, which markedly interfere with function. **Blepharospasm** is *the involuntary spasm of the orbicularis oculi muscles with forceful closure of the eyes.* Voluntary eye closure is performed normally. At first, the blinking occurs at widely spaced intervals, but the repetitive eye closure may become more frequent or even continuous, limiting vision. Corneal excoriation around the eyelids may be seen from repetitive blinking. Blepharospasm is not a sensory-evoked blink response, although bright lights, wind, reading, driving, or watching television may aggravate the condition. Some patients note that embarrassment or fatigue worsens it. Prolonged spasms can be overcome by forced opening with the fingers, forced jaw closure, yawning, or neck movements. The spasm disappears during sleep.

Oromandibular and orofacial dystonias are *involuntary spasms of the facial muscles, jaw muscles, tongue, and platysma that cause arrhythmic movements.* These dystonias may be provoked by attempts to talk or eat. Manifestations include forward protrusion of the tongue, drooling, opening of the mouth, clenching of the teeth, and pursing and retraction of the lips. Movements may occur in a repetitive pattern with spasms lasting from seconds to minutes; speech and swallowing may be affected.

In **spastic dysphonia,** *adductor muscles of the larynx are spasmodic.* Speech is tight and constricted, with the smooth flow of words broken up into an irregular pattern. This differs from voice tremor, in which the speech is normally regular but broken up by a tremor pattern. If the vocal cord and abductor are dystonic, a breathy dysphonia is produced, with the patient running out of words when speaking.

The cranial dystonias generally remain localized but in some instances occur in combination (eg, the combination of oromandibular dystonia with blepharospasm is referred to as **Meige's syndrome).** All these conditions must be differentiated from drug-induced and tardive dyskinesias as initial manifestations of more generalized neurologic disorders and psychiatric conditions.

Writer's Cramp

Spasms of the muscles of the hand and forearm occurring during the act of writing characterize this disorder. A typical posture results with pen grasped tightly and the distal segment of digits extended, the forearm pronated, and the wrist flexed. Tremor of the limb ensues, as when script writing is attempted. Surprisingly, symptoms are less profound when writing is attempted in the standing position (eg, writing with chalk on a board). In most individuals, symptoms are limited to writing, but they may progress to other coordinated acts, such as using a key to open a door.

Conditions similar to writer's cramp have been associated with other skilled acts, usually linked to occupational activities. Hence, typist's cramp, violinist's or cellist's cramps, and so forth, have been described. All seem to fall into a category for which cause and effective therapy are unknown.

SECONDARY DYSTONIA

Secondary dystonia may present as a pure dystonia or it may have additional neurologic abnormalities, eg, weakness, spasticity, ataxia, or reflex changes. Most cases begin with the movement at rest or with sustained posture. Those due to environmental causes, eg, head trauma and encephalitis, tend to remain stable without progression.

Numerous conditions have been identified as causing dystonia. As a rule, these conditions produce focal dystonic movements or postures that more frequently affect the upper limbs, particularly the hand. This applies especially to destructive lesions, such as tumors or arteriovenous malformations of the brain. *When focal dystonia is encountered in an adult, a complete study must be undertaken to determine causative factors.* TABLE 84–3 lists causes of secondary dystonia.

TABLE 84–3. CAUSES OF SECONDARY DYSTONIA

Genetic disorders
  Wilson's disease
  Huntington's chorea
  Hallervorden-Spatz syndrome
  GM_1 gangliosidosis
Viral encephalitis
Arteriovenous malformation
Tumors
Drugs
  Levodopa
  Neuroleptics
  Anticonvulsants
  Metoclopromide
Toxins—heavy metals

Treatment of dystonia is difficult. High doses of anticholinergics may be effective, but their side effects in older patients may preclude their use. Some patients may benefit from bromocriptine, baclofen, diazepam, clonazepam, or carbamezapine. Reserpine or tetrabenazine may also be of benefit. For blepharospasm and laryngeal dystonia, injection of botulinus toxin into the affected muscle provides temporary relief of the spasm that can last for several months but treatment is currently investigational.

Biofeedback through controlled relaxation methods suppresses spasmodic torticollis and dystonic writer's cramp in some patients. The benefits in more severe forms are limited. Surgical therapy can be considered after medical treatment has failed. Focal dystonia has responded to sectioning of peripheral nerves; however, regeneration of the nerve can result in recurrence of symptoms. More recently the injection of botulinus toxin, which blocks nerve conduction to the affected muscle, has been used.

In some cases, focal dystonia has developed in the contralateral muscle following section of the spinal accessory nerve or the anterior cervical root. Posterior cord or cerebellar stimulation by implanted electrodes has had inconsistent results; although some patients have responded well. Thalamotomy for contralateral limb dystonia should be reserved only for severely affected patients.

TARDIVE DYSKINESIA

*A syndrome of persistent, stereotyped, repetitive abnormal involuntary movements (**AIMs**) associated with chronic exposure to neuroleptic medications that block and bind with the dopamine (**DA**) receptor.* Higher dosage and prolonged treatment increase the likelihood of inducing the movements. The AIMs typically start while taking the medication and can be induced by *reducing* the dose or *discontinuing* the neuroleptic. *Reinstituting* the drug can alleviate the symptoms. The etiology is related to DA receptor supersensitivity. The prevalence of tardive dyskinesia increases with age and is more common in elderly women.

Classic oral tardive dyskinesia involves tongue movements and chewing, lip puckering, and lip smacking that differ from movements in chorea in that they are repetitive and predictable. Tardive dystonia and tardive akathisia are other expressions of this disorder. In **tardive dystonia,** the dystonic movements involve different regions of the body and are like those of the primary torsion dystonias. The face and neck are most often affected, and in older patients, the AIMs tend to remain focal. **Tardive akathisia** is a subjective state of motor restlessness or an aversion to being still. Objective motor signs are complex, stereotyped, and repetitive; they can include vocal, truncal, and appendicular movements. Repetitive rubbing or stroking parts of the body, crossing and uncrossing the arms or legs, picking at clothes, pacing, marching in place, swinging the legs, and moaning, grunting, or shouting are all manifestations of tardive akathisia.

Treatment of tardive dyskinesias includes, if possible, discontinuance of the DA antagonist. The orobuccal dyskinesias, if significant, can be treated with reserpine at a dosage of 0.25 mg/day and gradually increased to an average dosage of 5.0 mg/day. Tardive akathisia can also be treated with reserpine. Opiates, propranolol, and benzodiazepines can be helpful. Patients with tardive dystonia may also benefit from reserpine or from the anticholinergics trihexyphenidyl and ethopropazine.

HEMIBALLISMUS

A violent, involuntary movement that occurs when lesions involve the contralateral subthalamic nucleus (the corpus Luysii). The abnormal movements are seen if 20% of this nucleus is destroyed. However, the substantia nigra, pyramidal tract, and red nucleus must be intact for expression of this disorder. The subthalamic nucleus normally inhibits the globus pallidus. Although a variety of pathologic processes (eg, metastatic tumors, cysts, and infectious diseases) can be underlying causes, most cases result from vascular lesions, either hemorrhagic or occlusive. Consequently, they are seen in older patients, sometimes after a transitory hemiparesis. Often, the precipitating event is an acute cerebrovascular accident, accompanied by weakness or sensory deficit, or both.

As the neurologic signs clear or at a variable interval afterward, the ballistic movements begin. They do not occur during sleep, are localized to 1 side of the body, and involve the limbs in a forceful throwing movement, a result of almost continuous activity of the proximal musculature. The arm and leg may be equally involved, but usually 1 is more prominently involved than the other. The neck, tongue, or face may also be involved.

Initially, the violence of these movements may exhaust and incapacitate the patient to such an extent that death may ensue. However, in most instances, the initial intensity decreases gradually so that the movements become tolerable and can be suppressed somewhat or briefly interrupted by voluntary action. In about 6 to 8 wk, the movements stop spontaneously. **Pharmacologic treatment** has included haloperidol for postsynaptic blockade. Valproic acid and reserpine have also benefited some patients. **Surgical measures,** such as thalamotomy, are indicated only in life-threatening cases. In fact, hemiballismus has occurred following attempted thalamotomy for other extrapyramidal disorders, when poor localization has led to an inadvertent lesion in the corpus Luysii.

MYOCLONUS

Sudden, brief, involuntary single or repetitive contractions of a muscle or group of muscles. Myoclonus presents with a variable expression of amplitude, frequency, and distribution. The muscle jerks are often sensitive to stimuli, being induced by sudden noise, movement, light, or visual threat, and can be influenced by activity. The movements are caused by muscular contractions (positive myoclonus) or inhibitions (negative myoclonus) arising from hyperexcitable neurons in the spinal cord, medial reticular formation, or cerebral cortex. A primary metabolic abnormality with ionic-channel alteration or a decrease in inhibitory input from GABAergic, serotonergic, or glycinergic neurons may cause the neuron to be hyperexcitable. Myoclonus can be classified according to etiology. In the geriatric population, the major categories are those related to the dementias, metabolic or toxic encephalopathies, and focal CNS damage. Additional causes are listed in TABLE 84–4.

Myoclonus can be an early feature in **Creutzfeldt-Jakob disease (subacute spongiform encephalopathy).** The myoclonus can be elicited by a

TABLE 84–4. CAUSES OF MYOCLONUS

Physiologic myoclonus (normal)
    Sleep jerks (hypnic jerks)
    Anxiety induced
    Exercise induced
    Hiccups (singultus)
Symptomatic myoclonus
    Dementias
        Creutzfeldt-Jakob disease
        Alzheimer's disease
    Metabolic disorders
        Hepatic failure
        Renal failure
        Chronic hemodialysis
        Hyponatremia
        Hypoglycemia
        Nonketotic hyperglycemia
    Toxic encephalopathies
        Drugs, including levodopa
        Bismuth
        Heavy-metal poisons
        Methyl bromide, DDT
    Physical encephalopathies
        Posthypoxia
        Post-traumatic
        Heat stroke
        Electric shock
    Basal ganglia degenerations
        Wilson's disease
        Torsion dystonia
        Progressive supranuclear palsy
        Huntington's chorea
        Parkinson's disease
    Viral encephalopathies
        Subacute sclerosing panencephalitis
        Encephalitis lethargica
        Herpes simplex encephalitis
        Postinfectious encephalitis

stimulus or can occur spontaneously and is associated with a periodic synchronous discharge on the EEG. **In the later stages of Alzheimer's disease,** patients may exhibit myoclonus. The movements involve small, multifocal, distal muscle jerks or can involve a whole limb; rarely is the whole body involved. The EEG is slow, often with some epileptic activity that is not well correlated with the jerks. The event is shorter and more focal than that in Creutzfeldt-Jakob disease. The movement can be seen at rest, with voluntary activity, or with stimulation.

Myoclonus following a hypoxic insult is usually precipitated by voluntary motor action. Associated cerebellar ataxia, dysarthria, postural lapses, gait disturbances, and grand mal seizures can be seen. Decreased levels of 5-hydroxyindoleacetic acid in the CSF and improvement with 5-hydroxytryptophan suggest a disorder of serotonin metabolism. Treatment of posthypoxic myoclonus includes the administration of clonazepam or valproic acid or a combination of the 2 drugs. Other drugs that may alleviate the myoclonus are carbamazepine, levodopa, estrogens, 5-hydroxytryptophan, and piracetam.

Metabolic derangements, including uremia, hypercapnia, hepatic failure, hypoglycemia, hyponatremia, and need for chronic hemodialysis, may be complicated by multifocal, asymmetric, stimulus-sensitive myoclonus. Facial or proximal limb muscles are predominately involved. If the metabolic abnormality persists, generalized myoclonic jerks and, ultimately, generalized seizures may occur. The EEG shows a slow background with paroxysms of bifrontal, biphasic, and triphasic waves unrelated to the myoclonus.

Chronic levodopa treatment in some parkinsonian patients can induce myoclonus. Single, abrupt, symmetric jerks of the arms and legs usually occur during sleep, drowsiness, or at rest. A reduction in dose can alleviate the frequency and severity of the myoclonus. **Toxic doses of tricyclic antidepressants, lithium, valproic acid, carbamazepine, phenytoin, antihistamines, and monoamine oxidase inhibitors (MAOIs)** can also induce myoclonus.

High-dose infusion of penicillin or cephalosporins can induce nonrhythmic, asymmetric, and stimulus-sensitive myoclonus. High concentrations of the antibiotic in the CSF, especially in patients with renal failure or an impaired blood-brain barrier, account for the abnormal movements. Discontinuance of the drug leads to resolution of the myoclonus.

§3. ORGAN SYSTEMS: PSYCHIATRIC DISORDERS

Contents for **SKIN DISORDERS** begin on page 1025.

---

85. NORMAL CHANGES AND PATTERNS OF PSYCHIATRIC DISEASE

Gene D. Cohen

NORMAL CHANGES OF AGING

Failure to differentiate disease-related psychiatric changes from manifestations of normal aging have blurred the understanding of mental function in healthy older adults. Many decrements in capacity or performance viewed as age related—particularly those associated with cognition and behavior—have been found instead to reflect modifiable consequences of illness.

Cognitive Manifestations and Changes

Reports from a longitudinal study of cognitive capacity in a cohort of men followed since 1919 described increments in verbal ability and total score of intellectual performance as they moved from age 20 to age 50 yr, although mathematical ability showed a slight decline. As these men aged from 50 to 60 yr, there was little change in intellectual test scores.

These studies were among the first to raise serious doubts about the presumed normal decline in mental ability with advancing age that had been inferred from earlier cross-sectional research.

A 12-yr longitudinal study of men (median age, 71 yr) was conducted by the National Institute of Mental Health to examine a broad range of variables in individuals of advanced age in whom physical and psychiatric disease was absent or minimal. The goal was to separate the impact of aging from that of illness. As these healthy aging subjects moved from their 70s to their 80s, various intellectual functions declined, while others improved. For example, declines were noted in cognitive operations, quality of "draw-a-person" exercises, and quality of sentence completions. On the other hand, vocabulary and picture arrangement improved. This suggests that certain activities requiring a quick reaction time or a high degree of precision generally might not be completed as well by older adults, although the ability to understand one's situation and learn from new experiences is maintained.

Moreover, decrements in intellectual performance were significantly greater in subjects who developed arteriosclerotic cardiovascular disease than in those who remained healthy. The study illustrated the impact of illness on intellectual functioning, while showing that intellectual functioning is maintained in aging individuals who remain healthy. This research points out that significant changes in the intellectual performance of older individuals should not be dismissed as normal concomitants of aging but should be evaluated as potentially modifiable manifestations of disease (psychiatric as well as general medical). For example, both depression and hypothyroidism are treatable problems that can be covert and cause cognitive impairment.

Behavior and Personality Traits

Corresponding to the stereotype of inevitable, marked intellectual decline with aging are stereotypes of regressive behavior and increasing inflexibility of personality traits. However, these should also be seen more as a signal of psychiatric disturbance than as manifestations of aging. Consider the issue of caution. Research shows that older individuals are more cautious than younger adults about risk-taking in situations in which the "payoff" is predictable and at a constant level. If the size of the payoff depends upon the degree of risk, however, older individuals are not more cautious than younger ones.

Anxiety can result in cautiousness, causing delays in decision making and reactions. In other words, excessive cautiousness in the elderly may signal underlying anxiety or a related clinical disorder. On the other hand, it is entirely appropriate for a frail or disabled older person to be more careful in general. The difference lies in distinguishing an appropriate, adaptive response to reality from a maladaptive overcautiousness resulting from clinical anxiety.

When comparisons show older adults to be more rigid than younger ones, cohort differences (ie, generational differences that stem from having been brought up during different historic periods)—and not age differences—are more likely being described. Research shows not only that personalities remain stable with aging but that behavioral and psychologic adaptiveness continues and does not normally give way to regression or rigidity. Hence, if certain behaviors or traits grow increasingly exaggerated, maladaptive, and unmodifiable, neurosis rather than normal aging may be to blame. Treatment rather than acceptance is in order.

PATTERNS OF PSYCHIATRIC DISEASE

Epidemiology

Mental health problems in the elderly are significant in their frequency, their impact on mental status and emotional states, and their potential influence on the course of physical illness. Early epidemiologic studies documented the prevalence of seri~~~~~~~~~~~~ those ≥ 65 yr of age at 15 to 25%. Amo~~~~~~~~~~~~~~~~~~~~~~~~~~~ts, 27% are ≥ 65 yr of age.

Several studies have found that psychiatric problems are a primary or secondary diagnosis in 70 to 80% of nursing home residents; a recent study identified 94% of residents of a nursing home as having mental disorders, according to criteria defined in the *Diagnostic and Statistical Manual of Mental Disorders,* Third Edition **(DSM-III).** As a result of improvements in general medical care in the community, patients admitted to nursing homes today tend to be sicker, both mentally and physically, than in the past. Mental health problems, however, have always been numerous in nursing home patients, particularly because of the large percentage of those with organic mental disorders.

Such disorders (Alzheimer's disease being the most frequent) affect > 6% of those ≥ 65 yr of age. Significant depressive symptoms have been described in 15% of community-dwelling elderly persons, and schizophrenia, in 0.5 to 1.0%. The frequency of alcohol abuse is difficult to determine, but its prevalence is considered to be high. Suicide, more frequent in the elderly than in any other age group, is highest in white males.

The relationship between mental and physical health is particularly significant in the elderly. A growing body of scientific data corroborates the adverse effects of mental health problems on physical illness in later life. As a corollary, research is also demonstrating the positive effect of mental health interventions on general medical and surgical problems; psychiatric consultation significantly reduces length of stay and improves clinical outcome in hospitalized elderly cardiac and surgical patients. Given the frequency of mental health problems in seriously ill older patients, these findings become even more important. One study, for example, found that 24% of 406 elderly men with physical health problems in a primary-care setting complained of clinically significant depressive symptoms; other studies report even higher frequencies of depressive symptoms in such persons.

Primary vs. secondary depressions: One explanation for discrepancies in the prevalence of depression in the elderly is that different classifications of depression are being compared. Lower prevalences typically describe only primary depressions—ie, depressions occurring in the absence of physical disorders or drug side effects. Higher prevalences give a more accurate picture in that they include all depressions—both primary and secondary, with the latter representing those accompanying or resulting from somatic illness or adverse drug effects. The elderly are at greater risk for secondary depressions than other age groups because they have a much higher frequency of physical illness and the highest rate of drug use.

Symptoms and Signs

Psychiatric symptoms that develop in later life are often dismissed as normal manifestations of aging. Even symptoms of schizophrenia may be dismissed as eccentricity of old age or misdiagnosed as senility. Treatment cannot be planned if a problem is not acknowledged and identified.

Memory and intellectual difficulties: Significant changes in intellectual functioning are no longer readily dismissed, given heightened awareness of Alzheimer's disease. But the degree to which depression, anxiety, and other psychiatric disorders can interfere with cognition is still underappreciated. **Pseudodementia** (eg, depression or paraphrenia masquerading as dementia) is an extreme form of this interference.

Change in sleep pattern: An older person who complains of diminished sleep is commonly assured that this is a normal part of aging and told not to worry. However, this is not necessarily so. Although some studies have found that a reduction in total sleep time can occur in later life, other studies have not. Clinically, such changes should be viewed as a group characteristic that does not apply to all individuals. Furthermore, the reduction that does occur is typically gradual; consequently, sleep change should not be taken for granted, especially if it is of recent onset. An older person who reports noticeable reduction in sleeping (not just sleeping less at night because of daytime naps) should be evaluated.

Besides signaling potential medical problems (eg, of arthritic, urologic, or cardiologic origin), sleep changes can be a hallmark of psychiatric disorders. Early morning awakening may be an important clue to an underlying depression; difficulty in falling asleep or restless sleep with frequent awakenings may signal an anxiety disorder.

Change in sexual interest or capacity (see also Ch. 58, SEXUALITY, and Ch. 73, MALE HYPOGONADISM AND IMPOTENCE): As with sleep pattern changes, group characteristics of sexual changes should be separated from individual cases. Even as a group, healthy older men and women with a past history of normal sexual activity and current opportunity, retain their interest and capacity for sexual experience. Significant changes, particularly of recent onset, call for diagnostic assessment. The focus should include medical and surgical factors, drug side effects, and psychiatric causes. Medical and drug influences more commonly affect men than women, since these factors can interfere with erectile and ejaculatory function.

Common medical causes of erectile dysfunction include atherosclerosis (especially in patients with diabetes mellitus), hypothyroidism, malnutrition, and Parkinson's disease. Among possible drug causes, alcohol consumption should be considered, since alcohol is not only a depressant in higher amounts, thereby negatively influencing sexual interest, but it can also interfere with erectile and ejaculatory capacity. Depression or anxiety can affect older men and women alike by lowering their motivation for romantic involvement and diminishing sexual satisfaction. Regardless of the cause, a substantial number of these problems can be ameliorated or eliminated with proper intervention.

Fear of death: Research shows that while the elderly frequently think about death, fear of death is less common in this group than in other age groups. Thinking or talking about death is not the same as fearing or dreading it. Ideas or conversations about death are naturally more common in the elderly, since they more likely have peers and older relatives who have died or are dying. To understand dread of death, one must examine its context. Dread of death is uncommon in persons who are not dying or experiencing some major loss. The presence of a terminal illness, an underlying depression, or other emotional conflict—not the awareness of aging itself—predisposes certain elderly individuals to death anxiety.

Interestingly, the dread of death has been described as normal and more common in middle age, when individuals suddenly perceive how little time is left. At this stage, people find themselves confronting an existential awareness of their own mortality; with further aging, they adapt to this realization.

However, confronting mortality is different when one has a terminal illness or is suffering from depression. A terminal illness brings an awareness of dying that can lead to despondency. Eventually, most people come to terms with their fate and develop a reasonable acceptance of their condition. Depression at any age clouds one's thinking and often increases thoughts about death. Hence, an elderly patient's noticeable and persistent uneasiness about death should be evaluated as potentially signaling an underlying depression that could benefit from treatment.

Atypical Presentations

Just as infection may present atypically in the elderly (eg, without fever or an elevated WBC count), psychiatric illness may be manifested in atypical forms (eg, vague physical decline and multiple somatic complaints).

Vague physical decline: In later life, this does not always indicate physiologic aging or the subtle progression of underlying physical illness. Rather, psychosocial factors may aggravate medical problems, at times precipitating a latent physical disorder. The nature and rate of physiologic decline, under the influence of depression, can reflect the will to live or die. For example, deterioration of overall health because of heart failure may actually represent despair and loss of hope, resulting in self-termination of medication. Covert suicidal behavior can be missed.

Multiple somatic complaints: Depressed older persons have many concerns about their bodies. In 1 study of depressed patients > 60 yr of age, somatic concerns were found in $> 60\%$ of both men and women. Physical symptoms and multiple somatic complaints require diligent medical attention, including a search for underlying psychogenic factors.

Depression can lead to social withdrawal or isolation, which is a greater risk in the elderly; in the process, energy previously invested in interpersonal interactions can be turned inward, with an exaggerated focus on self and magnification of every ache and pain. Isolated older people may be reluctant to get into conflicts; they may have trouble dealing with rage, fearing they will drive away the few people to whom they can relate if they express their true feelings, turning the anger inward where it manifests itself as physical instead of emotional pain. The elderly are at increased risk for diverse losses (eg, loss of spouse, economic status, physical health, overall independence); such losses can lead to diminished self-esteem and depression, to a disturbing loss of control over one's life, resulting in physical symptoms that represent maladaptive efforts to control others, gain attention, or signal for help.

Suicide

Depression is one of the most common reasons for suicide. While data show that suicide rates among those 18 to 24 yr of age increased significantly from 1970 to 1980, the highest rates in the USA occur in those ≥ 65 yr old. The differences are most striking among white men. Suicide is nearly 25% more common in white men 65 to 74 yr of age and $> 70\%$ more common in those 75 to 84 yr old, compared with those 18 to 24 yr of age. Furthermore, different cohorts of elderly persons appear to have different suicide rates in old age as well as during other phases of life. (See also Ch. 89.)

Some recent data suggest that the elderly do not seek help or respond to offers of help designed to prevent suicide as well as younger patients. Also, elderly persons make fewer "gestures" of suicide and more often "succeed."

In addition to direct or overt suicidal acts in the elderly, there are indirect or covert forms of suicidal behavior. These can make the assessment of suicidal potential difficult; an example of covert suicidal behavior is provided below, under the paradigms for examining relationships between mental and physical health in the elderly.

Interactions Between Mental and Physical Health

There is increasing recognition of the impact of mental health status on the overall course of physical health and illness. Many elderly persons living in the community have the same degree of physical disability as those in nursing homes. What accounts for the difference? Clearly, the availability of family members or other types of social support works in their favor. However, significantly underappreciated and overlooked is the role of a concomitant psychiatric disorder that can destroy the individual's capacity to maintain independence.

The influence of cognitive, affective, and behavioral problems on the course of overall health in later life is a public health issue of enormous proportions. Consider the situation, for example, of a frail older person taking multiple drugs for various physical ailments; add depression or psychosis, and the individual's ability to think clearly enough to manage these drugs may become so impaired that potentially serious consequences to overall health status ensue.

Clinical concerns pertaining to the mental health aspects of physical illness can be framed in a number of ways. A few models follow.

Paradigms for Examining Relationships Between Mental and Physical Health

The impact of psychologic stress on physical health. Example—Anxiety → GI symptoms: Accurate diagnosis of GI symptoms can be very difficult, with research showing that up to 5 out of 9 elderly persons with GI complaints actually may be experiencing psychologic problems that led to their physical discomfort.

The effect of physical disorder on psychiatric disturbance. Example—Hearing loss → onset of delusions: Twenty-nine percent of elderly persons have hearing impairment; a sensory-deprivation phenomenon may be the cause of psychotic symptoms in certain vulnerable individuals.

The interplay of coexisting physical and mental disorders. Example—Heart failure + depression → further cardiac decline: Cardiac disorder and depression are 2 of the most common health problems in the elderly. A covert depression can bring about indirect suicidal behavior, as when the patient fails to follow a proper drug schedule; this could result in a further deterioration in cardiac function.

The impact of psychosocial factors on the clinical course of physical health problems. Example—Diabetic with infected foot, living alone → increased risk of gangrene: One in 3 older women and 1 in 7 older men live alone. The absence of people to help with medical management and follow-up poses the risk of complications and poorer outcome in elderly persons with chronic illnesses.

There are, of course, many other ways in which mental and physical health interact to affect overall health, but the above examples reflect the potential magnitude of public health problems brought about by such an interplay. They reflect, too, the role of mental health factors with aging in that elusive "whole person."

Is the problem mental or physical? Making the correct diagnosis can be especially challenging when differentiating psychologic from physical causes. Consider GI complaints, which represent an area of competing stereotypes. One stereotype holds that most GI complaints in the elderly are of psychogenic origin—a psychosomatic explanation. The opposing stereotype holds that if one looks hard enough, a physical basis for most GI symptoms will be found in older patients.

In an attempt to evaluate these views, a study was conducted of 300 patients > 65 yr of age with GI complaints who were followed comprehensively for at least 1 yr after their initial visit to the outpatient department of a medical center. Final diagnoses were as follows: 10%, GI malignancy; 8%, gallbladder disease; 6%, duodenal ulcer; 3%, gastric ulcer; 3%, diverticulosis of the colon; 14%, a wide variety of problems with an organic basis; and 56%, GI distress of a purely psychogenic nature. The physical problems of these last patients included irritable colon, spastic colitis, gastritis, heartburn, nausea, diarrhea, constipation, and other psychophysiologic disorders.

In short, the study revealed that the initial question (mental or physical) is inappropriate, as both psychogenic (56%) and physical (44%) factors play major roles in patients with GI problems. This makes it incumbent on the primary-care physician or psychiatrist to simultaneously incorporate both comprehensive general medical *and* psychiatric evaluation in the evaluation of GI complaints in older patients.

Treatment

After differentiating illness from aging and psychiatric from physical disease, the process of treatment planning begins. Clinicians today have access to improved psychotherapeutic, psychopharmacologic, and social interventions. However, with chronic mental illness, as in chronic physical illness, it is important to remember that both remissions and exacerbations can occur.

Psychotherapy: Many doubt the place of psychotherapy in geriatric medicine, but recent research has demonstrated its efficacy in many older patients, especially those with reactive depression, in whom psychosocially induced stress is prominent.

Further, as the average life expectancy increases, **time** is less likely to be considered an obstacle to psychotherapy. A 65-yr-old may have 20 more yr of life—ample time to undergo treatment and reap its benefits. Researchers have also reported that the elderly are **less resistant** to unpleasant insights compared with younger patients, thus increasing the opportunity for resolution of conflicts. Moreover, today's elderly are considerably **more receptive** to psychiatric intervention than were prior cohorts of older adults.

Pharmacologic interventions: After cardiovascular drugs, psychotropics are the most frequently prescribed for older patients. Psychotropics include antidepressants, anxiolytics, antipsychotics (neuroleptics), hypnotics, lithium (for the mania of bipolar depressive disorders), and those drugs that enhance cognitive function (primarily memory).

In an older patient, a psychotropic drug usually takes longer to work, remains in the body longer, and produces a greater effect than it would at the same dosage in a younger person. Thus, the advice generally has been to "start low, go slow," ie, to begin with a reduced dosage and to increase it gradually, if necessary. Attention to this dictum, as well as to potential drug interactions in those taking other medications, is prudent. (See also Ch. 18.)

There are 5 major areas of pharmacokinetic change with aging: (1) **absorption**, (2) **distribution**, (3) **metabolism**, (4) **excretion**, and (5) **CNS sensitivity** to the drug at receptor sites in the brain.

Absorption: Most psychotropic drugs taken orally by older adults are absorbed through the intestinal mucosa. Although aging does not significantly alter absorption, many older persons take other prescribed or OTC drugs that can interfere with how efficiently or quickly the psychotropics are absorbed. Consequently, more attention must be directed to the timing of psychotropic administration (eg, an hour before going to bed, to allow enough time for a hypnotic to be absorbed and induce sleep).

Distribution: With aging, body fat tends to increase, while lean body mass (muscle) and total body water diminish. Many psychotropic drugs (eg, long-acting benzodiazepines) are lipid (fat) soluble; only lithium is water soluble. The increased proportion of fat in the aging body results in the storage of lipid-soluble psychotropic agents, making a routine dosage more likely to accumulate to toxic levels. This risk is even greater in older women, since they have proportionately more body fat than older men. The risk can be mitigated by reducing the dose or frequency of administration. While this may result in a longer time for a therapeutic effect to be realized, the slower onset results in greater safety. Similarly, because the amount of body water decreases with aging, less lithium is required in the elderly than in younger adults to achieve comparable therapeutic effects.

Metabolism: Except for lithium, most psychotropic medications are metabolized by the liver. With advancing age, metabolism may slow for some drugs because of altered activity of hepatic enzymes. In such cases, the drug tends to remain available and active in the body for a longer period, leading to an increased risk of accumulation and toxicity unless the dosage is also reduced. Age-related differences in hepatic metabolism of the various psychotropic drugs may be important clinically. For example, antianxiety agents, such as diazepam and chlordiazepoxide, are generally metabolized 3 times more slowly in older persons than in younger ones. This is in addition to prolonged $t_{1/2}$ from larger distribution volumes. Oxazepam and lorazepam, on the other hand, are metabolized at essentially the same relatively fast rates, regardless of age. Therefore, the latter 2 are often preferred when anxiolytics are indicated in the elderly. However, drugs that are rapidly metabolized must often be taken more frequently, which can create a problem in patients with memory impairment. For such patients, a drug that can be taken once a day may be preferable. This is an issue of clinical judgment—specifically, balancing the risks and benefits, with emphasis on *individualization* in older patients.

Excretion: Whereas liver metabolism is the primary mechanism for deactivating lipid-soluble psychotropic agents, renal excretion is the primary pathway for water-soluble lithium. Since renal function is reduced with aging, excretion of lithium takes longer in the elderly, once again setting the stage for accumulation if dosage is not adjusted downward.

CNS sensitivity: Increased receptor sensitivity may also explain why dosage reduction of psychotropic drugs may be needed to achieve therapeutic benefit in the elderly. Prescribing the same dosage of drug as for younger patients risks adverse effects.

Choice of psychotropic drug as a factor of physical health status: Each psychotropic category has several drugs from which to choose, all with typically similar efficacy. The choice of agent for an elderly patient is often determined by efforts to avoid side effects. Tricyclic antidepressants, for example, vary in the degree to which they induce anticholinergic effects—untoward reactions that can aggravate glaucoma, urologic dysfunction, or memory impairment. Desipramine and nortriptyline are the tricyclics typically selected for elderly patients, since they are lowest in anticholinergic potential.

The choice of drug also may depend on the presence or absence of other medical problems. For example, all antipsychotic agents have the potential to lower BP. If an older schizophrenic has episodes of hypotension, a neuroleptic that is less likely to lower BP may be a better choice. Unfortunately, a drug that is less likely to cause one type of side effect may be more likely to cause another. Geriatric psychotropic therapy is, actually, a matter of trade-offs within the broader benefit-vs.-risk framework.

Conclusion

Whether the focus is on normal aging or on psychiatric disorder, the physician must maintain a proper perspective on the capacity for change and the influence of time in the elderly. The paradox surrounding change and time in later life was poignantly captured by Somerset Maugham: "When I was young, I was amazed at Plutarch's statement that the elder Cato began at the age of 80 to learn Greek. I am amazed no longer. Old age is ready to undertake tasks that youth shirked because they would take too long."

86. GERIATRIC PSYCHIATRIC CONSULTATION SERVICES

Robert J. Nathan

Biomedical considerations alone are often insufficient for prevention, diagnosis, or treatment of serious medical problems, particularly in aged patients. These individuals often have multiple medical diagnoses, frequently live in unstable social situations with the potential for rapid change, and may have functional problems (eg, depression) or diminished cognition. The interrelationships among physiologic, psychologic, and social factors are complex. Recognition of the importance of these relationships has led to the establishment of specialized geriatric psychiatric consultation **(GPC)** services, using a team approach within the general hospital setting.

The **multidisciplinary** nature of the GPC team enables it to carry out the diverse tasks necessary for diagnosis and treatment and provides continuing education of the medical and nursing staffs. A key member is the **psychiatrist** skilled in geriatrics, whose role is to evaluate, diagnose, and treat the patient with psychotherapy, and make recommendations on medications and avoidance of unwanted drug-drug interactions. Recognizing drug overuse leading to delirious or dementia-like states can be critical in elderly patients, who take an average of 3 major nonpsychiatric agents concomitantly. Similarly, high doses of anticholinergic drugs (eg, diphenhydramine for sedation) can lead to confusion. A **family therapist** addresses problems involving the patient and his family, and a **psychiatric nurse specialist** addresses practical issues of nursing care with nurses in the hospital and care givers at home. When indicated, a **geriatric psychiatric social worker** may be enlisted to assist with patient placement and agency referrals, although frequently this can be done through the hospital social services department.

An elderly patient admitted to a general hospital experiences a multitude of stresses (eg, pain, anxiety, and fear of the unknown, as well as separation from familiar surroundings and people). Special efforts are required to reduce these stresses and to prevent or modify adverse reactions to the hospital milieu. Additionally, the possibility that medical illness may initiate or exacerbate psychiatric disturbances must always be considered. The **threshold phenomena of delirium and dementia** ("brain failure") can be seen most dramatically in the hospitalized elderly patient. For example, the patient admitted with a broken hip, who is in pain and immobilized, subjected to sensory deprivation or overload, isolated from familiar objects, and separated from important individuals, may well become confused and disoriented and perhaps suffer from hallucinations and agitation, even though he seemed stable prior to admission. Nonpharmacologic attempts to reduce the patient's level of anxiety and depression, together with early ambulation, frequent family visits, and bringing familiar objects into the hospital setting may help effect rapid resolution of the delirium.

Unfortunately, delirium frequently goes undetected unless agitation is part of the symptom complex. The clearly disoriented patient who screams and pulls out IVs rapidly receives a psychiatric consultation. In contrast, the delirious patient who lies immobile in bed, smiling and responding to auditory or visual hallucinations, too often is not perceived to be in distress. The distinction between physical and mental illness may be further obscured in very sick patients—eg, a severely cachectic, dehydrated, depressed individual who lives alone, is discovered and brought to the hospital for emergency admission. In such a patient, it is difficult to differentiate an occult neoplasm, perhaps with brain metastasis, from a major depressive reaction.

Recent studies have indicated that the most common reasons for GPC in a general hospital are depression, questions of adequacy of judgment, organic brain syndrome, and anxiety. Formal psychiatric diagnosis revealed that 40% of these patients had either dementia or delirium, 21% had affective disorders, and 22% had adjustment disorders. Of course, these findings apply to only a small percentage of elderly patients admitted to general hospitals. Numerous studies have indicated a lack of general medical awareness of mild dementia, even in its potentially reversible forms. Frequently, early signs are dismissed as "just old age." In addition, there appears to be an attitude of hopelessness among many physicians concerning treatment of obvious dementia. Dementia and delirium are discussed in Chs. 9, 80, 81, and 82.

AFFECTIVE DISORDERS

A major category of hospitalized elderly patients seen in psychiatric consultation includes those with a **major affective disorder** or an **adjustment disorder with depression.** Most patients referred for behavioral problems ultimately are diagnosed as having adjustment disorders, usually of the depressive type. This subset of patients has responded to acute or chronic physical illness by developing psychiatric symptoms. Intervention should be broader than simply encouraging compliance with medical procedures. Patients frequently can be helped by support and psychotherapy (eg, formal intervention between family and patient to discuss the illness). Family therapy can defuse the tension between patient, family, nurses, and house staff.

In the case of the dying patient, similar technics can be used; however, not every dying patient needs psychologic or psychiatric treatment. (See also Ch. 26.)

Small dosages of alprazolam (0.25 mg bid for up to a week) or oxazepam (10 mg tid) or use of tricyclic antidepressants can be a helpful therapeutic adjunct in this situation, but long-term effects are problematic. Certain psychostimulants (methylphenidate and, rarely, dextroamphetamine) can be used to predict the probable response to tricyclics and to provide a short-term elevation of mood.

In treating a major depressive disorder in medically ill individuals, one must exercise great care. Although both the tricyclic antidepressants and the monoamine oxidase **(MAO)** inhibitors are safe when used judiciously in medically stable elderly people, patients with cardiac disease or unstable BP (eg, a tendency toward orthostatic hypotension) require special attention. Many internists and cardiologists are apprehensive about using these drugs for fear of cardiac side effects. However, these drugs are reasonably safe when properly used in individuals without serious heart disease. The dilemma, of course, is that a patient who is experiencing a major depressive disorder will not thrive until the depressive disorder is substantially reduced. The inability to respond to rehabilitative efforts and the patient's and family's fear of chronic invalidism become proportionately greater with longer hospitalization. Frequently, patients with depression are viewed as hopeless: Their hopelessness spreads to the medical staff, and less attention is paid to them. Modification of the patient's environment by nursing staff and family can be of help, but the depressive process itself also needs modification, usually through pharmacotherapy.

The use of **ECT** in depressed patients on the medical floor has proved problematic because of resistance from either the patient, members of the family, or medical house staff. However, when proper attention is given to its relative contraindications and ECT is given under optimal conditions, it is frequently the fastest and most efficient form of antidepressant treatment.

A small percentage of elderly patients seen for evaluation are schizophrenics or have long-standing personality disorders and present special problems to the consulting psychiatrist. Once again, the GPC team approach produces better results than individual psychiatric treatment using drugs alone.

---

87. ANXIETY DISORDERS

Dan G. Blazer, II

The *Diagnostic and Statistical Manual of Mental Disorders* **(DSM-III)** delineates 3 broad categories of anxiety disorders: **phobic disorders, posttraumatic stress disorder,** and **anxiety states.** Although phobic disorders affect some older adults, the more severe phobias (eg, agoraphobia and social phobia) begin early in life and are more common in children and younger adults. There are few data regarding their course through adulthood into late life.

Post-traumatic stress disorder is a relatively new nosology, even though the impact of severe stress during childhood or young adulthood on future psychologic functioning has been known for many years. Most current research and therapy directed toward this disorder are derived from stress syndromes associated with war experiences and sexual abuse. Onset generally occurs in childhood or young adulthood; little is known about the continuance of this disorder into later life.

In contrast, **generalized anxiety disorder** is common in later life. The prevalence in community samples of older adults reaches 5%, making it one of the more frequent psychiatric problems experienced by the elderly. **Obsessive-compulsive disorder,** another anxiety state, also is common in later life, although severe symptoms (eg, compulsive hand washing) are not usually prominent. **Panic disorder** usually begins in late adolescence or early adult life, and the symptoms generally recede by later life. Some older adults report episodes of panic, but these are usually less severe than those occurring earlier in life and are often complicated by depressive symptoms or physical illness (eg, postural hypotension).

Diagnosis

A number of medical conditions present as anxiety and therefore are mistaken for generalized anxiety disorder. Hyperthyroidism with atypical presentation can be missed unless adequate laboratory screening for thyroid function is performed. Cardiac arrhythmias that produce palpitations and shortness of breath are common in later life and symptomatically may resemble a generalized anxiety disorder with periodic exacerbations and remissions. Pulmonary emboli may present as shortness of breath and feelings of anxiety.

Drugs may contribute to anxiety states. Caffeine ingestion is a frequent cause, as are OTC sympathomimetic drugs (eg, ephedrine). Anticholinergic agents may subtly impair memory, thereby producing secondary anxiety. Withdrawal from certain drugs, especially alcohol, anxiolytic agents, and sedative-hypnotics, may cause anxiety symptoms.

A number of psychiatric disorders may be associated with secondary anxiety. Delirium (acute organic brain syndrome) is often coupled with moderately severe anxiety and agitation, especially if the patient is in unfamiliar surroundings. Major depression also may be associated with anxiety and agitation. The elderly frequently complain of fear and anxiety that border on panic in the early morning, especially if they awaken in the dark, when others in the house are asleep. These symptoms tend to remit as the day progresses. Hypochondriasis may be accompanied by moderately severe generalized anxiety, although anxiety in the older hypochondriac is generally intermittent and less severe than in older persons with other psychiatric disorders.

Possibly the most common cause of secondary anxiety in the elderly is primary degenerative dementia. Early recognition of cognitive dysfunction and memory loss in individuals with continued social demands frequently leads to generalized anxiety, with periodic episodes of panic. This, in turn, contributes to social withdrawal and isolation. The severe and traumatic behavioral changes that result from this anxiety syndrome frequently mask the underlying dementia.

Occasionally, the anxiety reported by patients is actually **fear** (possibly appropriate). The syndrome may exhibit itself only in situations that threaten security. For example, some elderly persons fear being mugged while walking along the street, fear losing their way to the doctor's office or some other appointment, or fear driving on busy, crowded highways. When these stressful experiences are avoided, such individuals rarely complain of anxiety and, therefore, do not truly suffer from a generalized anxiety syndrome.

Once external causes of anxiety are eliminated, further history will help rule out other possible causes. For example, episodic anxiety reported by an older patient may resemble panic disorder. However, further questioning may reveal a syndrome that resembles postural hypotension, which can be verified by checking sitting and standing BPs. Other older adults may suffer from hypoglycemia, which can be confirmed by a 5-h glucose tolerance test. In some cases, agitation (ie, the inability to remain still) may resemble anxiety. However, the agitated older adult does not report the sense of impending doom and dread that characterizes anxiety.

To establish the diagnosis of generalized anxiety, one must determine that the patient manifests symptoms from at least 3 of 4 DSM-III categories: (1) **motor tension** (shakiness, jumpiness, trembling, inability to relax); (2) **autonomic hyperactivity** (sweating, palpitations, dry mouth, dizziness, hot or cold spells, frequent urination, or diarrhea); (3) **apprehensive expectation** (worry or anticipation of personal misfortune); and (4) **vigilance and scanning** (distractability, poor concentration, insomnia, "edginess"). Anxiety should persist at least 1 mo to qualify for diagnosis (and probably will require 6 mo in further revisions of the psychiatric nomenclature).

Treatment

Successful management of generalized anxiety in older adults requires a strong physician-patient relationship, counseling, family support, appropriate medication, and, of course, an accurate diagnosis. Once the diagnosis is made, the physician must intervene to correct potential organic causes; eg, if postural hypotension contributes to a sense of panic, an effort should be made to withdraw nonessential drugs that may contribute to hypotension. If BP is normal at baseline, more salt in the diet may assist in correcting the problem (see also Ch. 31).

Appropriate intervention for concurrent psychiatric disorders may alleviate symptoms of anxiety. For example, the treatment of major depression with an effective dose of an antidepressant is usually sufficient to eliminate any associated anxiety and agitation. If a more structured environment is provided for the mildly to moderately demented patient, the associated anxiety may also be corrected. If residual anxiety persists, however, the decision to prescribe an anxiolytic agent must be predicated upon the following: (1) suitability of the pharmacologic agent for generalized anxiety and (2) avoidance of drug interactions between currently prescribed therapeutic agents and the anxiolytic.

Pharmacologic treatment, a major component of the management of generalized anxiety, is often the source of difficulties for both patient and clinician. In general, the response of older adults to anxiolytic drugs is satisfactory but not exceptional. Most experience relief but not elimination of tension and agitation, and many symptoms persist. In addition, elderly persons often complain of the side effects associated with anxiolytic agents.

The drugs of choice are the benzodiazepines, unless a tricyclic antidepressant or monoamine oxidase **(MAO)** inhibitor is being prescribed for panic disorder. In general, elderly persons respond better to short-acting agents (eg, alprazolam or oxazepam) than to longer-acting agents (eg, diazepam). The dosage usually can be set at a lower level than for younger patients (eg, alprazolam 0.25 mg orally bid or tid). Unless the older person takes only 1 or 2 doses a day, it is better to use a fixed dosage schedule than to prescribe the medication prn.

If it is made clear from the outset that the drug is to be used for only a brief period, discontinuance is easier. Once benzodiazepines are used continuously for an extended time, discontinuance may be difficult. Nevertheless, periodic efforts should be made to withdraw the drug or at least to reduce the dose.

Clinicians must be especially vigilant for development of drug **side effects.** Patients should be monitored closely for drowsiness, ataxia, slurred speech, sleep disturbances, and depressive symptoms. Poor concentration and memory loss also may result from anxiolytics. Even if hospitalization is necessary to effect withdrawal, drug discontinuance is essential to control these side effects.

Antipsychotic agents (neuroleptics) should *not* be prescribed for generalized anxiety, except when symptoms are secondary to delusions or other signs of psychosis. Such drugs may produce side effects (eg, tremulousness, restlessness and agitation, especially akathisia) that can complicate the symptoms of generalized anxiety. The most serious side effect, however, is tardive dyskinesia, which is usually irreversible.

In addition to personal support, direct psychotherapeutic approaches are sometimes useful in correcting generalized anxiety. **Intensive psychotherapy,** unfortunately, is not as successful as might be hoped, and psychoanalysis has little to recommend it. Short-term, insight-oriented therapy, however, may be of some benefit, particularly in the elderly patient suffering from anxiety secondary to grief. Bereavement may be related to the loss of a loved one, or it may be associated with a sudden decline in physical health and a sense of loss of control over one's environment. **Supportive psychotherapy** may be an important adjunct in treating generalized anxiety in isolated and physically impaired older adults, whereas **structured cognitive therapy** has shown some benefit in alleviating panic attacks (in young adults). If anxiety is associated with specific phobic experiences and panic, **behavioral therapy** may be indicated.

Biofeedback may enable selected older patients to develop some control over symptoms of anxiety. In addition, a **paced exercise program**

can be especially helpful in those sensing loss of control over other areas of life.

---

88. HYPOCHONDRIASIS

Dan G. Blazer, II

The third edition of the *Diagnostic and Statistical Manual of Mental Disorders* as revised **(DSM-III-R)** lists 4 psychiatric disorders whose essential features are physical symptoms suggesting a physical disorder. They are, therefore, classified as somatoform disorders. These are **somatization disorders** (recurrent and multiple somatic complaints of several years' duration with onset at an early age), **conversion disorder** (hysterical neurosis, conversion type), **somatoform pain disorder** (pain in the absence of adequate findings of an organic etiology and with evidence of contributing psychologic factors), and **hypochondriasis** (morbid anxiety about health, usually with symptoms that cannot be attributed to organic disease).

Hypochondriasis is the somatoform disorder of most relevance to the elderly, with as many as 15% reporting their perceived impairment to be greater than their actual impairment. Many such complaints can be successfully managed by intermittent care. Although psychogenic pain disorder, which typically arises in mid-life, may persist into later years, pain generally remits somewhat with aging. Chronic low back pain may be more common in later life, but older patients are less likely to be found in pain-management clinics.

Symptoms, Signs, and Diagnosis

The major disturbance in hypochondriasis is the individual's misinterpretation of clinically insignificant physical symptoms or sensations as reflections of a disease state. As a result, the patient becomes preoccupied with these symptoms or sensations. A thorough physical and laboratory evaluation provides no evidence of an organic disease that might account for the nature or perceived severity of the complaints. Despite medical reassurance, unrealistic fears or beliefs persist about the existence of disease, causing impairment in the patient's social, occupational, and even recreational functioning.

Although hypochondriasis may be the sole disorder afflicting an older adult, hypochondriacal symptoms are reported by elderly persons suffering from depression, anxiety, dementia, and even a schizophrenia-like illness. To meet DSM-III-R criteria for hypochondriasis, however, the somatic complaints must not be secondary to any of these disorders.

By history, the clinician must determine the duration of the patient's symptoms, their pattern of occurrence (continuous or episodic), and the past history of medical or psychiatric illness. Because the hypochondriac is prone to prescription drug abuse, a thorough current and past medication history is essential.

Social functioning and self-care capacity also should be assessed to determine the extent to which the symptoms interfere with the patient's usual daily activities. The mental status examination **(MSE)** allows for the assessment of affect and degree of suffering or discomfort secondary to the physical symptoms. Because interference with functioning may be secondary to somatic preoccupation, repeated evaluations (especially for an inpatient) are indicated. Given the association of hypochondriacal complaints with suicide, the presence of suicidal ideation should be investigated during the interview.

A complete physical evaluation should include a rectal and pelvic examination during the initial visit. BP, both sitting and standing, must also be measured. Neurologic evaluation should include a thorough sensory examination of areas in which pain is reported, plus an assessment of possible frontal lobe signs, especially if the patient exhibits evidence of a dementing illness.

Laboratory testing should be kept to a minimum. Routine screening tests, eg, a chemical analysis, Hct, and urinalysis, are sufficient unless specific historical and physical findings indicate a need for additional laboratory data. A thorough medical record review prevents the duplication of expensive tests and procedures.

The distinction between hypochondriasis and depressive illness can be made by observing the patient over time and obtaining adequate historical information. Several distinctions exist. Despite reporting numerous symptoms, the hypochondriac does not appear to suffer as severely as the depressed patient. Furthermore, hostility in the depressed person is usually directed inward, whereas hostility in the hypochondriac is directed outward. Although both the hypochondriacal and the depressed older adult may exhibit social withdrawal, acute withdrawal is usually more pronounced in the latter.

Depressed persons retrospectively report far fewer somatic symptoms in mid-life (except if clearly associated with a physical disorder) than the hypochondriacal patient, especially if the depression began late in life. Depressive episodes (and their associated physical symptoms) also tend to be episodic, whereas hypochondriacal symptoms are more persistent. Finally, depressed patients tolerate the side effects of antidepressant drugs better than hypochondriacal patients do.

The older adult with mild-to-moderate dementia may present with somatic symptoms. However, these are usually reported as episodic problems, unlike the persistent complaints of hypochondriacal patients. Furthermore, the poor performance of hypochondriacs on the MSE is usually related to somatic preoccupation and, therefore, improves with repeated testing, in contrast to the consistently poor performance of demented individuals. Also, hostility, although often observed in hypochondriacs, is much less common in demented patients.

Treatment

Hypochondriacs should be recognized as being "ill," insofar as they truly experience either real or imagined pain and discomfort. Despite the frustration of working with such patients, empathy on the part of the clinician is essential to developing a therapeutic relationship. The expression of professional interest also is essential to the development of a consistent treatment plan.

Clinicians will better serve hypochondriacal patients and alleviate undue strain on the health care system if they commit themselves to working with these individuals rather than referring them indiscriminately to multiple specialists. *The most important treatment element is the development of a comfortable, long-term, doctor-patient relationship.* A structured approach to the care of these patients renders their care less troublesome than is usually imagined.

Clinicians should agree to see hypochondriacal patients on a regular basis. It may be necessary initially to schedule an appointment every other week, but usually the frequency of visits can be reduced to $\leq 12/yr$. A specified amount of time, usually about 20 min, should be allotted per visit and, as far as possible, appointments should be begun and terminated promptly. Such regular visits can meet the patient's need to be heard and to have control over his life.

During the visit, the clinician should obtain an interval history and perform a brief (5-min) physical examination. This examination usually includes determination of sitting and standing BPs, pulse rate, cardiac auscultation, and abdominal palpation. During the remainder of the visit, the patient should be encouraged to discuss personal and social issues that go beyond physical concerns.

Clinicians should avoid venturing a diagnosis or prognosis. Although hypochondriacs seek "an answer" to their problems, they rarely accept a diagnosis, either somatic or psychiatric. Most have had involvement with many physicians and either praise or criticize them to the current clinician. The physician must avoid either defending or criticizing these colleagues, focusing the patient's attention instead on his own frustrations, anxieties, and fears.

Promises to cure the patient's illness must also be avoided, since they are unrealistic. The hypochondriacal patient is chronically ill and improves only gradually. When therapeutic promises are not kept, both the patient and the clinician becomes frustrated. At such times, it is tempting to refer the patient elsewhere. Referrals should be made with reluctance, as they expose the patient to unnecessary costs and the risks of tests and treatments by specialists who do not know the patient as well as the primary care physician.

Finally, the clinician should avoid statements such as "It is all in your head." Hypochondriacs rarely benefit from such interpretations, even if they recognize some truth in them. Rather, such comments are likely to topple an already unsteady therapeutic relationship.

A number of therapeutic adjuncts are available for managing the elderly hypochondriacal patient. An exercise program, physical therapy, and massage may be very effective for patients with poor health habits, eg, lack of exercise and its attendant adverse effects on muscles and joints. Physical therapy for the hospitalized patient may also be very rewarding. If pain and tension are primary complaints, biofeedback may be especially helpful. For the homebound patient, nutritional programs, eg, Meals on Wheels or lunch programs at senior centers, can break the cycle of social isolation.

If specific psychologic issues emerge in the course of management, hypochondriacal patients may be referred for individual psychotherapy. These referrals do not replace management by the primary care physician, however, especially since hypochondriacs usually do not respond to relief from an emotional problem with dramatic improvement in somatic complaints.

Drug use must be carefully monitored. Many hypochondriacs are already taking multiple pharmacotherapeutic agents when they arrive at the next clinician's office. Immediate withdrawal of these drugs usually is impossible. Rather, the physician should begin with small adjustments (eg, slowly decreasing the dose of those drugs to which tolerance can develop). Hypochondriacal patients are usually willing to allow gradual withdrawal if the physician remains firm in the conviction to eliminate these drugs and is willing to withdraw them slowly. Whenever possible, potentially addicting hypnotics, antianxiety agents, and analgesics should be avoided. Rather, drugs such as L-tryptophan can be prescribed for sleep, and non-narcotic analgesics can be used for relief of pain.

If drugs are a major contributing factor to dysfunction, hospitalization may be necessary to achieve withdrawal. Use of antidepressant and antianxiety agents is reserved for specific symptoms that are targeted for improvement. If the drugs are not effective, they should be discontinued promptly.

---

89. DEPRESSION

Dan G. Blazer, II

Depressive disorders constitute one of the most frequent psychiatric problems experienced by older adults. The incidence of depressive symptoms in older persons in the community, when measured by traditional scales, ranges between 10 and 15%. The institutionalized elderly experience an even higher prevalence of symptoms. On the other hand, the prevalence of major depression in later life is lower than at other times. The risk for suicide, however, is higher for elderly white males than for any other age, sex, or racial group.

These findings, which have surprised both clinicians and epidemiologists, probably reflect a cohort effect: Specifically, the current cohort between the ages of 65 and 85 yr have, throughout adult life, experienced fewer severe depressive disorders than the cohorts that preceded them. Nevertheless, considering that the number of older persons has increased, the number of cases of depression has not fallen appreciably. Furthermore, the risk of suicide continues to be highest in the elderly (TABLE 89–1). We can expect a substantial increase in cases over the next 20 to 30 yr as younger cohorts, who have a higher prevalence of depression, advance in age.

Symptoms, Signs and Diagnosis

Depression is best understood as a group of disorders of variable severity. Many elderly persons suffer from **chronic** and **persistent dyspho-**

TABLE 89–1. SUICIDE AND AGING: SUICIDES/100,000 POPULATION BY AGE AND SEX (1979–1980)

Age (yr)	Male (%)	Female (%)
5–14	0.6	0.2
15–24	20.2	4.3
25–34	25.0	7.1
35–44	22.5	8.5
45–54	22.5	9.4
55–64	24.5	8.4
65–74	30.4	6.5
75–84	42.3	5.5
85+	50.6	5.5

Risk factors for suicide
Age > 55 yr
Male sex
Presence of painful or disabling physical illness
Solitary living situation
History of prior suicide attempts
Family history of suicide
History of drug or alcohol abuse
Depression, especially associated with agitation, excessive guilt, self-reproach, and insomnia
Debt or decreased income
Bereavement
Suicidal preoccupation and talk
Well-defined plans for suicide
Persistence of low mood toward the end of depressive illness, even though energy has returned

(Reprinted with permission from the American Geriatrics Society, "Suicide in late-life: Review and commentary," by D.G. Blazer, J.R. Bachar, and K.G. Manton, *Journal of the American Geriatrics Society*, Vol. 34, pp. 519–525, 1986.)

ria *(restlessness or malaise)*. However, the symptoms do not meet the criteria for **dysthymic disorder** listed in the third edition (revised) of the *Diagnostic and Statistical Manual of Mental Disorders* **(DSM-III-R)**: depressed mood and 3 additional symptoms, eg, sleep problems, decreased appetite, suicidal ideation, and lethargy. Rather, these individuals report a depressed mood with generally few accompanying symptoms. The dysphoric elderly have been labeled "the worried well," as they rarely require or benefit from traditional modes of therapy.

Some older persons suffer from a chronic, persistent, and moderately severe dysthymic disorder. Symptoms must persist for at least 2 yr to meet the DSM-III-R criteria for this diagnosis. Some sleep disturbance, anorexia, and lethargy may be present, but these symptoms are not severe enough to constitute a major depressive episode.

Other elderly persons may report severe symptoms that persist over brief periods, but these usually can be explained by obvious difficulties in adjustment or by bereavement. Adjustment to a severe or ultimately fatal chronic illness and the loss of a spouse are among the more common causes of such symptoms. Affected persons recover with time or when the stressor is removed.

Elderly persons may experience other depressive disorders that are not well codified in DSM-III-R. Although best labeled as **depressive disorders, not otherwise specified,** these episodes may be quite common in older adults. Specifically, they involve moderately severe depressive symptoms that are consistent with DSM-III-R criteria, except for their duration (2 wk). Although the symptoms have no clear etiology and resolve spontaneously, affected patients may experience these brief episodes in increasingly rapid cycles. Other persons experience mild-to-moderate depressive symptoms that otherwise meet the criteria for dysthymic disorder, except that the asymptomatic periods last for months and, therefore, 2 yr of persistent symptoms are never reported.

A small number of elderly persons experience frank, major depression with or without melancholia. **The core symptoms of major depression** include dysphoric mood plus at least 4 of the following symptoms: (1) sleep disturbance (usually decreased sleep), (2) appetite disturbance, (3) weight loss, (4) psychomotor retardation, (5) suicidal ideation, (6) poor concentration, (7) feelings of guilt, and (8) lack of interest in usual activities. **Melancholic depression** exists if these symptoms are accompanied by a total lack of interest in the environment, diurnal variation, and psychomotor agitation or retardation. In a few individuals, major depression is characterized predominantly by psychotic thinking, especially delusions of illness or guilt regarding the past. Generally, the symptoms are similar in older and younger populations. Exceptions include a relative increase in psychotic symptoms and a decrease in sense of self-worth and in guilt in older adults.

The differential diagnosis of major depression includes the many medical and psychiatric illnesses that may present in later life as depression. For example, an idiopathic primary sleep disorder, while mimicking the sleep difficulties found in depression, can result in a reactive (secondary) depressive affect due to sleep deprivation. During the early stages of primary degenerative or multi-infarct dementia, a depressive affect may predominate. *Major depression and dementia often coexist,* with the usual course entailing remission of the depressive symptoms but persistence or worsening of the cognitive deficit.

Hypochondriacal symptoms are also often associated with a depressive affect. The gradual onset of the syndrome, coupled with the hypochondriac's lack of apparent distress, helps confirm the diagnosis of this somatoform disorder. Certain **physical illnesses** (eg, hypothyroidism and occult malignancy, especially carcinoma of the pancreas) frequently present as depressive symptoms. Depression secondary to pharmacologic treatment of hypertension is also frequently encountered.

The diagnosis of depression hinges on a thorough history and physical examination. A review of presenting symptoms against the patient's lifestyle and previous medical and psychiatric history often permits the physician to make an accurate diagnosis. If the patient is retarded or uncommunicative, a history obtained from the family is essential. The physical examination must include a complete neurologic evaluation. Presence of frontal lobe signs (eg, the palmomental reflex) helps to differentiate dementia from depression.

The laboratory serves an adjunctive role in the evaluation of depressed patients. Although not diagnostic, the **dexamethasone suppression test (DST)** may help to identify the specific depressive subtype. A positive DST, ie, a post-dexamethasone cortisol of > 5 μg/dL, is highly suggestive of endogenous or melancholic depression. **Polysomnography,** when available, can help identify melancholia as well. Decreased sleep time with shortened rapid eye movement **(REM)** latency provides diagnostic support.

Treatment

Treatment of the major melancholic depressions is primarily pharmacologic. Discovery of the tricyclic antidepressants in the late 1950s (first imipramine, then amitriptyline) marked a milestone. Although numerous antidepressants have been developed since then, the increased therapeutic efficacy of the newer agents is marginal. The choice of agent depends primarily on which drug produces fewer or less severe side effects rather than on any unique therapeutic property of the drugs. Older adults have difficulty tolerating the anticholinergic effects of these agents or the postural hypotension they are inclined to induce. Nortriptyline has relatively few side effects and has been used increasingly in the treatment of late-life depression. Desipramine and doxepin are also widely used. Monoamine oxidase **(MAO)** inhibitors are less frequently used.

Usual starting doses in otherwise healthy elderly are lower than in younger persons. For example, the daily starting dose for amitriptyline is 50 to 70 mg; for nortriptyline, 25 to 50 mg; for desipramine, 25 to 50 mg; and for doxepin, 50 to 75 mg. If possible, the entire dose should be given before bedtime to avoid daytime drowsiness. Although the dose can be increased gradually, the maintenance dose again is usually lower than that required in mid-life. Some drugs, eg, amitriptyline, nortriptyline, and desipramine, can be monitored effectively by plasma levels. A significant response usually occurs in 2 to 3 wk, and a total response in 5 to 6 wk. Sleep improves immediately. In recurrent unipolar depression and recurrent bipolar disorder, lithium carbonate (300 to 900 mg daily) may be prescribed prophylactically.

Some severely depressed patients respond only to **electroconvulsive therapy (ECT)**. These individuals typically include patients who have previously responded to ECT, who demonstrate significant psychotic symptoms or self-destructive behavior, or who do not tolerate or respond to tricyclic antidepressants. ECT is safest when performed with multiple-channel monitoring (EEG, ECG, BP, pulse, and respiratory function) under the supervision of an anesthetist or anesthesiologist and a psychiatrist. Improvement with ECT in persons who do not respond to antidepressant drugs reaches 80% in most studies, and is the same in the elderly as in younger patients.

Although some persistent memory loss can develop following ECT, the nature and extent of this problem remain to be elucidated. The acute amnesia that accompanies ECT is often most disturbing to the older patient who is already preoccupied with cognitive and somatic functioning.

Psychotherapy also is effective in the treatment of depression. Common sense and numerous empiric studies suggest that psychotherapy is most effective in those persons experiencing major nonmelancholic depression. Behavioral and cognitive therapies are considered more effective than nondirected or analytically oriented therapies. Psychotherapy may have a beneficial effect, even in persons with severe depression. Initial efficacy may be as great in inpatients as in outpatients. Finally, psychotherapy may be especially valuable in preventing relapses of episodic depression.

90.   ALCOHOL ABUSE AND DEPENDENCE

Dan G. Blazer, II

As the older population increases, more adults are at risk for developing significant alcohol-related problems. Such problems in the elderly are likely to increase with the aging of currently middle-aged persons who have used more alcohol throughout their adult lives than previous cohorts. The current prevalence of alcohol abuse and dependence in persons > 65 yr of age ranges from 2 to 5% for men and to about 1% for women. This prevalence is lower than that for younger persons, in whom abstinence is less common than in the elderly (with > 50% of older men and women reporting abstinence in a national survey). The risk factors for alcohol-related disorders, however, are similar in both populations: genetic predisposition, male sex, poor education, low income, and a history of psychiatric disorders, especially depression.

Growing concern about alcohol consumption in the elderly relates not to patterns of use but to physiologic changes that accompany aging and pose problems in the presence of regular alcohol consumption. Given the relatively complete absorption of alcohol by the older adult, the smaller volume of distribution, and increased organ dysfunction, older adults with persistent drinking patterns are subject to more toxic effects.

Secondary Problems

Malnutrition may result from chronic alcohol use, especially in heavy drinkers. **Cirrhosis** is one of the 8 leading causes of death in the > 65-yr-old population. The elderly chronic alcoholic who develops compromised hepatic function may also develop **osteomalacia** because of compromised metabolism of vitamin D. Alcohol abuse can also contribute to the development of **cardiomyopathies** and **atrophic gastritis.** Probably the most frequent and serious problem, however, is the associated **decline in cognitive status.** Acute alcohol abuse is associated with a variety of neuropsychologic and cognitive deficits. Although intelligence remains relatively unaffected, memory and information processing may decline remarkably with chronic alcohol intake. The cumulative effect of these physical and cognitive changes is marked impairment in most individuals who survive beyond middle age.

The central clinical problem in the older alcoholic, however, is the potential for **addiction and tolerance** to alcohol, with concomitant **withdrawal symptoms.** The relatively "quiet" use of alcohol over many years desensitizes the individual and his family to these problems. Therefore, the addiction may not be recognized. Interactions with other agents, especially benzodiazepines, leading to CNS depression, is of major clinical concern. Typically, addiction becomes evident when the older patient is placed in a setting where alcohol is not readily available. The patient exhibits increased anxiety, sleep problems, nausea, and weakness, secondary to a lower blood-alcohol level. If withdrawal continues without intervention, anxiety and agitation progress to a tremulous state within 1 to 2 days, followed by the onset of more severe symptoms, including hallucinations and, in some cases, withdrawal seizures (ie, delirium tremens).

Diagnosis

The diagnostic assessment hinges on a thorough **history.** Although specifics about drinking behavior should be obtained initially from the patient, such information must be supplemented by family members, preferably from at least 2 generations. Unfortunately, however, many older alcoholics have little or no social network (eg, the so-called skid-row alcoholic) and historic information is limited.

Information should be obtained first about the form in which alcohol is consumed and how often the patient drinks (ie, continually or in binges). While tolerance for binges decreases with age, guilt or concern about drinking also becomes less common. Frequently, patients may not recognize the connection between new symptoms and drinking habits that have been present for decades.

Psychiatric symptoms that may accompany alcohol abuse should be reviewed in detail. For example, major depression and alcohol abuse frequently coincide. Paranoid ideation involving relatives or friends is not uncommon in the elderly alcoholic. It is critical that suicidal ideation be documented, given the increased risk of suicide in both elderly persons and alcoholics.

If evidence of cognitive abnormalities emerges on the **mental status examination,** additional assessment is indicated. The clinician must make every effort to keep the patient abstinent for 2 to 3 wk prior to the detailed psychologic evaluation. Although scores may reveal little or no impairment, this evaluation provides a baseline for monitoring future changes in mental status.

During the **physical examination,** the clinician must screen for medical problems that may aggravate the effects of alcohol abuse or vice versa, and note direct signs of alcoholism, such as neglect of personal hygiene. A detailed neurologic examination should be performed, with attention directed to the evaluation of peripheral neuropathy. Traditional signs of chronic alcohol abuse (eg, flushing, injected conjunctiva, tremors, and malnutrition) often merge with the normal signs of aging or poor general health.

Laboratory evaluation should include standard liver function studies (LDH, AST [SGOT], ALT [SGPT], and alkaline phosphatase). Because electrolyte imbalance is common in the chronic alcoholic, a chemical screen with attention to glucose and Mg is also important. The ECG may suggest the presence of cardiomyopathy, which may be associated with arrhythmias, especially atrial fibrillation.

Treatment

Initial treatment is focused on restoring fluid and electrolyte balance during withdrawal from chronic alcohol use. Complaints of thirst and dry mucous membranes may suggest a diagnosis of dehydration, when in fact the drying may result from exhaled alcohol. To avoid overhydration, the clinician should begin administering 500 to 1000 mL 0.45% NaCl solution while awaiting results of blood chemistry studies. Glucose solutions should be *avoided,* since the older alcoholic may have been subsisting on a diet high in carbohydrates as well as on alcohol. In such cases, stress from glucose can produce clinically significant hyperglycemia. Dietary intake must be supplemented with IV vitamins, especially B vitamins. Chronic alcoholics also may suffer from Mg deficiency. A deep IM injection of 50% $MgSO_4$ solution in a dose of 0.1 to 0.15 mL/kg is an important adjunct to initial therapy.

After fluids are begun, the clinician must give medications that are cross-tolerant with alcohol. Chlordiazepoxide was preferred in the past because of its relatively extended half-life and clear cross-tolerance with alcohol. **Diazepam,** however, is probably the current drug of choice, given its high therapeutic-to-toxic effects ratio. Doses, based on the patient's height and weight, should be carefully monitored during the first 1 to 2 days of withdrawal. The usual starting dose is between 10 and 40 mg diazepam/day, divided into 4 equally spaced doses. Adequate dosing is confirmed by the elimination of delirium, agitation, and hallucinations without excessive sedation. Although most patients withdrawing from alcohol should be hospitalized, outpatient withdrawal is possible if there are no major medical problems and if symptoms are monitored daily by the clinician and responsible family members.

Following detoxification and withdrawal, treatment focuses on the long-term goal of **abstinence.** Therapeutic support helps to maintain abstinence, as does the use of prophylactic **disulfiram.** This drug should be prescribed only in healthy patients and, if used, a contract must be established between the physician, the patient, and usually 1 family member. All three agree that the family member is responsible for giving disulfiram, the patient for taking it, and the physician for prescribing it. If this is not possible, the local emergency room can provide the disulfiram each day.

Self-help groups provide essential long-term support for abstinent alcoholics. **Alcoholics Anonymous (AA)** has proved to be the most effective of these groups in encouraging ongoing abstinence. Older persons, however, frequently resist participating in the program, partly because they continue to deny their problem or believe themselves capable of correcting it alone. The self-sufficient attitude of many older adults reinforces this negative view of support groups. Nevertheless, if the patient can be encouraged to participate in such groups, the opportunity for success is improved dramatically.

---

91. SCHIZOPHRENIA AND SCHIZOPHRENIFORM DISORDERS

Dan G. Blazer, II

Suspiciousness, persecutory ideation, and paranoid delusions are frequently seen in cognitively impaired or emotionally distressed older adults. Between 2 and 5% of elderly persons in the community exhibit excessive suspiciousness and persecutory ideations. The prevalence of delusions and hallucinations reaches 4 to 5% in older persons, and these symptoms are frequently disabling. Nevertheless, the prevalence of schizophrenia, as defined by the *Diagnostic and Statistical Manual of Mental Disorders* **(DSM-III),** is only around 0.1% in later life. The primary reason for this is that DSM-III diagnostic criteria require that psychotic symptoms have their onset at an early age; ie, < 45 yr. If the age criterion is removed (as in DSM-III-R, the revised version), the prevalence is somewhat higher, although accurate prevalence estimates are not available.

Although current nomenclature does not help in the differential diagnosis of schizophrenic-like symptoms in the elderly, investigators and clinicians who have worked with older adults generally agree upon 4 relatively distinct syndromes: (1) abnormal suspiciousness, (2) transitional paranoid reactions, (3) late-life paraphrenia *(severe paranoid illness without deterioration of other cognitive or affective processes)* or paranoia associated with schizophrenia of late onset, and (4) acute paranoid reactions secondary to affective illness.

Symptoms, Signs, and Diagnosis

Most older adults who exhibit **abnormal suspiciousness** do not come into contact with mental health professionals. However, they frequently have medical problems and are often seen by the primary-care physician or geriatrician. These patients offer vague complaints of external forces controlling their lives. Occasionally, these beliefs become focal, often addressed toward their children; eg, such older persons believe they have been deserted by their children or that the children have plotted to obtain control of their finances or property. Perception of a loss of control, coupled with an inability to evaluate the social milieu, provides sufficient grounds for the development of this suspicious behavior.

Clinicians also encounter **suspiciousness associated with memory loss and attention deficits.** Institutionalized persons suffering from dementia are often suspicious of both family and staff. Their accusations are usually disjointed, unfocused, and unaccompanied by sustained emotional distress. Complaints about objects being stolen, medicines being swapped, and the misbehavior of attendants are common. Symptoms derive from the patient's inability to organize environmental stimuli and comprehend the frequently confusing activities of the hospital or long-term care facility. Whether an underlying paranoid personality contributes to excessive paranoid behavior in persons with dementia is not known.

Transitional paranoid reactions are narrow, focal, and situational. They are usually manifested in women who live alone and believe in plots against them. The focus of their hallucinations and delusional thinking usually moves gradually from outside the home to inside it, from complaints of noises in the basement and attic to reports of physical abuse or molestation. Hence, a transition can be observed from external threats to total violations of property and person. Social isolation and perceptional difficulties contribute to transitional paranoia.

Paraphrenia is not accepted by all investigators as a distinct syndrome. Those who do distinguish the syndrome emphasize that the condition **is primary and not secondary to an affective illness nor to an organic men-**

tal disorder. In addition, the gross disturbances of affect, volition, and function experienced by the schizophrenic patient are not prominent. Nevertheless, paranoid delusions and hallucinations are almost invariably present. The course of paraphrenia in later life may be chronic, but deterioration to the extent observed in schizophrenia or Alzheimer's disease is not characteristic. The boundaries blur not only between late-life paraphrenia and classic paranoid schizophrenia, but also between the transitional paranoid state and paraphrenia.

Persons suffering from late-onset paraphrenia often report plots against them, their focus once again being on family members. In contrast to mild suspiciousness, these plots are persistent, extreme, and elaborated. No cognitive impairment is noted. Although the paraphrenic is physically independent (diet and hygiene are rarely compromised), social functioning and cooperation with health care providers is greatly impaired. Such a person rarely speaks for long without referring to the symptoms of concern.

Clear association of late-onset paraphrenia with the female sex, social isolation, or previous personality type has not been established. Nevertheless, paraphrenics usually *are* female, live alone, and have exhibited evidence of difficult social interactions earlier in life. In contrast to schizophrenics, however, these persons are warm, friendly, and trusting, especially when they are interviewed in their own home and are not threatened with the diagnosis of a psychiatric disorder.

Treatment

The clinician caring for the paranoid older adult must establish a trusting and supportive relationship. Displays of respect, a willingness to listen to complaints and fears, and availability by telephone are essential. Most elderly persons do not abuse telephone privileges and are generally willing to wait for the physician to return a call.

Effective management also requires **antipsychotic drug therapy.** Initial dosages may range from 10 to 25 mg/day of thioridazine, 2 to 4 mg/day of thiothixene, or 1 to 3 mg/day of haloperidol. The choice of agent is determined by the side effects the clinician wishes to avoid. Thioridazine is especially troublesome in patients with postural hypotension, whereas haloperidol may create significant problems in those inclined to develop parkinsonian symptoms. Although each of these agents can cause tardive dyskinesia, those that are less likely to produce parkinsonian side effects are thought to be also less provocative of this problem.

Most elderly persons are willing to take an antipsychotic drug if told that the drug will help to improve sleep and decrease anxiety. Compliance is often problematic but less so in later life than earlier. Even paranoid elderly persons are usually trusting of their clinicians and willing to adhere to therapy. If objections occur, the family may be able to help. A strong objection to medication or other interventions may suggest the need for hospitalization if symptoms are severe.

The clinician must establish a relationship with key persons in the patient's social environment. Family members are often the first to notice a deterioration in the patient's condition and, therefore, the first to contact the physician when a problem arises. Police officers, neighbors, and pharmacists also can serve as valuable allies. If these persons understand the paranoid behavior, they will contact the physician or family when appropriate but will not overreact to such problems. However, physicians clearly must maintain standards of privilege and confidentiality when talking to family, neighbors, and friends.

The clinician should not—at least initially—confront the patient with the lack of reason and false assumptions inherent in paranoid ideation. Such an attack is of no value and may disrupt the therapeutic relationship. On the other hand, the clinician must not deceive the patient by pretending to agree with the paranoid beliefs. Rather, a desire should be expressed to better understand what is troubling to the patient and to work together despite any disagreement as to the source of the problem. A desirable goal is to develop a level of confidence that permits an examination of the patient's beliefs.

§3. ORGAN SYSTEMS: SKIN DISORDERS

---

92. SKIN CHANGES AND DISORDERS

Tania J. Phillips and *Barbara A. Gilchrest*

Numerous changes occur in the skin and skin appendages of aging individuals. Some changes are due to the aging process itself, and others, to the cumulative effects of exposure to sunlight or environmental factors. These changes often cause common skin disorders.

AGE-ASSOCIATED CHANGES IN NORMAL SKIN AND SKIN DERIVATIVES

The structural and functional changes that occur with age are summarized in TABLES 92–1 and 92–2.

Hair Changes

Gray hair is seen in approximately 50% of the population at age 50 yr. However, the widespread availability of color rinses and permanent dyes may make this figure seem lower.

Frontotemporal hair loss (androgenic alopecia) in men can start in the 3rd decade; by the 7th decade, 80% are substantially bald. In women, the same pattern of hair loss may be seen after the menopause.

TABLE 92–1. STRUCTURAL CHANGES IN THE AGING SKIN

Epidermis	Flattening of dermal-epidermal junction Variation in size, shape, and staining properties of basal cells Decreased number of Langerhans cells Decreased number of melanocytes
Dermis	Decreased thickness Decreased cellularity and vascularity Degeneration of elastin fibers
Appendages	Decreased number and distorted structure of sweat glands Loss of hair bulb melanocytes

TABLE 92–2. FUNCTIONAL CHANGES IN AGING SKIN

Altered skin permeability
Decreased inflammatory reactions
Decreased immunologic responsiveness
Impaired wound healing
Decreased eccrine sweating
Decreased elasticity
Decreased vitamin D production
Impaired sensory perception

Diffuse alopecia can be caused by iron deficiency or hypothyroidism, so these conditions should be excluded when indicated. Certain drugs, chronic renal failure, hypoproteinemia, and severe inflammatory skin disease such as erythroderma, can also cause diffuse alopecia.

Hair loss with scarring is not associated with aging alone. It can be caused by deep bacterial or fungal infections; by granulomatous disorders, eg, sarcoidosis, tuberculosis, or syphilis; and by inflammatory disorders, eg, lichen planus and cutaneous LE. Cicatricial pemphigoid is a chronic bullous eruption that affects mucous membranes and sometimes the scalp. Biopsy of the scalp is usually necessary to make any of these diagnoses.

Treatment: Topical minoxidil solution, applied to the bald areas of the scalp daily, causes hair regrowth in 25 to 30% of balding patients. However, cosmetically significant regrowth occurs in < 10%. Hair transplantation can be performed by a variety of technics, including one that involves the transplantation of punch grafts from the occipital hair-bearing areas to the bald temporal areas. The cosmetic results of this procedure can be enhanced by scalp reduction.

Excessive facial hair occurs in many older women. In fair-skinned women, these hairs can be bleached; they also can be removed by tweezing, waxing, or electrolysis. Men frequently have too much facial hair in the nares, eyebrows, or helix of the ear. Trimming the hairs with iris scissors usually produces adequate cosmetic results.

Nail Changes

Nails change with age in quality, shape, and color. They become dry and brittle and perhaps flat or concave instead of convex in cross section. Color can vary from yellow to gray. Occasionally, the nails become grossly thickened and distorted, a condition known as **onychogryposis.**

Treatment: For the patient's comfort, a podiatrist should trim thickened toenails with an electric drill and burrs or a CO_2 laser. Gloves should be worn during housework and laundry to protect brittle fingernails. Nails should be kept short, and use of nail polish removers, which dehydrate the nail, should be minimized. Brittle or discolored nails cannot be treated effectively.

PATTERNS OF CHANGE AND DISEASE

Skin changes in the elderly result from a combination of aging and the effects of cumulative environmental damage. In the USA, most visible cosmetic changes are due to chronic ultraviolet irradiation in sunlight and hence occur in areas that are habitually exposed. Skin of nonexposed areas, such as the buttocks, usually looks younger than that of habitually exposed areas, such as the face; older individuals whose pigmentation or life-style protects them from sun damage are often said to look younger than their chronologic age. Similarly, skin cancer in the elderly is photodistributed, being most common on the face and neck in both sexes and on the helix of the ear and the bald scalp in men.

Other skin diseases common in the elderly tend to occur in chronically occluded areas, where skin-skin apposition leads to compromised barrier function.

PHOTOAGING

Aging of the skin caused by chronic exposure to sunlight.

Prevention of photoaging is most successful if preventive measures are begun in childhood, but anecdotal evidence suggests that considerable clinical improvement can be achieved by avoidance of sun exposure and regular use of sunscreens, even after marked actinic damage has occurred.

Patients concerned with their appearance should be advised to avoid going outdoors unprotected when ultraviolet irradiation is the strongest, around midday. Sunscreens with a sun protection factor $\geq$ 15 should be applied liberally over all exposed skin and reapplied after swimming or washing. Patients should be encouraged to apply sunscreen as part of their daily routine, eg, after brushing their teeth in the morning. Because sunscreens also block ultraviolet-induced vitamin D formation in the skin, patients should be advised to consume dairy products or vitamin D supplements to prevent osteomalacia.

Treatment: Preliminary studies suggest that topical tretinoin (all-*trans*-retinoic acid) can partially reverse the structural damage caused by excessive exposure to sunlight and may, therefore, be useful in the treatment of photoaging. New capillary formation, new collagen synthesis, decreased elastosis (dermal collections of abnormal elastin), regularization of epidermal melanin distribution, and the disappearance of premalignant actinic keratoses have all been observed in volunteer subjects after 6 to 9 mo of daily tretinoin application. Clinically, more improvement is seen in patients with slight to moderate sun damage than in those with severe photoaging.

Initial treatment is with tretinoin cream 0.05%, applied once daily for 8 to 12 mo. The patient should be warned that erythema and peeling of treated areas will occur. If necessary, frequency of application can be reduced to every other day. Tolerance usually develops after 4 to 6 wk. After 8 to 12 mo, a maintenance regimen of applications on weekends only has been recommended. Further treatment of photoaging (TABLE 92–3) should be supervised by a dermatologist or plastic surgeon.

COMMON SKIN DISORDERS

Many common skin conditions affect younger and older adults equally, while others are restricted to children and young adults. Certain inflammatory diseases, infections, and neoplasms of the skin increase in prevalence with age. The disorders discussed here occur commonly but not exclusively in the elderly.

Management Principles

The patient should be questioned about topical home remedies, such as alcohol and detergents that may be causing or exacerbating the skin condition. Additionally, it is often helpful to ascertain the patient's concept of the condition and expectation of therapy.

Management of skin conditions must be tailored to individual patients and their physical capabilities. Many elderly patients live alone, have substantial limitation of motion because of neurologic impairment or arthritis, and often find it difficult to bathe and apply topical medications. Regimens that are virtually trouble free for younger patients, such as the use of oil in bath water, may be dangerous for the elderly.

Physicians should prescribe treatment regimens that are as simple as possible, since according to some surveys, 25 to 50% of elderly patients fail to take prescribed medication and 59% make medication errors. Moreover, the elderly are 2 to 3 times more likely to experience adverse reactions to antihistamines and corticosteroids, drugs that are often used to treat skin disorders. These agents should be prescribed with caution.

TABLE 92–3. TREATMENT OPTIONS FOR PHOTOAGING CHANGES

Skin Change	Treatment
Wrinkles	Collagen injections; chemical peels (phenol or trichloroacetic acid); rhytidectomy (face lift)
Solar lentigines Pigmented macules on sun-exposed areas (liver spots, age spots)	Light freezing with liquid N; hydroquinone 5% (bleaching cream); low-dose CO_2 laser or argon laser
Poikiloderma of Civatte Reddish-brown reticular pigmentation on the face, neck, and upper chest	—
Cutis rhomboidalis nuchae Thickened, yellow, furrowed skin on the back of the neck	—
Nodular elastoidosis Thickened, yellow skin with large comedones and follicular cysts	Comedo expression with extractor; curettage or excision of cysts
Senile purpura Large persistent bruises from minimal trauma	—
Vascular lesions **Venous lakes** Purplish macules or plaques on the face, lips, or ears	Electrocautery or argon laser
Senile angiomas Bright red papules that blanch easily on pressure	As above
Telangiectasia Dilated, tortuous superficial capillaries	As above
Sebaceous hyperplasia Soft, yellowish facial papules	Excision or cautery

Most agents used to treat dermatologic conditions are applied topically, and the choice of **base** in which the active agent is present is important. **Ointments,** *greasy preparations containing little water,* are most useful in treating conditions in which the skin is dry, scaly, or thickened. These agents are rarely irritating but may cause maceration of occluded areas. **Creams** are *semisolid emulsions of water in oil.* They are more cosmetically appealing than ointments, since they tend to vanish when rubbed into the skin. Because they tend to dry the skin, they are often useful in treating exudative conditions but may irritate inflamed skin. Most creams contain stabilizers or preservatives that can induce allergic sensitization when applied to broken skin. **Lotions** are usually *suspensions of fine powder in an aqueous base.* They are useful in cooling and drying the skin, especially when there is acute inflammation or oozing. **Soaks or compresses,** consisting of *gauze soaked in water, saline, aluminum acetate, or magnesium sulfate solution,* are useful in soothing and drying acutely "weeping" lesions.

BENIGN TUMORS

Many benign skin tumors are commonly seen in the elderly. They must be distinguished from malignant tumors, and the psychologic distress they often cause must also be recognized.

Seborrheic keratoses (seborrheic warts): These common, waxy, raised, verrucous lesions vary in color from flesh tones to dark brown or black and in size from barely perceptible papules to large verrucous plaques. **Dermatosis papulosa nigra** is a variant of seborrheic keratoses occurring exclusively in blacks, in which the face may be studded with numerous small dark papules that may be pedunculated.

Curettage and light cautery constitute one treatment modality. Freezing the warts with liquid N for 15 to 20 sec is another. Sometimes, light freezing of seborrheic keratoses prior to curettage makes them easier to remove.

Acrochordons (skin tags) are small, benign papillomas commonly found on the neck, axillae, and trunk in middle-aged and elderly people. They are flesh colored or pigmented, soft, and often pedunculated. They may be removed with sharp scissors or a scalpel or by an electrocautery cutting current.

Keratoacanthomas present as rapidly enlarging nodules, smooth in outline, with a central keratin plug. If not treated, they usually resolve spontaneously but may leave a scar. Further, they may be difficult to differentiate from squamous cell carcinoma.

Although the characteristic appearance and histology of the keratoacanthoma identify it as a benign lesion, most authorities believe it should be managed as a well-differentiated squamous cell carcinoma. The tumor is usually removed by curettage and cautery or by excision, especially if squamous cell carcinoma is suspected.

PREMALIGNANT CONDITIONS

Actinic keratosis appears as well-defined, scaly, sandpaper-like patches on sun-exposed areas of the body. If the diagnosis is doubtful, a skin biopsy is warranted, since actinic keratosis may evolve into squamous cell carcinoma. However, there is a long latent period, and the squamous cell carcinoma that develops usually grows very slowly and has little metastatic potential.

The patient should be advised to avoid sun exposure and to use a high-potency (SPF 15) sunscreen when outside. Cryotherapy with liquid N for 10 to 15 seconds or curettage and light cautery of lesions under local anesthesia are useful treatment methods if lesions are not numerous. Topical 5-fluorouracil **(5-FU)** can also be used, especially when there are multiple lesions. A 1 or 2% 5-FU solution or 1% 5-FU cream can be used for lesions on the face. Stronger concentrations of 5-FU cream (5%) can be applied to lesions on the trunk. The cream or solution should be applied once or twice a day, and care should be taken to avoid the eyes and mucous membranes.

The patient should be informed that treatment with 5-FU is not acceptable to all because it produces prolonged erythema and burning sensations. The usual response to treatment is increasing erythema, vesiculation, and finally ulceration after 2 to 4 wk, followed by reepithelialization over an additional 2 wk. Treatment should be discontinued once ulceration occurs. Application of a topical steroid cream may reduce the acute inflammation. Complete healing usually occurs by 2 mo.

Pain and burning sensations may be decreased, especially on sensitive areas such as the face, by first applying a 1 or 2% 5-FU solution and then applying a moderate-potency steroid cream 15 to 20 min later. This procedure can be repeated daily for 3 wk. Tretinoin cream can be combined with 5-FU, especially if lesions are present on more resistant areas such as the limbs or trunk.

Bowen's disease presents as a persistent, erythematous, scaly plaque with well-defined margins. It can occur anywhere on the skin or mucous membranes. The patient may have a history of arsenic exposure (either medicinal or occupational) in youth. Multiple lesions have been associated with an increased incidence of internal malignancies and mandate close follow-up.

Treatment consists of cryotherapy with liquid N for 15 to 20 sec or curettage and cautery. Topical 5-FU, applied as for actinic keratoses, is another option.

Radiotherapy can also be used, but full-tumor doses are necessary.

MALIGNANT SKIN TUMORS

Basal and squamous cell carcinomas are the most common malignant skin tumors. Both are strongly associated with environmental exposure to ultraviolet light, although ionizing radiation and chemical carcinogens are also predisposing factors.

BASAL CELL CARCINOMA (BCC)

The typical BCC or "rodent ulcer" has a pearly appearance, rolled edges, and telangiectasia on its surface. Other types include the so-called superficial or multicentric BCC, which is a scaly plaque with a raised pearly edge. Pigmented BCCs are sometimes mistaken for malignant melanoma. If not detected and treated early, BCC may invade deep tissues and ulcerate, possibly destroying bone and cartilage, especially around the eyes, nose, and ears. However, BCCs rarely metastasize. More than 90% of these lesions are found on the head and neck, although they can occur on any part of the body that has been exposed to ultraviolet light, irradiation, or other predisposing factors.

Treatment

The size of the carcinoma, depth of invasion, and the patient's history determine treatment modality. All BCCs should be confirmed histologically, preferably prior to the initiation of therapy.

Curettage and cauterization can be used to treat small tumors. The tumor should be curetted and cauterized at least twice to ensure complete removal. Cryotherapy is also effective in treating small lesions; usually, 2 freeze-thaw cycles are used.

The **tumor can be excised,** with primary closure or a split-thickness skin graft, if necessary, to cover the defect. Moh's chemosurgery can be used for large, recurrent, or high-risk BCCs. With this technic of staged excision, the entire tissue margins are examined histologically as surgery proceeds, ensuring complete tumor removal and permitting maximum sparing of noninvolved tissues.

Radiotherapy can be used in elderly patients in whom surgery might be undesirable or in cases of carcinoma recurrence following surgery. **Topical 5-FU** can be used to treat superficial BCCs under extraordinary circumstances, such as when tumors are extremely numerous. Recurrence rates following this type of treatment are high, and close follow-up is warranted to ensure that no carcinoma remains.

All patients with BCC should be closely followed for recurrence or development of new lesions for at least 5 yr. Statistically, patients stand a 1-in-3 chance annually of developing recurrence.

SQUAMOUS CELL CARCINOMA

These tumors usually arise in sun-damaged skin, although up to ¼ occur in sites of chronic inflammation, persistent ulceration (eg, long-standing lupus vulgaris, chronic venous ulcers, and SLE), or radiodermatitis. Fair-skinned people, who are not protected by melanin, have a higher incidence of the tumor. The earliest signs of malignant change are usually erythema and induration. The overlying epidermis may become scaly or hyperkeratotic, and ulceration occurs later.

Squamous cell carcinomas may also present as persistent nonhealing ulcers. In addition, such lesions of the vermilion border of the lip, the pinna, and the genitalia are more likely to metastasize than those found elsewhere, eg, on the face and limbs.

Treatment

The diagnosis must be confirmed by biopsy. Well-differentiated tumors are generally treated surgically or by local destructive measures, while poorly differentiated tumors are treated by radiotherapy. Although radiotherapy may be more suitable for elderly patients who cannot tolerate anesthesia, it usually entails multiple treatments that might present problems for those with limited mobility.

Surgical excision, extending at least 5 mm beyond the tumor borders, is used to treat small, well-differentiated tumors. Squamous cell carcinomas that recur in sites previously treated with another modality (eg, radiotherapy) can also be excised surgically.

Cryotherapy, which does not require anesthesia, can also be used to treat small tumors. The tumor, together with a margin of normal tissue, should be frozen, and 2 freeze-thaw cycles should be used. Although cryotherapy is useful in fair-skinned patients with small multiple lesions, healing can be prolonged in elderly patients.

Radiotherapy is generally used for poorly differentiated tumors of the head and neck and for tumors that recur after surgery. Although the cosmetic results of radiotherapy may be inferior to those obtained with surgery, it may be preferable for elderly patients in whom surgery is contraindicated. Radiotherapy is not used to treat tumors on the dorsa of the hand, since it may leave friable scars.

MALIGNANT MELANOMAS

Lentigo Maligna (Hutchinson's Freckle) and Lentigo-Maligna Melanoma

Lentigo maligna is *a pigmented macular lesion, often > 1 cm in diameter, with an irregular border, predominantly on sun-exposed areas (most commonly, the cheeks and forehead).* Pigmentation is characteristically varied, with brown, black, red, and white areas often found in a single lesion. Lentigo maligna enlarges, becoming progressively irregularly pigmented over time.

Development of nodules signifies invasion and conversion to lentigo maligna melanoma. This form of melanoma appears to be relatively indolent and is usually diagnosed as a comparatively thin lesion associated with favorable survival. In patients with lentigo maligna, the risk of developing melanoma by age 75 yr is estimated to be 1.2%. The case fraction of lentigo maligna melanoma among all melanomas is 5 to 10%, with a mean age of 67 yr at diagnosis.

A biopsy is necessary to confirm the diagnosis. If a nodule is present, it should be included in the specimen. Multiple biopsies, simultaneously or sequentially, are often indicated.

Treatment of lentigo maligna melanoma usually consists of a wide local excision, with a skin flap or split-thickness skin graft to repair the defect. The patient with lentigo maligna should be followed regularly to detect any changes (eg, irregular pigmentation, nodularity, or bleeding) that might signify malignant development. Some authorities recommend prophylactic surgical excision; others suggest cryotherapy or argon laser therapy to decrease the number of abnormal melanocytes, although high recurrence rates are associated with the latter technics.

Superficial Spreading Melanoma

This lesion accounts for about 60% of all melanomas. Although the incidence of this melanoma peaks in middle age, its age-specific incidence increases at least through the 8th decade. It can occur on any part of the body and presents as a pigmented plaque with an irregular border and variable pigmentation. Like all melanomas, it is usually asymptomatic. Itching and bleeding are associated with advanced lesions.

Nodular Melanoma

This melanoma accounts for about 15% of all melanomas and occurs in a wide age range of patients. It can be seen on any body site and is often diagnosed as a small but enlarging, darkly pigmented papule. Rarely, the melanoma may be amelanotic and therefore pink.

A deep excisional or incisional biopsy should be performed whenever melanoma is suspected. Histologic interpretation should be performed by an experienced dermatopathologist, and confirmed cases should immediately be referred to a dermatologist or other physician experienced in melanoma management.

Current treatment recommendations for superficial spreading or nodular melanoma are as follows: for low-risk lesions, excision with 1- to 2-cm margins; for intermediate to high-risk lesions, excision with 3-cm margins and removal of at least 1 cm of underlying subcutaneous fat. Removal of all palpably enlarged lymph nodes has also been recommended, but prophylactic lymphadenectomy appears to be without benefit. Close long-term follow-up of patients with melanoma is essential; they should be seen every 6 or 12 mo for life. The **prognosis** for patients with all types of melanoma depends primarily on the tumor's depth of invasion, not on the histologic type (TABLE 92–4).

KAPOSI'S SARCOMA

The typical presentation is an indolent tumor most commonly seen in elderly patients of central European origin, especially men of Jewish or

TABLE 92–4. PROGNOSIS FOR PATIENTS WITH MELANOMA
(ALL TYPES)

Melanoma Depth*	Prognosis
<0.85 mm	Highly curable; 99% of patients disease free at 8 yr
0.85–1.69 mm	Low risk of metastasis; 93% of patients disease free at 8 yr
1.70–3.64 mm	Moderate risk of metastasis; 67% of patients disease free at 8 yr
>3.65 mm	High risk of metastasis; 35% of patients disease free at 8 yr

* Measured from skin surface to point of deepest tumor invasion as evaluated in vertical cross sections.

Italian ancestry. One or more purple or dark blue macules appear on the legs and slowly enlarge to become nodules or ulcers. Histologically, the tumor cells are of endothelial origin; proliferating vessels and connective tissue cells are also present.

Simple excision or radiotherapy can be performed if the lesions are symptomatic. In the elderly, this tumor grows slowly and seems to be benign. **The lymphadenopathic form of Kaposi's sarcoma,** an aggressive tumor with a poor prognosis, is associated with acquired immune deficiency syndrome **(AIDS).**

PRURITUS

(Itching)

Itching is a common complaint in the elderly. Patients should be examined for inconspicuous primary skin lesions that might be causing symptoms. Systemic disorders that may be associated with generalized pruritus in which primary lesions are absent include liver and renal disease, iron deficiency anemia, lymphomas, leukemias, and polycythemia rubra vera. Some drugs (eg, barbiturates) can also cause itching. Other disorders associated with itching include diabetes mellitus, hyperthyroidism, and solid tumor malignancies. In research studies, an underlying disorder has been identified in up to $1/2$ of patients presenting with generalized pruritus. However, underlying conditions are less likely to be the cause of pruritus in most patients seen in clinical settings.

Treatment

The elderly pruritic patient who has no obvious skin disease should be examined for clinical clues to systemic disorders, such as lymphadenopathy, hepatosplenomegaly, jaundice, or anemia. Relevant screening tests include a CBC, ESR, electrolyte and urea levels, and liver function tests. Urine should be tested for glucose, and if indicated by history or examination, stool should be tested for blood, ova, and parasites. Suspicion should be highest and laboratory evaluation most thorough when symptoms are severe, unrelenting, and sudden in onset.

All patients complaining of pruritus should be treated for xerosis (dry skin), since even mild dryness can exacerbate itching of any etiology. Patients should also be advised to avoid very hot baths or showers, as well as bath additives and major tranquilizers, since these may pose dangers to the elderly and are rarely of sufficient benefit to justify the risk.

XEROSIS

(Dry Skin)

This is a common cause of pruritus in the elderly. Symptoms are often worst in the winter, when central heating decreases humidity indoors and skin is exposed to cold and wind outdoors.

Clinically, the skin is scaly, especially over the lower legs, forearms, and hands. The stratum corneum barrier may be compromised by fissures or excoriations, allowing environmental irritants to penetrate the skin and progressively worsen the condition. This complication of xerosis is called **erythema craquelé** or **asteatotic eczema.**

Treatment

Patients should be advised to keep the air in their home as humid as possible. They should avoid using strong soaps, rubbing alcohol, detergents, and other drying agents whenever possible. Bathing should be restricted to once a day, and a mild soap should be used. Potentially irritating materials next to the skin (such as wool) should also be avoided.

Emollients should be applied frequently and liberally, especially after bathing, when the skin is still moist. A wide variety of lubricating agents is available, from cosmetically elegant lotions to greasy ointments. White petrolatum jelly is an inexpensive and effective lubricant.

A mild topical corticosteroid ointment is useful in treating eczematous dry skin. It should be applied bid or at night with an occlusive dressing. Creams containing urea or lactic acid are also often helpful in keeping the skin hydrated and preventing symptoms.

SKIN INFECTIONS

The decline of the immune function that occurs with age is reflected in a higher incidence of certain chronic skin infections, such as tinea pedis. The compromised tissue perfusion and inherently slower healing of wounds in aging skin may explain the increased tendency toward bacterial superinfection of wounds in older persons.

BACTERIAL INFECTIONS

Impetigo

A superficial skin infection caused by staphylococci or streptococci. Vesicles or pustules in the early stages break down to form golden brown crusts that often adhere to the underlying skin. If the infection is extensive, malaise, fever, and lymphadenopathy may also be present. Impetigo often occurs as a secondary infection in conditions characterized by a broken cutaneous barrier to microbes (eg, eczema, senile pruritus, pediculosis, nodular prurigo, and herpes zoster).

Treatment

Single small lesions can often be managed by soaking them for 10 min with drying agents such as Burow's solution (aluminum acetate 5%). Extensive lesions require systemic antibiotics to reduce the risk of glomerulonephritis and to prevent this contagious condition from spreading. A skin swab should be taken for microbial culture and sensitivity assays.

Patients with **streptococcal pyoderma** should be treated with penicillin V 250 to 500 mg orally qid for 10 days. If the patient cannot be relied upon to take oral medication, it may be necessary to administer long-acting penicillin G benzathine 1.2 million u. IM. If the patient is allergic to penicillin, erythromycin 250 to 500 mg orally qid can be given. Patients with **staphylococcal pyoderma** should receive dicloxacillin 250 to 500 mg orally qid for 10 days.

Staphylococcal Scalded Skin Syndrome (SSSS)
(Lyell's Syndrome)

A severe, extensive bullous condition caused by staphylococcal infection of the skin, in which the epithelium lifts off in sheets to leave large denuded areas. Although this is generally a disease of young children, the condition is increasingly reported in immunocompromised adults. In elderly patients, staphylococci can usually be cultured from the skin as well as from the blood, and death usually occurs from septicemia. **Toxic epidermal necrolysis (TEN)**, a drug reaction that can produce an identical clinical picture, must be considered in the differential diagnosis.

Both these conditions are life threatening and require hospitalization. In differentiating between SSSS and TEN, the level of cleavage should be determined by taking a skin scraping or skin biopsy, which can be examined by frozen section. In SSSS, there is cleavage within the epidermis, just below the granular layer. In TEN, there is subepidermal blister formation, with damage of the basal cells. Differentiation between the 2 conditions is important because SSSS must be treated immediately with penicillinase-resistant antistaphylococcal antibiotics.

Treatment

Therapy is the same as for severe burns, with immediate replacement of fluid and electrolytes. Systemic antibiotics (oxacillin 250 to 500 mg qid, orally in the early stages, but IV for severe cases) should be given promptly. The source of infection may be difficult to isolate, but cultures should be taken from skin, blood, nares, and any other suspected sites. Topical silver sulfadiazine cream may help prevent cutaneous superinfection with gram-negative bacteria. The prognosis is poor.

Erysipelas

A superficial infection of the skin caused by Group A or Group C hemolytic streptococci. The organisms can enter the skin through minor cuts, wounds, or insect bites.

Swelling and erythema of the affected area may be seen. Lesions have well-defined margins that advance as the infection spreads. Vesicles or bullae may be present, and in the elderly, hemorrhage may occur. Fever, malaise, and lymphadenopathy may also develop.

Treatment

Penicillin V or erythromycin 250 to 500 mg orally qid should be given for 2 wk. Because the infection continues to spread during the first 12 to 24 h of oral therapy, patients with facial lesions often require hospitalization and IV antibiotics to prevent cavernous sinus thrombosis.

Cellulitis

A deep infection of the skin, most frequently caused by Group A streptococci, although gram-negative organisms have also been implicated. In the elderly, cellulitis most commonly occurs as a complication of an open wound, such as a venous ulcer. It also develops in areas of intact skin where edema is present, such as the lower limbs. Erythema, tenderness, swelling, and warmth of the affected area may be noted; lymphadenopathy may also be present.

Treatment

Penicillin or erythromycin 250 to 500 mg orally qid should be given for 2 wk. In some patients, cellulitis is slow to respond to antibiotics, and prolonged treatment is required.

FUNGAL INFECTIONS

Chronic fungal infections are common in the elderly, and the age-related diminution of cutaneous immunologic responses discussed earlier in this chapter may be partly responsible for this.

Tinea Pedis
(Athlete's Foot)

An infection usually caused by the dermatophytes Trichophyton mentagrophytes *and* T. rubrum. Infection usually begins in the interdigital spaces and may spread to the plantar surface and the toenails. The patient may complain of itching and scaly skin in the affected areas, or the condition may be asymptomatic. Web space maceration is common, and the risk of secondary cellulitis caused by gram-negative organisms merits therapy.

Diagnosis is made by scraping scale from an affected area and placing it on a glass slide with a drop of 20% potassium hydroxide (KOH) solution under a cover slip to observe the characteristic greenish fungal hyphae.

Treatment

Miconazole 2% or clotrimazole 1% creams can be used topically. Treatment may be required for several months or indefinitely to prevent recurrence. Nails will not respond to therapy with antifungal creams. Oral griseofulvin is effective but rarely indicated because it occasionally causes GI upsets, skin rashes, leukopenia, headaches, and vertigo.

Good foot care is important. Interdigital spaces should be dried well after the feet are washed. Patients should be encouraged to wear open footwear and to apply medicated powder or cotton pledgets between the toes to absorb the moisture that predisposes them to the infection.

Tinea Unguium

A fungal infection, usually caused by T. rubrum *or* T. mentagrophytes, *that affects the toenails more often than the fingernails.* The nails may become grossly thickened and so enlarged that wearing shoes may become painful.

Treatment

Fungal nail infection treatment is prolonged and rarely warranted. However, the fingernails may be treated with griseofulvin 500 to 1000 mg/day for 6 to 9 mo, while toenails require 12 to 18 mo of therapy. The overall cure rate is 40 to 70%. Although fingernails are more likely to respond to treatment than toenails, recurrence within 1 yr is common. In elderly patients whose main problem is discomfort, conservative management—ie, periodic clipping and trimming of the nails by a podiatrist—may be the most practical approach.

Tinea Cruris

A cutaneous fungal infection of the groin. Elderly patients are commonly affected. Predisposing factors include clothing made of synthetic fabrics that do not "breathe," obesity, and immobility.

The patient usually complains of itching, and examination may reveal scaly erythematous areas with well-defined margins. Maceration, lichenification, and secondary candidal or bacterial infection are common. A KOH smear, as described above, should be performed for diagnosis.

Treatment

Topical miconazole 2% cream or clotrimazole 1% cream should be used bid or tid. Affected areas should be kept as clean and as dry as possible.

YEAST INFECTIONS

Candidiasis

An infection caused by the yeast Candida albicans, *which thrives in warm, moist areas such as the groin, the axilla, and the submammary region.* Patients receiving systemic antibiotic therapy, diabetics, and those who are immunosuppressed are at increased risk. Because the organism may be carried asymptomatically in the bowel, mouth, and vagina, these sites may be sources of reinfection of treated sites.

Candidal vulvovaginitis presents with pruritus vulvae, vulvar erythema and edema, and a creamy vaginal discharge. Patients with these signs should be tested for glycosuria.

Oral candidiasis (thrush) is characterized by creamy white plaques on the tongue or buccal mucosa; the plaques can be scraped off easily.

Perlèche (angular cheilitis) is *a mixed bacterial and candidal infection of the corners of the mouth.* The skin appears moist, cracked, and fissured. Predisposing factors include deep folds at the corner of the mouth, poorly fitting dentures, and retention of saliva and food particles in the affected areas.

Treatment

Clotrimazole 1% or miconazole 2% cream can be applied tid for **vulvitis.** For **vulvovaginitis,** a 100-mg clotrimazole tablet can be inserted intravaginally once a day for 7 days. Nystatin vaginal suppositories can also be used (2 tablets of 100,000 u. each inserted high into the vagina each night for 14 nights). Nystatin cream should then be applied to the labia, perineum, and perineal area, after which the hands should be washed thoroughly.

To treat perlèche, or oral candidiasis, both nystatin and amphotericin B, available as mouthwashes or lozenges, can be used qid. Dentures, if worn, should be soaked in nystatin suspension, since they are invariably contaminated with *Candida albicans.* Miconazole 2% or nystatin cream tid for 1 wk usually produces rapid local improvement.

Intertrigo

Dermatitis, usually caused by yeasts, that occurs between 2 folds of skin, eg, between the buttocks, the thighs, the scrotum and the thigh, etc. Intertrigo often presents as moist, red, and sometimes scaly and pruritic areas in the flexures. The patient may complain of intense itching or soreness of the skin from the groin to the perineum, inner thighs, and intergluteal cleft. Contributing factors include obesity, poor personal hygiene, and clothing made of synthetic fabrics that do not "breathe."

Intertrigo is often accompanied by superinfection with *Candida,* and direct examination with KOH may reveal the characteristic budding yeasts and pseudohyphae.

Treatment

Affected areas should be kept as dry as possible. Topical antifungal creams (eg, clotrimazole 1% or miconazole 2%) should be applied tid. Nystatin cream, another anticandidal agent, is not effective against dermatophytes. Where inflammation is severe, a mild topical steroid cream (eg, hydrocortisone 1%) can be applied tid. Some available commercial preparations combine a topical corticosteroid cream with an antifungal agent.

TINEA INCOGNITO
(Steroid-Modified Tinea)

Fungal infections modified by topical or systemic corticosteroids.

Fungal infections appear to improve if treated with topical corticosteroids, in that inflammation is suppressed and there is loss of scaling. However, attempts to discontinue the steroid result in flares. With prolonged use of steroids, striae, atrophy, and telangiectasia may be superimposed on the original dermatitis. KOH preparations are floridly positive.

Treatment

Topical antifungal agents are used, as above. If a potent topical corticosteroid has been used, it may be necessary to progressively wean the skin by gradually reducing the number of corticosteroid applications to minimize the rebound flushing and fixed vasodilation seen in steroid-dependent skin.

VIRAL INFECTIONS

Herpes Zoster
(Shingles)

An acute eruption caused by reactivation of latent varicella virus in the dorsal root ganglia of a partially immune host.

Herpes zoster may occur at any age, but the peak incidence occurs between ages 50 and 70 yr and the age-specific incidence increases throughout life. It usually affects otherwise healthy individuals, but immunosuppressed patients are at higher risk. The major difference between herpes zoster in the elderly and in the young adult is the incidence of postherpetic neuralgia, which increases sharply with age to approximately 40% in those $\geq$ 60 yr of age. Significantly, the duration and severity of discomfort increase even more markedly with age than does incidence.

Symptoms and Signs

The patient may develop prodromal symptoms of chills, fever, malaise, and GI disturbance, as well as paresthesia or pain along the affected dermatome. Rarely, prodromal symptoms persist for 5 to 7 days, leading to a variety of misdiagnoses, from herniated disk to acute abdomen. Usually, within 3 days red papules are seen along a dermatome. These rapidly develop into vesicles, which vary in size and may be hemorrhagic. The eruption may be extremely painful. After about 5 days, the vesicles begin to dry and form scabs, with gradual healing occurring over the next 2 to 4 wk. Persistent hyperpigmentation or true scarring may result, particularly in the elderly.

In about 50% of patients with uncomplicated herpes zoster, some vesicles are present outside the affected dermatologic area. However, *if there is widespread severe dissemination, one should suspect and look for an underlying lymphoma or other causes of immune deficiency.*

Ophthalmic herpes zoster results from involvement of the ophthalmic division of the trigeminal nerve. Conjunctivitis, iridocyclitis, and keratitis may occur, and an ophthalmologic consultation should always be sought in these cases. Lesions on the tip of the nose indicate involvement of the nasociliary and ophthalmic nerves.

Geniculate zoster (Ramsay Hunt syndrome) results from involvement of the geniculate ganglion. Facial paralysis (usually temporary) occurs, and pain develops in the ear on the affected side, with loss of taste in the anterior ²/₃ of the tongue. Vesicles are present on the soft palate, fauces, and external auditory meatus on the affected side. Consultation with a neurologist is advisable.

Diagnosis

Biopsy or the presence of multinucleate giant cells on a cytologic smear of a vesicle confirms the diagnosis. The virus can be identified by electron microscopy and by vesicle fluid cultures, although false-negative results are common with the latter.

Treatment

Systemic corticosteroids (prednisone 40 to 60 mg/day), initiated within the first week of the eruption, appear to reduce both acute symptoms and the risk of postherpetic neuralgia in elderly patients. Corticosteroids are the treatment of choice in patients with geniculate herpes (Ramsay Hunt syndrome).

If the patient is seen early in the course of the eruption, preferably within 3 days of onset, IV or oral acyclovir is appropriate. This drug has been shown to reduce both the development of new vesicles and the duration of viral shedding and discomfort. It does not appear to influence the risk of postherpetic neuralgia. The recommended oral dosage is 400 to 800 mg 5 times daily for 7 days. The IV dosage is 5 mg/kg q 8 h for 5 days.

Analgesia is usually necessary to relieve the pain. Simple analgesics, such as aspirin, given regularly q 4 h, may be sufficient, but some patients require much more potent medications. The use of opiates should be avoided, if possible, especially in the elderly, because of the increased risks of adverse reactions and medication errors.

Topical treatment consists of soaking the affected areas in Burow's solution (aluminum acetate 5%) to clean away vesicle crusts, decrease oozing, and dry and soothe the skin. *The aluminum acetate solution is diluted 1:20 to 1:40 for use.* Gauze dressings are soaked in the solution, applied to the affected areas, and loosely bandaged. The dressings are removed after 2 or 3 h and then reapplied. If impetigo develops, systemic antibiotics should be given (see under BACTERIAL INFECTIONS, above).

PARASITIC INFESTATIONS

Scabies

An eruption caused by a mite, Sarcoptes scabiei. The female mite burrows into the skin and deposits eggs, which hatch into larvae in a few days. Scabies is easily transmitted by skin-to-skin contact and can be rapidly spread between members of the same household, nursing home, or institution.

Symptoms and Signs

The patient experiences intense pruritus. On examination, the skin is usually excoriated. The characteristic sign is the burrow—a linear ridge with a vesicle at one end—where the mite is usually found. Burrows are commonly found in the interdigital webs, the flexor aspects of the wrists, the axillae, and the umbilicus; around the nipples; and on the genitalia. Erythematous papules or nodules in the same areas are even more common.

In the elderly, scabies may present less typically, especially if it has been untreated for a long time. The condition may mimic eczema or exfoliative dermatitis, because widespread thick crusted lesions are present. The patient may have erythroderma and generalized lymphadenopathy.

Diagnosis

The mite at one end of a burrow can be excavated with a needle or a scalpel blade and examined under a microscope. However, in long-standing cases with widespread excoriations, a mite may be impossible to find. Therefore, treatment based on a presumptive diagnosis may be the best option.

Treatment

A lotion or cream containing lindane 1% (eg, Kwell®) should be applied to the entire body, from the neck down. The patient must understand that no areas can be missed and that assistance will be required in applying the medication. After 24 h, the patient should bathe; all clothes and bed linens should be machine-laundered in hot water or dry cleaned. Any household member or close personal contact should also be treated. In a nursing home, *all* clinical staff and patients and their household contacts should be treated, to avoid spreading scabies to individuals as yet asymptomatic.

A second application of the cream or lotion, also left on the body for 24 h, is indicated 7 days later to ensure that any newly hatched larvae are killed. The itching may not subside for 1 to 2 wk after the patient has been treated. However, itching can be effectively treated with topical corticosteroids or, in very severe cases, with a tapering course of oral corticosteroids.

Pediculosis

(Lice)

Lice may infest the head *(Pediculus humanus capitis)*, the body *(P. humanus corporis)*, or the genital area *(Phthirus pubis)*. Elderly people who have little interest in personal hygiene or who live in overcrowded surroundings are at risk for head and body lice.

Pediculosis capitis is transmitted through personal contact or through shared hairbrushes and head wear. The patient develops severe itching of the scalp, often with secondary eczematous changes and impetiginization. Cervical lymphadenopathy may also be present. On examination, small gray-white nits (ova) are seen on the hair shafts. Unlike scales, they cannot be easily removed. Adult lice are not usually found on the scalp.

Pediculosis corporis produce intense generalized itching. The patient frequently develops eczematous changes, severe excoriations, and secondary bacterial infection. Lice or nits may be found in the seams of the patient's clothing.

Pediculosis pubis is usually transmitted by sexual contact, but can be transferred on clothing or towels. Lice and their eggs should be carefully searched for at the base of pubic hairs. Sometimes dark brown particles (louse excreta) may be seen on underclothes.

Treatment

For head lice, shampoo containing lindane 1% is applied to the scalp and left in place for 4 min. After rinsing, the hair should be combed with a fine-tooth comb. The procedure should be repeated in 10 days to destroy any remaining nits. Combs and brushes should be soaked in the shampoo for 1 h.

For pubic lice, 1% lindane shampoo is applied to the pubic area for 4 min, then rinsed off. This treatment should be repeated in 10 days.

For body lice, the patient's clothing should be boiled, dry cleaned, or washed in a machine (hot cycle). The seams of the clothing should be pressed with a hot iron. Alternatively, the clothing can be disinfected with an insecticidal powder such as DDT 10% or malathion 1%. Eczema and/or infection should be treated appropriately.

DERMATITIS

(Eczema)

The terms *eczema* and *dermatitis* are often used interchangeably or in combination. Both imply *superficial inflammation of the skin due to irritant exposure, allergic sensitization (delayed hypersensitivity), and/or genetically determined idiopathic factors.* Pruritus, erythema, and edema of the skin are present, progressing to vesiculation, oozing, crusting, and scaling. If the process persists, the skin may eventually become thickened or lichenified, with prominent skin markings.

Surveys of skin conditions in the elderly have shown that dermatitis of unknown etiology is a common diagnosis (specific types are discussed separately, below). The patient complains of pruritis. The skin is often excoriated, and there may be papules and lichenified areas. The skin frequently is dry, with fine scaling.

Treatment

Patients should avoid any practice or product that might irritate the skin, such as excessive use of soaps and detergents. Clothing made of nonirritating fabrics such as cotton should be worn next to the skin. Emollients should be used liberally, especially after bathing. (See XERO-SIS, above.)

Corticosteroid ointments of moderate potency should be applied tid to affected areas. This helps relieve pruritus and control inflammation. Emollients should be applied between applications of steroid ointments if the skin remains dry. Once symptoms are alleviated, use of the topical corticosteroid can be reduced and often discontinued in favor of emollients alone.

Antihistamines may reduce pruritus and help the patient sleep. However, these agents must be used with caution in elderly patients, since they sometimes produce paradoxical agitation. Phototherapy with ultraviolet light in the 290- to 320-nm range (UV-B) or PUVA is sometimes effective but is often inconvenient for the patient. Therefore, it is not usually considered as a treatment option until all other modalities have failed.

DERMATITIS VARIANTS

Nummular Dermatitis
(Discoid Eczema)

Intensely itchy, annular, scaly patches that first appear on the limbs before becoming widespread. Discoid, or nummular, eczema occurs in middle-aged and elderly patients. There is no apparent precipitating cause.

Lichen Simplex Chronicus
(Neurodermatitis)

A localized pruritic condition resulting from repeated scratching. This condition is common in the elderly. The patient complains of itching, and the sites affected are readily accessible for scratching, eg, the lateral part of the ankle, dorsum of the foot, shin, back of the neck, forearm, and elbows. Clinically, the affected sites are well circumscribed, lichenified, or thickened, and have accentuated skin surface markings.

Treatment

Topical corticosteroids of moderate-to-strong potency are often required to control symptoms, after which the potency can be reduced.

Intralesional corticosteroids, such as triamcinolone 5 mg/mL (2 to 5 mg total dose) are often helpful for the more troublesome lesions. Tar-containing preparations (eg, Estar®Gel, Zetar®Emulsion) also may relieve symptoms.

Lesions at some sites, such as the forearms or legs, can be occluded for a week at a time with an Unna's boot. This helps to break the itch-scratch-itch cycle, producing considerable improvement after 1 wk. Phototherapy may alleviate symptoms when other treatments have failed.

SEBORRHEIC DERMATITIS

A scaly, erythematous eruption that affects the central part of the face, eyebrows and eyelids, nasolabial folds, postauricular and beard area, scalp, and body flexures. The central chest and interscapular areas can also be affected. Seborrheic dermatitis affecting the eyelids causes a blepharitis and sometimes an associated conjunctivitis. Despite its name, seborrheic dermatitis appears to have nothing to do with sebum.

Treatment

Seborrheic dermatitis of the scalp can be effectively treated with various shampoos. Active ingredients include sulfur (eg, Selsun®, Exsel®), zinc pyrithione (eg, Head and Shoulders®), salicylic acid and sulfur (eg, Sebulex®), and tar (eg, T-Gel®, Zetar®, Sebutone®). The scalp should be shampooed frequently, daily if necessary, and the product left in contact with the scalp for the recommended interval, usually 5 min. Elderly patients for whom shampooing is inconvenient or physically impossible can use topical steroid lotions instead. Such lotions applied to the scalp bid are helpful in severe cases. Hydrocortisone 1% lotion is often sufficient, but many fluorinated corticosteroid preparations are available as well.

For seborrheic dermatitis of the face and trunk, hydrocortisone 1% cream applied bid or tid is usually effective. Preparations containing sulfur and those containing salicylic acid are also helpful. **Seborrheic blepharitis** can be treated with hydrocortisone 1% cream. If there is associated conjunctivitis requiring treatment with sulfur/prednisolone suspensions (eg, Cetapred®, Blephamide®), ophthalmologic supervision to monitor intraocular pressures may be helpful.

CONTACT DERMATITIS

Skin inflammation caused by contact with irritant or allergenic substances.

Irritant Contact Dermatitis

This is the most common form of contact dermatitis, resulting from contact of the skin with strong chemicals or other irritants. Although the elderly have a less-pronounced inflammatory response to standard irritants than do younger patients, chronic irritant dermatitis is frequently seen in the older age group. This may be because of slower, muted cutaneous reactions that are less obviously related to the contactant, thereby encouraging repeated exposure.

Allergic Contact Dermatitis

Patients may develop delayed, cell-mediated hypersensitivity to a variety of substances that come into contact with the skin. Although older persons are less readily sensitized to experimental allergens, such as dinitrochlorobenzane, they can develop allergic contact dermatitis. Common sensitizers include nickel (found in jewelry), chromates (used in tanning leather), wool fats (particularly lanolin, which is found in many moisturizers and skin creams), rubber additives, topical antibiotics (typically, neomycin), and topical anesthetics, such as benzocaine or lidocaine. Areas of eczema appearing at the site of contact with the irritant or allergen may be acute, with vesiculation and edema, or more often chronic, with scaling and erythema.

Treatment

The patient should avoid contact with strong soaps, detergents, solvents, bleaches, etc. The involved skin should be lubricated frequently with emollients. A thorough history should be obtained, since it may reveal unrecognized exposures to irritants or allergens.

Acute eczema with blistering should be treated with soaks of aluminum acetate (Burow's solution) in a 1:20 dilution qid. Topical corticosteroid creams or lotions are helpful once the blistering subsides. For more chronic eczema, the patient should use emollients frequently and apply a moderately potent corticosteroid ointment tid (see DERMATITIS, above).

If contact dermatitis is suspected, the patient should be referred to a dermatologist. A detailed history and careful examination may be helpful in identifying the offending allergen. If necessary, **patch testing** can be performed to identify the causative agent. This involves applying a battery of standard potential allergens and other suspected allergens the patient may be using (eg, cosmetics) to the skin on the back. These test patches are left in situ for 48 h; the skin is then examined 20 min after the patches have been removed and 4 days later. A positive test is indicated by erythema, edema, and often vesiculation at the test site appearing 2 days after the patch has been applied and persisting for 4 days. Particularly in the elderly, however, clinical changes may not be apparent until 4 days after testing.

Once the agent causing the reaction has been identified, it should be avoided as far as possible. All documented cutaneous allergies should be carefully noted on the patient's chart since systemic exposure (eg, via prescription drugs) to chemically related compounds may result in systemic allergic reactions.

IDIOPATHIC HAND ECZEMA

Persistent erythema and scaling of the palms or lateral digits in the absence of an obvious precipitating factor. Skin scrapings should be examined for mycelia to exclude a fungal infection. Patch tests should be performed if contact dermatitis is suspected.

The patient should be advised to wear gloves whenever possible, especially when performing household tasks. Emollients should be used liberally and frequently. A moderate-to-strong potency topical corticosteroid ointment should be used. Overnight occlusion with plastic or rubber gloves greatly enhances steroid absorption and may be necessary in severe cases.

STASIS DERMATITIS

(Gravitational Eczema, Varicose Eczema)

Inflammation occurring as a result of venous hypertension in the lower leg. It usually coexists with edema, hemosiderin pigmentation, and dilation of superficial venules around the ankles. The cause is uncertain, but it is exacerbated by edema, contact dermatitis caused by medicaments, and scratching.

Well-fitting support stockings or firm bandages should be worn to control the edema, and the patient should be encouraged to rest and keep the limb elevated as much as possible. Mild topical corticosteroids, eg, hydrocortisone 1% ointment, may help relieve symptoms. Any possible contact allergens (eg, neomycin ointment) should be avoided.

EXFOLIATIVE DERMATITIS

(Erythroderma)

A generalized, severe dermatitis. The patient develops erythema, which rapidly becomes generalized, and may also suffer rigors because of uncontrolled cutaneous heat loss. The skin becomes red, scaly and thickened. (It does not lift off in sheets to leave denuded areas, as in staphylococcal scalded skin syndrome and toxic epidermal necrolysis.) Extensive skin scaling occurs, and lymphadenopathy is often present. In severe cases, hair and nails may be shed. The most common causes of erythroderma are specific dermatoses (such as eczema and psoriasis), drug-caused eruptions (due to use of allopurinol, gold, hydantoin, sulfonamides), and underlying malignancy (lymphoma, leukemia).

Severe exfoliative dermatitis is a life-threatening condition, and the patient should be admitted to the hospital. There is substantial loss of heat, fluid, and protein through the skin. The patient should be kept in a warm room to minimize heat loss, and core temperature should be monitored. Oral or IV fluid replacement is necessary, and positive fluid balance is essential. Topical emollients (eg, petrolatum ointment) should be used liberally and frequently. If a drug is implicated, it should be discontinued. Systemic prednisone 40 to 60 mg/day should be given early and continued until suppression of erythroderma has been achieved; the dosage can then be tapered gradually.

DRUG-CAUSED ERUPTIONS
Eruptions of the skin that appear after administration of a drug. Many rugs can cause skin eruptions. The most commonly seen rash is a airly symmetric maculopapular pattern. Eruptions typically begin 1 to 0 days after the patient first takes the drug and last for approximately 4 days after the drug is discontinued.

The most commonly implicated drugs are penicillins, sulfonamides, old, phenylbutazone, and gentamicin. However, all oral medications, ncluding OTC preparations and sporadically used agents, can cause ruptions.

Erythema Multiforme
An inflammatory eruption characterized by symmetric erythematous, dematous, or bullous lesions of the skin or mucous membranes. In about 0% of cases, no etiology can be determined. In the others, the disorder ppears to be a hypersensitivity reaction that can be triggered by almost ny drug and a wide variety of infections. Infections are more common 1 children and young adults (especially herpes simplex) and penicillin, ulfonamides, and barbiturates are the most common drugs implicated.

The severity varies from characteristic target lesions with a red periph- ry and cyanotic center, occurring in crops on the limbs, to a severe orm marked by extensive erosion of the skin and bullae on mucous nembranes; eg, the mouth, pharynx, anogenital region, and conjunctiva Stevens-Johnson syndrome).

Treatment: If a cause can be found, it should be removed if possible. Localized eruptions should be treated symptomatically. Patients with se- ere involvement require hospitalization. Close monitoring of fluid bal- nce and of ophthalmologic (corneal ulceration is common), renal, and ulmonary status is essential. The use of systemic corticosteroids is con- oversial and not a routine practice. If recurrent severe erythema ultiforme is preceded by herpes simplex, acyclovir 200 mg orally 5 mes/day may prevent attacks.

Toxic Epidermal Necrolysis (TEN)
A severe eruption that begins with general malaise, skin tenderness, and rythema and rapidly progresses to blistering and erosion of the skin. ikolsky's sign is positive, ie, application of a lateral force to the skin auses the overlying necrotic epidermis to shear off. The etiology in bout 1/3 of cases is a drug; the most frequently implicated include sul- onamides, hydantoin, barbiturates, NSAIDs, and penicillins.

TEN is a life-threatening condition with high mortality. The patient hould be managed in a burn unit (as in cases of staphylococcal scalded kin syndrome), and possible causative agents should be eliminated. All enuded areas of dermis should be covered with a biologic dressing, uch as a pigskin xenograft, or with an antibacterial agent such as silver ulfadiazine cream. Meticulous eye care with close supervision by an ophthalmologist is necessary. Use of systemic corticosteroids is widespread but controversial; they do not appear to influence the course of the disease and increase the risk of sepsis.

PSORIASIS

A disorder characterized by well-defined, erythematous plaques covered with a silvery scale. Although any area of the body can be involved, usual sites are the extensor surfaces (especially knees and elbows), scalp, and buttocks. Psoriatic lesions often appear at sites of trauma such as surgical scars or scratch marks **(Koebner's phenomenon).** Nail involvement produces pitting of the nail, with thickening, discoloration, and onycholysis (separation of the distal edge of the nail plate from the nail bed).

About 3% of patients acquire the condition after age 60 yr; 43% of patients between the ages of 60 and 74 yr first develop psoriasis after the age of 45. A detailed drug history should be taken since many drugs, especially β-blockers, can exacerbate the psoriasis.

Psoriatic arthritis typically involves the distal interphalangeal joints, with fusiform swelling and tenderness. Other types of arthritis can also occur: monoarthritis, sacroileitis, and a seronegative arthritis that is otherwise indistinguishable from rheumatoid arthritis. **Exfoliative dermatitis** can occur with psoriasis (see above in this chapter). **Pustular psoriasis, a** rare variant, is characterized by sterile pustules; they may be localized to the hands and feet or they may become generalized.

Treatment

The extent of the psoriasis and the mobility of the patient determine the treatment, which must be individually tailored. Application of topical preparations tid is not practical in elderly patients whose motion is limited by neurologic impairment or arthritis.

Coal tar has been used for many years to treat psoriasis. However, crude coal tar ointments (1 to 5%) can stain clothing, are messy, and have an unpleasant odor. More current and cosmetically acceptable formulations (Estar®, T/Derm®) are available in combination with other topical agents.

Anthralin (dithranol) cream or paste can be effective for thick, scaly plaques, but it has to be applied carefully because it can irritate normal skin. The patient also should be warned that anthralin stains clothing and skin. There are 2 methods of treatment: (1) lower-strength anthralin cream (0.1% increasing to 0.4%) is applied to psoriatic plaques at night and removed in the morning; (2) short-contact anthralin cream (0.4% to 1%) is applied to psoriatic plaques for 20 min and then removed. As long as there is no skin irritation, treatment time is gradually increased.

Topical corticosteroids may be used alone or in conjunction with coal tar or anthralin. They are especially effective when used under an occlusive dressing. Initial treatment may require the short-term use of a potent topical steroid ointment, such as betamethasone dipropionate 0.05%

)r triamcinolone acetonide 0.1%. As the psoriatic plaques respond to reatment, the strength of the ointment should be reduced until only lu->ricants are used topically. For small, localized lesions, flurandrenolide-mpregnated tape (Cordran® tape) can be applied and left on overnight. Topical steroids should be used cautiously to prevent long-term side ef-ects (atrophy, striae, telangiectasia). Because withdrawal may cause a ebound flare of psoriasis, the use of systemic corticosteroids is essen-ially prohibited.

Mild scalp involvement can be treated with a **tar-based shampoo** (see 5EBORRHEIC DERMATITIS, above). For thick scaling, **keratolytic gel** Keralyt® gel) can be applied to the scalp at night under an occlusive vrap. The gel can be washed out with a tar-based shampoo the next norning, and a steroid solution or gel can be applied to the scalp for he rest of the day. Resistant scalp patches can be **injected with triam-:inolone acetonide suspension** (2.5 mg/mL).

Phototherapy with **ultraviolet B (UV-B) light** in a whole-body treatment :abinet 3 times a week is highly effective. The patient should apply lu->ricants to the skin prior to treatment. An advantage of phototherapy is hat the side effects associated with frequent topical treatments are ivoided. Regular sun exposure is often equally helpful but requires a fa-vorable climate and appropriate sunbathing facilities.

Photochemotherapy with PUVA (psoralens plus UV-A) is useful for se-vere, widespread cases of psoriasis. A photoactive drug, usually me-hoxsalen (0.6 mg/kg), is taken orally 2 h before treatment. The patient s then exposed to UV-A light at a dosage based on the skin type or on he experimentally determined minimum phototoxic dose. Lesions usu-lly disappear after 20 to 25 treatments. Maintenance treatment every 2 vk is often necessary to prevent flare-ups.

Methotrexate may be used in patients who have been unresponsive to)ther treatments. It is an antimetabolite that interferes with DNA syn-hesis and is especially useful in widespread pustular psoriasis, exfolia-ive psoriasis, and disabling psoriatic arthritis. In elderly patients with lisabling psoriasis who are unable to use topical agents, methotrexate losages as low as 2.5 or 5 mg/wk are capable of controlling the disease :ompletely. Close supervision by a dermatologist is recommended. He->atic and renal function, including creatinine clearance, must be nonitored.

BULLOUS DISORDERS

BULLOUS PEMPHIGOID

A chronic, benign bullous eruption occurring predominantly in elderly)ersons. It is characterized by the development of tense bullae on nor-nal or erythematous skin. Lesions may be localized or generalized and nucous membranes are involved in approximately 50% of cases. The irst symptom, which develops before the onset of blistering, may be)ruritus. The disease tends to have a relapsing and remitting course. Men and women are equally affected.

Histologically, there are subepidermal bullae. Immunofluorescent staining reveals deposition of C3 in all patients and IgG in many patients along the dermal-epidermal junction in both lesional and perilesional skin. Circulating anti-basement membrane-zone antibodies can be found in about 45% of patients with bullous pemphigoid.

The differential diagnosis includes pemphigus vulgaris, dermatitis herpetiformis, erythema multiforme, benign mucosal pemphigoid, and drug eruptions.

Treatment: For patients with localized disease, topical intralesional corticosteroids can be used. Patients with disseminated disease require oral corticosteroid treatment, 40 to 60 mg prednisolone daily initially. This may need to be increased to 100 mg or more daily in young patients with active disease. Azathioprine 50 to 150 mg daily in divided doses may be added as a steroid-sparing agent.

Prognosis: Bullous pemphigoid tends to run a chronic course, but disseminated disease can be fatal in about $1/3$ of patients if untreated. Once the condition is controlled with corticosteroids, patients often go into prolonged remissive phases, allowing tapering and discontinuance of the drugs.

PEMPHIGUS VULGARIS

A rare, potentially life-threatening dermatologic condition characterized by intraepidermal bullae on the skin or mucous membranes. Although the peak incidence is in middle age, many patients are $\geq$ 60 yr of age.

Pemphigus presents with flaccid bullae that rupture easily and leave superficial erosions on the trunk, limbs, and mucous membranes. The surrounding skin looks normal. Many patients present with a painful mouth; oral lesions may dominate the clinical picture, especially early in the course of the disease. Blistering can become widespread, and patients are at high risk for secondary infection and sepsis. **Nikolsky's sign** is often positive (see TOXIC EPIDERMAL NECROLYSIS, above). The disease usually progresses from a localized to a generalized form, and long-term treatment and follow-up are necessary. Histology shows an intraepidermal blister; immunofluorescence reveals intercellular deposits of immunoglobulin and complement.

Differential diagnosis includes bullous pemphigoid, benign mucous membrane pemphigoid, toxic epidermal necrolysis, drug eruptions, and erythema multiforme.

Prognosis: Before the advent of corticosteroids, the mean survival time was only 14 mo. Mortality is now about 25%.

Treatment

Mild bullous pemphigoid can often be controlled with potent topical steroids alone. Widespread bullous pemphigoid or pemphigus may require hospitalization. Prednisone 60 to 100 mg/day then may be needed to bring the disease under control. High-dose corticosteroid therapy in elderly patients requires careful monitoring. A chest x-ray should be performed to rule out reactivation of old TB, and urine should be tested daily for glycosuria. An H_2 antagonist is often given as prophylaxis against GI bleeding.

After the skin lesions have resolved, the corticosteroid dosage is decreased to approximately 60 mg/day over a 1-mo period, and then more gradually. To minimize adrenal suppression, the total dose can be given every morning or every other morning.

About 50% of patients with bullous pemphigoid have complete remission after several months of systemic treatment, after which they require no medication. In pemphigus, which usually requires life-long treatment, the patient should be observed for any sign of recurrence as the dosage of prednisone is reduced.

Because of the risks of prolonged corticosteroid therapy in the elderly, immunosuppressive agents are usually given concomitantly for their steroid-sparing effect. Azathioprine can be given in dosages of 50 to 150 mg/day; methotrexate can be given orally or IM in a dosage of 25 to 35 mg/wk; and cyclophosphamide can be initiated at a dosage of 2 to 3 mg/kg/day and then reduced to a maintenance dose of 100 mg/day. Because immunosuppressive agents do not take effect for 6 to 8 wk, the steroid dosage cannot be reduced immediately. Side effects of immunosuppressants include bone marrow depression and hepatotoxicity.

DECUBITUS ULCERS
(Pressure Sores)
(See Ch. 13)

VENOUS ULCERS

These are a major source of morbidity in elderly patients. Etiologic factors include incompetent superficial veins and perforators, as well as postphlebitic syndrome. These factors result in persistent venous hypertension and a corresponding rise in capillary pressure, with leakage of fibrinogen into the tissues. Pericapillary fibrin cuffs form, limiting the diffusion of O_2 and other nutrients to the skin.

Venous ulcers commonly occur on the medial or lateral aspect of the lower limbs. Edema, hyperpigmentation (due to hemosiderin deposition), eczematous changes, and induration are often present in the surrounding skin. Sharply demarcated sclerotic atrophic white plaques (atrophie blanche) stippled with telangiectasia and surrounded by hyperpigmentation are distinctive scars also commonly found in patients with venous insufficiency.

All patients with venous ulceration should be examined for systemic disorders, eg, heart failure, hypoalbuminemia, and nutritional deficiencies, since they may contribute to the condition. Peripheral neuropathy, diabetes mellitus, and arterial insufficiency should also be excluded.

Treatment

Edema reduction is the cornerstone of therapy in venous insufficien The patient should be advised to elevate the affected limb whene possible, especially at night when in bed or when sitting. Compressi stockings and graduated pressure bandages or Unna's boots, a from toe to knee, are effective in reducing limb edema.

Ulcer dressings should be kept as simple as possible. Frequent applications of wet-to-dry dressings with normal saline may help diminish debris and slough over the ulcer. If the wound is infected with *Pseudomonas,* frequent application of compresses with acetic acid 5% reduces the bacterial count.

Systemic antibiotics do not enhance wound healing unless cellul present. However, if there are signs of cellulitis, with erythema, swelling and tenderness around the ulcer, the patient should be treated with pe icillin V 250 to 500 mg qid or dicloxacillin 250 to 500 mg qid for 7 10 days. If the patient is allergic to penicillin, erythromycin can be substituted.

Patients with venous ulceration and stasis dermatitis are at considerable risk for developing allergic contact dermatitis to topical antibiotics or other potential sensitizers applied to the broken skin surface. Chronic low-grade delayed hypersensitivity reactions may impede ulcer healing and increase local pruritus and edema. Neomycin ointment, wood alcohols, and balsam of Peru are among the most commonly implicated allergens. When allergy is suspected, topical therapy should be discontinued for at least 2 wk and the ulcer treated with wet-to-dry saline compresses. Patch testing should be performed, if possible.

In patients with very deep or nonhealing ulcers, surgical intervention may be required. Split-thickness skin grafts or pinch grafts, if successful, can reduce healing time significantly. In the elderly, however, postoperative immobilization increases the risks of deep venous thrombosis and may slow the healing of split-thickness skin graft donor sites.

§3. ORGAN SYSTEMS: EYE DISORDERS

Contents for EAR, NOSE, AND THROAT DISORDERS begin on page 1083.

---

93. OPHTHALMOLOGIC DISORDERS

Carl Kupfer

ANATOMY AND PHYSIOLOGY OF THE AGING EYE

Evaluation of the symptoms and signs associated with disorders of the aging eye and visual axis must be based on an understanding of anatomy and physiology. FIG. 93–1 depicts the structures that undergo anatomic or physiologic changes with aging.

OCULAR STRUCTURES

Conjunctiva

The conjunctiva is the thin mucous membrane covering the sclera. Its goblet cells produce mucin, essential for lubricating eyelid movement as well as providing a protective layer to slow evaporation of the tear film. With aging, mucous cells decrease in number, either as a result of **kera-**

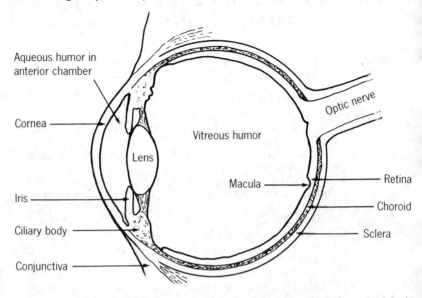

Fig. 93–1. **Structures of the eye that undergo anatomic and/or physiologic changes with aging.**

titis sicca (with or without Sjögren's syndrome) or nonspecifically. These changes contribute to the **"dry eye" syndrome** (see also under Lacrimal Gland and Tear Drainage, below), manifested by a scratchy sensation and chronic irritation, often with increased redness due to conjunctival vascular dilatation. Diagnosis is confirmed by examining the cornea with slit-lamp biomicroscopy, and treatment is usually methylcellulose eyedrops (artificial tears) or some variant thereof.

The conjunctiva can also undergo metaplasia and hyperplasia. This may lead to an accumulation of tissue at the temporal junction of the sclera and cornea (the temporal limbus), called a **pinguecula,** or at the nasal limbus, a **pterygium,** which can invade the cornea superficially (see Fig. 93–2). If the pterygium continues to grow and reaches the center of the cornea, it can interfere with vision. Pterygia are usually seen in individuals who spend much time outdoors, especially in dusty and windy environments. Although pingueculas are frequent in women and may be a cosmetic problem, they rarely require removal; however, pterygia should be followed and, at first evidence of corneal involvement, surgical excision should be considered.

Sclera

The sclera is seen more clearly when there is thinning of the overlying conjunctiva. Deposition of calcium and cholesterol salts at the limbus

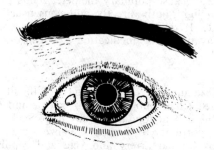

Fig. 93–2. Pinguecula. The conjunctiva can undergo metaplasia and hyperplasia, leading to an accumulation of tissue at the temporal junction of the sclera and cornea (the temporal limbus). Pingueculas appear almost uniformly with aging and are harmless. (From B. Bates, *A Guide to Physical Examination and History Taking,* ed. 4. Copyright 1987 by J. B. Lippincott Company. Used with permission of J. B. Lippincott Company and the author.)

arcus senilis) is a common finding in those > 60 yr of age. Efforts to link this sign to systemic disease have failed except rarely in cases of **systemic hyperlipoproteinemia.** Physicians should also look for jaundice.

Cornea

Arcus senilis can also occur in the cornea, just inside the limbus for a distance of 1 to 2 mm, but it will not progress to the point of interfering with vision. The major age-related change of the cornea is the propensity of the endothelial cells lining its inner surface to undergo degeneration, which if progressive can eventually result in failure to keep the cornea free of extracellular fluid. The resultant corneal edema and accompanying hazy appearance will interfere with vision and may require corneal transplantation. The hazy appearance of the cornea requires referral to an ophthalmologist.

Iris

The iris contains 2 sets of muscles that regulate the size of the pupil and its reaction to light. With age, the pupil tends to become smaller, reacts more sluggishly to light, and dilates more slowly in the dark. Thus, elderly persons may complain that objects are not as bright (a smaller pupil allows less light to enter the eye), that they are dazzled when going outdoors (slow pupillary constriction), and that they experience difficulty when going from a brightly lit environment to a darker one (slow pupillary dilation). If visual acuity is normal, reassurance is in order.

Relative pupillary size and reaction to light can be evaluated in a dimly lit room by shining a penlight obliquely into each eye and observing the brisk constriction of the pupil in both the illuminated eye and the contralateral eye. Because pupillary diameter tends to decrease with age, the reaction to light both directly and consensually tends to be smaller in magnitude. If the pupillary response is very sluggish or absent, the patient may be taking medication that causes constriction or dilation of the pupil.

Retina

Ophthalmoscopic examination of the retina is difficult in elderly patients because of their small pupils, eye movement, and opacities. Providing a target for the patient to stare at may help. Such examination is, however, the only opportunity to directly visualize a cranial nerve (optic nerve), blood vessels (retinal artery and vein and capillary bed), and that portion of the retina responsible for the highest level of visual acuity (the macula). It is important, therefore, to recognize age-related changes in the appearances of these structures. **The optic nerve** tends to have less distinct margins and may appear slightly paler because of loss of capillaries resulting from small-vessel disease secondary to atherosclerosis. **The macula,** which in young persons usually has a bright central foveal light reflex, may not demonstrate any foveal reflex. In addition, yellowish-white spots often appear in the macular area **(drusen),** and some disruption may occur in the pattern of pigmentation (see AGE-RELATED MACULOPATHY, below). Unless these changes in the macula are accompanied by distortion of objects seen or a frank decrease in visual acuity unexplained by other causes, they are not clinically important.

The arteries also demonstrate atherosclerotic changes, including slight narrowing and an increased light reflex from thickened vessel walls. The veins may show marked venous indentation (nicking) at the arteriovenous crossings, with slight proximal distention. In general, the retina, which glistens in younger individuals, becomes duller with aging.

EXTRAOCULAR STRUCTURES

Lids

The close apposition of the lids to the eyeball tends to diminish with age so that the lid margin (especially that of the lower lid) falls away from the globe. This is usually caused by a decrease in the strength of the orbicularis oculi muscles, which squeeze the lids tightly shut. If the lower lid margin is no longer in contact with the globe **(ectropion),** the punctum of the medial lower lid is no longer in contact with the eyeball, and tears cannot drain properly from the conjunctival sac into the lacrimal sac (see FIG. 93–3). Complaints of excess tear production and tears draining onto the face follow (see also Lacrimal Gland and Tear Drainage, below).

With decreased orbicularis oculi action, the lids may not close completely during sleep, resulting in drying of the cornea and secondary abrasion, redness, and irritation **(superficial punctate keratitis).** On the other hand, spasm of the orbicularis oculi muscle may cause the lid margin (especially that of the lower lid) to turn in **(entropion),** bringing

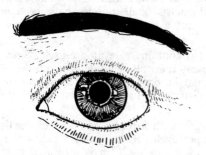

Fɪɢ. **93-3. Ectropion** occurs if the lower lid margin is no longer in contact with the globe. In this situation, the punctum of the medial lower lid no longer is in contact with the eyeball, and tears cannot drain properly from the conjunctival sac into the lacrimal duct. (From B. Bates, *A Guide to Physical Examination and History Taking,* ed. 4. Copyright 1987 by J. B. Lippincott Company. Used with permission of J. B. Lippincott Company and the author.)

the eyelashes at the lid margin in contact with the eyeball, causing rubbing of the globe with each lid blink, resulting in chronic irritation (see Fɪɢ. 93-4). Over time, scarring of the cornea and conjunctiva may result if this condition **(trichiasis)** is not corrected surgically.

For reasons not understood, some individuals manifest intermittent or, in some cases, constant severe spasms of the orbicularis oculi muscles bilaterally so that the eyelids are shut tightly for periods varying from seconds to minutes. This **blepharospasm** can incapacitate an individual, and often must be treated by partial surgical denervation of the or-

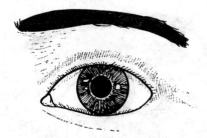

Fɪɢ. **93-4. Entropion** occurs when spasm of the orbicularis oculi muscle causes the lid margin (especially that of the lower lid) to turn in, bringing the eyelashes at the lid margin in contact with the eyeball, causing rubbing of the globe with each lid blink, and resulting in chronic irritation. (From B. Bates, *A Guide to Physical Examination and History Taking,* ed. 4. Copyright 1987 by J. B. Lippincott Company. Used with permission of J. B. Lippincott Company and the author.)

bicularis oculi muscles. More recently, small injections of botulinus toxin into the orbicularis oculi muscles have been used with some encouraging results, but a controlled clinical trial has not yet been conducted.

The upper lid also contains a levator muscle. Since this muscle holds the upper lid against the pull of gravity, some decrease in muscle tone can result in a slight **lid droop,** with a decrease in the size of the palpebral fissure (the distance between the margins of the upper and lower lids).

Loss of skin turgor with atrophy and loss of elasticity may cause the lid skin of the upper eyelid to hang down below the margin of the upper lid. Excision of the excess skin is indicated only if vision is interfered with.

A protrusion of fat through the orbital fascia, which forms a septum between the lid and orbital contents, can cause a localized or diffuse swelling of the eyelid. The fat can be palpated and surgical repair of the septum is based on cosmetic considerations.

Seborrheic dermatitis usually begins in childhood but often becomes more severe in the older patient. The signs are dilated blood vessels at lid margins, loss of lashes, and scaling at the base of the remaining lashes. A chronic conjunctivitis is often present. The most severe cases of blepharitis occur in patients with rosacea. Treatment consists of cleaning the eyelid margin, frequent shampooing of the scalp and, if indicated, local application of antibiotic ointment.

With age, a variety of lesions appear on the lids, including **xanthelasma** (see FIG. 93–5), often on the inner portion of both upper and lower lids; these are rarely of clinical significance. **Basal cell carcinoma** (see FIG. 93–6), and to a much lesser extent, **squamous cell carcinoma** are, of course, quite significant.

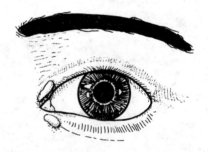

FIG. 93–5. Xanthelasma. Slightly raised, yellowish, well-circumscribed plaques typically appear along the nasal portion of 1 or both eyelids. They may accompany lipid disorders but may also appear in normal individuals. (From B. Bates, *A Guide to Physical Examination and History Taking,* ed. 4. Copyright 1987 by J. B. Lippincott Company. Used with permission of J. B. Lippincott Company and the author.)

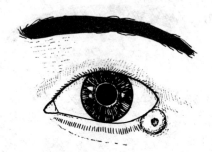

Fig. 93–6. **Basal cell carcinoma** usually involves the lower lid when it occurs near
ιe eye. It appears as a papule with a pearly border and a depressed or ulcerated cen-
r. (From B. Bates, *A Guide to Physical Examination and History Taking*, ed. 4. Copy-
ght 1987 by J. B. Lippincott Company. Used with permission of J. B. Lippincott Com-
ιny and the author.)

acrimal Gland and Tear Drainage

Abnormalities of the lacrimal system may result in either decreased
:ar production or overflow of tears because of faulty drainage. Tear
roduction by the lacrimal gland may decrease with age, with fewer
:ars available to keep the surface of the eye (especially the cornea) well
ιoistened. This incipient **dry eye** condition may result in a chronic
ɔreign-body sensation and is made worse by weakness of the orbicularis
:culi muscles, resulting in incomplete lid closure during sleep. Use of
rtificial tears is indicated. If actual disease involves the lacrimal gland,
s in Sjögren's syndrome, more aggressive surgical intervention (eg, par-
al tarsorrhaphy of the lids) may be indicated.

Severe tearing (with overflow of tears) is a frequent complaint; it usu-
lly represents a loss of apposition between the lacrimal puncta and the
yeball, so tears cannot drain properly from the conjunctival sac into
ιe lacrimal system, causing them to roll down the face (see Lids,
bove). This worsens in cold weather, when there is a slight increase in
:ar production. The patient should be reassured that excess tearing is
referable to a dry eye condition and is not a cause for concern (but a
andkerchief should be used liberally). If severe ectropion exists, causing
xcess tearing and recurrent low-grade inflammation, surgical correction
indicated.

Occasionally, excessive tearing is caused by puncta that have become
ccluded from recurrent chronic bacterial infection resulting in **da-
ryocystitis** (see Fig. 93–7). This situation is the exception rather than
ιe rule.

Tear production can be measured with the **Schirmer's test** by suspend-
ιg a 20-mm strip of filter paper from the lower conjunctival sac. The
xtent (in millimeters) of wetting on this strip after 5 min is measured.

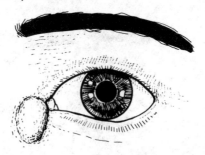

FIG. 93–7. **Dacryocystitis,** a recurrent, chronic bacterial infection, results in exces
sive tearing caused by an occluded punctum. Swelling between the lower eyelid an
nose suggests inflammation of the lacrimal sac. Pressure on the sac expresses materia
through the punctum. (From B. Bates, *A Guide to Physical Examination and History Tak
ing,* ed. 4. Copyright 1987 by J. B. Lippincott Company. Used with permission of J. E
Lippincott Company and the author.)

If it is $\geq$ 10 mm, tear production is adequate, but if it is $<$ 10 mr
and the patient complains of a scratchy sensation or foreign-body feel
ing, referral to an ophthalmologist is indicated. If the patient complain
of excess tears and the punctum of the lower lid is not in contact wit
the eyeball, referral is also indicated.

Orbit

The orbit undergoes age-related changes, with loss of periorbital fat of
ten leading to a sinking of the eyeball into the orbit **(enophthalmos).** Al
though asymptomatic, enophthalmos often is a cosmetic problem an
may require the attention of a surgeon.

SYMPTOMS AND SIGNS ASSOCIATED WITH AGING

COMPLAINTS RELATED TO EYE COMFORT

FOREIGN-BODY SENSATION

A "false" foreign-body sensation may be related to a dry eye condi
tion, entropion, chronic fatigue of the eye muscles due to lack of sleep
poor health, a latent eye muscle imbalance, or excessive close vision (eg
reading when extremely tired). It is, however, always important to rul
out a true foreign body.

HEADACHE

Three general types of headache can be distinguished in the elderly pa
tient.

Tension headache is related to any cause of increased muscle tone, eg
stress, presence of arthritic pain, fatigue, or anxiety. These condition:

may lead to chronic spasm of the scalp, face, or 6 extraocular muscles that provide eye movements. Over time, the muscles may go into spasm and produce lactic acid, which stimulates local pain receptors, resulting in headache. Such tension headache is usually described as a tight band about the head, or pressure, and in most cases can be related to a specific activity. The headache worsens with continuation of the activity and is often relieved by muscle relaxants or analgesics, but occasionally the pain is truly debilitating.

Eye muscle pain often presents as a brow ache, first appearing on awakening, especially if the patient had been reading or watching television late the previous night. The pain can take the form of a throbbing, dull ache localized behind one or both eyes or across the brow or the entire forehead. It can involve either side of the head. Other symptoms include redness, burning, and tearing, especially after prolonged close-range work or reading at night when fatigued.

A major cause of this type of headache is related to a tendency with aging for the eyes to turn outward **(exophoria),** due to a gradual, bilateral decrease in the tone of the medial rectus muscle, which serves to turn the eye inward when reading or focusing on objects within 1 to 10 ft.

Exophoria is **diagnosed** by asking the patient to look at a flashlight approximately 1 ft away through reading glasses while alternately covering each eye, never allowing the light to be seen by both eyes at the same time. Each eye is observed as soon as it is uncovered. If the eye moves inward to look at the light, it must have drifted outward while it was covered, suggesting an exophoria.

Headache associated with exophoria can often be rendered asymptomatic by advising the patient to rest more or do close-range work in the early part of the day. Exophoria can be counteracted by increasing the contractile tone of the medial rectus muscles through **exercise therapy.** The patient holds the index finger of 1 hand approximately 12 in. from the nose and aligns this finger with the index finger of the other hand held 18 in. from the nose. Looking only at the closer finger, the patient moves this finger slowly toward the nose while keeping the farther finger in a fixed position. The more distant finger appears as a double image and the distance between the 2 images widens as one follows the closer finger's movement to the nose. Doing this simple exercise 3 times/day for approximately 5 min each session usually provides symptomatic relief in 4 to 6 wk.

Migraine headache usually develops in the early 20s or 30s but may occur at a later age in some individuals. It is often preceded by an aura of flashing bright lights in the form of a vertical zigzag or picket-fence configuration, either to the far left or far right of the visual field, and is always unilateral. This aura may be followed by severe pain on the opposite side of the head. The pain is pounding and relentless, made worse by bright lights or movement, and made better by lying down in the dark. The aura is due to marked cerebral vasoconstriction involving vessels of the visual cortex, and the subsequent pain is due to marked secondary vasodilation (with associated stretching of perivascular nerve endings).

Treatment is most effective when administered at the first sign of the aura, to abort the attack by pharmacologically maintaining vasoconstriction with ergotamine. Once headache supervenes, analgesics and rest are indicated. Prophylaxis with a variety of medications may prevent the attack by blocking the antecedent vasoconstriction.

COMPLAINTS RELATED TO VISION

GLARE

Decreased visual perception related to glare is a frequent complaint. As the eye ages, changes in both the lens and vitreous result in increased scattering of light in the ocular media. Lens opacities at the periphery, while not directly interfering with vision, can increase the scattering of light passing through the lens, especially at night or in low levels of illumination, when the pupil is slightly dilated. Thus, it is not unusual for the elderly patient to complain of the glare of oncoming headlights while driving at night. As long as visual **acuity** is still normal, the patient should be advised to *curtail driving at night or avoid looking directly at oncoming headlights.*

Decreased visual perception due to daytime glare is also common. With aging, opacities may appear in various portions of the lens, such as the nucleus and cortex. Such opacities may interfere little with visual acuity, but when they appear in the region of the central cortex just beneath the posterior lens capsule **(posterior subcapsular lens opacities),** they tend to scatter light to a greater extent. This occurs because the opacities are closer to the focal point of the lens, through which all light rays must pass on the way to the retina. Although these opacities may eventually increase in size or density and interfere with visual acuity **(posterior subcapsular cataract),** their earliest manifestation is the scattering of light and increased glare, especially in high levels of illumination.

Some temporary relief may result from mild dilation of the pupil with mydriatic drops and by wearing sunglasses so that it may be possible to see "around" the opacity. However, these strategies should be used only under appropriate ophthalmologic care. Early nuclear opacities may actually improve close vision in the elderly (see REFRACTIVE CHANGES, below). Cataracts are discussed further, below.

HAZINESS, FLASHING LIGHTS, AND MOVING SPOTS

Decreased visual perception due to opacities in the ocular media are most often attributed to vitreous floaters or to the lightning flashes of Foster Moore. The vitreous humor is a gelatinous-like material that fills the back of the eye between the posterior surface of the lens and the anterior surface of the retina. The vitreous is normally clear, but with age, changes may occur that can be categorized as either discrete opacities or structural changes leading to a general haziness. By focusing the ophthalmoscope, using +10 to +2 lenses, it may be possible to distinguish between lens opacities, best seen with a +10 lens, and vitreous opacities, best seen with a +2 lens. Although these changes are not serious, they do upset the patient and an explanation and reassurance are necessary. However, when there is a shower of opacities, often accompanied by flashing lights in the peripheral visual fields, referral to rule out retinal detachment is indicated.

The vitreous is firmly attached to the most anterior peripheral portion of the retina and posteriorly at the optic nerve. With age, the vitreous undergoes liquefaction and, as a result, eye movements place the vitreous attachment to the retina under intermittent tension. This tugging tends to stimulate the peripheral retina mechanically, causing vertically oriented flashing lights almost always in the far temporal visual field. Unlike the aura in migraine, these flashing lights occur in only 1 eye at a time. If they are not accompanied by decreased vision or other changes in visual function, they can be disregarded and the patient reassured. *However, if they persist and there is the sense of a "veil" over the eye or a decrease in the visual field, the patient should be referred immediately for a thorough ophthalmologic examination to exclude retinal detachment.*

In patients who are nearsighted (myopic), as well as many others in their late 50s and early 60s, opacities in the form of lines, spots, webs, and clusters of dots often move slowly across the field of vision. Usually, they move more rapidly with eye movements and may become stationary when the eye is not moving. These opacities represent bits of vitreous that have coalesced to form visible opacities or vitreous that has broken off from its attachment to the peripheral or central portion of the retina and now float freely in the vitreous cavity **(floaters).** Such symptoms are annoying but usually have no clinical importance. If, after appropriate examination, the patient is reassured and encouraged to ignore the symptoms, they gradually become less noticeable. Only when there is a shower of opacities, often accompanied by flashing lights in the peripheral visual field, is referral indicated to rule out retinal detachment. Floaters may also occur in uveitis.

REFRACTIVE CHANGES

A universal age-related change in lens physiology, beginning in the 50s, is the **loss of accommodation (presbyopia);** when one wishes to see an object closer than 1 or 2 ft ($\frac{1}{3}$ to $\frac{2}{3}$ m), the lens must increase its thickness, thereby providing additional refractive power to focus the light from a near object on the retina.

If one is farsighted **(hyperopic),** the presbyopic condition tends to occur at a slightly earlier age. If one is nearsighted **(myopic),** removing one's glasses usually makes it possible to read small print, although the material may need to be held quite close, depending on the degree of myopia. Presbyopia is corrected both in nearsighted and farsighted individuals by prescribing either separate reading glasses or bifocal glasses. Since accommodation is lost progressively from approximately 45 to 65 yr of age, the reading lens must be changed and increased in strength every 2 or 3 yr.

Refractive changes resulting from **cataracts** are discussed below.

DIAGNOSTIC PROCEDURES

TESTS FOR VISUAL ACUITY

A visual acuity chart set at 20 ft (10 ft if a mirror is used) and well illuminated is used for testing distance vision, while a **reading card** with various print sizes should be available to test near vision. Adequate lighting of the distance-acuity chart is ensured by using a 60-watt bulb 3 ft from the chart; the bulb is shielded from the patient by a lamp housing to prevent glare. If the 20/40 line on the chart cannot be read, even when the patient is wearing his distance eyeglasses, the patient should look through a pinhole (literally, the opening made by a pin pushed through a piece of thin cardboard). If the decreased acuity is due to a need for glasses or a change in the current prescription, acuity should improve to at least 20/30 when the pinhole is used. If the decreased acuity is due to other causes, use of the pinhole will not improve the vision. Immediate referral is indicated since inability to improve vision with a pinhole suggests the presence of serious eye disease.

Near vision can also be tested by the ability to read ordinary newsprint. If the patient cannot do this, yet has good distance vision, only a change in reading glasses is indicated.

VISUAL FIELD EXAMINATION

Assessment of visual fields by the **confrontational method** involves the examiner and patient directly facing each other with eyes directly engaged. The examiner swings his outstretched arm in a circle and determines if the patient can detect a moving finger. This method may detect gross visual field defects, but in view of the clinical importance of such defects, definitive determination of visual field status should be done **quantitatively** by experts.

OPHTHALMOSCOPIC EXAMINATION

Ophthalmoscopic examination of the lens, vitreous, and retina is best accomplished through a pupil dilated to at least 6 mm in diameter. Dilation is achieved by using a phenylephrine 2½% ophthalmic solution, applying 1 drop to each eye twice, 10 min apart. If the anterior chamber is very shallow and the patient is prone to develop angle-closure glaucoma, dilation with phenylephrine 2½% may precipitate an acute attack. Although this is rare, the patient should be informed that intraocular pressure may rise, causing discomfort, and may require immediate treatment that is very successful in curing the underlying condition. The advantages of a careful examination of the retina far outweigh the rare precipitation of an attack of angle-closure glaucoma, which, if diagnosed early, can be cured.

The ophthalmoscope should have a halogen bulb for greater brightness, especially when used for viewing the retina through a less-than-optimally dilated pupil. To begin, a +10 diopter (blue number) lens should be used in the viewing aperture, and the pupillary space should be filled with a bright red reflex reflected back from the blood-filled choroid beneath the retina. If dark areas are blocking this red reflex, opacities are present in the cornea, lens, or vitreous. If these opacities interfere with visualizing the retina, they can also interfere with the patient's vision, thus suggesting decreased visual acuity. If opacities are not present, the examiner should slowly focus on the retina by progressively decreasing the lens power until details of the retinal blood vessels come into view.

The posterior retina should be scanned slowly until the optic nerve head is seen. The examiner should record the color (it should be pink), the size of the optic cup as a fraction of the optic nerve head diameter, and most important, the presence of a flat rim of optic nerve surrounding the cup. If this rim slopes down to the cup or if it is notched, glaucoma should be suspected. Comparing the appearance of the right and left optic nerves is of particular value, since asymmetry in optic cup size can be important in identifying damage due to elevated intraocular pressure.

Next, the examiner should move temporally across the retina about 2 or 3 mm to evaluate the macular area and the adjacent posterior retina. Diabetic or hypertensive retinopathy and other vascular changes most often occur in these areas. In addition, lesions of the macular area, especially age-related maculopathy, can cause decreased vision. Finally, the branches of the central retinal artery and vein should be examined for changes in caliber and presence of adjacent hemorrhages, exudates, or microaneurysms. Any such changes should prompt referral for definitive diagnosis.

AGE-RELATED EYE DISEASES

CATARACT

An opacity of the lens that reduces visual acuity to 20/30 or less. An opacity of the lens outside the visual axis (central region of the lens) is not considered a cataract, since it does not interfere with vision, although it may cause glare (see GLARE, above).

The lens is normally clear until after age 40, when nonspecific opacities may be noted. Since age is the major risk factor for the development of cataract, almost all individuals will develop clinically significant cataract if they live long enough. The cause is thought to be oxidative damage to the lens proteins, reducing solubility and eventually forming insoluble opacities in an otherwise transparent tissue.

Types of Cataract

There are 4 types of age-related cataract, categorized according to the location of the opacity within the lens. These are cortical, nuclear, and posterior subcapsular cataracts **(PSC),** and a combination of $\geq$ 2 of the above. Idiopathic PSC usually occurs at an earlier age and probably has a genetic basis. However, treatment with local or systemic corticosteroids should be ruled out as a cause.

Symptoms and Signs

With the development of lens opacities, especially in the nucleus, visual acuity is relatively unaffected for a time, but the refractive index, and hence the refractive power, of the lens increases—ie, it shifts toward myopia. This increase in refractive power can partially compensate for the loss in accommodation and temporarily corrects presbyopia. Thus, in some individuals 60 to 70 yr of age, early nuclear lens changes may induce myopia and allow the individual to read again without glasses. This condition is referred to as **"second sight."**

An early symptom of PSC may be the complaint of glare from bright lights at night or even during the day—the result of rays of light being scattered by the opacities (see GLARE, above). Over time, however, the lens opacities progress and eventually interfere with vision so that reading becomes difficult even with glasses. The hallmark of all cataracts is painless, progressive loss of vision, but the rate of visual loss is nonlinear and variable. It is important to measure visual acuity near and far.

Lens opacities can be seen easily when the pupil is dilated by observing the red reflex of the retina and choroid with the ophthalmoscope, using a +10 diopter lens in the viewing aperture. Any lens opacity will show in silhouette as a black area.

Treatment

Cataract surgery involves removal of the lens from the eye. Removal of the entire lens in toto, including its capsule, is referred to as an **intracapsular cataract extraction.** However, removal of the central portion of the anterior capsule and aspiration of the contents of the lens, so that an intact posterior lens capsule remains, is termed an **extracapsular cataract extraction.** The latter procedure is most common, since it allows for the placement of a posterior-chamber intraocular lens **(IOL).**

In 1986, approximately 1 million cataract extractions were performed in the USA and approximately 90% of these procedures involved an IOL. In the majority of cases, the IOL was placed behind the iris—ie, in the posterior chamber. In a small percentage of cases, the IOL was

placed in the anterior chamber. Posterior-chamber placement is considered safer and results in fewer postoperative complications, but anterior-chamber placement is easier to perform. Anterior-chamber IOL placement is expected to decrease even further in the future.

Cataract surgery is an elective procedure, requiring ample justification that the potential benefits outweigh the possible complications and discomfort of undergoing the procedure. The decision resides primarily with the patient. If activities such as performing one's job, reading, driving a car, or watching television can no longer be performed, and the surgeon is confident that successful cataract surgery will result in vision of 20/30 or better, surgery should be considered. The concept of waiting until the cataract matures is no longer valid. Cataract surgery can be performed at any stage of cataract maturation, depending only on the patient's visual disability. If, despite some decrease in vision, the patient can continue to perform all desired activities, surgery can be postponed.

Rarely, a very advanced cataract may swell and the capsule may become leaky. Lens material leaking into the anterior chamber may cause secondary glaucoma. This can be readily diagnosed and successfully treated by surgical removal of the cataract.

Cataract extraction should be approached with caution if there is associated eye disease. Age-related maculopathy and severe diabetic retinopathy or other retinal diseases jeopardize the prospect for successful cataract extraction. Surgery should be deferred until there is reasonable assurance that the postoperative result will be acceptable to the patient. Even though most cataract surgery is performed under local anesthesia, special consideration should be given to the patient with severe respiratory or cardiovascular difficulties that may preclude his lying supine for the 30 to 60 min necessary for preoperative preparation and surgery.

In good hands, **complication** rates are low. **Major complications** resulting from surgery are faulty wound closure, with leakage of aqueous humor; prolapse of the iris into the corneal wound; and intractable secondary glaucoma. The most serious complication is inflammation of the eye **(endophthalmitis)**, which is usually noted 24 to 48 h following surgery. Immediate hospitalization and aggressive treatment with IV antibiotics and steroids is mandatory to prevent possible loss of the eye. Fortunately, this complication is rare, occurring in approximately 1 in 5000 cases. Cataract surgery is one of the most successful of surgical procedures, with excellent visual results in approximately 95% of patients.

GLAUCOMA

Disorders characterized by increased intraocular pressure that can lead to irreversible damage to the optic nerve, with attendant impairment in visual function. The glaucomas account for approximately 10% of all blindness in the USA.

ANGLE-CLOSURE GLAUCOMA (ACG)

(Narrow-Angle Glaucoma)

ACG accounts for only about 10% of all glaucomas in the USA but is particularly important because it is the only form that can be cured; thus prompt diagnosis is essential. The anterior chamber of the eye is bounded anteriorly by the cornea and posteriorly by the lens. A major risk factor for this type of glaucoma is an anatomically shallow anterior chamber, especially at the periphery. The chamber becomes even more shallow with advancing age, since the lens continues to grow and thicken throughout life, tending to move the iris forward. Patients who are farsighted (hyperopic) tend to have smaller eyes and thus may be predisposed in later life to ACG. The potential for angle closure is suspected on slit lamp examination and best assessed by gonioscopic examination of the angle structures using special corneal contact lenses.

The elevation of intraocular pressure (IOP) occurs when, after many years, the base of the iris is pushed forward and seals off the trabecular meshwork of the outflow channels. Since aqueous humor is continuously being produced in the eye and circulates through the anterior chamber before leaving via the outflow channels in the anterior chamber angle, the inability of aqueous humor to leave the eye can result in a rapid increase (within a matter of hours) in the IOP to levels as high as 50 to 60 mm Hg (normal values range from 15 to 20 mm Hg). This is the etiology of acute glaucoma and usually presents in one eye. However, the fellow eye is similarly disposed.

Symptoms, Signs, and Diagnosis

The rapid rise in IOP is accompanied by redness and pain in or about the eye, severe headache, nausea, vomiting, and blurring of vision, often preceded by seeing halos around lights (see FIG. 93–8). The latter symptom results from edema of the cornea; the small droplets of fluid cause the patient to see colored halos similar to those seen surrounding oncoming automobile headlights at night when viewed through a wet windshield. In an acute glaucomatous attack, the eye is tender and, if gently palpated, feels particularly firm compared with the contralateral eye. The pupil is fixed in mid-dilation. As the IOP continues to rise, nausea and vomiting can become so severe that an acute abdomen may be suspected. Within 48 to 72 h, depending on the extent of IOP elevation, vision may be irreversibly damaged. *Thus, an attack of ACG constitutes an emergency requiring immediate referral to an ophthalmologist.* Although the IOP can usually be reduced with drugs, surgical intervention (laser iridotomy) is the only intervention that will effect a cure.

Treatment

When an ophthalmologist is not available, emergency measures include local instillation of 2% pilocarpine q 5 min × 6 or 250 mg oral administration of acetazolamide or 40 mL of oral glycerin. Immediate hospitalization and referral are indicated.

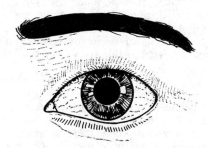

Fɪɢ. 93–8. **Angle-closure glaucoma** is characterized by a rapid rise in intraocular pressure accompanied by redness and pain in or about the eye, severe headache, nausea, vomiting, and blurring of vision, often preceded by halos of light. (From B. Bates, *A Guide to Physical Examination and History Taking,* ed. 4. Copyright 1987 by J. B. Lippincott Company. Used with permission of J. B. Lippincott Company and the author.)

For all practical purposes, ACG should be treated surgically to effect a cure. A small opening is made at the base of the iris (iridotomy) to allow the IOP to equalize on either side of it and prevent the iris from obstructing the outflow channels. Other procedures are available, but iridotomy with a laser can be performed in the ophthalmologist's office in only a few minutes. If surgical intervention is accomplished before permanent adhesions develop between the iris and outflow channels (usually within the first 24 h), cure is likely and further attacks will be prevented.

OPEN-ANGLE GLAUCOMA (OAG)

OAG accounts for about 80% of all glaucomas in the USA. It differs from ACG by being asymptomatic until very late, causing slow loss of visual field over years, affecting both eyes simultaneously, and occurring more commonly in blacks, who rarely have ACG. Although it cannot be cured, OAG can usually be controlled with topical and systemic therapy. Onset is insidious and it is usually asymptomatic; even the progressive loss of visual field may not be noticed by the patient until late in the course of the disease. Routine IOP monitoring and examination of the optic nerve head may detect OAG in the absence of symptoms. Diagnosis depends on the presence of an anatomically normal anterior-chamber angle and outflow channels (as viewed by gonioscopy), increased resistance to aqueous humor outflow (as measured by tonography), and the presence of characteristic visual-field defects (measured by quantitative perimetry).

Although in OAG, the IOP usually is > 21 mm Hg (considered the upper limit of normal), it can be within the normal range but for unknown reasons may be too high for that particular eye to tolerate. With time, optic atrophy expressed as cupping and pallor of the nerve head is noted, indicating advanced disease. When the IOP is > 21 mm Hg but no visual-field defect is demonstrable, the diagnosis is considered to be **ocular hypertension**. The optic nerve usually appears normal. Such patients should be seen at least q 6 mo for visual-field testing, but treatment is usually not indicated at this stage.

Prevention

All patients > 40 yr old, especially those in high-risk groups (eg, those who have a parent or sibling with glaucoma or who are receiving chronic corticosteroid therapy), should have routine measurement of IOP. OAG is more prevalent among blacks, while ACG appears to be more prevalent among Orientals, especially Chinese. Measurement of IOP alone will detect approximately $1/2$ the patients with glaucoma. This measurement as well as examination of the optic nerve for excavation of the nerve head from elevated IOP increases the detection rate to approximately 80%.

IOP is measured with the Schiotz or the applanation tonometer. After instillation of a topical anesthetic (eg, proparacaine 0.5%), the Schiotz tonometer foot plate is gently placed directly on the center of the cornea while the patient is in the supine position, looking at his thumb held straight ahead and up at arm's length. The reading in absolute units on the tonometer (reflecting the indentation of the cornea by the tonometer's plunger) is recorded and converted, with the use of a chart, to mm Hg of IOP. If the practitioner plots the absolute units for each patient measured against the patient's age, a range of normal values for each age group in an individual practice can be developed. This can be helpful, since IOP measurements falling outside this normal range probably represent abnormal values and should prompt referral to an ophthalmologist.

Treatment

Whether or not the patient has symptoms, medication is necessary to reduce the IOP to a level that will prevent irreversible damage to the optic nerve and thus the loss of peripheral visual field. Treatment should be undertaken only by an ophthalmologist, since each medication has specific indications and numerous side effects. The need for lifetime treatment necessitates expert care.

Topical medications include pilocarpine, a parasypathomimetic drug that can cause brow ache following instillation; epinephrine, which may be irritating to the eye and may lead to an allergic lid reaction; and timolol, a β-blocker that may cause cardiopulmonary symptoms in susceptible individuals. **Systemic medication** consists of carbonic anhydrase inhibitors, such as acetazolamide and methazolamide, which may cause slight nausea, tingling, paresthesias, and mental changes. With chronic administration, systemic acidosis or kidney stones (in predisposed individuals) may occur. Since these medications can have adverse side effects and interact with other medications, and since the patient with glaucoma needs to be examined periodically, these medications should only be prescribed by eye care specialists competent to monitor the patient.

Since OAG can be controlled but not cured, medication is continued indefinitely. An IOP ≥ 22 mm Hg requires referral. A visual-field examination should be performed q 6 mo. If medication fails to control the progression of the glaucoma, as evidenced by the development and progression of a visual-field defect, surgery is recommended to lower the IOP to a level at which the disease can be slowed or halted.

SECONDARY GLAUCOMA

Secondary glaucoma, which accounts for 10% of glaucoma cases in the USA, is characterized by the presence of a pathologic process in the eye that anatomically or functionally blocks the outflow channels. Diabetes and occlusion of the central retinal vein can result in a fibrovascular membrane growing over and sealing off the outflow channels. Uveitis, or ocular inflammation, can cause obstruction of the outflow channels by inflammatory cells or debris. Ocular tumors may obstruct outflow channels either by direct pressure from the tumor located in the anterior-chamber angle or by tumor cells blocking the drainage channels. Patients with secondary glaucoma usually present with a red, uncomfortable eye, often chronically painful and usually accompanied by decreased vision.

Treatment

Treatment is difficult and is directed first to removing the underlying cause, eg, treating uveitis with anti-inflammatory drugs or removing a tumor. In addition, antiglaucoma drugs may be tried to reduce elevated IOP. If those fail, surgery is needed to create a new outflow pathway for the aqueous humor to leave the eye.

Drug treatment for other disorders may have an adverse impact on incipient or recognized glaucoma.

Hypotensive drugs: Damage to the optic nerve may be related in part to the relationship between the BP within the optic nerve (perfusion pressure) and the IOP. When the perfusion pressure adequately exceeds the IOP, the optic nerve receives sufficient nutrition. Increased IOP reduces the perfusion pressure. If a hypertensive patient with glaucoma is being treated with antihypertensive medication, the ophthalmologist should be informed so that visual fields can be monitored while the BP is being lowered. The glaucoma medication may need to be increased to reduce the IOP further.

Psychotropic drugs: Drugs with anticholinergic (atropine-like) effects may be dangerous, primarily in patients predisposed to angle-closure glaucoma (by causing chronic pupillary dilation) and possibly in patients with open-angle glaucoma (by antagonizing the antiglaucoma medication).

DIABETIC RETINOPATHY (DR)

DR is the third leading cause of adult blindness, accounting for almost 7% of blindness in the USA. Its incidence is primarily associated with the duration of diabetes; therefore, its prevalence will increase, presenting a major public health problem as the population ages and diabetic patients live longer.

Etiology and Pathophysiology

The etiology of DR is related to the development of diabetic microaneurysms. Retinal capillaries have 2 types of cells—endothelial cells lining the capillary and intramural pericytes or mural cells embedded within the basement membrane of the capillary. For every endothelial cell, there is a mural cell. The first change consistently observed within the retina is a selective loss of mural cells.

The initial loss of these cells sets in motion a series of events culminating in the development of DR. The present hypothesis to explain the mural cell loss involves an enzyme, aldose reductase, which is present in mural but not in endothelial cells. As glucose concentration increases in diabetes, glucose in the mural cells is converted by aldose reductase to its sugar alcohol, sorbitol, which is metabolized slowly and diffuses poorly across cell membranes. Thus, the sorbitol concentration increases within the cell and water moves down its osmotic gradient into the mural cell, which swells, eventually ruptures, and disappears. It is postulated that this mechanism may be the cause of neuropathy and nephropathy, because aldose reductase is localized in the Schwann cells and axoplasm of peripheral nerves and in the kidney.

Since mural cells appear to have contractile properties, their loss results in capillary dilation. The dilated capillaries tend to carry more and more blood, because they are wider than adjacent capillaries that still contain a full complement of mural cells. With mural cell loss and the capillaries carrying more blood, endothelial cells proliferate and form outpouchings, which become **microaneurysms,** while the adjacent capillaries, carrying less and less blood, eventually carry no blood, becoming ghost vessels with loss of all cellular components. Thus, next to clusters of microaneurysms are areas of nonperfused retina.

Eventually, shunt vessels appear between adjacent areas of microaneurysms, and the clinical picture of early DR with microaneurysms and areas of nonperfused retina is seen. The microaneurysms leak and capillary vessels may hemorrhage so that exudates and hemorrhages appear. Thus, the initial stages of background DR are established and progress over a period of years, in some cases to form proliferative DR **(PDR).**

Symptoms, Signs, and Diagnosis

Annual ophthalmoscopic examination with pupillary dilation is indicated in all diabetic patients to detect macular edema and evidence of PDR, indicating impending loss of vision. *Since laser photocoagulation can prevent or slow down visual loss at the early stages of these conditions, early diagnosis is of paramount importance.*

Usually, there is little or no evidence of DR until about 3 to 5 yr after the onset of diabetes. Symptoms may be subtle, eg, early and minimal visual loss from macular edema, a shower of spots, or clouding of vision due to a small vitreous hemorrhage. The first appearance of DR is characterized by microaneurysms, seen as red spots with sharp margins about the width of a vein, at the disk margin. These lesions disappear after 3 to 6 mo, to be replaced by fresh microaneurysms. Over time, the next stage of **nonproliferative DR (NPDR)** is seen, with the addition of punctate, flame-shaped (linear) or blot-shaped **retinal hemorrhages, soft exudates, hard exudates,** and **intraretinal microvascular abnormalities,** the latter appearing as small areas of dilated capillaries.

An important aspect of NPDR is the pooling of edema fluid in the macula with resultant macular elevation. This **macular edema** is a major cause of reduced vision in NPDR and, if allowed to persist, can result in an irreversible loss of vision.

Over time, all the above lesions increase, while some areas of retina continue to lose their capillary vessels and become nonperfused. Eventually, approximately 5% of NPDR cases proceed to PDR with the appearance of new vessels on the disk and elsewhere on the retina. These new blood vessels grow into the vitreous and, because they are friable, tend to bleed easily. Thus, they progress to preretinal hemorrhages, and in advanced PDR to massive vitreous hemorrhage, which may fill a major portion of the vitreous cavity.

The end stage of DR is recurrent vitreous hemorrhage, often accompanied by retinal detachment or secondary glaucoma due to proliferating new vessels obstructing the outflow channels in the anterior chamber angle (see TABLE 93–1).

Treatment

In the presence of clinically significant macular edema, focal laser treatment of the leaking microaneurysms surrounding the macular area reduces vision loss in 50% of cases, compared to no treatment. Early di-

TABLE 93–1. CLASSIFICATION OF DIABETIC RETINOPATHY (DR)

Description	Definition
No DR	Absence of all DR-related lesions
Early DR	≤ 5 microaneurysms in each eye
Nonproliferative DR (NPDR)	Hard exudates, soft exudates, retinal hemorrhages, and intraretinal microvascular abnormalities
Proliferative DR (PDR)	New vessels on the disk and elsewhere on the retina, preretinal hemorrhages, and vitreous hemorrhage

agnosis and treatment—before significant loss of vision occurs—is important. In the case of PDR, the laser scatters several thousand tiny burns throughout the retina (sparing the macular area); this panretinal laser treatment reduces rates of blindness by 60%.

If vitreous hemorrhage is severe enough to preclude the use of laser therapy because of poor visualization of the retina, vitrectomy can be performed to restore vision, especially in young juvenile diabetics soon after the vitreous hemorrhage occurs. Vitrectomy can also benefit diabetic patients with impending retinal detachment.

Although the effect of blood glucose levels on the development or progression of DR is difficult to determine, there is evidence that good control benefits general health and well-being. Therefore, stringent monitoring and regulation of blood glucose should be continued.

Clinical trials are being conducted to determine whether the development of DR and diabetic neuropathy can be prevented or slowed by limiting the accumulation of sorbitol with aldose reductase inhibitors; results should be available within the next few years. Studies are also under way to determine whether laser therapy can prevent the progression of NPDR to PDR. If so, the laser could be even more beneficial if used earlier, ie, in the NPDR stage.

AGE-RELATED MACULOPATHY

Immediately beneath the sensory retina lies a single layer of cells called the **retinal pigment epithelium.** These cells provide nourishment to the portion of the retina in immediate contact with them—the **photoreceptor cells** that contain the visual pigments. For unknown reasons, the maintenance of this contact is threatened in the macula of the aging eye. Any disruption of this close apposition of retinal pigment epithelial cells and photoreceptor cells in the macular region results in an initial distortion of vision and, if persistent, a loss of central visual acuity. Two major processes can occur in the macula and disrupt the retinal pigment epithelium-sensory retina interface; hence there are 2 types of age-related maculopathy.

A small hemorrhage may break through the retinal pigment epithelium from the underlying choroid, which contains a rich vascular bed. Blood accumulates between the retinal pigment epithelium and sensory retina and, if bleeding resolves quickly, no permanent harm results. However, if new blood vessels grow from the choroid into the clot, these new vessels will continue to leak, causing more separation of the retinal pigment epithelium–sensory retina interface. This will lead to disruption of the photoreceptor cells' nutrition and to their death, with attendant loss of central visual acuity.

This type of age-related maculopathy results from a subretinal neovascular membrane and is referred to as the **wet type** because of the leaking vessels and edema or blood that detaches the sensory retina from the retinal pigment epithelium. The **dry type** consists of disintegration of the retinal pigment epithelium with secondary loss of the overlying photoreceptor cells because of nutritional loss. The wet type accounts for only 10% of cases of age-related maculopathy but results in 90% of cases of legal blindness (visual acuity of 20/200 or less). The dry type reduces vision but usually to levels of 20/50 to 20/100.

Symptoms, Signs, and Diagnosis

The patient may notice distortion of central vision as objects appear larger or smaller, or straight lines appear distorted, bent, or missing a central segment. If this occurs in only 1 eye, the patient is unlikely to notice any change in vision. However, if a comparison is made by viewing a grid of fine lines with each eye alternately, any distortion in 1 eye can be quickly perceived. Therefore, individuals considered at high risk for age-related maculopathy are given a grid to view each morning. Following onset of distortion, visual acuity may decrease concomitantly, possibly within days. The signs of age-related maculopathy correlate poorly with the level of visual acuity.

In the dry type, a disturbance of the pigmentation pattern with the presence of drusen may be noted in the macular area. Drusen are excrescences of the basement membrane of the retinal pigment epithelium that protrude into the cells, causing them to bulge anteriorly. Through the ophthalmoscope, they appear as small, rounded, yellow-white areas with an indistinct border. Their specific role in age-related maculopathy is still unclear.

In the wet type, a small detachment of the sensory retina in the macular area may be noted, but the definitive diagnosis of a subretinal neovascular membrane requires fluorescein angiography.

Treatment

There is no treatment for the dry form of age-related maculopathy. However, laser treatment to obliterate the neovascular membrane in the wet form may prevent further loss of vision in approximately 50% of patients. Therefore, in high-risk patients (eg, those who already have an age-related maculopathy in 1 eye or have a family history of the condition), daily viewing of a grid to detect early distortion in central vision may help identify cases that may benefit from early laser treatment.

Although age-related maculopathy affects central visual acuity and therefore restricts such activities as reading and driving a car, the remaining sensory retina are unaffected. Thus, the patient can be assured he will never be completely blind and will be able to continue to perform many everyday activities.

For near-vision tasks (eg, reading and watching television), magnifying lenses and high-intensity lighting matched for daylight are of some help to most patients with loss of central visual acuity (see also AIDS FOR THE VISUALLY HANDICAPPED in Ch. 21). Driving a car requires vision of 20/40 or better in at least 1 eye. Although a telescopic lens may produce that level of vision, it limits the ability to use side vision, precluding driving. However, this type of lens may help the patient identify street signs and perform other visual tasks that facilitate travel. Some optometrists and ophthalmologists specialize in the fitting of such optical aids.

VASCULAR DISEASES

OCCLUSION OF THE CENTRAL RETINAL ARTERY (CRA)

Occlusion of the CRA produces sudden blindness in the affected eye. The usual cause in older patients is atheromata, broken off usually from the wall of the carotid artery. The atheroma occludes the CRA in the deeper portion of the optic nervehead and thus cannot be seen. Within 1 h after vision loss, the spasm of the CRA has ceased and some blood flow is restored to the retina, giving the ophthalmoscopic picture of a relatively normal retina. However, within several hours, the retina becomes edematous and gray in appearance due to the death of retinal ganglion cells. Since the retina in the foveal area contains no ganglion cells, the reddish color of the underlying choroid will still be visible, accounting for the characteristic central cherry red spot surrounded by gray retina. By 2 to 3 wk, the cherry red spot disappears and as the ganglion cells and their axons die, the optic nerve becomes white, the hallmark of primary optic atrophy.

When an atheroma breaks off and passes through the CRA to lodge in one of the branches of the retinal artery, it can usually be seen as a refractile object in the branch and is referred to as a Hollenhorst plaque. Such a finding is evidence of embolic activity, usually from the carotid system. The portion of the retina supplied by the occluded vessel will lose its function and a field defect, which may not affect central vision, will result.

If the effects of occlusion are to be prevented, intervention is necessary within a few minutes after occlusion to prevent the death of retinal cells. Acutely reducing IOP by paracentesis combined with vasodilators may abort the sequelae.

OCCLUSION OF THE CENTRAL RETINAL VEIN (CRV)

Retinal vein occlusion is probably the most common vascular accident in the eye. Even after CRV occlusion, some vision remains. The ophthalmoscopic picture is typical. The veins are distended and tortuous, with massive retinal hemorrhages and edema throughout the retina. The margins of the optic nerve become blurred and the disk swollen. Resorption of the hemorrhages and edema may take months to years to complete. In the older patient, prognosis in terms of vision is poor. In addition, about 25% of patients will develop a fibrovascular membrane that seals the aqueous humor outflow channels in the anterior chamber, resulting in a neovascular glaucoma within 3 to 6 mo. It is painful, and elevation of the IOP is marked. It is difficult to treat but if the IOP remains elevated, blindness results in a matter of weeks. About 10% of patients having an occlusion of the CRV will have the same event in the other eye. Thus, prompt referral is indicated.

Branch vein occlusion is also seen when one of the branches of the CRV becomes obstructed, most often the superior temporal branch. The characteristic picture of extensive exudates and hemorrhages is confined to the involved quadrant of retina with an attendant field defect. Vision is usually unaffected unless the retinal swelling impinges on the macula. A recent clinical trial has demonstrated the beneficial effect of laser photocoagulation in the treatment of branch vein occlusion with respect to preservation of vision. Fortunately, the development of neovascular glaucoma is much less common in branch vein occlusion.

ISCHEMIC OPTIC NEUROPATHY
(Temporal Arteritis or Atheromatosis)

Ischemic optic neuropathy, regardless of etiology, almost always occurs over the age of 60. Partial or complete loss of vision occurs suddenly accompanied by swelling of the optic nervehead, often with a hemorrhage or 2 and an altitudinal visual field defect (loss of half the visual field with horizontal demarcation). With **temporal arteritis,** there can be tenderness along the course of the temporal artery, headache, pain in the jaw while chewing, and fever. Symptoms are almost always accompanied by an elevated sedimentation rate. Since the fellow eye can become affected in a matter of weeks, prompt diagnosis and referral for treatment with corticosteroid therapy is of the utmost importance. When **atheromatosis** is thought to be the cause of the ischemic optic neuropathy, there is often no pain and the decrease in vision is soon followed by pallor of the optic disk. The loss of vision of the fellow eye may occur months or years later and once the ischemic episode has occurred, treatment is of no avail. In selected older patients with a history of blackouts (amaurosis fugax) suggestive of atheromatosis, long-term anticoagulant therapy may be of help.

BLACKOUTS
(Amaurosis Fugax)

Unilateral blackouts suggest either retinal or optic nerve ischemia. The blackout may present as a dimming of vision with slow recovery after 5 to 10 min. The restoration of clear vision occurs in the reverse order from the pattern of onset. Although several episodes of amaurosis may precede an attack of ischemic optic neuropathy, episodes may occur for years without serious sequelae. However, such patients should be under medical care. The blackout can be bilateral if associated with low blood pressure.

Unilateral blackouts are characteristic of carotid artery narrowing, usually at the bifurcation of the common carotid artery. Since atheroma is the major cause of vessel narrowing, patients over the age of 50 are most susceptible. Obstruction of the left carotid is 6 times more frequent than the right. When amaurosis fugax is accompanied by a hemiplegia on the side opposite the affected eye (transient ischemic attack), carotid stenosis on the side of the affected eye should be strongly suspected. Early recognition of serious carotid stenosis is important since a large number of affected patients will develop loss of vision or hemiplegia. Appropriate medical and surgical intervention may provide a cure in suitable patients.

The aortic arch syndrome may also be suspected if the increasingly frequent blackouts are related to changes in posture such as sitting up or standing suddenly.

OCCIPITAL LOBE VASCULAR ACCIDENT

A vascular lesion of the occipital lobe is usually characterized by the sudden onset of a homonomous hemianopsia, usually the result of a posterior cerebral artery infarction. This infarction in 1 or both occipital lobes may result from local atheromatous disease, vascular insufficiency or emboli to the vertebral-basilar system. Total blindness occurs suddenly, with some vision returning within minutes in the ipsilateral homonomous visual field. Bilateral posterior cerebral occlusions usually occur simultaneously. Thrombosis of the basilar artery will also produce a bilateral homonomous hemianopsia. In almost all cases of cortical blindness, some return of vision is expected.

MISCELLANEOUS EYE CONDITIONS

ACUTE DOUBLE VISION

The **3rd cranial nerve** innervates the medial, superior, and inferior recti muscles, the inferior oblique muscle, and the levator muscle and also carries the parasympathetic nerves constricting the pupil and controlling accommodation. A complete 3rd nerve palsy results in a ptosis of the upper lid, a divergence of the eye when looking straight ahead, a dilated fixed pupil, and a lack of upward, inward, and downward movement of the eye. The main causes of isolated 3rd nerve palsy are intracranial aneurysm, trauma, and diabetic neuropathy. Whereas the 3rd nerve palsy due to diabetes will clear spontaneously within 6 to 12 wk, that due to intracranial aneurysm and trauma need immediate diagnostic and, if indicated, therapeutic intervention.

The **4th cranial nerve** innervates the superior oblique muscle and palsy is invariably due to a small hemorrhage in the roof of the midbrain, usually from arteriosclerosis. Recovery occurs spontaneously after several weeks.

The **6th cranial nerve** innervates the lateral rectus muscle and since it has the longest intracranial course, is often affected by meningitis, skull fractures, and increased intracranial pressure. When affected by diabetes, there is spontaneous recovery within 6 to 12 wk.

DIABETIC OPHTHALMOPLEGIA

Severe pain in the eye or over the forehead followed by a 3rd nerve palsy with sparing of the pupil should be considered a manifestation of diabetic neuropathy.

INTRACRANIAL TUMOR

An intracranial space-occupying mass is often accompanied by increased intracranial pressure and severe headache. Ophthalmoscopy may show papilledema. Prompt referral for a neurosurgical diagnostic workup is indicated.

MYASTHENIA GRAVIS

Any combination of extraocular muscle palsies, which may vary in severity during a period of days or weeks, in the presence of a normal pupillary response to light and accompanied by a history of fatigue that waxes and wanes during the day should raise the possibility of myasthenia gravis. An edrophonium chloride (Tensilon®) test should help establish the diagnosis.

§3. ORGAN SYSTEMS: EAR, NOSE, AND THROAT DISORDERS

94. EAR DISORDERS

A. Julianna Gulya

HEARING LOSS

Hearing loss may result from dysfunction of any component of the auditory system. In **conductive hearing loss,** the dysfunction affects the orderly transmission of sound from the external environment to the inner ear and may involve any of the structures lateral to the oval window; eg, the tympanic membrane or stapes. **Sensorineural hearing loss** is due to dysfunction of the sensory elements (hair cells) or neural structures (fibers of the cochlear nerve). In a cochlear sensorineural hearing loss, the structures within the cochlea are affected. A retrocochlear hearing loss refers specifically to disorders of the cochlear nerve, particularly in the internal auditory canal or cerebellopontine angle **(CPA)**, although the general definition is a dysfunction of any element of the auditory system medial to the cochlea. A **mixed hearing loss** combines both sensorineural and conductive elements. In **central hearing loss,** the dysfunction is localized to the higher auditory centers of the brain.

TESTS OF AUDITORY FUNCTION

Clinical Evaluation

A rough estimate of a patient's ability to hear can and should be obtained in a general office setting. The **Weber test** is performed by placing a vibrating 512-Hz tuning fork on the midline of the forehead. Normally, the vibratory sound is perceived as equally loud on each side. With conductive hearing loss, the vibratory sound is perceived as being louder on the affected side. In the **Rinne test,** the stem of a vibrating tuning fork is placed on the mastoid tip (with firm pressure) and then the tines are held just in front of the external auditory canal. Normally, the vibratory sound is perceived as being louder at the external auditory canal (ie, air conduction is greater than bone conduction). The reverse indicates a significant conductive hearing loss.

A **whisper test,** using a Bárány box to mask the contralateral ear, can provide a crude estimate of auditory thresholds. Also, an **audioscope,** which combines both otoscopic visualization and the capacity to estimate frequency-specific auditory thresholds, is now available. Any complaint of hearing loss or any abnormality on office screening tests should be followed up with a complete audiogram.

The **complete audiogram** (FIG. 94–1) comprises a sophisticated battery of tests that evaluate pure tone and speech reception thresholds and tympanometry. Thresholds for pure tones varying by 1-octave intervals are ordinarily obtained for frequencies from 250 to 8000 Hz. Testing is done both by air conduction (using earphones) and bone conduction (placing an oscillator directly on the mastoid). The **pure tone average** is the average threshold, in dB, for the frequencies 500, 1000, and 2000 Hz.

The **speech reception threshold (SRT)** test measures the intensity at which the patient can correctly identify 50% of a series of spondees (words of 2 syllables, equally accented; eg, *cowboy*). The SRT should be within 10 dB of the pure tone average. The **speech discrimination score** is determined by presenting a list of spondees 40 dB above the patient's SRT and having the patient repeat them; the score is the percentage correctly identified by the patient.

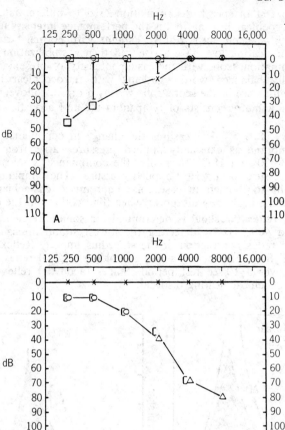

			Unmasked	Masked
AUDIOGRAM	Right Ear (AD)	Air	○	△
		Bone	<	[
CODE	Left Ear (AS)	Air	×	□
		Bone	>	]
	No Response		↓	↓

FIG. 94–1. **Audiograms in patients with hearing loss.** A: Top panel, a left, low-frequency, conductive hearing loss; the right ear has normal hearing. The air-bone gap between the air curve (□ and ×) and the bone curve (]) is indicated by (⊢–⊣). B: Bottom panel, the left ear is normal, but the right ear has a downward-sloping, sensorineural hearing loss. (Adapted from *Quick Reference to Ear, Nose, and Throat Disorders* by W. R. Wilson and J. B. Nadol, Jr. Copyright 1983 by J. B. Lippincott Company. Used with permission.)

A specialized test of speech discrimination used to differentiate cochlear from retrocochlear hearing loss is the **performance intensity function for phonetically balanced words (PIPB)**. Patients with normal hearing or with a cochlear hearing loss have a rise and then a stabilization in the speech discrimination score with increasing intensity of presentation of the phonetically balanced words. Patients with retrocochlear hearing loss have an initial rise in the score, followed by a dip (a rollover).

Impedance audiometry consists of tympanometry and acoustic (stapes) reflex measurements.

Tympanometry (FIG. 94–2) measures the change in compliance of the tympanic membrane as externally applied pressure varies from -400 mm H_2O to $+400$ mm H_2O. Normally, the compliance is maximal at atmospheric pressure (0 mm H_2O applied pressure). The tympanometric curve may shift to the left in cases of compromised eustachian tube function, while the peak may disappear when fluid collects in the ear.

The **acoustic reflex threshold** is determined for sound frequencies between 500 and 4000 Hz by detecting the lowest sound intensity that will produce a reflex contraction of the stapedius muscle. Reflex decay is an abnormal finding involving a decrease of the original reflex amplitude $\geq 50\%$ over a 10-sec test period. Stapes (acoustic) reflex decay suggests a retrocochlear hearing disorder.

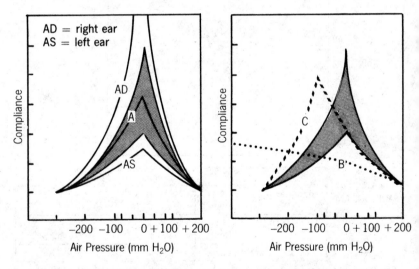

FIG. 94–2. Tympanogram tracings, at left, with normal middle ear pressure. AS is a "stiffened" curve, indicative of reduced tympanic compliance. AD is a "deep" curve, seen with either a flaccid tympanic membrane or ossicular discontinuity. At right, curve C is seen with negative middle ear pressure, while curve B is a nonpeaking curve, suggestive of middle ear fluid. (Adapted from *Quick Reference to Ear, Nose, and Throat Disorders* by W. R. Wilson and J. B. Nadol, Jr. Copyright 1983 by J. B. Lippincott Company. Used with permission.)

If auditory thresholds are ambiguous, or if the possibility of a retro-cochlear disorder exists, appropriate testing includes evaluation of the **auditory brainstem response (ABR)**. In this test, recording electrodes are attached to the patient's earlobes and vertex and are connected to an averaging computer. The activity of the auditory system in response to a sound stimulus (a click) is analyzed by the computer and generally results in the delineation of 5 sequential waves (FIG. 94–3). Waves I and II are thought to originate from the peripheral and central auditory nerve, while Wave III emanates from the cochlear nuclei and Wave IV arises from activity in the superior olivary nucleus. The lateral lemniscus is thought to give rise to Wave V. The intensity of the click needed to elicit the characteristic wave forms is an indication of the auditory thresholds, which can be determined for each ear individually.

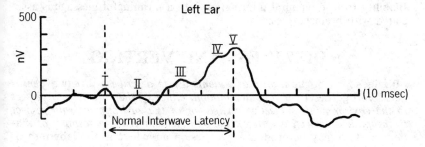

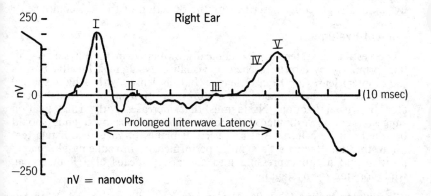

FIG. 94–3. Normal auditory brainstem response (ABR) for the left ear at top and abnormal ABR for the right ear at bottom. A vestibular schwannoma was subsequently confirmed surgically. (Adapted from *Quick Reference to Ear, Nose, and Throat Disorders* by W. R. Wilson and J. B. Nadol, Jr. Copyright 1983 by J. B. Lippincott Company. Used with permission.)

In addition, the time at which each wave appears after the sound stimulus (latency) has diagnostic implications. A delay in onset of the entire sequence of wave forms suggests a conductive hearing loss; a delay in onset of Wave V strongly suggests a retrocochlear hearing loss.

Special tests to determine central auditory function are also available but the results may be invalidated by the presence of a concurrent peripheral hearing loss. In general, these tests evaluate a patient's ability to synthesize distorted or degraded speech signals divided between the 2 ears, or to detect a specific message in 1 ear while a competing message is presented via the other ear.

The term **contralateral ear effect** describes the tendency of a cortical (temporal lobe) lesion to cause poor performance in the ear contralateral to the lesion in response to tests using distorted or degraded messages. Inability to fuse binaural information into a meaningful message is associated with brainstem lesions.

DIZZINESS AND VERTIGO

Dizziness is a *vague term that patients use to describe a variety of sensations.* **Vertigo** describes *a rotary motion, either of the patient with respect to the environment (subjective vertigo) or of the environment with respect to the patient (objective vertigo); the key element is the perception of motion.* Vertigo may be produced by a lesion anywhere in the labyrinth or its CNS connections. **Nystagmus,** specifically jerk nystagmus, results from stimulation of the vestibular system. The slow phase of nystagmus is related to the direction of the endolymph flow, while the quick, jerk-like corrective movement is controlled by the CNS. The direction of the nystagmus is generally described by the direction of the fast component.

Clinical Evaluation

The vestibular system can be clinically evaluated in the physician's office, primarily by efforts to elicit or visualize nystagmus. Ideally, Bartels (20-diopter) lenses or Frenzel lenses (Bartels lenses with a light source) should be used to eliminate the suppression of nystagmus usually created by visual fixation. Nystagmus that increases with visual fixation suggests central vestibular dysfunction. Spontaneous nystagmus should be sought in both horizontal and vertical planes of gaze. The **fistula test** (or testing for **Hennebert's sign**) is performed by introducing alternately positive and negative pressure into an ear by means of a Politzer bag while looking for nystagmus.

Positioning testing (FIG. 94-4) also can be easily performed. With the patient in the sitting position and the head turned to one side, rapidly lower the patient to the supine position with his head hanging over the edge of the table; note any nystagmus. Repeat this procedure with the patient's head turned to the opposite side, as well as with his head hanging straight back. **Caloric testing,** using cool or ice water, can also be performed in the office and provides information concerning the symmetry of vestibular function.

Laboratory Evaluation

Vestibular testing to determine the severity or location of dysfunction lacks the diagnostic precision of auditory system testing, partly because of the complexity of the functional interconnections of the vestibular

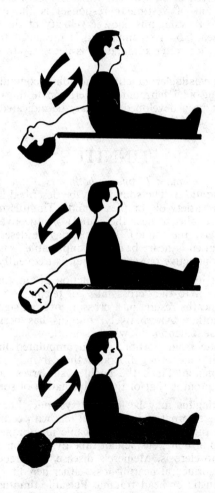

FIG. 94–4. Hallpike positioning testing; each position should be held for at least 10 sec. (Adapted from *Quick Reference to Ear, Nose, and Throat Disorders* by W. R. Wilson and J. B. Nadol, Jr. Copyright 1983 by J. B. Lippincott Company. Used with permission.)

system. **Electronystagmography (ENG)** is the most commonly available vestibular test; electrodes are placed around the patient's eyes, and eye movements are recorded on an ECG-like tracing by measurement of the corneoretinal potential. ENG usually consists of tests for horizontal and vertical gaze, pendulum tracking, opticokinetic nystagmus, positional and positioning nystagmus, and caloric stimulation. Each ear is stimulated with 250 mL of warm (44 C [111 F]) and then cool (30 C [86 F]) water, each delivered in 40 sec. The less responsive ear (canal paresis, a unilateral reduction of vestibular response) is the ear that shows a shorter duration of nystagmus, slower velocity of the slow component, or a lower frequency of nystagmus and is presumed to be the diseased ear. Occasionally, ice water stimulation is necessary to elicit a vestibular response.

Newer tests of vestibular function, including computerized rotational chair testing (sinusoidal harmonic acceleration testing) and posturography testing, have been developed and may be indicated in special cases; however, they are not widely available.

TINNITUS

The perception of a sound in one or both ears in the absence of an externally applied stimulus. The sound may be described as a ringing, hissing, whistling, or variety of complex sounds. Tinnitus may be subjective (only the patient is able to hear the sound) or objective (the examiner is also able to perceive the sound). Tinnitus may be described as pulsatile, paralleling the patient's heart beat, or nonpulsatile. An associated hearing loss, either conductive or sensorineural, is frequently present.

The mechanism involved in the production of tinnitus is not known. One theory likens it to the "cross talk" of telephone wires; patchy loss of their myelin sheaths results in a crossing over of signals from 1 auditory fiber to another. Alternatively, tinnitus has been likened to the phantom-limb phenomenon, in which sensations such as pain are perceived to originate from portions of an amputated limb; loss of hair cells and/or their innervating fibers in the ear may produce a similar phantom phenomenon. Since the cochlea subserves auditory function, the resulting symptom is that of the hallucination of sound, or tinnitus.

The causes of tinnitus may be local or systemic. Local causes include obstruction of the external auditory canal (eg, with cerumen or a foreign body); infections of the ear canal, tympanic membrane, middle ear, inner ear, or temporal bone; eustachian tube dysfunction; conductive hearing losses (eg, otosclerosis, Meniere's disease, or cerebellopontine angle tumors); and sensorineural hearing loss, either hereditary, noise induced, or related to acoustic or head trauma. Pulsatile tinnitus may be related to a glomus tumor of the middle ear or mastoid; other causes include vascular obstruction, aneurysmal dilatation, or vascular malformation. Palatal myoclonus may be associated with a perception of repetitive clicking sounds, whereas a patulous eustachian tube results in the perception of breath sounds in the ear. The latter condition often follows loss of fat deposits around the tube, as occurs after significant weight loss.

Systemic causes of tinnitus include syphilis, meningitis, arachnoiditis, drug-induced ototoxicity (eg, resulting from aminoglycoside antibiotics, salicylates, or quinine and its derivatives), hypertension, anemia, hypothyroidism, and cardiovascular diseases, including arteriosclerosis.

Evaluation of the patient after a careful history and thorough physical examination requires a complete audiogram and appropriate hematologic testing (eg, CBC, ESR) to rule out systemic causes. Unilateral or asymmetric tinnitus demands further evaluation, auditory brainstem response **(ABR)** testing and/or radiologic investigation of the head and brain (eg, with CT scanning or MRI). Pulsatile tinnitus requires evaluation of the vascular system; 4-vessel cerebral angiography may be indicated.

Treatment of tinnitus begins with management of potentially reversible causes. In many instances, eg, tinnitus associated with bilateral sensorineural hearing loss, reassurance that there is no serious underlying disorder may be helpful. Many clinicians recommend that patients with tinnitus avoid such stimulants as caffeine and chocolate, as well as alcohol, cigarettes, stress, and fatigue. With an associated hearing loss, treatment of the hearing loss or amplification may reduce the perception of tinnitus. Tinnitus maskers have *not* proven helpful. Since many patients complain that the tinnitus is most troublesome at night when they are trying to fall asleep, playing an FM radio, particularly on interband frequencies, may mask the tinnitus.

Some patients are driven to distraction by their tinnitus. Psychologic studies suggest that depression is a common underlying theme. Treatment with biofeedback, antidepressant medication, or both may be helpful. The American Tinnitus Association is a helpful support group.

OTALGIA

Ear pain may result from an otologic process or may be referred along neural pathways, including the trigeminal, glossopharyngeal, vagus, and cervical nerves. Inflammation of the pinna, external auditory canal, tympanic membrane, or middle ear results in a clinically obvious cause of the otalgia. With eustachian tube obstruction, negative pressure in the middle ear may produce a painful retraction of the tympanic membrane.

A complaint of otalgia without a clearly identified otic source demands complete examination of the head and neck. Pain in the temporomandibular joint **(TMJ)** may be referred to the ear. More ominously, tumors of head and neck structures, eg, the larynx, pharynx, esophagus, nose, and base of the tongue, as well as tumors of the base of the skull may present initially with referred otalgia. Thus, examination for otalgia should include visualization of the nasopharynx and hypopharynx and palpation of the base of the tongue and tonsillar fossae. Radiographic evaluation of the skull base may be indicated.

Treatment is related to the underlying cause.

SPECIFIC DISEASES

EXTERNAL EAR

Gout and **rheumatoid arthritis (RA)** may be associated with lesions of the pinna. The nodules of RA may be painful and can develop an area of central necrosis. Gouty tophi, most commonly found on the helix, also may be painful, occasionally discharging monosodium urate crystals. In both disorders, treatment is related to the underlying systemic disease.

Winkler's disease (chondrodermatitis nodularis chronicus helicis), particularly prevalent in older men, is characterized by the presence of exquisitely painful, firm nodules on the periphery of the pinna. Injection of hydrocortisone acetate (25 mg/mm diameter) may provide some relief from pain, or a local excision may be necessary.

MALIGNANT TUMORS

Squamous Cell Carcinoma

The most common malignant tumor of the pinna, squamous cell carcinoma, is predominantly a disease of older men. The posterior-superior aspect of the pinna is most frequently involved in men, but in women these tumors tend to occur closer to the external auditory canal. The lesions are generally painless, and biopsy is required for diagnosis. Treatment consists of wide local excision by standard technics or by Mohs' chemosurgery. The prognosis is good with small lesions of the helix, but tumors approaching the opening of the external auditory canal have a much graver prognosis.

Basal Cell Carcinoma

The second most common malignant tumor of the pinna, basal cell carcinoma, also is most prevalent in older men and appears as a nodule with pearly, heaped-up borders. Biopsy is required for definitive diagnosis. Wide excision is the therapy of choice.

Basal cell and, particularly in patients with a history of chronic otitis media, squamous cell carcinoma, may involve the external auditory canal. The initial manifestation may be an unrelenting infection that, with extension of disease, produces facial nerve paralysis. If the middle ear and facial nerve are not involved, lateral temporal bone resection (removal of the external auditory canal, tympanic membrane, malleus, and incus) is performed, followed by radiation therapy. More extensive lesions have a poor prognosis.

EXTERNAL OTITIS
(Swimmer's Ear)

A painful infection of the external auditory canal, external otitis is usually precipitated by maceration of the ear canal skin by retained water or self-inflicted trauma associated with attempts to clean the canal. This disorder is particularly significant in elderly diabetics, in whom it may progress to a potentially life-threatening *Pseudomonas* osteomyelitis of the temporal bone, commonly referred to as **malignant external otitis.** Immunodeficiency and diabetic angiopathy may promote the development of an invasive process.

An early examination may disclose only an acute external otitis, but attention should be paid to the posterior-inferior aspect of the external auditory canal. The appearance of granulation tissue in this region is an ominous sign, demanding further investigation and aggressive therapy. Once the infection penetrates the external auditory canal epithelial barrier, it tends to spread along vascular and fascial planes, resulting in numerous complications, including facial nerve paralysis, lateral venous sinus thrombosis, paralysis of cranial nerves IX through XII, and extension to the contralateral temporal bone.

Laboratory evaluation begins with a culture (which almost always reveals the presence of *Pseudomonas aeruginosa*) and sensitivity testing. **Mastoid x-rays** may demonstrate clouding of the mastoid air cell spaces and suggest a more invasive disorder than ordinary external otitis. A **technetium 99m diphosphonate bone scan** provides early detection of temporal bone osteomyelitis, while **scanning with gallium 67 citrate** monitors antibiotic response. **Temporal bone CT scanning** and, more recently, **MRI** are other diagnostic adjuncts. **Biopsy of the granulation tissue** is helpful in distinguishing malignant external otitis from other inflammatory processes.

Treatment involves hospitalization and the initiation of IV antibiotic therapy with a combination of aminoglycoside antibiotics (eg, gentamicin, tobramycin, or amikacin) and the synthetic penicillin, ticarcillin. Ticarcillin is generally administered in dosages of 3 gm IV q 4 h. Alternative therapies include ticarcillin with potassium clavulanate or third-generation cephalosporins such as ceftazidime. Several weeks of treatment may be required.

Curettage of the granulation tissue with insertion of antibiotic-containing wicks, as well as hyperbaric O_2 therapy, may be useful. Surgery is reserved for cases not responsive to medical therapy. Meticulous management of diabetes is an essential part of total patient care.

ACCUMULATION OF CERUMEN

Massive accumulation of cerumen resulting from years of inattention may be seen in the elderly. The accumulation may be rock-hard and, particularly in older men, may contain a generous admixture of exfoliated hairs. The patient may complain of hearing loss and a feeling of fullness in the ear. Obstruction of the external canal is obvious on examination. Because the adnexal elements responsible for the production of cerumen are located in only the lateral 2/3 of the canal, the extension of impaction to the medial portion suggests manipulation with instruments such as cotton-tipped applicators.

The cerumen should be removed as gently as possible. In some cases, this may be accomplished with a cerumen spoon, along with good visualization and use of an aural speculum. The skin of the external auditory canal can easily be traumatized and is exquisitely sensitive to manipulation. Thus, with hard accumulations, topical therapy for several days to a week may be necessary to soften the debris so it may be removed atraumatically.

Application of an antibiotic otic solution 4 drops qid in the affected ear softens the wax and quells any smoldering infection. When adequately softened, the wax can be easily removed, either with the cerumen spoon or by water irrigation. *Irrigation is contraindicated in the presence of a tympanic membrane perforation, since it may provoke an infection.* To avoid perforating the tympanic membrane, the irrigation force should be gentle and directed along the canal wall, *not* directly at the eardrum.

MIDDLE EAR

SEROUS OTITIS MEDIA

An effusion in the middle ear, usually related to obstruction of the eustachian tube but also seen in the course of resolving acute otitis media. The fluid generally is not grossly purulent but may contain low levels of pathogenic organisms. Unilateral serous otitis media in the elderly adult has different implications from that in a young child. The former demands evaluation for and exclusion of a nasopharyngeal mass; such lesions commonly present with unilateral serous otitis media due to obstruction of the eustachian tube at its nasopharyngeal orifice.

The patient perceives a sensation of aural fullness and hearing loss. On physical examination, amber fluid can be visualized medial to the tympanic membrane, causing the malleus handle to appear whiter than usual. Occasionally, air bubbles or an air-fluid level may also be seen. The nasopharynx should be examined by mirror or fiberscope to assess the eustachian tube orifice. CT scanning or MRI may be indicated to visualize a more lateral obstruction.

Treatment of any mass lesion depends on the information provided by biopsy. If serous otitis media is accompanied by upper respiratory tract infection or allergy, antibiotic or local vasoconstrictive therapy, or both, may be helpful. Nasal sprays, eg, oxymetazoline HCl 0.05%, can provide local decongestion but should not be used > 5 days in succession. In some cases, myringotomy with aspiration of fluid and, possibly, insertion of a ventilation tube may be necessary.

CHRONIC OTITIS MEDIA

A chronic middle ear infection generally associated with a tympanic membrane perforation and intermittent, purulent otorrhea. Chronic otitis media is not specifically a disorder of the elderly but may present or recur in this age group. Polypoid hypertrophy of the middle ear mucosa may progress to the extent that it presents as an ear canal mass.

The patient may have a history of previous ear surgery and generally complains of ear drainage and hearing loss. The complaint of dizziness is ominous, suggesting erosion of the bone of the labyrinth. Facial nerve paralysis, another ominous sign, suggests extensive disease.

A complication of chronic otitis media is the development of **cholesteatoma**, *the accumulation of keratin debris in the middle ear or mastoid.* This debris originates from keratinizing squamous epithelium that has entered these areas from the external auditory canal, generally through a tympanic membrane marginal perforation. Symptoms are produced by progressive erosion of middle and inner ear structures. The cholesteatoma may extend through the tegmen into the brain or may involve the lateral venous sinus, further complicating the disorder.

Physical examination may disclose that the external auditory canal is occluded by purulent debris; this should be gently aspirated and submitted for culture. Otoscopic examination, supplemented by microscopic visualization, can document the presence of a tympanic membrane perforation and the status of the middle ear mucosa. In other cases, polypoid granulation tissue, representing hypertrophied middle ear mucosa, may preclude adequate examination. An evaluation of the postauricular area may show a scar and depression, indicating previous mastoid surgery.

Plain films of the mastoids can give some idea of the extent of mastoid air cell system development and can indicate whether a lytic lesion is present and whether surgery was previously performed. **CT scanning** with a specific bone-imaging algorithm visualizes more clearly the status of the middle ear and mastoid structures, as well as the integrity of the tegmen and the otic capsule.

Manual removal of accumulated debris to the extent safely possible is the initial therapeutic step. Irrigation with 2 oz 1.5% acetic acid tid helps mechanically debride the remaining debris and restore the normal acidic pH of the auditory canal. A topical antibiotic solution should be instilled after each irrigation session and in the evening.

Preparations containing neomycin, which is ototoxic, should be avoided. A commercially available ophthalmic preparation containing sulfacetamide sodium and prednisolone has not been documented to have any ototoxic properties and does not produce a burning sensation upon instillation. Topical therapy can often reduce the size of hypertrophied mucosal lesions.

Polypoid tissue may be gently excised for biopsy. Avulsion of such lesions must be avoided, since their medial attachments may include the stapes or facial nerve. Depending upon the etiology of the chronic otitis media and the general condition of the patient, surgery may be recommended.

OTOSCLEROSIS

A disease of the bone of the otic capsule and the most common cause of progressive conductive hearing loss in the adult with a normal tympanic membrane.

This disease, unique to the human otic capsule, is reported to occur in 10% of the temporal bones of white persons. Approximately 10% of affected persons actually develop clinically significant conductive hearing loss. A family history of otosclerosis is seen in 50 to 60% of cases.

The disease is characterized by irregular areas of bone resorption and new bone formation, occurring predominantly at the oval window and eventually resulting in ankylosis of the stapes. In addition to causing conductive hearing loss, otosclerosis occasionally causes sensorineural hearing loss when the cochlea is involved.

Otosclerosis generally is diagnosed before old age. Surgical bypass of the stapes can correct the conductive component of the hearing loss in most cases. Although a hearing aid is an acceptable alternative for many persons, occasionally a patient with mixed hearing loss can benefit from stapedectomy. In some cases, closure of the air-bone gap brings the patient's hearing threshold to a level that can be more amenable to hearing aid fitting.

TUMORS

Tumors of the middle ear and mastoid are rare. Of these, the most common benign tumors are **paragangliomas,** which are derived from paraganglion tissue (eg, the carotid body). Patients with these lesions, otherwise known as **glomus tumors,** generally present with a conductive hearing loss and pulsatile tinnitus. Tumors originating in the middle ear **(glomus tympanicum)** are clinically evident even when small, whereas tumors arising in the jugular vein at the mastoid **(glomus jugulare)** become clinically apparent at relatively late stages and may produce symptoms such as paralysis of cranial nerves IX through XII.

Physical examination may reveal a pulsatile red mass in the middle ear. The integrity of the cranial nerves should be assessed. Audiometric evaluation usually documents a conductive hearing loss, but in more widespread tumors, an additional sensorineural component may also be detected. Because of the multicentricity of these lesions, 4-vessel cerebral angiography may reveal additional, occult growths. Glomus tumors have also been associated with catecholamine production, resulting in intermittent hypertension.

Therapy depends upon the size of the tumor as well as the general medical condition of the patient. In the healthy patient, small tumors can be removed relatively easily. Extensive tumors in the infirm patient are probably best managed more conservatively. Relatively low-dose radiation therapy and arteriographic embolization are palliative and may be more appropriate in the elderly.

Squamous cell carcinoma may occur in the middle ear, generally associated with a chronic ear infection. The treatment of choice is surgery, consisting of wide-field resection of the temporal bone, followed by radiation therapy.

INNER EAR

PRESBYCUSIS

A bilaterally symmetric, sensorineural hearing loss that occurs as a part of normal aging. Hearing loss of some sort affects approximately ⅓ of all adults between 65 and 74 yr of age and approximately ½ of those between 75 and 79. It is estimated that in the USA, > 10 million elderly people have a hearing impairment.

The presence, progression, and severity of presbycusis varies among individuals and depends upon a variety of factors. Men typically have a more severe impairment than women of the same age. Noise exposure, diet, and hypertension, as well as metabolic and hereditary factors, play a role. Age-related changes in the inner ear and CNS, including cellular loss, reduced activity, and depletion of neurotransmitters, may be aggravated by vascular lesions that result in hypoperfusion.

Usually, presbycusis initially affects the very high frequencies, which do not interfere with speech understanding. When the hearing loss involves the higher speech frequencies that affect consonant discrimination, individuals begin noting difficulty understanding speech. Patients characteristically complain of having difficulty understanding persons with higher-pitched voices (eg, women and young children) and conversations in large groups or with background noise, as in restaurants or bars. As the hearing loss progresses, communication requires increasing effort. The embarrassment of misunderstanding can precipitate withdrawal from social contacts, leading to loneliness, depression, and paranoia.

Four pathophysiologic types of presbycusis have been described (see FIG. 94–5). **Sensory presbycusis** is marked by atrophy of the organ of Corti, worst at the basal end of the cochlea. The hearing loss generally begins in middle age and progresses slowly. A loss of cochlear neurons parallels the loss of the organ of Corti. The audiogram generally shows an abrupt, high-frequency hearing loss with good discrimination.

Neural presbycusis, usually manifested in the later years of life, is ascribed to a loss of cochlear neurons with a relative preservation of the organ of Corti. The degeneration of the neural population is apparently related to genetic factors. Audiometric evaluation shows a predominantly high-frequency hearing loss with very poor discrimination; a progressive loss of speech discrimination (phonemic regression) occurs, but pure tone thresholds are maintained. Rapidly progressing neural pres-

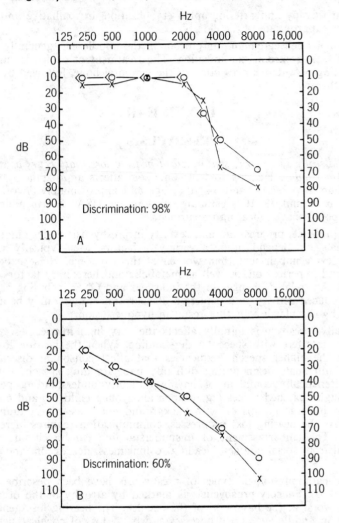

FIG. 94–5. **Audiograms in patients with presbycusis.** A: Abrupt, bilaterally symmetric, high-frequency hearing loss typical of sensory presbycusis. Discrimination is excellent. B: Downward-sloping sensorineural hearing loss with poor discrimination; characteristic of neural presbycusis. (See audiogram code on page 1085 for key to symbols.)

bycusis may be accompanied by other signs of CNS degeneration, including intellectual deterioration, memory loss, and motor incoordination.

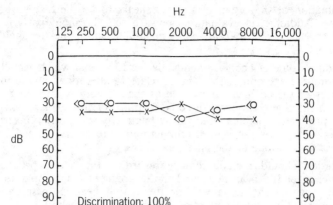

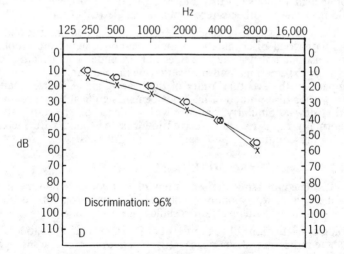

C: Flat sensorineural hearing loss, as seen in metabolic presbycusis. Discrimination is unaffected. D: Bilaterally symmetric, downward-sloping, sensorineural hearing loss with excellent discrimination; consistent with cochlear conductive presbycusis. (Adapted from *Quick Reference to Ear, Nose, and Throat Disorders* by W. R. Wilson and J. B. Nadol, Jr. Copyright 1983 by J. B. Lippincott Company. Used with permission.)

A third type is **metabolic presbycusis.** This type of hearing loss has a familial tendency, with onset in middle age and slow progression. Patchy atrophy of the stria vascularis, which affects the electrophysiologic function of the organ of Corti, appears to be the histopathologic correlate. Audiometric evaluation shows a flat threshold pattern, with normal speech discrimination scores maintained until the thresholds exceed 50 dB.

The fourth type is **cochlear conductive presbycusis,** which usually begins in middle age and is thought to relate to alterations in the motion mechanics of the cochlear duct, such as that caused by stiffening of the basilar membrane. However, there is no proof of this explanation. This type of presbycusis is characterized by bilaterally symmetric, linearly descending thresholds; speech discrimination is inversely related to the steepness of the slope of the pure tone curve.

Evaluation should include inquiry regarding the onset, progression, and severity of the hearing loss. Tinnitus frequently accompanies presbycusis. Asymmetric, unilateral, or fluctuating hearing losses are not characteristic. Physical examination generally is unrevealing.

The minimal diagnostic evaluation comprises a complete audiogram, including pure tone, speech, and tympanometric testing. Any asymmetry in the audiogram or retrocochlear signs should be pursued with an auditory brainstem response **(ABR)** and a CT scan or MRI to rule out an acoustic neuroma or other cerebellopontine angle **(CPA)** tumor.

Treatment of presbycusis generally relates to the audiometric pattern; patients with good discrimination should readily benefit from amplification. A sensorineural hearing loss does not preclude benefit from a hearing aid. The expectations and motivation of the patient have a considerable impact on the eventual utility of the hearing aid. However, patients with very poor discrimination may not benefit significantly from an amplification device. Similarly, patients with evidence of "recruitment" (ie, an abnormally rapid rise in perceived loudness of sound with increased volume of presentation) require carefully fitted devices.

DYSEQUILIBRIUM OF AGING

Dizziness, encompassing the sensations of vertigo, dysequilibrium, and unsteadiness, is a nearly uniform complaint elicited from up to 90% of patients seen in outpatient geriatric clinics (see also Ch. 6).

Histologic evaluation of temporal bones from elderly patients has given some indication of the degenerative changes associated with aging. Loss of hair cells appears to be particularly predominant in the cristae of the semicircular canal but also occurs in the maculae of the otolithic organs. Losses may also occur in the innervating fibers of the hair cells as well as among the neurons in Scarpa's ganglion. Degenerative changes in the otoconia predominate in the saccule and are observed only occasionally in the utricle.

Accumulation of lipofuscin appears to progress within the labyrinth as in the cochlea. Because of the complexity of the vestibular system and its diffuse interconnections, it is difficult to correlate the observed clinical picture with the described histopathologic findings as readily as has been done in the case of the cochlea; nonetheless, 4 distinct types of dysequilibrium of aging have been described, as follows:

1. Cupulolithiasis of aging (benign paroxysmal positional vertigo of aging) is characterized by *brief, intense episodes of true spinning vertigo upon assumption of a particular head position.* Most commonly, the patient notes that rolling over in bed to 1 side or the other (but not both) precipitates the symptoms. Occasionally, patients note that a sudden movement of the head to the left or right, as well as rapid head extension or (less frequently) flexion, also precipitates symptoms. Although head injury, ear infection, neurologic disease, ear surgery, or viral infection may precipitate symptoms of cupulolithiasis, usually no specific cause is found. Degeneration of the labyrinth (especially otoconial degeneration) may result in the generation of high specific gravity deposits that tend to settle on the cupula of the posterior semicircular canal (FIG. 94–6). The disorder is generally self-limited but occasionally may recur over months or years.

Because of their reduced muscle strength and reflex speed, older persons are particularly prone to falls when afflicted with dizziness. Positioning nystagmus testing (see above) demonstrates a horizontal-rotary nystagmus toward the lowermost ear that appears within a few seconds of assumption of the provocative position. The nystagmus lasts < 30 sec, and often a complementary nystagmus occurs with resumption of the sitting position. Immediate repetition of the provocative head position elicits a reduced response, if any; this loss of response is referred to as fatigability. Electronystagmography **(ENG)** generally shows a normal caloric response bilaterally.

Treatment consists of avoiding the provocative position until the process remits spontaneously. In patients debilitated by this disorder, sectioning of the nerve to the posterior semicircular canal, using a middle ear approach, may be helpful.

2. Ampullary dysequilibrium of aging consists of *vertigo associated with rotational head movements.* Patients note a persistent sensation of motion a few seconds after rapidly turning their head to the right or left; extension or flexion of the head may also precipitate this symptom. A subsequent sensation of unsteadiness may linger for several hours. The histopathologic correlate is not clearly defined but appears to be related to a degenerative change in the ampullae of the semicircular canals.

Physical examination may not document the brief flash of nystagmus precipitated by sudden head rotation. Response to caloric stimulation may be reduced, as documented by ENG. Treatment consists of avoiding abrupt head movements.

3. Macular dysequilibrium of aging is *the onset of vertigo upon changes of head position with respect to gravity.* Typically, patients complain that they can no longer jump out of bed, but instead must sit on the side of the bed and steady themselves for a few seconds, after which they carry on without further problems. The histopathologic correlate appears to

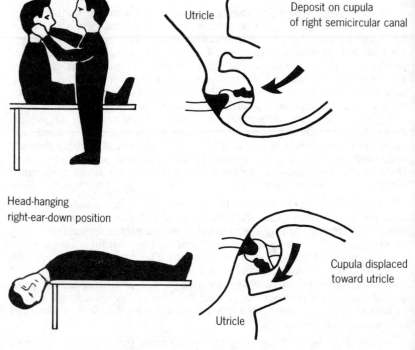

FIG. 94–6. **The pathophysiology of cupulolithiasis (of aging).** (Adapted from *Quick Reference to Ear, Nose, and Throat Disorders* by W. R. Wilson and J. B. Nadol, Jr. Copyright 1983 by J. B. Lippincott Company. Used with permission.)

lie in degenerative changes in the otolithic membranes or sensory hair cells of the otolithic organs. Physical examination should seek to exclude possible hypotension. ENG testing generally shows normal caloric responses. There is no specific treatment.

4. Vestibular ataxia of aging consists of *a constant sensation of imbalance with ambulation.* The patient has no difficulty with posture while sitting but hesitancy and frequent side stepping are manifested upon attempting to walk. This dysequilibrium may relate to dysfunction of the reflex control of the vestibular system over the lower limbs. Vestibular testing is nondiagnostic, and no treatment is available.

The absence of effective medical therapy for the dysequilibria of aging must be emphasized. Vestibular depressants (eg, meclizine or diazepam) do not suppress the burst of vertigo encountered in cupulolithiasis. Worse yet, they may depress the protective reflexes of elderly patients, rendering them more prone to falls. Providing handrails and adequate lighting, particularly at night, may allow the patient to maximize appropriate proprioceptive and visual orientational clues and thus ambulate more safely.

OCCLUSION OF THE ANTERIOR VESTIBULAR ARTERY

The anterior vestibular artery supplies the lateral and superior semicircular canals as well as the utricle. Acute obstruction results in the sudden onset of severe vertigo without other otologic or CNS manifestations. As in the vertigo of acute viral labyrinthitis, recovery occurs over several weeks. However, positional vertigo develops and may persist for years. Anterior vestibular artery obstruction is thought to cause necrosis of the supplied structures, resulting in the deposition of necrotic debris on the cupula of the otherwise unaffected posterior semicircular canal. This disorder is in other ways identical to cupulolithiasis. Aspirin prophylaxis may be indicated in such patients.

VESTIBULAR SCHWANNOMA
(Acoustic Neuroma)

A benign tumor that develops from the Schwann cells forming the sheaths of the vestibular nerves. These tumors most commonly arise in or immediately medial to the internal auditory canal; with growth, they present as a cerebellopontine angle **(CPA)** mass.

Patients usually complain of a unilateral hearing loss accompanied by tinnitus and, occasionally, dysequilibrium. Large tumors may also affect 5th and lower cranial nerves and produce hydrocephalus. Since **physical examination** may disclose only a unilateral or asymmetric hearing loss, inspection of cranial nerve function is mandatory.

A complete **audiogram** generally shows an asymmetric sensorineural hearing loss with disproportionately poor speech discrimination scores. The acoustic reflex may be absent or decayed, and rollover may be found on PIPB (phonetic balance) testing. Auditory brainstem response **(ABR)** testing shows abnormalities consistent with a retrocochlear lesion. **Radiologic investigation** consists of CT scanning with contrast or MRI directed toward the CPA and the internal auditory canals.

Treatment of acoustic tumors in the elderly is controversial. Complete surgical excision, as performed in younger patients, is recommended by some surgeons, while others believe that a palliative subtotal resection is wiser. The size of the tumor, its associated symptoms, and the overall medical condition of the patient should be considered when deciding on appropriate therapy.

METASTATIC LESIONS

Hematogenous dissemination of cancer may seed the temporal bone with metastatic foci. **The most common primary tumors metastasizing to the temporal bone,** in descending order of frequency, are those of the breast, kidney, lung, stomach, larynx, prostate, and thyroid.

Symptoms depend upon the location of involvement within the temporal bone. Conductive hearing loss and pain are associated with involvement of the external auditory canal, middle ear, mastoid, or eustachian tube. Sensorineural hearing loss, vertigo, and facial paralysis are more characteristic of internal auditory canal involvement.

Appropriate evaluation includes radiographic documentation and confirmation by biopsy. Therapy depends upon the lesion detected.

VERTEBROBASILAR INSUFFICIENCY

The blood supply to the inner ear is derived from the internal auditory artery, which arises as a branch of the anterior inferior cerebellar artery or directly from the basilar artery. Patients with disordered perfusion of the vertebrobasilar system may complain of episodes of dizziness, usually associated with dysarthria, visual disturbances, or syncope.

The most common cause is atherosclerosis of the vertebrobasilar system, but in some cases, cervical compression of the vertebral artery causes the insufficiency. The **thyrocervical steal syndrome,** resulting from blockage of the subclavian artery proximal to the vertebral artery, may also be associated with vertebrobasilar insufficiency.

Vestibular tests are nonspecific, and arteriography is often indicated. Therapy depends upon the cause and site of the lesion. Control of hypertension is indicated, and anticoagulant therapy may be a consideration.

OTOTOXICITY

Drugs particularly notorious for ototoxicity include the aminoglycoside antibiotics (streptomycin, kanamycin, neomycin, gentamicin, and viomycin); salicylates; the diuretics ethacrynic acid and furosemide; and quinine or its synthetic analog, chloroquine. Although both the vestibular and auditory portions of the inner ear can be affected, streptomycin, gentamicin, and viomycin are particularly toxic to the vestibular system, while neomycin, kanamycin, and amikacin are more toxic to the auditory system.

Salicylates in large doses can cause a reversible hearing loss, tinnitus, and vertigo. The symptoms generally appear with plasma concentrations approximating 35 mg/dL. Ethacrynic acid, when administered IV, is associated with permanent hearing loss; concomitant aminoglycoside administration appears to be an aggravating factor. Furosemide is associated with temporary hearing loss. Quinine and its synthetic analogs are associated with both permanent and temporary hearing losses, the former occurring with large doses. Chemotherapeutic agents, particularly nitrogen mustard and cisplatin, are implicated in sensorineural hearing loss.

The elderly, especially those with hearing loss or renal dysfunction, should not be treated with ototoxic drugs unless no suitable alternative exists. If such a drug must be used, a baseline audiogram should be obtained prior to the initiation of treatment, and the patient should be monitored daily until treatment is completed. The vestibular effects may be more insidious, particularly when patients are bedridden. A bedside test of the vestibulo-ocular reflex has been proposed and may be helpful in early detection of vestibular dysfunction.

Although the perilymph of the inner ear may tend to concentrate and retain certain ototoxic drugs, regular monitoring of serum for therapeutic blood levels should help avoid ototoxicity.

AMPLIFICATION AND AUDITORY REHABILITATION

The goal of rehabilitation is to achieve the best hearing possible in the patient by using a combination of amplification, speech reading, and auditory training.

Assistive Listening Devices (ALDs)

ALDs comprise a group of devices used to help hearing-impaired persons overcome problems associated with use of the telephone, TV, or radio, and communication in small or large groups.

Portable and nonportable amplifiers boost the telephone speaker output, while special signaling devices produce either a louder ring or a flashing light alert. Other devices can sufficiently amplify TV and radio signals for the hearing-impaired person, while family members continue to listen at normal volume levels. Telecaptioning may benefit those with good vision whose residual hearing is not sufficient to benefit from amplified sound signals.

For small-group communication (eg, in card games), relatively inexpensive devices with portable microphone, amplifier, and headset are available. For large-group communication (eg, in a concert hall or church), many public facilities have installed group amplification systems, such as infrared transmission. The individual can borrow a special, portable receiver so that he can tune in.

Hearing Aids

Amplification with hearing aids can be helpful in persons with conductive or sensorineural hearing losses. Although hearing aids vary in size and power, they share certain common features. A microphone receives the sound, transforms it into electrical energy, and sends this signal to an amplifier that increases its energy. The degree of amplification of the incoming signal as manifested in the output of the hearing aid speaker is known as **gain**. The earmold channels the hearing aid output into the ear canal.

For a time, the most widely used type of hearing aid was the **behind-the-ear or postauricular version**. In this type, the bulk of the device is hooked above and posterior to the auricle; it is connected to the earmold by flexible tubing. However, the growing popularity of **in-the-ear**

(ITE) aids has now made these the most common type. These aids are retained entirely within the ear canal and concha; in-the-canal aids are even smaller devices contained solely within the ear canal. Generally, the smaller the device, the less powerful it is and the poorer the fidelity of sound it transmits.

The popularity of eyeglass-mounted aids has diminished, perhaps because of the combined visual and auditory deficits precipitated by their frequent need for repair. For high-frequency hearing losses, a modification of the mold, termed **venting**, may selectively amplify the frequencies the patient is missing.

The contralateral routing of signals (CROS) aid is used in a unilateral, total hearing loss with preservation of relatively normal hearing in the contralateral ear. A microphone directs sound from the poorer-hearing to the better-hearing ear. If the better-hearing ear is also impaired, the signal from the poorer-hearing ear can be amplified; this type of device is called a **BiCROS aid.** Originally, the 2 devices were connected by cords, but newer models can incorporate FM signal transmission.

A body aid, the most powerful type available (ie, possessing the highest gain), may be concealed in a pocket or worn with a body strap and is connected by wiring to the earpiece, which is connected to the earmold. For the elderly, particularly those with impaired fine motor skills, the controls of a body aid may be more easily managed. Alternatives include geriatric molds, designed for easier handling, and remote controls similar to a credit card to facilitate adjusting settings.

Hearing aids are now available with a variety of sophisticated modifications. The T switch enables the user to hear telephone communications through the hearing aid. Circuitry modifications include automatic gain control **(AGC),** automatic signal processing **(ASP),** and multiple signal processing **(MSP).** AGC automatically dampens or amplifies incoming loud or soft sounds so they are perceived at about the same volume; such control is especially helpful in patients with "recruiting" ears, in whom sounds too much greater than their thresholds can be painful. ASP and MSP attempt to improve the signal (human speech)-to-noise ratio and thus improve hearing ability in the presence of environmental sound.

In contrast to air-conduction aids, which require an earmold, the oscillator of the **bone-conduction aid** is placed in direct contact with the head, usually over the mastoid, with a type of headset. This type of aid may be appropriate when an ITE aid is contraindicated, as in persistent, uncontrollable otorrhea or canal atresia.

A more recent advance is the development of an **implantable bone-conduction device.** A magnet is implanted posterior-superior to the mastoid bone in a minor surgical procedure. An overlying component, similar to a behind-the-ear aid, receives and transmits signals to the magnet, causing it to vibrate; the vibrations are transmitted to the skull and the inner ear structures. Currently, this device is indicated only for conductive hearing losses.

The hearing aid evaluation requires matching the patient's auditory thresholds across the frequency band and speech discrimination ability with the type of hearing aid recommended for those characteristics. The social stigma as well as the expense of the hearing aid may be difficult barriers to overcome. Important factors in determining whether a patient will be a successful hearing aid user include motivation, the need to communicate, and the appropriateness of expectations as to what can be achieved with the hearing aid.

The patient should be taught how to adjust the device as well as how to keep it clean and functional. Some patients with relatively normal pure-tone thresholds demonstrate very poor speech discrimination; they are not likely to benefit from a hearing aid. Similarly, some patients have hearing loss associated with recruitment so severe that stimulation above threshold may be painful.

Cochlear Implants

The cochlear implant is approved for use in the profoundly deaf adult who obtains no benefit from the most powerful hearing aid. This device includes a microphone that picks up the incoming sound signal and sends it to a speech processor; the processor modifies the signal and transmits it to external circuitry, which then relays the information to the receiver circuitry in the implanted device. From the internal circuitry, an electrode or a series of electrodes implanted in the cochlea stimulates the remaining neural elements of hearing. Implantation of the device generally requires mastoid surgery and brief hospitalization.

The device is expensive, and insurance coverage is variable. Although the population it may help is limited, the cochlear implant can make a tremendous difference in the life of an otherwise isolated person.

Vibrotactile Devices

These devices are alternative modes of rehabilitation of the profoundly deaf; they transform speech and environmental sounds into vibrations that can be perceived on the skin by vibrators placed either on the wrist or sternum or around the waist. With appropriate training, patients can learn to identify and localize sounds as well as to use the vibrotactile information to improve their communication skills.

Speech Reading

The term **speech reading** has replaced the older term **lip reading** in accordance with the concept that linguistic information can be obtained not only by watching the speaker's lips but also by following facial expressions and gestures. Such visual cues may be an adjunct or an alternative to hearing aid use. Factors that may mitigate against mastering speech reading are decreasing visual acuity and poor short-term memory.

Auditory Training

Auditory training is often combined with amplification to maximize the benefit from a particular device. Auditory training attempts to help patients discriminate between distinctly differing sounds with hearing alone, eventually enabling them to develop schemes for making fine distinctions, particulary between similar speech sounds. In essence, such training makes the patient more aware of subtle auditory clues.

With auditory training, as with any aspect of auditory rehabilitation, having interested family members accompany the geriatric patient is helpful. Family members not only can provide encouragement and support but also may prompt the older patient when short-term memory fails.

General Considerations

Certain guidelines are helpful in attempting to communicate with any hearing-impaired individual. Communication is most effective when competing environmental sound is absent or minimal. The speaker must first make sure that his face is well illuminated and that the listener is attentive. Speech should be slow, clear, and presented at an optimal distance of approximately 3 ft from the listener's better or aided ear. Shouting is not necessary. If the person misunderstands a statement, it should not be repeated word for word; instead, the original statement should be paraphrased.

95. NOSE AND THROAT DISORDERS

William R. Wilson

NOSE AND PARANASAL SINUSES

In general, conditions that affect the nose and throat in the younger adult also appear in the elderly. However, only conditions that occur either more commonly or exclusively in the elderly and are associated with aging are discussed here.

NASAL OBSTRUCTION SECONDARY TO GRAVITATIONAL EFFECTS

The nose gradually changes over a lifetime. Most apparent are gravitational effects, resulting in an increased droop of the nasal tip. Usually, the angle between the columella of the nose and the upper lip is 90° in a man and 110° in a woman. With time, this angle gradually decreases because of laxity of the skin and thinning and softening of the alar cartilage. When this effect is pronounced, nasal obstruction may result.

Elongation of the nose results in narrowing, and many elderly patients have nasal obstruction due to closure of the softened ala against the septum during inspiration. This form of obstruction can be diagnosed by manually elevating the nasal tip with the examiner's thumb; this should produce immediate improvement. The nasal airway can be opened further by placing gentle traction on the cheek. When sufficiently severe, the problem can be corrected surgically by lifting the tip, shortening the nasal septum, and correcting the laxity of the skin.

DISORDERS DUE TO AGING OF THE NASAL MUCOUS MEMBRANE

The mucous membrane becomes thinner, with a decrease in elastic fibers and submucosal tissues and atrophy of the mucus-secreting structures. The result is a decrease in mucus production and some dryness of the nose. Treatment consists of prn use of buffered saline nasal sprays.

RHINORRHEA

The elderly may complain of excessive watery, dripping nasal secretions associated with eating, particularly hot or spicy foods. The rhinorrhea necessitates frequent wiping of the nose during a meal. This condition is probably due to altered function of the parasympathetic vasomotor secretory fibers in the nose; no satisfactory treatment is available.

Drugs that are generally innocuous in younger populations when routinely prescribed for nasal congestion or rhinorrhea can cause serious side effects in the elderly. Sympathomimetic amines (eg, pseudoephedrine), which can cause agitation and confusion, more commonly cause urinary retention. Antihistamines may produce excessive sedation, hypotension, vertigo, syncope, and disturbances of coordination.

EPISTAXIS
(Nosebleed)

Atrophic changes in the mucous membrane and increased susceptibility of the nasal vasculature to rupture because of thinning of vessel walls make epistaxis relatively common in the elderly. It occurs in 2 forms: anterior and posterior.

Anterior epistaxis is commonly due to ulceration of the mucosa overlying old septal spurs or deviations, particularly in patients taking anticoagulants (eg, daily aspirin following MI). Any coagulopathy should be corrected, at least temporarily, to allow a thrombus to form and the mucous membranes to heal. For treatment of acute epistaxis, oxymetazoline has long-acting vasoconstricting properties and no significant systemic effects. It can be applied with cotton to the bleeding site, which is then compressed externally until the bleeding stops. Bleeding sites also can be cauterized and protected with a petroleum-based ointment until healed.

Posterior epistaxis is more serious. Most commonly, it is caused by the rupture of a branch of the sphenopalatine artery in the region of the posterior tip of the inferior turbinate. Nasal packing is usually required to control the bleeding, particularly in hypertensive individuals. The nose should be anesthetized with a lidocaine-based spray followed by a vasoconstricting spray (eg, oxymetazoline). Next, a commercially available epistaxis balloon (Nasostat®) should be placed in the nose and expanded with water, rather than air (to prevent softening), until the bleeding is controlled. The balloon should be left in place for approximately 5 days and a prophylactic antibiotic administered to prevent sinusitis.

Gauze packing has the disadvantage of causing nasal obstruction and often depresses the palate, resulting in partial obstruction of the oral airway. In younger individuals, this packing generally is tolerated without difficulty, but in the elderly, hypoxia and CO_2 retention can occur. Elderly patients with posterior nasal packing should be hospitalized for monitoring of respiratory status and arterial blood gas levels.

If epistaxis persists despite the above procedure, 1 of 2 additional therapeutic approaches may be used, depending upon the medical expertise available and the patient's condition. The first is transantral ligation of the sphenopalatine artery in the pterygomaxillary space. The second is angiography and embolization of the internal maxillary artery and sphenopalatine artery. After the epistaxis has been treated, the patient should have a full set of sinus x-rays to determine if sinusitis has developed or if an underlying tumor is the cause of the bleeding.

NASAL FRACTURES

Nasal fractures are relatively common in the elderly, the result of falls and age-related thinning of bony facial structures. Treatment by closed reduction usually suffices; ie, elevation and positioning of the bony fragments with a small, nonobstructing nasal packing for about 1 wk (until the fracture has stabilized). As noted above, all nasal packings should be accompanied by antibiotic administration to prevent sinus infection.

ORAL CAVITY
(See also Ch. 44)

VARICOSITIES

Varicosities in the floor of the mouth, the ventral surface of the tongue, and the hypopharynx are common in the elderly. However, they rarely, if ever, bleed.

LOSS OF DENTITION

The edentulous elderly suffer subsequent resorption of the alveolar bone portion of the upper and lower jaw. Nevertheless, upper dentures with a large surface area on the hard palate can usually be adjusted to fit satisfactorily. Occasionally, the alveolar surface may be insufficient for proper fitting of lower dentures. New dental post technics have alleviated this situation by providing anchorage for lower dentures. Loose or absent dentures may cause angular cheilitis from drooling of saliva due to decreased skin or muscle tone. Angular cheilitis occasionally is caused by nutritional insufficiency, which results from poorly fitting dentures.

XEROSTOMIA
(Dry Mouth)

This common disorder in the elderly results from atrophy of the major and minor salivary glands. It is also a side effect of many drugs, especially diuretics. Salivary flow is necessary for a healthy mouth and teeth. Reduction of flow results in an increase in dental caries and loss of teeth.

BURNING-TONGUE SYNDROME

This common complaint is related to many factors, including atrophy of the oral mucous membrane, poor oral hygiene, decreased saliva, poor nutrition, and vitamin deficiencies.

SIALADENITIS

Inflammation of a salivary gland. Decreased salivary flow and chronic mild dehydration are responsible for the increased incidence of parotid and submandibular sialadenitis in the elderly. Clinical features include swelling, pain, and erythema over the affected gland, associated with fever. Leukocytosis is common. Palpation of the gland expresses from the ducts a purulent discharge that can be Gram stained and cultured; the most common organism is *Staphylococcus aureus.* Treatment consists of rehydration and antibiotic administration. Occasionally, an abscess requires surgical drainage.

Temporomandibular joint (TMJ) syndrome (see Ch. 44) presents as an aching pain overlying the joint and in the ear, pain and tenderness on pressure over the joint or pterygoid muscles, and pain on chewing. Crepitus often is associated with joint movement. Therapy includes a soft diet, anti-inflammatory drugs, muscle relaxants, and moist heat.

Temporal arteritis (see Ch. 63) must be differentiated from TMJ pain. This condition occurs in individuals over 50 yr of age and is manifested by a tender temporal artery on palpation and an elevated ESR. The condition can lead to blindness if not treated. Diagnosis is made by biopsy, which should include at least a 3-cm segment of the palpable portion of the temporal artery.

DISORDERS OF SMELL AND TASTE

With aging, the ability to smell and taste gradually diminishes because of neural degeneration and, perhaps, years of cigarette smoking. (See also Risk Factors for Malnutrition in Ch. 2 and GUSTATORY DYSFUNCTION in Ch. 44.) Occasionally, patients complain of **dysgeusia,** *a sensation of an unpleasant taste,* or **dysosmia,** *a sensation of an unpleasant* *smell.* These may be idiopathic or, more rarely, due to a CNS disorder or undiagnosed pharyngeal or esophageal cancer. A **Zenker's diverticulum** develops because of a gradual weakening of the cricopharyngeal muscle, resulting in collection of food, regurgitation of undigested food particles, and an offensive odor and taste (see Ch. 47). Diagnosis is made by barium esophagogram.

The elderly have a diminished gag reflex, which makes examination of the oropharynx and hypopharynx relatively easy in this age group. However, in many patients, the diminished gag reflex leads to silent, chronic aspiration that may result in episodes of pneumonia.

LARYNX

ATROPHIC LARYNGITIS

In addition to a loss of minor salivary gland tissue and moisture in the larynx, elderly persons experience muscle atrophy, with decreased vibratory mass, loss of fibrous tissue support, and squamous metaplasia. These changes may cause a chronic "tickle" in the throat and a constant urge to clear it. Treatment is symptomatic. Lozenges or sugar-free, citrus hard candies can stimulate salivary flow.

Elderly men often complain of a high, trembling, weakened voice, which is associated with frailty but can occur prior to apparent changes in the rest of the body. They may have a bowing of the vocal cords related to a decrease in elasticity and muscle mass, which allows increased air escape with phonation. A weakened voice may also be caused by a decrease in pulmonary volume and expiratory effort. Patients can be instructed to take a deep breath before they speak. This will transiently correct the condition and confirm the diagnosis. A speech therapist may be able to help.

REFLUX LARYNGITIS

This condition becomes more common with advancing age, because older persons are more likely to have impaired esophageal peristalsis and weakened esophageal sphincter tone. Patients who sleep in the recumbent position may experience a burning sensation (heartburn) in the hypopharynx and larynx because of the nocturnal reflux of gastric juice, which must be differentiated from angina. Sleeping with the head elevated often corrects the condition. An H_2 blocker (eg, ranitidine) or a smooth muscle agonist (eg, metoclopramide) may be beneficial.

CRICOARYTENOIDITIS

Inflammation of the cricoarytenoid joint. This condition occurs in the elderly arthritic patient, usually becoming symptomatic only in those with the severest forms of arthritis, and resulting in chronic pain on swallowing and speaking. Laryngeal examination discloses swelling over the arytenoid and fixation of the joint so that the vocal cords abduct poorly. This can result in respiratory distress and may necessitate correction, either by arytenoidectomy or tracheostomy.

ESOPHAGUS
(See also Ch. 47)

Motility disorders may occur as a consequence of aging (presbyesophagus), but also occur in association with other disorders of aging (eg, Parkinson's disease, senile dementia). Diagnosis is by esophagogram and manometric studies.

Mechanical obstruction is most commonly due to carcinoma of the esophagus; however, webs or benign strictures occasionally are found on esophagogram; these may be treated by dilatation.

Cervical osteophytes ("spurs") are a common finding on cervical x-rays but rarely, if ever, cause dysphagia.

Esophageal foreign bodies occur commonly in the elderly because of their poor vision and decreased ability to feel foreign objects in the mouth (especially bones in meat) while wearing dentures. Sometimes, bridgework becomes an esophageal foreign body in this age group.

PAIN SYNDROMES DUE TO AGING

Elongation of the styloid process and calcification of the stylohyoid ligament can result in an intermittent, sharp pain along the distribution of the glossopharyngeal nerve (ie, in the hypopharynx and base of the tongue). Glossopharyngeal neuralgia may be secondary to scarring of the tonsillar bed following an old tonsillectomy **(Eagle's syndrome),** but tonsillectomy is usually not a precondition in the elderly. When treatment is required, resection of the elongated styloid process is curative.

Carotodynia, *a neck pain associated with carotid bulb tenderness,* is intensified by palpation and head movement. This is a self-limited disorder that may last for months. It responds to anti-inflammatory analgesics.

Cervical arthritis is often responsible for chronic neck and occipital pain along the distribution of C-2 and C-3. Analgesia and a cervical collar are helpful. However, in the elderly, angina pectoris may be atypically manifested by intermittent, intense, exercise-related pain in the neck, throat, or jaw.

§4. SPECIAL ISSUES

96. EPIDEMIOLOGY AND DEMOGRAPHICS

Jacob A. Brody and *Victoria W. Persky*

In the USA, life expectancy has increased dramatically throughout this century, with an acceleration since 1968 augmented by a decline in mid-fe mortality from coronary artery disease **(CAD).** The proportion of persons > 65 yr of age has risen concomitantly. In 1900, only 25% of the population lived beyond the age of 65, compared with 70% in 1985 (with 30% living beyond 80). In 1900, persons ≥ 65 yr of age made up 4% of the population, compared with 12% in 1985, of whom 40% are ≥ 75 yr of age (expected to increase to 50% by the year 2000). With further reductions in cardiovascular mortality, continued increases in life expectancy can be anticipated.

The increase in the size of the elderly population has been accompanied by a substantial and growing increase in health care expenditures. Nursing home costs alone are expected to increase from over $20 billion in 1980 to nearly $40 billion by the year 2020, assuming a fixed value of the dollar.

Elderly women in the USA greatly outnumber elderly men. In 1982, there were 1.5 women for each man > 65 yr of age, and nearly 3 times as many women as men between the ages of 95 and 99 yr. Sex differences in mortality are generally highest in industrialized societies, partly because of differences in CAD, smoking, alcohol intake, and accidents. These differences are increasing, with men currently surviving 7 yr less than women and having higher death rates than women at all ages.

Ninety-one percent of the elderly population is white, compared with 86% of the total population, reflecting higher mortality rates in blacks at younger ages. Although blacks represent a smaller proportion of the elderly population, blacks who survive to age 65 live at least as long as whites. The largest proportion of older persons is in metropolitan and rural nonfarm areas, as a result of emigration from the farm to local towns.

In 1981, among persons ≥ 75 yr of age, almost 50% of women lived alone, compared with 20% of men. This reflects the female survival advantage and the fact that women marry men who are, on average, 7 yr older than they. Numbers of nursing home residents of both sexes have risen dramatically from < 800,000 in 1969 to 1½ million in 1982, or 5.8% of the population aged ≥ 65 yr.

Mortality

TABLE 96–1 lists the 10 major causes of death in persons ≥ 65 yr of age and FIG. 96–1 shows the time trends in mortality among older persons.

Cardiovascular disease: The major cause of death in the elderly, as in the total population, is cardiovascular disease, with CAD alone accounting for 44% of the deaths in those ≥ 65 yr of age (see TABLE 96–1). Death rates for cardiovascular disease (see FIG. 96–2) show increases with age. Men have considerably higher rates than women, especially at younger ages.

CAD death rates have declined dramatically in all age groups, including those ≥ 65 yr, since the late 1960s (see FIG. 96–3), but CAD has remained the most important cause of death in the elderly. Thus, by

TABLE 96-1. LEADING CAUSES OF DEATH BY AGE IN 1982
(Rates/100,000)

Cause of Death	Age (yr)			
	65+	65–74	75–84	≥85
All causes	5049	2885	6330	15,048
Diseases of the heart	2224	1156	2801	7342
Malignant neoplasms	1022	825	1239	1599
Cerebrovascular disorders	506	194	675	2001
Chronic obstructive pulmonary disease	177	131	236	278
Pneumonia and influenza	153	48	183	748
Atherosclerosis	95	21	103	563
Diabetes mellitus	94	60	125	212
Accidents	86	51	104	256
Nephritis, nephrotic syndrome, and nephrosis	54	26	70	183
Chronic liver disease	35	40	31	18

(Adapted from J. A. Brody, D. B. Brock, and T. F. Williams: "Trends in the health of the elderly population," in *Annual Review of Public Health,* Vol. 8, pp. 211-234, 1987. Used with permission.)

some estimates, if all deaths from cardiovascular disease were eliminated, the gain in life expectancy at age 65 would be 11 yr, whereas if all cancer deaths were eliminated, the gain would be only 1½ yr.

The decline in CAD death rates in the USA has been duplicated in many but not all countries and is thought primarily to reflect changes in risk factors for CAD as well as improved therapy. Since the peak of the CAD epidemic in the early 1960s, serum cholesterol levels have decreased about 10%; 20% fewer middle-aged males are smokers; and the proportion of hypertensive persons whose BP is controlled has increased from 16 to 57%. With continued improvement in diet, cessation of smoking, and BP control, the decline in the prevalence of CAD should continue to increase life expectancy in the USA.

Major risk factors for CAD in younger persons—smoking, hypertension, hypercholesterolemia, and diabetes—are also associated with risk in the elderly, although less consistently. Hypertension remains an important risk factor in all age groups, with systolic BP being as predictive as diastolic BP. In the Framingham study, cigarette smoking, diabetes, and hypercholesterolemia were less consistent as risk factors in the elderly than in younger persons (see also Ch. 74). Cigarette smoking predicted CAD mortality in men but not in women, whereas diabetes predicted CAD in women but not in men.

Cancer is the second most common cause of mortality in the elderly (see TABLES 96-1 and 96-2), currently causing about 20% of deaths in

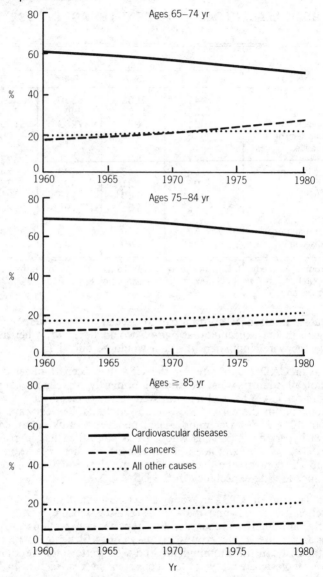

Fig. 96–1. Percent of total mortality for cardiovascular diseases, cancer, and all other causes by age in the USA, 1960-1980. (From J. A. Brody, D. B. Brock, and T. F. Williams: "Trends in the health of the elderly population," in *Annual Review of Public Health*, Vol. 8, pp. 211-234, 1987. Used with permission.)

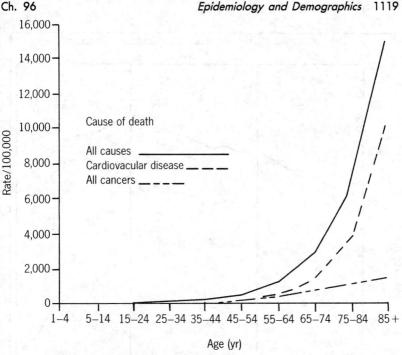

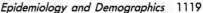

FIG. 96–2. Death rate by age for all causes, cardiovascular disease, and cancer.
(From. J. A. Brody, D. B. Brock, and T. F. Williams: "Trends in the health of the elderly
population," in *Annual Review of Public Health,* Vol. 8, pp. 211-234, 1987. Used with
permission.)

persons aged $\geq$ 65 yr, compared with 16% in 1970; the mortality rate
increased from 923 to 1022/100,000 over the same period. However, the
increase in percent deaths is related more to the decline in CAD mortality than to an absolute increase in cancer mortality.

Cancer incidence and mortality rates increase with age until the 84th
yr, when they plateau and may even decline slightly. Thus, in the oldest
group of persons, those > 84 yr of age, cancer is responsible for a
smaller proportion of deaths than in younger age groups (see FIG. 96–2).
Cancers that exhibit the most consistent increases in rate with age
are leukemia and cancers of the digestive system, breast, prostate, and
urinary tract. Between 1969 and 1976, age-adjusted cancer incidence
rates increased annually by an average of 1.3% for men and 2% for
women. Much of this increase was caused by a rise in the lung cancer
rate, which has leveled off for men in recent years. During the same period, mortality associated with cervical and stomach cancer declined and
mortality associated with most other cancers was fairly stable.

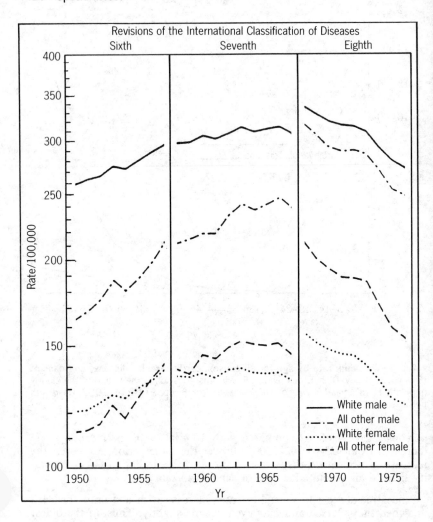

FIG. 96–3. **Age-adjusted death rates for ischemic heart disease in the USA, by color and sex, 1950-1976.** Discrepancies between panels are due to diagnostic differences among the 6th, 7th, and 8th revisions of the *International Classification of Diseases.* The decline in deaths from ischemic heart disease since 1967 is clearly evident and is continuing. (From *Proceedings of the Conference on the Decline in Coronary Heart Disease Mortality,* edited by R. J. Havlik and M. Feinlieb. U.S. Department of Health, Education, and Welfare, Public Health Service, National Institutes of Health. NIH Publication No. 79-1610, May 1979.)

TABLE 96–2. AVERAGE ANNUAL AGE-SPECIFIC CANCER INCIDENCE, SELECTED SITES, ALL RACES, BOTH SEXES, 1978–1981 (Rates/100,000)

Site	Age (yr)				
	65–69	70–74	75–79	80–84	≥ 85
All sites	1410.8	1771.5	2067.2	2267.0	2361.7
Lung and bronchus	265.6	294.7	279.7	236.3	175.7
Breast	161.9	186.0	210.1	226.5	265.6
Prostate	161.2	247.6	318.5	354.0	342.4
Colon	148.5	216.3	285.1	364.3	403.5
Rectum	67.0	91.0	107.2	121.0	129.8
Corpus uteri	60.3	57.8	56.9	49.3	41.4
Stomach	37.6	51.0	70.1	88.9	103.6
Non-Hodgkin's lymphomas	38.8	49.0	63.5	67.8	64.0
Leukemias	29.9	46.2	56.4	80.9	94.1

(Adapted from J. A. Brody, D. B. Brock, and T. F. Williams: "Trends in the health of the elderly population," in *Annual Review of Public Health,* Vol. 8, pp. 211-234, 1987. Used with permission.)

Cerebrovascular disease is the third leading cause of death in the elderly in the USA (TABLE 96–1). Specific causes of stroke include thrombosis (which accounts for between 50 and 75% of all stroke deaths), emboli (16%), and hemorrhage, including intracerebral bleeding and subarachnoid hemorrhage (15 to 25%). There is a modest increase in stroke prevalence among the elderly; 1 study showed a rate of 4.5% in persons between ages 65 and 74 yr, and a rate of 7.3% in persons > 75 yr of age. Strokes continue to be far more common in blacks than in whites, with two- to three-fold differences in mortality.

International differences are substantial; eg, the highest rates of stroke mortality are seen in Bulgaria, Japan, Czechoslovakia, and Hungary. Patterns of thrombotic vs. hemorrhagic stroke also vary; eg, Japan has a higher proportion of hemorrhagic stroke than western Europe.

Consistent declines in stroke mortality rates in the USA since the early 1900s (with an accelerated decline since the late 1960s for all sex and race groups) support the hypothesis that exogenous factors contribute to the disease. Similar declines have been seen throughout many developed western countries, with more recent declines in Japan. Studies of Japanese immigrants in Hawaii show that their stroke rates approximate those seen in the host country, again suggesting the etiologic importance of environmental factors.

Data on incidence and type of stroke are limited because of variations in diagnostic criteria among different populations; eg, the Framingham study noted that in 40% of deaths due to stroke this cause was not mentioned on the death certificate, and in those cases in which stroke was recorded, 21% could not be verified. Nevertheless, incidence data for 1945 to 1979 parallel mortality data in showing overall decreases in cerebral infarction and intracerebral hemorrhage. In general, there has been no overall change in the rate of subarachnoid hemorrhage, although recent data from New Zealand and Finland suggest that there may be some slight decline in those countries.

Elevation of BP (both systolic and diastolic) is a strong risk factor for all types of stroke. Diabetes and smoking are less consistent risk factors; diabetes has a stronger relationship to thrombotic than to nonthrombotic stroke and to stroke in women than to stroke in men. Alcohol and cholesterol have inconsistent relationships to stroke; alcohol appears to be a risk factor for hemorrhagic but not nonhemorrhagic stroke, and serum cholesterol levels are positively associated with thrombotic and negatively associated with hemorrhagic stroke. Atrial fibrillation also increases the risk of stroke and stroke recurrence, particularly embolic stroke. The risk of stroke recurrence is 50% between 3 and 6 mo after the first stroke in persons with atrial fibrillation vs. 20% in those with a negative history. Other risk factors for stroke include prior cardiac disease, history of transient ischemic attacks, carotid bruits, and oral contraceptive use.

Accidents are the eighth leading cause of death in the elderly (see TABLE 96–1), with 24% of all deaths from unintentional injuries occurring in the 11% of the population aged $\geq$ 65 yr. An overall decline in deaths due to accidents has occurred since the 1950s. Falls, fires, contact with hot substances, and vehicular crashes account for 75% of all injury deaths. Death associated with falls (50% of all injury deaths in this age group) is more common in urban populations, in women, in persons living alone, in persons with multiple medical problems, and in those receiving multiple medications. Factors contributing to the risk of falling are disorders of vision, the vestibular system, and proprioception, as well as deficits in brain perfusion, structural CNS changes, and environmental hazards (particularly those involving foot-ground contact).

Seven percent of all injury deaths in the elderly involve contact with fire or hot water (with such deaths occurring more often in men and in nonwhites), and 23% involve motor vehicle deaths. Predominant causes of motor vehicle accidents involving the elderly are disregarding traffic signals and failing to yield right of way. Risk factors for vehicular accidents include diabetes, epilepsy, cardiovascular disease, alcoholism, and mental illness. Pedestrian fatalities are also more frequent in persons > 65 yr of age, with men, nonwhites, and widows at greatest risk.

Other causes of death: Chronic obstructive pulmonary disease, for which smoking is the major risk factor, is the fourth leading cause of death in the elderly (see TABLE 96–1). The combination of pneumonia and influenza follows and was responsible for 3% of deaths in that population in 1982. In general, the pattern of pneumonia and influenza mortality follows that of cardiovascular disease. Atherosclerosis, as a diagnosis, is the sixth leading cause of death in the elderly. Mortality associated with diabetes, the seventh leading cause of death in 1978, has declined since 1970. Finally, although suicide is not a major cause of death in the elderly, suicide rates in men are strongly age related and warrant additional research.

Morbidity

The central issues in the epidemiology of aging include morbidity as well as mortality. It is currently estimated that for each functionally active year gained, about 3.5 functionally compromised years have been added. The future challenges are not only to increase life expectancy but also to increase the duration of independence and to improve the quality of life.

The extent of morbidity in the older population varies according to the measurement technic used. Most current data come from medical records and surveys that rely on self-reporting. There is increasing interest, however, in observational studies in the home. In national surveys, arthritis is the most frequently reported chronic condition in the elderly; hypertension, heart disease, decreased hearing, and decreased vision are also prominent (see TABLE 96–3). Noninstitutionalized persons have fewer diseases than institutionalized persons, with some studies noting several-fold differences in heart disease, stroke, and dementia. The proportion of persons institutionalized is heavily age related, rising from only 1.5% between ages 65 and 74 yr, to nearly 7% between ages 75 and 84 yr, and to > 21% in those ≥ 85 yr of age.

Osteoarthritis (OA) is increasingly recognized as an important cause of disability in the elderly. Studies of OA, however, are limited by methodologic problems and inconsistencies in disease definition. Symptoms and x-ray changes frequently do not correlate with each other, and hos-

TABLE 96–3. NUMBER OF SELECTED REPORTED CHRONIC CONDITIONS/1000 PERSONS IN THE USA BY AGE, 1982

Type of Condition	Total 65+ yr	65–74 yr	≥ 75 yr
Arthritis	495.8	507.8	476.0
Hypertension	390.4	384.3	400.4
Hearing impairment	299.7	262.0	362.2
Heart disease	256.8	224.7	310.0
Deformity or orthopedic impairment	168.5	172.7	161.5
Chronic sinusitis	151.7	159.1	139.6
Visual impairment	101.1	80.7	134.8
Diabetes	88.9	96.6	76.3
Varicose veins	77.7	79.3	75.2
Hernia of abdominal cavity	75.5	87.8	55.2

(Adapted from J. A. Brody, D. B. Brock, and T. F. Williams: "Trends in the health of the elderly population," in *Annual Review of Public Health,* Vol. 8, pp. 211-234, 1987. Used with permission.)

pital discharge diagnoses often fail to mention OA. From the limited data available, it appears that about 24 million persons in the USA have OA; it is more common in women and has a strong age association. Physical examination data indicate that the prevalence of OA increases from 4% in persons aged 40 to 59 yr to between 20 and 40% in persons aged > 60 yr. Similarly, x-ray data from 2 national studies indicate that prevalence is < 1% in persons aged 35 to 44 yr, between 1 and 6% in those aged 65 to 74 yr, and between 5 and 50% in persons aged ≥ 75 yr, depending on which joints are x-rayed.

In general, risk factors are thought to reflect wear and tear on the joints and include obesity, occupation, life-style, and genetic predisposition.

The cost in terms of morbidity is large; OA is thought to be responsible for the total incapacitation of 1 million persons > 55 yr of age.

Hip fractures and osteoporosis: About 225,000 hip fractures occur each year in the USA. This figure is expected to increase to 350,000 by the year 2000 and to 650,000 by 2050. The average age of persons with hip fractures is 79 yr. The incidence increases exponentially after age 40 yr, with a doubling of the rate every 6 yr. Although women have a considerably higher incidence of hip fractures than men, the rate rises similarly in both groups; however, the increase in women precedes that in men by about 6 yr. Whites in the USA and Japanese living in Japan have higher rates than blacks in the USA and South African Bantus, while data on Hispanics and other ethnic groups in the USA are limited.

Although hip fractures cause the greatest disability of all fractures in the elderly, fractures of the radius, ulna, humerus, and vertebral column also cause considerable morbidity.

It is estimated that osteoporosis is a major contributory factor in 1,200,000 fractures per year that occur in the USA. Radiographic determination of osteoporosis is often inaccurate, because a substantial portion of bone mass must be lost before the condition can be seen on x-ray. Measurements of cortical bone thickness, while more reliable, are still only poorly correlated with other factors associated with bone strength. Recently, photon absorptiometry has become the method of choice. Estimates, however, are complicated by varying bone composition in different sites. Vertebral bone is about $2/3$ trabecular, while femoral bone is about $2/3$ cortical. Single photon absorptiometry is fairly inexpensive and suitable for peripheral appendicular bone but is of limited use when soft tissue is prominent around the bone.

In whites, 34% of men and 44% of women aged 65 to 74 yr may have measurable osteoporosis. However, age-specific prevalence data are sparse. Risk factors for osteoporosis are age, female sex, white race, thin and tall body habitus, lack of weight-bearing exercise, smoking, low Ca intake, and, apparently, nonuse of postmenopausal estrogen replacement therapy. The effect of hormones on osteoporosis has not been completely delineated, but the increase in osteoporosis with age, the large difference in bone density between men and women, and the protective effect of exogenous estrogens, all imply a strong hormonal causal link in females. However, the increase in risk begins before menopause, and men also have exponential increases in risk that begin later than in women. This suggests that there may be age-related risk factors unrelated, or indirectly related, to hormonal status.

Dementia: In 1980, there were about 2 million persons with Alzheimer's disease **(AD)**, with a mean age of 80 yr. It is estimated that by the year 2000, this number will rise to almost 4 million, and by the year 2050, to 8 ½ million.

The epidemiology of dementia has been limited by difficulties in diagnosis and classification. Some parameters of cognitive function appear to decline with age and are related to a multitude of psychosocial factors. Persons of higher socioeconomic and educational status generally do better on tests, and large cross-cultural differences exist, making tests difficult to standardize. In addition, declining vision and hearing, as well as concurrent diseases and medications common in older persons render measurement difficult. Overall estimates of prevalence of dementia in noninstitutionalized persons aged 60 to 65 yr range between 1 and 2% and in persons aged $\geq$ 65 yr, between 3 and 9%; the rate doubles every 5 yr to 32% at age 85. Annual incidence rates for AD in 1 study were estimated to be 0.33% at age 70, 1.3% at age 80, and 5.4% at age 90. Survival is, generally, inversely related to age at onset and from 5 to 10 yr following diagnosis.

Between 15 and 30% of dementia in the elderly has a vascular or multi-infarct cause. In a small proportion of patients (10 to 15%), the causes are reversible: depression, drug intoxication, hypothyroidism, anemia, alcohol abuse, metabolic disturbance, chronic subdural hematoma, and normal pressure hydrocephalus. A few patients have nonreversible causes: Parkinson's disease, Pick's disease, multiple sclerosis, and Jakob-Creutzfeldt disease. The largest proportion of dementia cases (between 50 and 75%) is associated with neuropathologic evidence of AD.

Risk factors for multi-infarct dementia are presumed to include hypertension, atrial fibrillation, and heart disease, since these are associated with thromboembolism. The factors most consistently associated with AD are family history of dementia and history of head trauma, but even these associations have been questioned. Risk factors less consistently associated with AD include older maternal age at the time of birth of the propositus and a family history of Down's syndrome. On Guam, associations have been suggested between an AD-like syndrome and neurotoxins as well as between AD and metallic cations, including calcium, aluminum, manganese, and silicon.

Cross-cultural comparisons are severely limited by different diagnostic criteria, low autopsy rates, and diagnostic misclassification. In Japan, overall dementia rates are reported to be similar to those in the USA, but with a greater proportion secondary to cerebrovascular disease and a prevalence of AD about half that in the USA. Preliminary studies suggest no racial difference in prevalence of AD between blacks and whites in the USA. Thus, current data indicate that AD is strongly related to age, with perhaps a genetic component. Environmental contributions to the disease process have yet to be delineated, although research in this area is rapidly expanding.

Hearing: Hearing loss is strongly age related and, according to 1 national study, thought to be the single most prevalent impairment in the elderly. Some studies have noted that 80% of older persons have some hearing impairment and that up to 20% of those 80 to 84 yr of age use hearing aids. The most common diagnosis of hearing loss is presbycusis, with degenerative changes of the cochlear mechanism, 8th nerve changes, and CNS alterations in sound perception also contributing to hearing disability. Other associated problems are cerumen impaction, changes in the external auditory canal, diminished mechanical responsiveness of the tympanic membrane, and arthritic changes in the ossicles of the middle ear.

Risk factors for hearing loss include age, associated illness, a history of noise exposure, a family history of hearing loss, Meniere's disease, diabetes, hyperlipidemia, smoking, and hypertension. Causes of presbycusis remain obscure.

Vision: Some 90% of older persons require glasses, and up to 20% of those > 80 yr old are unable to read newspapers, even with glasses. In the Framingham study, estimates of legal blindness (ie, visual acuity < 20/200) in 1 or both eyes reached 16% by age 75 to 84 yr. The most common visual problems are cataracts and retinal vascular changes, each prevalent in 20 to 40% of all persons between the ages of 65 and 74 yr. Other common diseases are age-related macular degeneration (previously called senile macular degeneration), corneal guttata, healed corneal opacities, neoplasms, and glaucoma. Estimates of prevalence vary but each of these diseases probably affects between 5 and 20% of the population between 65 and 74 yr of age.

Cataracts reportedly account for 9, 15, and 22% of all blindness in the USA, Canada, and Great Britain, respectively. Fortunately, cataracts, for which over ½ million people ≥ 65 yr of age were hospitalized in the USA in 1983, are usually amenable to surgical intervention. Factors associated with cataracts include age, female sex, diabetes, hypertension, steroid use, electromagnetic radiation exposure, and myopia.

Retinal vascular changes are strongly related to age and to prevalence of diabetes (particularly the duration of diagnosed diabetes). Of those ≥ 75 yr of age, 50% of those with > 15 yr of diagnosed diabetes have retinopathy, compared with 28% with 10 to 15 yr of disease and 18% with < 5 yr of disease.

Open-angle glaucoma accounts for up to 22% of all blindness in the USA and is also associated with decreased life expectancy. Prevalence in adults of all ages varies from 0.5 to 4%. Although in Iceland there is some evidence that prevalence of glaucoma is decreasing, substantial trends over time have not been noted in the USA. Risk factors include race (with blacks more often affected than whites), age, use of cortico-steroids, family history of glaucoma, diabetes, and hypertension.

Macular degeneration is strongly age related, with prevalence rates rising to 22% by age 75. Numerous other risk factors have been suggested, including sex (women are more often affected than men), family history of macular degeneration, occupational exposure to chemicals, blue or medium-pigmented eyes, cardiovascular disease, decreased hand grip, hyperopia, smoking, increased diastolic BP, left ventricular hypertrophy, short height, decreased vital capacity, and history of pulmonary infection.

97. SOCIAL ISSUES

Terrie Wetle

The social context of geriatric care influences the risk of disease, the experience of illness for the older person, and the physician's ability to deliver timely and appropriate care. The social status of the elderly, the changing demographics of health and illness, and evolving social values exert complex pressures on the patchwork of policies, programs, and services that constitute the continuum of care available to older individuals. Thus, the successful practice of geriatric medicine requires an understanding of the broader context in which illness occurs and care is provided.

USE OF SERVICES

Older individuals are more likely to use health care services than are younger persons. While they make up only 12% of the population, older persons account for 39% of the total acute hospital bed-day census, use 25% of all prescription drugs dispensed, and are responsible for 30% of the overall $425 billion health care expenditure and > 50% of the $124 billion federal health budget. This large use of health resources is neither unfair nor unjustified. The escalating burden of disease accompanying aging produces the accelerated need for and use of health care services. Moreover, the chronic nature of many of these diseases results in repeated contact with the health care system.

Use of institutional services, eg, hospitals and nursing homes, is also more frequent among older persons. The availability of family members to provide care at home decreases with age. Older individuals, particularly women, are likely to be widowed, and when they become very old, their children may be elderly themselves. Divorce and geographic separation may weaken family ties, and the entry of women (particularly those of middle age) into the paid labor force has reduced their availability to provide home care. These factors, along with increased prevalence of disease, increase the demand of older persons for institutional services.

SOCIAL SUPPORTS AND FAMILY CARE GIVING

Social supports are an important factor in predicting use of health services. The availability of family care givers plays a salient role in delaying, if not preventing, institutionalization of the chronically ill older person.

Although the concept of social supports encompasses neighbors and friends, family members are usually responsible for most care giving, providing substantial physical, emotional, social, and economic support. The amount of involvement and the nature of the services provided depend on economic resources, family structure, quality of relationships, and other competing demands on family time and energy. Approximately 80% of home health care is provided as informal support (as opposed to purchased services) by family members. This care is provided to elderly persons living with adult children as well as to those living in their own home. The amount of care that the family provides can range from minimal assistance (eg, periodic checking in) to elaborate full-time care. Women are more likely to be both receivers and givers of such care.

Spouses are major providers of care for the frail elderly. While adult children frequently provide care to mildly or moderately impaired older individuals, the severely disabled elderly are more likely to be cared for by a spouse. As a group, "care-giving" couples are disproportionately poor, with the care giver usually in poor health. Spouse care givers experience considerable stress and suffer associated health problems.

Supportive services for family care givers may enhance their willingness and ability to provide care. These supportive services are of 2 types: those that *support* family care givers (technical assistance in learning new skills, counseling, family mental health services, or personal supports) and those that *supplement* family care giving (personal care, home health care, adult day care, meals programs, and social services).

Social supports also have an impact on health status. Social isolation or lack of support is associated with increased mortality risk. On the other hand, social supports are claimed to buffer the elderly from the negative effects of life transitions, such as the departure of children, retirement, and widowhood.

EFFECTS OF LIFE TRANSITIONS

For most elderly, late life is a period of transition and adjustment to loss. Transitions include retirement; relocation; death of spouse, family members, or friends; and loss of former levels of physical health and function.

Retirement is frequently the first major transition faced by older persons. It is estimated that about ⅓ of retirees have difficulty adjusting to such aspects of retirement as reduced income and change in social role. However, the circumstances surrounding the retirement influence the existence and severity of adjustment problems. Some persons choose to retire and look forward to quitting unpleasant work; others are forced to retire because of health reasons or job loss. These factors explain, to some degree, the different physical and mental health outcomes experienced by retirees. Appropriate preparation for retirement and the availability of counseling for families and individuals who experience difficulties ameliorate most associated problems.

Relocation is another transition faced by many older persons. An individual or family may experience several housing transitions in later years, including sale of the family residence and subsequent move to smaller quarters, a move into senior-citizen or retirement housing to minimize the burden of upkeep, and finally a move into a nursing home. "Relocation trauma" continues to arouse controversy. Those who respond poorly to a move are more likely to be male, living alone, socially isolated, poor, and depressed.

However, 2 important factors mediate the stress of moving—the degree of perceived control over the event and the degree of predictability of the new environment. Families should be encouraged to acquaint the older person with the new setting well in advance of moving. For the cognitively impaired elderly, a move away from familiar surroundings may trigger a substantial increase in functional dependence and disruptive behavior. Awareness of the increased vulnerability of those with dementia may help families and staff cope during the period of adjustment.

Bereavement is a complex phenomenon that changes many aspects of the elderly person's life. Loss of companionship upon the death of a spouse may be accompanied by reduction in financial resources, loss of caretaker, decline in social interaction, and change in social status. Loss of a spouse has different effects on men and women. Men tend to have higher mortality rates in the 2-yr period following the death of a spouse than do women. On the other hand, elderly men are much more likely to remarry after the death of a spouse than are women.

Health care providers should be alert to symptoms of stress and depression during the grieving period. A hasty attempt to treat feelings of sadness with antidepressant drugs should be avoided because of potential interference with the process of grieving and adjustment. On the other hand, counseling and supportive services, such as "widow-to-widow" groups, may ease difficult transitions and enhance adjustments to new roles and life circumstances. Prolonged and pathologic grief usually requires psychiatric evaluation and treatment.

CONTINUUM OF CARE
(See also Ch. 20)

The array of health services needed by older persons is complex and fragmented. Specific types of services have different funding sources, regulatory agencies, eligibility requirements, and geographic distribution. Nonetheless, there is general agreement regarding the basic components of the continuum of care. FIG. 97–1 presents a breakdown of the service system that exists in most communities and serves as a framework for the following discussion of specific services.

Acute care hospitals are the final common pathway for most older people requiring care. Clinicians should be alert to several risks for hospitalized elderly, including acute confusional states (as a result of unfamiliar surroundings, sleep deprivation, and abrupt changes in medication). Efforts to shorten hospital stays have resulted in concerns that patients are released "sicker and quicker." Many elderly are fearful of being sent home too soon with inadequate support.

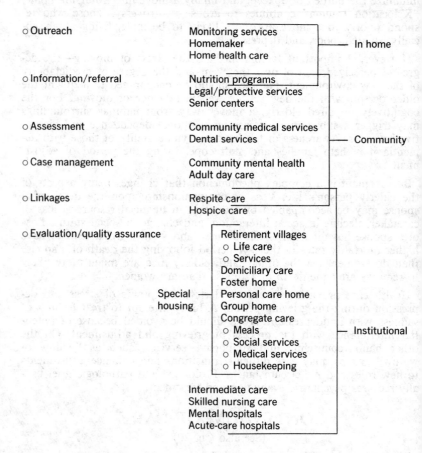

FIG. 97–1. **Continuum of geriatric care.** (Adapted from S. J. Brody and C. Masciocchi: "Data for long-term care planning by health systems agencies," in *American Journal of Public Health,* Vol. 70, pp. 1194–1198, 1980. Used with permission of American Public Health Association, Inc. and the authors.)

Mental hospitals were once a major source of care for the elderly, particularly those suffering from dementing illness. Implementation of a policy of deinstitutionalization has led to major reductions in the populations of such facilities over the past decade. Unfortunately, for many mentally ill older persons, deinstitutionalization has translated into "reinstitutionalization" as patients have been transferred from state mental hospitals to nursing homes, which have been termed the "new back wards." For others, deinstitutionalization has meant release into the community, with the only available care coming from poorly coordinated and underfunded—if extant—community-based programs.

Nursing homes are defined as facilities whose primary function is to provide nursing care. They tend to be classified according to their certification status as providers of care in the Medicare and Medicaid programs. Since the passage of the Medicaid legislation in 1965, the rate of nursing home use by the elderly has doubled from 2.5% in 1966 to the current 5% of those > 65 yr of age. The typical nursing home resident is elderly, white, female, and widowed.

Special housing for the elderly varies widely. Life-care communities are the most comprehensive type, providing a range of services from independent living in apartments to skilled nursing care. While most life-care communities have a single campus, some models provide services at a variety of sites. **Congregate care** refers to housing arrangements in which older persons live in individual apartments or rooms with selected services provided. This arrangement differs from life-care communities in that the residents do not own their units and there is no commitment to provide care over time as their needs change. **Foster, domiciliary, and personal-care homes** generally offer room, board, and some supervision. These housing options, particularly those that provide supervision, are woefully inadequate in most communities.

Hospice care is a set of services intended to improve the quality of life for terminally ill patients. A major goal of hospice care is to enable such patients to live the remainder of their lives as comfortably and peacefully as possible. Many aspects of hospice care are being adopted by care providers in the general health system. This type of care has also been suggested for patients with certain other illnesses (eg, Alzheimer's disease), even when death is not imminent.

Respite care refers to services that allow family members time away from care giving responsibilities. Services range from an in-home visit of a few hours by a volunteer or paid worker to institutional stays of several weeks. The importance of this service, given the considerable stress of providing care to an aged spouse, sibling, or parent, cannot be overestimated.

Community mental health centers provide ambulatory psychiatric care and other services to residents in specified catchment areas. These centers tend to provide services to the elderly in much lower proportions than population statistics indicate they are needed, but several centers have special outreach programs, nursing home consultation, and other services targeted toward geriatric clients.

Adult day care takes 2 basic forms: the adult day hospital and multipurpose social day care center. Both types are designed for individuals who require supervision or medical services during the day but who can spend evenings with family members or in other supportive environments.

Senior centers provide opportunities for social contact and recreational activities. They also serve as a convenient site for health screening, nutrition and education programs, and outreach activities. Most offer meals on weekdays, and some have extensive health and social services programs, including adult day care.

Nutrition programs provide 2 types of services—congregate or group meals and home-delivered meals. Congregate meals not only contribute to nutritional health but also provide opportunity for social contact, educational programs, and outreach efforts. **Meals for the homebound** or "Meals on Wheels" are an important resource for individuals who are unable to shop, prepare meals, or follow special dietary regimens.

Home health care includes a wide range of services, eg, skilled nursing; occupational, physical, and speech therapy; medical social services; physician care; nutritional/dietary services and meals; homemaker services; home health aide services; respiratory and IV therapy; and medical supplies, including drugs and medical appliances.

Monitoring services keep health care systems in touch with chronically impaired or frail persons living at home and include organized services, such as telephone networks and friendly visitors; these can be a secondary function of other services.

Access to services occurs through a variety of mechanisms. **Outreach programs** are designed to identify individuals with unmet needs. **Information and referral** services are offered by a variety of community agencies to answer service-related questions, to make appropriate referrals to service providers, and ideally, to follow up on the referrals and determine whether appropriate services have been received. **Comprehensive assessment** is crucial for matching older persons with the appropriate services. While health and illness may be the primary focus of the physician, other factors are important in determining the most appropriate service package. **Case management** entails the development of an individualized care plan based on comprehensive assessment. The case manager coordinates the delivery of the services and follows up to determine that the client received them.

FINANCING HEALTH CARE
(See also Ch. 104)

The services needed and used by the elderly are financed by an array of federal, state, and private programs. The cost of geriatric health care is a substantial burden for public programs and for the elderly themselves. Frequently, several sources will contribute to reimbursement of a single type of service, as well as to the multiple services required by many older persons. The major programs that support geriatric care are described below.

Medicare is the principal public health insurance for those ≥ 65 yr of age. Hospital Insurance (Part A) and Supplementary Medical Insurance (Part B) are the 2 parts of the Medicare program. Part A covers 4 kinds of care: (1) inpatient hospital care, (2) medically necessary inpatient care in a skilled nursing facility, (3) home health care, and (4) hospice care. Payment for **hospital services** is based on a prospective payment system, using diagnosis related groups **(DRGs)**, implemented in 1983. Payment for inpatient care in a certified *skilled* **nursing facility** has restrictive requirements, which are described in detail in Ch. 104.

Home health services—part-time or intermittent skilled nursing care, physical therapy, and speech therapy—are covered if the patient is homebound and if a physician develops and certifies a plan of care. **Hospice services** are covered if a physician certifies that the patient is terminally ill *and* the patient chooses to receive hospice care instead of standard Medicare benefits *and* care is provided by a Medicare-certified hospice program.

Part B, a voluntary program, pays a portion of the cost of physician services, outpatient hospital care, outpatient physical and speech therapy services, and some home health care services and supplies not covered by Part A. There are restrictions on the types of outpatient care and therapists covered. Payment for services is made either directly to the patient or to the physician. In either case, the patient is liable for a $75 annual deductible fee as well as a 20% copayment. If payment is not made directly to the physician (assignment), the patient may also be billed for amounts above the 20% of "reasonable allowable costs."

Health maintenance organizations (HMOs) provide an alternative type of care for enrolled Medicare patients. For each Medicare enrollee, the HMO receives 95% of the adjusted average per capita cost for its geographic region. Some authorities believe the HMO has the potential to improve on the fragmented care provided in the fee-for-service sector by improving management of care and offering a wider array of services.

Medicaid, a federal-state partnership, provides payment for health services for the aged poor, the blind, the disabled, and low-income families with dependent children. Services required under the federal guidelines are (1) inpatient and outpatient hospital care, (2) laboratory and x-ray services, (3) physician services, and (4) skilled nursing care and home health services for persons > 21 yr of age. States may also choose to provide certain optional services, including prescriptions, dental services, eyeglasses, and intermediate-level nursing home care. Eligibility requirements are determined by each state but must include cash-assistance recipients (eg, supplemental security income), as well as certain groups of poor children and pregnant women.

Medicaid is the major public payer for long-term care, contributing about 42% of the $35.2 billion spent for nursing home services in 1985. To qualify for Medicaid reimbursement for such services, older persons must "spend down" (ie, pay for care from their own resources until they meet stringent income and asset-related eligibility requirements for the state in which they live). Although the Medicaid program was intended to serve the poor, the high cost of long-term care rapidly brings a majority of the elderly who require chronic care into this category.

Veterans Administration (VA) health care services are provided without charge on a space-available basis, with priority going to veterans with service-connected disabilities. The VA operates 172 hospitals, 16 domiciliary facilities, and > 100 nursing homes, and contracts for care in community hospitals and nursing homes. The VA has also launched several innovative geriatric programs, including geriatric assessment units **(GAUs)**, Geriatric Research, Education and Clinical Centers **(GRECCs)**, and hospital-based home health care programs.

Private insurers have recently begun to pay more attention to the large market segment comprising those > 65 yr of age. A wide array of private insurance policies are available to elderly individuals, most taking the form of "Medigap" insurance, which pays for some or all of Medicare deductibles and copayments. Very few of these policies cover services such as long-term home health or nursing home care because benefits tend to be tied to Medicare definitions of eligibility and covered services. Recently, a number of private insurers have begun to offer long-term care insurance. However, it remains to be seen whether the elderly or their family members will be willing to pay the relatively high premiums required, or alternatively, to enroll at younger ages (when lower premiums would be available) far in advance of probable need for services.

Other federal programs also provide services for the elderly. Since its enactment in 1965, the **Older Americans Act** has evolved from a program of small grants and research projects to a network of 57 state units on aging (including US territories and Indian tribes), more than 600 area agencies on aging, and thousands of community agencies. Its primary purpose is to coordinate and deliver the following services at the community level: information and referral, outreach, transportation, senior centers, nutritional programs, advocacy, protective services, senior employment, ombudsman programs, and supportive services. In addition, the Older Americans Act funds research and training. **Title XX** of the Social Security Act authorized reimbursements to states for social services, including a variety of home health and homemaker services of benefit to the frail elderly. These funds have been shifted to the Social Services Block Grant **(SSBG)** program, which is designed to "prevent or reduce inappropriate institutional care by providing for community-based care."

Although **Social Security** is not usually considered a health program, as a basic pension system, it provides resources to the elderly that are frequently used to pay for many health care needs. There are 2 types of payments to the elderly: **Old Age and Survivors Insurance (OASI)** (Title II) and **Supplementary Security Income (SSI)** (Title VI). SSI provides a guaranteed minimal income to aged, blind, and disabled persons. For the elderly, SSI replaced the state-run old-age assistance programs, which varied widely across the country by eligibility and benefits.

---

98. MISTREATMENT

Ronald D. Adelman and *Risa Breckman*

Each year, about 1 million older Americans are injured physically, debilitated psychologically, or neglected by a family member, according to a study conducted in 1986 by the Family Research Laboratory at the University of New Hampshire. Elderly men and women, with or without impairments or dependency on family care, are vulnerable to mistreatment. In addition to suffering physical injuries, these victims often develop overwhelming feelings of fear, isolation, and anger and need extensive counseling to regain independence. Given the present incidence of mistreatment and the projected growth of this segment of the population, it is imperative that health care providers who care for the elderly learn to recognize and intervene on behalf of victimized patients. However, it must be recognized that the information base about abuse and neglect of the elderly is limited, and more research is needed to better understand the causes and prevention of this problem, as well as ways to intervene.

In defining abuse and neglect of the elderly, the following questions must be considered: **(1) Who is being abused or neglected?** Although definitions of "elderly" vary, one of the common determinants is being 65 yr of age or older. The victim may be competent or incompetent, healthy or frail, male or female. **(2) Who is doing the abusing or neglecting?** Abuse or neglect may be family mediated (eg, spouse, child, grandchild), may be inflicted by a hired care giver, or at the hands of unrelated perpetrators. **(3) Where is abuse or neglect occurring?** Abuse or neglect can occur in the elderly person's home, in the perpetrator's home, in a shared living arrangement, or in an institution. This chapter primarily addresses family-mediated mistreatment occurring in the community. **(4) What is the pattern of abuse or neglect?** Although a 1-time act of violence can be damaging, abuse or neglect of the elderly is commonly characterized by a pattern of violence increasing in severity and incidence over time. **(5) What types of abuse or neglect are occurring?** Abuse or neglect can include physical, psychological, or financial mistreatment. **(6) Is the mistreatment intentional or unintentional?** In some cases, abusers deliberately mistreat to cause harm; in other cases, the resulting harm is nondeliberate, and interventions should vary according to the intent to harm. For example, mismedicating a relative because of poor understanding of the physician's directions may result in drug toxicity. Clearer instructions can remedy this unintentional mistreatment. However, deliberate mismedication of an older relative to control his ability to function independently requires more intensive interventions.

A historic perspective on this form of family violence is instructive. In the 1960s, the phenomenon of child abuse was fully recognized, and in the 1970s, a new awareness of spouse abuse occurred. Both of these derive primarily from family-mediated violence. The awareness of abuse of the elderly grew out of a preexisting interest and appreciation of these forms of violence in the family. In the late 1970s, a seminal work entitled *Behind Closed Doors,* by Straus and Steinmetz, explored domestic violence in the USA. Abuse of the elderly was not mentioned, indicating that it is a relatively recent and still-emerging phenomenon. It has since, however, come to the attention of the public and has spurred appropriate legislation.

About 100 yr passed between awareness of the problem of child abuse and the enactment of legislation, while about 10 yr passed between awareness of spouse abuse and passage of legislation. In the case of abuse of the elderly the awareness and legislation came almost simultaneously. In 43 states, reporting is mandatory when abuse occurs in the home, and in all states, it is mandatory when abuse is detected within institutions. Thus, physicians need to become familiar with their state laws. No research has been done to indicate whether legislation has been effective.

Etiology

A poor understanding of the aging process and negative attitudes toward aging may contribute to abuse and neglect of the elderly. An ageist world, in which negative attitudes toward aging and old people are common, encourages development of an environment in which mistreatment of the elderly may readily occur. Isolation works as a barrier to detection of such behavior. Further isolation is created through mandatory retirement and underutilization in a society that values youth as well as power and status, which are often defined by jobs.

The 5 major theories most often used to explain abuse and neglect of the elderly are psychopathology of the abuser, stress, transgenerational violence, dependency, and isolation.

Psychopathology of the abuser: A number of abusers have had a series of hospitalizations for serious psychiatric disorders (eg, schizophrenia and other psychoses). Many of them abuse alcohol or other drugs.

When an adult child has a mental illness requiring inpatient psychiatric assistance, the parents' home is often the discharge site of last resort. Out of concern that the child will be homeless or have to stay in a shelter, or just out of love, parents often agree to take the child back into their home. With the trend toward deinstitutionalization, psychiatrists who discharge a dependent adult child to the parents' home must be cognizant of possible effects on the older parents. Patients who are not violent within the institution may be violent in the home. When the potential for domestic violence is not carefully scrutinized and provisions for follow-up are not made, a situation may be created in which abuse of the elderly is a likely outcome.

Stress: Family violence researchers report that financial problems, caregiving responsibilities, and other tensions may create frustration and anger that may be expressed by some people through acts of abuse.

Transgenerational violence: Sometimes, abusers were abused when they were children—either by the older victim or by the victim's spouse. A spirit of retaliation is suggested in response to previous abuse; there may even be tacit complicity on the part of the older victim. Some experts believe that because the abuser has experienced maltreatment, the violent behavior is transmitted transgenerationally and mirrors how the individual has learned to express anger and frustration. This theory has been hard to substantiate, because information from elderly abuse victims about prior abuse of their spouse or children is difficult to obtain. Most people do not readily admit to having been violent, and individuals who maltreat family members may not define it as such or may not remember themselves or their spouses as being abusive.

Dependency: Often, abusers are dependent on their elderly relatives for financial support, emotional support, and housing. In some cases, a mutual dependency exists. For example, the older person may be dependent on the abuser for socialization or for performing activities of daily living, while the abuser may be dependent on the victim for housing or money.

Isolation: Several studies have found that elderly abuse victims are more isolated than their nonabused counterparts. This isolation may provide increased opportunities for mistreatment.

Epidemiology

The epidemiology of abuse or neglect of the elderly has been better understood since results of a 1986 survey conducted by the Family Research Laboratory at the University of New Hampshire of 2020 randomly selected elderly people living in the Boston metropolitan area were reported. Thirty-two of every 1000 people 65 yr of age and older reported being abused. Abuse was defined as **physical abuse,** which included hitting, slapping, and pushing; **neglect,** which involved depriving a person of something needed for daily living; and **chronic verbal aggression,** which included verbal threats and insults.

The investigators found that most abuse is committed by one spouse against another. Of the abuse cases, 65% were between spouses and only 23% involved an adult child abusing a parent. The study results also contradicted the previous impression that most elderly abuse victims are women. In this study, elderly husbands actually had twice the risk of being abused as did wives, although abused wives reported more serious injuries. Abuse occurred at all economic levels and in all age groups among the elderly. Another misconception corrected by the study was the belief that the person who perpetrates the abuse usually is a care giver. The study found the opposite to be true; abusers usually were dependent in some way on the individual they abused. It appears from the study that a significant risk factor for abuse and neglect is close proximity of living arrangements of victim and abuser. However, a clear profile of the abuser has not yet been determined.

Classification

The 3 general categories of abuse and neglect are psychologic, physical, and financial. All can be intentional or unintentional.

Psychologic abuse and neglect encompasses a range of behavior that causes emotional stress or injury to an older person. This behavior includes verbal abuse—threatening remarks, insults, or harsh commands—as well as being silent or ignoring the person. One form of psychologic abuse is infantilism (a form of ageism), whereby the elderly individual is treated as a child, which both patronizes and encourages the person to passively accept a dependent role.

Physical abuse and neglect produces a wide range of bodily injuries. Examples of this type of mistreatment include striking, shoving, shaking, beating, restraining, or improper feeding. Sexual assault, included in this category, requires special emphasis, since many providers find this form of violence inconceivable when an older individual is involved. Sexual assault refers to any form of sexual intimacy without consent or by force or threat of force.

Financial abuse is the misuse or exploitation of or inattention to an older person's possessions or funds. This form of mistreatment includes conning, pressuring the victim to distribute assets, or irresponsibly managing the victim's money.

Symptoms and Signs

Following are some of the symptoms and signs that, when clustered, suggest underlying abuse or neglect.

Psychological mistreatment may be indicated by insomnia, sleep deprivation, need for excessive sleep, unusual weight gain or loss, change in appetite, tearfulness, unexplained paranoia, low self-esteem, excessive fears, ambivalence, confusion, resignation, or agitation. **Physical mistreatment** may be indicated by bruises, burns, welts, lacerations, punctures, fractures, and dislocations; evidence of misuse of medications; malnutrition/dehydration, or hair pulling; unexplained venereal disease or unusual genital infections; signs of physical restraint or confinement against the patient's will (eg, rope burns); absence of eyeglasses, hearing aids, dentures, or prostheses; and unexpected or unexplained deterioration of health. **Financial abuse** indicators include sudden or unexplained: (1) inability to pay bills; (2) withdrawal of money from accounts; or (3) disparity between assets and satisfactory living conditions.

Diagnosis

The detection of abuse and neglect varies in difficulty, depending on whether the manifestations of underlying mistreatment are obvious or subtle. There are many impediments to identification of abuse and neglect. Misconceptions about aging (eg, the belief that all old people develop cognitive deficits) can lead to misattributions concerning cause and to missing the possibility that an older person might be harmed. Protectionist attitudes toward older people are widely held, yet in reality, not everyone is protective. Thus, the health provider should have a high index of suspicion for abuse and neglect, since the symptoms and signs may not be readily apparent.

Isolation of the elderly victim is common and is a formidable barrier to detection. Factors such as retirement, loss of friends and relatives through death and relocation, and disabilities that limit mobility conspire to leave older people generally more isolated than their younger counterparts. Isolation tends to increase when the person is being abused, since the abuser typically limits the victim's access to the outside world (eg, denying visitors, refusing telephone calls). Indeed, the health provider is often the only individual to whom the victim has access, which emphasizes the need for physicians to be aware of this form of domestic violence.

In addition to being isolated, victims may be deeply ashamed of their dilemma and tend to hide their problem. Often, victims feel an obligation to protect the abuser-relative or fear retaliation and fail to report mistreatment. Ageism is also a factor in the way society responds to older victims. Sometimes when elderly abuse victims do reach out for help, they are met with responses such as authorities unquestionably accepting a relative's statement that an elderly parent has Alzheimer's disease (supporting the stereotype that all people > 65 yr of age have some degree of dementia) or dismissing the possibility of abuse because they cannot believe that an 80-yr-old husband is capable of beating his 79-yr-old wife.

Health providers who are unaware of abuse and neglect of the elderly may miss obvious instances. For example, a patient may be brought to the emergency room with a fracture, and the relative accompanying the patient may attribute the problem to a fall caused by poor balance. Although falls and osteoporosis are common in the aging population, each new fracture must be thoroughly assessed, and the possibility of abuse must be considered. Medical personnel must probe the specifics of environmental conditions relating to injury and not misattribute conditions because of incomplete history taking or ageist stereotyping.

When interviewing an elderly patient, especially one who is always accompanied by a relative or care giver, *it is important that the health provider be alone with the patient at some time during the visit.* This provides an opportunity for the physician to inquire into the patient's life and establish the rapport and confidentiality that appear to be essential for accurate detection.

Since health providers usually receive little or no training in recognizing and intervening in abuse and neglect of the elderly, they often have little therapeutic optimism, which inversely correlates with efforts directed toward detection. The lack of exposure, protocols, and well-defined approaches to treating the elderly abuse victim contributes to poor skills in detection, misdiagnosis, and limited intervention strategies.

Several maxims of domestic violence derived from clinical impressions may be helpful in diagnosis. If the severity of the injury does not fit the explanation given by the relative, the physician must suspect abuse. The relative's resistance to outside intervention (eg, visiting nurse or home-maker services, physical therapy in the home) or reluctance to leave the older person alone with the health provider may indicate underlying mistreatment. When elderly victims say they are certain there will be no further victimization, the health provider can question this point of view and help the patient explore intervention alternatives.

Assessment and Intervention

Since there is no prototypical abuser of the elderly, the physician must evaluate the specific cause of abuse in every case. There may be an over-lap of causes, such as care giver stress coexisting with transgenerational violence. These etiologic factors provide a framework that can help guide the intervention and protect the victim. For example, intervention on behalf of a victim with a psychotic family member would be differ-ent from that on behalf of a victim recently stricken with a stroke whose care giver relative was under overwhelming stress. It is important to remember that many abusers are not care givers but family members who are dependent on the older relative for money, housing, or emo-tional support.

Before intervention can be carried out, a medical and psychosocial as-sessment of the victim should be obtained. The following questions should be addressed:

1. Is access to the victim a problem? Victims and abusers may be re-luctant to allow professional contact. Sometimes, abusers refuse to allow a professional to visit the house, or they may monitor the victim's con-tacts very closely to prevent disclosure of the mistreatment. In some cases, professionals may have to rely on ingenuity to gain access to the victim, and must also be conscious of possible threats to their own safety.

2. Is the mistreatment intentional or unintentional? The health provider should ask the victim why he or she thinks the abuse is occurring, when the abuse started, and what circumstances usually surround abusive be-haviors.

3. How severe is the abuse? If the pattern of mistreatment has esca-lated and the abuse, already severe, is occurring frequently, the victim may be in serious danger. This evaluation takes into account the kind of injuries the victim has sustained and whether weapons are being used, and how frequently the mistreatment is occurring.

4. Is the victim aware of the problem? Does the victim perceive the se-riousness of the problem? Does the victim deny the problem or ac-knowledge that abuse is occurring? The victim's responsiveness and awareness of the problem, and his level of self-blame, self-acceptance, and ambivalence to the intervention options presented help determine the degree to which the victim will participate in intervention plans.

Therefore, the determination of the victim's view of various options is essential.

5. What risk factors are present in the particular situation? Is the older person isolated? Does the victim have access to a phone or friends? Is there evidence of stress? Is there psychopathology on the part of the abuser? Is there a history of family mistreatment? Is there a family member who is dependent on the older person?

6. Who is inflicting the abuse? Is the suspected abuser a family member? Is the victim dependent on this person or is the abuser the dependent one? There may be more than one perpetrator; an accurate assessment is imperative to target appropriate interventions.

7. What is the victim's cognitive status? Is the older person competent? Does the victim have enough intellectual control to follow a plan of action if an abusive episode occurs? Some people may be competent enough to live independently, without guardianship, yet not be able to understand the risks and consequences of remaining in an abusive situation or to plan an escape if abuse recurs.

Often, living with considerable danger results in depression. Before writing off a victim as mentally impaired, one should rule out an underlying pseudodementia secondary to exogenous depression or other reversible causes of dementia. If a hospitalized victim is described by the accompanying care giver as confused or demented, the physician should observe the victim's behavior in the hospital and assess the victim's cognitive status. Is the older person still confused after receiving care and proper nutrition? A discrepancy between the care giver's account and what is observed in the hospital warrants further investigation.

8. What is the victim's health and functional status? Does the victim have a medical condition or mobility problem that will modify management?

9. What are the victim's resources? What are the financial resources? Are there supportive family members, concerned neighbors, and friends?

10. What community resources are available? Are respite-care options available (eg, temporary overnight shelters, day care, or foster care)?

11. Has any intervention been made in the past? Information about previous interventions (eg, court orders of protection) and why they failed should be obtained to avoid embarking on the same approach.

The health professional must decide whether emergency intervention is required. Circumstances that dictate immediate intervention include the urgent need for medical or psychiatric attention, abuse that is life-threatening or likely to result in permanent damage, and impairment of the abusing individual to the degree that he is unable to care for the victim.

Other interventions range from providing educational information (eg, teaching victims about abuse and available options and helping them to devise safety plans); psychologic support (eg, individual psychotherapy and support groups); emergency supports (eg, respite housing and help in getting immediate medical attention); legal aid (eg, obtaining orders of protection and advocacy on behalf of the victim in the criminal justice system); medical assistance; and alternative housing (ranging from sheltered senior housing to nursing home placement).

Abusers usually do not abuse continuously, and between episodes they may maintain fairly normal behavior. Unless there are persons who can fill the void in the life of the victim if the abuser is removed, it may be extremely hard for the victim to forgo contact with the abuser. Also, since counseling the elderly abuse victim usually requires several sessions, the health care provider should anticipate progress in incremental steps, rather than in rapid advances with short-term resolution.

With competent victims, the health care provider presents options and the victims decide how to proceed. With incompetent victims, decisions are made, ultimately by the courts. When working with a judgmentally impaired older victim, one usually should choose the least restrictive alternative. Before deciding whether the victim should be institutionalized, one should consider the victim's lifetime life-style choices and try to make decisions consistent with those choices. Although it may be difficult to reconcile, sometimes allowing the victim to remain in an abusive environment is better than admitting the person to a long-term care institution (eg, if it is known that the victim prefers to be at home).

With a cognitively impaired, incompetent victim, most decisions are better made by an interdisciplinary team. Decisions need to be made with a full awareness of the severity of the violence, the life-style choice history of the individual, and the legal ramifications. Often, there is no single correct decision, and each case must be carefully followed up. Because various state protective service laws govern intervention and reporting for incompetent victims, health care providers should be familiar with the laws and protective service resources available.

---

99. LEGAL ISSUES

Nancy Neveloff Dubler

The legal issues that surround the care of the elderly are both similar to and different from the legal concerns that guide care for all patients. An older person has the same legal rights and protections as any other adult patient who is not congenitally retarded and who has not been declared incompetent by a court of appropriate jurisdiction.

As a class, however, elderly patients are statistically more likely to possess characteristics that place them at risk for the abrogation of their legal rights. This vulnerability requires that providers proceed with en-hanced vigilance and sensitivity to identify and support the rights and interests of elderly patients and to guard against accidental or planned disempowerment.

Elderly persons are at increased legal risk because they are more likely to be alone and isolated, poor, demented, and institutionalized. They may be less able to be effective, strong advocates for their personal be-liefs and desires. They tend to have less available ancillary support from informal support networks.

An awareness of their legal rights and vigorous advocacy of their per-sonal interests are both critical in our adversary system of justice, which depends largely on individual redress of grievances. This awareness is especially crucial in the medical context, in which patients are often ill-informed or misled about the nature and extent of individual rights and liberties.

PATIENT RISKS AND BENEFITS

Because of their previously discussed vulnerabilities, elderly persons are at risk for **guardianship (committeeship)** or **limited guardianship (conser-vatorship)** actions. The former action is designed to prove incompetence; the latter attempts to demonstrate diminished functional ability to man-age property and personal-care decisions. The elderly are at enhanced risk for these actions, since many statutes stipulate that old age is one of the statutorily acceptable grounds for instituting such a lawsuit. (Physical addictions and mental illness are 2 other commonly stated bases.) Because of gradually increasing cognitive deficits, elderly persons are more likely to need support in managing financial and personal-care plans. They are also more likely to be legally challenged regarding plans and preferences that may seem strange or bizarre to others or that con-flict with the self-interest of prospective heirs or other affected persons.

The legal rights of elderly patients may also be at risk in medical set-tings. Physicians and all health care providers have been taught to diag-nose, cure, and comfort; their mission—to do good—encourages pater-nalism. They have been taught to pursue what is in the patient's "best interest," which may be at odds with the course of treatment the patient would choose. Thus, the patient's legally protected right to choose may be compromised by the physician's benevolently motivated commitment to what is seen as appropriate care.

Older patients are at even greater risk for disempowerment in acute-care settings, in which the toxic reactions to illness, the effects of drugs, postsurgery delirium, or temporary dementia can remove the patient en-tirely from discussions about preferred care. These possibilities require that geriatricians discuss patterns of preference and possible future op-tions for care with a patient when that person is capable of formulating a choice and communicating the decision. The patient's expressed pref-

erence should be noted in the medical record (see ADVANCE DIREC-
TIVES, below).

The geriatric practitioner should be aware that **elderly patients are often the targets of unscrupulous schemes to defraud them of property or
money.** Often, these plots can be defeated by timely and effective legal
intervention by lawyers knowledgeable about or dedicated to the legal
problems of the elderly. Offices that provide legal services for elderly
persons are generally available and can be located by calling the local
Agency on Aging. Where available, these services can be of incalculable
support in defending against fraud and pursuing individual rights and
benefits. Medical practitioners often become aware of the problems first
and should refer the patient for legal assistance.

In most jurisdictions, older patients are eligible for a range of age-
based and needs-based entitlements. In every state, the elderly are eligible for Medicare (see FINANCING HEALTH CARE in Ch. 97 and Ch.
104). The type of physician and hospital visits and the range of services
(ie, eyeglasses, medications, hearing aids) that Medicare will or will not
reimburse changes regularly with new statutory and regulatory amend-
ments. It is important for physicians to know the basic contours of the
rules, to have materials available that describe the range and extent of
benefits, and to be able to refer patients to knowledgeable legal and social service resources, if any exist, for further counseling and support.

The denial of a patient's claim is often reversible by using a "fair hearing" administrative forum to challenge bureaucratic denials of payment
under Medicare. Many benefit denials can be reversed by prompt individual challenge supported by administrative appeal via a fair hearing.

Elderly poor may also be entitled to further medical benefits under
Medicaid. Although only about one third of elderly patients will possess
sufficiently limited income and assets to qualify, additional support in
these cases may be critical. Levels of resources and income that qualify
a patient for Medicaid vary among states. State departments of social
services, local Medicaid offices, and legal services for the elderly or the
poor are good sources of information, materials, support, and individual
representation.

In addition, many states and localities have a bewildering array of special benefits and programs for the elderly, which range from subsidies
for transportation, housing, heating bills, telephone, and food expenses
to discounts at movies. Physicians should have explanatory materials on
these benefits and programs displayed prominently and referral resources available. Medical providers are responsible for educating elderly patients about and providing access to benefits and entitlements
that could be important to the patients' physical well-being or mental
health. Physicians should not attempt to be lawyers, but they should
develop an expanded definition of care that includes enhanced sensitivity
to the legal risks and benefits of being old.

DECISION-MAKING IN MEDICAL CARE AND TREATMENT

INFORMED CONSENT AND THE RIGHT TO REFUSE

Since the early 20th century, the concept that "every patient of adult years and sound mind shall have a right to decide what shall be done with his own body" has gradually become the rule. This theme, which lawyers call **self-determination** and philosophers label **autonomy,** is the foundation of the legal and ethical aspects of the concept of informed consent.

Historically, the basis of medicine was considered to be "touching." Consent in advance to that touching defeated a subsequent action for assault and battery. In the past century, however, negligence replaced assault and battery as the legal rubric governing medicine, and that imposed certain positive duties of care on practicing medical professionals. One of these duties was the responsibility to provide information and to outline the risks and benefits of alternative treatments so that the patient could exercise this right to self-determination, or to choose in an informed manner.

The constitutional right to privacy, given its first modern articulation in the Supreme Court cases that legalized contraception and used as the basis for a woman's right to an abortion, also supports the right of persons to choose individually appropriate medical care plans. Further, concepts of personal liberty and restraints on state behavior that interfere with independent action and choice also support the legal rights of the person who is capable of making health care decisions to choose among medical care options.

Physicians must, therefore, inform patients of the diagnosis, the prognosis, the available alternative interventions, the risks and benefits of those options, and the risk and probable outcome of nonintervention. *The patient then has the right to informed choice,* ie, to consent to or refuse care, even if the likely outcome of refusal is death. *The physician has an obligation to communicate this right to choose*—to help to empower the unaware, uninformed, or unsophisticated.

The doctrine of informed consent does not require that the physician be a mere passive conduit for technical information. It does require that information be disclosed in a language and manner appropriate to the individual patient so that the patient may fashion a personal, albeit idiosyncratic, comfortable choice. The patient's right to choose can be a legal reality only with a physician's support and counsel.

These requirements mean that patients have a legal right to make decisions, even those that, in the physician's judgment, are unwise or foolish. A refusal does not necessarily mean that the patient is "incompetent" or "crazy." Physicians must be aware, however, that *the single greatest reason for a patient's refusal of suggested care is misunderstanding or miscommunication between the patient and physician.*

A patient's refusal of care is not an attempted suicide. Courts distinguish between a suicide, which is characterized by behavior commenced by and under the control of the person (the inception) and intended (the intent) to cause death, and refusal of care. Thus, courts readily distinguish between jumping out of a 20-story window and refusing further painful and uncomfortable chemotherapy that might or might not arrest or reverse the progress of a malignancy. Courts regularly protect the right of an adult Jehovah's Witness (who has no minor children or disabled dependents) to refuse blood transfusions, which are prohibited by his religious teaching, even when they are necessary for effective medical care in the judgment of the attending physician. The individual's right to choose almost always outweighs the physician's responsibility to deliver usual and customary medical care when these 2 come into conflict.

Some states do recognize an exception to the informed consent process, called the **"therapeutic privilege."** *This allows a physician to withhold information when, in the judgment of the physician, the patient would suffer direct and immediate harm as a result of the disclosure* and provides a limited exception to the usual rules governing the physician's responsibility to disclose and the patient's right to choose. This doctrine is appropriate very infrequently. Mere upset or anguish over a grim situation does not qualify. The patient's state of mind should be reevaluated frequently to ensure that disclosure is made to the patient as soon as, in the judgment of the physician, the risk of serious adverse effects has sufficiently abated.

THEORY AND REALITY

The theory of informed consent and the rights of patients are regularly violated by well-meaning and benevolent physicians, often acting in concert with concerned family members. The patient is often ill and frightened, and it appears reasonable, even kind, to involve loving family members in difficult discussions and decisions. This may be valid, but **family involvement should occur only with the patient's agreement and permission.**

Involving the family without the patient's consent is a violation of the patient's right to choose and the patient's right to confidential care. Some patients prefer that decisions be made by family or physician; some, however, refuse to involve the family. Nevertheless, all patients should be given the choice.

Ethical oaths and specific statutes protect confidentiality within the doctor-patient relationship in every state. The relationship is also protected by the doctrine of "privilege," which provides that the patient has the right to exclude otherwise appropriate, relevant, and admissible testimony in a court of law; this privilege can only be raised by the patient. Additionally, most states have professional licensing statutes that incorporate professional oaths, and make their strictures a clear part of professional practice.

An elderly patient is entitled to confidential care—to have his secrets protected unless and until he gives permission for disclosure or unless it is clear beyond question that he is no longer able to express a preference (eg, the patient is in a deep coma). Even then personal secrets should be guarded although decisions about care may need to be discussed with appropriate surrogates. When a patient is no longer capable of making health care decisions, prior expressed preferences should be respected.

COMPETENCE OR DECISIONAL CAPACITY
(See also Ch. 100)

Competence is a societal judgment as well as a legal concept. Historically, persons became "competent" at age 21, at which time they were entitled to vote, to sign binding contracts, and to otherwise participate in the workings of society. The concept of competence thus reflects a societal determination to include or exclude certain persons from full participation. It does not reflect any focused inquiry into the abilities or disabilities of an individual person.

The term **"decisional capacity"** more accurately captures the notion of individual capability, which is at stake in examination of a patient's mental status, judgment, and short-term memory. Decisional capacity **(de facto competence)** is a prerequisite for providing legally adequate and morally sufficient informed consent or refusal. The President's Commission for the Study of Ethical Problems in Medicine and Biomedical and Behavioral Research stated: "Decision-making capacity requires, to greater or lesser degree: (1) possession of a set of values and goals; (2) the ability to communicate and to understand information; and (3) the ability to reason and to deliberate about one's choices."

Many legal scholars, bioethicists, and psychiatrists—in comments that tend to mix normative and descriptive language—have asserted that the greater the risk of the proposed intervention, the greater the degree to which a patient's capabilities to consider must be finely honed. Thus a patient may be capable of choosing between relatively benign alternatives (that may have few serious consequences), yet may not be capable of evaluating and choosing alternatives in a life-threatening circumstance. All states require—by a combination of statute, common law, and regulation—that informed consent of the competent patient precede medical intervention. Yet many elderly patients who are not truly capable of understanding and evaluating alternatives are treated as if they are capable because they nod agreement or do not actively oppose a proposed intervention. Since it is in no one's interest to question this "consent," it is rarely contested. In many cases, however, this lack of individual scrutiny means that no one is exercising the important right of the patient to evaluate and choose the individually most appropriate medical care plan (see SURROGATE DECISION-MAKING, below).

A patient need not be equally aware at all times in order to provide legally adequate informed consent. Patients with fluctuating ability who are intermittently confused may, in their more lucid moments, be perfectly capable of providing legally adequate informed consent. A **"window of lucidity"** may exist in a patient who exhibits "sundowning" (enhanced confusion in the evening) or who is somewhat confused from time to time.

Similarly, a patient with compromised short-term memory may nonetheless be able to judge the individual appropriateness of a suggested intervention despite memory deficit. This is especially true if there is a long-standing pattern of choice **(a sedimented life preference) that the patient has exhibited and that is supported by the corroborating statements of others.**

Alternatively, the patient may have deficits in understanding or reasoning of such severity that the average person would not want that patient to bear responsibility for the choice he proposes to make (or for any choice).

Judgments regarding decisional capacity are, in most instances, properly made by the care team. In both acute-care institutions and long-term care facilities, the nursing staff is often most aware of a patient's range of abilities and can provide critical testimony on how momentary capabilities reflect overall functioning.

Formal mental status testing can help determine whether a patient should be considered competent. However, *a score on a standard examination does not dictate a conclusion about competence.*

Care providers must inform patients of alternatives, risks, and benefits and elicit their choice; however, this does not mean that the physician should or even may accept the first sign of reluctance as a refusal of care. A physician is not a neutral conduit for the passage of information. He is an active participant, able, and indeed ethically required to encourage acceptance of the treatment judged to be in the patient's best interest. Advocacy, however, must stop short of coercion, duplicity, or deceit. Most patient refusals of care will be reversed with attention, extended discussion, and even some cajoling. Some refusals are adamant, however; these must be respected and can only be reversed by petition to a court. Physicians must not deprive patients of their rights; only a court, after full adversary argument, can order care over a patient's clear and consistent refusal. The fact that a patient is refusing care is not, in and of itself, evidence of diminished ability or compromised capacity (ie, "This patient is refusing, therefore this patient must be crazy").

ADVANCE DIRECTIVES

If a patient can no longer provide the emotional and intellectual scrutiny the law demands for informed consent, the first appeal to an alternative should be to any specific documents or empowerments executed while the person was capable of choosing and intended to direct and determine care at some point in the future. These documents, living wills and durable powers of attorney for health care decisions, provide the closest approximation to the contemporaneous individual evaluations of risks and benefits.

A regular power of attorney (in most states) is a way for a competent person to delegate some of his rights to someone else (eg, the right to sell a car or manage stocks), but this power lapses if the person granting it becomes incompetent. A durable power of attorney specifies that the appointee's power begins or continues with the onset of incompetence. In most states, the legal requirements are so simple that an attorney is not needed to execute such documents.

The schema of most advance directives is usually as follows: (1) a statement of present capacity to decide; (2) specification of possible trigger events in the future (ie, hopeless or terminal state, no possibility of returning to sapient existence, inability to relate to others); and (3) a litany of interventions that would not be desired (eg, use of a ventilator, dialysis, intensive care, antibiotics). In theory, advance directives could be used by someone to request all care to be provided in the future. In fact, they are used almost exclusively to ward off unwanted care—to facilitate what has been labeled "death with dignity."

The formal requirements and binding power of living wills and durable powers of attorney vary from state to state. All states now recognize (at least by common law and often by statute) the right of a patient to provide informed consent prior to a medical intervention. Most states recognize statements made when the patient was capable as evidence of prior preference that can be applied by others in the future. Some states have passed statutes that stipulate the form and the formal measures with which an advance directive must comply before it is effective and binding. Many of these statutes provide immunity for physicians who withhold or withdraw care in compliance with properly executed and witnessed directives. Other states have developed case law that not only supports written directives but also permits care givers and others to honor oral statements by the patient that are explicit and clear.

Without specific statutes that indicate when directives may or must be followed, the effectiveness of the instruction depends greatly on the clarity, specificity, and applicability of the directive; the consequences of following the prior communication; and the legal climate of the locality. A document that attempts to refuse "heroic" care provides vague and insufficient guidance for care givers. Clear statements are more likely to be directive and thus more likely to be followed.

Advance directives are not a perfect substitute for contemporaneous patient evaluation of a particular situation. It can always be claimed that in this circumstance the patient would or might feel differently, which might be true. Nonetheless, these prior statements, albeit flawed, are legally and morally far superior to the alternative, ie, a decision by others based on their own standards rather than those of the patient.

As more patients become disinclined to permit the extension of organ function beyond sapient and relational existence, physicians must assume responsibility for raising these sorts of issues with their patients and providing forms and models of advance directives, either required or most respected by state law. They should also document on the patient's chart discussions about advance directives and specific decisions. These discussions, acknowledgedly difficult, are best done when the patient is not in crisis.

The objection is often made that such discussions will depress and dispirit the patient. But as society and the media increasingly focus on these issues, many more persons will have already considered them. The physician is the best person to explain life-sustaining technologies and interventions to the patient and to assist in developing a specific advance directive that reflects the patient's preference and describes, to the extent possible, the future preferred contours of care.

SURROGATE DECISION-MAKING

If the patient is not capable of making a choice and no advance directive provides an alternative basis for consent or refusal, some other person or persons must provide the direction and legally adequate oversight for care. In the past, elderly patients were cared for by their physician and family, guided by personal conceptions or beneficence and respect. This sort of unreviewed and unsupervised surrogate decision-making, although still the norm, is increasingly circumscribed by growing legal awareness of the problems involved and the development of rules and regulations to guide and constrain the decisions.

In the past decade, courts and legislatures have fashioned rules holding that persons who cannot decide about care do not lose their right to consent or refuse. These rights may be exercised by others, based on specific legal standards with procedural safeguards and stipulated possibilities for review.

There is a basic lack of symmetry in the discussion of surrogate decision-making. When consent to provide care is sought, most hospitals and physicians accept the authorization of a broad spectrum of relatives, close friends, and professionals. The consent of a spouse, child, member of the clergy, or even a distant and uninvolved relative is usually sufficient to provide care. In most states, none of these persons is actually legally empowered to consent on behalf of another. By tradition, however, and based on the supposition that a close relative would care and know most about the patient (despite the known facts about family conflict and ambivalence), it makes practical and ethical sense to accept the judgment of involved family members and friends over that of total strangers. This reasoning falls apart when the formalistic permission of a distant, uninvolved, or estranged relative is secured as the basis for care. When hospital, physician, and family agree, however, that agreement—except in exceedingly rare circumstances—is a generally accepted (although often not formally adequate) basis for care.

For elderly people who have outlived family and friends, **a court-appointed guardian,** who is often uninterested and actually serves a perfunctory role, may be the only alternative. Some institutions and regions are experimenting with **public guardians** and **patient advocates,** which may prove appropriate and cost-effective.

When surrogates attempt to refuse care or the decision involves withholding or withdrawing care (an often articulated distinction without any substantial legal or ethical difference), there is often increased legal concern, since the natural, inevitable outcome of these actions is death. Inasmuch as all courts agree that the state has a fundamental interest in the preservation of life, these decisions are often legally problematic.

The first questions in these circumstances are, Who decides? and, On what basis is the decision made? Answers vary widely among the states. In New Jersey, a specially appointed guardian may opt for a refusal that, it is thought, will permit death after a hospital ethics committee (actually a prognosis committee) has determined that the prognosis is hopeless and after the state Office of the Ombudsman has determined that the decision does not constitute "abuse." The decision of the surrogate is supposed to be based on the legal standard of substituted judgment, ie, What would this patient want if he could tell us? In Massachusetts, such decisions are reserved for a court, after full adversary argument on the issues of patient prognosis, patient preference, and state interest. Other states have formal or informal mechanisms that balance the interests of the state in preserving life, preventing suicide, protecting innocent third parties, and protecting the integrity of the medical profession against the prior wishes of the patient, the desires of family, and the abstract notions of best interest and respect for persons.

In most states, the firmest substantive basis for decision, absent an explicit advanced directive, is **substituted judgment.** If insufficient information is known or can be surmised about the patient and if a decision crisis has been reached, care givers, family, and sometimes the courts appeal to notions of **"best interest."** These discussions often focus on the intrusiveness and burden of the intervention, the benefit it is likely to produce, the suffering of the patient, and the ultimate possibility of recovery. As burden and intrusiveness rise and as benefit and prognosis dim, the care is less likely to be morally or legally mandatory.

Certain sorts of decisions present special problems — eg, the decision to discontinue artificial hydration and nutrition. Care providers, legislators, judges, clergy, and scholars from law, medicine, religion, and ethics (among others) are now struggling to analyze the issues and to propose acceptable solutions regarding such life-sustaining interventions. All courts that have considered the issues have held that the mechanical provision of food and fluid is a medical treatment and thus is subject to the same strictures that guide other medical decisions.

In sum, a surrogate decider can be a person appointed specially by the patient under a proxy designation or a durable power of attorney, a statutorily designated other, an informally identified close family member, or a friend in concert with the physician or the court. The protocol for decision-making is the prior explicit statement of the patient when decisionally capable, inference from patterns of preference and from observed statements and behavior (ie, substituted judgment), or some notion of best interest, which precludes unjustified suffering when the treatment is invasive and intrusive, the benefit speculative, and the prognosis hopeless. All courts that have considered the issues have found that under certain circumstances, permitting death is not incompatible with a patient's best interest and with the state's interest in life.

These decisions are complex for all parties: patient, family, provider, institution, state, legislature, court, and special interest groups, eg, religious groups or single issue constituencies. The legal interests of the patient are in self-determination, dignity, and privacy. The family has no legal interest if not specially appointed as proxy or designated by statute, although its emotional, moral, and often financial stakes are weighty. Providers have an interest in professional integrity, in providing legally adequate care, and in avoiding later civil or criminal challenge (although the latter almost never occurs). Institutions are also concerned about possible future liability. The state must safeguard the lives and the values of its various individual citizens and heterogeneous cultures, and it must be cognizant of its disparate special interests.

DISCHARGE AND PLACEMENT

There has been almost no legal focus and only scant scholarly analysis regarding discharge planning and placement decisions for elderly patients. Many physicians and family members assume responsibility for these decisions without adequate discussion with the patient and often over a patient's objection. Just as patients have the right to consent to or refuse treatment, they also have the right to consider and choose the living arrangements and type of care they want in the future. This right, however, is not as exclusive to the patient as are the rights of informed consent and refusal of treatment. The legal, practical, and quality-of-life interests of family and neighbors may be compromised by the patient's return home to a community setting or to the home of a family member.

The fact that a community placement may entail more risk than a residential placement in a long-term care facility does not a priori mean that this choice is unavailable to the patient. Patients may assume the risks of placement just as they may choose a risk-laden treatment alternative. Many elderly persons choose to return home when care givers are convinced that residential treatment is medically and socially preferable. Some patients even choose to return home when the likely result may be death. *If the patient is decisionally capable, this decision, like a refusal of arguably needed care, is legally adequate.* A decisionally capable patient cannot be placed in a residential facility over his objection without a court order. Elderly patients have a right to be obstinate and foolish unless the rights or interests of others are clearly compromised.

Overriding a patient's discharge preference may require petitioning the court for a guardian or a limited guardian. Overriding a treatment decision can often be accomplished by the appointment of a special guardian designated for that specific and limited purpose. The ongoing supervision of an elderly person, however, requires a person with sustained powers and commitment. Unfortunately, many states provide insufficient education, training, and supervision of such court-appointed guardians, who often opt for the least burdensome alternative for themselves rather than the least restrictive alternative for the patient.

DO-NOT-RESUSCITATE ORDERS
(See also Ch. 26)

For the last decade, scholars have discussed and institutions have experimented with policies governing special categories of care, especially **resuscitation**. Many hospitals—and with increasing frequency, long-term care facilities—have policies to guide decisions about resuscitation. These policies vary widely and range from those that categorize this as a decision reserved for the physician to those that clearly empower patients or, if they are unable, designated surrogates to make the decision. One state, New York, has legislated the patient's right to decide on resuscitation status.

Legally, it is clear that decisions about resuscitation are like other decisions about future care and, whenever possible, should be brought to the patient's attention when he is lucid. *Whoever decides, some system should exist for recording, communicating, and reviewing the decision.* There has been no legal case in which either a physician or an institution has been found liable for respecting an order not to resuscitate when the order was arrived at after an appropriate discussion with patient and family that was duly noted on the patient's chart.

LONG-TERM CARE
(See also Chs. 20 and 97)

Legal scrutiny of long-term care institutions is increasing. This stems primarily from the exposés during the past decade of the neglectful and abusive care provided to vulnerable, often demented, elderly institutionalized patients. The nature and degree of abuse offended legal, moral, and civic sensibilities. This resulted in a network of federal and state regulations that prescribe staffing patterns, record keeping, and many aspects of institutional practice. Increasingly, long-term care facilities are being challenged regarding policies that automatically apply life-sustaining technologies to the unknowing and unaware with no provision for stopping. Practitioners should be aware of developments as states struggle to define and constrain these decisions.

This legal climate is a crucial background for discussions with patients and families about possible future care. Many long-term care facilities are adding to their postadmission discussions information about future preference for care and resuscitation status.

Federal law and state regulations also govern long-term care financing (see also Chs. 97 and 104). Most long-term care is funded by Medicaid, the needs-based cooperative federal and state health reimbursement program. Very little long-term care is funded by Medicare, the age-based federal medical program for the elderly. Most elderly patients, couples, and families do not understand the complex rules that require "spending down" their income and assets to a level of poverty before Medicaid will assume the cost of long-term care. **In most states, knowledgeable legal advocates can protect a surviving spouse from impoverishment by appeal to state regulations that permit segregation of funds.** If that is not possible, an attorney may institute a suit for support in the Family Court or other appropriate state forum. Every state has a long-term care ombudsman whose office is funded by Medicare. These offices can provide information about some of the rights and protections available to residents of long-term care facilities.

LEGAL RISKS FOR PHYSICIANS AND CARE GIVERS

The structure of the US legal system ensures that physicians will rarely be sued for malpractice over an incident relating to the care of an elderly patient. The primary reason is that the measure of recovery—mainly, lost earnings—is very low for elderly persons, who generally have ended their economically productive work life. Since most malpractice cases are arranged on a contingent fee basis, the prospective calculation of lost earnings is very low, the award low, and the percentage available for a lawyer's fee low; the whole enterprise is therefore unattractive to the negligence bar.

Legal activity is more likely to occur around the propriety of discontinuing treatment and issues of surrogate decision-making. Also, legal focus is emerging on suits in assault and battery for not discontinuing treatment when treatment is refused by a debilitated but decisionally capable patient. In addition, some nursing home actions have found criminal negligence based generally on patterns of disregard that violate specific regulations for institutional behavior.

LEGAL ISSUES FOR THE AGING FAMILY

As a family ages, the physician should recommend they seek **legal "family planning,"** so that sufficient funds are available for adequate health care or long-term care in the future. Someone, preferably a person who is close and available, must have a durable power of attorney over finances, so that in the event of disability, bills can be paid and money expended to support care.

In the event of increasing dementia, the affected person and family should consider possible assignment or transfer of assets so that in the future the patient can qualify for Medicaid funding of long-term care without risking the impoverishment of the spouse. Arrangements should be made, if possible, to support the care of adult dependent or retarded children by legal appointment of a guardian. If any assets are at stake, the person should execute a will and, if the person has strong feelings about the use of life-sustaining care, a living will. For those with substantial assets, trust funds permit the allocation and protection of property.

For many older persons, the physician is the only professional with whom they have frequent contact. The physician must be aware, therefore, of the ancillary legal factors that affect present and future well-being and be able to direct and refer the patient to available resources.

---

100. ETHICAL ISSUES

Lila T. McConnell, Joanne Lynn, and *Jonathan D. Moreno*

In caring for older individuals, legal and ethical concerns arise with unusual frequency, offering special challenges. The most common problems are assessing competence, determining the range of treatment options, developing advance directives, and anticipating death. In addition, ethical dilemmas are influenced by concerns about allocation of resources and control of costs.

Generally, the approach to solution of ethical problems is the same for older as for younger people, since the 2 groups are more alike than different. However, older people vary more in their physiologic, psychologic, and social reserves. Thus, in discussing ethical issues, inclusion of the category "elderly" in the rationale requires careful deliberation.

For some purposes, an age-based definition may be adequate (eg, "Those > 80 yr of age have done so much for the country, they should be given adequate housing"). For others, age is merely a substitute for the real rationale (eg, "Those > 80 yr of age are often multiply handicapped; multiply handicapped people are usually poor surgical candidates; therefore, surgery for those > 80 yr should be severely restricted"). In such a circumstance, articulation of the underlying rationale may be more accurate and effective; ie, a robust 80-yr-old with excellent physiologic, psychologic, and social reserves who could benefit from surgery should not have that option withheld only because of age. Conversely, there might be valid reasons for advising a less-well 80-yr-old not to undergo a potentially beneficial surgical procedure, and these reasons should be clearly identified, understood, and agreed upon by the patient.

MEDICAL DECISION-MAKING

Ethical dimensions are often overlooked in making medical decisions. Rarely is a decision so simple that it depends only on technical and empiric information, especially in persons with chronic illness and disability. Medical goals should not focus exclusively on correcting abnormal physiology. The purpose of medical care is to determine what alternatives will preserve and promote the patient's well-being *in accordance with the patient's perspectives, beliefs, and goals.* To enhance future well being from the patient's point of view requires both informing and being informed by the patient. The physician's knowledge and clinical experience and the patient's preferences ordinarily are not in opposition, so decisions usually can be made with mutual accord.

While medical decision-making ordinarily requires accurate diagnosis and treatment, these are not the only means of providing the best possible future for the patient. For patients with chronic disability and illness, there may be no possibility of cure or even improvement in overall condition. Specific diagnostic or therapeutic interventions may even be contraindicated. Thus, one must determine the length and nature of the life the person is likely to live, based on consideration of burdens, disabilities, and costs arising from the illness and any proposed diagnostic and therapeutic interventions. For example, diagnosis and treatment of infection might have little to do with beneficial future for a patient in a nursing home with severe dementia, intractable heart failure, and contractures. Instead, this patient might best be treated with antipyretics and meticulous skin care. In essence, physicians should treat patients, not merely their illnesses.

In some cases, disagreement may arise concerning the choice of an alternative. If the physician believes the patient is making a poor choice because of lack of knowledge or information, the physician is obliged to inform the patient more fully. If it appears the patient is incompetent, the physician must initiate more formal review and designation of a surrogate to protect the patient (see also COMPETENCE OR DECISIONAL CAPACITY in Ch. 99). However, a competent patient can always abandon medical care (although a physician cannot abandon a patient). A competent patient's choice will almost invariably be upheld in court in the event of conflict.

Honoring self-determination limits the times that the physician may make choices without informing or consulting the patient. Making decisions for patients without their collaboration often leads to erroneous decisions—courses of care that reflect the physician's preferences but may not optimally advance the patient's interests. More serious, perhaps, is that making choices without involving the patient can be demeaning and infantilizing to the patient.

Nevertheless, a physician is not required to honor a patient's treatment choice if he strongly disagrees with it, even if the patient is competent. If such issues cannot be resolved, the physician can consider withdrawing from the case after examining the risks and benefits of each treatment option, the patient's right to self-determination, and the physician's own commitment to current practice standards and professional integrity. If the physician decides to withdraw, the patient should be notified, perhaps by certified mail, and care should be terminated only upon referral to another physician or after providing ample opportunity for the patient to find another physician.

THE PHYSICIAN AND THE LAW
(See also Ch. 99)

While physicians may wish they could simply ask if some course of action is legal and resolve difficult problems on this ground alone, the law is not so directive. Only a few things (eg, violent killing, outright fraud) are always wrong, and only a few (eg, informing a patient, referring to another well-qualified physician for consultation) are always legally safe. Nearly everything else is sometimes protected, sometimes penalized, and often ambiguous. Especially in any emotionally charged area of medicine, legal precedents are likely to be in conflict or to be uncertain in application to a particular case. This is because all that the law can do well is to regulate the "coarse adjustment" of behavior—to define those things that are clearly beyond the boundaries.

In any difficult area, disagreement arises as to what is considered unreasonable behavior, and legal developments reflect the disagreement. However, one generalization currently holds in the USA: *What is considered by professionals and society to be the best of medical and ethical practice has ordinarily been permitted when tested in court.* In other words, if one proceeds with due care, good documentation, and understanding of the local legal risks, legal considerations do not bar good medical practice. Physicians should know the law affecting their practice and should seek to learn about it through reliable sources. Most of the "you can't do that because of the law" statements heard in hospital corridors are probably not true.

COMPETENCE

Assessing competence is an ethical as well as a legal issue (see also Ch. 99). The need for a decision as to competence always arises from a specific state of affairs. It must be determined whether a patient is capable of making a specific choice at a given time. When faced with a particular alternative, a person may be judged competent if he can choose among various therapeutic goals, understand and communicate relevant information, and demonstrate an ability to reason and to apply that information to the pursuit of those goals.

A very disoriented person may have periods during which these general conditions are met and can, therefore, be considered competent in making particular decisions. In contrast, an elderly individual might live in a life-care facility, be pleasant and sociable, and perform activities of daily living (eg, dressing, eating, and walking) but have a cognitive impairment that so hampers comprehension he might not be able to formulate a decision about a preferred future.

A patient declared legally incompetent may actually be either competent or incompetent to make a particular choice, as may one who is legally considered competent. If a court has determined that a person is legally incompetent but the physician and others feel the patient is actually competent to make a particular decision, both the patient and the court-appointed surrogate (guardian) must agree on a course to follow, since one has ethical and the other legal authority. If they cannot agree, the issue will have to be presented to court again.

A physician's disagreement with a patient's decision never establishes that the patient is incompetent. While professional value judgments might never be entirely absent from determinations of competence, the criteria that a physician uses in deciding competence must take into consideration the patient's values and well being. Patients may have different value systems, which must be respected. In difficult situations where some substantial issue is at stake, consultation with others (eg, family members and hospital ethics committees) and referral to court may be necessary.

An awareness that older people may have certain sensory or emotional problems that can adversely affect decision-making is crucial. The physician should be aware that maximizing a patient's capacity to make decisions is essential in assessing competence. For example, untreated medical conditions and treatments themselves might affect cognitive capabilities and must be mitigated if possible. Mood disturbances do not necessarily render an individual incompetent but may seriously affect judgment. Hearing and visual disorders can affect the *perception* of competence and should be evaluated and corrected, if possible.

INFORMED CONSENT

The process of obtaining informed consent is the formal component of cooperative decision-making by physician and patient (see also Ch. 99). Unfortunately, the various documents developed by institutions to formally record the process are often substituted for the process itself. Informed consent embodies certain conditions that must be satisfied; ie, adequate information, freedom from coercion, and sufficient mental competence. Ensuring fulfillment of these conditions is generally the physician's responsibility.

The physician should ensure that the patient's level of comprehension is at least as great as would be desirable for any other similarly important life choice. Facts about the patient's medical condition and available interventions, including their risks and benefits, should be explored and understood. Not all minor or rare risks or benefits need be identified; however, those that could be expected to affect a particular patient's choice need to be explained. Limiting or forgoing treatment and the consequential risks and benefits might also be discussed. The patient's life-style, the functional outcome of any choice, and psychosocial factors will affect what the patient needs to know.

Certain attributes of informed consent are especially germane to the older individual. One must ensure that the patient is free of undue coercion, such as imposition of the physician's or family's goals and values, and that the patient is not acquiescing to please others or because of perceived loss of self-determination (as may occur if the patient is institutionalized or profoundly dependent at home). Communication with an older patient may require more time because of sensory deficits or slowing of cognition.

RANGE OF TREATMENT OPTIONS

Developing a list of treatment options for a particular patient is a central component of good decision-making. Suboptimal choices are guaranteed if the optimal choice is not even considered. Two assumptions are helpful in developing options for a particular patient: First, although society's financial concerns are an issue, the choices made with *this* patient must be assumed to have negligible effects upon society as a whole, neither greatly changing costs nor depleting other resources. For example, choosing to dialyze an elderly, disabled patient must be assumed to have no major effect upon the availability of dialysis to others. Second, all potential options that can be envisioned for the patient should be considered, including that of forgoing specific treatment. Thus, a patient with an embolic stroke will have at least the options of (1) having no further interventions, (2) having further diagnostic studies to better assess risks, or (3) receiving anticoagulation therapy. Proceeding directly to full diagnosis and treatment without considering the merits relative to forgoing specific treatment can result in a suboptimal choice.

Decision-making may be inappropriately simplified by assembling several categories of dichotomous decisions, one of each pair being an unacceptable solution (eg, the claim that one cannot discontinue a ventilator even though one would have been correct not to have started it, or the claim that one must always provide "ordinary" treatments but that "extraordinary," or "heroic," endeavors need not be applied). Thus, one can "allow to die" but cannot "kill."

The language to which professionals are accustomed often hinders clear thinking, particularly when unexamined assumptions underlie the use of certain words. An example of this tendency is the reliance upon these either/or categories that misleadingly reduce a complex situation to simple moral alternatives. They are poor substitutes for the more correct mandate to ensure that choices be made to advance the patient's best interests, as the *patient* defines them. This may involve stopping a treatment; deciding not to use ordinary interventions, such as antibiotics or feeding tubes; or giving medications that may lead to an earlier death as well as to relief of the symptoms.

Appeal to the common distinction between ordinary and extraordinary is made in cases in which some question exists about whether there is an obligation to treat. This use of the distinction raises 2 problems: First, from an empiric standpoint, rapidly changing technologies and views about what practices are indicated undermine references to ordinary care. Second, and more serious from an ethical point of view, although a practice may be common, it is not necessarily morally right.

The terms ordinary and extraordinary are often used in conflicting and confusing ways, reflecting such aspects as usualness, complexity, artificiality, expense, or availability of care. Care that is in fact extraordinary in the sense that it is rarely, if ever, provided might turn out to be care that is morally required for a limited time in an unusual case. For example, a patient might wish to buy extra time by being kept on a ventilator to survive beyond the birth of a grandchild. Ordinary and extraordinary are useful terms to express one's *conclusions* about the ethical evaluation of a situation, but they do not provide the evaluation. The terms designate useful concepts only if used to indicate whether the burdens imposed on the patient by a treatment are disproportionate to its benefits. Thus, in certain cases, even treatment with antibiotics might be considered as extraordinary as a major surgical procedure.

Many physicians express reservations about *withdrawing* treatment in instances in which, all other things being equal, they would not have had doubts about *withholding* treatment. There are often powerful psychologic inhibitions against stopping a course of action, but there does not seem to be any moral difference between treatment and cessation of treatment. Having tried a treatment may make it easier to conclude that it is without net benefit, which could not have been predicted with certainty before the trial. Admitting that the treatment is not achieving the desired benefits is more painful (and stopping it often entails more documentation than not starting it would have), but such problems can usually be mitigated by having planned end points of therapeutic trials. Such planning is as necessary for the use of nasogastric feeding tubes as it is for more sophisticated interventions (eg, dialysis or repeated blood transfusions); in each case, the best decision cannot be known until after treatment has been initiated. Simply put, one need not persist in a course of treatment that is not working merely because one has undertaken that course.

Certain prudent steps should be taken whenever the care plan for the patient involves physician action that may shorten life (eg, administering high-dose narcotics for pain or respiratory distress, forgoing antibiotics or feeding tubes, or agreeing to withhold a life-sustaining transfusion or radiation treatment). (1) One must be very sure that the course chosen is correctly assessed, ie, there should be no serious deficiency in the empiric data. (2) Respected colleagues (including nurses, social workers, and clergy) can be asked to evaluate the situation. If they disagree with the plan, it should be reassessed and implementation delayed. (3) One can try to ascertain that the patient agrees or would have agreed with the plan if competent. (4) The process by which the decision was made should be carefully documented. (5) One can arrange for a formal review by an ethics or patient care committee or for a court review. The last step is emotionally and financially costly and usually unnecessary if the first 4 steps are followed.

ADVANCE DIRECTIVES

If a patient becomes incompetent and no advance directives have been discussed, there is a strong tradition that the "next of kin" (often a child or spouse who is likely to know and share the patient's values) assume the role of decision-maker for the patient. However, sometimes the next of kin is emotionally distant or hostile, and another person (eg, a friend) may be a better surrogate. When someone other than the next of kin is designated surrogate, the reasons for the choice should be documented.

Often, the surrogate for an elderly person is a group of children (and their spouses), who may seriously disagree with one another. Undesirable motivations (eg, guilt over past inattention or a desire to inherit) may surface. If the controversy threatens to obstruct what seems to be the best course of action, the physician must seek outside review and enable appropriate persons to file for court-appointed guardianship. (See also Ch. 99).

ALLOCATION OF RESOURCES

Health care in modern society is held to a stronger demand to be distributed equitably than are most goods and services. The unfairness of being denied needed health services is more serious than being denied transportation or agricultural assistance. Also, having the population at large share the costs of health care is more widely accepted than sharing similar costs for most other goods and services.

The concern is not whether the special status of health care is defensible but that the value accorded to an equitable allocation of health care has recently led to major upheavals in medical practice. When costs escalated to a level at which businesses and government thought it would be necessary to reduce commitments to other priorities, only 2 corrective actions were possible: (1) Certain people (or health care interventions) could be eliminated as potential recipients, or (2) access to health care could be limited for most people so that all could be guaranteed a minimal level. The first action is more politically appealing; the second is difficult in practice but morally more justifiable.

In the near future, physicians must either accept or reject a major role in allocation decisions. Each patient generally trusts that the physician tries to achieve maximal benefit to the patient. If the physician must limit that advocacy by being responsible for stewarding public funds, conflicts for the physician abound and the trust of the patient is jeopardized.

The need to control expenditures so as to be more equitable is counterbalanced by a substantial and conflicting body of ethics and negligence law, requiring that all efforts possible be made on behalf of each patient. Malpractice litigation and such regulatory practices as the recent federal involvement in "Infant Doe" come close to demanding that nonresisting patients be treated maximally without regard to cost or quality of life.

The divergent demands of cost control and maximal treatment have profound implications for care of the elderly—an issue that has received inadequate attention. Those concerned about the poor financial health of Medicare would like physicians to avoid seeking long-term, low-yield, costly treatment, especially for patients whose life-style is already profoundly limited. For example, they might not want to dialyze a 94-yr-old diabetic with dementia and disability due to multiple strokes. On the other hand, those who fear the devaluing of the dependent elderly (or even systematic and abusive discrimination against them) want any such case to be treated without regard to cost or, especially, to "productivity" or the cognitive abilities of the patient. Physicians vary widely in their responses to these inconsistent value positions. Probably the best resolutions in this interim period are marked by a general physician advocacy for their patients (especially if they are at special risk for discriminatory practices); a willingness to limit treatments with very few benefits; and open, honest communications with patients and families.

101. LIVING ALONE

Robert N. Butler and *Kathryn Hyer*

Of the nearly 28 million noninstitutionalized elderly in the USA, > 8 million live alone. Providing medical care to these people requires sensitivity as well as recognition of their nonmedical needs, because living alone complicates the aging experience and efforts at medical intervention. They lack social support from a spouse, and > ¼ of them have no living children. Although most of those who do have children see them once a week, almost 20% see their children only once a year or less. Elderly persons living alone are more vulnerable to a decline in health and well-being, and this decline is frequently quite rapid.

The process of beginning to live alone is frequently the death of a spouse. Studies of mortality after conjugal bereavement suggest an immediate increase in mortality for both men and women, and a long-sustained but slight increase in mortality among men. In the first week after the death of a spouse, a Finnish study showed a doubling of the expected mortality rate, primarily from ischemic heart disease. A Swedish study found a 48% increased mortality among widowers > 65 yr of age and a 22% increased mortality for widows compared to married people in the first 3 mo after bereavement. The rate of death among widowed men from infectious diseases, accidents, and suicide remains higher than expected for up to 10 yr after the death of a spouse.

Health care providers to the elderly who have lost a spouse need to be watchful and supportive without overemphasizing adverse effects. For frail elderly, it is important to identify social support and interaction and to secure access to vital services. Referral to self-help groups such as Widow-to-Widow may provide the support necessary to deal with the loss.

Seventy-seven percent of the elderly living alone are women. Most are widowed, older, frailer, and poorer than elderly men. More than ½ of those who live alone are > 75 yr of age. The poverty rate is 19% (see FIG. 101–1), almost 5 times the rate for couples. Many widows become poor only after illness depletes savings and the husband's death results in the loss of his pension benefits.

The "safety net" of Medicaid does not ensure access to medical care. Fully ⅔ of those who are poor do not qualify for Medicaid benefits, because income and assets eligibility is determined by state governments

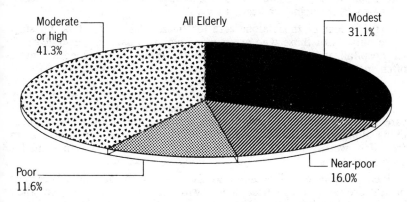

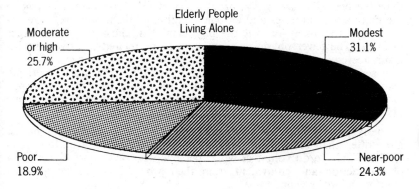

Income levels (expressed as percentages above or below poverty line):

Poor = < 100%   Modest = 150% – 299%
Near-poor = 100% – 149%   Moderate or high = ≥ 300%

FIG. 101–1. Poverty distribution of the elderly, 1987. (From Commission on Elderly People Living Alone: *Medicare's Poor.* Based on ICF Estimates in *Old, Alone and Poor*, 1987. Copyright 1987 by The Commonwealth Fund. Used with permission.)

(see Chs. 97 and 104). The poor elderly without Medicaid spend $1/4$ of their income on medical expenses (an average of $815 per capita). Therefore, poverty rates of those living alone rise from 19 to 27% when medical expenses are deducted from income.

When the "near poor" are considered, fully 45% of the elderly living alone survive on < $154/wk. While the median annual income for couples is $20,000, for those who live alone it is $9400. Furthermore, as age increases, the likelihood of poverty rises. Twenty-seven percent of women > 85 yr of age are poor. With limited income and high medical care costs, these frail individuals often must choose which basic necessities—food, medicine, or heat—they will receive.

Forty percent of those alone care for themselves after a hospital stay, while only $1/4$ of those who are married claim to care for themselves after hospitalization. At all age and income levels, those alone are more often institutionalized, especially when a serious illness occurs. Without a social network or community support, they are at the greatest risk for permanent institutionalization and loss of independent life-style if they suffer a decline in health. Access to social service networks and home-care services may be critical to their recuperation. Almost $1/4$ of those living alone report they have no one they could count on to help them for a few weeks, and 13% indicate they have no one to help them for even a few days.

Elderly people who live alone are more likely to face serious chronic health problems than those living with others, and 43% view their health as fair or poor (see FIG. 101–2). Of those living alone, 53% are hypertensive, 42% have vision problems, and 63% have arthritis. Despite the more severe illnesses and chronic conditions, those who have low incomes are less likely to visit the physician than those who have larger incomes. The fewer physician visits seem to be related to private health insurance coverage. Those who have only Medicare coverage use physician services less frequently than those who have supplementary private insurance. They are also hospitalized less frequently than those with private insurance or Medicaid coverage. This suggests that low-income older persons face a financial barrier to getting health care.

Elderly people living alone attend senior centers, especially for meals, more often than those living with others. Although those who live alone are less likely to do volunteer work, persons who do, report higher rates of satisfaction and enjoyment from their work than married persons who do volunteer work.

Loneliness is a serious problem for 60% of those $\geq$ 75 yr of age. Depression is also common (see Ch. 89). More than $1/3$ of those living alone report feelings of depression, and almost $1/2$ of those who live alone and are poor admit to feeling depressed. Although common, depression should not be ignored; such feelings should routinely be explored with elderly patients who live alone.

Despite the hardships faced, almost 90% of those living alone express a keen desire to maintain their independent life-style. For many, the greatest fear is too much dependence on others, and, despite the loneliness, they want to continue to live alone.

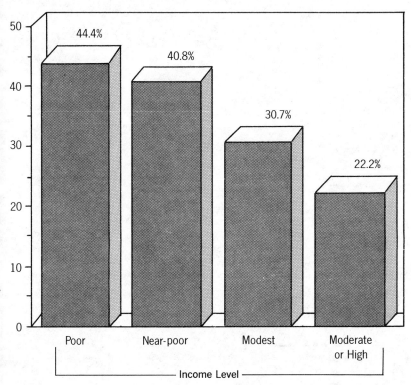

Fig. 101–2. Percent of elderly people reporting fair or poor health by income, 1984. (From Commission on Elderly People Living Alone: *Medicare's Poor*. Based on estimates from the 1984 National Health Interview Survey and Supplement on Aging. Copyright 1987 by The Commonwealth Fund. Used with permission.)

§5. REFERENCE GUIDES

102. CHANGES IN LABORATORY VALUES

Eugene Coodley

The compilation of normal laboratory values in the elderly is complicated by latent or overt disease, multisystem disease, physiologic and anatomic changes associated with aging, and the effect of diet and malnutrition on a number of laboratory factors, which preclude many elderly individuals from serving as normals in determining reference laboratory values. Diet is particularly important, since a large percentage of these patients have some degree of malnutrition.

Many studies have been conducted on the efficacy of laboratory tests in screening for disease, made possible by the development of large-volume, automated instruments. However, automated methods tend to be more susceptible to error from interfering substances and technical factors (eg, residual, trace amounts of a previous specimen remaining in the instrument). In addition, biologic sources of variability include differences in demographics, diet, drugs, and the presence of covert disease, both within an individual and between persons.

The **normal value** for a biochemical test is *the mean value for the test in a population of healthy individuals, $\pm$ 2 SD*. Thus, in practice, 5% of results from normal persons are mistakenly reported as abnormal, and if one assumes that each test in the battery is independent of the others, the probability of a normal individual having completely normal test results is relatively low.

Specific to the elderly, a recent study of 150 individuals 65 to 80 yr of age and 150 subjects > 80 yr, carefully selected by history and physical examination to exclude apparent disease, showed most hematologic and biochemical tests fell within the normal range. Glucose, chloride, and triglycerides were elevated in just over 10% of women in one or both age groups. Deviations in the 5 to 10% category included a low Hct in women > 80 yr, elevated Ca levels in women 65 to 80 yr, reduced serum P concentrations, and elevations of LDH and alkaline phosphatase levels in both sexes at both age levels. In addition, the likelihood of a disease being present when an abnormal test result is obtained depends on test sensitivity and specificity, as well as the pretest probability of the disease.

Laboratory values are often expressed in SI (Système International) units. Conversion factors for currently used values to SI units are shown in TABLE 102–1.

PHYSIOLOGIC CHANGES

Age-associated declines in cardiac, pulmonary, renal, and metabolic function correlate with changes in normal laboratory values. Heart size increases, and coronary disease becomes more frequent. Diet may affect nutritional status. Vital capacity, forced expiratory volume at 1 sec, and maximal breathing capacity decrease progressively with age, while systolic BP increases. Auditory and visual acuity, muscle strength, cardiovascular response to standard exercise, glucose tolerance, nerve conduction velocity, and creatinine clearance decrease.

However, the average change over time in the functional performance of different organ systems proceeds at different rates. Nerve conduction velocity diminishes by only about 10% between the ages of 30 and 70 yr, while renal function may decrease by 50% over the same time span. In addition, an individual's organ systems may vary in levels of performance. Nomograms have been developed to illustrate the serial changes in various physiologic functions with age. Some functions change consistently with progressing age, while others change specifically in certain decades. Therefore, no single standard performance level can be assigned for physiologic age.

Similarly, while **average values** of laboratory tests can be determined, these will not apply to all older individuals. The effects of age can be determined for specific performance levels, but the predictive value of such findings for future performance levels is very low. In general, the same principle applies to the use and interpretation of laboratory tests in detecting disease.

LABORATORY SCREENING TESTS

An assessment of the value of biochemical profiles for screening asymptomatic individuals indicates that **fasting blood glucose** is useful and relatively inexpensive. Also, the value of **serum cholesterol** determination is worth the cost, considering the risk for atherosclerosis produced by an elevated cholesterol level and evidence that lowering the level may reduce the incidence of cardiovascular morbidity and mortality (see also Ch. 74). However, the sensitivity of **creatinine** and **BUN** levels as an indicator of mild to moderate degrees of renal insufficiency is relatively poor. Serum creatinine tends to be lower in the elderly; therefore, a "normal" value may not reflect the extent of renal disease. Thus, a creatinine clearance determination is required to assess renal function (see also Ch. 54).

Measurement of **serum Ca** as a screening test is controversial. The diagnosis of primary hyperparathyroidism has increased since automated biochemical study has become widespread and with the frequent use of diuretics in the elderly. These drugs increase serum Ca and may unmask hyperparathyroidism.

Analysis of the value of **biochemical profiles** shows that most diseases detected by such laboratory measurements present with sufficient clinical symptoms and signs so that the biochemical markers rarely have significant diagnostic value. An elevated serum level of lactate dehydrogenase is associated with several conditions, but these conditions are rarely seen in elderly patients with unremarkable histories and physical examinations. In addition, asymptomatic increases in lactate dehydrogenase levels are only weakly predictive of underlying disease.

The sensitivity of a test or the rate of detection is probably more significant. For example, the total serum protein level is not very sensitive diagnostically for any of the conditions in which it may be altered; on the other hand, elevated serum cholesterol or blood glucose levels are virtually always detected in the presence of familial hypercholesterolemia or diabetes mellitus, respectively. Measurement of alkaline phosphatase is probably useful, since a number of treatable disease entities are associated with its elevation. Screening for uric acid is probably not worthwhile in the absence of clinical evidence of gout. Routine screening of electrolytes and hepatic enzymes is probably not indicated in the absence of a specific clinical indication or a drug history that might affect such tests.

An abnormal finding requires that the test be repeated or additional tests be performed, leading to increased costs with a relatively low yield. It has been estimated that most screening tests yield $< 5\%$ unanticipated or potentially important findings. In general, the prevalence of unsuspected disease is higher in patients admitted to the hospital than in those undergoing office screening; therefore, the pretest probability for detecting disease is considerably higher in the former setting.

TABLE 102–1. SYSTÈME INTERNATIONAL CONVERSION FACTORS FOR FREQUENTLY USED LABORATORY COMPONENTS

System*	Component	Present Reference Intervals (Examples)[†]	Present Unit	Conversion Factor	SI Reference Intervals[†]	SI Unit Symbol	Significant Digits[‡]	Suggested Minimum Increment
	Hematology							
(B) Ercs	Erythrocyte sedimentation rate							
	Female	0–30	mm/h	1	0–30	mm/h	XX	
	Male	0–20	mm/h	1	0–20	mm/h	XX	
B	Hematocrit							
	Female	33–43	%	0.01	0.33–0.43	1	0.XX	
	Male	39–49	%	0.01	0.39–0.49	1	0.XX	
B	Hemoglobin							
	Mass concentration							
	Female	12.0–15.0	gm/dL	10	120–150	gm/L	XXX	
	Male	13.6–17.2	gm/dL	10	136–172	gm/L	XXX	
	Substance concentration (Hb[Fe])							
	Female	12.0–15.0	gm/dL	0.6206	7.45–9.31	mmol/L	XX.XX	
	Male	13.6–17.2	gm/dL	0.6206	8.44–10.67	mmol/L	XX.XX	

(B) Ercs	Mean corpuscular hemoglobin					
	Mass concentration	27–33	pg	1	27–33	pg	XX
	Substance concentration (Hb[Fe])	27–33	pg	0.06206	1.68–2.05	fmol	X.XX
(B) Ercs	Mean corpuscular hemoglobin concentration						
	Mass concentration	33–37	gm/dL	10	330–370	gm/L	XX0
	Substance concentration (Hb[Fe])	33–37	gm/dL	0.6206	20–23	mmol/L	XX
(B) Ercs	Mean corpuscular volume						
	Erythrocyte volume	76–100	μm^3	1	76–100	fL	XXX

(Continued)

Fe = iron; mmol = millimole; μm^3 = cubic micrometer; fmol = femtomole; pmol = picomole; nmol = nanomole.

* P represents plasma; B, blood; S, serum; U, urine; Sf, spinal fluid; Ercs, erythrocytes; and Lkcs, leukocytes.

† These reference values are not intended to be definitive since each laboratory determines its own values. They are provided for illustration only.

‡ "Significant digits" refers to the number of digits used to describe the reported results. XX implies that results expressed to the nearest whole number are meaningful; XX0, that results are only meaningful when rounded to the nearest 10, and that results reported to lower numbers or decimal points are beyond the sensitivity of the procedure.

(Adapted from JAMA, Vol. 260, pp. 2136–2138, October 14, 1988. Copyright 1988, American Medical Association. Used with permission of JAMA.)

TABLE 102-1. SYSTÈME INTERNATIONAL CONVERSION FACTORS FOR FREQUENTLY USED LABORATORY COMPONENTS *(Cont'd)*

System*	Component	Present Reference Intervals (Examples)†	Present Unit	Conversion Factor	SI Reference Intervals†	SI Unit Symbol	Significant Digits‡	Suggested Minimum Increment
B	Red blood cell count (erythrocytes)							
	Female	3.5-5.0	$10^6/\mu L$	1	3.5-5.0	$10^{12}/L$	X.X	
	Male	4.3-5.9	$10^6/\mu L$	1	4.3-5.1	$10^{12}/L$	X.X	
(Sf) Ercs	Red blood cell count	0	$/\mu L$	1	0	$10^6/L$	XX	
B	Reticulocyte count (adults)	10,000-75,000	$/\mu L$	0.001	10-75	$10^9/L$	XX	
	Number fraction	1-24	0/00 (No. per 1000 erythrocytes)	1	1-24	10^{-3}	XX	
		0.1-2.4	%	10	1-24	10^{-3}	XX	
B	Thrombocytes (platelets)	150-450	$10^3/\mu L$	1	150-450	$10^9/L$	XXX	
B Lkcs	White blood cell count	3200-9800	$/\mu L$	0.001	3.2-9.8	$10^9/L$	XX.X	
	Number fraction (differential)	...	%	0.01	...	1	0.XX	

(Sf) Lkcs								
S	White blood cell count	0–5	/µL		0–5	10^6/L	XX	1 u./L

Clinical Chemistry

S	Alanine aminotransferase (ALT)	0–35 (37C)	u./L	1.00	0–35	u./L	XX	1 u./L
			Karmen u./mL	0.482	...			
S	Albumin	4.0–6.0	gm/dL	10.0	40–60	gm/L	XX	1 gm/L
S	α_1-Antitrypsin	150–350	mg/dL	0.01	1.5–3.5	gm/L	X.X	0.1 gm/L
P	Ammonia As ammonia (NH_3)	10–80	µg/dL	0.5872	5–50	µmol/L	XXX	5 µmol/L
	As ammonium (NH_4^+)	10–85	µg/dL	0.5543	5–50	µmol/L	XXX	5 µmol/L
	As nitrogen (N)	10–65	µg/dL	0.7139	5–50	µmol/L	XXX	5 µmol/L
S	Amylase, enzymatic	0–130 (37C)	u./L	1.00	0–130	u./L	XXX	1 u./L
	Somogyi/ Caraway	50–150	Somogyi u./dL	1.850	100–300	u./L	XX0	10 u./L

(Continued)

TABLE 102–1. SYSTÈME INTERNATIONAL CONVERSION FACTORS FOR FREQUENTLY USED LABORATORY COMPONENTS *(Cont'd)*

System*	Component	Present Reference Intervals (Examples) †	Present Unit	Conversion Factor	SI Reference Intervals †	SI Unit Symbol	Significant Digits ‡	Suggested Minimum Increment
S	Aspartate/amino-transferase (AST)	0–35 (37C)	u./L	1.00	0–35	u./L	XX	1 u./L
			Karmen u./mL	0.482	. . .	u./L	XX	1 u./L
S	Bilirubin Total	0.1–1.0	mg/dL	17.10	2–18	μmol/L	XX	2 μmol/L
	Conjugated	0.0–0.2	mg/dL	17.10	0–4	μmol/L	XX	2 μmol/L
S	Calcium Male	8.8–10.3	mg/dL	0.2495	2.20–2.58	mmol/L	X.XX	0.02 mmol/L
	Female <50 yr	8.8–10.0	mg/dL	0.2495	2.20–2.50	mmol/L	X.XX	0.02 mmol/L
U	Calcium, normal diet	<250	mg/24 h	0.02495	<6.2	mmol/day	X.X	0.1 mmol/day
B, P, S	Carbon dioxide content (bicarbonate + CO_2)	22–28	mEq/L	1.00	22–28	mmol/L	XX	1 mmol/L
S	Chloride	95–105	mEq/L	1.00	95–105	mmol/L	XXX	1 mmol/L

P	Cholesterol <29 yr	<200	mg/dL	0.02586	<5.20	mmol/L	X.XX	0.05 mmol/L
	30–39 yr	<225	mg/dL	0.02586	<5.85	mmol/L	X.XX	0.05 mmol/L
	40–49 yr	<245	mg/dL	0.02586	<6.35	mmol/L	X.XX	0.05 mmol/L
	>50 yr	<265	mg/dL	0.02586	<6.85	mmol/L	X.XX	0.05 mmol/L
P	Cholesterol esters, as a fraction of total cholesterol	60–75	%	0.01	0.60–0.75	1	X.XX	0.01
S	Complement, C3	70–160	mg/dL	0.01	0.7–1.6	gm/L	X.X	0.1 gm/L
S	Copper	70–140	µg/dL	0.1574	11.0–22.0	µmol/L	XX.X	0.2 µmol/L
U	Copper	<40	µg/24 h	0.01574	<0.6	µmol/day	X.X	0.2 µmol/day
P	Corticotropin (ACTH)	20–100	pg/mL	0.2202	4–22	pmol/L	XX	1 pmol/L
S	Creatine Male	0.17–0.50	mg/dL	76.25	10–40	µmol/L	X0	10 µmol/L
	Female	0.35–0.93	mg/dL	76.25	30–70	µmol/L	X0	10 µmol/L

(Continued)

1176

TABLE 102–1. SYSTÈME INTERNATIONAL CONVERSION FACTORS FOR FREQUENTLY USED LABORATORY COMPONENTS *(Cont'd)*

System*	Component	Present Reference Intervals (Examples) †	Present Unit	Conversion Factor	SI Reference Intervals †	SI Unit Symbol	Significant Digits ‡	Suggested Minimum Increment
U	Creatine Male	0–40	mg/24 h	7.625	0–300	μmol/day	XX0	10 μmol/day
	Female	0–80	mg/24 h	7.625	0–600	μmol/day	XX0	10 μmol/day
S	Creatine kinase (CK)	0–130 (37C)	u./L	1.00	0–130	u./L	XXX	1 u./L
S	Creatine kinase isoenzymes, MB fraction	> 5 in myocardial infarction	%	0.01	> 0.05	1	X.XX	0.01
S	Creatinine	0.6–1.2	mg/dL	88.40	50–110	μmol/L	XX0	10 μmol/L
U	Creatinine	Variable	gm/24 h	8.840	Variable	mmol/day	XX.X	0.1 mmol/day
S, U	Creatinine clearance ¶	75–125	mL/min	0.01667	1.24–2.08	mL/sec	X.XX	0.02 mL/sec
U	Cystine	10–100	mg/24 h	4.161	40–420	μmol/day	XX0	10 μmol/day
P	Digoxin, therapeutic	0.5–2.2	ng/mL	1.281	0.6–2.8	nmol/L	X.X	0.1 nmol/L
		0.5–2.2	μg/L	1.281	0.6–2.8	nmol/L	X.X	0.1 nmol/L

P	Diphenylhydantoin, therapeutic	10–20	mg/L	3.964	40–80	µmol/L	XX	5 µmol/L
P	Ethyl alcohol	>100	mg/dL	0.2171	>22	nmol/L	XX	1 mmol/L
P	Fibrinogen	200–400	mg/dL	0.01	2.0–4.0	gm/L	X.X	0.1 gm/L
P	Follicle-stimulating hormone (FSH)							
	Female	2.0–15.0	mIU/mL	1.00	2–15	IU/L	XX	1 IU/L
	Peak production	20–50	mIU/mL	1.00	20–50	IU/L	XX	1 IU/L
	Male	1.0–10.0	mIU/mL	1.00	1–10	IU/L	XX	1 IU/L
U	Follicle-stimulating hormone (FSH)							
	Follicular phase	2–15	IU/24 h	1.00	2–15	IU/day	XXX	1 IU/day
	Midcycle	8–40	IU/24 h	1.00	8–40	IU/day	XXX	1 IU/day
	Luteal phase	2–10	IU/24 h	1.00	2–10	IU/day	XXX	1 IU/day
	Menopausal women	35–100	IU/24 h	1.00	35–100	IU/day	XXX	1 IU/day
	Male	2–15	IU/24 h	1.00	2–15	IU/day	XXX	1 IU/day

(Continued)

¶ Creatinine clearance (corrected for body surface area) $= \dfrac{\mu mol/L\ (urine\ creatinine)}{\mu mol/L\ (serum\ creatinine)} \times mL/sec \times \dfrac{1.73}{A}$, where A is the body surface area in square meters.

TABLE 102–1. SYSTÈME INTERNATIONAL CONVERSION FACTORS FOR FREQUENTLY USED LABORATORY COMPONENTS *(Cont'd)*

System*	Component	Present Reference Intervals (Examples) [†]	Present Unit	Conversion Factor	SI Reference Intervals [†]	SI Unit Symbol	Significant Digits [‡]	Suggested Minimum Increment
S	γ-Glutamyl transferase (GGT)	0–30 (30C)	u./L	1.00	0–30	u./L	XX	1 u./L
P	Glucose	70–110	mg/dL	0.05551	3.9–6.1	mmol/L	XX.X	0.1 mmol/L
B	Hemoglobin							
	Male	14.0–18.0	gm/dL	10.0	140–180	gm/L	XXX	1 gm/L
	Female	11.5–15.5	gm/dL	10.0	115–155	gm/L	XXX	1 gm/L
S	Immunoglobulins							
	IgG	500–1200	mg/dL	0.01	5.00–12.00	gm/L	XX.XX	0.01 gm/L
	IgA	50–350	mg/dL	0.01	0.50–3.50	gm/L	XX.XX	0.01 gm/L
	IgM	30–230	mg/dL	0.01	0.30–2.30	gm/L	XX.XX	0.01 gm/L
	IgD	<6	mg/dL	10	<60	mg/L	XX0	10 mg/L
	IgE							
	0–3 yr	0.5–1.0	u./mL	2.4	1–24	µg/L	XX	1 µg/L
	3–80 yr	5–100	u./mL	2.4	12–240	µg/L	XX	1 µg/L
S	Iron							
	Male	80–180	µg/dL	0.1791	14–32	µmol/L	XX	1 µmol/L
	Female	60–160	µg/dL	0.1791	11–29	µmol/L	XX	1 µmol/L
S	Iron-binding capacity	250–460	µg/dL	0.1791	45–82	µmol/L	XX	1 µmol/L

S	Lactate dehydrogenase (L → P)	50-150 (37C)	u./L	1.00	50-150	u./L	XXX	1 u./L
S		Wroblewski u./mL	0.482	. . .	u./L	XXX	1 u./L
S	Lactate dehydrogenase isoenzymes							
	LD$_1$	15-40	%	0.01	0.15-0.40	1	X.XX	0.01
	LD$_2$	20-45	%	0.01	0.20-0.45	1	X.XX	0.01
	LD$_3$	15-30	%	0.01	0.15-0.30	1	X.XX	0.01
	LD$_4$	5-20	%	0.01	0.05-0.20	1	X.XX	0.01
	LD$_5$	5-20	%	0.01	0.05-0.20	1	X.XX	0.01
	LD$_1$	10-60	u./L	1	10-60	u./L	XX	1 u./L
	LD$_2$	20-70	u./L	1	20-70	u./L	XX	1 u./L
	LD$_3$	10-45	u./L	1	10-45	u./L	XX	1 u./L
	LD$_4$	5-30	u./L	1	5-30	u./L	XX	1 u./L
	LD$_5$	5-30	u./L	1	5-30	u./L	XX	1 u./L

(Continued)

TABLE 102–1. SYSTÈME INTERNATIONAL CONVERSION FACTORS FOR FREQUENTLY USED LABORATORY COMPONENTS *(Cont'd)*

System*	Component	Present Reference Intervals (Examples) †	Present Unit	Conversion Factor	SI Reference Intervals †	SI Unit Symbol	Significant Digits ‡	Suggested Minimum Increment
B	Lead, toxic	>60	μg/dL	0.04826	>2.90	μmol/L	X.XX	0.05 μmol/L
			mg/dL	48.26	. . .	μmol/L	X.XX	0.05 μmol/L
U	Lead, toxic	>80	μg/24 h	0.004826	>0.40	μmol/day	X.XX	0.05 μmol/day
P	Lipids, total	400–850	mg/dL	0.01	4.0–8.5	gm/L	X.X	0.1 gm/L
P	Lipoproteins Low-density (LDL), as cholesterol	50–190	mg/dL	0.02586	1.30–4.90	mmol/L	X.XX	0.05 mmol/L
	High-density (HDL), as cholesterol Male	30–70	mg/dL	0.02586	0.80–1.80	mmol/L	X.XX	0.05 mmol/L
	Female	30–90	mg/dL	0.02586	0.80–2.35	mmol/L	X.XX	0.05 mmol/L
S	Magnesium	1.8–3.0	mg/dL	0.4114	0.80–1.20	mmol/L	X.XX	0.02 mmol/L

		Reference Range	Units	Factor	SI Reference Range	SI Units		SI Increment
P	Phosphatase, acid (prostatic)	0–3	King-Armstrong u./dL	1.77	0–5.5	u./L	X.X	0.05 u./L
			Bodansky u./dL	5.37	0–16.1	u./L	X.X	0.5 u./L
S	Phosphatase, alkaline	30–120	u./L	1.00	30–120	u./L	XXX	1 u./L
			Bodansky u./dL	5.37	161–644	u./L	XXX	1 u./L
			King-Armstrong u./dL	7.1	213–852	u./L	XXX	1 u./L
S	Phosphate (as phosphorus)	2.5–5.0	mg/dL	0.3229	0.80–1.60	mmol/L	X.XX	0.05 mmol/L
S	Potassium	3.5–5.0	mEq/L	1.00	3.5–5.0	mmol/L	X.X	0.1 mmol/L
P	Progesterone Follicular phase	<2	ng/mL	3.180	<6	nmol/L	XX	2 nmol/L
	Luteal phase	2–20	ng/mL	3.180	6–64	nmol/L	XX	2 nmol/L
S	Protein, total	6–8	gm/dL	10.0	60–80	gm/L	XX	1 gm/L
Sf	Protein, total	<40	mg/dL	0.01	<0.40	gm/L	X.XX	0.01 gm/L

(Continued)

TABLE 102–1. SYSTÈME INTERNATIONAL CONVERSION FACTORS FOR FREQUENTLY USED LABORATORY COMPONENTS *(Cont'd)*

System*	Component	Present Reference Intervals (Examples) †	Present Unit	Conversion Factor	SI Reference Intervals †	SI Unit Symbol	Significant Digits ‡	Suggested Minimum Increment
U	Protein, total	<150	mg/24 h	0.001	<0.15	gm/day	X.XX	0.01 gm/day
S	Sodium	135–147	mEq/L	1.00	135–147	mmol/L	XXX	1 mmol/L
U	Sodium	Diet dependent	mEq/24 h	1.00	Diet dependent	mmol/day	XXX	1 mmol/day
U	Steroids							
	Hydroxycortico-steroids (as cortisol)							
	Female	2–8	mg/24 h	2.759	5–25	μmol/day	XX	1 μmol/day
	Male	3–10	mg/24 h	2.759	10–30	μmol/day	XX	1 μmol/day
U	17-Ketogenic steroids (as dehydroepian-drosterone)							
	Female	7–12	mg/24 h	3.467	25–40	μmol/day	XX	1 μmol/day
	Male	9–17	mg/24 h	3.467	30–60	μmol/day	XX	1 μmol/day

U	17-Ketosteroids (as dehydroepiandrosterone)						
	Female	6–17	mg/24 h	3.467	20–60	μmol/day	XX	1 μmol/day
	Male	6–20	mg/24 h	3.467	20–70	μmol/day	XX	1 μmol/day
U	Ketosteroid fractions Androsterone						
	Female	0.5–3.0	mg/24 h	3.443	1–10	μmol/day	XX	1 μmol/day
	Male	2.0–5.0	mg/24 h	3.443	7–17	μmol/day	XX	1 μmol/day
	Dehydroepiandrosterone						
	Female	0.2–1.8	mg/24 h	3.467	1–6	μmol/day	XX	1 μmol/day
	Male	0.2–2.0	mg/24 h	3.467	1–7	μmol/day	XX	1 μmol/day
	Etiocholanolone						
	Female	0.8–4.0	mg/24 h	3.443	2–14	μmol/day	XX	1 μmol/day
	Male	1.4–5.0	mg/24 h	3.443	4–17	μmol/day	XX	1 μmol/day
B	Sulfonamides, as sulfanilamide, therapeutic	10.0–15.0	mg/dL	58.07	580–870	μmol/L	XX0	10 μmol/L
P	Testosterone						
	Female	<0.6	ng/mL	3.467	<2.0	nmol/L	XX.X	0.5 nmol/L
	Male	4.0–8.0	ng/mL	3.467	14.0–28.0	nmol/L	XX.X	0.5 nmol/L

(Continued)

TABLE 102–1. SYSTÈME INTERNATIONAL CONVERSION FACTORS FOR FREQUENTLY USED LABORATORY COMPONENTS *(Cont'd)*

System*	Component	Present Reference Intervals (Examples) †	Present Unit	Conversion Factor	SI Reference Intervals †	SI Unit Symbol	Significant Digits ‡	Suggested Minimum Increment
S	Triiodothyronine (T_3)	75–220	ng/dL	0.01536	1.2–3.4	nmol/L	X.X	0.1 nmol/L
S	Urea nitrogen	8–18	mg/dL	0.3570	3.0–6.5	mmol/L of urea	X.X	0.5 mmol/L
U	Urea nitrogen	12–20 (diet dependent)	gm/24 h	35.70	430–700	mmol/day of urea	XX0	10 mmol/day
U	Urobilinogen	0–4.0	mg/24 h	1.693	0.0–6.8	µmol/day	X.X	0.1 µmol/day
S	Zinc	75–120	µg/dL	0.1530	11.5–18.5	µmol/L	XX.X	0.1 µmol/L
U	Zinc	150–1200	µg/24 h	0.0153	2.3–18.3	µmol/day	XX.X	0.1 µmol/day

With a 1% disease prevalence, the probability of a patient having that disease after an abnormal test result is only 16%; thus, there is an 84% likelihood that such a patient is free of the disease. In general, markedly abnormal test values are more predictive of disease than minimally abnormal values. *In assessing the value of a specific test for a disease entity, it is important to consider the discrimination property of that test at each level of abnormal results, to be aware of all of the diseases that might yield an abnormal result, and to know the probability of different diseases coexisting in a particular person.*

BIOCHEMICAL CHANGES

Although the data reported are not entirely consistent, it appears that the ranges of common biochemical test results in the elderly are not very different from those in younger patients, with very minor exceptions. In interpreting findings of laboratory tests, one must know whether the results should be modified according to age. A weakness of cross-sectional studies is that test results are obtained at 1 point in patients' growth and do not demonstrate serial changes. For this reason, most current studies are longitudinal, and data have been accumulated over successive 1-, 2-, or 5-yr periods. Proper studies provide a distribution of values that allow the derivation of mean and standard deviations. Reference ranges are determined on the basis of appropriate population samples obtained under precisely defined conditions.

Good health is frequently determined by history and physical examination alone, which may be misleading. Major problems have been exclusion of patients with subclinical disease, exclusion of patients whose laboratory test results may have been altered by pretest diet, and inclusion of healthy elderly persons taking drugs that might affect laboratory values. Automated procedures show a 5 to 10% incidence of abnormal values in all patients; several studies have shown an incidence of 15% in the elderly. Some of these abnormalities were directly attributable to aging (eg, decline in renal function and increase in alkaline phosphatase occasionally associated with osteoporosis).

Serum electrolyte values are rarely abnormal because of age alone. **Alkaline phosphatase** values approaching 140 u./L may be found in up to 5% of healthy patients of all ages who test outside a normal reference range of 35 to 120 u./L. An elevation exceeding 20% of the normal reference level is usually required to suspect disease. This enzyme increases with age, with secondary osteoporosis, with drugs (eg, narcotics), and following a fatty meal. An elevation of another liver enzyme, **γ-glutamyl transpeptidase (GGTP)**, suggests that the alkaline phosphatase is of hepatic rather than osseous origin. Bone abnormalities that may elevate alkaline phosphatase include tumors, hyperparathyroidism, Paget's disease, a healing bone fracture, osteomalacia, and renal osteodystrophy. However, the positive predictive value of the alkaline phosphatase level is only 5% in patients with no prior diagnosis of liver disease, malignancy, or bone disease.

Serum Ca, phosphate, alkaline phosphatase, and electrophoretic protein pattern are usually normal in patients with primary osteoporosis. Alkaline phosphatase is frequently increased in patients with metastatic cancer and almost always in those with osteomalacia. Transient increases, which do not usually exceed normal limits, have been noted in osteoporotic women after hip fractures. Some studies have not shown a high incidence of hypocalcemia; a low albumin may have artificially created low Ca levels in prior studies.

There are no significant changes in hematologic values associated with aging, except for a minimal decrease in **serum iron**. A decrease in **serum albumin** has been described in many older persons, but this may be related to diet. One study was unable to substantiate a significant decrease in serum albumin in healthy elderly persons.

A gradually progressive decrease in **glucose tolerance** occurs with age, but there is no significant change in **fasting blood glucose**. The decrease in glucose tolerance is particularly evident in the nonfasting state after a glucose challenge or during a cortisone-glucose tolerance test.

DRUG EFFECTS

Older patients use drugs disproportionately. One survey found that patients $\geq$ 65 yr of age average 10.8 prescriptions annually; those in hospitals often receive $\geq$ 6 drugs, while 95% of nursing home residents receive $\geq$ 1 medications. Drugs may alter laboratory tests by pharmacologic or toxic actions or by interference with the testing procedure. Examples of test interference are false-positive urine glucose reactions associated with isoniazid, levodopa, morphine, nalidixic acid, and penicillin G. Levodopa may also produce false increases in serum bilirubin and uric acid. The possibility of an adverse drug effect or test interference should always be considered when unexplained laboratory abnormalities are encountered.

SEDIMENTATION RATE

A study of 111 ambulatory retirement-home residents indicated that *age per se had no influence on the ESR*. An elevation of the Westergren ESR > 20 mm/h correlated with the presence or absence of clinical disorders. The sensitivity of an elevated ESR in identifying the presence of a clinical disorder was 0.55; however, the specificity was 0.96, and the positive predictive value of an elevated ESR being associated with a clinical disorder was 0.93. The presence of a monoclonal gammopathy or elevated fibrinogen is probably the major cause of elevated ESRs in patients having no other obvious cause. The influence of plasma fibrinogen, total protein, serum globulins, and immunoglobulins on the ESR in older persons is similar to that in younger adults. It appears that any age-related changes in ESR are best explained by disease rather than by aging itself. The presence of severe anemia or hypoalbuminemia limits the utility of the ESR.

HORMONES

The decrease in plasma testosterone in the elderly may be due entirely to aging, or it may be influenced by environmental factors (eg, stress, minor illness, and physical activity). There is an age-dependent decrease in morning and mean 24-h plasma testosterone; free testosterone levels are less affected. Gonadotropin levels increase moderately. Smokers have higher testosterone levels than nonsmokers in all age groups, but this is not significant in the elderly.

Serum testosterone levels tend to increase more in younger than in older patients in response to stress. A marked decrease in testosterone occurs only after the 7th decade. Testosterone levels are not altered by institutionalization when compared with home living. Diet does not seem to influence testosterone levels significantly at any age. (See TABLE 102–2 for specific data regarding plasma testosterone and free testosterone according to age groups.)

In general, pituitary and adrenal function decrease slightly, and decreases in serum renin, endorphins, and calcitonin occur with aging. Serum concentrations of immunoreactive and bioactive parathyroid hormone increase with age.

TABLE 102–2. PLASMA TESTOSTERONE AND FREE TESTOSTERONE CONCENTRATION LEVELS AND BODY MASS INDEX ACCORDING TO AGE GROUPS

Age	T (ng/dL)	AFTC (ng/dL)	BMI
20–39 yr Mean 26 ± 5 (n=70)	683 ± 209	10.75 ± 2.68	23.0 ± 2.8
40–59 yr Mean 45 ± 5 (n=54)	599 ± 167	11.93 ± 3.70	25.5 ± 2.9
60–69 yr Mean 65 ± 3 (n=41)	575 ± 134	6.23 ± 2.58	26.6 ± 4.5
70–79 yr Mean 74 ± 1 (n=51)	428 ± 128	5.28 ± 2.22	26.2 ± 4.3
80–89 yr Mean 84 ± 3 (n=76)	434 ± 174		24.6 ± 4.4
90–101 yr Mean 93 ± 3 (n=9)	391 ± 189	4.72 ± 1.24	25.2 ± 5.4

All values are mean ± SD.

T = testosterone; AFTC = free testosterone concentration; BMI = body mass index.

(Adapted from J. P. Deslypere and A. Vermeulen: "Leydig cell function in normal men: Effect of age, lifestyle, residence, diet, and activity," in *Journal of Clinical Endocrinology and Metabolism,* Vol. 59, No. 5, pp. 955-962, 1984. © by The Endocrine Society. Used with permission of the Society and the authors.)

Urinary estrogen increases in elderly men, resulting in an increased estrogen/testosterone ratio. The source of this estrogen appears to be androstenedione, which is metabolized to estrogen by peripheral tissues. An increase in luteinizing hormone **(LH)** and follicle-stimulating hormone **(FSH)** concentration in blood begins at approximately 50 yr of age in men but is much less pronounced than in postmenopausal women. The increase in FSH is usually more prominent than the increase in LH in both sexes. Increased gonadotropin secretion in older men may be the result of decreased testosterone secretion. The response of the pituitary to luteinizing-hormone–releasing hormone is less marked in elderly men, as is the release of LH. A progressive increase in serum prolactin has also been described in aging men, which may be related to the gradual increase in serum estrogen. Dehydroepiandrosterone **(DHEA)** and its ester, the major secretory products of the adrenal gland, also decrease with age.

PROTEINURIA

Trace proteinuria has been reported to occur with an incidence of 40% at age 16, decreasing to 2% in the 3rd decade, and rising to 30% in old age. This is based on an upper limit for normal of 80 mg protein $\pm$ 25 SD/24 h. Glomerular and interstitial nephritis are rare in patients with protein excretion $<$ 400 mg/24 h.

The magnitude of proteinuria can be estimated by measuring protein/ creatinine ratios in single-voided urine samples. These correlate with determinations of 24-h urinary proteins and are particularly useful in elderly patients when 24-h specimens are difficult to obtain. Protein/creatinine ratios $>$ 3.0 indicate massive proteinuria ($>$ 3.5 gm), while ratios $<$ 0.2 indicate insignificant protein excretion.

MONOCLONAL GAMMOPATHIES

A study using agarose gel electrophoresis and immunofixation demonstrated a 10% incidence of monoclonal gammopathy in apparently healthy patients ranging in age from 62 to 95 yr. The incidence is 6% in patients $<$ 80 yr of age and 14 to 19% in patients $>$ 90 yr of age. An unexplained elevation in the ESR in the elderly warrants investigation for the presence of a monoclonal gammopathy, which occurs in approximately 50% of such individuals. These gammopathies may be indicators of a dysregulation of the immune system occurring with age (ie, impaired T cell or B cell function).

Serum levels of the major subsets of immunoglobulins (eg, IgG, IgM, and IgA) do not show clinically significant changes with age. A decline in T cell function is the most consistent age-related change in the immune system.

103. ASSESSMENT INSTRUMENTS

Laurence Z. Rubenstein

The goal of **geriatric assessment,** which may be defined as *a multidisciplinary, diagnostic process designed to quantify an elderly individual's medical, psychosocial, and functional problems and capabilities,* is to develop a comprehensive plan for therapy and long-term follow-up. Such multidimensional functional assessment (see Ch. 15) plays a pivotal role in geriatric care because of the complexity of frail elderly patients and their numerous unmet needs. Also, such assessment increasingly has been shown to improve health care outcomes in elderly patients.

Although specific forms or scales (instruments) are not essential for performing geriatric assessment per se, the use of easily administered, well-validated instruments that encompass the major assessment domains makes the process more reliable and considerably easier. These forms also facilitate transmission of clinically relevant information among health care providers and permit tabulation of clinical data and measurement of therapeutic progress over time.

The major components (domains and subdomains) of geriatric assessment are listed in TABLE 103–1. Each of the 4 major domains—physical health, functional ability, psychologic health, and socioenvironmental factors—comprises several subdomains.

Most health care professionals **quantify a patient's physical health** by compiling a traditional problem list of defined diagnoses and symptom

TABLE 103–1. MEASURABLE DIMENSIONS IN GERIATRIC ASSESSMENT

Physical health
  Traditional problem list
  Disease severity indicators
  Quantification of services used
  Disease-specific scales (eg, gait, parkinsonism, dementia)
Overall functional ability
  Activities of daily living (ADL) scales
  Instrumental ADL (IADL) scales
Psychologic health
  Cognitive (mental status) tests
  Affect (depression) scales
Socioenvironmental factors
  Social interactions network
  Social support resources and special needs
  Environmental adequacy and safety

complexes. Beyond this documentation, there are only a few severity indicators that most clinicians are aware of (eg, the New York Heart Association 4-point functional scale, which can help clarify and communicate the degree of disability resulting from a cardiac condition). Documenting the number of days of hospitalization and disability and the use of related health care services can also be helpful in defining severity of health problems.

A number of detailed, disease-specific scales are also available for quantifying levels of function, dysfunction, disability, and handicap attributable to particular diseases. These are similar in principle to the New York Heart Association's scale. Some, such as measurements made in a pulmonary function or physiology laboratory, are purely quantitative; others, such as a quality-of-life scale, are purely qualitative; and still others include both kinds of information, such as a dementia-disability scale. Well-established disease-related scales exist for dementia, depression, parkinsonism, gait and balance dysfunction, and multiple sclerosis.

Functional ability, sometimes called role functioning, is usually measured separately from physical health, although there may be overlap. Included in this domain are the measurable aspects of basic activities of daily living **(ADLs)** and the more advanced instrumental ADLs **(IADLs).** Measurement of basic ADLs focuses on the skills needed to attend to everyday personal necessities, such as eating, moving from bed or chair to sitting or standing, bathing, and dressing—things a person must be able to do independently so that the constant presence of a nurse or attendant is not required. Measurement of IADLs focuses on skills (beyond the basic ADLs) needed to live independently in the community; eg, the ability to cook, shop, use the telephone, and handle finances. Several validated instruments are available for measuring these abilities.

Psychologic health measurement includes the 2 major quantifiable subdomains of cognition (mental status) and affect. Sometimes other psychologic aspects, such as the presence of specific psychiatric symptoms (eg, paranoia, delusions, behavior abnormalities) are included, but these are less easily quantified and are rarely given a rating scale. Many scales are available for measuring both cognition and affect: these range from brief, 10-item screening scales to complex tests that require ≥ 1 h to administer. For multidimensional geriatric assessment, intermediate scales that have between 10 and 30 items are appropriate. (See also Ch. 80).

The socioenvironmental domain is complex and currently the least well quantified, probably because of the heterogeneity of its components. These include the concepts of a network of everyday social interactions, available social support resources and special needs, and environmental adequacy. A number of instruments are available for documenting this domain, but a quantitative scale has yet to be perfected.

Selection of an Assessment Instrument

Before an assessment instrument is selected for a given patient population, several issues need to be considered. These include the reliability and validity of the instrument, patient acceptability, time and personnel required for administering the tests, and the relevance and usefulness of the data to be collected. These issues are usually addressed in the development and testing of an assessment instrument, but not always; therefore, caution must be exercised.

Following are examples of some of the most useful, most widely used, and best validated instruments for the major assessment domains. The exclusion of others should not be considered a negative judgment of their value. Rather, the former were chosen because of the author's familiarity with them and their wide applicability to large numbers of geriatric patients and to a wide variety of measurement situations, as well as for their value in both initial assessments and repeated measurements to demonstrate change over time.

These instruments include the Katz Activities of Daily Living **(ADL)** Index (FIG. 103–1), the Lawton Instrumental ADL Scale (FIG. 103–2), the Folstein Mini-Mental State Examination (see Ch. 80), and the Yesavage Geriatric Depression Scale (FIG. 103–3).

	Independent Yes	No
1. **Bathing** (sponge bath, tub bath, or shower) Receives either no assistance or assistance in bathing only 1 part of body	☐	☐
2. **Dressing** Gets clothes and dresses without any assistance except for tying shoes	☐	☐
3. **Toileting** Goes to toilet room, uses toilet, arranges clothes, and returns without any assistance (may use cane or walker for support and may use bedpan/urinal at night)	☐	☐
4. **Transferring** Moves in and out of bed and chair without assistance (may use cane or walker)	☐	☐
5. **Continence** Controls bowel and bladder completely by self (without occasional "accidents")	☐	☐
6. **Feeding** Feeds self without assistance (except for help with cutting meat or buttering bread)	☐	☐

Total ADL score: ☐ (Number of "yes" answers, out of possible 6)

FIG. 103–1. **Basic Activities of Daily Living (ADLs).** (Modified from S. Katz, T.D. Downs, H.R. Cash, et al: "Progress in the development of the index of ADL," in *Gerontologist*, Vol. 1, pp. 20–30, 1970. Copyright by The Gerontological Society of America. Used with permission.)

A. Ability to use telephone
1. Operates telephone on own initiative; looks up and dials numbers, etc   1
2. Dials a few well-known numbers   1
3. Answers telephone but does not dial   1
4. Does not use telephone at all   0

B. Shopping
1. Takes care of all shopping needs independently   1
2. Shops independently for small purchases   0
3. Needs to be accompanied on any shopping trip   0
4. Completely unable to shop   0

C. Food preparation
1. Plans, prepares, and serves adequate meals independently   1
2. Prepares adequate meals if supplied with ingredients   0
3. Heats, serves, and prepares meals or prepares meals but does not maintain adequate diet   0
4. Needs to have meals prepared and served   0

D. Housekeeping
1. Maintains house alone or with occasional assistance (eg, heavy work, domestic help)   1
2. Performs light daily tasks such as dish washing, bed making   1
3. Performs light daily tasks but cannot maintain acceptable level of cleanliness   1
4. Needs help with all home-maintenance tasks   1
5. Does not participate in any housekeeping tasks   0

E. Laundry
1. Does personal laundry completely   1
2. Launders small items, rinses stockings, etc   1
3. All laundry must be done by others   0

F. Mode of transportation
1. Travels independently on public transportation or drives own car   1
2. Arranges own travel via taxi but does not otherwise use public transportation   1
3. Travels on public transportation when accompanied by another   1
4. Travel limited to taxi or automobile with assistance of another   0
5. Does not travel at all   0

G. Responsibility for own medications
1. Is responsible for taking medication in correct doses at correct time   1
2. Takes responsibility if medication is prepared in advance in separate doses   0
3. Is not capable of dispensing own medication   0

H. Ability to handle finances
1. Manages financial matters independently (budgets, writes checks, pays rent and bills, goes to bank), collects and keeps track of income   1
2. Manages day-to-day purchases but needs help with banking, major purchases, etc   1
3. Incapable of handling money   0

Score: ☐ (Out of possible 8)

FIG. 103–2. Instrumental Activities of Daily Living Scale (IADLs) (Modified from M.P. Lawton and E.M. Brody: "Assessment of older people: Self-monitoring and instrumental activities of daily living," in *Gerontologist,* Vol. 9, pp. 179-186, 1969. Copyright by The Gerontological Society of America. Used with permission.)

Choose the best answer for how you felt this past week.

* 1.	Are you basically satisfied with your life?	YES	NO
2.	Have you dropped many of your activities and interests?	YES	NO
3.	Do you feel that your life is empty?	YES	NO
4.	Do you often get bored?	YES	NO
* 5.	Are you hopeful about the future?	YES	NO
6.	Are you bothered by thoughts you can't get out of your head?	YES	NO
* 7.	Are you in good spirits most of the time?	YES	NO
8.	Are you afraid that something bad is going to happen to you?	YES	NO
* 9.	Do you feel happy most of the time?	YES	NO
10.	Do you often feel helpless?	YES	NO
11.	Do you often get restless and fidgety?	YES	NO
12.	Do you prefer to stay at home, rather than going out and doing new things?	YES	NO
13.	Do you frequently worry about the future?	YES	NO
14.	Do you feel you have more problems with memory than most?	YES	NO
*15.	Do you think it is wonderful to be alive now?	YES	NO
16.	Do you often feel downhearted and blue?	YES	NO
17.	Do you feel pretty worthless the way you are now?	YES	NO
18.	Do you worry a lot about the past?	YES	NO
*19.	Do you find life very exciting?	YES	NO
20.	Is it hard for you to get started on new projects?	YES	NO
*21.	Do you feel full of energy?	YES	NO
22.	Do you feel that your situation is hopeless?	YES	NO
23.	Do you think that most people are better off than you are?	YES	NO
24.	Do you frequently get upset over little things?	YES	NO
25.	Do you frequently feel like crying?	YES	NO
26.	Do you have trouble concentrating?	YES	NO
*27.	Do you enjoy getting up in the morning?	YES	NO
28.	Do you prefer to avoid social gatherings?	YES	NO
*29.	Is it easy for you to make decisions?	YES	NO
*30.	Is your mind as clear as it used to be?	YES	NO

*Appropriate (nondepressed)
answers = yes, all others = no

Score: ☐ (Number of "depressed" answers)

Norms

Normal	5 ± 4
Mildly depressed	15 ± 6
Very depressed	23 ± 5

FIG. 103–3. Geriatric Depression Scale (GDS). (Reprinted with permission from *Journal of Psychiatric Research*, Vol. 17, J. Yesavage, T. Brink, et al, "Development and validation of a geriatric screening scale: A preliminary report," Copyright 1983, Pergamon Press PLC.)

Proper interpretation of the scores from these tests is gained from experience, but some guidelines are possible. For example, a top score of 6 on the Katz ADLs indicates that the person has full basic function—usually implying that nursing home care would be inappropriate. A score of 2 usually indicates intact feeding and continence (since the scale is hierarchical in its scoring) but impairment of the more advanced items—implying that a care giver or nursing home would be required for survival. Similarly, on the IADL scale, a high score indicates independence and a low score a need for assistance.

Two newer instruments that have not yet been evaluated as thoroughly as those listed above but appear to be useful in assessing 2 other areas of importance among the older population are the Tinetti Balance and Gait Evaluation (FIG. 103–4) and the National Safety Council Home Safety Checklist (FIG. 103–5). TABLE 103–2 provides a brief summary of the general features of these assessment instruments.

BALANCE		
Instructions: Subject is seated in hard armless chair. The following maneuvers are tested.		
1. **Sitting balance**		
	Leans or slides in chair	= 0
	Steady, safe	= 1 _____
2. **Arises**		
	Unable without help	= 0
	Able but uses arms to help	= 1
	Able without use of arms	= 2 _____
3. **Attempts to arise**		
	Unable without help	= 0
	Able but requires more than 1 attempt	= 1
	Able to arise with 1 attempt	= 2 _____
4. **Immediate standing balance** (first 5 sec)		
	Unsteady (staggers, moves feet, marked trunk sway)	= 0
	Steady but uses walker or cane or grabs other objects for support	= 1 _____
	Steady without walker or cane or other support	= 2 _____

(Continued)

FIG. 103–4. Tinetti Balance and Gait Evaluation.

BALANCE *(Cont'd)*

5. **Standing balance**
    Unsteady   = 0
    Steady but wide stance (medial heels more
        than 4 in. apart) or uses cane, walker, or
        other support   = 1
    Narrow stance without support   = 2   _____

6. **Nudged** (subject at maximum position with feet as
        close together as possible, examiner pushes lightly
        on subject's sternum with palm of hand 3 times)
                                        Begins to fall   = 0
                                        Staggers, grabs, but
                                            catches self   = 1
                                        Steady   = 2   _____

7. **Eyes closed** (at maximum position No. 6)
                                        Unsteady   = 0
                                        Steady   = 1   _____

8. **Turning 360°**
                                        Discontinuous steps   = 0
                                        Continuous   = 1   _____

                                        Unsteady (grabs,
                                            staggers)   = 0
                                        Steady   = 1   _____

9. **Sitting down**
                                        Unsafe (misjudged distance, falls into
                                            chair)   = 0
                                        Uses arms or not a smooth motion   = 1
                                        Safe, smooth motion   = 2   _____

Balance score: _____/16

GAIT

Instructions: Subject stands with examiner; walks down hallway or across room,
                first at his "usual" pace, then back at "rapid, but safe" pace (using
                usual walking aid such as cane, walker).

10. **Initiation of gait** (immediately after told to "go")
                        Any hesitancy or multiple attempts to start   = 0
                        No hesitancy   = 1   _____

(Continued)

FIG. 103–4. Tinetti Balance and Gait Evaluation.

GAIT *(Cont'd)*

11. **Step length and height**
    a. Right swing foot

Does not pass left stance foot with step	= 0
Passes left stance foot	= 1
Right foot does *not* clear floor completely with step	= 0
Right foot completely clears floor	= 1

    b. Left swing foot

Does not pass right stance foot with step	= 0
Passes right stance foot	= 1
Left foot does *not* clear floor completely with step	= 0
Left foot completely clears floor	= 1

12. **Step symmetry**

Right and left step length not equal (estimate)	= 0
Right and left step appear equal	= 1

13. **Step continuity**

Stopping or discontinuity between steps	= 0
Steps appear continuous	= 1

14. **Path** (estimated in relation to floor tiles, 12-in. diameter; observe excursion of 1 foot over about 10 ft of the course)

Marked deviation	= 0
Mild/moderate deviation *or* uses walking aid	= 1
Straight without walking aid	= 2

15. **Trunk**

Marked sway or uses walking aid	= 0
No sway but flexion of knees or back or spreads arms out while walking	= 1
No sway, no flexion, no use of arms, and no use of walking aid	= 2

16. **Walking stance**

Heels apart	= 0
Heels almost touching while walking	= 1

Gait score: _____/12
Total score: _____/28

FIG. 103–4. **Tinetti Balance and Gait Evaluation.** (Modified with permission from the American Geriatrics Society, "Performance-oriented assessment of mobility problems in elderly patients," by M. Tinetti, *Journal of the American Geriatrics Society*, Vol. 34, pp. 119-126, 1986.)

		Yes	No
Housekeeping			
1.	Do you clean up spills as soon as they occur?		
2.	Do you keep floors and stairways clean and free of clutter?		
3.	Do you put away books, magazines, sewing supplies, and other objects as soon as you're through with them and never leave them on floors or stairways?		
4.	Do you store frequently used items on shelves that are within easy reach?		
Floors			
5.	Do you keep everyone from walking on freshly washed floors before they're dry?		
6.	If you wax floors, do you apply 2 thin coats and buff each thoroughly or else use self-polishing, nonskid wax?		
7.	Do all small rugs have nonskid backings?		
8.	Have you eliminated small rugs at the tops and bottoms of stairways?		
9.	Are all carpet edges tacked down?		
10.	Are rugs and carpets free of curled edges, worn spots, and rips?		
11.	Have you chosen rugs and carpets with short, dense pile?		
12.	Are rugs and carpets installed over good-quality, medium-thick pads?		
Bathroom			
13.	Do you use a rubber mat or nonslip decals in the tub or shower?		
14.	Do you have a grab bar securely anchored over the tub or on the shower wall?		
15.	Do you have a nonskid rug on bathroom floor?		
16.	Do you keep soap in an easy-to-reach receptacle?		
Traffic lanes			
17.	Can you walk across every room in your home, and from one room to another, without detouring around furniture?		
18.	Is the traffic lane from your bedroom to the bathroom free of obstacles?		
19.	Are telephone and appliance cords kept away from areas where people walk?		
Lighting			
20.	Do you have light switches near every doorway?		
21.	Do you have enough good lighting to eliminate shadowy areas?		
22.	Do you have a lamp or light switch within easy reach from your bed?		
23.	Do you have night lights in your bathroom and in the hallway leading from your bedroom to the bathroom?		

(Continued)

Fig. 103–5. Home Safety Checklist.

		Yes	No
Lighting *(Cont'd)*			
24.	Are all stairways well lighted?	____	____
25.	Do you have light switches at both the tops and bottoms of stairways?	____	____
Stairways			
26.	Do securely fastened handrails extend the full length of the stairs on each side of stairways?	____	____
27.	Do rails stand out from the walls so you can get a good grip?	____	____
28.	Are rails distinctly shaped so you're alerted when you reach the end of a stairway?	____	____
29.	Are all stairways in good condition, with no broken, sagging, or sloping steps?	____	____
30.	Are all stairway carpeting and metal edges securely fastened and in good condition?	____	____
31.	Have you replaced any single-level steps with gradually rising ramps or made sure such steps are well lighted?	____	____
Ladders and step stools			
32.	Do you have a sturdy step stool that you use to reach high cupboard and closet shelves?	____	____
33.	Are all ladders and step stools in good condition?	____	____
34.	Do you always use a step stool or ladder that's tall enough for the job?	____	____
35.	Do you always set up your ladder or step stool on a firm, level base that's free of clutter?	____	____
36.	Before you climb a ladder or step stool, do you always make sure it's fully open and that the stepladder spreaders are locked?	____	____
37.	When you use a ladder or step stool, do you face the steps and keep your body between the side rails?	____	____
38.	Do you avoid standing on top of a step stool or climbing beyond the second step from the top on a stepladder?	____	____
Outdoor areas			
39.	Are walks and driveways in your yard and other areas free of breaks?	____	____
40.	Are lawns and gardens free of holes?	____	____
41.	Do you put away garden tools and hoses when they're not in use?	____	____
42.	Are outdoor areas kept free of rocks, loose boards, and other tripping hazards?	____	____
43.	Do you keep outdoor walkways, steps, and porches free of wet leaves and snow?	____	____
44.	Do you sprinkle icy outdoor areas with deicers as soon as possible after a snowfall or freeze?	____	____
45.	Do you have mats at doorways for people to wipe their feet on?	____	____
46.	Do you know the safest way of walking when you can't avoid walking on a slippery surface?	____	____

(Continued)

FIG. 103–5. **Home Safety Checklist.**

Footwear	Yes	No

47. Do your shoes have soles and heels that provide good traction? ___ ___

48. Do you wear house slippers that fit well and don't fall off? ___ ___

49. Do you avoid walking in stocking feet? ___ ___

50. Do you wear low-heeled oxfords, loafers, or good-quality sneakers when you work in your house or yard? ___ ___

51. Do you replace boots or galoshes when their soles or heels are worn too smooth to keep you from slipping on wet or icy surfaces? ___ ___

Personal precautions

52. Are you always alert for unexpected hazards, such as out-of-place furniture? ___ ___

53. If young grandchildren visit, are you alert for children playing on the floor and toys left in your path? ___ ___

54. If you have pets, are you alert for sudden movements across your path and pets getting underfoot? ___ ___

55. When you carry bulky packages, do you make sure they don't obstruct your vision? ___ ___

56. Do you divide large loads into smaller loads whenever possible? ___ ___

57. When you reach or bend, do you hold onto a firm support and avoid throwing your head back or turning it too far? ___ ___

58. Do you always use a ladder or step stool to reach high places and never stand on a chair? ___ ___

59. Do you always move deliberately and avoid rushing to answer the phone or doorbell? ___ ___

60. Do you take time to get your balance when you change position from lying down to sitting and from sitting to standing? ___ ___

61. Do you hold onto grab bars when you change position in the tub or shower? ___ ___

62. Do you keep yourself in good condition with moderate exercise, good diet, adequate rest, and regular medical checkups? ___ ___

63. If you wear glasses, is your prescription up to date? ___ ___

64. Do you know how to reduce injury in a fall? ___ ___

65. If you live alone, do you have daily contact with a friend or neighbor? ___ ___

FIG. 103–5. **Home Safety Checklist.** This checklist is used to identify fall hazards in the home. After identification, hazards should be eliminated or reduced. One point is allowed for every *no* answer. A score of 1 to 7 is excellent, 8 to 14 is good, 15 or higher is hazardous. (Developed by the National Safety Council in cooperation with the National Retired Teachers Association and the American Association of Retired Persons. From "Falling—The Unexpected Trip." A Safety Program for Older Adults, Program Leader's Guide. By the U.S. National Safety Council in cooperation with the American Association of Retired Persons, 1982. Reprinted with permission from the National Safety Council, 444 North Michigan Avenue, Chicago, IL 60611.)

TABLE 103–2. GUIDELINES FOR USE OF SELECTED GERIATRIC ASSESSMENT INSTRUMENTS

Instrument	Who Administers	Who Answers	Score Range (bad to good)	Time Required to Administer (min)
Katz ADL Index	I	CP, NP	0-6	2-4
Lawton IADL Scale	I	S,CP,NP	0-8	3-5
Folstein Mini-Mental State Examination	I	S	0-30	5-15
Yesavage Geriatric Depression Scale	I, SA	S	30-0	5-15
Tinetti Balance/Gait Evaluation	I	S	0-28	5-15
National Safety Council Home Safety Checklist	SA	S,CP	0-65	10-20

ADL = Activities of daily living; IADL = Instrumental activities of daily living; I = Interviewer; S = Subject; SA = Self-administer; CP = Care giver proxy; NP = Nurse proxy.

104.   HEALTH INSURANCE

(See also FINANCING HEALTH CARE in Ch. 97)

Mal Schechter

PERSPECTIVE

In the USA, insurance programs for chronic care are weak and disorganized compared with those for acute care. The concept of insured, comprehensive geriatric services, including long-term care in the community as well as the nursing home, has only begun to be tested operationally through a variant of prepaid group practice (see below). Private indemnity coverage, also a relatively recent option, is directed chiefly at nursing home expenses. Medicare is public insurance derived from an acute-care model with features antagonistic to the office-based practice of geriatric medicine (eg, fee scales favoring procedures by specialists over "cognitive" services). Medicaid, a welfare program for the poor rather than an insurance program, provides for long-term as well as acute care but has restrictions on eligibility, scope of services, and provider payment.

Medicare and Medicaid spending for the elderly in 1987 was estimated at $86 billion; private insurance supplemental to Medicare, at $5 to $10 billion; and private long-term care insurance, at $300 million. These sources spent almost $100 billion in a $500 billion health care economy. No overall monetary equivalent has been given for the "informal providers" of the overwhelming bulk of long-term care—family members. However, patients and family members paid $1/2$ of the nation's $35 billion nursing home bill.

Medicare does not cover individuals $\geq$ 65 yr at work in organizations with $\geq$ 20 employees in which the employer offers health benefits. In this situation, employers provide primary coverage and Medicare provides secondary coverage. However, older workers may reject the employer's health plan and choose to receive Medicare coverage.

Because Medicare and other types of insurance have spurred inflation in the health care economy, expenses, such as deductibles and uncovered items of service, that individuals and families must pay have risen. In 1987, Medicare was estimated to have paid for only 45% of the average health care expenses of the elderly. In 1984, out-of-pocket expenses for the elderly averaged $1705 per person, of which $700 was attributed to nursing home expense alone. Even with benefits from Medicare, Medicaid, and Medicare supplemental policies, the elderly still must pay $1/4$ of the health care bill out of pocket. The growth of uncovered expenses, particularly for the poorly insured, long-term care sector, seriously affects those with limited income, especially the very old, who may be unable to purchase outpatient prescribed drugs as well as professional services.

Some 12% of the older population lives in poverty as defined by federal standards, which actually characterize severe deprivation. By other standards, 2 of every 5 older persons are poor. In 1984, 18.8% of elderly households and 55.4% of older individuals living alone had annual incomes < $10,000. The official poverty rate for persons > 85 yr of age exceeds 20%.

Proposals to extend Medicare coverage for acute care (essentially, very long hospital stays) ignore the leading cause of impoverishment from health care expenses, ie, long-term care in nursing homes and at home. Moreover, attempts to control Medicare hospital payments through prospective payment arrangements, using diagnosis related groups (DRGs), have resulted in shorter hospitalizations and greater need for at-home services (for which Medicare may not pay). Increasingly, gaps in insurance coverage and in available, affordable long-term care services in the community confront both physicians and elderly patients with difficult problems in achieving therapeutic goals.

MEDICARE

Medicare is the principal health insurance system for persons $\geq$ 65 yr of age in the USA. In many respects, it is supplemented by Medicaid, a federal-state program for poor elderly and other persons. Medicare is an outgrowth of the social insurance (Social Security) and public assistance

(Welfare) provisions of the 1935 Social Security Act. An objective of social insurance is to prevent poverty in old age. The poverty-inducing effect of medical and hospital expenses was recognized in 1935, but because of opposition by organized medicine, health insurance was not added to the broad spectrum of social insurance until the 1960s.

The structure of Medicare was conditioned by politics and the evolution of employment-based health insurance. Hence, what was enacted in 1965 as Medicare contained benefits suited to younger breadwinners in the work force. Long-term care benefits were not included then and are still not included.

To secure physician cooperation, legislators agreed that Medicare would encompass a basic hospital benefit program as compulsory social insurance and a voluntary major medical plan supported by premiums and federal general revenues, providing direct or indirect payment for almost all physician services. The hospital portion of Medicare is called Part A and the major medical portion, Part B. Since almost all Medicare beneficiaries opt for Part B coverage, both parts of the program are almost universal. Physicians would be well advised to have on hand office copies of *Your Medicare Handbook,* an official publication for beneficiaries available from Social Security offices or Medicare carriers.

The absence of coverage for long-term care, preventive medicine, and outpatient prescribed drugs represented legislators' fears in 1965 of embarking on a program that would be too costly and administratively unwieldy. Deductibles and coinsurance amounts were applied in various ways to hold down costs to government. This cost sharing, the noted exclusions, and allowances for physicians to bill what they desired still left patients exposed to risk of impoverishment.

Over the ensuing decades, as health care costs and service intensity increased, this risk grew. The shield against financial catastrophe weakened not only in Medicare but in private insurance programs. Difficulties experienced by older persons and by state Medicaid programs generated campaigns for remedial federal action. Thus, some members of Congress introduced legislation to expand Medicare coverage for long-term care, while others and administration officials awaited developments in private insurance that might blunt the Medicare expansion drive.

Medicare was expanded legislatively in 1988 to protect further against financial catastrophe from acute care and other medical expenses. Protection was introduced against very high annual expenses of outpatient prescription drugs. In a bow to long-term care needs, a respite care benefit was initiated for families.

The same legislation required states to pay for Medicare premiums for older persons below the federal poverty level and eased "spend down" requirements that tended to impoverish the spouse (who remains in the community) of a Medicaid nursing-home resident. The Medicare "catastrophic" insurance act required private insurance policies designated as

Medicare supplements to be revised to eliminate any overlap with the new statutory provisions and the associated fraction of premiums.

The legislation was notable not only for transforming major portions of the Medicare superstructure but also for financing the expansion entirely from levies on beneficiaries (ie, a premium addition paid by all beneficiaries, plus a surcharge on income taxes paid by the relatively wealthy beneficiaries). As this departure from the broader sharing of the health care costs of the elderly hit their pocketbooks, demands for repeal swelled in volume. The description below applies to the program as amended in 1988, which was under reconsideration by Congress at press time. Refer to the most recent *Your Medicare Handbook* for current coverage.

PART A: HOSPITAL INSURANCE

After a deductible (less than $600 in 1989), the patient is covered for hospitalization at no further expense for the calender year. There is no limit on number of inpatient hospital days covered, except for a long-standing, 190-day lifetime limit for psychiatric hospital care.

There is no coinsurance for inpatient hospital services at any time. (In the past, copayments began after the 60th hospital day, and a second deductible was applicable for patients who had been out of the hospital for at least 30 days.) Part A does not cover services billed by private physicians in the hospital; these are covered under Part B.

Among the hospital services covered by Part A is rehabilitation (eg, physical and occupational therapy and speech pathology). Part A also pays for (1) medically necessary inpatient care in a skilled nursing facility, (2) home health care, and (3) hospice care. Bills (net of cost sharing by patients) are paid directly to institutions and agencies.

In 1983, Medicare began paying hospitals prospectively according to a schedule based on the principal diagnosis for each hospital stay (diagnosis related groups, or DRGs). A DRG payment may be adjusted, to an extent, for age and comorbidity. Although intended to permit a hospital to recover costs for the Medicare population it serves, this payment pattern has been criticized as not adequately supporting sound geriatrics and as promoting premature discharge.

Contrary to past policy, a patient may be admitted directly to an approved skilled nursing facility **(SNF)** without having previously been hospitalized. Medicare pays for all covered SNF services for up to 150 days, subject to a coinsurance payment (about $20/day in 1989) for the first 8 days only. To qualify for the SNF services, the patient's physician must certify the need for and receipt of acute skilled nursing or rehabilitation services. In both the hospital and SNF, the coverage can be withdrawn by a utilization review committee or peer review organization on a finding that the stay is unnecessary.

A critical point for physicians and patients is the definition: **Skilled care** is *care that can be performed only by or under the supervision of li-*

censed nurses or professional therapists pursuant to a doctor's orders. If these services are required occasionally rather than daily or if they can be provided outside the SNF, they are not covered by Part A. Nor does Part A cover services that are no longer improving the patient's condition; ie, the patient has been stabilized and needs only custodial care.

Hospice care is covered if the following conditions are met: (1) The physician certifies that the patient is terminally ill; (2) the patient chooses to receive care from a hospice, defined as an organization primarily engaged in providing pain relief, symptom management, and supportive services to the terminally ill and their families; and (3) care is provided through a Medicare-certified hospice program (most services are provided in the patient's house). By selecting hospice coverage, the patient forgoes standard Medicare benefits for the terminal illness. Part A covers 210 hospice days (with extension possible). There are no deductibles or copayments except for part of the cost of outpatient drugs and inpatient **respite care,** *a short inpatient stay (no more than 5 consecutive days) to relieve the care giver at home.* For a condition unrelated to the terminal illness, Medicare pays benefits for services covered under the standard program.

Hospice services encompass nursing; drugs (including outpatient drugs for pain relief and symptom management); physical, occupational, and speech therapy; home health aide and homemaker services; medical social services; medical supplies and appliances; short-term inpatient care; and counseling. (Medicare Part B pays for services of the attending physician, if that person is not working for the hospice program.)

PART B: SUPPLEMENTARY MEDICAL INSURANCE

This portion of Medicare covers (1) physician services, (2) outpatient hospital care, (3) outpatient physical and speech therapy, (4) home health care, (5) certain services and supplies not covered by Part A, such as independent clinical laboratory services, and (6) outpatient prescribed drugs, starting Jan. 1, 1991.

Effective Jan. 1, 1990, the program will pay 100% of all approved expenses after the beneficiary has paid a certain amount (about $1400 in 1990) in deductibles, premiums, and copayments during the year. Physician charges above the amounts Medicare deems reasonable do not count toward the ceiling. The beneficiary is to be notified when the ceiling has been reached.

A special deductible and coinsurance apply to outpatient drugs; the program pays for half the approved cost of prescribed drugs, once the beneficiary has met a $600 deductible.

The program begins reimbursing patients (or pays physicians directly if the patient assigns them the right to collect) after $75 in approved charges have been incurred in the calender year. Part B generally pays 80% of approved or "reasonable" charges.

Actual payments by the program depend on its definition of "reasonable charges," which tend to be less than actual billing amounts. The determination of approved charges is highly complex. Attempts to control program costs for physician fees in 1985–86 led to "freezes" and other maneuvers, under which the physician could not legally collect fees in excess of amounts calculated from fees in a base period. A physician who accepts assignment for all claims agrees to the amounts Medicare approves, receives payments directly, is listed in a special directory available to the public, and may display an emblem or certificate designating this affiliation.

Part B covers major physician services normally included under medical insurance. Excluded are routine physical examinations, routine foot care, vision or hearing examinations for prescribing or fitting glasses or hearing aids, immunizations (except for pneumococcal vaccination or those for an injury or immediate risk of infection), and cosmetic surgery, except for that needed because of accidental injury or for functional improvement of a body malformation.

Other Part B benefits are (1) outpatient treatment of mental illness (up to $1100/yr, or half of allowed physician charges, whichever is less, but the limit does not apply for physician services to adjust medications) and partial hospitalization through a day program (with institutional costs covered until the limit on physician reimbursement is reached); (2) chiropractic services—specifically, manual manipulation of the spine to correct a subluxation demonstrable on x-ray but only when done by a Medicare-certified chiropractor; (3) podiatric services, including removal of plantar warts, treatment of fungal infections, and foot care required in management of severe diabetes; (4) dental care for surgery of the jaw and setting fractures but not for care of teeth; (5) optometric examination for aphakia; and (6) mammography screening every other year (up to an approved charge).

Part B also covers outpatient surgical services and comprehensive outpatient rehabilitation facility services upon referral by a physician. Independent laboratory services are covered if the laboratory accepts assignment and is certified for the services prescribed. Ambulance transportation is covered to bring the patient to or from a hospital or an SNF. Portable diagnostic x-ray services, prosthetic devices, durable medical equipment, and medical supplies are generally covered.

Home health care benefits are closely circumscribed. Payment is made only if all 4 of the following requirements are met: (1) The care needed includes part-time or intermittent skilled nursing, physical therapy, or speech therapy; (2) the patient is confined to home; (3) the physician certifies that home health care is needed and sets up a plan for the patient; and (4) the agency providing the care is certified by Medicare.

When skilled nursing is no longer needed, Part B still covers home visits for occupational therapy. Since July 1, 1987, a patient discharged from an SNF can receive occupational therapy at home for uninterrupted treatment.

Because Congress found that Medicare administrators tend to construe home-care limits too narrowly, the 1988 legislation defined the part-time or intermittent nature of home care to allow services for up to 7 days/wk and for up to 38 days in any given period (instead of 5 days/wk for up to 2 or 3 wk).

The home health benefit excludes general household services, meal preparation, shopping, assistance in bathing and dressing, and other personal or domestic needs. (These services, however, may be available under state Medicaid or programs of the Older Americans Act, depending on the patient's eligibility.)

A novel benefit addition, perhaps a token of future long-term care benefits, is payment for respite care in the home provided by a home care agency. For a beneficiary who (1) is dependent on a volunteer care giver for assistance with 2 activities of daily living and (2) who has reached the "catastrophic" ceiling, the program will pay for up to 80 h/yr. The program also covers in-home IV drug therapy, including immunosuppressive drugs and antibiotics.

COMBINED HOSPITAL AND PHYSICIAN BENEFITS: HMO PROVISION

The Part A and Part B spectrum of benefits may be furnished through a health maintenance organization (HMO). Medicare pays the HMO a lump sum (capitation) based on average expenditures for Medicare patients in the vicinity. A portion of any savings realized by the HMO must be shared with its elderly members in the form of additional services not covered by Medicare (eg, preventive medical services or long-term care). The patient who joins a Medicare-participating HMO may be required to use the HMO for all regular services; emergency services provided elsewhere may be covered by the HMO under its Medicare contract.

Under authority to conduct demonstrations, Medicare is supporting 4 social and health maintenance organizations (SHMOs). These provide regular Medicare benefits, preventive medicine services, outpatient drugs, and long-term care in a nursing home or in the patient's home. They have latitude to combine Medicare, Medicaid, and patient payments to cover a complete spectrum of care, managed by nurses, social workers, and physicians. The SHMO is at some financial risk for the cost of services and, therefore, like other HMOs, has a stake in economic care.

MEDICAID

Medicaid is the name given to the state programs that receive federal aid for meeting the health care expenses of people in certain categories of need. All Medicaid programs cover the poor who are aged, blind, and disabled and poor families with dependent children. Each state sets its own definition of poor in terms of income and assets. States may also cover certain groups of individuals not in these categories, as well as those in the foregoing categories who are in danger of becoming poor because of health-related expenses, ie, the medically needy. State Medicaid programs determine the payment, duration, and scope of covered services.

State programs vary in the services they cover under Medicaid beyond those required by the federal government. Required services include inpatient and outpatient hospital care and the services of physicians, laboratories, and SNFs for adults. States have the option to cover prescribed drugs, care in an intermediate-care facility, physical therapy, and dental care.

About 10% of the elderly receive Medicaid, and they account for 39% of all Medicaid spending. A patient enrolled in the federal Supplemental Security Income **(SSI)** program is automatically eligible for Medicaid benefits. SSI is for the low-income elderly, blind, and disabled. A person who falls into ≥ 1 of these categories but has income and assets higher than acceptable for SSI may become eligible for Medicaid after "spending down" to the medically needy level.

Under SSI, the elderly are defined as persons > 65 yr of age; the blind, as individuals with ≤ 20/200 vision with use of a corrective lens in the better eye or with tunnel vision of ≤ 20°; and the disabled, as persons unable to engage in any substantial gainful activity by reason of a medically determined physical or mental impairment that is expected to result in death or that has lasted or may last for at least 12 consecutive months.

VETERANS BENEFITS

By 1990, there will be 8 million American veterans, and 1 of every 2 elderly American men will be eligible for Veterans Administration **(VA)** benefits, such as medical and long-term care, without charge. The system operates hospitals, nursing homes, domiciliary facilities, and outpatient clinics. Contract care is provided in non-VA hospitals and in community nursing homes, and the VA pays a fee for service for visits to non-VA physicians and dentists.

With many veterans eligible for Medicare as well as for VA benefits, the demand for care through 1 program depends on restrictions in the other. VA services are available subject to capacity, with priority given to disabled and poor veterans. The VA also provides hospital-based home care, adult day health care, and community residential care. Comprehensive evaluations are offered at 45 geriatric assessment units in medical service or intermediate care wards.

PRIVATE INSURANCE

Because Medicare covers only 45% of all health care expenses of the elderly, there is a demand for both private insurance and an expansion of Medicare. Over ⅔ of Medicare beneficiaries have private insurance (and 10% are poor enough to qualify for Medicaid, which may pay for Part B on their behalf). Often called **"Medigap" insurance,** the private policies generally supplement Medicare by paying deductibles and coinsurances. They do not usually extend beyond Medicare benefits and exclude coverage for long-term care, preventive medicine, and physician fees above the Medicare-approved amounts.

Most states have adopted a model regulation governing policies sold as "Medicare supplements," requiring insurers to pay out benefits averaging at least 60% of the individual and 75% of the group policy price. Policies must cover expenses for preexisting illnesses within 6 mo of purchase. However, these restrictions do not apply to policies that avoid the Medicare-supplement label.

The greatest single threat to the financial security of the elderly is the cost of long-term care. Until recently, virtually no private **long-term care insurance** was available. In 1988, approximately 500,000 policies had been issued; these should be considered experimental as insurers evaluate their experience.

In the aggregate, about ½ the expenses of nursing home care are met by individuals and families out of pocket, and almost ½ by Medicaid. Private policies tend to focus on nursing home expenses, although polls show a public preference for home care. The capacity of private insurance to forestall poverty and to promote sound geriatric care remains untested. Currently, most private-pay patients become Medicaid patients in < 1 yr after entering a nursing home.

The unaffordability of financial protection older persons need against the costs of health care challenges government and private long-term care insurance resources. Few individuals can cope with institutional expenses of $25,000 to $40,000/yr for long-term care. Yet, the absence of secure funding for community-based and institutional services for the chronically ill is a deterrent to the development of private insurance.

Private policies generally offer indemnity benefits in SNFs for up to $50/day. Premiums are scaled to age, waiting periods, and amount of indemnity desired. Preexisting conditions may be excluded or made the basis for additional waiting periods before eligibility for payment commences. Mental illness, including Alzheimer's disease, may not be covered. The policies may provide for home care at a reduced daily indemnity, often only after an institutional stay.

A means of unifying housing, health care, and other services under packaged financing and management is the **life care community** or **continuing care retirement community.** With disability-oriented housing, eating, and recreational facilities, as well as clinics and even nursing facilities on campus, the most extensive of these communities respond to wealthy retirees seeking security who are willing to sign long-term contracts and pay a substantial entrance fee and monthly mortgage-type payments.

Some life care communities have failed because service expenses exceeded income as populations aged. Newer communities provide minimal services but offer opportunities to buy additional services separately. Under study is an alternative to a defined campus; the **life care at home** concept provides long-term care and other services to subscribers living in conventional neighborhoods.

Several state programs, notably in Oregon, have amalgamated governmental funds into comprehensive long-term care programs that allow individually tailored continuums of care to be formed for frail individuals. Such efforts help overcome the personally destructive and demoralizing fragmentation of programs that have differing eligibility criteria, benefit clusters, medical and social service orientations, and social and economic purposes.

INDEX

Page numbers followed by *f* indicate **FIGURE**; by *t*, **TABLE**

Androgenic hormones, and bone homeostasis, 711
Androgens
    in male hypogonadism, 843
    in myelodysplasia, 663
    and sexuality, 639 *t*, 640 *t*
Androstenedione, aging effects, in men, 776 *t*
Androsterone, aging effects
    in men, 776 *t*
    in women, 775 *t*
Anemia, **644**, 646 *t*
    aplastic, 646 *t*, **652**, 678 *t*
        and drugs, 652 *t*
    chronic disease and, **648**
    in chronic renal failure, 606
    and folate deficiency, 646 *t*, **654**
    hemolytic, 646 *t*, **649**
        drugs causing, 650 *t*
    iron-deficiency, **645**, 646 *t*
        and diet, 7
        diagnosis, 646
        pathophysiology, 645
        treatment, 647
    macrocytic, 646 *t*, **652**
    microcytic, 645, 646 *t*, 648
    normocytic, 646 *t*, 648
    pernicious, 501, 653
        and dementia, 945
    refractory, 660
    sideroblastic, 648
    and syncope, 48
    thalassemia minor, 648
    unexplained, 649
    vitamin B$_{12}$ deficiency, 653
Anesthesia
    preoperative evaluation, 230
    during surgery, 232
Aneurysms
    arterial, **396**
        aortic
            abdominal, **397**
                prognosis and treatment, 399
                symptoms, signs, and diagnosis, 398
            dissecting, **400**
                diagnosis, 402
                and mediastinal compression, 401
                symptoms and signs, 400
                treatment, 403
            thoracic, 396
        carotid, 400
        femoral, 400
        popliteal, **399**
    gastric (cirsoid or racemose), 558
Angina pectoris, **353** (*see also* Coronary artery disease)
    and coronary bypass surgery, 418
    and sleep dysfunction, 139
    treatment, **355**

Angiodysplasia, 19
    colonic, **512**, 558
    gastric, 504
Angiography
    in aortic dissection, 402
    in cerebral ischemia, 963
    coronary, 335, 335 *t*
    digital subtraction, 336
    in gastrointestinal bleeding, 555
    pulmonary, in pulmonary embolism, 454
Angioplasty
    coronary, percutaneous transluminal (PTCA), 357, **419**
    in peripheral vascular diseases, 392
Angiotensin
    aging effects on, 183, 600
    converting enzyme (ACE) inhibitors
        in heart failure, 384 *t*, 386
        and hyperkalemia, 183
        in hypertension
            mode of action, 340
            treatment with, 345, 346 *t*, 347 *t*
Angle-closure glaucoma, **1070**, 1071 *f*
Angular cheilitis, 1040
Ankle/brachial index, 389
Ankylosis, and therapeutic exercises, 252
Anorectal disorders, **579**
    abscesses, 583
    carcinoma (*see* Carcinoma)
    fissures, 582
    fistula, 584
    hemorrhoids, 581
    incontinence, 508
    prolapse and procidentia, 584
    pruritus ani, 580
Anorexia, **4**
    diagnosis, 10
    in diabetes mellitus, 793
    in dying patient, 292
    treatment, 11
Anoscopy, **493**
Anoxia
    and delirium, 939
    and non-Alzheimer dementia, 945
Anserine bursitis, 698
Antacids, and peptic ulcer, 502
Anterior vestibular artery occlusion, 1103
Anterograde amnesia, 942
Anthralin, in psoriasis, 1050
Antianginals, and bladder function, 610 *t*
Antiarrhythmics (*see* Arrhythmias, treatment; and under specific agents)
Antibiotics, **894**
    amdinocillin (mecillinam), **899**
        pivoxil (pivmecillinam), **899**
    aminoglycosides, **896**
    amoxicillin, **898**
    ampicillin, **898**
    antipseudomonal penicillins, **899**
    and aplastic anemia, 652, 652 *t*

H

THE MERCK MANUAL OF GERIATRICS is set in 10-point Times Roman with sideheads and key words in News Gothic Bold. Figure legends and tables are set in 8-point News Gothic. The text was typeset by International Computaprint Corporation, Fort Washington, Pennsylvania, and the index was typeset by Alexander Typesetting, Inc., Indianapolis, Indiana. The book was printed by web offset on 30-pound Bible paper at National Publishing Company, Philadelphia, Pennsylvania.

NOTES

NOTES

NOTES

NOTES

NOTES

NOTES

NOTES